Yoshiki Oshida

Magnesium Materials

Also of interest

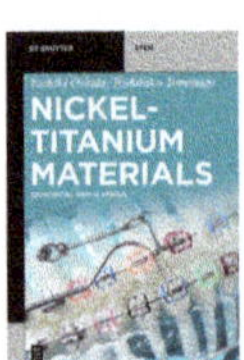

Nickel-Titanium Materials.
Biomedical Applications
Oshida, Tominaga, 2020
ISBN 978-3-11-066603-8, e-ISBN 978-3-11-066611-3

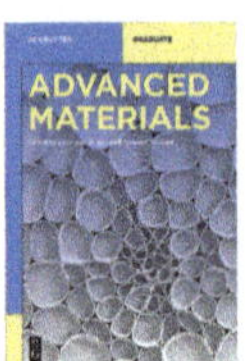

Advanced Materials
van de Ven, Soldera (Eds.), 2019
ISBN 978-3-11-053765-9, e-ISBN 978-3-11-053773-4

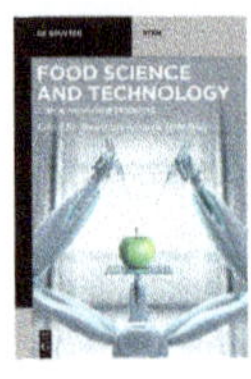

Food Science and Technology.
Trends and Future Prospects
Ijabadeniyi (Eds.), 2020
ISBN 978-3-11-066745-5, e-ISBN 978-3-11-066746-2

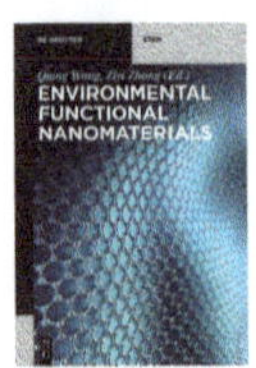

Environmental Functional Nanomaterials
Wang, Zhong, 2020
ISBN 978-3-11-054405-3, e-ISBN 978-3-11-054418-3

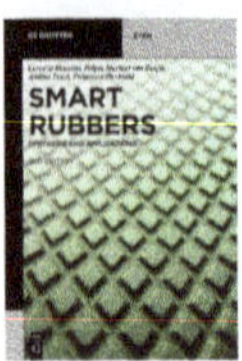

Smart Rubbers.
Synthesis and Applications
Polgar, van Essen, Pucci, Picchioni, 2019
ISBN 978-3-11-063892-9, e-ISBN 978-3-11-063901-8

Yoshiki Oshida

Magnesium Materials

From Mountain Bikes to Degradable Bone Grafts

DE GRUYTER

Author
Dr. Yoshiki Oshida, MS PhD.
Adjunct Professor
University of California San Francisco School of Dentistry
Professor Emeritus
Indiana University School of Dentistry
Visiting Professor
University of Guam School of Science
408 Wovenwood
Orinda, California, 94563
USA

ISBN 978-3-11-067692-1
e-ISBN (PDF) 978-3-11-067694-5
e-ISBN (EPUB) 978-3-11-067713-3

Library of Congress Control Number: 2020952137

Bibliographic information published by the Deutsche Nationalbibliothek
The Deutsche Nationalbibliothek lists this publication in the Deutsche Nationalbibliografie; detailed bibliographic data are available on the Internet at http://dnb.dnb.de.

Cover image: RickLeePhoto/iStock/Getty Images Plus
Typesetting: Integra Software Services Pvt. Ltd.

www.degruyter.com

Contents

Prologue

This book was prepared and written based on a review of about 4,000 carefully selected articles, and presents itself as a typical example of evidence-based learning (EBL). Evidence-based literature reviews can provide foundation skills in research-oriented bibliographic inquiry, with an emphasis on such review and synthesis of applicable literature. Information is gathered by surveying a broad array of multidisciplinary research publications written by scholars and researchers.

In order for EBL to be used effectively, the content of every publication must be critically evaluated in terms of its degree of reliability. There is an established protocol for ranking the reliability of sources – this is an especially useful tool in the medical and dental fields. The ranking from the most to least reliable evidence source is as follows: (i) clinical reports using placebo and double-blind studies; (ii) clinical reports not using placebo, but conducted according to well-prepared statistical test plans; (iii) study reports on time effect on one group of patients during predetermined period of time; (iv) study/comparison reports, at one limited time, on many groups of patients; (v) case reports on a new technique and/or idea; and (vi) retrospective reports on clinical evidence. Unfortunately, the number of published articles increases in this descending reliability order. The greatest advantage of the EBL review is that it helps identify common phenomena in a diversity of fields and literature. It is then possible to create synthetic inclusive hypotheses that deepen and further our understanding. As important as the diversity of source material is to the EBL review, it can pose unique challenges. The sources used in this review are mainly journal articles published in the medical/dental and engineering fields. These two groups' studies have very different analytical criteria and inherent issues.

In medical/dental journals, authors typically present statistically analyzed results; this lends these studies a high degree of reliability. Though we may be confident in the conclusions drawn from statistical analysis, it can be difficult to develop generalized ideas from this literature. Some controversy exists in the medical and dental fields on the relationship between in vitro and in vivo test results. This situation is further complicated and confusing because among the various in vivo tests exists a wide variety of animal model species. The in vitro studies are also not without weakness – it is almost impossible to broadly extrapolate in vitro test results, since it is very rare to find articles where identical test methods were employed. In contrast to medical/dental studies, the data presented in the engineering journals are normally not subjected to statistical analysis. The characterization of data is considered more important to interpretation results because researchers try to explain phenomena, mechanisms and kinetics.

Discoveries in the engineering realm are vitally important to the advancement of medicine and dentistry: the materials and most of the technologies currently employed in medical and dental fields were originally developed in the engineering field. In this book, the author draws upon his unique experience in both fields to

https://doi.org/10.1515/9783110676945-203

bridge the gap between medical/dental and engineering research and tried to put together individual information in the transdisciplinary manner.

About 4,000 carefully selected articles cited in this book have been extracted from about 350 journals. For those who might be interested in literature survey in similar scope of this book, a lengthy list of journals is given as follows:

ACS Applied Materials & Interfaces
ACS Biomaterials Science & Engineering
ACS Nano
Acta Biomaterialia
Acta Crystallographica B
Acta Materialia
Acta Metallurgica Sinica (English Letters)
Additive Manufacturing
Advanced Cardiology
Advanced Drug Delivery Reviews
Advanced Engineering Materials
Advanced Healthcare Materials
Advanced Material Process
Advanced Materials Research
Advanced Powder Technology
Advances in Colloid and Interface Science
Advances in Dental Research
Advances in Orthopedic Surgery
Advances in Science and Materials Engineering
American Ceramic Society
American Heart Journal
American Journal of Dentistry
American Journal of Orthodontics
American Journal of Orthodontics and Dentofacial Orthopedics
American Journal of Roentgenology
Analytical Chemistry
Annals of Biomedical Engineering
Annual Review of Materials Research
Annual Review of Materials Science
Angle Orthodontist
Applied and Environmental Microbiology
Applied Physics Letters
Applied Surface Science
Archives of Civil and Mechanical Engineering
Archives of Foundry Engineering
ASM International
Bioactive Materials

Biochemical and Biophysical Research Communication
Biochemistry
Bioelectrochemistry
Biomaterials
Biometals
Biomedical Materials
BioNano Materials
Breast Cancer
British Journal of Pharmacology
British Medical Journal
Bulletin of Alloy Phase Diagrams
Calcified Tissue International
Calphad
Carbon
Cardiology in the Young
Casting Engineering
Catalysis Today
Catheterization and Cardiovascular Interventions
Cell
Ceramics International
Chemical Engineering Journal
CIRP Annals: Manufacturing Technology
Clinica Chimica Acta
Clinical Implant Dentistry and Related Research
Clinical Materials
Clinical Oral Implants Research
Clinical Oral Investigations
Clinical Orthopaedics and Related Research
Coatings
Cochrane Database System Review
Colloids and Surfaces A: Physicochemical and Engineering Aspects
Colloids and Surfaces B: Biointerfaces
Composite Structures
Composites Part B: Engineering
Composites Science and Technology
Comprehensive Materials Processing
Computational Materials Science
Contact Dermatitis
Corrosion
Corrosion of Magnesium Alloys
Corrosion Prevention of Magnesium Alloys
Corrosion Science

Current Applied Physics
Current Opinion in Solid State and Materials Science
Current Pharmaceutical Design
CRC Critical Reviews in Biocompatibility
Critical Reviews in Oral Biology & Medicine
Data in Brief
Defence Technology
Dental Materials Journal
Der Orthopäde
Die Casting Engineer.
Digest Journal of Nanomaterials and Biostructures
Electrochimica Acta
Electrochemistry Communications
Emerging Materials Research
Energy
Engineering Failure Analysis
Engineering Fracture Mechanics
Epidemiology
European Heart Journal
Expert Review of Precision Medicine and Drug Development
Faraday Discuss
Fatigue & Fracture of Engineering Materials & Structures
Finite Elements in Analysis and Design
Frontiers in Materials: Structural Materials
Future Cardiology
General Dentistry
Heart
Heat Treatment of Metals
Implant Dentistry
Intech Open
Intermetallics
International Archives of Allergy and Immunology
International Dental Journal
International Journal of Adhesion and Adhesives
International Journal of Advanced Manufacturing Technology
International Journal of Artificial Organs
International Journal of Biomedical Science
International Journal of Bioprinting
International Journal of Corrosion Process and Corrosion Control
International Journal of Electrochemical Science
International Journal of Engineering Trends and Technology
International Journal of Fatigue

International Journal of Heat and Mass Transfer
International Journal of Hydrogen Energy
International Journal of Lightweight Materials and Manufacture
International Journal of Materials Research
International Journal of Medical Sciences
International Journal of Molecular Sciences
International Journal of Nanomedicine
International Journal of Oral & Maxillofacial Implants
International Journal of Oral Surgery
International Journal of Plasticity
International Journal of Prosthodontics
International Journal of Thermophysics
Interventional Medicine and Applied Science
International Molecular Science
Iron and Steel Institute of Japan, International
Journal of Acute Disease
Journal of Adhesion
Journal of Adhesion Science and Technology
Journal of Alloys and Compounds
Journal of the American Ceramic Society
Journal of the American Dietetic Association
Journal of Applied Biomaterials
Journal of Applied Biomaterials & Functional Materials
Journal of Applied Oral Science
Journal of Applied Physics
Journal of Arthroplasty
Journal of the Association for the Advancement of Medical Instruments
Journal of Bacteriology
Journal of Bioactive and Compatible Polymers
Journal of Biochemical and Biophysical Method
Journal of Biomaterials and Tissue Engineering
Journal of Biomaterials Science, Polymer Edition
Journal of Biomechanics
Journal of Bio-Medical Materials and Engineering
Journal of Biomedical Materials Research A
Journal of Biomedical Materials Research B: Applied Biomaterials
Journal of Biomimetics, Biomaterials, and Tissue Engineering
Journal of Bioscience and Bioengineering
Journal of Bone and Joint Surgery – American Volume
Journal of Bone and Mineral Research
Journal of Cardiovascular Research
Journal of Chronic Diseases

Journal of Clinical Investigations
Journal of Clinical Pathology
Journal of Colloid and Interface Science
Journal of Composite Materials
Journal of Cranio-Maxillofacial Surgery
Journal of Crystal Growth
Journal of Dental Research
Journal of Electroanalytical Chemistry
Journal of Electroceramics
Journal of Electrochemical Society
Journal of Electronic Packing
Journal of Engineering Tribology
Journal of Experimental Medicine
Journal of Functional Biomaterials
Journal of Geophysical Research
Journal of Immunology
Journal of Industrial and Engineering Chemistry
Journal of International Academy of Periodontology
Journal of Invasive Cardiology
Journal of Investigative Dermatology
Journal of Iron and Steel Research, International
Journal of Japan Institute of Light Metals
Journal of the Less-Common Metals
Journal of Magnetism and Magnetic Materials
Journal of Manufacturing Processes
Journal of Materials at High Temperatures
Journal of Materials Chemistry B
Journal of Materials Engineering
Journal of Materials Engineering and Performance
Journal of Materials Processing Technology
Journal of Materials Research and Technology
Journal of Materials Science
Journal of Materials Science Letters
Journal of Materials Science & Technology
Journal of Materials Science: Materials in Medicine
Journal of Magnesium and Alloys
Journal of Magnetic Resonance Imaging
Journal of Metals
Journal of Mechanical Behavior of Biomedical Materials
Journal of Minerals & Materials Characterization & Engineering
Journal of Nanomaterials
Journal of Nanoscience and Nanotechnology

Journal of Nanotechnology
Journal of Non-Crystalline Solids
Journal of Oral Implants
Journal of Oral Rehabilitation
Journal of Orofacial Orthopedics
Journal of Orthopaedic Translation
Journal of Orthopaedics and Traumatology
Journal of Phase Equilibria and Diffusion
Journal of Porous Materials
Journal of Power Sources
Journal of Prosthetic Dentistry
Journal of Prosthodontics
Journal of Rare Earths
Journal of Rehabilitation Research and Development
Journal of Science: Advanced Materials and Devices
Journal of Solid State Chemistry
Journal of Supercritical Fluids
Journal of the Taiwan Institute of Chemical Engineers
Journal of Vacuum Science & Technology
Journal of Wound and Care
JSciMed Dental Surgery
Key Engineering Materials
Lancet
Langmuir
Magnesium Research
Magnetic Resonance Imaging
Materialia
Materials
Materials (Basel)
Materials Characterization
Materials Chemistry and Physics
Materials and Corrosion
Materials & Design
Materials Horizons
Materials Letters
Materials and Manufacturing Processes
Materials Performance
Materials Research Express
Materials Research Innovations
Materials Science and Applications: Scientific Research
Materials Science & Engineering A: Structural Materials: Properties, Microstructure and Processing

Materials Science & Engineering B: Advanced Functional Solid-State Materials
Materials Science & Engineering C: Materials for Biological Applications
Materials Science and Engineering Technology
Materials Science Forum
Materials and Technology
Materials and Technology: Advanced Performance Materials
Materials Today: Proceedings
Materials Transaction
Materials World
Materialwissenshaft und Werkstofftechnik
Medical Devices and Technology
Medical News Today
Medical Progress Through Technology
Medical Science Monitor
Metal Science and Heat Treatment
Metallic Bone Foam
Metallurgy of the Light Metals
Metallurgical and Materials Transactions A
Metallurgical and Materials Transactions B
Metals
Micro & Nano Letters
Micron
Mineral, Metals and Materials Society
Molecular Biology of the Cell
Nano Energy
Nanomedicine
Nanotechnology
Nature
Nature Communications
Nature Materials
Neuroradiology
Neurotoxicology
Nano Letters
Nonstructured Materials
Optical Materials
Optics & Laser Technology
Oral Microbiology and Immunology
Oral Surgery Oral Medicine Oral Pathology Oral Radiology Endodontics
Orthopedic Clinic of North America
Orthopedics
Oxidative Medicine and Cellular Longevity
Philosophical Magazine: Journal of Theoretical Experimental and Applied Physics

Physica C: Superconductivity
Physical Chemistry Chemical Physics
Physical Metallurgy
Physical Review Letters
Physics and Chemistry of Liquids
Physics of the Earth and Planetary Interiors
Physics of Metals and Metallography
PLoS One
Polymer
Powder Technology
Procedia Chemistry
Procedia Engineering
Procedia Materials Science
Procedia Structural Integrity
Progress in Materials Science
Progress in Natural Science: Materials International
Progress in Organic Coatings
Proceedings of the Royal Society B: Biological Sciences
Quintessence International
Quintessence Journal of Dental Technology
Radiology
Rare Metal Materials and Engineering
Regenerative Biomaterials
Renewable Energy
Results in Physics
Reviews on Advanced Materials Science
Royal Society of Chemistry Advances
Scandinavian Journal of Plastic and Reconstructive Surgery
Scanning
Science
Science Bulletin
Science and Technology of Advanced Materials
Science and Technology of Welding and Joining
Scientific Reports
Scientific World Journal
Scripta Metallurgica et Materialia
Scripta Materialia
SN Applied Sciences
Solar Energy Materials and Solar Cells
Solid State Ionics
Superlattices and Microstructures
Surface and Coatings Technology

Surfaces and Interfaces
Surgery
Surgery, Gynecology & Obstetrics
Surface and Interface Analysis
Surface Technology
Surface Treatment
Technologies
Thin Solid Films
Thermochimica Acta
Theoretical and Applied Mechanics Letters
Tissue Engineering
Total Materia
Toxicology
Transactions of the Electrochemical Society
Transactions of Nonferrous Metals Society of China
Transactions of the Society of Biomaterials
Tribology in Industry
Tribology International
Tribology Letters
Ultrasonics Sonochemistry
Vacuum
Virtual and Physical Prototyping
Wear
Welding Journal
Welding Research Supplement
Weld World
Welkstoffe und Korrosion
Wire Journal International

The author would like to express sincere respect and gratitude to author(s) of individual publications who contributed indirectly to this book, to journal editorial board members for providing them a publication opportunity and to review members to their acceptance evaluations.

Chapter 1
Introduction

Magnesium is named after the Greek "Magnesia region" which is also known as a production area of "magnesium-rich steatite," although nowadays dolomite ($CaMg(CO_3)_2$) and/or carnallite ($KMgCl_3 \cdot 6H_2O$) are used as Mg ores. Magnesium is the ninth most abundant element in the universe and is as strong as some types of steels, but 33% lighter than aluminum, 60% lighter than titanium and 75% lighter than steel. Magnesium is the lightest common structural metal with a density of 1.74 g/cm^3 in its solid state. Magnesium has a hexagonal closed pack crystalline structure that resists the slip to parallel basal planes and, therefore, magnesium cannot be plastically deformed at room temperature, due to the facts that the work-hardening rate is high and ductility is low. Therefore, magnesium alloys are formed above 226 °C with a range of 343–510 °C as the slip process becomes easier at elevated temperatures [1].

Although magnesium overwhelms the amount of underground (including underwater) reserves of 1.8×10^{11} tons over Fe (8×10^{10}), Al (2.8×10^{10}), Cu (6×10^8) and Ti (6×10^8), there is still a need for recycling against the limited natural resources. The ratio of energy required to produce fresh ingot to the required energy to reproduce ingot (in other words, recycling energy ratio) for Ti is estimated to be 77.1, 40.7 for Fe, 10.5 for Ni and 4.9 for Al, while for Mg, it is estimated to be 3.3, indicating that Mg is the most cost-efficient metallic material among important metallic elements to be recycled – excellent recyclability [2, 3].

Table 1.1 compares typical properties among three popular alloys, indicating that the lightweight of Mg materials is emphasized in terms of specific strength as well as specific rigidity [4].

Table 1.1: Brief comparison of major properties among three common alloys.

Property\material	Mg–9Al–1Zn	Al–3Cu–8Si	Ti–6Al–4V
Density (g/cm^3)	1.82	2.70	4.42
Melting point (°C)	596	595	1,600
Tensile strength (MPa)	280	315	1,000
Specific strength	153.8	116.7	226.2
Elongation (%)	8	3	15
Modulus of elasticity (GPa)	45	71	113
Specific rigidity	24.7	26.3	25.6

https://doi.org/10.1515/9783110676945-001

As one of the lightest engineering materials, magnesium alloys have exhibited quite special properties including high specific strength, high thermal conductivity, excellent electromagnetic interference shielding, good excellent machinability, good vibration and shock absorption, high damping capacity, good weldability under the controlled ambient and excellent castability. All these characteristics lead to specific applications such as automotive, communication, electronics, sports equipment and other industries [5–8]. In the aerospace industry, magnesium can be found in the thrust reversers of airliners and the transmission casings of helicopters. It is also used in missiles. Electronic assemblers should be included such as the strength, durability and lightweight of magnesium. Magnesium also dissipates heat and shields against electromagnetic and radio frequency interference. The housings for cameras, cell phones, laptops and portable media players are commonly made from magnesium. Magnesium parts can be found in sporting goods, such as golf clubs, bicycle frames and in-line skates, as well as household goods, such as vacuums, power tools, chain saws and lawn mowers. Besides these non-medical applications (for details, refer to Chapter 16), versatile applications in medical and dental areas will be discussed in Chapter 19.

Poor corrosion resistance associated with Mg materials can be reversely employed as a beneficial property in industries. Magnesium along with zinc are well known to serve as a sacrificial anode cathodic protection material to protect important components such as underground pipelines, rudder and screw for large-scale ocean-going ships and tankers. Poor corrosion resistance (or fast degradation) can be also utilized in medical field. In recent years, the paradigm about the metal with improved corrosion resistance for application in surgery and orthopedy has been shifted. The new class of biodegradable (degradation in biological environment) metal emerges as an alternative for biomedical implants. These metals corrode gradually with an appropriate host response and release of corrosion products. Magnesium serves this aim best; it plays the essential role in body metabolism and should be completely excreted within a few days after degradation. Magnesium-based alloys – particularly Mg materials designed as a biodegradable class, can serve for cardiovascular and orthopedic medical device applications, and as a temporary scaffold when placed in vivo, which is desirable for treatments when temporary supportive structures are required to assist in the wound healing process (detailed discussion on managing degradation rate will be found in Chapter 18).

Such popularity of Mg materials can be recognized by counting manuscripts published in various peer-reviewed journals, most of which are cited in this book. Referring to Figure 1.1, each mark represents accumulated publication numbers for 5 years, so that data on year 2000 indicate total number of publications from 1996 through 2000. There are three groups of marks in the figure: triangle blues are for titanium materials and red marks are for magnesium materials, in which red circle marks represent numbers for total magnesium materials and square red marks are

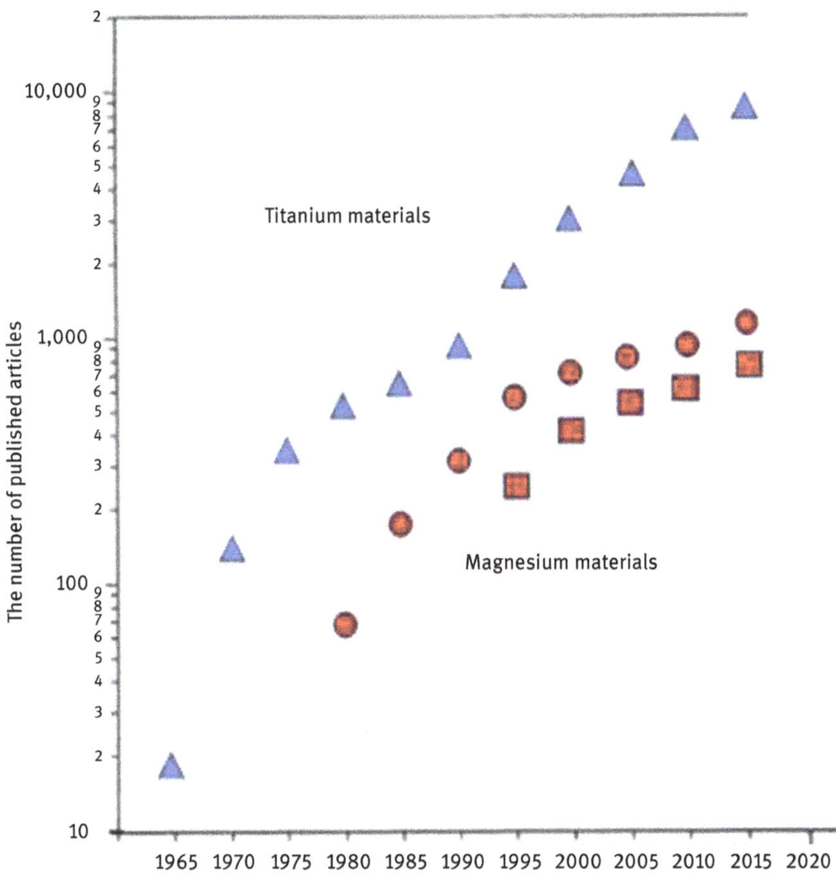

Figure 1.1: Cumulative publications of titanium and magnesium materials. Blue triangles: titanium materials; red circles: magnesium materials, in which red squares are sum of AZ31 and AZ91 Mg-based alloys.

for sum of AZ31 (Mg–3Al–1Zn) and AZ91 (Mg–9Al–1Zn) alloys only. The reason why AZ31 + AZ91 are presented is that these two alloys are considered as typical biodegradable Mg-based alloys. It can be mentioned that (i) publications on Ti materials are roughly ten times (one decade) larger than Mg materials due to the degree of versatility of Ti materials, and (ii) even both materials are considered to exhibit high specific strengths, their (in vitro and in vivo both) corrosion behaviors are quite different from each other. It can be speculated that data points for both materials in 2020 (cumulative from 2016 through 2020) should jump high due to advanced technology in tissue engineering in medical industry; particularly, biodegradable Mg materials should increase publications, since during the preparation of this book, the author had already noticed remarkable numbers of publication on this area in 2016, 2017, 2018, 2019 and first half of 2020.

Formability
– Super plasticity
– SPF/DB
Rolling
Extrusion
Forging
Severe plastic working
ECAP
FSP
Machining
Joining
Shapes
– Rods/bars
– Ribbon/wire
– Sheets
– Tube/pipe
– Powders
– Foam
– Amorphous
Powder metallurgy
Casting
Wrought
Primary process
Hot/cold working
Secondary process
To other alloys
Binary alloys
Ternary alloys
Quaternary alloys
Composites
Glassy
Hybrids
Intermetallics
Alloying elements
Mg
Mg Biomaterials
Engineering applications in
– Automobiles
– Aircrafts
– Housing for electronics
– Sacrificial anode
– Battery anode
Characteristic
– Lightweight
– High specific strength
– Heat conductivity
– Electromagnetic shielding
– Damping capacity
– Mechanical properties
– Physical properties
– Chemical properties
Microstructures
– Heat treatments
– Grain refining
– DRX
– LPSO
– Dislocation
– Slip/twinning
Supporting technologies
– NNS forming
– Dislocation engineering
– Thixo-technology
– Tissue engineering
– 3D printing
– Additive manufacturing
– Functional gradation
Characteristics
– Poor corrosion resistance
– Controlled degradation
– Compatibilities (bio-, cyto-, hemo-)
– Hydrophobicity
– Wettability
Modification
– Heat treatment
– Shot peening
– Coatings
– MAO,PEO
Medical applications
– Temporary implants
– Stents
– Scaffolds
– Sutures
– Drug delivery

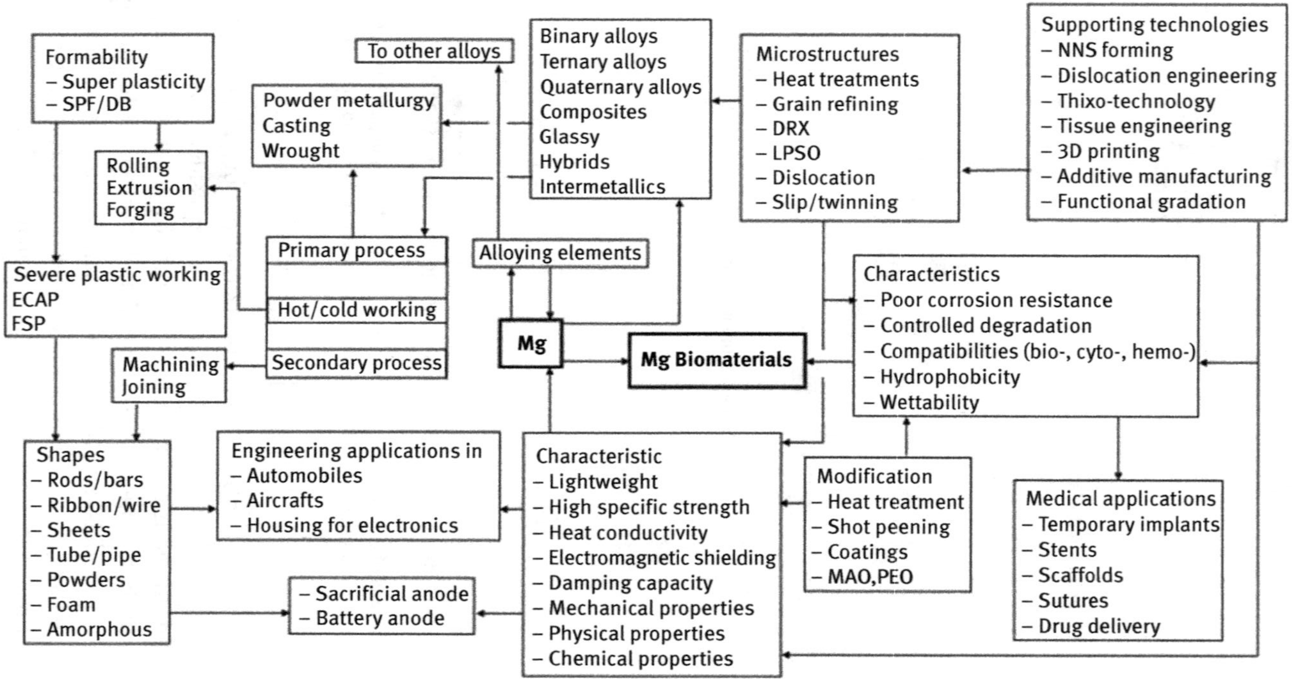

Figure 1.2: Magnesium map, exhibiting interconnecting fabrications, forming, modification, alloying and characterization toward development of practical applications with various supporting technologies and engineering.

There should be numerous tasks and technologies, science and engineering involved, which are interrelated in the most complicated manners to make a material to a useful stage. Mg material is not an exception and rather it possesses more complicity due to its unique metallurgical nature and chemical behavior as well. These characters are just few among many elements influencing Mg materials. Figure 1.2 depicts the interacting magnesium map of various disciplines and elements involved in magnesium materials and most of these individual elements are covered in this book.

References

[1] Cooke KO, Alhazaa A, Atieh AM. Dissimilar Welding and Joining of Magnesium Alloys: Principles and Application. IntechOpen. 2019, DOI: 10.5772/intechopen.85111.

[2] Ohnishi T. Recycling of Aluminum Alloys. Casting Engineering. 1997, 69, 995–1002.

[3] The Japan Magnesium Association. Basic Information and Properties; magnesium.or.jp/property/.

[4] The Japan Magnesium Association. Current Status of Magnesium Industry. 2015; https://www.meti.go.jp/policy/nonferrous_metal/strategy/magnesium02.pdf.

[5] Luo AA. Magnesium Development as a Lightweight Material - In Competition with Other Structural Materials. In: Solanki K. et al. ed., Magnesium Technology. 2017. The Minerals, Metals & Materials Series. Springer, 2017, 7.

[6] Atrens A, Song G-L, Liu M, Shi Z, Cao F, Dargusch MS. Review of recent developments in the field of magnesium corrosion. Advanced Engineering Materials. 2015, 17, 400–53.

[7] Kang Z, Li W. Facile and fast fabrication of superhydrophobic surface on magnesium alloy by one-step electrodeposition method. Journal of Industrial and Engineering Chemistry. 2017, 50, 50–6.

[8] La M, Zhou H, Li N, Xin Y, Sha R, Bao S, Jin P. Improved performance of Mg-Y alloy thin film switchable mirrors after coating with a superhydrophobic surface. Applied Surface Science. 2017, 403, 23–8.

Chapter 2
Positioning of magnesium

Magnesium has atomic number 12. Magnesium is the ninth most abundant element in the universe, as shown in Figure 2.1, and is the eleventh most abundant element by mass in the human body. It is also believed that (i) magnesium, like most pure metallic elements, is not sufficiently strong in its pure form so that it must be alloyed with other materials in order to gain higher strength-to-weight ratio (in other words, specific strength), (ii) susceptibility to corrosion (which is sometimes beneficial if it works as a protective sacrificial anode) can be reduced by alloying (by mostly aluminum, zinc, manganese) and (iii) ductility of Mg-based alloys is also higher than pure Mg because alloying increases the number of active slip planes within the material. In this chapter, examining several comparative charts and diagrams is the goal to grab reasonable idea of magnesium's position among many other competitive materials in terms of mostly mechanical properties and chemical/electrochemical behaviors.

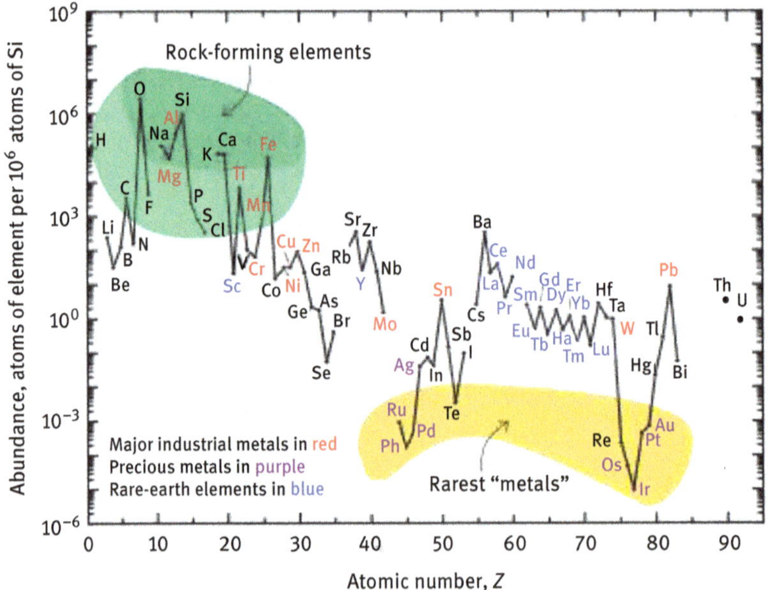

Figure 2.1: Abundance (atom fraction) of the chemical elements in earth's upper continental crust as a function of atomic number [1].

https://doi.org/10.1515/9783110676945-002

2.1 Mechanical properties

To evaluate and compare mechanical properties of Mg materials with various types of other materials, there are valuable charts and diagrams available. Figure 2.2 provides a general idea on grouping material kinds with respect to the relationship between density (specific weight) and modulus of elasticity (or stiffness) [2]. It is obvious that metal group is located at zone of high specific modulus. Within such metal group, Mg can be identified at the lightest side of the metal envelope, indicating that Mg materials exhibit the highest value of specific modulus. Figure 2.3 explains the same trend when individual material's name is inserted [3]. Furthermore, Figure 2.4 plots relationship between density and strength at fracture [3]. It is again indicated that Mg materials can be found at the highest specific strength (or left side of the metal group zone).

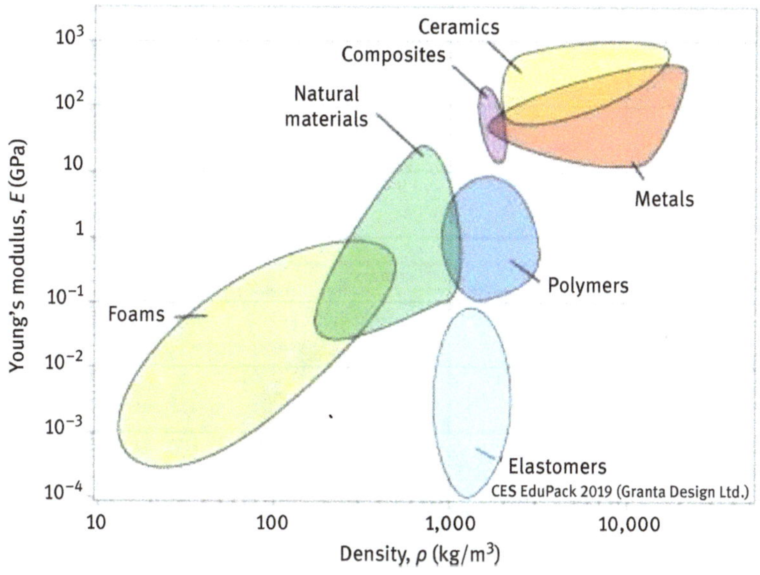

Figure 2.2: Density versus Young's modulus of different kinds of materials [2].

In the generalized variation of Hooke's law, it states that the strain/deformation of an elastic object or material is proportional to the stress applied to it. It may be expressed mathematically as $\sigma = E \cdot \varepsilon$. Hence, Young's modulus of elasticity, E, is linearly related to stress (σ). Accordingly, as shown in Figure 2.5, these two mechanical parameters are linearly related. As will be discussed in later chapter(s), since pure Mg element is not strong enough to serve as any structural component, Mg is normally alloyed with various metallic elements (which varies widely in terms of their

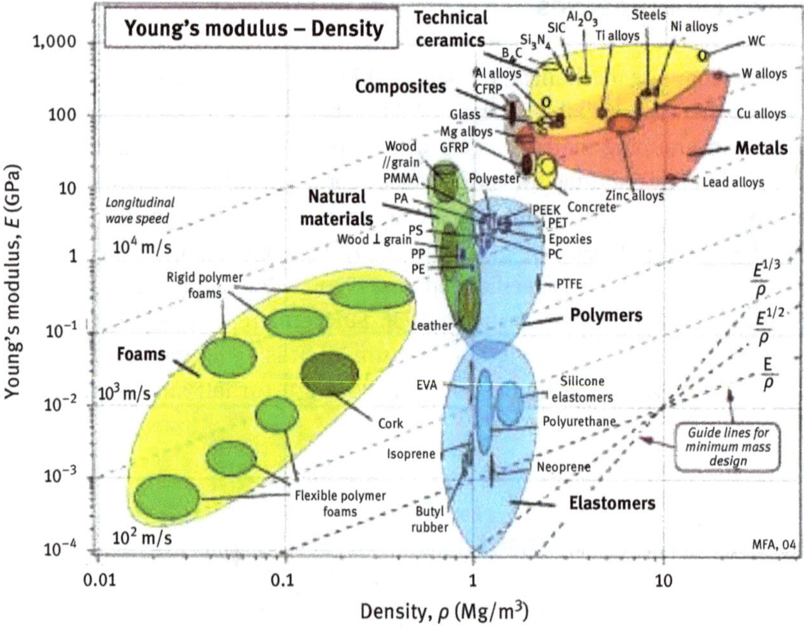

Figure 2.3: Density versus Young's modulus of various materials [3].

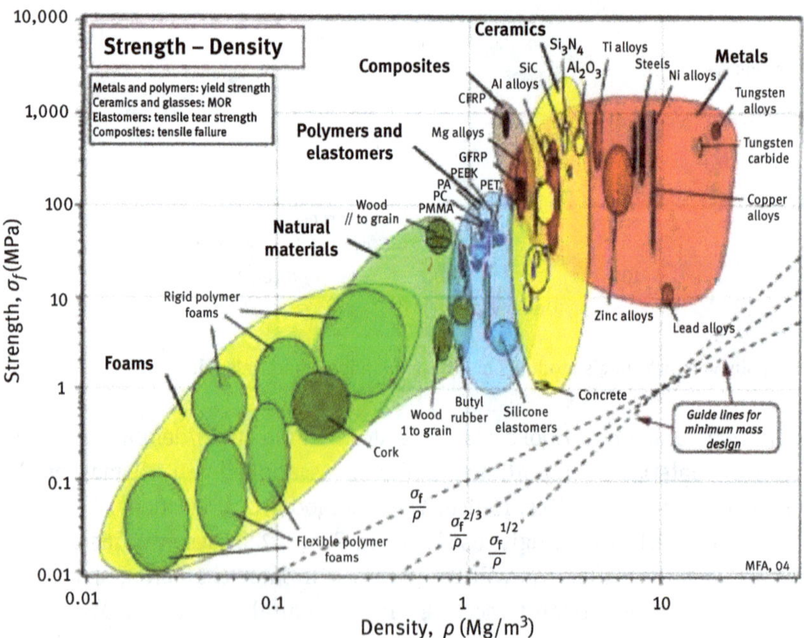

Figure 2.4: Density versus strengths of various materials [3].

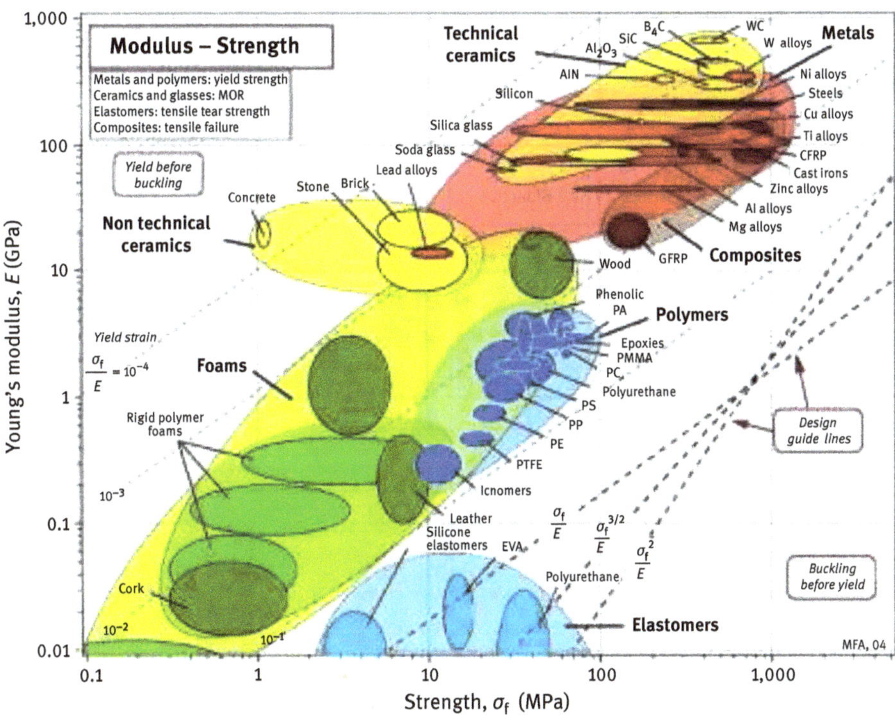

Figure 2.5: Strength versus Young's modulus of elasticity of various materials [3].

density, resulting in the Mg zone within the metal group being stretched along the density axis).

Figure 2.6 shows the similar relationship between modulus of elasticity and yield strength of biomaterials in log–log plot, where P represents polymeric materials; B, the bone; HSP the high-strength polymer (Kelvar, Kapton, PEEK, etc.); D, the dentin; TCP, the tricalcium phosphate; HAP, the hydroxyapatite; E, the enamel; TI, the commercially pure titanium (all unalloyed grades); TA, the titanium alloys (e.g., Ti-6Al-4V, Ti-6Al-7Nb); S, the stainless steels (e.g., 304-series stainless steels); A, the alumina; PSZ, the partially stabilized zirconia; CF, the carbon fiber; and MG, the magnesium materials [4]. It is particularly important to see any material close to (implant)-receiving hard tissue (bone) when the successful implant fixation (or osseointegration) is required owing to excellent biomechanical compatibility. It is noticed, accordingly, that Mg material with the red square mark is closer to the bone than any other metallic biomaterials.

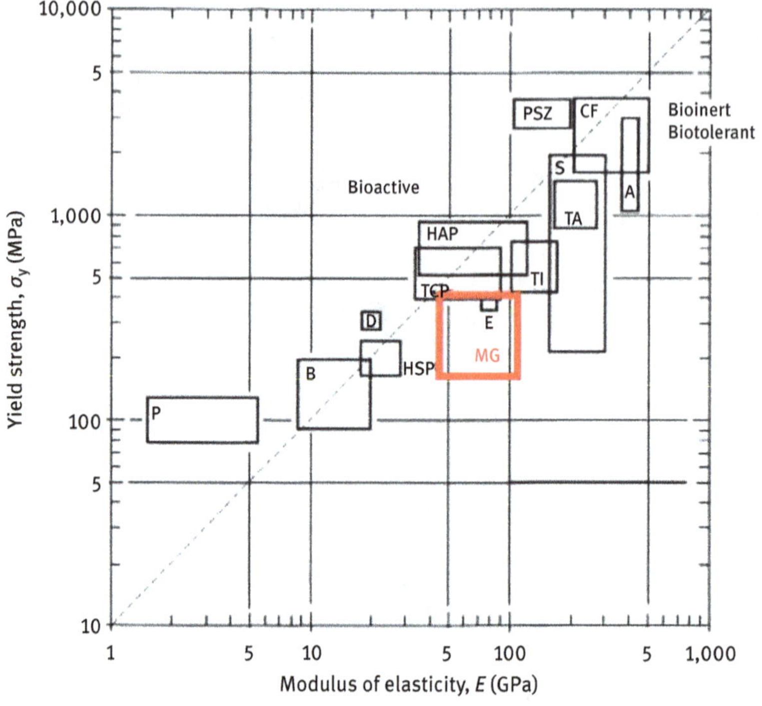

Figure 2.6: Relationship between modulus of elasticity and yield strength of typical biomaterials [4].

2.2 Chemical/electrochemical properties

An electromotive force (EMF) series, listing chemical species (atoms, molecules and ions) in the order of their tendency to gain or lose electrons (be reduced or oxidized, respectively), is expressed in volts and measured with reference to the hydrogen electrode, which is taken as a standard and arbitrarily assigned the voltage of zero. The more positive the potential, the more noble the element. In a case of dissimilar metal (element) coupling exposed to an electrolyte, the galvanic cell has been established and less noble metal behaves as an anode and tends to be corroded. This is a way why Mg materials (along with zinc) are so important in engineering since Mg (or Zn) can serve as a cathodic protecting sacrificial anode. It is also indispensable to mention here that Mg materials are biodegradable (ability of controlled degradation in biological environment) [6], so that there are versatile medical applications including bone grafting, scaffolds, stents and sutures.

Figure 2.7 compares EMF (or galvanic) series of practical metallic materials in seawater (meaning less oxygen content aqueous atmosphere) for practical metals and alloys [5]. It should be noted that Mg is located at far less-noble potential than other metallic materials.

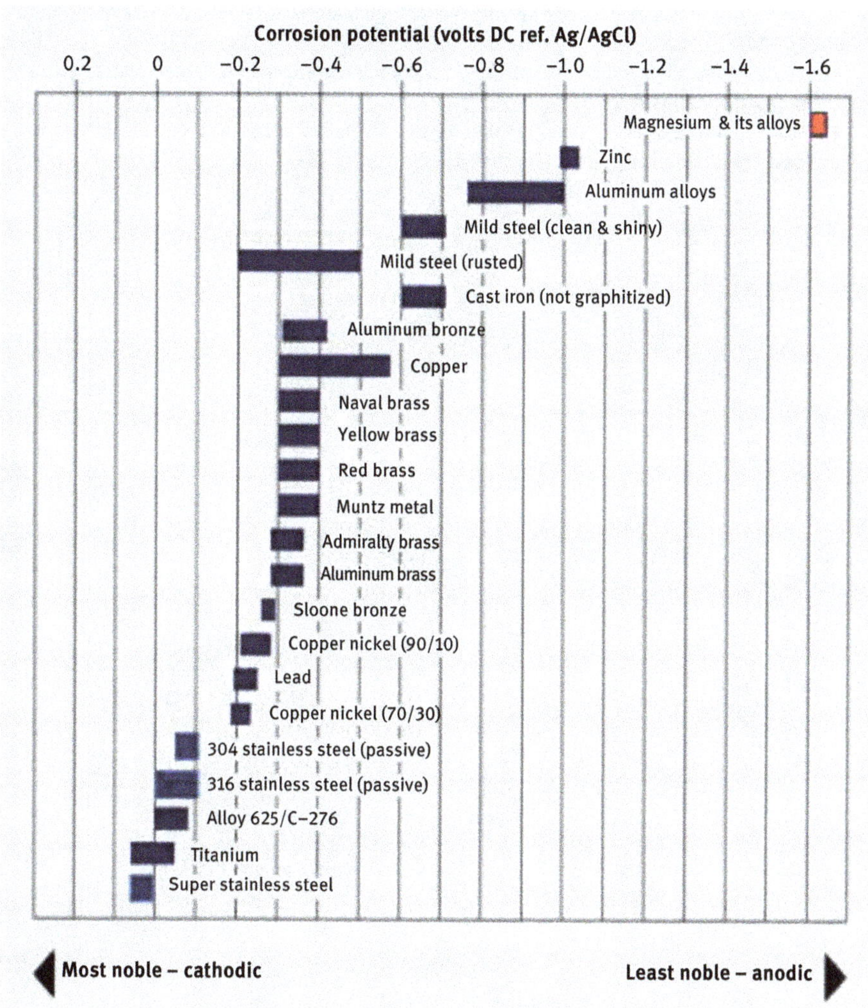

Figure 2.7: Galvanic series of practical metals and alloys in seawater [5].

References

[1] Anderson DL. Chemical composition of the mantle. Journal of Geophysical Research. 1983, 88, B41–B52.

[2] Materials Property chart; https://grantadesign.com/education/students/charts/.

[3] Ashby MF. Materials Selection in Mechanical Design: Material Property Charts. 55th edition, 2016. Elsevier, Butterworth-Heinemann.

[4] Oshida Y. Bioscience and Bioengineering of Titanium Materials. 1st edition, Elsevier, Oxford UK, 2007.
[5] https://www.imoa.info/molybdenum-uses/molybdenum-grade-stainless-steels/architecture/avoid-galvanic-corrosion.php.
[6] Manivasagam G, Suwas S. Biodegradable Mg and Mg based alloys for biomedical implants. Journal of Materials Science and Technology. 2014, 30, 515–20.

Chapter 3
Mg-based alloys

Like other alloys, magnesium alloys have excellent practical applications. At the same time, Mg element is an important alloying element to other metallic alloy systems. In this chapter, we discuss the Mg-based alloy classification and designation, alloying element to form Mg-based alloys and Mg as an alloying element to other alloy systems.

3.1 Alloy classification and alloy designation

Normally Mg-based alloys are produced in either casting alloys or wrought alloys. The common magnesium alloys employed for casting purposes usually contain varied percentages of aluminum, manganese and zinc. Nearly all the casting alloys may be heat treated to improve the mechanical properties. On the other hand, several magnesium alloys have been developed especially for the manufacture of wrought products. As casting alloys, the principal added elements in the wrought compositions are aluminum, manganese and zinc. Furthermore, Mg-based alloys for wrought products are classified as nonheat treatable and heat treatable. The principal wrought manufactures that are commercially available in magnesium alloys include sheet and other flat rolled products, extrusions (bars, rods, solid shapes, hollow shapes and tubing) and forgings [1]. There are three main groups of Mg-based alloys (in both cast and wrought): (1) Mg–Al–Zn alloy systems, manufactured by die casting, sandcasting, permanent mold casting, forging and extrusion, and the alloys are heat treatable; (2) Mg–Mn alloy systems, exhibiting good weldability and suitable for manufacturing thin plates; and (3) Mg–Zn–Zr alloy systems, possessing high impact toughness, good corrosion resistance and machinability, and the alloys are heat treatable [1–3].

Mg-based alloys are designated by group of alphabets and numerical numbers and practically composed of four parts as follows [4–7]:

(1) The first part indicates the two principal alloying elements and consists of two code letters representing the two main alloying elements arranged in the order of decreasing percentage (or alphabetically if percentages are equal) (e.g., AZ81A-T4):
A – aluminum
B – bismuth
C – copper
D – cadmium
E – rare earth element
F – iron

https://doi.org/10.1515/9783110676945-003

G – magnesium
H – thorium
J – strontium
K – zirconium
L – lithium
M – manganese
N – nickel
P – lead
Q – silver
R – chromium
S – silicon
T – tin
V – gadolinium
W – yttrium
X – calcium
Y – antimony
Z – zinc

(2) The second part indicates the amounts of the two principal alloying elements and consists of two numbers corresponding to rounded-off percentages of the two main alloying elements and arranged in same order as alloy designations in first part (e.g., AZ81A-T4)
(3) The third part distinguishes between different alloys with the same percentages of the two principal alloying elements and consists of a letter of the alphabet assigned in order as compositions become standard, normally starting alphabet letters A, B and C (except letters I and O), for example, AZ81A-T4
(4) The fourth part indicates condition (temper) and consists of a letter followed by a number (e.g., AZ81A-T4):
F: as fabricated
O: annealed, recrystallized (wrought products only)
H: strain hardened
Subdivision of the "H" tempers:
H1: plus one or more digits for strain hardened only
H2: plus one or more digits for strain hardened and then partially annealed
H3: plus one or more digits for strain hardened and then stabilized
W: solution heat treated, unstable temper
T: thermal treated to produce stable tempers other than F, O or H
Subdivisions of the "T" tempers:
T1: cooled and naturally aged
T2: annealed (cast products only)

T3: solution heat treated and then cold worked
T4: solution heat treated
T5: cooled and artificially aged
T6: solution heat treated and artificially aged
T7: solution heat treated and stabilized
T8: solution heat treated, cold worked and then artificially aged
T9: solution heat treated, artificially aged and then cold worked
T10: cooled, artificially aged and cold worked

Consider, for example, AZ81A-T4, the first part of the designation, AZ, indicates that aluminum and zinc are the two principal alloying elements; the second part of the designation, 81, means the rounded-off percentages of aluminum and zinc (8 and 1 wt%, respectively); the third part, A, indicates that it is the fifth alloy standardized with 8% Al and 1% Zn as the principal alloying additions; and the fourth part, T4, denotes that the alloy is solution heat treated.

3.2 Alloying elements to Mg-based binary alloys

Refined magnesium almost always normally possesses other impurity elements, which result from the natural composition of magnesium found within the earth, as well as the casting and refining processes. The degree of impurities after the refining process is dependent upon the efficiency of the refining process itself. Elements currently found within the magnesium include: Cu (100–300 ppm), Be (4 ppm), Ni (20–50 ppm) and Fe (35–50 ppm) [8, 9]. The main aim of alloy's development is the improvement in mechanical properties, corrosion resistance and other properties. The alloy properties also depend on intermetallic compound and microstructural effect based on the processing route. It is generally believed that the major alloying effects of each element as follows [10–13]:

Al increases solid solution and/or precipitation hardening, hardness, strength and improves the castability.

Zn is an important alloying element with a relatively high solubility in Mg up to 6.2 wt%. Zn content that is up to 4 wt% significantly increases the ultimate tensile strength (UTS) and elongation (EL) of as-cast Mg–Zn alloys, but any higher percentage of Zn would lead to the reduction of both properties and decrease the corrosion resistance of the alloy (to which nickel and iron impurities assist to improve the corrosion resistance). The mechanical and degradation properties being the main concerns, the Mg–Zn alloys with low Zn content (<4 wt%) were further alloyed by adding the third alloying elements, including Ca, Mn, Sr, Y and Zr to form ternary alloys.

Mn increases saltwater corrosion resistance within some aluminum containing alloys and increases creep resistance.

Ca contributes to solid solution and/or precipitation hardening and also acts to some extent as a grain refining agent and additionally contributes to grain boundary strengthening. Also, it reduces surface tension.

Sr is normally used in conjunction with other elements to enhance creep performance.

Y enhances high temperature strength and creep performance when combined with other rare earth (RE) metals, acts as a good grain refining element, and increases elevated temperature tensile strength and creep resistance.

Ni increases both yield and ultimate strength at room temperature, but negatively impacts ductility and corrosion resistance, and it can assist easily forming metallic glasses.

Ce improves corrosion resistance and also increases plastic deformation capability, magnesium EL and work-hardening rates, but it reduces yield strength (YS).

Nd improves material strength.

Cu assists in increasing both room and high temperature strength and also increases castability and can assist easily in forming metallic glasses, but it shows detrimental influence on corrosion resistance.

Sn improves ductility and reduces tendency to crack during processing, when used with aluminum.

Based on these alloying elements with well-established alloying effects, there are major eleven Mg-based binary alloy systems: Mg–Al, Mg–Zn, Mg–Mn, Mg–Ca, Mg–Sr, Mg–Y, Mg–Ni, Mg–Ce, Mg–Nd, Mg–Cu and Mg–Sn. As listed in Table 3.1, each alloying element exhibits its unique alloying function to magnesium. These binary alloy systems provide the bases for ternary alloys, as seen later; while there are still minor alloying elements as listed in Table 3.2.

Table 3.1: Alloying elements to Mg binary alloys.

	Al	Zn	Mn	Ca	Sr	Y	Ni	Ce	Nd	Cu	Sn
Mechanical properties	[14–18]	[15, 19, 20]		[21–24]	[25]	[26–29]					[30]
Castability	[14–16]		[31]								[16]
Flammability	[32]					[32]					
Corrosion resistance		[20, 33–35]	[36]	[22, 37]	[38–41]			[42]	[43]	[44]	
Formability			[45]			[45]					[46, 47]
Cell viability				[48]							
Grain refining				[49, 50]	[38]						
Biocompatibility					[51]				[52, 53]		
Antibacterial reaction					[54]					[55–58]	
Damping property						[26]	[59]				
Microstructure						[60–62]					[47]
Optical							[63]				
Hydrogen storage							[64, 65]				
Ductility								[66]			

Table 3.2: Minor alloying elements to magnesium binary alloys.

	Ag	Cd	Co	Dy	Ga	Gd	Pd	RE	Sc	Si	Sm	Ti
Antibacterial reaction	[67]				[54]							
Corrosion resistance	[67]			[68]				[18]				[69, 70]
Mechanical property	[67]	[71]		[68]		[29, 72, 73]	[74]				[75]	
Grain refining		[71]										[76]
Hydrogen storage			[77]								[78]	
Hardness						[72]						
Formability								[79, 80]				
Shape memory effect									[81]			
Damping property										[82]		[83]

3.3 Alloying elements to Mg-based ternary alloys

In the above-mentioned Mg-based binary alloys, each element is alloyed to form ternary alloys as shown in the following tables along with phase diagrams [13].

3.3.1 Mg–Al alloy system

This is the most important Mg-based binary alloy because Al is added to Mg in most of the commercial types of Mg alloys.

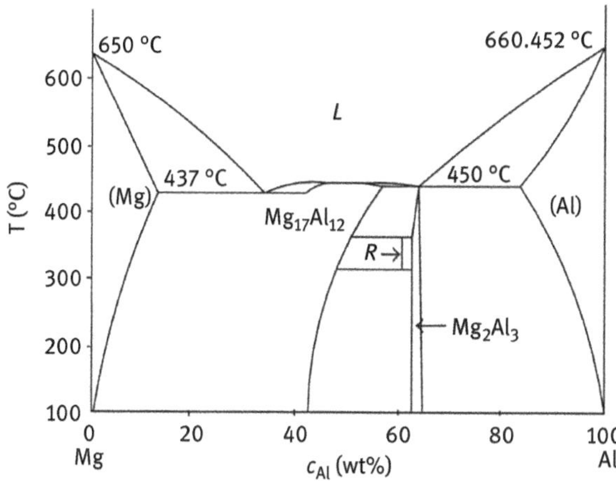

	Al	Zn	Mn	Ca	Sr	Y	Ni	Ce	Nd	Cu	Sn
Twinning		[84, 85]									
Mechanical property		[86]		[23, 87]		[88]	[89]	[90]	[91]	[92]	[93]
Ductility			[18]			[88]					
Grain refining			[94–96]	[97–99]	[100, 101]						
Corrosion resistance			[18, 102]					[103]			
Hydrogen storage							[104]				
Biocompatibility								[103]			
Biological reaction										[92]	
Electrochemical reaction											[105]

3.3.2 Mg–Zn alloy system

Zn is commonly alloyed with Mg in AZ, EZ, ZK and in smaller amounts in AM and AE series.

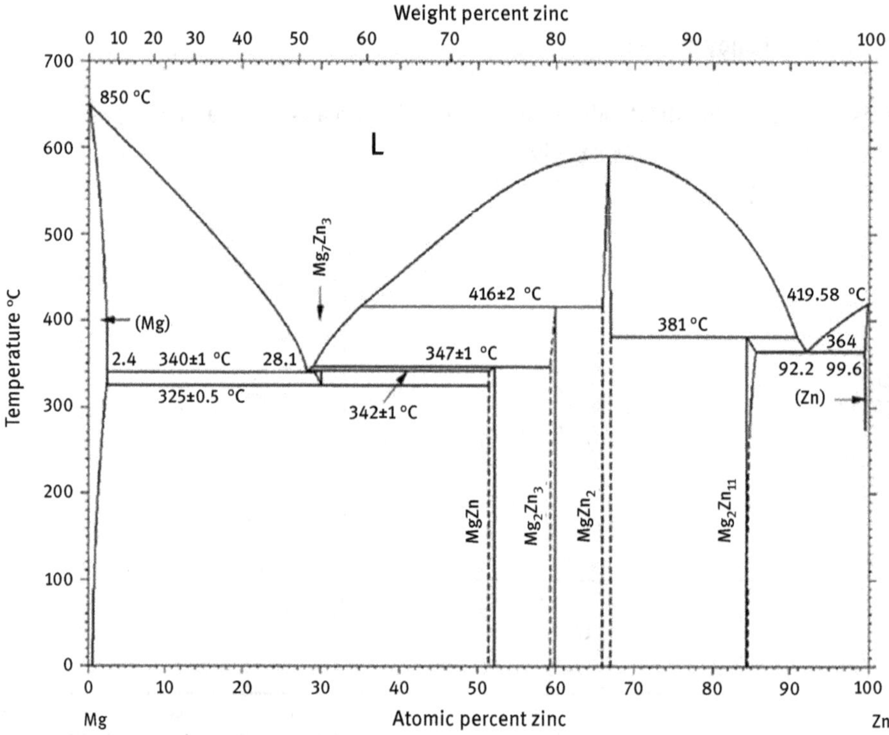

3.3.3 Mg–Mn alloy system

Mg–Mn system is characterized by a wide miscibility gap in the liquid and is characterized with limited solid solubility of Mn in Mg.

	Al	Zn	Mn	Ca	Sr	Y	Ni	Ce	Nd	Cu	Sn
Twinning	[106]										
Mechanical property	[107]		[108]	[109–113]	[100]	[114–116]		[112, 115]	[111]	[117–119]	[120]
Microstructure				[109–113]	[100]	[114–116, 121]		[112, 115]	[111]		[120]
Machinability	[122]										
Corrosion resistance	[34]		[18]		[101]						[123]
Ductility				[124]							
Formability				[125]	[125]						
Damping capacity						[126]					
Hydrogen storage							[127]				

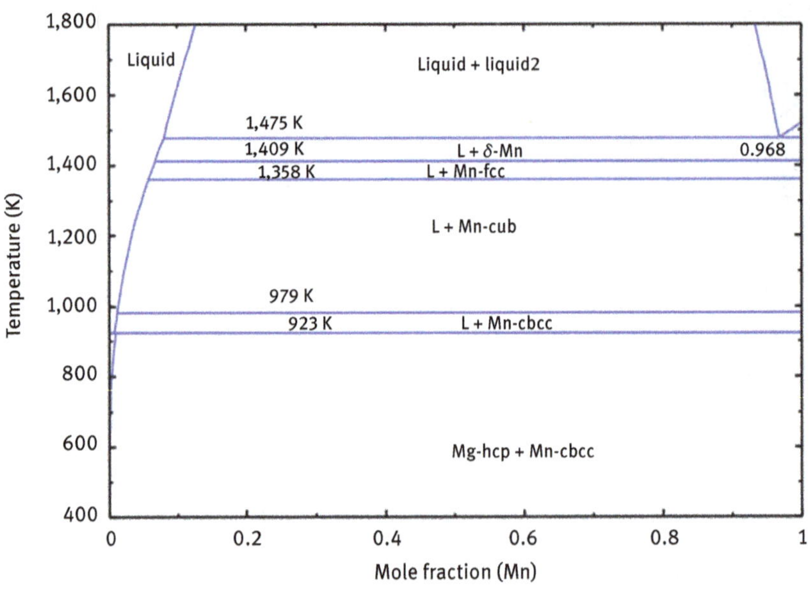

	Al	Zn	Mn	Ca	Sr	Y	Ni	Ce	Nd	Cu	Sn
Electromagnetic properties	[128]										
Mechanical property		[36, 129, 130]		[131, 132]	[133]	[134]		[135–138]	[139]	[140]	[141, 142]
Corrosion resistance		[130]		[132, 143]							[142]
Microstructure				[131]	[133]	[134]		[135–138]	[139]	[140]	[141]
Creep resistance						[144]					
Hydrogen storage							[145]				
Thermal conductivity								[138]			
Damping capacity										[140]	

3.3.4 Mg–Ca alloy system

In this alloy system, the solubility of Ca in Mg is limited.

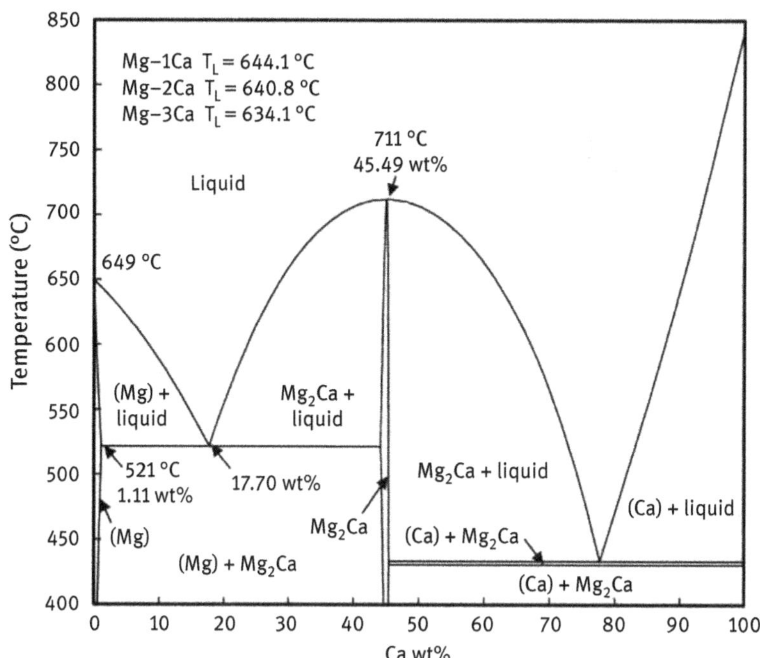

	Al	Zn	Mn	Ca	Sr	Y	Ni	Ce	Nd	Cu	Sn
Mechanical property	[146]	[147, 148]									
Microstructure	[146]	[147]					[149]				
Hardening	[150]	[151]									
Corrosion resistance		[147]	[152]		[153]	[154, 155]					
Fracture toughness		[148]									
Flammability								[156]			

3.3.5 Mg–Sr alloy system

The solid solubility of Mg in Sr is limited.

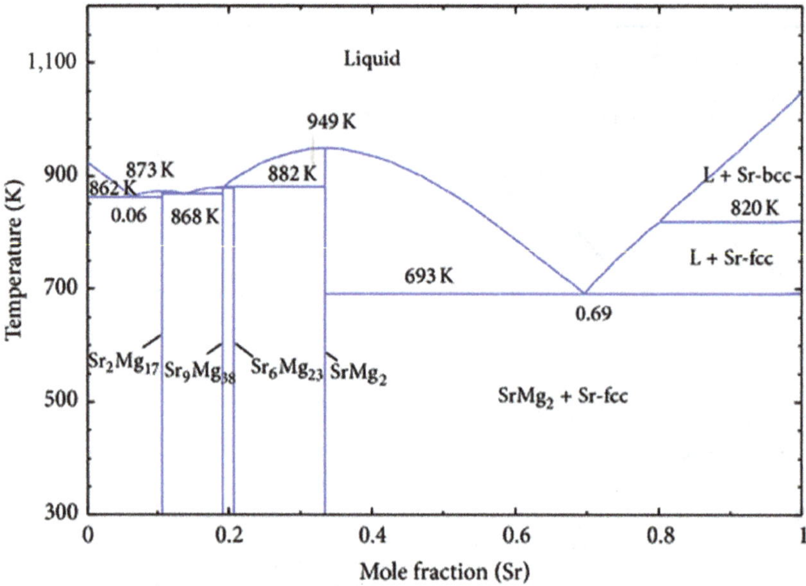

	Al	Zn	Mn	Ca	Sr	Y	Ni	Ce	Nd	Cu	Sn
Microstructure	[157, 158]			[159]		[160, 161]	[158]		[162]		
Creep behavior			[163–165]								
Mechanical properties				[159]		[160, 161]					
Ductility											
Corrosion resistance				[166]							
Flammability				[167]							

3.3.6 Mg–Y alloy system

The maximum primary solid solubility of Y in Mg is 2.63 at% Y at the eutectic temperature (575 °C).

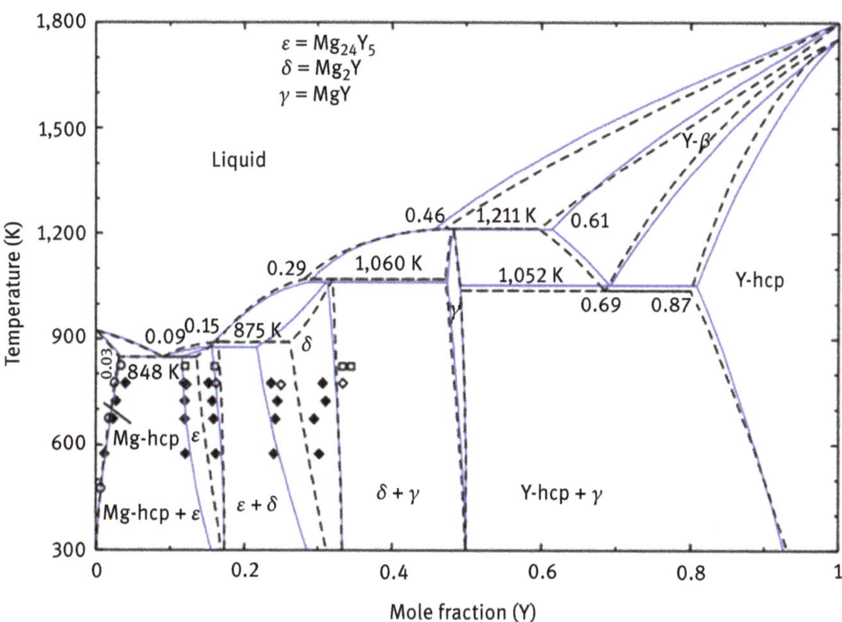

	Al	Zn	Mn	Ca	Sr	Y	Ni	Ce	Nd	Cu	Sn
Microstructure	[168, 169]	[170–173]	[174]								
Mechanical properties		[170–173]							[175]	[176]	
Ductility				[177]							
Corrosion resistance					[178]				[179]		
Electrochemical property							[180]			[181]	
Oxidation behavior								[182]			[183]
Precipitation strengthening									[184, 185]		
Thermal stability										[176, 181]	

3.3.7 Mg–Ni alloy system

There are two eutectic and one peritectic reactions in the Mg–Ni system.

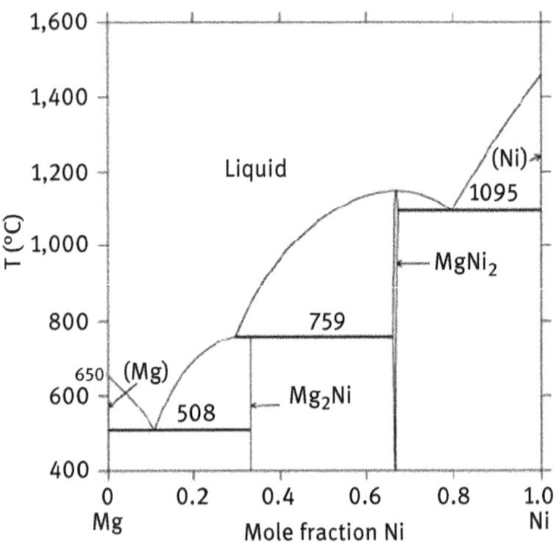

	Al	Zn	Mn	Ca	Sr	Y	Ni	Ce	Nd	Cu	Sn
Microstructure		[186, 187]		[188]	[189]	[190, 191]			[192, 193]	[194]	[195–197]
Mechanical properties				[198]		[191, 199]				[194]	
Internal friction, damping						[199]					
Hydrogen storage								[200, 201]	[64, 192, 193]	[194, 202]	[203]

3.3.8 Mg–Ce alloy system

There are three intermetallic compounds $CeMg_{12}$, $CeMg_3$ and Ce_5Mg_{41} formed peritectically in the Mg-rich corner.

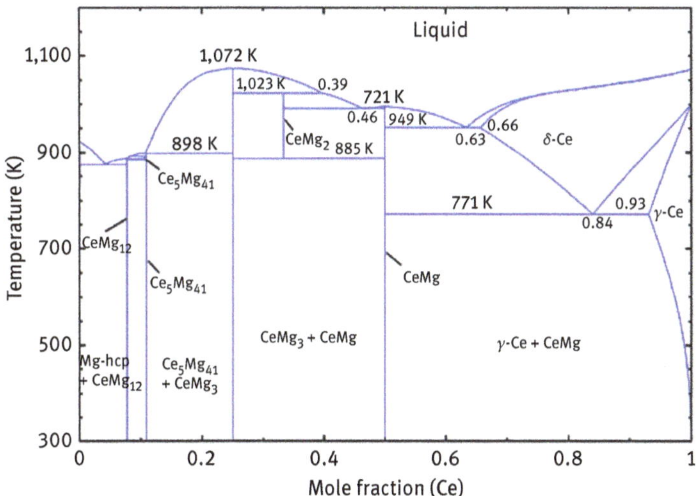

	Al	Zn	Mn	Ca	Sr	Y	Ni	Ce	Nd	Cu	Sn
Microstructure	[204]		[205, 206]		[207]				[208]	[209]	
Mechanical properties	[204]						[210]				
Age hardening	[211]										
Plastic deformation		[212]									
Electrochemical reaction		[213]									
Precipitation			[206]								
Creep resistance			[206]								
Ductility							[210]				
Hydrogen storage							[214, 215]				

3.3.9 Mg–Nd alloy system

The terminal solid solubility of Nd in Mg is 0.1 at% Nd.

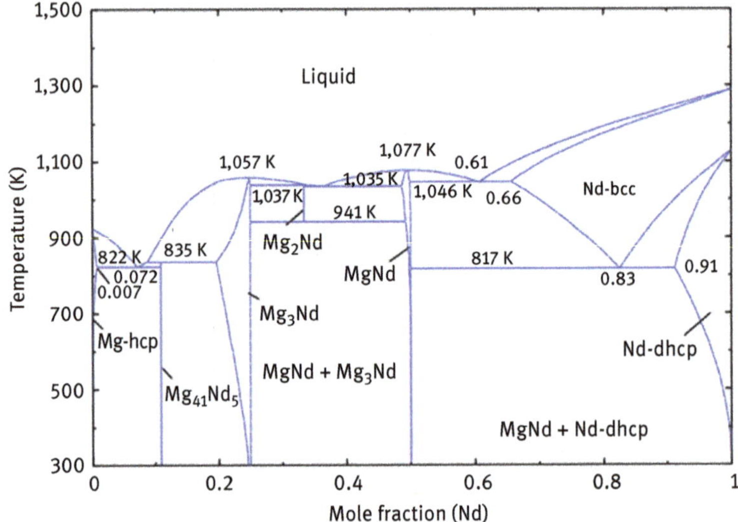

	Al	Zn	Mn	Ca	Sr	Y	Ni	Ce	Nd	Cu	Sn
Microstructure		[216–218]			[219, 220]	[221, 222]					
Mechanical properties		[217, 218]									
Corrosion behavior		[223, 224]			8	[225]					
Plastic deformation				[226]							

3.3.10 Mg–Cu alloy system

Limited terminal solubility of Cu in Mg as well as Mg in Cu has been reported and the solubility of Cu in Mg increases from about 0.1 at% Cu at room temperature to about 0.4–0.5 at% Cu at 485 °C.

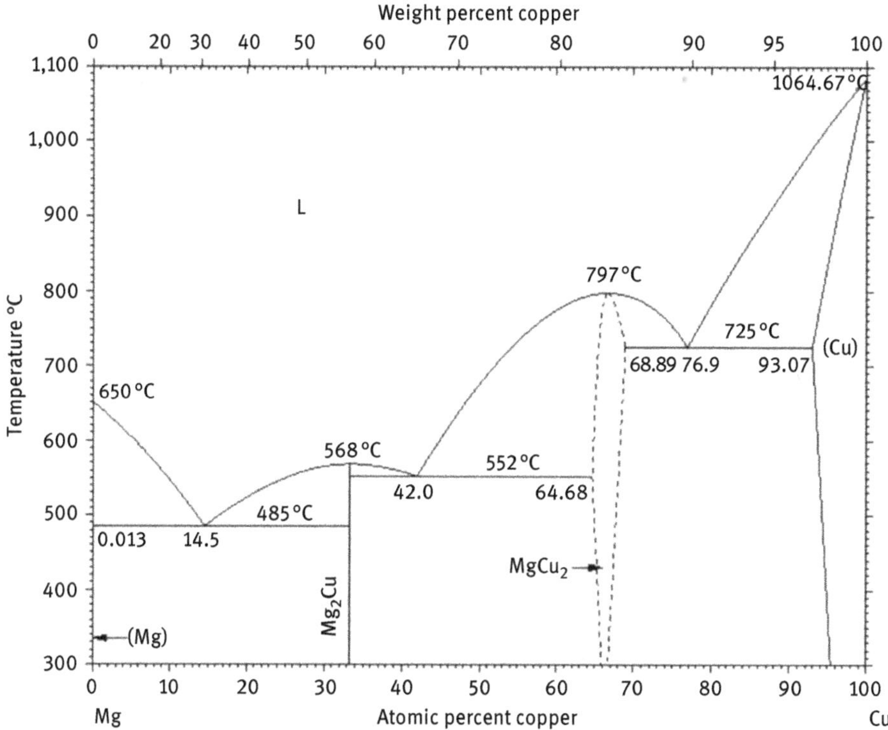

	Al	Zn	Mn	Ca	Sr	Y	Ni	Ce	Nd	Cu	Sn
Microstructure		[227]				[228, 229]			[230]		[231]
Mechanical properties		[232]	[233]			[229, 234]					
Damping capacity			[233, 235]								
Hydrogen storage							[236]				

3.3.11 Mg–Sn alloy system

There is a very narrow solid solubility range of Mg and Sn in Mg_2Sn at high temperature.

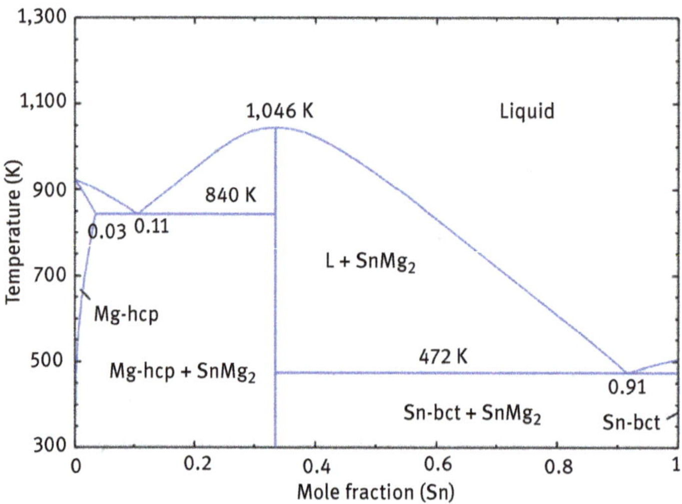

	Al	Zn	Mn	Ca	Sr	Y	Ni	Ce	Nd	Cu	Sn
Microstructure	[237, 238]	[239–241]	[242–244]	[239, 245–248]	[249–251]	[252, 253]		[254–256]	[257]	[258, 259]	
Mechanical properties	[238]	[239–241, 260, 261]	[244, 262]	[239, 246–248], 263, 264]	[249]			[255, 256]	[257]	[258, 259]	
Age hardening	[238, 265]	[266, 267]	[262, 268]								
Superplasticity	[269]										
Creep resistance	[270]			[248, 271]							
Corrosion behavior			[272]	[264, 271, 273]				[256]			
Ductility						[274]					

3.4 Mg-based quaternary alloy systems and other Mg-based alloys

3.4.1 Mg–Li alloy system

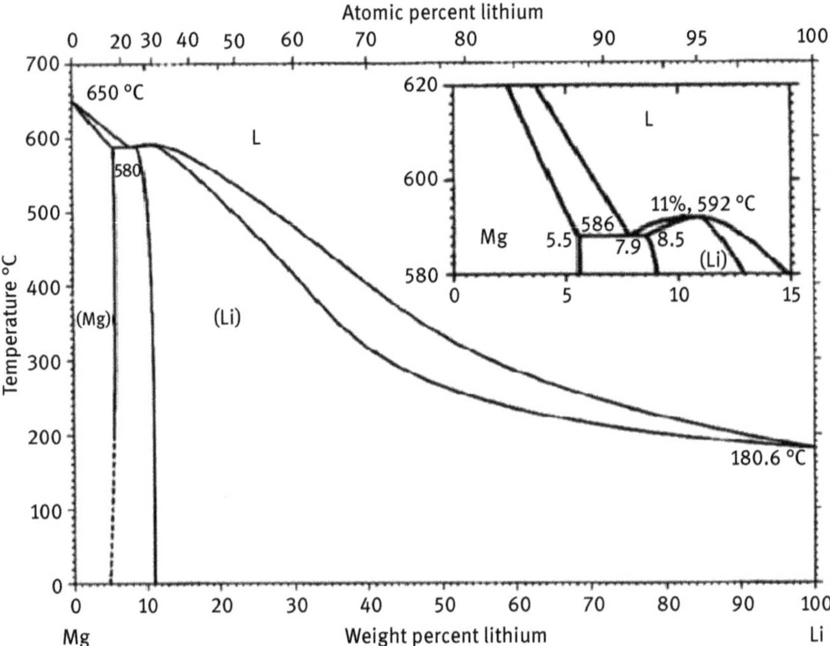

According to the Mg–Li phase diagram [275], the alloys exhibit two phase structures of α (hexagonal close packed: HCP) Mg-rich and β (body-centered cubic: BCC) Li-rich phases at room temperature when 5–11% Li is added to magnesium. Further additions of Li (more than 11%) can transform the HCO α-Mg solid solution into highly workable, BCC alloys. In Mg–Li alloy systems, there are researches in the range from relatively small concentration of Li from 3 wt% with Sc addition [276], 4 wt% with Al + Si additions [277] and 5 wt% Al alloy with Y + Nd addition [278, 279] or 5 wt%Al–Zn alloy with Sn + Y addition [280, 281] or with Cu addition [282], showing improved mechanical strength and hardness. These improvements are attributed to the synergistic effects of precipitation strengthening as well as solid solution strengthening and grain refinement strengthening. In a group of Mg–8Li alloy systems there are alloying elements such as addition of Ce-rich RE [283], Nd [284], Y [285] and Al [286]. There are quite a number of developed Mg–9Li alloy systems with further additions of mischmetal (La + Ce) [287], Sn + Y [288–290], Y + Ce [291–293] and Ca [294]. All these alloying element exhibits effective function to improve the mechanical properties due to precipitation hardening. There are still Mg–Li alloy systems possessing higher Li concentration: 10 Li with Zn + Er [295], Al + Sn + Ca [296], Sr [297] and Al + Y + Sr [298]. It is reported that all these developed complicate Mg–Li alloy systems exhibit optimum combination of tensile properties with the UTS, YS and EL.

3.4.2 Mg–Y alloy system

In Mg–Y alloy systems, there seems to be limited concentration in the development of alloys, due to the solubility limit of Y into Mg matrix, which is about 4 at% Y (see attached Mg–Y phase diagram [299]). Accordingly, there are research works on Mg–4Li alloy systems with addition of Mn + Zn [300], Zn + Zr [301], Nd + Zr + Dy [302], Gd [303], Dy + Zr [304] and RE + Zr [305] showing improved mechanical properties of solid solution hardening and refined microstructure.

Before introducing other types of Mg–Y alloy systems with higher Y concentration, it is necessary to briefly discuss the long-period stacking ordered (LPSO) structure specified with Mg–Y–Zn alloy, which exhibits high YS and EL compared to ordinally extruded Mg alloy [306]. Kawamura et al. [307] reported that the mechanical properties of $Mg_{97}Zn_1Y_2$ (at%) alloy has the tensile yield strength (TYS) of 610 MPa and EL of 5% which was prepared by rapid solidification processing and hot extrusion. These improvements should be ascribed to the dispersed nanoscale LPSO phases. Since then, Mg-Zn-Zr-RE and Mg–TM–RE (TM = Zn, Cu, Ni; RE = Y, La, Ce, Pr, Sm, Nd, Dy, Ho, Er, Gd and Tm) alloys have been investigated and developed. Normally, these alloys are also recognized for excellent corrosion resistance [306, 308]. There are still Mg–Y alloy systems with higher Y concentrations such as Mg-6Y-Zn-Sn [309] and Mg-7Y-Sm-Zr [310, 311] accompanied with improved mechanical properties. It was reported that (i) after solution treatment, LPSO phase precipitated only at grain boundaries in Zn-containing alloy, while RE-containing cuboid compound appeared in both alloys (Zn-free and Zn-containing) and (ii) the strength improvement after Zn addition is mainly attributed to the synergistic contribution of LPSO structure, γ' precipitates and β'-phase [311].

3.4.3 Mg–Ti alloy system

For searching materials exhibiting excellent corrosion, hydrogenation and switchable mirror performance, Mg–Ti alloy systems have been developed through various manufacturing processes including magnetron sputter deposition [312], mechanical alloying (MA) [78] or laser welding [313]. It was reported that (i) MA of Mg and Ti results in a nanocrystalline Mg–Ti alloy and an extended solubility of Ti in Mg, due to the favorable size factor and the isomorphous structure of Mg and Ti and (ii) in the case of Mg–20Ti (at%), about 12.5% Ti is dissolved in the Mg lattice when the MA process reaches a stable state.

3.4.4 Mg–Zr alloy system

Addition of Zr is a powerful grain refiner for Mg alloys, which results in improved ductility, smoothened grain boundaries and enhanced corrosion resistance. It is usually used in alloys containing Zn, RE, Y and thorium, and it cannot be used together with Al and Mn as they form stable compounds with Zr [314, 315]. Mg-based alloys have been extensively considered for their use as biodegradable implant materials. However, controlling their corrosion rate in the physiological environment (in other words, biodegradation rate) is still a significant challenge. One of the most effective approaches to address this challenge is to carefully select alloying compositions with enhanced corrosion resistance and mechanical properties when designing the Mg alloys, including Al, Ca, Li, Mn, Zn, Zr, Sr and RE elements on the corrosion resistance and biocompatibility of Mg alloys, from the viewpoint of the design and utilization of Mg biomaterials, and the REs include Ce, Er, La, Gd, Nd and Y [316, 317]. Recently, the Mg–Zr alloys had attracted considerable attention because of their high-specific damping capacity (around 80%), which may help to suppress the vibrations generated during movement and stress at the implant/bone interface [318]. It was indicated that 1 wt% of Zr addition in Mg resulted in significant improvement of the strength and ductility of the metal and reduced the degradation rate by 50%, and coaddition of Sr and Sn could effectively reduce the degradation of as-cast Mg–Zr–Ca alloy [317]. Some authors investigated alloys with a wide range of Zr content 1–5 wt % and showed that the degradation rate increased with increasing Zr content [319].

3.4.5 Mg–Co alloy system

Mg-based metal hydride systems along with Mg–Co–H alloy are potential high-temperature heat storage media [320]. It was reported that (i) the systems Mg/MgH_2, Mg–Ni/Mg_2NiH_4, Mg–Fe/Mg_2FeH_6 and Mg–Co–H alloy showed cyclic stability in certain temperature ranges and (ii) the thermal energy which is released by these systems covers a temperature range from 250 to 550 °C. Zhang et al. [77] synthesized Mg–Co alloy by MA and reports that the most of Mg–Co BCC alloys absorbed hydrogen at 100 °C under 6 MPa of hydrogen pressure and (ii) the $Mg_{60}Co_{40}$ alloy showed the highest hydrogen absorption capacity, about 2.7 mass% hydrogen. As-cast and as-extruded Mg-x at% Co–6 at%Y (x = 0, 1, 2, 4) alloys were prepared [321]. It was reported that (i) the tensile strength of the as-cast Mg–x at% Co–6 at%Y (x = 0, 1, 2, 4) alloys reached the peak value of ~246 MPa with the addition of 1 at% Co; (ii) additionally, the tensile strength of the as-extruded Mg–x at% Co–6 at% Y (x = 0, 1, 2, 4) alloys reached the peak value of ~369 MPa with the addition of 1 at% Co and (iii) the LPSO phase played a highly important role in the strengthening mechanism of the as-cast and as-extruded Mg–x at% Co–6 at% Y (x = 0, 1, 2, 4) alloys.

3.4.6 Mg–Ni alloy system

Fang et al. [322] investigated the effect of Al and Zn additives on the grain size of Mg–3Ni–2MnO$_2$ alloy. The nanostructured Mg–3Ni–2MnO$_2$ and Mg-3Ni-2MnO$_2$-3Al-Zn were made by ball milling process under hydrogen atmosphere. It was reported that adding beneficial elements to nanostructured magnesium alloys can form excellent hydrogen storage materials. Yang et al. [323] studied the evolution of phase constituent of $Mg_{99.0\text{-}x}Ni_xY_{1.0}$ ($x = 0.2, 0.5, 0.8, 1.0, 1.5$ at%) alloys. It was found that (i) apart from the α-Mg phase, the secondary phases in these ternary alloys mainly consist of LPSO structure, $Mg_{24}Y_5$ phase or Mg_2Ni phase, which depend on the atomic ratio of Ni and Y; (ii) the amount of LPSO structure in the alloys increases first and then decreases with the increase of Ni level, but the change in the amount of LPSO structure is not proportional to that of Ni level; (iii) the tensile properties of different alloys are tested and the changing trend of strength is similar to that of the amount of LPSO structure; and (iv) when the Ni content is 0.5 at%, the UTS, yield stress and EL are 208 MPa, 93 MPa and 8.0%, respectively, which are the optimal properties among these alloys.

3.4.7 Mg–Cu alloy system

Alloying effects of Cu and Mn to form Mg–3Cu–1Mn (CM31) alloy were subjected to study microstructure, mechanical properties and damping capacity [324] and it was reported that (i) Cu and Mn additions remarkably reduce the grain size of Mg–Cu–Mn alloy, but have little influence on phase composition and solute atoms concentration and (ii) the tensile properties increase obviously and the internal friction of Mg–Cu–Mn alloy decreases with grain refining. Wang et al. [325] investigated the effects of Y and Zn additions and reported that with the increase of Y and Zn contents, the secondary dendrite arm spacing of alloys is reduced; meanwhile, the YS is increased. In low-strain amplitude, the damping capacity of alloys with Y and Zn addition is lower than that of CM31 alloy; however, in strain amplitude over 5×10^{-3}, the damping capacity of alloy with a trace of Y and Zn addition (1% Y and 2% Zn, mass fraction) increases abnormally with the increase of strain amplitude and is near to that of pure Mg, probably due to the increase of dislocation density caused by the precipitation of secondary phase.

3.4.8 Mg–Ag alloy system

Magnesium-based alloys gained great interest for medical biodegradable applications. Limitations arise from high corrosion rates and mechanical properties of the Mg-based alloys. Hence, it is required to develop promising Mg-based alloy which exhibits controlled corrosion rate in biological environment (or biodegradation rate). A solubility of low concentration of Ag (<15 wt% Ag) in Mg is theoretically achievable according to the Mg–Ag phase diagram [326].

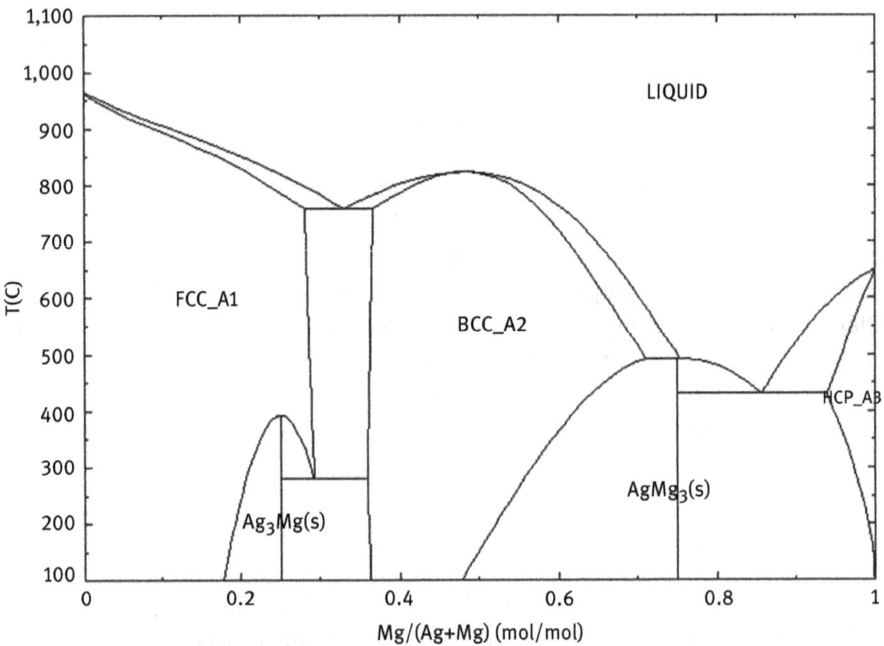

The alloys of the Mg–Ag system are interesting for the use as an implant material because in this system, the biodegradable properties of Mg are combined with the antibacterial properties of Ag [327, 328]. The Mg–Ag bulk alloys with up to 6 wt% showed a decrease in the corrosion rate compared to Mg and Mg–Ag alloys without any solution heat treatment [329, 330]. Tie et al. [331] found the lowest corrosion rate for in vitro test obtained for Mg–2Ag measured in Dulbecco's modified Eagle's medium. At higher concentrations of Ag, precipitates were formed, which led to an increased corrosion rate [330]. Another important criteria for biodegradable metallic implants are their mechanical properties, namely, the strength as well as EL at fracture. The modulus of elasticity of Mg alloys is about 70 ± GPa (see Figure 2.6) which is closer to that of bone (15 ± GPa), when compared to other metals, for example, Fe with 200 ± GPa, For this reason, Mg is considered as a promising material for orthopedic applications, because the likelihood of stress shielding is minimized [332, 333]. Tie et al. [334] conducted the mechanical and electrochemical measurements on three casting Mg–Ag alloys under cell culture conditions, indicating that in cell culture media, Mg–Ag alloys show higher but still acceptable general corrosion rates while less susceptibility to pitting corrosion than pure Mg with increasing content of silver. Jessen et al. [335] fabricated thin-film dog-bone-shaped samples with a thickness of 20 µm of Mg–Ag alloys with Ag content varied from 2 to 10 wt%. It was reported that (i) the YS is approximately doubled for Ag containing samples than pure Mg samples; (ii) for films with a Ag concentration up to 8 wt%, the EL at fracture reaches a value of ~7%; and (iii) further increase of the Ag concentration leads to lower EL at fracture, indicating that especially due to the low corrosion rate, Mg–6Ag shows the optimum of all investigated alloys, with a YS of ~310 MPa and an EL at fracture of ~6%.

3.4.9 Mg–Zn alloy system

There are numerous alloys for Mg–Zn–based ternary, quaternary or much higher systems.

3.4.9.1 Mg–Zn–Al

The effects of Sn element (from 0.5 to 6 wt%) to Mg–4Zn–1.5Al [336], Mg–6Zn–2Al [337] and Mg–7Zn–5Al [338] were investigated and it was reported (i) 2 wt% Sn addition had optimal mechanical properties and (ii) excessive Sn addition led to the coarsening of Mg_2Sn particles, resulting in decrease of strength and plasticity.

Studying the alloying effects of Sr and Ca to Mg-12Zn-4Al-0.3Mn alloy, Xiaofeng et al. [339] mentioned that a small amount of calcium addition to the base alloy results in decrease of ultimate strength as well as ductility, whereas addition of strontium causes increase of both ultimate and YS but decrease of ductility.

Zhu et al. [340] investigated alloying effects of Cu (0.5–1.5 wt%) Mg–6Zn–4Al alloy and mentioned that (i) compared with Mg–6Zn–4Al alloy, the Cu-containing alloys exhibit improved age-hardening response during single-aging treatment, (ii) in addition, high-density fine precipitates are formed in the matrix during double-aging treatment, resulting in remarkable improvement of the tensile strength, (iii) the double-aged Mg-6Zn–4Al–0.5Cu alloy shows the relatively optimal tensile properties and (iv) the YS, UTS and EL are 202 MPa, 312 MPa and 7%, respectively, which is attributed to the combined effects of fine grains and the uniform distribution of high-density fine precipitates.

The effects of Sr on the microstructure and mechanical properties of Mg–5Zn–2Al alloy are studied [341]. It was reported that (i) the as-cast ZA52 alloy mainly consists of α-Mg matrix, τ-$Mg_{32}(Al, Zn)_{49}$ and MgZn phases; (ii) Sr addition results in the precipitation of Al_4Sr and suppression of MgZn phase; (iii) in high Sr-containing alloys, the $Mg_5Zn_2Al_2$ phase can also be observed; and (iv) both the dendrite and grain size of the alloys can be refined by 1.0% Sr addition; however, the 0.2% Sr addition results in the grain coarsening in the alloy due to the decrease of contribution of Al and Zn solutes on the grain refinement.

Wang et al. [342] studied effects of RE alloy element on the microstructure and mechanical properties of Mg–8Zn–4Al (ZA84) alloy. It was reported that (i) a new quaternary precipitate $Mg_3Al_4Zn_2RE$ forms during the solidification and its phase transformation temperature point is 413 °C in RE-containing ZA84 alloys and (ii) the room-temperature and high-temperature tensile properties of as-cast and aged ZA84 alloys can be improved by RE addition.

The influences of different La and Ca combinations on the microstructure and mechanical properties of Mg-4Zn-4Al-*x*La-yCa ($x + y = 4$) alloys have been investigated [343]. It was found that (i) the tensile strengths at both room temperature and 175 °C increased with increasing Ca addition, while the ductility is decreased due to the increased formation of networked $Ca_2Mg_6Zn_3$ phase and (ii) the Mg-4Zn-4Al-2La-2Ca alloy shows the optimal tensile properties at both room temperature and high temperature.

The effects of Ce on the microstructure and mechanical properties of the Mg-20Zn-8Al-*x*Ce ($x = 0–2$ wt%) alloys were investigated [344]. It was found that (i) the dendrite as well as grain size were refined by the addition of Ce, and the best refinement was obtained in 1.39% Ce containing alloy and (ii) the addition of Ce improved the mechanical properties of the alloys with grain refinement and compound reinforcement.

Luo et al. [345] investigated the effects of combined addition of 0.6 wt% Nd and 0.4 wt% Y on the microstructure and mechanical properties of Mg–7Zn–3Al alloy. It was reported that (i) the Nd and Y addition led to obvious dendrite coarsening; however, it could modify the morphology and distribution of τ-$Mg_{32}(Al, Zn)_{49}$ intermetallics, (ii) after ageing treatment, the alloy with the Nd and Y addition exhibited better precipitation strengthening effects by forming finer $MgZn_2$ and $Mg_{32}(Al, Zn)_{49}$ precipitates into the α-Mg matrix and (iii) the yield and ultimate strength of Mg-7Zn-3Al-0.6Nd-0.4Y alloy could be increased to 182 and 300 MPa by peak-ageing treatment.

3.4.9.2 Mg–Zn–Zr

The effects of Y (yttrium) to Mg–4.9Zn–0.7Zn [346] and Mg-5.5Zn-*x*Y-0.8Zr [347] were studied and it was reported that (i) yttrium addition promoted nucleation of recrystallization during hot rolling process, (ii) the grain size of Mg–4.9Zn–0.7Zr alloy samples grew significantly with annealing temperature (300–400 °C) and holding time (0–120 min), while the microstructure of the alloy with yttrium addition remained unchanged and fine, (iii) the alloy with Y content of 1.08 wt% had the superior tensile strength, but its ductility was the lowest and (iv) when Y content reached 1.97 or 3.08 wt%, the tensile strength of the alloys decreased obviously, but the ductility had a little improvement.

The effects of neodymium (Nd) and ytterbium (Yb) on the microstructures and tensile properties of Mg–5.5Zn–0.6Zr alloy were investigated [348]. It was reported that (i) an addition of Nd or Yb both brings about the precipitation of a new γ (Mg, Nd) Zn_2 or γ (Mg, Yb) Zn_2 eutectic phase and results in a refinement in dendritics; however, the combination addition of Nd and Yb has an opposite effect on dendritics and leads to the formation of γ (Mg, Nd + Yb) Zn_2 eutectic phases in the shape of network-like, even the lamellar eutectics are somehow thickened and (ii) the tensile strength, YS and the EL are about 255.6 MPa, 163.6 MPa and 17.4%, respectively, at room temperature, due to mainly combined strengthening factors induced by Yb addition. Wang et al. [349] studied the effect of Nd and Dy (dysprosium) to Mg–1Zn–0.6Zr alloys. It was found that (i) with the addition of Nd or Dy, obvious grain refinement and texture weakening effect were obtained compared with the alloy free of RE element, (ii) notable improvement in ductility was got by adding Nd or Dy in the alloy, (iii) the enhanced ductility may be attributed to finer grain structure and weaker texture and (iv) YS of the alloy was also enhanced by adding RE.

Alloying effect of Sm (Samarium) was studied on Mg–6Zn–0.4Zr [350], Mg–6.0Zn–0.5Zr [351] and Mg–0.5Zn–0.5Zr [352]. The common findings are (i) the addition of Sm could obviously refine the as-cast grains, modify the eutectic morphology and affect the mechanical properties of the alloys, (ii) the maximum values of UTS (214 MPa) and EL (7.42%) were simultaneously obtained from the alloy with 2% Sm; however, Sm addition had no obvious effects on the fracture behavior of the alloys, namely, the fracture pattern of Mg–6Zn–0.4Zr alloy belonged to intergranular and brittle modes while the fracture regimes of all the Sm-containing alloys were dominated by the mixture of intergranular and transgranular modes and (iii) Sm addition can significantly enhance the strength of the as-extruded Mg–0.5Zn–0.5 Zr alloy at room temperature, with the optimal dosage of 3.5 wt%. The optimal YS and UTS are 368 MPa and 383 MPa, which were enhanced by approximately 23.1% and 20.8% compared with the Sm-free alloy, respectively.

3.4.9.3 Mg–Zn–Mn

The effects of Ce addition to Mg–2Zn–1Mn [353] and Mg–6ZN–1Mn [354] were investigated. It was reported that the thermal conductivity of as-cast ZM21–0.2Ce alloy was higher than that of as-cast ZM21 and ZM21–0.6Ce alloys, while thermal conductivity of as-extruded alloys increased unconventionally with the Ce content increasing [353], and the improved tensile properties of as-extruded ZM61–0.5Ce alloy were due to the finer grain sizes as compared to ZM61 alloy; however, the UTS and YS decreased severely and the EL increased when ZM61–0.5Ce was treated by T6 and T4 + two-step aging [354].

Zhou et al. [355] investigated the effects of Sn addition (0–1.5 mass%) on dynamic recrystallization of Mg–5Zn–1Mn alloy during high strain rate deformation by hot compression testing. It was reported that (i) with a higher Sn addition, the strain corresponding to the maximum softening rate and the critical strain corresponding to the onset of dynamic recrystallization decrease at first and (ii) then increase and the Mg-5Zn-1Mn-0.9Sn alloy shows the biggest recrystallization extent. Qi et al. [356] examined the microstructure and mechanical properties of Mg–6Zn–1Mn alloys with varying Sn contents (0, 1, 2, 4, 6, 8 and 10 wt%). It was found that among them, the 4 wt% Sn containing sample with double-peak aging after solution treatment had the highest strengths and moderate EL. Hu et al. [357] studied the alloying effects of Nd to Mg-6Zn-1Mn-4Sn alloy and reported that (i) α-Mg, α-Mn, Mg_7Zn_3, Mg_2Sn and MgSnNd phases are found in the as-cast Nd-containing alloys and (ii) the ZMT614–1.5Nd alloy under the extruded and aged states exhibits higher strength, because of the fine grains after extruding and high number density of rod-shaped β1′ precipitates in the α-Mg matrix after aging, respectively.

3.4.9.4 Mg–Zn–Y

The effect of 0–1 wt% Ca addition on solidification pathway of Mg–5Zn–1Y alloy and its solidification characteristics such as nucleation transformation and intermetallics formation temperatures was investigated [358]. It was reported that (i) the presence of three peaks in the first derivative curve of the ternary Mg–5Zn–1Y alloy, including to the formation of α-Mg primary phase and intermetallics $Mg_3Zn_3Y_2$ (W-phase) and Mg_3YZn_6 (I-phase), (ii) one more peak, corresponding to the formation of intermetallic $Ca_2Mg_6Zn_3$ phase, appeared in that of the quaternary Mg-5Zn-1Y-*x*Ca alloy when Ca content exceeds 0.1 wt%, (iii) the cooling curves showed that increasing Ca content from 0 to 1 wt% results in reducing the liquidus temperature from 659 to 636 °C and the average grain size from 2.8 to 1.7 mm in the Mg–5Zn–1Y alloy and (iv) the increase in Ca content also decreased the formation temperature of $Ca_2Mg_6Zn_3$ phase significantly, about 29 °C, while it increased the solidus temperature from 219 to 233 °C. Kwak et al. [359] studied the effect of adding 0.3 wt% Ca to a Mg–9.5Zn–2.0Y alloy with icosahedral phase (I-phase: Mg_3Zn_6Y). It was mentioned that (i) the upper limit of hot workability temperature decreased to 325 °C, which is lower than that of the Mg–9.5Zn–2.0Y alloy by −148 °C and (ii) the cast Mg-9.5Zn-2.0Y-0.3Ca alloys prepared using the two different routes exhibited high similarity in ignition temperature, chemical composition, microstructure, hot compressive behaviors and processing maps, indicating that the use of CaO is as effective as the use of Ca in producing the same quality of Ca-containing Mg alloys.

The addition effect of Mn to $Mg_{95.21}Zn_{1.44}Y_{2.86}Mn_{0.49}$ alloy with a Zn/Y ratio of 0.5 [360] and Mn + Ca to $Mg_{94}Zn_{2.5}Y_{2.5}Mn_1$ alloy [361] was examined. It was reported that (i) when the Zn/Y ratio is constant, the as-extruded $Mg_{95.21}Zn_{1.44}Y_{2.86}Mn_{0.49}$ alloy has the best mechanical properties, exhibiting a tensile strength of 421 MPa, a YS of 333 MPa and an EL of 5.85%; and (ii) the high strength is mainly due to the strengthening by the refinement of α-Mg matrix grains through an increase in the amount of X-phase [360]. By further adding Ca, it was mentioned that (i) Ca induced the formation of LPSO structure while discouraged that of $Mg_3Zn_3Y_2$ eutectic structure and (ii) with Ca addition, the microstructures were refined, and the mechanical properties were enhanced [361].

Hao et al. [362] investigated the effects of Ti to microstructure and mechanical properties of Mg-2.5Zn-2.5Y-1Mn and found that the addition of 0.3 at% Ti yielded the best strength. Medina et al. [363] studied the effect of Ca, Mn and Ce mischmetal additions on the mechanical properties of the extruded Mg–6Zn–1Y (wt%) alloy. It was mentioned that (i) the highest yield stress value corresponds to the material modified with cerium-rich mischmetal and (ii) Mn addition leads to the best balance between strength and ductility while calcium addition has a negligible effect on the mechanical properties of ternary alloy.

3.4.9.5 Mg–Zn–Sn

Effects of minor Sr addition (0, 0.2, 0.4, 0.6 and 1.0 mass%) on microstructure and mechanical properties of the as-cast Mg-4.5Zn-4.5Sn-2Al-based alloy system are investigated [364]. It was reported that minor Sr addition can effectively refine grains, dendrites and grain boundary compounds, and this effect is more obvious with a higher Sr addition; however, a smaller amount of grain boundary compounds and a larger amount of the intracrystalline intermetallics are detected with a higher Sr addition. The as-cast alloy with 0.2% Sr addition exhibits the best combined mechanical properties at ambient temperature with the UTS and EL of 238 MPa and 12.1%, respectively; however, excessive Sr addition results in the decline of strength and plasticity. Furthermore, the Sr addition in the range of 0.2% and 1.0% has no obvious beneficial effect on the UTS of the as-cast alloys and leads to plasticity loss at 175 °C. Wei et al. [365] studied effects of minor Ca addition (0, 0.2, 0.4 and 0.6 mass %) on microstructure and mechanical properties of the as-cast and the as-rolled Mg-4.5Zn-4.5Sn-2Al-based alloy system. It was found that (i) the as-cast alloy with 0.2% Ca addition exhibits a fairly good roll-forming ability and the optimal combined mechanical properties, with the UTS and EL of 243 MPa and 13.9%, respectively, (ii) the 0.2% Ca addition plays important roles in refining twins and dynamic recrystallization grains, increasing twinning density and promoting precipitations in the as-rolled alloy, contributing to the enhanced strength and (iii) the as-rolled Mg-4.5Zn-4.5Sn-2Al-0.2Ca alloy exhibits the UTS of 406 MPa and the YS of 285 MPa, about 18% and 26% higher than the Ca-free alloy; however, the 0.2% Ca addition reduces the plasticity of the as-rolled alloy.

Son et al. studied the effects of Ag addition on the microstructure and mechanical properties of hot-extruded Mg-6Zn-2Sn-0.4Mn-based alloys [366] and Li addition to Mg-3Zn-1Sn-0.4Mn alloys [367]. It was reported that (i) Ag addition resulted in grain refinement and weaker basal texture in the alloys, (ii) Ag-containing extruded alloys had better mechanical properties than the alloys without Ag and (iii) the UTS and EL of alloys containing 1 wt% Ag were 352 MPa and 19%, respectively. As to the effect of Li element, it was mentioned that (iv) by Li addition from 5 wt% to 8 and

11 wt%, the ductility was significantly increased from 18.1% to 30.9% and 49.3% at room temperature due to transformation from HCP to BCC crystal structure and formation of a weaker basal texture of the α-Mg phase region, (v) the UTS was decreased from 252.0, 201.1 and 148.7 MPa as Li content increased from 5 to 8 and 11 wt% and (vi) on the other hand, the tensile strength of Sn containing alloys was remarkably increased compared to the alloys without Sn addition due to the presence of the fine $MgLi_2Sn$ intermetallic compounds.

3.4.9.6 Mg–Zn–Ca

The effect of Mn addition on grain refinement of a biodegradable as-cast Mg alloy, Mg-4Zn-0.5Ca-*x*Mn ($x = 0$, 0.4, or 0.8 wt%), was investigated [368]. It was found that the grain sizes of the Mg–4Zn–0.5Ca, Mg-4Zn-0.5Ca-0.4Mn and Mg-4Zn-0.5Ca-0.8Mn alloys were 124, 72 and 46 μm, respectively, indicating that adding Mn to the alloy Mg–4Zn–0.5Ca causes gradual grain refinement, which is related to undercooling. Tong et al. [369] investigated the effect of trace Mn addition on the microstructure, texture and mechanical properties of the as-cast and as-extruded Mg–5.25 wt%Zn–0.6 wt%Ca (ZX51) alloys. It was reported that (i) Mn addition had a negligible effect on the grain size of the as-cast ZX51 alloy; however, the addition of Mn led to the obvious decrease of grain size in the as-extruded Mg-5.25 wt%Zn-0.6 wt%Ca-0.3 wt%Mn (ZXM510) alloy, because the Mn addition restricted the grain growth during the hot extrusion process and (ii) both TYS and UTS were increased in the as-extruded ZXM510 alloy, while the ductility was slightly decreased, due to combined effects of the grain refinement and texture strengthening.

Ding et al. [370] evaluated the effects of Ca addition on five Mg alloys: Mg–2Zn, Mg–0.5RE, Mg–0.5Ca, Mg–2Zn–0.5Ca and Mg–2Zn–0.5RE (wt%) alloys. It was reported that the ductility increase through the addition of Ca to Mg is related to the texture weakening of extruded Ca-containing alloys. Wang et al. [371] extruded Mg-*x* Zn-0.2Ca-0.2Ce ($x = 0.5$, 1.0, 1.5 and 2.0, wt%) alloys and evaluated the effects of Zn addition on the mechanical properties and texture characteristics. It was mentioned that (i) both the strength and plasticity were improved with the increasing Zn addition, by solid solution hardening, solid solution softening and the enhanced cohesion of grain boundaries, while further Zn addition deteriorated the plasticity, because of the dominant solid solution hardening and (ii) Mg-Zn-Ca-Ce magnesium alloys received the best comprehensive mechanical properties when Zn addition reached 1.5 wt%, with tension YS and tension fracture EL about 131.0 MPa and 42.4%, respectively.

To Mg–3.8Zn–2.2Ca alloy, Yang et al. added Sn element (0, 0.5, 1 and 2, wt%) [372] and Gd element (0, 0.36, 0.88, 1.49 and 2.52 wt%) [373] and evaluated microstructure, tensile and creep properties. With Sn element, it was reported that (i) the grains of the Sn-containing alloys are effectively refined, and the grains of the alloy with 0.90 wt% Sn are the finest, (ii) compared with the ternary alloy, the tensile and creep properties of the alloys with the additions of 0.46 wt% and 0.90 wt% Sn are effectively improved; however, the UTS and EL of the alloy with 1.88 wt% Sn are decreased though its YS and creep properties are improved and (iii) among the three Sn-containing alloys with the additions of 0.46, 0.90 and 1.88 wt% Sn, the alloy with 0.90 wt% Sn exhibits relatively optimal tensile and creep properties; while as to alloying effect of Gd element, it was found that (i) the additions of 0.36–2.52 wt% Gd to the Mg–3.8Zn–2.2Ca ternary alloy can refine the grains of the alloy, and an increase in Gd content from 0.36 to 2.52 wt% causes the grain size to gradually decrease, (ii) the additions of 0.36–2.52 wt% Gd to the Mg–3.8Zn–2.2Ca ternary alloy can also improve the tensile properties of the alloy, and the alloy with the addition of 1.49 wt% Gd exhibits the best tensile properties, (iii) the additions of 0.36–2.52 wt% Gd to the Mg–3.8Zn–2.2Ca ternary alloy do not change the creep mechanism of the alloy; however, the creep properties of the Gd-containing alloys are improved, and an increase in Gd content from 0.36 to 2.52 wt% causes the creep properties to gradually increase and (iv) among the Gd-containing alloys with the additions of 0.36, 0.88, 1.49 and 2.52 wt% Gd, the alloy with the addition of 1.49 wt % Gd exhibits the relatively optimal tensile and creep properties.

3.4.9.7 Mg–Zn–RE

In this section, several RE elements will be reviewed in terms of their effective alloying function to Mg–Zn-based alloy systems.

Addition of La to Mg–6Zn was studied and reported that (i) La addition weakened the texture and gave rise to the formation of nonbasal texture component, attributing to the existence of La in the form of solute atoms in matrix, (ii) the ductility was enhanced significantly by adding La to Mg–6 wt%Zn alloy, while the strength was reduced and (iii) the Mg–6Zn–0.2La (wt%) alloy exhibited a superior ductility with the EL to fracture up to 35%; however, with further increasing of La content to 1 wt%, the strength of the as-extruded Mg–Zn–La alloys was not improved but the ductility was reduced, suggesting that small addition of La is preferred for the improvement of mechanical properties [374].

Fu et al. [375] studied the influence of Ca addition on the as-cast microstructure, casting fluidity and mechanical properties of the Mg-4.2Zn-1.7Ce-0.5Zr (wt%) alloy. It was reported that (i) the as-cast alloys consisted of α-Mg matrix, Ca-contained T-phase and $Mg_{51}Zn_{20}$ phase, (ii) addition of 0.2–0.6 wt% Ca led to effective grain refinement and enhanced the fluidity of the alloys; (iii) when the content of Ca was 0.2 wt%, the alloy exhibited the finest grain size of 35.9 µm, and the filling length was increased by approximately 55.4% compared with the quaternary alloy; and (iv) with an increase in Ca content, the YS increased gradually, whereas the UTS and EL showed a decreasing tendency.

The microstructures and mechanical properties of Mg–2.0Zn–1.0Mn (ZM21) alloys with certain amount of Ce and Nd additions were investigated [376]. The results indicated that (i) the addition of Nd and Ce can refine the grains in ZM21 alloy and (ii) the average grain size of ZM21 alloy with the additions of 0.4 wt% Nd and Ce reached 6 ± 3 µm and 13 ± 2 µm, respectively.

There are several studies on allying effect of Gd element to Mg–Zn-based alloy systems, including Mg–2Zn–(0.1 and 0.3%) Gd [377], Mg-2Zn-0.5Zr-(0.5–1%) Gd [378], Mg–4.0Zn–2.0Gd alloys with (0–1.0%) Ca [379], Mg–4.5Zn– (0, 0.5, 1.0 and 1.5 wt%) Gd [380] and Mg-7Zn-5Gd-0.6Zr [381]. Noticeable alloying effects of Gd element: (i) the room-temperature tensile testing demonstrated that the annealed Mg–2.0Zn–0.3Gd sheet showed a high EL to failure of 35% while the annealed Mg–2.0Zn–0.1Gd sheet showed a low ductility of about 20% which were due to different textures [377]; (ii) the good degradation resistance and mechanical properties of as-cast Mg-2Zn-1Gd-0.5Zr alloy makes it outstanding for biomedical application [378]; (iii) after extrusion, the grains are refined and the large precipitates in as-cast state are cracked to fine and dispersive particles, and all these changes are helpful to the improvement of tensile properties [379]; (iv) the strengths were greatly improved with Gd additions, and the highest strength level was obtained in the Mg–4.5Zn–1.5Gd alloy, in which the UTS and YS were 231 and 113 MPa, respectively [380]; and (v) a high-performance I-phase containing Mg-7Zn-5Gd-0.6Zr alloy is prepared by conventional casting and subsequent hot extrusion and it owns an ultimate and YS of 350 MPa and 285 MPa, respectively, and its EL is 13.6% [381], exhibiting ultimate strength of 350 MPa, YS of 285 MPa and EL of 13.6% [381].

3.4.10 Mg–Al alloy system

3.4.10.1 Mg–Al–Si

Hu et al. [382] modified the commercially used Mg–3Al–1Si (AS31) alloy with B and Sn additions, followed by the hot rolling. It was reported that (i) simultaneous addition of B and Sn resulted in large grains and coarse Mg_2Si phase in the as-cast alloy, which showed the highest tensile strength of 231 MPa and ductility of 19.5%; (ii) for the hot-rolled alloys, B or Sn addition distinctly refined the grains of AS31 sheet, while their combination severely retarded dynamic recrystallization, leading to much unrecrystallized structure; and (iii) the AS31–2Sn sheet exhibited the best YS of ~260 MPa with desirable ductility of ~15%, due to the solid solution strengthening, grain boundary strengthening, texture strengthening and dislocation strengthening.

3.4.10.2 Mg–Al–Zn

Basically, there are several works on modifications of the commercially used AZ31, AZ61, AZ62, AZ82 and AZ91 with various alloying elements. Shang et al. [383] modified AZ31 with Ca, Sr and Ce (0.2 wt% for each element). It was mentioned that the results of electron probe microanalysis showed the existence of phases other than

$Mg_{17}(Al, Zn)_{12}$ and Al_8Mn_5 in AZ31 alloy, namely Al_2Ca, Al_2Sr, $Al_{11}Ce_3$, Al_8CeMn_4 and $Al_2(Ca Sr)$, and these new phases were thermally stable at 450 °C for 10 h. Wang et al. [384] investigated the microstructure and tensile properties of Mg-*x*Al-*y*Zn-2Ca ($x + y = 8$ wt%) alloys with various Al and Zn contents. It was reported that (i) two Laves phases, that is, C36 and C15, Q phase and/or $Ca_2Mg_6Zn_3$ isomorphs phases were observed in as-cast alloys, (ii) the majority of second phase was C36 in high Al-containing alloys, (iii) by decreasing Al content, the C36 was transformed to C15 Laves phase and $Ca_2Mg_6Zn_3$ isomorphs phase, (iv) the tensile strength and ductility of Mg-Al-Zn-Ca alloys were greatly dependent on the category and the morphology of second phases and (v) the alloy containing the majority of networked C36 phase shows optimal mechanical properties at both room temperature and elevated temperature.

In AZ61 alloy, effects of Pd (0–6 wt%) [385], Ti (0.01–0.02 wt%) [386] and Sm (0.5–2.0 wt%) [387] were studied. It was reported that (i) at room temperature, the tensile strength increased with increasing Pd addition up to 2 wt% Pd, and the EL to fracture decreased with a concomitant increase in the aggregation of the coarse Al_4Pd phase, while at 150 °C, the tensile strength increased with the addition of Pd. Therefore, the room- and elevated-temperature tensile properties of as-cast Mg–6Al–1Zn alloys can be improved by Pd addition [385], (ii) The addition of a larger amount of Ti (0.02 wt%) increased the corrosion rate, but the AZ61 alloy with 0.02 wt% Ti exhibited a much better corrosion resistance than the AZ61 alloy with 0.01 wt% Ti [386] and (iii) Sm can dramatically improve the YS and tensile strength of the alloy at 20–175 °C and with 0.5–2.0 wt% Sm addition, the microstructure of alloy is remarkably refined [387]. Additionally, Bae et al. [388] studied the effects of Sn addition (2.4 and 8 wt%) to AZ62 alloy and reported that (i) the tensile and compressive YS of the extruded alloy improve gradually with an increase in the Sn content, which is attributed mainly to the enhancement of the grain boundary hardening and precipitate hardening effects and (ii) the tensile EL decreases slightly up until the addition of 4 wt% Sn and then deteriorates considerably upon the addition of 8 wt% Sn because of the presence of large undissolved Mg_2Sn particles in the AZT628 alloy.

AZ82 was modified with Sn [389], while AZ91 was modified with B [390], Sc [391] or Sm [392]. The main results are as follows: (i) the UTS improves with Sn addition of up to 4 wt%, but deteriorates beyond that point due to premature fracture caused by crack initiation at large particles [389]; (ii) the addition of boron in the form of Al–4B master alloy significantly refines the grain size of AZ91 alloy [390]; (iii) the microstructure is mainly composed of α-Mg matrix, β-$Mg_{17}Al_{12}$ phase and Mg_5Al_4Sc intermetallic compound when 0.3% Sc was added, and Sc (scandium) addition improves the morphology and distribution of $Mg_{17}Al_{12}$ phase, which substantially improves the mechanical properties of the alloy at both room temperature and high temperature [391]; and (iv) preferential segregation of Sm with Al, leading to the formation of Al_2Sm, was found and formation of Al_2Sm in AZ91 resulted in a morphology change of β-$Mg_{17}Al_{12}$ phase, from a coarse, mesh structure to a fine short rod structure – reducing the overall β-$Mg_{17}Al_{12}$ phase area fraction [392].

There are still researches on Mg–Al–Zn alloys with higher Al contents: 10 wt% Al modified with Si [393] and 20 wt% Al modified with La element [394].

3.4.10.3 Mg–Al–Mn

Alloying effects of Sm to AM50 [395] or potassium fluoride (KF) [396] and Ca [397] or Sr [398] to AM60 were investigated. It was reported that tensile results showed that Mg-5Al-0.3Mn-2Sm alloy exhibited the highest tensile properties at both room temperature and 150 °C, compared with UTS, YS and EL (ε) of Mg–5Al–0.3Mn alloy, UTS, YS and ε of Mg-5Al-0.3Mn-2Sm alloy were enhanced by 30%, 45% and 35% at room temperature and by 17%, 48% and 96% at 150 °C, respectively, mainly due to the decreased amount of β-$Mg_{17}Al_{12}$ and its refined morphology and high thermal stable $Al_{11}Sm_3$ and Al_2Sm precipitates [395]. The addition of KF plays a key role in the formation of in situ sealing pores and KF can change the initial film and promote the film growth rate [396]. Calcium addition can substantially improve creep properties by substituting β-$Mg_{17}Al_{12}$ phase with an interconnected and thermally stable Al_2Ca phase; unlike β-$Mg_{17}Al_{12}$ particles that crack during creep, the network of lamellar Al_2Ca phase withstands deformation at high temperatures, and thus, improves creep resistance and (iv) addition of strontium element modified the structure and refined the grain size and the hardness and YS of the alloys increased continuously with increasing strontium content, while the EL was gradually decreased, and the tensile strength value of the based alloy was increased by adding Sr up to 1 wt%. After more addition of Sr, the tensile strength starts to diminish.

3.4.10.4 Mg–Al–Ca

Nakata et al. [399] studied the effect of Mn content on the mechanical properties and microstructures of extruded Mg-1.1Al-0.24Ca-based alloys. It was found that (i) in a solution-treated condition, tensile yield stress is enhanced to 200 MPa with increasing Mn content up to 0.68 wt% and the compressive yield stress is also improved to 164 MPa with increasing Mn content up to 1.0 wt% due to grain size refinement (ii) after an artificial aging, the tensile and compressive yield stresses are increased by 70 and 30 MPa regardless of the Mn content; consequently, the peak-aged 1.1Al–0.24Ca–1.0Mn alloy, AXM1021, exhibits high tensile and compressive yield stresses of 263 and 197 MPa with a good yield asymmetry of 0.74 (a ratio of compressive yield stress to tensile one). The commercially used AXJ alloy (Mg-Al-Ca-Sr) was subjected to study the effects of Sr addition [400] and it was mentioned that Sr addition leads to the coarsening of α-Mg matrix; however, with the Sr content increasing from 0.1% to 0.5%, the grain size decreases from 83.9 to 65.8 μm and the addition of Sr ranging from 0.1% to 0.3% refines the Al_2Ca phase.

Using Mg-Al-Ca-Mn alloy, the effect of Ca/Al ratio was investigated on microstructure and mechanical properties [401, 402]. It was the common observation that Ca/Al ratio shows a direct relationship with the total amounts of Laves intermetallics and the amount of the C36 phase and an indirect relationship with the amount of C14 phase. It was also reported that (i) the as-cast Mg-Al-Ca-Mn alloys with Ca/Al mass ratios less than 0.50 contain divorced and lamellar eutectic $(Mg,Al)_2Ca$; (ii) when Ca/Al ratio is greater than 0.90, fine lamellar Mg_2Ca phase is formed in the as-cast Mg-Al-Ca-Mn alloys; (iii) the hardness and room temperature yield and UTS increase while the ductility at all temperatures decreases with increasing Ca/Al ratio; (iv) the strength of the as-extruded Mg-Al-Ca-Mn alloys increases significantly with increasing Ca/Al ratio and the as-extruded Mg-2.7Al-3.5Ca-0.4Mn (wt%) alloy exhibits a tensile proof strength of 438 MPa and an UTS of 457 MPa; and (v) at elevated temperatures, the UTS has a relationship with the dissolved amount of Ca and Mn in the α-Mg phase and creep strain was found to decrease from 0.35% to 0.05% as Ca/Al increases from 0.6 to 0.9 and as the amount of the C36 phase which can strengthen grain boundaries increases.

3.4.10.5 Mg–Al–Sn

Suh et al. [403] investigated the effect of Sn (tin) element to Mg–3Al ally and found that (i) AT31 (Mg–3Al–1Sn) shows a much higher stretch formability than AZ31 alloy, and (ii) on the other hand, AZ31 alloy shows the development of intense shear bands during stretch forming, and these shear bands act as crack propagating paths, limiting the stretch formability of AZ31 alloy.

Mg–4Al–2Sn (AT42) alloy was modified by Ca/Sr [404] and RE [405]. It was reported that (i) the creep and corrosion resistance were improved by adding Ca and Sr [404] and (ii) the best result (yield of 70 MPa, tensile strength of 168 MPa and EL of 14%) could be achieved by aging the AT42 + 1RE alloy at 170 °C for 8 h; however, mechanical properties of AT42 + 1RE alloy starts to decrease after exceeding its optimum aging conditions due to the coarsening of intermetallics [405].

Kim et al. [406] studied Li alloying effect (2, 5, 8 and 11 wt%) to Mg-6Al-2Sn-0.4MN alloy and found that (i) compression YS was increased from 212 to 235, 242 and 239 MPa as Li content was increased from 2% to 5%, 8% and 11%, respectively, (ii) EL was remarkably increased above 60% in 11% Li alloy and (iii) it is probable that Li-containing phases play a significant role in the enhanced mechanical properties by Li addition.

Miao et al. [407] investigated the effect of Ag to age-hardening response of Mg–7Al–2Sn ally. It was found that (i) segregation of Ag atoms was observed at the interphase boundary between continuous $Mg_{17}Al_{12}$ precipitate and magnesium matrix in Mg–7Al–2Sn alloy with 0.7 wt% Ag addition and (ii) substantial grain size refinement and increased number density of $Mg_{17}Al_{12}$ precipitates may be responsible for the enhanced age-hardening response in Mg–7Al–2Sn alloy with Ag addition.

Jiang et al. [408] and Wang et al. [4–13, 78, 77, 275–409] examined the alloying effect of Zn to Mg–8Al–2SN alloy and found that (i) addition of Zn promoted the age-hardening response and precipitation of the $Mg_{17}Al_{12}$ phases through high grain boundary migration and the increase of the nucleation rate of $Mg_{17}Al_{12}$ phases and (ii) the YS of the Mg-8Al-2Sn-1Zn alloy was increased by 24% after the aging treatment. The peak-aged AZT812 alloy exhibited mechanical properties that included YS, UTS and EL of 296 MPa, 408 MPa and 7%, respectively.

In Mg–9Al–2Sn alloy, Zhu et al. [410] examined the effect of Mn addition and Liu et al. [411] studied the effect of Zn addition and reported that Mn addition has less influence on the fracture behavior of Mg–9Al–2Sn alloy, while the fracture pattern is mainly determined by the thermal conditions. Mg-9Al-2Sn-0.1Mn alloy has the best combination of strength and EL when aged at 200 °C for 8 h and the YS, UTS and EL are 154 MPa, 292 MPa and 5%, respectively [410] and Zn additions can remarkably increase the alloy hardness in the as-quenched condition and the peak hardness value of the Mg–9Al–6Sn alloy increases from 90 ± 0.87 HV to 103 ± 3.83 HV, when the Zn addition is 3 wt%, which is the highest among the magnesium casting alloys that are free of RE elements; these improvement being attributable to an increased volume fraction of smaller Mg_2Sn particles in the solution-treated condition and the formation of $[0001]_{Mg}$ $Mg_{17}Al_{12}$ rods and $Mg_{21}(Zn, Al)_{17}$ precipitates in the peak-aged condition [411].

3.4.10.6 Mg–Al–RE

In Mg–3Al alloy, alloying effect of SM was examined [412] and reported that the grain refinement was observed when 2.1 wt% Sm is added due to the formation of potent Al_2Sm nucleant particles prior to the solidification of α-Mg. Kumar et al. [413] added La and studied its alloying effect. It was reported that (i) the grain size of Mg–3Al was significantly reduced by the addition of La and it was minimum for 2.5 La-containing alloy (~5.8 μm, 25% of pure Mg grain size); (ii) the TYS, UTS and ductility for Mg–3Al–2.5La alloy are the best (TYS ~ 160 MPa, UTS ~ 249 MPa and fracture strain ~22%); (iii) results of damping measurement revealed an increase in damping of Mg–3Al alloy due to the presence of La (2.5%); and (iv) compression results show that the addition of La to Mg–3Al caused gradual decrease in compression YS and EL.

In Mg–4Al–RE (AE42) alloy, Wu et al. [414] added Ca and examined its alloying effect. It was found that (i) by increasing Ca content, the microstructure changed from dendrite crystal to equiaxed grain, and the grains were refined continuously; (ii) the Al_2Ca phase which has higher heat resistance was formed, replacing the original $Al_{11}Sm_3$ phase, and the formation of $Mg_{17}Al_{12}$ phase was effectively inhibited; (iii) the addition of Ca significantly improved the YS of AE42 alloy at both room and elevated temperatures; and (iv) the tensile strength of AE42 alloy at elevated temperature was improved significantly. Similarly, Zhang et al. [415] studied the alloying effect of Ca and Sr to Mg–4Al–RE (AE41) alloy. It was reported that (i) the compressive creep rates of AE41 alloys are decreased with increasing duration in the primary creep stage, and the steady-state compressive creep rates decreased with increasing Ca and Sr concentrations and (ii) the compressive creep resistance of Mg-Al-RE-Ca and Mg-Al-RE-Ca-Sr alloys is improved by the grain refinement, and the granular Al_2Nd, bone $(Mg, Al)_2Ca$ and fish-bone Al_4Sr hinder the dislocation climbing and grain boundary sliding. Wei et al. [416] investigated the effect of Gd on the microstructures and mechanical properties of Mg–4Al–5RE (wt%) and reported that (i) the average grain size is dramatically decreased from 493.9 to 205.8 µm, and the acicular $Al_{11}RE_3$ phase is modified to rod-like shape with a pronouncedly decreased average length from 22.0 to 3.8 µm; (ii) the modified microstructures are attributed to the formation of $Al_2(Gd, RE)$ particles, which act as nucleation sites for both α-Mg and $Al_{11}RE_3$; and (iii) the modified alloy exhibits dramatically enhanced YS, UTS and EL at about 12%, 23% and 48%, respectively.

In Mg–5Al–5Re (AME505) alloy, the influence of Ti particles was examined [417]. It was reported that the composite exhibited higher examined mechanical properties in comparison with the pure AME505 matrix alloy.

3.4.11 Mg–Sn alloy system

In the Mg–2Sn system, Ca and Zn additions were tested as an alloying element to wrought Mg–2Sn alloys [418]. It was reported that (i) the Mg–2Sn–1Ca wt% (TX21) alloy exhibited YS of 269 MPa, UTS of 305 MPa, while those of the TX21 alloy extruded at 300 °C decreased to be 207 MPa and 230 MPa, respectively; (ii) for Mg-2Sn-1Ca-2Zn wt% (TXZ212) alloy, MgSnCa, MgZnCa and $MgZn_2$ phases were observed, and the average grain size increased to be ~5 µm and the YS and UTS of TXZ212–260 alloy evolved to be 218 MPa and 285 MPa, respectively, and the EL reached as high as 23%; and (iii) the high EL of 23% in TXZ212 alloy was consistent with the high work-hardening rate, which was attributed to the larger grain size, more high angular grain boundaries, presence of more nanoparticles and the weaker texture.

In Mg–3Sn–2Ca alloy, Yang and Pan [419] investigated the effects of Y addition on the as-cast microstructure and mechanical properties. It was mentioned that adding 0.5 wt% Y to the Mg–3Sn–2Ca alloy does not cause the formation of any new phases; however, the MgSnY phase is formed in the Mg–3Sn–2Ca alloys added 1.0 or 1.5 wt% Y. Adding 0.5–1.5 wt% Y to the Mg–3Sn–2Ca alloy not only can suppress the formation of the CaMgSn phase but can also refine the CaMgSn phase. Adding 0.5–1.5 wt% Y to the Mg–3Sn–2Ca alloy can effectively improve the tensile and creep properties of the alloy, and these improvements attribute to the refinement of the CaMgSn phase. Alloying effect of Ti was also studied in Mg–3SN–2Sr alloy [420]. It was reported that (i) after the additions of 1.0% Ce, 1.0% Y and 1.0% Gd to the Mg–3Sn–2Sr alloy, the $Mg_{12}Ce$, YMgSn, GdMgSn and/or $Mg_{17}Sr_2$ phases are formed, respectively; (ii) at the same time, the formation of the primary SrMgSn phase is suppressed and the coarse needle-like primary SrMgSn phase is modified and refined; (iii) in addition, the additions of 1.0% Ce, 1.0% Y and 1.0% Gd to the Mg–3Sn–2Sr alloy can simultaneously improve the tensile and creep properties of the alloy; and (iv) among the Ce-, Y- and Gd-containing alloys, the tensile properties of the Ce-containing alloy are relatively higher than those of the Y- and Gd-containing alloys. Chen et al. [421] investigated the effect of Zn to Mg–3Sn-based alloy on microstructure and mechanical properties. It was found that for Mg-3Sn-*x*Zn-1Al alloys, (i) the grain size was basically similar, and the amount of fine Mg_2Sn particle increases markedly as the Zn content increases and (ii) the better mechanical property is attributed to the finer grains and an amount of fine Mg_2Sn particles due to the recrystallization accompanied by dynamic precipitation, that is, an UTS of 290 MPa and an EL of 12.2% at room temperature.

In Mg–4.5Sn alloy, the microstructure and tensile properties of the as-cast and as-rolled Mg–4.5Sn–5Zn alloys by adding various Sc content were investigated [422]. It was mentioned that (i) improvement of the tensile properties in as-cast Sc-containing alloys is attributed to the grain refinement and modification of secondary phase morphology; (ii) further increasing the Sc addition rate to 0.4 wt%, however, resulted in the clustering of the Sc-rich phases and was found to reduce the tensile properties of the alloy, especially the EL; (iii) the as-rolled Mg-4.5Sn-5Zn-0.3Sc alloy exhibits an optimum combination of tensile properties and (iv) the UTS, YS and EL are 293.0 MPa, 164.2 MPa and 21.5%, respectively, and the EL is about 68% higher than that of Sc-free alloy.

In Mg–5Sn alloy, Shi et al. [423] tested the Mg-5Sn-1Ca-*x*Gd ($x = 0$, 1) alloys to investigate the change in solidification paths, phase formation and mechanical properties. It was found that (i) the microstructure of as-cast Mg–5Sn–1Ca alloy is composed of α-Mg, Mg_2Sn and CaMgSn phases (ii) with the addition of Gd, the formation of the Mg_2Sn phase is impeded and the CaMgSn phase is refined, whereas the UTS and EL decrease. Nayyeri et al. [424] studied the effects of Ca and Sb additions to Mg–5Sn alloy system, including Mg–5Sn, Mg–5Sn–1.4Ca and Mg–5Sn–0.4Sb alloys. It was reported that (i) creep resistance and shear strength of the base alloy were significantly enhanced with the addition of Sb and Ca, due to the concurrent formation of Mg_2Sn particles with the more thermally stable CaMgSn or Mg_3Sb_2 phases, which strengthen both matrix and grain boundaries during deformation and (ii) mechanical properties and creep resistance of the aged alloys were much better than those of the as-cast materials, due to the higher volume fraction of Mg_2Sn, Mg_3Sb_2 and CaMgSn precipitates distributed homogeneously in the microstructure of the aged materials. Keyvani et al. [425] studied the effects of 1–3 wt % Bi, 0.15–0.70 wt% Sb and 0.7–2 wt% Ca additions on the high-temperature hardness of a cast Mg–5Sn alloy in the temperature range 25–250 °C. It was reported that (i) small amounts of Bi, Sb and Ca additions increase the hardness of Mg–5Sn alloy at both room and elevated temperature, (ii) compared to the base alloy, the ternary alloys can better retain their hardness at elevated temperatures, due to their more stable microstructures and due to the formation of thermally stable second phase particles, such as Mg_3Bi_2, Mg_3Sb_2 and CaMgSn in the Bi-, Sb- and Ca-containing alloys, respectively and (iii) the Mg–5Sn–2Ca alloy exhibits the highest hot hardness values among all tested materials, due to a refined microstructure and the high volume fraction of the thermally stable CaMgSn phase. The effect of trace additions of Ag (0.175 wt%) and Cu (0.035 wt%) on the microstructural evolution and mechanical behavior of extruded Mg–5Sn alloy was investigated [426]. It was mentioned that (i) compared to pure Mg, all the alloys showed significant improvement in hardness, tensile and compressive strength values, with Ag and Cu trace additions contributing to enhanced tensile ductility and (ii) the effect of trace additions of Ag and Cu on the material behavior was identified based on structure–property correlation. Kimm et al. [427] studied the effect of Al addition to Mg–5Sn–1Zn alloy and reported that (i) the addition of 1–4.5 wt% Al to Mg–5Sn–1Zn alloy results in grain refinement and a significant decrease in yield asymmetry in the extruded condition and (ii) the Mg–5Sn–1Zn alloy with 4.5 wt% Al showed nearly symmetric yielding behavior at room temperature, exhibiting a compressive-to-TYS ratio of 0.99.

In Mg–6Sn alloy system, the effect of Zn addition was investigated [428]. It was mentioned that in Mg–6Sn–*x*Zn ($x = 0$, 2 and 4 wt%), (i) the Young's modulus increased with increasing Zinc content up to 2% and reached a maximum value of 40 GPa for the Mg–6Sn–2Zn alloy. In the case of the cast/heat treated condition, the UTS and EL to rupture increased with the Zn content, reaching maximum values of 189.7 MPa and 7.15%, respectively and (ii) the maximum strength of the alloys in the rolled conditions was achieved for Mg–6Sn–4Zn alloy with a value of 253 MPa with 12.32% EL while in the extruded conditions, the Mg–6Sn–4%Zn alloy exhibited a maximum combination of strength and EL of 276.33 MPa and 23.1%, respectively.

In Mg–7Sn ally system, Kim et al. [429] investigated the effects of Ce addition to Mg-7Sn-1Al-1Zn (TAZ711). It was found that (i) a Ce_3Sn_5 phase forms along the grain boundaries and within grains; the volume fraction of this phase also increased with Ce content and (ii) the tensile strength gradually decreased with increasing Ce content, which was mainly attributed to a decrease in the number of precipitates and the EL of the alloy was increased by a decrease in the fraction of coarse undynamic recrystallized grains in which microcracking can be easily initiated. Kim et al. [430] studied the effects of Al (4 wt%) addition to Mg–7Sn–1Zn alloy and reported that (i) the Al addition dramatically increases the area fraction of the dynamically recrystallized grains of the extruded alloy, due to the particle-stimulated nucleation effect induced by undissolved Mg_2Sn particles, the increased amount of grain boundaries owing to grain refinement of the billet and the increase in stress applied during extrusion, (ii) the tensile and compressive strengths of the extruded alloy considerably improved with Al addition, which is due to the combined effects of Al solute atoms, undissolved Mg_2Sn particles, more Mg_2Sn precipitates and reduced grain size and (iii) the grain size reduction caused by the Al addition suppresses the formation of twins (which can act as cracking sites) during tensile deformation; this results in a considerable increase in the tensile EL of the extruded alloy.

In Mg–8Sn alloy systems, Cheng et al. [431], using Mg-8%Sn-1%Zn-X (X = Al, Mn and/or Ce) system, studied the efficiency of various alloying elements such as Al, Mn and Ce. It was reported that (i) combined addition of Al and Mn shows features distinct from separate addition of Al or Mn, (ii) additions of 1% Al and 1% Mn to base alloy result in the formation of massive Al–Mn phase in α-Mg matrix grains, (iii) addition of Ce element can refine the second eutectic precipitates and form intermetallic compounds with Sn and (iv) the effects of alloying elements on Vickers microhardness and indentation size effect of base alloy were examined. Liu et al. [432] examined the role of Ce addition to Mg-8Sn-1Al-1Zn-Ca alloy. It was reported that (i) the average grain size of studied alloys decreased from 79 to 52 μm with increasing Ca content, (ii) after Ca addition, the new phases of CaMgSn and Mg_2Ca can be found, with the CaMgSn phase presenting needle-like or particle-like shape, (iii) the corrosion resistance of the studied alloys increased first and then decreased as the Ca content increased and (iv) the Mg-8Sn-1Al-1Zn-1Ca alloy exhibited the best corrosion resistance behavior with the corrosion rate of 8.1 mm/year.

3.4.12 Mg–RE alloy system

The last but not least important there are still valuable Mg–RE-based alloys as listed in Table 3.3.

Table 3.3: Alloying elements to minor Mg-based alloy systems.

	Mg–RE	Mg–Ce	Mg–Nd	Mg–Sm	Mg–Nd	Mg–Ho	Mg–Er
Ag	[433]			[434]	[435–439]		
Zn	[433]	[440]	[441–443]	[444, 445]	[436–453]	[454]	[455]
Ca	[456]	[440, 457]			[439, 451]		
Sn	[458]						
Zr		[459]	[441–443]	[445]	[437, 439, 449, 451–453, 460–465]		
Sr		[459]			[461]		
Gd				[444]	[464]		

Table 3.3 (continued)

	Mg–RE	Mg–Ce	Mg–Nd	Mg–Sm	Mg–Nd	Mg–Ho	Mg–Er
Mn		[440, 459]			[448, 450, 452, 460, 461, 466]		
Sc		[457, 459]			[460, 461, 465]		
Y		[457]			[439, 448– 464, 467]		
Yb				[445]	[451]		
La					[463]		
Cu							[468]
V							[468]
Nd				[444]			
Ni					[448, 469]		
Ce					[449, 463]		
Si					[467]		

3.5 Mg as an alloying element to other alloys

As we have been discussing the addition effect(s) of various alloying elements to Mg-based binary, ternary, quaternary or higher alloy systems, Mg element itself plays an import role in enhancing and/or improving various properties in different alloy systems.

3.5.1 Al–Cu alloy system (2xxx series)

Al–Cu alloy typically contains between 2% and 10% Cu. The Cu provides substantial increases in strength and facilitates precipitation hardening and also reduces ductility and corrosion resistance. The influence of Mg along with Ag and Zn to Al–Cu–Li alloy was investigated and it was mentioned that when adding Mg, the precipitation kinetics are strongly accelerated, which is shown to be related to the dominant formation of T_1 precipitates [470]. Effects of Mg on the aging behavior of Al–4Cu alloy were investigated [471], and it was reported that (i) minor addition of Mg enhances the hardness values of Al4Cu powder metallurgy alloys and (ii) the highest hardness value was 118 HB obtained from 24 h aged Al–4Cu–2Mg alloy. Chen et al. [472] studied the effects of Cu/Mg ratio on microstructures and mechanical properties of Al-4.6Cu-Mg-0.5AG alloy. It was reported that (i) reducing the Cu/Mg ratio of the alloy by increasing the amount of Mg caused Ω phase to become the primary strengthening phase and increased the effect of solution and strain hardening and (ii) the hardness and strength of Al-4.6Cu-Mg-0.5Ag alloys tempered to T8 condition are increased by work hardening, but the ductility is decreased. Mondol et al. [473] developed a new Al–Cu-based ally by addition of small amounts of Sc and Mg to 2219 alloy (Al-6Cu-0.3Fe-0.3Mn-0.2Si). It was reported that by addition of small amounts of Sc (0.8 wt%) and Mg (0.45 wt%), remarkable improvement of room temperature strength occurs due to fine grain size, Al_3Sc and $Al_3(Sc,Zr)$ dispersoids.

3.5.2 Al–Si alloy system (4xxx series)

The addition of Si to Al reduces melting point and improves fluidity. Si alone in Al produces a nonheat-treatable alloy; however, in combination with Mg, it produces a precipitation hardening heat-treatable alloy. Salleh et al. [474] investigated the effects of different amounts of Mg (0.5, 0.8 and 1.2 wt%) on the microstructures and tensile properties of thixoformed Al–5%Si–Cu alloys. It was reported that (i) Mg was able to refine the size of α-Al globules and the eutectic silicon in the samples, (ii) a compact π-$Al_9FeMg_3Si_5$ phase was formed when the magnesium content was 0.8 and 1.2 wt%, (iii) the highest attainment was recorded by the alloy containing 1.2 wt% Mg with its UTS as high as 306 MPa, YS of 264 MPa and EL to fracture of 1.8% and (iv) the fracture of thixoformed alloy with a low Mg content (0.5 wt%) showed a combination of dimple and cleavage fracture, whereas in the alloy that contained the highest Mg content (1.2 wt%), cleavage fracture was observed. Tavitas-Medrano et al. [475] studied effects of Mg and Sr to 319 (Al–6Si–3.5Cu) alloy. It was found that (i) the best combination of properties is found in the Sr-modified alloy containing 0.4 wt% Mg (i.e., alloy 319 + Mg + Sr) and (ii) the optimum artificial aging temperature changes (150–240 °C, for periods of 2–8 h) when Mg is present in the alloy.

In Al–7Si-based alloy system, Kang et al. [476] studied synergistic effects of Ce and Mg to Al-7SI-0.3Mg-0.2Fe alloy and Fortini et al. [77, 78, 292–477] investigated combined effects of Mg and Mn to A356 (Al–7 wt% Si–0.5Mg) alloy. It was reported that (i) the combined addition of Mg and Ce significantly improved the strength and EL due to grain refinement and eutectic Si modification and the UTS, YS and EL reached 313 MPa, 227 MPa, 5.7%, respectively [476], and (ii) increasing the Mn/Fe ratios does not result in a significant increase of the tensile properties of the alloys; however the reduction of the Mg amounts leads to the decrease of yield stress, UTS and hardness combined with an increase in the EL to fracture [477].

3.5.3 Al–Mg alloy system (5xxx series)

The addition of Mg to Al increases strength through solid solution strengthening and improves their strain-hardening ability. Liu et al. [478] investigated the effects of Mg on Al–0.5Mg and Al–4.1Mg alloys. It was found that (i) slight solid solution strengthening by Mg addition is found in the as-cast alloys; while further significant strengthening effect is achieved in the alloys produced by high-pressure torsion, and (ii) an extraordinarily high strength of ~800 MPa is achieved in the Al–4.1Mg alloy, as a result of deformation-induced ultrafine grains, high-density stacking faults and Mg segregation. Goel et al. [479] studied effect of Mg on strain-hardening response of Al–Mg (2.5, 5 and 13 wt%)–Mn alloy and reported that Mg content and processing parameters have shown strong effect on the mechanical properties of Al-Mg-Mn-based alloys. Kim et al. [480] examined the high-temperature yield drop phenomenon in Al–Mg alloys with high contents of Mg (5–13 wt%) in a wide range of strain rates under compression. It was reported that the yield drop was highly pronounced when the added amount of Mg was beyond 10 wt%; for example, at 1/s strain rate and at 425 °C, the yield drop ratio between the upper yield stress and the lower yield stress was as high as 1.43 in the Al–13Mg alloy, while the yield drop ratios for the Al–5Mg, Al–7Mg and Al–10Mg alloys were 1, 1.1 and 1.1, respectively.

3.5.4 NiTi alloy

The effects of Mg (1, 3 and 5 wt%) on the microstructure and mechanical properties of NiTi shape-memory alloy was investigated [481]. The result indicated that (i) there was a significant reduction of the content of undesirable Ti_2Ni phase by the addition of magnesium and (ii) magnesium increased corrosion resistance and YS.

3.5.5 Nd-based alloy

A mixture of $(PrNd)_{29.9}Dy_{0.1}B_1Co_1Cu_{0.15}Fe_{bal}$ (wt%) powders with Mg (0.1–0.4 wt%) powders as grain boundary modifiers [482] was prepared. It was mentioned that with increase of Mg addition level, the magnet turns to have a higher corrosion potential and lower corrosion current density, the corrosion poverty is improved; however, temperature coefficient remained nearly unchanged with Mg addition. Zhang et al. [483] prepared $Nd_{1-x}Mg_xNi_3$ ($x = 0.10–0.50$) alloys as anode–electrode materials of nickel metal hydride batteries by powder sintering method. It was reported that (i) the content of Mg is a key factor that affects the phase structure and electrochemical properties for Nd–Mg–Ni-based alloy and (ii) less than or more than the maximum solid solubility value of Mg is disadvantageous to the cycling stability of the alloy due to the formation of impurity phase in the alloys.

References

[1] Avedesian M, Baker H. ASM Specialty Handbook: Magnesium and Magnesium Alloys, 1999, ASM International. ISBN: 978-0-87170-657-7.
[2] The Japan Magnesium Association. Current Status of Magnesium Industry. 2015; https://www.meti.go.jp/policy/nonferrous_metal/strategy/magnesium02.pdf.
[3] Kopeliovich D. Classification of magnesium alloys. 2012; https://www.substech.com/dokuwiki/doku.php?id=classification_of_magnesium_alloys.
[4] Sillekens WH, Hort N. Magnesium and Magnesium Alloys. In: Lehmhus et al., ed., Structural Materials and Processes in Transportation. 2013, Wiley-VCH; DOI: 10.1002/9783527649846.ch3.
[5] Introduction to Magnesium Alloys. In: Moosbrugger C, ed., Engineering Properties of Magnesium Alloys, 2017 ASM International; https://www.asminternational.org/documents/10192/22833166/05920G_SampleChapter.pdf/d1a641ad-e4e8-789d-c565-c9c690c1931e.
[6] https://www.totalmateria.com/page.aspx?ID=CheckArticle&site=ktn&NM=34.
[7] Magnesium Alloys and Temper Designations; https://www.totalmateria.com/page.aspx?ID=CheckArticle&site=ktn&NM=4.
[8] Witte F, Hort N, Vogt C, Cohen S, Kainer K, Willumeit R, Feyerabend F. Degradable biomaterials based on magnesium. Current Opinion in Solid State and Material Science. 2008, 12, 63–72.
[9] Revie R. Uhlig's Corrosion Handbook. 2nd Edition. NY, USA: John Wiley & Sons; 2000.
[10] Mezbahul-Islam M, Mostafa AO, Medraj M. Essential magnesium alloys binary phase diagrams and their thermochemical data. Journal of Materials. 2014; http://dx.doi.org/10.1155/2014/704283.
[11] Magnesium overview, 2013; http://www.intlmag.org/index.cfm.
[12] Magnesium Alloys. http://www.dierk-raabe.com/magnesium-alloys/.
[13] Magnesium Alloys Overview. International Magnesium Association, https://www.intlmag.org/page/design_mag_all_ima/Magnesium-Alloys-Overview.htm.
[14] Zhang L et al., Effect of Al content on the microstructures and mechanical properties of Mg–Al alloys. Materials Science and Engineering: A. 2009, 508, 129–33.
[15] Wang C et al., Effects of distributions of Al, Zn and Al+Zn atoms on the strengthening potency of Mg alloys: A first-principles calculations. Computational Materials Science. 2015, 104, 23–8.
[16] Dev A et al. Influence of solute elements (Sn and Al) on microstructure evolution of Mg alloys: An experimental and simulation study. Journal of Crystal Growth. 2018, 503, 28–35.
[17] Wu RZ et al., Reviews on the influences of alloying elements on the microstructure and mechanical properties of Mg-Li alloys. Review Advanced Material Science. 2010, 24, 35–43.
[18] Witte F et al., Degradable biomaterials based on magnesium corrosion. Current Opinion in Solid State & Materials Science. 2008, 12, 63–72.
[19] Němec M et al., Influence of alloying element Zn on the microstructural, mechanical and corrosion properties of binary Mg-Zn alloys after severe plastic deformation. Materials Characterization. 2017, 134, 69–75.
[20] Cai S et al., Effects of Zn on microstructure, mechanical properties and corrosion behavior of Mg–Zn alloys. Materials Science and Engineering: C. 2012, 32, 2570–7.
[21] Kannan MB et al., In vitro degradation and mechanical integrity of calcium-containing magnesium alloys in modified-simulated body fluid. Biomaterials. 2008, 29, 2306–14.
[22] Wan Y et al., Preparation and characterization of a new biomedical magnesium-calcium alloy. Materials & Design. 2008, 29, 2034–7.

[23] Zhang L et al., Microstructures and mechanical properties of Mg–Al–Ca alloys affected by Ca/Al ratio. Materials Science and Engineering: A. 2015, 636, 279–88.
[24] Zhu G et al., Improving ductility of a Mg alloy via non-basal slip induced by Ca addition. International Journal of Plasticity. 2019, 120, 164–79.
[25] Zhao C et al., Microstructure, mechanical properties, bio-corrosion properties and cytotoxicity of as-extruded Mg-Sr alloys. Material Science and Engineering C 2017, 70, 1081–8.
[26] Niu R-L et al., Effect of yttrium addition on microstructures, damping properties and mechanical properties of as-cast Mg–based ternary alloys. Journal of Alloys and Compounds. 2019, 785, 1270–8.
[27] Kim JI et al., Effect of Y addition on removal of Fe impurity from magnesium alloys. Scripta Materialia. 2019, 162, 355–60.
[28] Pei Z et al., The effect of yttrium on the generalized stacking fault energies in Mg. Computational Materials Science. 2017, 133, 1–5.
[29] Tang L et al., Alloying Mg with Gd and Y: Increasing both plasticity and strength. Computational Materials Science. 2016, 115, 85–91.
[30] Liu H et al., The microstructure, tensile properties, and creep behavior of as-cast Mg–(1–10)% Sn alloys. Journal Alloys and Compounds. 2007, 440, 122–6.
[31] Zhang J et al., Development of a T-Type Mg-Zn-Al Alloy: An Investigation of the Microstructure and Solidification Characteristics. Materials Science Forum. 2007, 123, 546–9.
[32] Prasad A et al., Influence of Al and Y on the ignition and flammability of Mg alloys. Corrosion Since. 2012, 55, 153–63.
[33] Yan Y et al., Effects of Zn concentration and heat treatment on the microstructure, mechanical properties and corrosion behavior of as-extruded Mg-Zn alloys produced by powder metallurgy. Journal of Alloys and Compounds. 2017, 693, 1277–89.
[34] Zhang S et al., Research on an Mg–Zn alloy as a degradable biomaterial. Acta Biomaterialia 2010, 6, 626–40.
[35] Huang J et al., *In vivo* study of degradable magnesium and magnesium alloy as bone implant. Front. Mater. Sci. China. 2007, 1, 405–9.
[36] Xu L et al., In vivo corrosion behavior of Mg-Mn-Zn alloy for bone implant application. Journal of Biomedicine Material and Research A. 2007, 83, 703–11.
[37] Wang HX et al., *In Vitro* Degradation and Mechanical Integrity of Mg-Zn-Ca Alloy Coated with Ca-Deficient Hydroxyapatite by the Pulse Electrodeposition Process. Acta Biomaterialia. 2010, 6, 1743–8.
[38] Li Y et al., Mg–Zr–Sr alloys as biodegradable implant materials. Acta Biomaterialia 2012, 8, 3177–88.
[39] Gu XN et al., In vitro and in vivo studies on a Mg–Sr binary alloy system developed as a new kind of biodegradable metal. Acta Biomaterialia. 2012, 8, 2360–74.
[40] Nam ND et al., Corrosion resistance of Mg–5Al–*x*Sr alloys. Corrosion Resistance of Mg–5Al–xSr Alloys. Journal of Alloys and Compounds 2011, 509, 4839–47.
[41] Gil-Santos A et al., Microstructure and degradation performance of biodegradable Mg-Si-Sr implant alloys. Material Science and Engineering C 2017, 71, 25–34.
[42] Ding Y et al., Effects of Alloying Elements on the Corrosion Behavior and Biocompatibility of Biodegradable Magnesium Alloys: A Review. Journal of Materials Chemistry. B 2014; https://pubs.rsc.org/en/content/articlelanding/2014/tb/c3tb21746a/unauth#!divAbstract.
[43] Seitz JM et al., Characterization of MgNd2 alloy for potential applications in bioresorbable implantable devices. Acta Biomaterialia. 2012, 8, 3852–64.
[44] Zhang E-L et al., Role of Cu element in biomedical metal alloy design. Rare Metals 2019, 38, 476–94.

[45] Somekawa H et al., Effect of alloying elements on room temperature stretch formability in Mg alloys. Materials Science and Engineering: A .2018, 732, 21–8.
[46] Zeng Y et al., Improved formability with theoretical critical shear strength transforming in Mg alloys with Sn addition. Journal of Alloys and Compounds. 2018, 764, 555–64.
[47] Zhao C et al., Preparation and characterization of as-extruded Mg–Sn alloys for orthopedic applications. Materials & Design. 2015, 70, 60–7.
[48] Kirkland NT et al., In vitro dissolution of magnesium–calcium binary alloys: clarifying the unique role of calcium additions in bioresorbable magnesium implant alloys. Biomedicine Material and Research B. 2010, 95, 91–100.
[49] Ali Y, et al., Influence of CaO Grain Refiner Addition on the Microstructure and Mechanical Properties of As-Cast Mg Alloys. In: Solanki K. et al., ed., Magnesium Technology 2017. The Minerals, Metals & Materials Series. Springer, 2017, 93–98.
[50] Andritsos EI et al., Effect of Ca on the Microstructure and Mechanical Properties in Mg Alloys. In: Orlov D. et al., ed., Magnesium Technology 2018. TMS 2018. The Minerals, Metals & Materials Series. Springer, 2018, 63–69.
[51] Bornapour M et al., Biocompatibility and biodegradability of Mg–Sr alloys: The formation of Sr-substituted hydroxyapatite. Acta Biomaterialia. 2013, 9, 5319–30.
[52] Hampp C et al., Research on the biocompatibility of the new magnesium alloy LANd442 – an invo study in the rabbit tibia over 26 weeks. Advance Engineering Materials 2012, 14, 28–37.
[53] Hampp C et al., Evaluation of the biocompatibility of two magnesium alloys as degradable implant materials in comparison to titanium as non-resorbable material in the rabbit. Material Science and Engineering C 2013, 33, 317–26.
[54] Gao Z et al., Improving in vitro and in vivo antibacterial functionality of Mg alloys through micro-alloying with Sr and Ga. Materials Science and Engineering: C. 2019, 104; https://doi.org/10.1016/j.msec.2019.109926.
[55] Li Y et al., Biodegradable Mg-Cu alloy implants with antibacterial activity for the treatment of osteomyelitis: *in vitro* and *in vivo* evaluations. Biomaterials. 2016, 106, 250–63.
[56] Yan X et al., Improvement of biodegradable and antibacterial properties by solution treatment and micro-arc oxidation (MAO) of a magnesium alloy with a trace of copper. Corrosion Science 2019, 156, 125–38.
[57] Liu C et al., Biodegradable Mg-Cu alloys with enhanced osteogenesis, angiogenesis, and long-lasting antibacterial effects. Scientific Reports. 2016, 6; https://doi.org/10.1038/srep27374
[58] Chen JX et al., Effect of copper content on the corrosion behaviors and antibacterial properties of binary Mg–Cu alloys. Materials and Technology. 2018, 33; https://doi.org/10.1080/10667857.2018.1432170.
[59] Hu XS et al., A study of damping capacities in pure Mg and Mg-Ni alloys. Scripta Materialia. 2005, 52, 1141–5.
[60] Socjusz-Podosek M et al., Effect of yttrium on structure and mechanical properties of Mg alloys. Materials Chemistry and Physics. 2003, 80, 472–5.
[61] Farzadfar SA et al., Role of yttrium in the microstructure and texture evolution of Mg. Materials Science and Engineering: A. 2011, 528, 6742–53.
[62] Du J et al., Effect of additional solute elements (X= Al, Ca, Y, Ba, Sn, Gd and Zn) on crystallographic anisotropy during the dendritic growth of magnesium alloys. Journal of Alloys and Compounds. 2019, 775, 322–9.
[63] Yoshimura K et al., Optical switching of Mg-rich Mg–Ni alloy thin films. Applied Physics Letters 2002, 81, 4709–10.
[64] Yin J et al., Improvement of Hydrogen Storage Properties of Mg-Ni Alloys by Rare-Earth Addition. Materials Transaction. 2001, 42, 712–6.

[65] Skripnyuk V et al., The effect of equal channel angular pressing on hydrogen storage properties of a eutectic Mg-Ni alloy. Journal of Alloys and Compounds. 2007, 436, 99–106.
[66] Sabat RK et al., The deciding role of texture on ductility in a Ce containing Mg alloy. Materials Letters. 2015, 153, 158–61.
[67] Tie D et al., In vitro mechanical and corrosion properties of biodegradable Mg-Ag alloys. Materials and Corrosion. 2014, 65, 569–76.
[68] Yang L et al., Mechanical and corrosion properties of binary Mg-Dy alloys for medical applications. Materials Science and Engineering: B. 2011, 176, 1827–34.
[69] Ai X. Effect of Ti on Mechanical Properties and Corrosion of Cast AZ91 Magnesium Alloy. The Open Mater Sci Journal. 2012, 6, 6–13.
[70] Ai XL. Effect of Ti on Corrosion of Cast AZ91 Magnesium Alloy. Advanced Mater Res. 2011, 311/313, 1457–61.
[71] Shan G et al., Effect of Cd Addition on Microstructure and Properties of Mg-Cd Binary Magnesium Alloy. Rare Metal Materials and Engineering. 2015, 44, 2401–4.
[72] Xu Y et al., Effects of Gd solutes on hardness and yield strength of Mg alloys. Progress in Natural Science: Materials International. 2018, 28, 724–30.
[73] Harmuth J et al., Wide Range Mechanical Customization of Mg-Gd Alloys With Low Degradation Rates by Extrusion, Frontiers in Materials: Structural Materials. 2019, 8; https://doi.org/10.3389/fmats.2019.00201.
[74] Yamaura S et al., Structure and properties of melt-spun Mg-Pd binary alloys. Materials Transactions. 2003, 44, 1895–8.
[75] Dritis ME et al., Mechanical properties of binary alloys of Mg-Sm system. Metal Science and Heat Treatment. 1986, 27, 7–8.
[76] Hemeimat R et al., Investigation on the effect of titanium (Ti) addition to the Mg-AZ31 alloy in the as cast and after extrusion conditions on its metallurgical and mechanical properties. Mater Sci Eng. 2016; http://iopscience.iop.org/1757-899X/146/012026.
[77] Zhang Y et al., The study on binary Mg-Co hydrogen storage alloys with BCC phase. Journal of Alloys and Compounds. 2005, 393, 147–53.
[78] Liang G et al. Synthesis of Mg-Ti alloy by mechanical alloying. Journal of Materials Science. 2003, 38, 1179–84.
[79] Jung I-H et al., Role of RE in the deformation and recrystallization of Mg alloy and a new alloy design concept for Mg–RE alloys. Scripta Materialia. 2015, 102, 1–6.
[80] Hidalgo-Manrique P et al., Precipitation strengthening and reversed yield stress asymmetry in Mg alloys containing rare-earth elements: A quantitative study. Acta Materialia. 2017, 124, 456–67.
[81] Natarajan AR et al., First-principles investigation of phase stability in the Mg-Sc binary alloy. Physical Review B. 2017, 95: https://doi.org/10.1103/PhysRevB.95.214107.
[82] Diqing W et al., High damping properties of Mg–Si binary hypoeutectic alloys. Materials Letters. 2009, 63, 391–3.
[83] Zhang Y et al., Effect of Ti and Mg on the damping behavior of in situ aluminum composites. Mater Letters. 2005, 59, 3775–8.
[84] Wang YN et al., The role of twinning and untwinning in yielding behavior in hot-extruded Mg-Al-Zn alloy. Acta Materialia. 2007, 55, 897–905.
[85] Myshlyaev MM et al., Twinning, dynamic recovery and recrystallization in hot worked Mg-Al-Zn alloy. Materials Science and Engineering: A. 2002, 337, 121–33.
[86] Razzaghi M et al., Unraveling the effects of Zn addition and hot extrusion process on the microstructure and mechanical properties of as-cast Mg–2Al magnesium alloy. Vacuum. 2019, 167, 214–22.

[87] Jiang H et al., The influence of Ca and Gd microalloying on microstructure and mechanical property of hot-rolled Mg-3Al alloy. Procedia Engineering. 2017, 207, 932–7.
[88] Wang J et al., The effect of Y content on microstructure and tensile properties of the extruded Mg-1Al-xY alloy. Materials Science and Engineering: A. 2019, 765; https://doi.org/10.1016/j.msea.2019.138288.
[89] Hou L et al., Microstructure and mechanical properties at elevated temperature of Mg-Al-Ni alloys prepared through powder metallurgy. Journal of Materials Science & Technology. 2017, 33, 947–53.
[90] Chaubey AK et al., Microstructure and mechanical properties of Mg-Al-based alloy modified with cerium. Materials Science and Engineering: A. 2015, 625, 46–9.
[91] Cheng W et al., Improved mechanical properties of ECAPed Mg–15Al alloy through Nd addition. Materials Science and Engineering: A. 2015, 633, 63–8.
[92] Safari N et al., Influence of copper on the structural, mechanical, and biological characteristics of Mg-1Al-Cu alloy. Materials Chemistry and Physics. 2019, 237; https://doi.org/10.1016/j.matchemphys.2019.121838.
[93] Park SH et al., Improving mechanical properties of extruded Mg-Al alloy with a bimodal grain structure through alloying addition. Journal of Alloys and Compounds. 2015, 646, 932–6.
[94] Cao P et al., Effect of manganese on grain refinement of Mg-Al based alloys. Scripta Materialia. 2006, 54, 1853–8.
[95] Kim YM et al., Grain refinement of Mg-Al cast alloy by the addition of manganese carbonate. Journal of Alloys and Compounds. 2010, 490, 695–9.
[96] Han G et al., Effect of manganese on the microstructure of Mg-3Al alloy. Journal of Alloys and Compounds. 2009, 486, 136–41.
[97] Du J et al., Improvement of grain refining efficiency for Mg-Al alloy modified by the combination of carbon and calcium. Journal of Alloys and Compounds. 2009, 470, 134–40.
[98] Du J et al., Poisoning-free effect of calcium on grain refinement of Mg-3%Al alloy containing trace Fe by carbon inoculation. Transactions of Nonferrous Metals Society of China. 2013, 23, 307–14.
[99] Nagasivamuni B et al., An analytical approach to elucidate the mechanism of grain refinement in calcium added Mg-Al alloys. Journal of Alloys and Compounds. 2015, 622, 789–95.
[100] Fan J et al., Effect of Sr/Al Ratio on Microstructure and Properties of Mg-Al-Sr Alloy. Rare Metal Materials and Engineering. 2012, 41, 1721–4.
[101] Du J et al., Effect of strontium on the grain refining efficiency of Mg-3Al alloy refined by carbon inoculation. Journal of Alloys and Compound. 2009, 470, 228–32.
[102] Metalnikov P et al., The relation between Mn additions, microstructure and corrosion behavior of new wrought Mg-5Al alloys. Materials Characterization. 2018, 145, 101–5.
[103] Ding Y et al., Effects of alloying elements on the corrosion behavior and biocompatibility of biodegradable magnesium alloys: a review. Journal Material and Chemistry B. 2014, 2, 1912–33.
[104] Xiao X et al., Microstructures and electrochemical hydrogen storage properties of novel Mg-Al-Ni amorphous composites. Electrochemistry Communications. 2009, 11, 515–8.
[105] Xiong et al., Effects of microstructure on the electrochemical discharge behavior of Mg-6wt% Al-1wt%Sn alloy as anode for Mg-air primary battery. Journal of Alloys and Compounds. 2017, 708, 652–61.
[106] Tahreen N et al., Influence of aluminum content on twinning and texture development of cast Mg-Al-Zn alloy during compression. Journal of Alloys and Compounds. 2015, 623, 15–23.

[107] Zhang Y et al., The influences of Al content on the microstructure and mechanical properties of as-cast Mg-6Zn magnesium alloys. Materials Science and Engineering: A. 2017, 686, 93–101.
[108] Pan F et al., Development of high-strength, low-cost wrought Mg-2.0mass% Zn alloy with high Mn content. Progress in Natural Science: Materials International. 2016, 26, 630–5.
[109] Song L et al., The effect of Ca addition on microstructure and mechanical properties of extruded AZ31 alloys. Vacuum. 2019, 168; https://doi.org/10.1016/j.vacuum.2019.108822.
[110] Zhang B et al., Effects of calcium on texture and mechanical properties of hot-extruded Mg-Zn-Ca alloys. Materials Science and Engineering: A. 2012, 539, 56–60.
[111] Ha C et al., Influence of Nd or Ca addition on the dislocation activity and texture changes of Mg-Zn alloy sheets under uniaxial tensile loading. Materials Science and Engineering: A. 2019, 761; https://doi.org/10.1016/j.msea.2019.138053.
[112] Du Y et al., Improving microstructure and mechanical properties in Mg-6 mass% Zn alloys by combined addition of Ca and Ce. Materials Science and Engineering: A. 2016, 656, 67–74.
[113] Lejček P et al., Effect of Ca-addition on dynamic recrystallization of Mg-Zn alloy during hot deformation. Materials Science and Engineering: A. 2013, 580, 217–26.
[114] Jiang HS et al., The partial substitution of Y with Gd on microstructures and mechanical properties of as-cast and as-extruded Mg-10Zn-6Y-0.5Zr alloy. Materials Characterization. 2018, 135, 96–103.
[115] Liu P et al., The effect of Y, Ce and Gd on texture, recrystallization and mechanical property of Mg-Zn alloys. Journal of Magnesium and Alloys. 2016, 4, 188–96.
[116] Xu DK et al., The influence of element Y on the mechanical properties of the as-extruded Mg-Zn-Y-Zr alloys. Journal of Alloys and Compounds. 2006, 426, 155–61.
[117] Buha J et al., Mechanical properties of naturally aged Mg-Zn-Cu-Mn alloy. Materials Science and Engineering: A. 2008, 489, 127–37.
[118] Buha J et al., Natural Aging in Mg-Zn(-Cu) Alloys. Metall and Mat Trans A 2008, 39, 2259–73.
[119] Pan H et al., High conductivity and high strength Mg-Zn-Cu alloy. Materials Science and Technology. 2014, 30, 759–64.
[120] Wei S et al., Effects of Sn addition on the microstructure and mechanical properties of as-cast, rolled and annealed Mg-4Zn alloys. Materials Science and Engineering: A. 2013, 585, 139–48.
[121] Su J et al., Study on alloying element distribution and compound structure of AZ61 magnesium alloy with yttrium. Journal of Physics and Chemistry of Solids. 2019, 31, 125–30.
[122] Akyuz B. Influence of Al content on machinability of AZ series Mg alloys. Transactions of Nonferrous Metals Society of China. 2013, 23, 2243–49.
[123] Jiang W et al., Effect of Sn addition on the mechanical properties and bio-corrosion behavior of cytocompatible Mg-4Zn based alloys. Journal of Magnesium and Alloys. 2019, 7, 15–26.
[124] Ding H et al., Texture weakening and ductility variation of Mg-2Zn alloy with Ca or RE addition. Materials Science and Engineering: A. 2015, 645, 196–204.
[125] Yuasa M et al., Effects of group II elements on the cold stretch formability of Mg-Zn alloys. Acta Materialia. 2015, 83, 294–303.
[126] Lan A et al., Effect of substitution of minor Nd for Y on mechanical and damping properties of heat-treated Mg-Zn-Y-Zr alloy. Materials Science and Engineering: A. 2016, 651, 646–56.
[127] Akiba E et al., Mg-Zn-Ni hydrogen storage alloys. Journal of the Less Common Metals 1991, 172/174, 1071–7.
[128] Collings EW et al., Magnetic and electrical properties of some ternary Mg-Mn-Al alloys at low temperatures. The Philosophical Magazine: Journal of Theoretical Exp and Applied Physics. 1964, 10, 159–67.

[129] Xu L et al., Phosphating treatment and corrosion properties of Mg-Mn-Zn alloy for biomedical application. Journal of Material Science and Material Medicine. 2009, 20, 859–67.
[130] Yin D-S et al., Effect of Zn on mechanical property and corrosion property of extruded Mg-Zn-Mn alloy. Transactions of Nonferrous Metals Society of China. 2008, 18, 763–8.
[131] Stanford N. The effect of calcium on the texture, microstructure and mechanical properties of extruded Mg-Mn-Ca alloys. Materials Science and Engineering: A. 2010, 528, 314–22.
[132] Sun X et al., Mechanical and corrosion properties of newly developed Mg-Mn-Ca alloys as potential biodegradable implant materials. International Journal of Corrosion Process and Corrosion Control. 2014, 49, 303–10.
[133] Borkar H et al., Effect of strontium on the texture and mechanical properties of extruded Mg–1%Mn alloys. Materials Science and Engineering: A. 2012, 9, 168–75.
[134] Qi F-G et al., Effect of Y addition on microstructure and mechanical properties of Mg–Zn–Mn alloy. Transactions of Nonferrous Metals Society of China. 2014, 24, 1352–64.
[135] Masoumi M et al., The influence of Ce on the microstructure and rolling texture of Mg-1%Mn alloy. Materials Science and Engineering: A. 2011, 528, 3122–9.
[136] Ma N et al. Effects of cerium on microstructures, recovery behavior and mechanical properties of backward extruded Mg-0.5Mn alloys. Materials Science and Engineering: A. 2013, 564, 310–6.
[137] Yang Q et al., Microstructure and mechanical behavior of the Mg-Mn-Ce magnesium alloy sheets. Journal of Magnesium and Alloys. 2014, 2, 8–12.
[138] Zhong L et al., Effect of Ce addition on the microstructure, thermal conductivity and mechanical properties of Mg-0.5Mn alloys. Journal of Alloys and Compounds. 2016, 661, 402–10.
[139] Ma N et al., Effects of Annealing on Microstructure and Mechanical Properties of Backward Extruded Mg-0.5Mn-1Nd Alloy. Key Engineering Materials. 2013, 575/576, 235–8.
[140] Chen S et al., Effects of Cu on microstructure, mechanical properties and damping capacity of high damping Mg-1%Mn based alloy. Materials Sciemce Engineering: A. 2012, 551, 87–94.
[141] Guan et al., Corrosion Optimization and Mechanical Properties of Mg-Al-Sn-Mn Alloys by Orthogonal Design. Materials. 2018, 11; doi.org/10.3390/ma11081424
[142] Yu Z et al., Effects of Sn content on the mechanical properties and corrosion behavior of Mg-3Al-xSn alloys. Mater Res Express. 2020, 7, doi:10.1088/2053-1591/aba149
[143] Bahmani A et al., Corrosion behavior of Mg-Mn-Ca alloy: Influences of Al, Sn and Zn. Journal of Magnesium and Alloys. 2019, 7, 38–46.
[144] Gröbner J et al., Selection of promising quaternary candidates from Mg-Mn-(Sc, Gd, Y, Zr) for development of creep-resistant magnesium alloys. Journal of Alloys and Compounds. 2001, 320, 296–301.
[145] Denys RV et al., New Mg-Mn-Ni alloys as efficient hydrogen storage materials. Intermetallics. 2010, 18, 1579–85.
[146] Chai Y et al., Role of Al content on the microstructure, texture and mechanical properties of Mg-3.5Ca based alloys. Materials Science and Engineering: A. 2018, 730, 303–16.
[147] Du H et al., Effects of Zn on the microstructure, mechanical property and bio-corrosion property of Mg-3Ca alloys for biomedical application. Materials Chemistry and Physics. 2011, 125, 568–75.
[148] Somekawa H et al., High strength and fracture toughness balance on the extruded Mg-Ca-Zn alloy. Materials Science and Engineering: A. 2007, 459, 366–70.
[149] Islam F et al., The phase equilibria in the Mg-Ni-Ca system. CALPHAD. 2005, 29, 289–302.
[150] Jayaraj J et al. Enhanced precipitation hardening of Mg-Ca alloy by Al addition. Scripta Materialia. 2010, 63, 831–4.

[151] Oh JC et al., TEM and 3DAP characterization of an age-hardened Mg-Ca-Zn alloy. Scripta Materialia. 2005, 53, 675–9.
[152] Zakiyuddin et al., Effect of a small addition of zinc and manganese to Mg-Ca based alloys on degradation behavior in physiological media. Journal of Alloys and Compounds. 2015, 629, 274–83.
[153] Berglund ID et al., Synthesis and characterization of Mg-Ca-Sr alloys for biodegradable orthopedic implant applications. Journal of Biomedicine Materials Research B: Applied Biomaterials. 2012, 100B, 1524–34.
[154] Liu Y et al., Influence of biocompatible metal ions (Ag, Fe, Y) on the surface chemistry, corrosion behavior and cytocompatibility of Mg-1Ca alloy treated with MEVVA. Colloids and Surfaces. B, Biointerfaces. 2015, 133, 99–107.
[155] Li CY et al., Biodegradable Mg-Ca and Mg-Ca-Y Alloys for Regenerative Medicine. Materials Science Forum. 2010, 654/656, 2192–2195.
[156] Meng XK et al., Study on Interfacial Tension and Flammability of Mg-Ca-Ce Alloy Melt. Advanced Materials Research. 2011, 418/420, 383–6.
[157] Chang YW et al., Research and Development of Mg-Al-Sr Alloys. Advanced Materials Research. 2007, 26/28, 115–7.
[158] Liu Z-R et al., Stability and formation of long period stacking order structure in Mg-based ternary alloys. Computational Materials Science. 2015, 1–3, 90–6.
[159] Rameznzade S et al. Microstructure and mechanical characterizations of graphene nanoplatelets-reinforced Mg-Sr-Ca alloy as a novel composite in structural and biomedical applications. Journal of Composite Materials. 2000, 54: https://doi.org/10.1177/0021998319867464
[160] Gao J et al., A Study on Morphologies of Second Phases in the Mg-Sr and Mg-Sr-Y Alloys. Advanced Materials Research. 2010, 146/147, 336–9.
[161] Chen G et al., Effects of extrusion process on microstructure and mechanical properties of Mg-Sr-Y master alloy. Transactions of Materials and Heat Treatment. 2012: http://en.cnki.com.cn/Article_en/CJFDTotal-JSCL201206015.htm.
[162] Xu G et al., Thermodynamic database of multi-component Mg alloys and its application to solidification and heat treatment. Journal of Magnesium and Alloys. 2016, 4, 249–64.
[163] Celikin M et al., Microstructural investigation and the creep behavior of Mg-Sr-Mn alloys. Materials Science and Engineering: A. 2012, 550, 39–50.
[164] Celikin M et al., The role of α-Mn precipitation on the creep mechanisms of Mg-Sr-Mn. Materials Science and Engineering: A. 2012, 556, 911–20.
[165] Celikin M et al., Dynamic co-precipitation of α-Mn / $Mg_{12}Ce$ in creep resistant Mg-Sr-Mn-Ce alloys. Materials Science and Engineering: A. 2018, 719, 199–205.
[166] Svensson Berglund IE et al., Synthesis and characterization of Mg-Ca-Sr alloys for biodegradable orthopedic implant applications. Journal of Biomedical Materials Research. Part B, Applied Biomaterials 2012, 100, 1524–34.
[167] Villegas-Armenta LA et al. The Ignition Behavior of a Ternary Mg-Sr-Ca Alloy. Advanced Engineering Materials 2020, https://doi.org/10.1002/adem.201901318
[168] Al Shakhshir S et al. Computational thermodynamic model for the Mg-Al-Y system. Journal of Phase Equilibria and Diffusion. 2006, 27, 231–44.
[169] Drits ME et al., Phase equilibria in Mg-Y-Al alloys. Journal Russian Metallurgy. 1979, 3, 223–7.
[170] Oñorbe E et al., High-Temperature Mechanical Behavior of Extruded Mg-Y-Zn Alloy Containing LPSO Phases. Metallurgical and Materials Transactions A. 2013, 44, 2869–83.
[171] Tong LB et al., Effect of long period stacking ordered phase on the microstructure, texture and mechanical properties of extruded Mg-Y-Zn alloy. Materials Science and Engineering: A. 2013, 563, 177–83.

[172] Kim J-K et al., On the room temperature deformation mechanisms of a Mg-Y-Zn alloy with long-period-stacking-ordered structures. Acta Materialia. 2015, 82, 414–23.

[173] Chen B et al., Effects of yttrium and zinc addition on the microstructure and mechanical properties of Mg-Y-Zn alloys. Journal of Materials Science. 2010, 45, 2510–7.

[174] Chen J-M et al., Microstructure and heat treatment behavior of Mg-Y-Mn-Sc alloy as-casting. Heat Treatment of Metals. 2006; researchgate.net/publication/293343339.

[175] Zhu SM et al., Serrated flow and tensile properties of a Mg-Y-Nd alloy. Scripta Materialia. 2004, 50, 51–5.

[176] Amiya K et al., Thermal Stabilities and Mechanical Properties of Mg-Y-Cu-M (M = Ag, Pd) Bulk Amorphous Alloys. Material Transactions JIM. 2000, 41, 1460–2.

[177] Zhou N et al., High ductility of a Mg-Y-Ca alloy via extrusion. Materials Science and Engineering: A. 2013, 560, 103–10.

[178] Hwang L-F. Bio-corrosion studies of biodegradable alloys in the Mg-Y-Sy and Mg-Zn-Sy system. MS thesis, University of Pittsburgh, 2019.

[179] Neubert V et al., Thermal stability and corrosion behaviour of Mg-Y-Nd and Mg-Tb-Nd alloys. Materials Science and Engineering A. 2007, 462, 329–33.

[180] Zhang Y-H et al., Properties of Mechanically Milled Nanocrystalline and Amorphous Mg-Y-Ni Electrode Alloys for Ni-MH Batteries. Acta Metall. Sin. 2015, 28, 826–36.

[181] Gebert A et al., Stability of the bulk glass-forming $Mg_{65}Y_{10}Cu_{25}$ alloy in aqueous electrolytes. Materials Science and Engineering: A. 2001, 299, 125–35.

[182] Fan JF et al., Surface oxidation behavior of Mg-Y-Ce alloys at high temperature. Metall and Mat Trans A. 2005, 36, 235–9.

[183] Yu X et al., High temperature oxidation behavior of Mg-Y-Sn, Mg-Y, Mg-Sn alloys and its effect on corrosion property. Applied Surface Science. 2015, 353, 1013–22.

[184] Gao Y et al., Simulation study of precipitation in an Mg-Y-Nd alloy. Acta Materialia. 2012, 60, 4819–32.

[185] Nie JF et al., Characterisation of strengthening precipitate phases in a Mg-Y-Nd alloy. Acta Materialia. 2000, 48, 1691–703.

[186] Komura Y et al., The relation between electron concentration and stacking variants in the alloy systems: Mg-Cu-Ni, Mg-Cu-Zn and Mg-Ni-Zn. Acta Crystallographica B. 1972, B28, 976–8.

[187] Bhan S et al., The Mg-Ni-Zn System (Magnesium-Nickel-Zinc). Journal of Phase Equilibria. 1997, 18: https://doi.org/10.1007/BF02647860.

[188] Laws KJ et al., Ultra magnesium-rich, low-density Mg-Ni-Ca bulk metallic glasses. Scripta Materialia. 2014, 88, 37–40.

[189] Yang X et al., Modification of LPSO Structure in Mg-Ni-Y Alloy with Strontium. Materials Science Forum. 2018, 941, 869–74.

[190] Liu C et al., A 12R long-period stacking-ordered structure in a Mg-Ni-Y alloy. Journal of Materials Science and Technology. 2018, 34, 2235–9.

[191] Itoi T et al., A high-strength Mg-Ni-Y alloy sheet with a long-period ordered phase prepared by hot-rolling. Scripta Materialia. 2008, 59, 1155–8.

[192] Yin J et al., Hydrogen-Storage Properties and Structure Characterization of Melt-Spun and Annealed Mg-Ni-Nd Alloy. Materials Transactions. 2002, 43, 417–20.

[193] Huang LJ et al., Hydrogen-storage properties of amorphous Mg-Ni-Nd alloys. Journal of Alloys and Compounds. 2006, 421, 279–82.

[194] Chen SQ et al., Effects of Cu on microstructure, mechanical properties and damping capacity of as-cast Mg–3%Ni alloy. Advanced Materials Research 2012, 463/464, 52–7.

[195] Nayeb-Hashemi AA et al., The Mg-Ni (Magnesium-Nickel) system. Bulletin of Alloy Phase Diagrams. 1985, 6, 238–44.

[196] Boudard M et al., Tetragonal phase in the Mg-Ni-Sn system. Journal of Alloys and Compounds. 2004, 370, 169–76.
[197] Boudard M et al., The structure of the Y-phase in the Mg-Ni-Sn system. Journal of Alloys and Compounds. 2004, 372, 121–8.
[198] Muthia T et al., Synthesis and Characterization of Mechanical Alloyed Mg-Ni-Ca and Mg-Cu-Ca Amorphous Alloys. Procedia Materials Science. 2015, 9, 428–34.
[199] Soifer YM et al., Internal friction and the Young's modulus change associated with amorphous to nanocrystalline phase transition in Mg-Ni-Y alloy. Nanostructured Materials. 1999, 12, 875–8.
[200] Xie L et al., Microstructure and hydrogen storage properties of Mg-Ni-Ce alloys with a long-period stacking ordered phase. Journal of Power Sources. 2017, 338, 91–102.
[201] Li J et al., Microstructure and absorption/desorption kinetics evolutions of Mg Ni Ce alloys during hydrogenation and dehydrogenation cycles. International Journal of Hydrogen Energy. 2018, 43; DOI:10.1016/j.ijhydene.2018.03.113.
[202] Li L et al., Hydriding combustion synthesis of hydrogen storage alloys of Mg-Ni-Cu system. Intermetallics. 2002, 10, 927–32.
[203] Oh SK et al., Fabrication of Mg-Ni-Sn alloys for fast hydrogen generation in seawater. International Journal of Hydrogen Energy. 2017, 12, 7761–9.
[204] Jiang Z et al., Role of Al modification on the microstructure and mechanical properties of as-cast Mg–6Ce alloys. Materials Science and Engineering: A. 2015, 645, 57–64.
[205] Kang Y-B et al., Critical Evaluation and Thermodynamic Optimization of the Binary Systems in the Mg-Ce-Mn-Y System. Journal of Phase Equilibria and Diffusion. 2007, 28, 342–54.
[206] Celikin M et al., Effects of manganese on the microstructure and dynamic precipitation in creep-resistant cast Mg-Ce-Mn alloys. Scripta Materialia. 2012, 66, 737–40.
[207] Sun S et al., Experimental investigation of the isothermal section at 400 °C of the Mg-Ce-Sr ternary system. Journal of Magnesium and Alloys. 2016, 4, 30–5.
[208] Gröbner J et al., Thermodynamic analysis of as-cast and heat-treated microstructures of Mg-Ce-Nd alloys. Acta Materialia. 2011, 59, 613–22.
[209] Liu Z-R et al., Stability and formation of long period stacking order structure in Mg-based ternary alloys. Computational Materials Science. 2015, 103, 90–6.
[210] Inoue A et al., New Amorphous Mg-Ce-Ni Alloys with High Strength and Good Ductility. Japanese Journal of Applied Physics. 1988, 27, 2248–51.
[211] Brar H et al., Age hardening response of Mg-Ce-Al alloys. 2008; https://www.researchgate.net/publication/288754543_Age_hardening_response_of_Mg-Ce-Al_alloys/references.
[212] Yu K et al., Plastic deformation behaviors of a Mg-Ce-Zn-Zr alloy. Scripta Materialia 2003, 48, 1319–23.
[213] Park KC et al., Electrochemical behaviour of Mg-Ce-Zn system. Materials Technology: Advanced Performance Materials. 2012, 27, 73–5.
[214] Lin HJ et al., Hydrogen storage properties of Mg-Ce-Ni nanocomposite induced from amorphous precursor with the highest Mg content. International Journal of Hydrogen Energy. 2012, 37, 14329–35.
[215] Wang XL et al., Hydrogen storage properties of nanocrystalline Mg–Ce/Ni composite. Journal of Power Sources. 2006, 1589, 163–6.
[216] Tolnai D et al., Phase Formation during Solidification of Mg-Nd-Zn Alloys: An In Situ Synchrotron Radiation Diffraction Study. Materials (Basel). 2018, 11: doi:10.3390/ma11091637.
[217] Wu D et al., Microstructure and mechanical properties of a sand-cast Mg-Nd-Zn alloy. Materials & Design. 2014, 58, 324–31.

[218] Dvorský D et al., Structure and mechanical characterization of Mg-Nd-Zn alloys prepared by different processes. 4th International Conference Recent Trends in Structural Materials IOP Publishing IOP Conf. Series: Materials Science and Engineering. 2017, 179: doi:10.1088/1757-899X/179/1/012018.
[219] Xu G et al., Experimental Investigation and Thermodynamic Modeling for the Mg-Nd-Sr System. Metallurgical and Materials Transactions A. 2013, 44, 5634–41.
[220] Zhang XB et al., Effects of Sr on microstructure and corrosion resistance in simulated body fluid of as cast Mg-Nd-Zr magnesium alloys. Int'l Journal of Corrosion Processes and Corrosion Control 2014, 49, 345–51.
[221] Rokhlin LL et al., Peculiarities of the phase relations in Mg-rich alloys of the Mg-Nd-Y system. Journal of Alloys and Compounds. 2004, 367, 17–9.
[222] Cao G et al., Microstructure evolution and mechanical properties of Mg-Nd-Y alloy in different friction stir processing conditions. Journal of Alloys and Compounds. 2015, 636, 12–9.
[223] Zhang X et al., Biocorrosion properties of as-extruded Mg-Nd-Zn-Zr alloy compared with commercial AZ31 and WE43 alloys. Materials Letters. 2012, 66, 209–11.
[224] Zong Y et al., Comparison of biodegradable behaviors of AZ31 and Mg-Nd-Zn-Zr alloys in Hank's physiological solution. Materials Science and Engineering: B. 2012, 177, 395–401.
[225] Argade GR et al., Corrosion Inhibition Study of Mg-Nd-Y High Strength Magnesium Alloy Using Organic Inhibitor. Journal of Materials Engineering and Performance. 2019, 28, 852–62.
[226] Abba SH. Effect of Extrusion Temperature and Isothermal Severe Plastic Deformation on Magnesium and its Alloys. MS Thesis, Graduate School of Seoul National University Department of Materials Science and Engineering, 2018.
[227] Men H et al., Bulk metallic glass formation in the Mg-Cu-Zn-Y system. Scripta Materialia. 2002, 46, 699–703.
[228] Hojvat R et al., Calculation of metastable free-energy diagrams and glass formation in the Mg-Cu-Y alloy and its boundary binaries using the Miedema model. Intermetallics. 2006, 14, 297–307.
[229] Kim J-M et al., Microstructure and mechanical properties of a thixocast Mg-Cu-Y alloy. Scripta Materialia. 2003, 49, 687–91.
[230] Keqiang Q et al., Glass-Forming Ability for Mg-Cu-Nd Alloys. Metallurgical and Materials Transactions A. 2008, 39, 1882–7.
[231] Somoza JA et al., An experimental and theoretical study of the glass-forming region of the Mg-Cu-Sn system. Journal of Materials Science. 1995, 30, 40–6.
[232] Zhang CM et al., Formation of high strength Mg-Cu-Zn-Y alloys. Materials Science and Engineering. A, Structural Materials: Properties, Microstructure and Processing. 2008, 491, 470–5.
[233] Nishiyama K et al., Damping properties of a sintered Mg-Cu-Mn alloy. Journal of Alloys and Compounds. 2003, 355, 22–5.
[234] Inoue A et al., Mg-Cu-Y Bulk Amorphous Alloys with High Tensile Strength Produced by a High-Pressure Die Casting Method. Materials Transactions. 1992, 33, 937–45.
[235] Zhang Z-Y et al., Effects of Cu and Mn on mechanical properties and damping capacity of Mg-Cu-Mn alloy. Transactions of Nonferrous Metals Society of China. 2008, 18, 55–8.
[236] Kalinichenka S et al., Microstructure and hydrogen storage properties of melt-spun Mg-Cu-Ni-Y alloys. International Journal of Hydrogen Energy. 2011, 36, 1592–600.
[237] Bowles AL. Microstructural investigations of the Mg-Sn and Mg-Sn-Al Alloy Systems. Magnesium Technology 2004 Edited by Alan A. Luo TMS (The Minerals, Metals & Materials Society). 2004, 307–10.
[238] Son H-T et al., Effects of Al and Zn additions on mechanical properties and precipitation behaviors of Mg-Sn alloy system. Materials Letters. 2011, 65, 1966–9.

[239] Chai Y et al., Effects of Zn and Ca addition on microstructure and mechanical properties of as-extruded Mg-1.0Sn alloy sheet. Materials Science and Engineering: A. 2019, 746, 82–93.
[240] Chen Y et al., Microstructure and mechanical properties of as-cast Mg-Sn-Zn-Y alloys. Journal of Alloys and Compounds. 2018, 740, 727–34.
[241] Chen Y et al., Microstructure, Texture and Mechanical Properties of Mg-Sn-Zn Alloy Sheets Processed by Extrusion and Hot Rolling. Key Engineering Materials. 2017,727, 196–203.
[242] Shi Z-Z et al., Characterization and interpretation of the morphology of a Mg_2Sn precipitate with irrational facets in a Mg-Sn-Mn alloy. Journal of Philosophical Magazine. 2012, 92, 1071–82.
[243] Güleç AE et al., Characterization of Ternary Mg-Sn-Mn Alloys. Conference: 5thThe International Advances in Applied Physics and Materials Science Congress (AMPAS2015), 2015.
[244] Zhang M-Y et al., Microstructural Characteristics and Mechanical Properties of a Novel Extruded Dilute Mg-Sn-Mn-Ca Alloy. Frontiers in Materials. 2019, 12; https://doi.org/10.3389/fmats.2019.00321.
[245] Kozlov A et al., Phase equilibria, thermodynamics and solidification microstructures of Mg-Sn-Ca alloys, Part 1: Experimental investigation and thermodynamic modeling of the ternary Mg-Sn-Ca system. Intermetallics. 2008, 16, 299–315.
[246] Suresh K et al., Microstructure and mechanical properties of as-cast Mg-Sn-Ca alloys and effect of alloying elements. Transactions of Nonferrous Metals Society of China. 2013, 23, 3604–10.
[247] Keyvani M et al., Effect of Bi, Sb, and Ca additions on the hot hardness and microstructure of cast Mg-5Sn alloy. Materials Science and Engineering: A. 2010, 527, 7714–8.
[248] Nayyeri G et al., The microstructure, creep resistance, and high-temperature mechanical properties of Mg-5Sn alloy with Ca and Sb additions, and aging treatment. Materials Science and Engineering: A. 2010, 527, 5353–9.
[249] Liu H et al., Effects of strontium on microstructure and mechanical properties of as-cast Mg–5wt%Sn Alloy. Journal of Alloys and Compounds. 2010, 504, 345–50.
[250] Zhou B-C et al., First-principles calculations and thermodynamic modeling of the Sn-Sr and Mg-Sn-Sr systems. Calphad. 2014, 46, 237–48.
[251] You J-H et al., Effect of Si and Ca Additions on Microstructure of As-Cast Mg-Sn-Sr Alloy. Effect of Si and Ca Additions on Microstructure of As-Cast Mg-Sn-Sr Alloy. In: Marquis F. ed., Proceedings of the 8th Pacific Rim International Congress on Advanced Materials and Processing. Springer, 2013.
[252] Zhao HD et al., Isothermal sections of the Mg-rich corner in the Mg-Sn-Y ternary system at 300 and 400 C. Journal of Alloys and Compounds. 2009, 481, 140–3.
[253] Zhao H-D et al., Microstructure and tensile properties of as-extruded Mg-Sn-Y alloys. Transactions of Nonferrous Metal. Society of China. 2010, 20, 493–7.
[254] Kozlov A et al., Phase Formation in Mg-Sn Alloys Modified by Ca and Ce. Journal of Phase Equilibria and Diffusion. 2014, 35, 502–17.
[255] Yarkadaş G et al., The effect of Cerium addition on microstructure and mechanical properties of high pressure die cast Mg-5Sn alloy. Materials Characterization. 2018, 136, 152–6.
[256] Özarslan S et al., Microstructure, mechanical and corrosion properties of novel Mg-Sn-Ce alloys produced by high pressure die casting. Materials Science and Engineering: C. 2019, 105; https://doi.org/10.1016/j.msec.2019.110064.
[257] Wang Q et al., Study on microstructure and mechanical properties of as-cast Mg-Sn-Nd alloys. Journal of Rare Earths. 2010, 28, 790–3.
[258] Jayalakshmi S et al., Effect of Ag and Cu trace additions on the microstructural evolution and mechanical properties of Mg-5Sn alloy. Journal of Alloys and Compounds. 2013, 565, 56–65.

[259] Pan H et al., Effect of Cu/Zn on microstructure and mechanical properties of extruded Mg-Sn alloys. Materials Science and Technology. 2016, 32, 1–9.
[260] Sasaki TT et al., A high-strength Mg-Sn-Zn-Al alloy extruded at low temperature. Scripta Materialia. 2008, 59, 1111–4.
[261] Hu T et al., Improving tensile properties of Mg-Sn-Zn magnesium alloy sheets using pre-tension and ageing treatment. Journal of Alloys and Compounds. 2018, 735, 1494–504.
[262] Liao H et al., Effects of Mn addition on the microstructures, mechanical properties and work-hardening of Mg-1Sn alloy. Materials Science and Engineering: A. 2109, 754, 778–85.
[263] Pan H et al., Enhancing mechanical properties of Mg-Sn alloys by combining addition of Ca and Zn. Materials & Design. 2015, 83, 736–44.
[264] Zhao C-Y et al., Microstructure, mechanical and bio-corrosion properties of as-extruded Mg-Sn-Ca alloys. Transactions of Nonferrous Metals Society of China. 2016, 26, 1574–82.
[265] Elsayed FR et al., Compositional optimization of Mg-Sn-Al alloys for higher age hardening response. Materials Science and Engineering: A. 2013, 566, 22–9.
[266] Sasaki TT et al., Effect of double aging and microalloying on the age hardening behavior of a Mg-Sn-Zn alloy. Materials Science and Engineering: A. 2011, 530, 1–8.
[267] Mendis CL et al., An enhanced age hardening response in Mg-Sn based alloys containing Zn. Materials Science and Engineering: A. 2006, 435/436, 163–71.
[268] Huang X-F et al., Improved age-hardening behavior of Mg-Sn-Mn alloy by addition of Ag and Zn. Materials Science and Engineering: A. 2012, 552, 211–21.
[269] Park SS et al., Low-temperature superplasticity of extruded Mg-Sn-Al-Zn alloy. Scripta Materialia. 2011, 65, 202–5.
[270] Kang DH et al., Development of creep resistant die cast Mg-Sn-Al-Si alloy. Materials Science and Engineering: A. 2005, 413/414, 555–60.
[271] Hort N et al., Properties and processing of magnesium-tin-calcium alloys. Kovove Mater 2011, 49, 163–77.
[272] Zhen Z et al., In Vitro Study on Mg-Sn-Mn Alloy as Biodegradable Metals. Journal of Material Science and Technology 2014, 30, 675–85.
[273] Abu Leil T et al., Microstructure and corrosion behavior of Mg-Sn-Ca alloys after extrusion. Transactions of Nonferrous Metals Society of China. 2009, 19, 40–4.
[274] Wang Q et al., A micro-alloyed Mg-Sn-Y alloy with high ductility at room temperature. Materials Science and Engineering: A. 2018, 735, 131–44.
[275] Białobrzeski A, Pezda J. Registration of Melting and Crystallization Process of Ultra-light Weight MgLi12,5 Alloy with Use of ATND Method. Archives of Foundry Engineering. 2012, 12, 143–6.
[276] Sha G, Sun X, Liu T, Zhu Y, Yu T. Effects of Sc Addition and Annealing Treatment on the Microstructure and Mechanical Properties of the As-rolled Mg-3Li alloy. Journal of Materials Science & Technology. 2011, 27, 753–8.
[277] Zhao Z, Sun Z, Liang W, Wang Y, Bian L. Influence of Al and Si additions on the microstructure and mechanical properties of Mg-4Li alloy. Materials Science and Engineering: A. 2017, 702, 206–17.
[278] Cui C, Wu L, Wu R, Zhang J, Zhang M. Influence of yttrium on microstructure and mechanical properties of as-cast Mg–5Li–3Al–2Zn alloy. Journal of Alloys and Compounds. 2011, 509, 9045–9.
[279] Zhu T, Sun J, Cui C, Wu R, Zhang M. Influence of Y and Nd on microstructure, texture and anisotropy of Mg–5Li–1Al alloy. Materials Science and Engineering: A. 2014, 600, 1–7.
[280] Xiang Q, Wu RZ, Zhang ML. Influence of Sn on microstructure and mechanical properties of Mg–5Li–3Al–2Zn alloys. Journal of Alloys and Compounds. 2009, 477, 832–5.

[281] Sun Y, Wang R, Peng C, Feng Y. Effects of Sn and Y on the microstructure, texture, and mechanical properties of as-extruded Mg-5Li-3Al-2Zn alloy. Materials Science and Engineering: A. 2018, 733, 429–39.
[282] Li J, Qu Z, Wu R, Zhang M. Effects of Cu addition on the microstructure and hardness of Mg–5Li–3Al–2Zn alloy. Materials Science and Engineering: A. 2010, 527, 2780–3.
[283] Peng X, Wu G, Xiao L, Ji H, Liu W. Effects of Ce-rich RE on microstructure and mechanical properties of as-cast Mg-8Li-3Al-2Zn-0.5Ndm alloy with duplex structure. Progress in Natural Science: Materials International. 2019, 29, 103–9.
[284] Li M, Hao H, Zhang A, Song Y, Zhang X. Effects of Nd on microstructure and mechanical properties of as-cast Mg-8Li-3Al alloy. Journal of Rare Earths. 2012, 30, 492–6.
[285] Zhao J, Zhang J, Liu W, Wu G, Zhang L. Effect of Y content on microstructure and mechanical properties of as-cast Mg–8Li–3Al–2Zn alloy with duplex structure. Materials Science and Engineering: A. 2016, 650, 240–7.
[286] Pugazhendhi BS, Kar A, Sinnaeruvadi K, Suwas S. Effect of aluminium on microstructure, mechanical property and texture evolution of dual phase Mg-8Li alloy in different processing conditions. Archives of Civil and Mechanical Engineering. 2018, 18, 1332–44.
[287] Li Y, Peng X, Hu F, Wei G, Wang X. Effect of Mischmetal on Microstructure and Mechanical Properties of Superlight Mg-Li Alloys. Rare Metal Materials and Engineering. 2017, 46, 1775–81.
[288] Guo J, Chang LL, Zhao YR, Jin YP. Effect of Sn and Y addition on the microstructural evolution and mechanical properties of hot-extruded Mg-9Li-3Al alloy. Materials Characterization. 2019, 148, 35–42.
[289] Jiang B, Zeng Y, Zhang M-X, Yin H-M, Pan F-S. Effects of Sn on microstructure of as-cast and as-extruded Mg–9Li alloys. Transactions of Nonferrous Metals Society of China. 2013, 23, 904–8.
[290] Chang L-L, Shi C-C, Chui H-W. Enhancement of mechanical properties of duplex Mg-9Li-3Al alloy by Sn and Y addition. Transactions of Nonferrous Metals Society of China. 2018, 28, 30–5.
[291] Ji Q, Ma Y, Wu R, Zhang J, Zhang M. Effect of Y and Ce addition on microstructures and mechanical properties of LZ91 alloys. Journal of Alloys and Compounds. 2019, 800, 72–80.
[292] Peng X, Li J, Li W, Yan Y, Wei Q. Effect of Y on Microstructure and Mechanical Properties as well as Corrosion Resistance of Mg-9Li-3Al Alloy. Rare Metal Materials and Engineering. 2013, 42, 1993–8.
[293] Yin H-M, Jiang B, Huang X-Y, Zeng Y, Pan F-S. Effect of Ce addition on microstructure of Mg–9Li alloy. Transactions of Nonferrous Metals Society of China. 2013, 23, 1936–41.
[294] Zeng Y, Jiang B, Huang D, Dai J, Pan F. Effect of Ca addition on grain refinement of Mg–9Li–1Al alloy. Journal of Magnesium and Alloys. 2013, 1, 297–302.
[295] Ji H, Liu W, Wu G, Ouyang S, Ding W. Influence of Er addition on microstructure and mechanical properties of as-cast Mg-10Li-5Zn alloy. Materials Science and Engineering: A. 2019, 739, 395–403.
[296] Kim JT, Park G, Kim YS, Hong SH, Park HJ, Suh J-Y, Son HT, Lee MH, Park JM, Kim KB. Effect of Ca addition on the plastic deformation behavior of extruded Mg-11Li-3Al-1Sn-0.4Mn Alloy. Journal of Alloys and Compounds. 2016, 687, 821–6.
[297] Jiang B, Zeng Y, Yin H, Li R, Pan F. Effect of Sr on microstructure and aging behavior of Mg–14Li alloys. Progress in Natural Science: Materials International. 2012, 22, 160–8.
[298] Li R-H, Pan F-S, Jiang B, Yin H-M, Liu T-T. Effects of yttrium and strontium additions on as-cast microstructure of Mg-14Li-1Al alloys. Transactions of Nonferrous Metals Society of China. 2011, 21, 778–83.
[299] Okamoto H. Mg-Y (Magnesium-Yttrium). Journal of Phase Equilibria and Diffusion. 2010, 31, 199.

[300] Yang M, Duan C, Li H, Guo T, Zhang J. Effects of minor Ca addition on as-cast microstructure and mechanical properties of Mg–4Y–1.2Mn–1Zn (wt.%) magnesium alloy. Journal of Alloys and Compounds. 2013, 574, 165–73.
[301] Zhang Z, Liu X, Hu W, Li J, Cui J. Microstructures, mechanical properties and corrosion behaviors of Mg–Y–Zn–Zr alloys with specific Y/Zn mole ratios. Journal of Alloys and Compounds. 2015, 624, 116–25.
[302] Liu H-H, Ning ZOL, Yi J-Y, Ma Q, Sun J-F. Effect of Dy addition on microstructure and mechanical properties of Mg-4Y-3Nd-0.4Zr Alloy. Transactions of Nonferrous Metals Society of China. 2017, 27, 797–803.
[303] Luo K, Zhang L, Wu G, Liu W, Ding W. Effect of Y and Gd content on the microstructure and mechanical properties of Mg–Y–RE alloys. Journal of Magnesium and Alloys. 2019, 7, 345–54.
[304] Kowalski K, Jurczyk MU, Wirstlein PK, Jakubowicz J, Jurczyk M. Influence of 45S5 Bioglass addition on microstructure and properties of ultrafine grained (Mg-4Y-5.5Dy-0.5Zr) alloy. Materials Science and Engineering: B. 2017, 219, 28–36.
[305] Li J, Chen R, Ma Y, Ke W. Effect of Zr modification on solidification behavior and mechanical properties of Mg–Y–RE (WE54) alloy. Journal of Magnesium and Alloys. 2013, 1, 346–51.
[306] Xu D, Han E-H, Xu Y. Effect of long-period stacking ordered phase on microstructure, mechanical property and corrosion resistance of Mg alloys: A review. Progress in Natural Science: Materials International. 2016, 26, 117–28.
[307] Kawamura Y, Hayashi K, Inoue A, Masumoto T. Rapidly Solidified Powder Metallurgy $Mg_{97}Zn_1Y_2$Alloys with Excellent Tensile Yield Strength above 600 MPa. Material Transactions 2001, 42, 1172–6.
[308] Abe E, Kawamura Y, Hayashi K, Inoue A. Long-period ordered structure in a high-strength nanocrystalline Mg-1 at% Zn-2 at% Y alloy studied by atomic-resolution *Z*-contrast STEM. Acta Materialia. 2002, 50, 3845–57.
[309] Gao J, Chen Y, Wang Y. Effect of Sn element on the formation of LPSO phase and mechanical properties of Mg-6Y-2Zn alloy. Materials Science and Engineering: A. 2018, 711, 334–42.
[310] Zhao Y, Wang Q-D, Gao Y. Effect of zinc addition on microstructure and mechanical properties of Mg–7Y–3Sm–0.5Zr Alloy. Transactions of Nonferrous Metals Society of China. 2012, 22, 1924–9.
[311] Lyu S, Xiao W, Li G, Zheng R, Ma C. Achieving enhanced mechanical properties in Mg-Y-Sm-Zr alloy by altering precipitation behaviors through Zn addition. Materials Science and Engineering: A. 2019, 746, 179–86. Mg-7Y-5Sm-0.3Zr alloy
[312] Song G-L, Haddad D. The topography of magnetron sputter-deposited Mg–Ti alloy thin films. Materials Chemistry and Physics. 2011, 125, 548–52.
[313] Baqer YM, Ramesh S, Yusof F, Manladen SM. Challenges and advances in laser welding of dissimilar light alloys: Al/Mg, Al/ Ti, and Mg/Ti alloys. The International Journal, Advanced Manufacturing Technology. 2018, 95, 4353–69.
[314] Ramsden DM, Allen DM, Stephenson DJ, Alcock JR, Peggs GN, Fuller G, Goch G. The Design and Manufacture of Biomedical Surfaces. CIRP Annual – Manufacturing Technology 2007, 56, 687–711.
[315] Friedrich HE, Mordike BL. Magnesium Technology – Metallurgy, Design Date, Applications. Springer-Verlag, Berlin – Heidelberg – New York, 2005.
[316] Zhang W, Li M, Chen Q, Hu W, Zhang W, Xin W. Effects of Sr and Sn on microstructure and corrosion resistance of Mg–Zr–Ca magnesium alloy for biomedical applications. Materials & Design. 2012, 39, 379–83.
[317] Ding Y, Wen C, Hodgson P, Li Y. Effects of alloying elements on the corrosion behavior and biocompatibility of biodegradable magnesium alloys: a review. Journal of Materials Chemistry B. 2014, 2, 1912–33.

[318] Tsai MH, Chen MS, Lin LH, Lin MH, Wu CZ, Ou KL, Yu CH. Effect of heat treatment on the microstructures and damping properties of biomedical Mg-Zr alloy. Journal of Alloys Compounds. 2011, 509, 813–9.
[319] Li Y, Wen C, Mushahary D, Sravanthi R, Harishankar N, Pande G, Hodgson P. Mg-Zr-Sr alloys as biodegradable implant materials. Acta Biomaterialia. 2012, 8, 3177–88.
[320] Reiser A, Bogdanović B, Schlichte K. The application of Mg-based metal-hydrides as heat energy storage systems. International Journal of Hydrogen Energy. 2000, 25, 425–30.
[321] Gao S, Liu Y, Zhao D, Zhuang Y, Wang J. Effect of different Co contents on the microstructure and tensile strength of Mg-Co-Y alloys. Materials Science and Engineering: A. 2019, 750, 91–7.
[322] Fang W, Sun H-F, Fang W-B, Wang B. Effect of Al and Zn additives on grain size of Mg-3Ni-2MnO2 alloy. Transactions of Nonferrous Metals Society of China. 2009, 19, 355–8.
[323] Yang X, WU S, Lü S, Hao L, Fang X. Effects of Ni levels on microstructure and mechanical properties of Mg-Ni-Y alloy reinforced with LPSO structure. Journal of Alloys and Compounds. 2017, 726, 276–83.
[324] Zhang Z-Y, Peng L-M, Zeng X-Q, Ding W-J. Effects of Cu and Mn on mechanical properties and damping capacity of Mg-Cu-Mn alloy. Transactions of Nonferrous Metals Society of China. 2008, 18, 55–8.
[325] Wang J-F, Wei W-W, Li L, Liang H, Pan F-S. Effects of Y and Zn on mechanical properties and damping capacity of Mg-Cu-Mn alloy. Transactions of Nonferrous Metals Society of China. 2010, 20, 1846–50.
[326] ASM International. Alloy Phase Diagrams, 10th ed., Materials Park, OH: ASM International, 1992.
[327] Lansdown ABG. Silver I: its antibacterial properties and mechanism of action. J. Wound Care. 2002, 11, 125–30.
[328] Mijnendonckx K, Leys N, Mahillon J, Silver S, Van Houdt R. Antimicrobial silver: Uses, toxicity and potential for resistance. BioMetals. 2013, 26, 609–21.
[329] Maier P, Zimmermann F, Rinne M, Szakács G, Hort N, Vogt C. Solid solution treatment on strength and corrosion of biodegradable Mg6Ag wires, mater. Corrosion. 2018, 69, 178–90.
[330] Liu Z, Schade R, Luthringer B, Hort N, Rothe H, Müller S, Liefeith K, Regine Willumeit R, Feyerabend F. Influence of the microstructure and silver content on degradation, cytocompatibility, and antibacterial properties of magnesium-silver alloys *in vitro*. Oxidative Medicine and Cellular Longevity. 2017; doi: 10.1155/2017/8091265.
[331] Tie D, Feyerabend F, Müller W, Schade R, Liefeith K, Kainer KU. Antibacterial biodegradable Mg-Ag alloys. European Cell Materials 2013, 25, 284–98.
[332] Staiger MP, Pietak AM, Huadmai J, Dias G. Magnesium and its alloys as orthopedic biomaterials: a review, Biomaterials. 2006, 27, 1728–34.
[333] Oshida Y. Surface Engineering and Technology for Biomedical Implants. Momentum Press, New York NY, 2014.
[334] Tie D, Feyerabend F, Hoeche D, Kainer KU, Willumeit R, Mueller WD. In vitro mechanical and corrosion properties of biodegradable Mg-Ag alloys. Materials and Corrosion. 2014, 65, 569–76.
[335] Jessen LK, Zamponi C, Quandt E. Mechanical Properties of Magnetron Sputtered Free Standing Mg-Ag Alloy Films. Frontiers in Materials. 2019, 6;https://doi.org/10.3389/fmats.2019.00236.
[336] Wang B, Chen X, Pan F, Mao J. Effects of Sn addition on microstructure and mechanical properties of Mg-Zn-Al alloys. Progress in Natural Science: Materials International. 2017, 27, 695–702.
[337] Chen J, Chen Z, Yan H, Zhang F, Liao K. Effects of Sn addition on microstructure and mechanical properties of Mg–Zn–Al alloys. Journal of Alloys and Compounds. 2008, 461, 209–15.

[338] Xiao W, Jia S, Wang L, Wu Y, Wang L. Effects of Sn content on the microstructure and mechanical properties of Mg–7Zn–5Al based alloys. Materials Science and Engineering: A. 2010, 527, 7002–7.

[339] Xiaofeng W, Yangshan S, Feng X, Jing B, Weijian T. Effects of Sr and Ca on the microstructure and properties of Mg–12Zn–4Al–0.3Mn alloy. Materials Science and Engineering: A. 2009, 508, 50–8.

[340] Zhu S, Luo T, Zhang T, Li Y, Yang Y. Effects of Cu addition on the microstructure and mechanical properties of as-cast and heat treated Mg-6Zn-4Al magnesium alloy. Materials Science and Engineering: A. 2017, 689, 203–11.

[341] Chen Y, Gao J, Song Y, Wang Y. The influences of Sr on the microstructure and mechanical properties of Mg-5Zn-2Al alloy. Materials Science and Engineering: A. 2016, 671, 127–34.

[342] Wang Y, Guan S, Zeng X, Ding W. Effects of RE on the microstructure and mechanical properties of Mg–8Zn–4Al magnesium alloy. Materials Science and Engineering: A. 2006, 416, 109–18.

[343] Zhang W, Xiao W, Wang F, Ma C. Development of heat resistant Mg-Zn-Al-based magnesium alloys by addition of La and Ca: Microstructure and tensile properties. Journal of Alloys and Compounds. 2016, 684, 8–14.

[344] Xiao W, Jia S, Wang J, Wu Y, Wang L. Effects of cerium on the microstructure and mechanical properties of Mg–20Zn–8Al alloy. Materials Science and Engineering: A. 2008, 474, 317–22.

[345] Luo J, Qiu K, Jie W, Dong X, Li F. Microstructure and mechanical properties of Mg-7Zn-3Al alloy with Nd and Y additions. Journal of Rare Earths. 2012, 30, 486–91.

[346] Fang X, Yi D, Luo W, Wang B, Zheng F. Effects of yttrium on recrystallization and grain growth of Mg-4.9Zn-0.7Zr alloy. Journal of Rare Earths. 2008, 26, 392–7.

[347] Xu DK, Tang WN, Xu YB, Han EH. Effect of Y concentration on the microstructure and mechanical properties of as-cast Mg–Zn–Y–Zr alloys. Journal of Alloys and Compounds. 2007, 432, 129–34.

[348] Xu C, Wang X, Zhang J, Zhang Z. Effect of Nd and Yb on the Microstructure and Mechanical Properties of Mg-Zn-Zr Alloy. Rare Metal Materials and Engineering. 2014, 43, 1809–14.

[349] Wan YC, Jiang SN, Liu CM, Wang BZ, Chen ZY. Effect of Nd and Dy on the microstructure and mechanical property of the as extruded Mg–1Zn–0.6Zr alloy. Materials Science and Engineering: A. 2015, 625, 158–63.

[350] Zhang Y, Huang X, Li Y, Ma Z, Hao Y. Effects of samarium addition on as-cast microstructure, grain refinement and mechanical properties of Mg-6Zn-0.4Zr magnesium alloy. Journal of Rare Earths. 2017, 35, 494–502.

[351] Guan K, Li B, Tang Q, Qiu X, Meng J. Effects of 1.5 wt% samarium (Sm) addition on microstructures and tensile properties of a Mg–6.0Zn–0.5Zr alloy. Journal of Alloys and Compounds. 2018, 735, 1737–49.

[352] Guan K, Meng F, Qin P, Yang Q, Meng J. Effects of samarium content on microstructure and mechanical properties of Mg–0.5Zn–0.5Zr Alloy. Journal of Materials Science & Technology. 2019, 35, 1368–77.

[353] Peng J, Zhong L, Wang Y, Yang J, Pan F. Effect of Ce addition on thermal conductivity of Mg–2Zn–1Mn alloy. Journal of Alloys and Compounds. 2015, 639, 556–62.

[354] Zhang D-F, Qi F-G, Lan W, Shi G-L, Zhao X-B. Effects of **Ce** addition on microstructure and mechanical properties of Mg-**6**Zn-1Mn alloy. Transactions of Nonferrous Metals Society of China. 2011, 21, 703–10.

[355] Zou J, Chen J, Yan H, Xia W, Wu Q. Effects of Sn addition on dynamic recrystallization of Mg-5Zn-1Mn alloy during high strain rate deformation. Materials Science and Engineering: A. 2018, 735, 49–60.

[356] Qi F, Zhang D, Zhang X, Xu X. Effect of Sn addition on the microstructure and mechanical properties of Mg–6Zn–1Mn (wt.%) alloy. Journal of Alloys and Compounds. 2014, 585, 656–66.
[357] Hu G, Zhang D, Tang T, Shen X, Pan F. Effects of Nd addition on microstructure and mechanical properties of Mg–6Zn–1Mn–4Sn alloy. Materials Science and Engineering: A. 2015, 634, 5–13.
[358] Naghdaki S, Jafari H, Malekan M. Cooling curve thermal analysis and microstructure characterization of Mg-5Zn-1Y-xCa (0–1 wt%) alloys. Thermochimica Acta. 2018, 667, 50–8.
[359] Kwak TY, Lim HK, Kim WJ. Effect of Ca and CaO on the microstructure and hot compressive deformation behavior of Mg–9.5Zn–2.0Y alloy. Materials Science and Engineering: A. 2015, 648, 146–56.
[360] Qi F, Zhang D, Zhang X, Xu X. Effects of Mn addition and X-phase on the microstructure and mechanical properties of high-strength Mg–Zn–Y–Mn alloys. Materials Science and Engineering: A. 2014, 593, 70–8.
[361] Wang J, Zhang J, Zong X, Xu C, Nie K. Effects of Ca on the formation of LPSO phase and mechanical properties of Mg-Zn-Y-Mn alloy. Materials Science and Engineering: A. 2015, 648, 37–40.
[362] Hao J, Zhang J, Xu C, Zhang Y. Effects of Ti addition on the formation of LPSO phase and yield asymmetry of Mg-Zn-Y-Mn alloy. Materials Science and Engineering: A. 2018, 735, 99–103.
[363] Medina J, Pérez P, Garcés G, Adeva P. Effects of calcium, manganese and cerium-rich mischmetal additions on the mechanical properties of extruded Mg-Zn-Y alloy reinforced by quasicrystalline I-phase. Materials Characterization. 2017, 129, 195–206.
[364] He X, Chen J, Yan H, Su B, Zhang G, Miao C. Effects of minor Sr addition on microstructure and mechanical properties of the as-cast Mg–4.5Zn–4.5Sn–2Al-based alloy system. Journal of Alloys and Compounds. 2013, 579, 39–44.
[365] Wei J, Chen J, Yan H, Su B, Pan X. Effects of minor Ca addition on microstructure and mechanical properties of the Mg–4.5Zn–4.5Sn–2Al-based alloy system. Journal of Alloys and Compounds. 2013, 548, 52–9.
[366] Son H-T, Kim D-G, Park JS. Effects of Ag addition on microstructures and mechanical properties of Mg–6Zn–2Sn–0.4Mn-based alloy system. Materials Letters. 2011, 65, 3150–3.
[367] Son H-T, Kim Y-H, Kim D-W, Kim J-H, Yu H-S. Effects of Li addition on the microstructure and mechanical properties of Mg–3Zn–1Sn–0.4Mn Based Alloys. Journal of Alloys and Compounds. 2013, 564, 130–7.
[368] Cho DH, Nam JH, Lee BW, Cho KM, Park IM. Effect of Mn addition on grain refinement of biodegradable Mg4Zn0.5Ca Alloy. Journal of Alloys and Compounds. 2016, 676, 461–8.
[369] Tong LB, Zheng MY, Xu SW, Kamado S, Lv XY. Effect of Mn addition on microstructure, texture and mechanical properties of Mg–Zn–Ca alloy. Materials Science and Engineering: A. 2011, 528, 3741–7.
[370] Ding H, Shi X, Wang Y, Cheng G, Kamado S. Texture weakening and ductility variation of Mg–2Zn alloy with Ca or RE addition. Materials Science and Engineering: A. 2015, 645, 196–204.
[371] Wang G, Huang G, Chen X, Deng Q, Pan F. Effects of Zn addition on the mechanical properties and texture of extruded Mg-Zn-Ca-Ce magnesium alloy sheets. Materials Science and Engineering: A. 2017, 705, 46–54.
[372] Yang M, Guo T, Li H, Duan C, Zhang J. Effects of Sn Addition on as-Cast Microstructure and Mechanical Properties of Mg-3.8Zn-2.2Ca Magnesium Alloy. Rare Metal Materials and Engineering. 2013, 42, 1541–6.
[373] Yang M, Guo T, Li H. Effects of Gd addition on as-cast microstructure, tensile and creep properties of Mg–3.8 Zn–2.2Ca (wt%) magnesium alloy. Materials Science and Engineering: A. 2013, 587, 132–42.

[374] Du Y, Zheng M, Qiao X, Peng W, Jiang B. Effect of La addition on the microstructure and mechanical properties of Mg–6wt% Zn alloys. Materials Science and Engineering: A. 2016, 673, 47–54.
[375] Fu Y, Wang H, Liu X, Hao H. Effect of calcium addition on microstructure, casting fluidity and mechanical properties of Mg-Zn-Ce-Zr magnesium alloy. Journal of Rare Earths 2017, 35, 503–9.
[376] Lv B, Peng J, Peng Y, Tang A. The effect of addition of Nd and Ce on the microstructure and mechanical properties of ZM21 Mg alloy. Journal of Magnesium and Alloys. 2013, 1, 94–100.
[377] Luo J, Yan H, Chen R-S, Han E-H. Effects of Gd concentration on microstructure, texture and tensile properties of Mg–Zn–Gd alloys subjected to large strain hot rolling. Materials Science and Engineering: A. 2014, 614, 88–95.
[378] Chen J, Tan L, Yu X, Yang K. Effect of minor content of Gd on the mechanical and degradable properties of as-cast Mg-2Zn-xGd-0.5Zr alloys. Journal of Materials Science & Technology. 2019, 35, 503–11.
[379] Wen Q, Deng K-K, Shi J-Y, Zhang B-P, Liang W. Effect of Ca addition on the microstructure and tensile properties of Mg–4.0Zn–2.0Gd alloys. Materials Science and Engineering: A. 2014, 609, 1–6.
[380] Yang J, Xiao W, Wang L, WU Y, Zhang H. Influences of Gd on the microstructure and strength of Mg–4.5Zn alloy. Materials Characterization. 2008, 59, 1667–74.
[381] Yin S, Zhang Z, Liu X, Le Q, Cui J. Effects of Zn/Gd ratio on the microstructures and mechanical properties of Mg-Zn-Gd-Zr alloys. Materials Science and Engineering: A. 2017, 695, 135–43.
[382] Hu T, Wang F, Zheng R, Xiao W, Ma C. Effects of B and Sn additions on the microstructure and mechanical property of Mg-3Al-1Si alloy. Journal of Alloys and Compounds. 2019, 796, 1–8.
[383] Shang L, Jung IH, Yue S, Verma R, Essadiqi E. An investigation of formation of second phases in microalloyed, AZ31 Mg alloys with Ca, Sr and Ce. Journal of Alloys and Compounds. 2010, 492, 173–83.
[384] Wang F, Hu T, Zhang Y, Xiao W, Ma C. Effects of Al and Zn contents on the microstructure and mechanical properties of Mg-Al-Zn-Ca magnesium alloys. Materials Science and Engineering: A. 2017, 704, 57–65.
[385] Kim B, Park K, Park Y, Park I. Effect of Pd on microstructures and tensile properties of as-cast Mg–6Al–1Zn alloys. Materials Letters. 2011, 65, 122–5.
[386] Choi JY, Kim WJ. Significant effects of adding trace amounts of Ti on the microstructure and corrosion properties of Mg–6Al–1Zn magnesium alloy. Journal of Alloys and Compounds. 2014, 614, 49–55.
[387] Li K-J, Li Q-A, Jing X-T, Chen J, Zhang Q. Effects of Sm addition on microstructure and mechanical properties of Mg–6Al–0.6Zn Alloy. Scripta Materialia. 2009, 60, 1101–4.
[388] Bae SW, Kim S-H, Lee JU, Jo W-K, Park SH. Improvement of mechanical properties and reduction of yield asymmetry of extruded Mg-Al-Zn alloy through Sn addition. Journal of Alloys and Compounds. 2018, 766, 748–58.
[389] Park SH, Jung J-G, Yoon J, You BS. Influence of Sn addition on the microstructure and mechanical properties of extruded Mg–8Al–2Zn alloy. Materials Science and Engineering: A. 2015, 626, 128–35.
[390] Suresh M, Srinivasan A, Ravi KR, Pillai UTS, Pai BC. Influence of boron addition on the grain refinement and mechanical properties of AZ91 Mg alloy. Materials Science and Engineering: A. 2009, 525, 207–10.
[391] Xiao DH, Song M, Zhang FQ, He YH. Characterization and preparation of Mg–Al–Zn alloys with minor Sc. Journal of Alloys and Compounds. 2009, 484, 416–21.

[392] Hu Z, Liu RL, Kairy SK, Li X, Birbilis N. Effect of Sm additions on the microstructure and corrosion behavior of magnesium alloy AZ91. Corrosion Science. 2019, 149, 144–52.
[393] Wang H, Zhou B, Zhao Y, Zhou K, Kiang W. Effect of Si addition on the microstructure and mechanical properties of ECAPed Mg–15Al alloy. Materials Science and Engineering: A. 2014, 589, 119–24.
[394] Singh K, Mittal R. The effect of lanthanum on Microstructure & Mechanical properties of stir casted Mg alloy. Materials Today Proceedings. 2018, 5, 6360–9.
[395] Wang J, Wang L, Wu Y, Wang L. Effects of samarium on microstructures and tensile properties of Mg–5Al–0.3Mn alloy. Materials Science and Engineering: A. 2011, 528, 4115–9.
[396] Liu F, Yu J, Song Y, Shan D, Han EH. Effect of potassium fluoride on the in-situ sealing pores of plasma electrolytic oxidation film on AM50 Mg alloy. Materials Chemistry and Physics. 2015, 162, 452–60.
[397] Kondori B, Mahmudi R. Effect of Ca additions on the microstructure and creep properties of a cast Mg–Al–Mn magnesium alloy. Materials Science and Engineering: A. 2017, 700, 438–47.
[398] Şevik H, Kurnaz SC. The effect of strontium on the microstructure and mechanical properties of Mg–6Al–0.3Mn–0.3Ti–1Sn. Journal of Magnesium and Alloys. 2014, 2, 214–9.
[399] Nakata T, Xu C, Ajima R, Matsumoto Y, Kamado S. Improving mechanical properties and yield asymmetry in high-speed extrudable Mg-1.1Al-0.24Ca (wt%) alloy by high Mn addition. Materials Science and Engineering: A. 2018, 712, 12–9.
[400] Lou Y, Bai X, Li L-X. Effect of Sr addition on microstructure of as-cast Mg-Al-Ca alloy. Transactions of Nonferrous Metals Society of China. 2011, 21, 1247–52.
[401] Li ZT, Zhang XD, Zheng MY, Qiao XG, Kamado S. Effect of Ca/Al ratio on microstructure and mechanical properties of Mg-Al-Ca-Mn alloys. Materials Science and Engineering: A. 2017, 682, 423–32.
[402] Ali Elamami H, Incesu A, Korgiopoulos K, Pekguleryuz M, Gungor A. Phase selection and mechanical properties of permanent-mold cast Mg-Al-Ca-Mn alloys and the role of Ca/Al ratio. Journal of Alloys and Compounds. 2018, 764, 216–25.
[403] Suh B-C, Kim JH, Bae JH, Hwang JH, Kim NJ. Effect of Sn addition on the microstructure and deformation behavior of Mg-3Al alloy. Acta Materialia. 2017, 124, 268–79.
[404] Kim BH, Park KC, Park YH, Park IM. Effect of Ca and Sr additions on high temperature and corrosion properties of Mg–4Al–2Sn based alloys. Materials Science and Engineering: A. 2011, 528, 808–14.
[405] Majd AM, Farzinfar M, Pashakhanlou M, Nayyeri MJ. Effect of RE elements on the microstructural and mechanical properties of as-cast and age hardening processed Mg–4Al–2Sn alloy. Journal of Magnesium and Alloys. 2018, 6, 309–17.
[406] Kim Y-H, Son H-T. Effects of Li addition on microstructure and mechanical properties of Mg–6Al–2Sn–0.4Mn alloys. Transactions of Nonferrous Metals Society of China. 2016, 26, 697–703.
[407] Miao J, Sun W, Klarner AD, Luo AA. Interphase boundary segregation of silver and enhanced precipitation of Mg17Al12 Phase in a Mg-Al-Sn-Ag alloy. Scripta Materialia. 2018, 154, 192–6.
[408] Jiang L, Huang W, Guo F, Zhang Y, Lium Q. Effects of Zn addition on the aging behavior and mechanical properties of Mg8Al2Sn wrought alloy. Materials Science and Engineering: A. 2019, 752, 145–51.
[409] Wang H-Y, Rong J, Liu G-J, Zha M, Jiang Q-C. Effects of Zn on the microstructure and tensile properties of as-extruded Mg-8Al-2Sn alloy. Materials Science and Engineering: A. 2017, 698, 249–55.
[410] Zhu T, Fu P, Peng L, Hu X, Ding W. Effects of Mn addition on the microstructure and mechanical properties of cast Mg–9Al–2Sn (Wt.%) Alloy. Journal of Magnesium and Alloys. 2014, 2, 27–35.
[411] Liu C, Chen H, He C, Zhang Y, Nie J-F. Effects of Zn additions on the microstructure and hardness of Mg–9Al–6Sn alloy. Materials Characterization. 2016, 113, 214–21.

[412] Hu X, Fu P, St John D, Peng L, Zhang M. On grain coarsening and refining of the Mg–3Al alloy by Sm. Journal of Alloys and Compounds. 2016, 663, 387–94.
[413] Kumar A, Meenashisundaram GK, Manakari V, Parande G, Gupta M. Lanthanum effect on improving CTE, damping, hardness and tensile response of Mg-3Al alloy. Journal of Alloys and Compounds. 2017, 695, 3612–20.
[414] Wu X, Zhao C, Liu X. Effect of Ca addition on the microstructure and tensile property of AE42 alloy. Materials Letters. 2019, 252, 150–4.
[415] Zhang Y, Yang L, Sai J, Guo G, Liu Z. Effect of Ca and Sr on microstructure and compressive creep property of Mg–4Al–RE alloys. Materials Science and Engineering: A. 2014, 610, 309–14.
[416] Wei J, Wang Q, Zhang L, Yin D, Ding W. Microstructure refinement of Mg-Al-RE alloy by Gd addition. Materials Letters. 2019, 246, 125–8.
[417] Braszczyńska-Malik KN, Przełożyńska E. The influence of Ti particles on microstructure and mechanical properties of Mg-5Al-5RE matrix alloy composite. Journal of Alloys and Compounds. 2017, 728, 600–6.
[418] Pan H, Qin G, Xu M, Fu H, Song B. Enhancing mechanical properties of Mg–Sn alloys by combining addition of Ca and Zn. Materials & Design. 2015, 83, 736–44.
[419] Yang M, Pan F. Effects of Y addition on as-cast microstructure and mechanical properties of Mg–3Sn–2Ca (wt.%) magnesium alloy. Materials Science and Engineering: A. 2009, 525, 112–20.
[420] Yang M, Li H, Duan C, Zhang J. Effects of minor Ti addition on as-cast microstructure and mechanical properties of Mg–3Sn–2Sr (Wt.%) Magnesium Alloy. Journal of Alloys and Compounds. 2013, 579, 92–9.
[421] Chen Y, Jin L, Song Y, Liu H, Ye R. Effect of Zn on microstructure and mechanical property of Mg–3Sn–1Al alloys. Materials Science and Engineering: A. 2014, 612, 96–101.
[422] Wang P, Guo E, Wang X, Kang H, Wang T. The influence of Sc addition on microstructure and tensile mechanical properties of Mg–4.5Sn–5Zn Alloys. Journal of Magnesium and Alloys. 2019, 7, 456–65.
[423] Shi B-Q, Chen R-S, Ke W. Effect of element Gd on phase constituent and mechanical property of Mg-5Sn-1Ca alloy. Transactions of Nonferrous Metals Society of China. 2010, 20, 341–5.
[424] Nayyeri G, Mahmudi R, Salehi F. The microstructure, creep resistance, and high-temperature mechanical properties of Mg-5Sn alloy with Ca and Sb additions, and aging treatment. Materials Science and Engineering: A. 2010, 527, 5353–9.
[425] Keyvani M, Mahmudi R, Nayyeri G. Effect of Bi, Sb, and Ca additions on the hot hardness and microstructure of cast Mg–5Sn alloy. Materials Science and Engineering: A. 2010, 527, 7714–8.
[426] Jayalakshmi S, Sankaranarayanan S, Koh SPX, Gupta M. Effect of Ag and Cu trace additions on the microstructural evolution and mechanical properties of Mg–5Sn alloy. Journal of Alloys and Compounds. 2013, 565, 56–65.
[427] Kim R, Baek S-M, Jeong HY, Lee JG, Park SS. Grain refinement and reduced yield asymmetry of extruded Mg–5Sn–1Zn alloy by Al addition. Journal of Alloys and Compounds. 2016, 660, 304–9.
[428] El Mahallawy N, Ahmed Dia A, Akdesir M, Palkowski H. Effect of Zn addition on the microstructure and mechanical properties of cast, rolled and extruded Mg-6Sn-xZn alloys. Materials Science and Engineering: A. 2017, 680, 47–53.
[429] Kim S-H, Jung J-G, You BS, Park SH. Effect of Ce addition on the microstructure and mechanical properties of extruded Mg-Sn-Al-Zn alloy. Materials Science and Engineering: A. 2016, 657, 406–12.
[430] Kim S-H, Lee JU, Kim YJ, Jung J-G, Park SH. Controlling the microstructure and improving the tensile properties of extruded Mg-Sn-Zn alloy through Al addition. Journal of Alloys and Compounds. 2018, 751, 1–11.

[431] Cheng WL, Park SS, Tang WN, You BS, Koo BH. Influence of alloying elements on microstructure and microhardness of Mg-Sn-Zn-based alloys. Transactions of Nonferrous Metals Society of China. 2010, 20, 2246–52.
[432] Liu Q, Cheng W, Zhang H, Xu C, Zhang J. The role of Ca on the microstructure and corrosion behavior of Mg–8Sn–1Al–1Zn–Ca alloys. Journal of Alloys and Compounds. 2014, 590, 162–7.
[433] Wang J et al., Enhanced strength and ductility of Mg-RE-Zn alloy simultaneously by trace Ag addition. Materials Science and Engineering: A. 2018, 728, 10–9.
[434] Wang C et al., Effect of Al additions on grain refinement and mechanical properties of Mg–Sm alloys. Journal of Alloys and Compounds. 2015, 620, 172–9.
[435] Fang C et al., Significant texture weakening of Mg-8Gd-5Y-2Zn alloy by Al addition. Materials Science and Engineering: A. 2017, 701, 314–8.
[436] Gao X et al., Enhanced precipitation-hardening in Mg–Gd alloys containing Ag and Zn. Scripta Materialia. 2008, 58, 619–22.
[437] Li RG et al., Effect of Ag addition on microstructure and mechanical properties of Mg–14Gd–0.5Zr alloy. Materials Characterization. 2015, 109, 43–9.
[438] Zhang Y et al., A comparative study of the role of Ag in microstructures and mechanical properties of Mg-Gd and Mg-Y alloys. Materials Science and Engineering: A. 2018, 731, 609–22.
[439] Movahedi-Rad A et al., Effect of Ag addition on the elevated-temperature mechanical properties of an extruded high strength Mg–Gd–Y–Zr alloy. Materials Science and Engineering: A. 2014, 614, 62–6.
[440] Yang M et al., Effects of Ca addition on as-cast microstructure and mechanical properties of Mg–3Ce–1.2Mn–1Zn (wt.%) magnesium alloy. Materials & Design. 2013, 52, 274–83.
[441] Zhang X et al., Influence of silver addition on microstructure and corrosion behavior of Mg–Nd–Zn–Zr alloys for biomedical application. Materials Letters. 2013, 100, 188–91.
[442] Li J-H et al., Effect of gadolinium on aged hardening behavior, microstructure and mechanical properties of Mg-Nd-Zn-Zr alloy. Transactions of Nonferrous Metals Society of China. 2008, 18, 27–32.
[443] Zhou Y et al., Precipitation modification in cast Mg–1Nd–1Ce–Zr alloy by Zn addition. Journal of Magnesium and Alloys. 2019, 7, 113–23.
[444] Che C et al., The effect of Gd and Zn additions on microstructures and mechanical properties of Mg-4Sm-3Nd-Zr alloy. Journal of Alloys and Compounds. 2017, 706, 526–37.
[445] Zhang D et al., Improvement on both strength and ductility of Mg–Sm–Zn–Zr casting alloy via Yb addition. Journal of Alloys and Compounds. 2019, 805, 811–21.
[446] Hoseini-Athar MM et al., Effect of Zn addition on dynamic recrystallization behavior of Mg-2Gd alloy during high-temperature deformation. Journal of Alloys and Compounds. 2019, 806, 1200–06.
[447] Yuan J et al., Effect of Zn content on the microstructures, mechanical properties, and damping capacities of Mg–7Gd–3Y–1Nd–0.5Zr based alloys. Journal of Alloys and Compounds. 2019, 773, 919–26.
[448] Zhang R et al., Substitution of Ni for Zn on microstructure and mechanical properties of Mg–Gd–Y–Zn–Mn alloy. Journal of Magnesium and Alloys. 2017, 5, 355–61.
[449] Li B et al., Effects of 0.5 wt% Ce addition on microstructures and mechanical properties of a wrought Mg–8Gd–1.2Zn–0.5Zr alloy. Journal of Alloys and Compounds. 2018, 763, 120–33.
[450] Huna S et al., Effect of Gd and Y contents on the microstructural evolution of long period stacking ordered phase and the corresponding mechanical properties in Mg–Gd–Y–Zn–Mn alloys. Materials Science and Engineering: A. 2014, 612, 363–70.
[451] Li B et al., Influence of various Yb additions on microstructures of a casting Mg–8Gd–1.2Zn –0.5Zr alloy. Journal of Alloys and Compounds. 2019, 789, 720–9.

[452] Rong W et al., Effects of Zr and Mn additions on formation of LPSO structure and dynamic recrystallization behavior of Mg-15Gd-1Zn alloy. Journal of Alloys and Compounds. 2017, 692, 805–16.

[453] Fu W et al., Effects of Zr addition on the multi-scale second-phase particles and fracture behavior for Mg-3Gd-1Zn alloy. Journal of Alloys and Compounds. 2018, 747, 197–210.

[454] Liu J et al., Effects of Ho content on microstructures and mechanical properties of Mg-Ho-Zn alloys. Materials Characterization. 2019, 149, 198–205.

[455] Wang Q-F et al., Effect of Zn addition on microstructure and mechanical properties of as-cast Mg–2Er alloy. Transactions of Nonferrous Metals Society of China. 2014, 24, 3792–6.

[456] Zhang J-S et al., The effect of Ca addition on microstructures and mechanical properties of Mg-RE based alloys. Journal of Alloys and Compounds. 2013, 554, 110–4.

[457] Yang M-B et al., Effects of minor Ca on as-cast microstructures and mechanical properties of Mg-3Ce-1.2Mn-0.9Sc and Mg-4Y-1.2Mn-0.9Sc alloys. Transactions of Nonferrous Metals Society of China. 2014, 24, 1698–708.

[458] Lim HK et al., Effect of addition of Sn on the microstructure and mechanical properties of Mg–MM (misch-metal) alloys. Journal of Alloys and Compounds. 2008, 454, 515–22.

[459] Pan F et al., Effects of minor Zr and Sr on as-cast microstructure and mechanical properties of Mg–3Ce–1.2Mn–0.9Sc (wt.%) magnesium alloy. Materials Science and Engineering: A. 2011, 528, 4292–9.

[460] Fang XY et al., Effect of Zr, Mn and Sc additions on the grain size of Mg–Gd alloy. Journal of Alloys and Compounds. 2009, 470, 311–6.

[461] Yang M et al., Comparison about effects of minor Zr, Sr and Ca additions on microstructure and tensile properties of Mg-5Gd-1.2Mn-0.4Sc (wt%) magnesium alloy. Materials Science and Engineering: A. 2012, 545, 201–8.

[462] Wang J et al., Effect of Y for enhanced age hardening response and mechanical properties of Mg–Gd–Y–Zr alloys. Materials Science and Engineering: A. 2007, 456, 78–84.

[463] Peng Q et al., The effect of La or Ce on ageing response and mechanical properties of cast Mg–Gd–Zr alloys. Materials Characterization. 2008, 59, 435–9.

[464] Liu X et al., Effects of Nd/Gd value on the microstructures and mechanical properties of Mg–Gd–Y–Nd–Zr alloys. Journal of Magnesium and Alloys. 2016, 3, 214–9.

[465] Jafari Nodooshan HR et al., Effect of Gd content on high temperature mechanical properties of Mg–Gd–Y–Zr alloy. Materials Science and Engineering: A. 2016, 651, 840–7.

[466] Wang Y et al., Effects of Mn addition on the microstructures and mechanical properties of the Mg-15Gd-1Zn alloy. Journal of Alloys and Compounds. 2017, 698, 1066–76.

[467] Zhang X et al., Effects of Si addition on microstructure and mechanical properties of Mg–8Gd–4Y–Nd–Zr alloy. Materials & Design. 2013, 43, 74–9.

[468] Du XH et al., Effect of V on the microstructure and mechanical properties of Mg–10Er–2Cu alloy with a long period stacking ordered structure. Materials Letters. 2014, 122, 312–4.

[469] Wang D et al., Abundant long period stacking ordered structure induced by Ni addition into Mg–Gd–Zn alloy. Materials Science and Engineering: A. 2014, 618, 355–8.

[470] Gumbmann E, De Geuser F, Sigli C, Deschamps A. Influence of Mg, Ag and Zn minor solute additions on the precipitation kinetics and strengthening of an Al-Cu-Li alloy. Acta Materialia. 2017, 133, 172–85.

[471] Gökçe A, Fındık F, Kurt AO. Effects of Mg content on aging behavior of Al4CuXMg PM alloy. Materials & Design. 2013, 46, 524–31.

[472] Chen Y-T, Nieh G-Y, Wang J-H, Wu T-F, Lee S-L. Effects of Cu/Mg ratio and heat treatment on microstructures and mechanical properties of Al–4.6Cu–Mg–0.5Ag Alloys. Materials Chemistry and Physics. 2015, 162, 764–70.

[473] Mondol S, Alam T, Banerjee R, Kumar S, Chattopadhyay K. Development of a high temperature high strength Al alloy by addition of small amounts of Sc and Mg to 2219 alloy. Materials Science and Engineering: A. 2017, 687, 221–31.
[474] Salleh MS, Omar MZ, Syarif OJ. The effects of Mg addition on the microstructure and mechanical properties of thixoformed Al–5%Si–Cu alloys. Journal of Alloys and Compounds. 2015, 621, 121–30.
[475] Tavitas-Medrano FJ, Gruzleski JE, Samuel FH, Valtierra S, Doty HW. Effect of Mg and Sr-modification on the mechanical properties of 319-type aluminum cast alloys subjected to artificial aging. Materials Science and Engineering: A. 2008, 480, 356–64.
[476] Kang J, Su R, Wu DY, Liu CH, Narayanaswamy B. Synergistic effects of Ce and Mg on the microstructure and tensile properties of Al-7Si-0.3Mg-0.2Fe Alloy. Journal of Alloys and Compounds. 2019, 796, 267–78.
[477] Fortini A, Merlin M, Fabbri E, Pirletti S, GAragnani GL. On the influence of Mn and Mg additions on tensile properties, microstructure and quality index of the A356 aluminum foundry alloy. Procedia Structural Integrity. 2016, 2, 2238–45.
[478] Liu Y, Liu M, Chen X, Cao Y, Zhou H. Effect of Mg on microstructure and mechanical properties of Al-Mg alloys produced by high pressure torsion. Scripta Materialia. 2019, 159, 137–41.
[479] Goel R, Upadhyay M, Msulik O, Prasad YVSS, Kumar V. Effect of Magnesium on Strain Hardening Response of Al-Mg-Mn based alloys. Procedia Materials Science. 2014, 5, 1241–7.
[480] Kim WJ, Jeong HT. Pronounced yield drop phenomenon at high temperatures in Al-Mg alloys with high contents of Mg (5–13 wt%). Materials Science and Engineering: A. 2019, 743, 590–6.
[481] Školáková A, Novák P, Salvetr P, Moravec H, Šefl V, Deduytsche D, Detavernier C. Investigation of the Effect of Magnesium on the Microstructure and Mechanical Properties of NiTi Shape Memory Alloy Prepared by Self-Propagating High-Temperature Synthesis. Metallurgical and Materials Transactions A. 2017, 48, 3559–69.
[482] Li ZOJ, Wang X-E, Li J-Y, Li J, Wang H-Z. Effects of Mg nanopowders intergranular addition on the magnetic properties and corrosion resistance of sintered Nd-Fe-B. Journal of Magnetism and Magnetic Materials. 2017, 442, 62–6.
[483] Zhang L, Wang J, Du W, Ding Y, Fan Y. The influence of Mg substitution on the phase structure and electrochemical properties of Nd1–xMgxNi3 (x = 0.10–0.50) alloys. Journal of Alloys and Compounds. 2015, 653, 498–505.

Chapter 4
Mg-based composites, glassy materials and intermetallics

In general, a composite is considered to be any multiphase material that exhibits a combination of properties that makes the composite superior to each of the component phases. According to this principle of combined action, new properties, better property combinations and/or a higher level of properties are fashioned by the judicious combination of two or more distinct materials. In nature, it is not hard for us to see composite materials. Wood consists of strong and flexible cellulose fibers surrounded by and held together by stiffer materials called lignin. Bone is a composite of the strong yet soft protein collagen and the hard, brittle mineral apatite. The tooth structure is a composite of relatively soft-tissue dentin surrounded by the hard-tissue enamel. Many composite materials are composed of just two phases: one is termed the matrix, which is continuous and surrounded, and the other is often called the dispersed phase. Depending on the type of matrix materials, there are basically metal matrix composite (MMC), ceramic matrix composite and polymer matrix composite. In this chapter, we are dealing with M(Mg)MC. Overall, the properties of composites are a function of the properties of the constituent phases, their relative amounts (or loading percentage) and the geometry of the dispersed phase. In terms of compositing manner, there are mainly three distinct ways: (1) fine particle dispersing, (2) fiber reinforcing and (3) lamellae structuring [1–5].

In this chapter, we discuss Mg-based composites with metallic materials, Mg-based composites with polymeric materials and Mg-based composites with ceramic materials. In addition, we will also talk about the glassy Mg-based materials and Mg-involved intermetallic materials (or phases).

4.1 Mg-based composites with metallic materials

In a category of Mg-based composites with metallic materials, there are two major techniques to fabricate composites, that is, lamellae structuring and powder sintering.

4.1.1 Lamellae structuring

Feng et al. [6] investigated microstructure and mechanical behavior of a Mg/Al composite rod with a soft Mg AZ31 sleeve and an ultrahard Al 7050 core, with the aim to disclose the influence of Al core on microstructure and texture of Mg sleeve and

https://doi.org/10.1515/9783110676945-004

that of Al fraction on mechanical behavior. It was shown that when compared with extrusion of a monolithic Mg billet, coextrusion of the Mg/Al bimetal billets does not change the typical extrusion texture of Mg sleeve, but can effectively refine the grains in Mg sleeve. The Mg/Al composite has much higher tensile or compressive yield strengths than the monolithic Mg rod, meanwhile a similar plasticity. With the Al fraction up to 33.8%, the tensile yield strength increases by about 61% and compressive yield strength by about 214%. The Mg/Al rod also possesses a much lower tension–compression yield asymmetry than the monolithic Mg rod, a higher Al fraction further reduces this yield asymmetry. Both the inclusion of a hard Al core and the grain refinement in Mg sleeve contribute to the quite high strength and the much lower yield asymmetry in Mg/Al rod. It was also mentioned for the same lamellae composite that the experimental yield strength of the composite is slightly higher than that predicted by the rule of mixtures, while the predicted ultimate strength greatly differs from the experimental one, and the main reason lies in the fact that during tension of the Mg/Al composite, the Mg and the Al layers fracture before they reach their ultimate strength [7]. Hai et al. [8] studied the effects of intermetallic compounds on the fracture behavior of Mg/Al-laminated composite which was fabricated by accumulative roll bonding. It was reported that (i) massive cracked intermetallic compounds at the interface of the laminated Mg/Al composite was observed and (ii) obvious Mg/Al interface delamination is promoted by the cracked intermetallic compounds, and the cracks propagate into the softer Mg layer and lead to the rupture of Mg layer and these two factors result in the premature failure of the laminated Mg/Al composite.

Ham et al. [9] reported on Mg/Nb nanolayer composites that (i) as the individual thickness (ranging from 2.5 to 200 nm) height decreases, the hardness of multilayers increases and approaches a maximum of ~2.7 GPa at a few nm layer thickness and (ii) size-dependent strengthening in Mg/Nb multilayers is compared with that in Mg with various grain sizes, and Cu/Nb and Al/Nb multilayers. The deformation modes of Mg in a steel–Mg–steel multilayer composite were studied by step-by-step deformation and electron backscatter diffraction for the same region at 0%, 20% and 30% deformation [10]. It was mentioned that (i) the basal texture intensity significantly increases up to 20% deformation; however, from 20% to 30% deformation, activity of prismatic slip increases and the intensity of the overall basal texture is reduced and (ii) shear stress and Schmid factor analysis of the multilayer system showed the probability of prismatic slip increases up to 35% by increasing the stress ratio up to 0.4 and decreases afterward.

There are several studies on laminated Al/Mg/Al composite. Nie et al. [11, 12] fabricated Al/Mg/Al laminates by hot rolling at 400 °C and annealed at temperatures ranging from 200 to 400 °C for 1 to 4 h. It was reported that (i) microstructural examination revealed that brittle intermetallics identified as $Mg_{17}Al_{12}$ and Al_3Mg_2 (see Mg–Al phase diagram in Chapter 3) appeared at Mg/Al interface when annealing temperature exceeded 300 °C; (ii) Al layers in laminates annealed at 200 °C exhibited typical copper-type texture, which totally transformed to recrystallized cube texture at 400 °C with a higher intensity; (iii) recrystallization extent of Mg layer increased with the increase in annealing temperature and/or annealing time, and nuclei preferred to occur in grains near Mg/Al interface; (iv) grain size, texture type of matrix and thickness of intermetallic layers all influence mechanical properties of Al/Mg/Al laminates; (v) laminates annealed at 200 °C for 1–4 h exhibited better ultimate tensile strength (UTS) ranging from 223 to 240 MPa and elongation ranging from 21% to 26%; (vi) despite more extensive recrystallization of laminate annealed at 400 °C, thicker intermetallics greatly decreased its strength and plasticity because of crack initials and quickly propagates along Mg/Al interface or in the interior of intermetallics; and (vii) delamination appears during the tensile process of Al/Mg/Al laminate, and fractures mainly propagate among the intermetallics at Mg/Al interface. Habila et al. [13] studied the microstructure and texture of an Al1050/AZ31/Al1050-laminated composite fabricated by accumulative roll bonding at 400 °C up to five cycles. It was found that (i) the accumulative roll bonding processing led to microstructural refinement with equiaxed grain microstructure in AZ31 layers and to the development of elongated grains parallel to the rolling direction in Al1050 layers, (ii) no new phases formed at the bond interface after the first processing cycle while $Mg_{17}Al_{12}$ and Mg_2Al_3 phases appeared after subsequent cycles, (iii) the microhardness of Al1050/AZ31/Al1050-laminated composite increased with increasing processing cycles and almost saturated after five cycles, (iv) the yield strength and ultimate strength increased gradually between one and three cycles due to the strain hardening and grain refinement and they decreased with further increasing of the roll bonding cycles because of crack and failure of the Mg_xAl_y intermetallic compounds which developed during fourth and fifth cycles and (v) the deformation behavior of the laminated composite becomes rather similar to the behavior of AZ31 alloy that underwent a dynamic recrystallization during processing. Chen et al. [14] employed a porthole die coextrusion process to fabricate the Al/Mg/Al laminate. It was mentioned that (i) the laminate was successfully extruded without voids or cracks on the Al/Mg interface, (ii) the transition layer was formed and its thickness was increased with the increase of temperature, (iii) the near-complete extruded grain structure was observed in Mg layer, and the average grain size increases with increasing temperature, (iv) at lower extrusion temperature, both the Al and Mg matrixes exhibited higher hardness and (v) the hardness of Al/Mg interface is lower than that of the Al and Mg matrix.

Liu et al. [15] prepared a laminated Mg/Al/Mg composite with different reduction ratios via warm roll bonding. It was found that (i) microstructure and composition of the composite discovered refined grains in the Mg and Al layers with no intermetallic compounds at the interface, (ii) the tensile strengths of the laminated composite reached their peak values at 35% reduction ratio and (iii) the delamination mechanism in composite significantly improved the bending properties; however, this effect decreases with increasing reduction ratio.

There are some more complicated laminated composites. Nie et al. [16] used the hot rolling (at 450 °C, followed by annealing at 200 and 300 °C for 1 h) to fabricate the Ti/Al/Mg laminates. It was mentioned that (i) both Mg/Al and Ti/Al interfaces are well bonded, without cracks or pores, (ii) mechanical properties of laminate largely depends on the microstructure of Mg layer and (iii) rolled laminate stretched along rolling direction shows excellent UTS of 580 MPa and elongation of 38%, resulting from dynamic recrystallization of Mg grains near Mg/Al interface and twinning far away from Mg/Al interface. Wang et al. [17] fabricated Mg-3Al-1Zn/Mg-0.3Y (AZ31/WO)-laminated composite sheet porthole die extrusion. It was reported that (i) a tiny diffusion zone of ~0.35 μm and crystallographic interface were observed in the AZ31/WO interface, indicating that the AZ31/WO-laminated composite sheet had a well-bonding interface, (ii) the stretch formability at room temperature of the AZ31/WO-laminated composite sheet was apparently improved by ~71% and ~20%, respectively, as compared with the AZ31 sheet and WO sheet and (iii) the activation of more basal slip in the WO layer of the AZ31/WO-laminated composite sheet and the formation of extensive tensile twins in the AZ31 layer, which could effectively accommodate through-thickness strain during stretch forming, were assumed to be the main contribution to the stretch formability enhancement. Anne et al. [18] utilized the accumulative roll-bonding process to Mg–2%Zn/Ce/Al hybrid composite. It was found that (i) the grains are significantly reduced and reached up to 1 μm in Mg–2%Zn layer and 1.8 μm in Al layer having high angle misorientation of grain boundaries after being subjected to five passes of the process; (ii) the $Al_{17}Mg_{12}$, $AlMg_4Zn_{11}$ and $Al_{11}Ce_3$ intermetallic phases were observed through the X-ray diffraction (XRD) analysis; (iii) mechanical properties of the hybrid composite improved with increase in the number of roll-bonding passes which is attributed to work hardening, grain refinement and uniform distribution of Ce particles; (iv) presence of Ce in the hybrid composite restricts the phenomenon of dynamic recrystallization and prevents the grain growth during the process; and (v) the corrosion rate of Mg–Zn/Ce/Al hybrid composite (0.72 mm/year) improved about 3.3 times as compared to that of Mg–2%Zn alloy (2.37 mm/year).

4.1.2 Composites with particles

Braszczyńska-Malik et al. [19] fabricated an Mg–5Al–5RE (rare earth; AME505) matrix composite by the stir-casting method with 30 wt% pure spherical Ti particles. It was reported that (i) the fabricated composite was characterized by uniform distribution of the Ti particles within the matrix alloy, (ii) the composite microstructure was composed mainly of α-Mg and $Al_{11}RE_3$ phases but also revealed a higher volume fraction of Al_2RE phases than the unreinforced matrix alloy cast in the same conditions, which was located on the Ti particles that indicated heterogeneous nucleation of Al_2RE on the reinforcement, (iii) the tensile and compression strength as well as yield strength of the composite were examined in both uniaxial tensile and compression tests and (iv) the composite exhibited higher examined mechanical properties in comparison with the pure AME505 matrix alloy.

In order to add damping capacity function to Mg-based alloys, NiTi particles are composited to Mg-based alloys. Li et al. [20] developed a method combining pore-forming technique, powder sintering and pressureless infiltration of Mg to fabricate shape-memory NiTi-based composites (i.e., Mg/NiTi). It was reported that (i) the Mg/NiTi composites possess excellent mechanical and physical properties, such as high damping capacity, high fracture strength and low density, (ii) the composites show higher compressive strength than the porous NiTi alloys and exhibit excellent superelasticity over 2% and (iii) the damping performance of Mg/NiTi was noticed by synergistic effect of internal friction and modulus. Guo et al. [21] fabricated a NiTi/Mg composite using a method that combines top-down pore-forming and pressureless infiltration processes. It was found that the phase constituents of this simple composite are B2-NiTi, B19′-NiTi and Mg phases, with fine and homogeneous size and the distribution of the Mg phase. The composite has about 1.2-fold higher mechanical strength and 1.5-fold higher damping capacity than those of similar composite with different microstructures. Being generally attributed to the high damping capacity of Mg, the physical continuity of the composite and the homogeneous distribution of fine Mg phase, which generate more interfaces, contributing to the damping capacity, indicating that the composite is considered a good candidate for use as a damping material in engineering applications. Wakeel et al. [22] reinforced Mg with 2 wt% NiTi shape-memory alloy nanoparticles and studied the shape-memory alloy particle effect on the mechanical properties and microstructural evolution of monolithic magnesium. It was reported that (i) a near-dense Mg–2 wt% NiTi nanocomposite was obtained, (ii) the addition of NiTi nanoparticle resulted in a ~29% and ~73% enhancement in the microhardness and grain size of pure Mg, (iii) damping capacity and loss rate of pure Mg also had a superior enhancement of ~119% and ~2.6 times, respectively, due to the presence of NiTi nanoparticle and (iv) the compressive strength properties also exhibited a visible enhancement due to the presence of NiTi nanoparticle without compromising on the fracture strain of the material. With different aims, Aydogmus et al. [23] produced Mg/$Ti_{49.4}Ni_{50.6}$-interpenetrating composites via spark plasma sintering technique. It was mentioned that (i) interpenetrating matrix and the reinforcement networks were formed simply by adjustment of the particle sizes of the starting pure Mg and TiNi alloy powders, (ii) the microstructure of TiNi shape-memory alloy reinforcement material is highly sensitive to processing conditions especially to sintering time, (iii) room temperature yield and compressive strength of the composite samples were in the range of 53–113 MPa and 226–315 MPa respectively, depending on the reinforcement content (10–30 vol%) and the texture formation during processing, (iv) ductility of the composites on the other hand was in the range of 9.6–20%. 30% TiNi addition resulted in minimum ductility, whereas composite samples with 20% TiNi reinforcement exhibited the maximum ductility values, (v) Mg/TiNi composites displayed extraordinary mechanical properties at high temperatures and (vi) yield strength and elastic modulus of the composites increased with increasing temperature up to 150 °C due to the increase of transformation stress and the elastic modulus of TiNi shape-memory reinforcements with increasing temperature. Beyond 150 °C, both properties decreased with further temperature increase. Based on these findings, it was concluded that TiNi alloys seem to be promising candidates for reinforcement of pure Mg and Mg alloys to be used in automotive powertrain applications, and composites produced with 20% and 30% TiNi content meet the high strength and elastic modulus requirements at the service conditions of 150–200 °C and the stress levels of 50–70 MPa.

Further complicated composite systems have been developed using different particles via basic sintering accompanied with various additional methods. Vahid et al. [24] fabricated porous Mg–Nb and Mg–Ta composites via a combination of mechanical milling and powder metallurgy processes and studied the effect of Nb and Ta contents on the porosity, pore size and mechanical properties of the porous Mg composites. It was mentioned that (i) the microstructural observations show irregular cell shapes, including micro- and macropores in the porous materials; (ii) the number and size of macropores increased with an increase in the amount of reinforcement (Nb or Ta); (iii) the mechanical properties of the porous Mg composites increased with an increase in reinforcement contents up to 2 wt% and then decreased and the type, particle size and position of reinforcements influence the strength of porous composites; (iv) fractography of the compressed porous samples showed that in porous Mg–Nb and Mg–Ta composites, cracks are initiated from pores and gaps between Mg powders and propagated through cell walls and cell edges; and (v) the strength of these porous Mg composites is comparable to that of human bone; indicating that the biomechanical compatibility is confirmed. Tian et al. [25] investigated the microstructure, phase transformation and mechanical property of Ni–Mn–Ga particles/Mg composites with a strong interfacial reaction between the particles and the matrix, which was related to the large surface area and energy per unit volume of the flaky shape Ni–Mn–Ga particles that favor the reaction between the particles and matrix. It was reported that the martensitic transformation behavior was largely weakened due to the interfacial reactions and thus the reduced volume fraction of Ni–Mn–Ga particles. The composites exhibited an improved compressive strength and ductility in comparison with that of the Ni–Mn–Ga alloy. The compressive plasticity of the composites was decreased when the Ni–Mn–Ga particle content exceeded 40 wt%. In comparison with the Mg composites with large size Ni–Mn–Ga particles, the composites with small size particles would have a much stronger interfacial reactions, which was detrimental to the phase transformation and mechanical ductility of the composites, indicating that the results could provide a reference for the design and preparation of the particles reinforced metal matrix functional composites. Jayalakshmi et al. [26] synthesized and characterized $Ni_{60}Nb_{40}$ amorphous alloy particle-reinforced Mg composites with varying volume fractions via the microwave-assisted two-directional rapid sintering technique followed by hot extrusion. It was shown that (i) structural analysis indicated the retention of amorphous structure of the reinforcement in all the composites, (ii) the distribution of the reinforcement was strongly dependent on the volume fraction, (iii) the addition of $Ni_{60}Nb_{40}$ amorphous alloy particles modified the preferred crystal orientation of Mg, (iv) the composites showed significant improvement in hardness (increment up to 120%) and compressive strength (~85% increase at 5% volume fraction) and (v) comparison of mechanical properties of the developed composites with those of conventional Mg composites having ceramic/metallic reinforcements highlights the effectiveness of using amorphous particles as promising reinforcement materials.

4.2 Mg-based composites with polymeric materials

In order to improve mechanical properties and corrosion resistance, mainly polylactic acid (PLA), poly-L-lactic acid (PLLA). Poly-lactic-*co*-glycolic acid (PLGA) as well as carbon fiber-reinforced polymer (CFRP) are incorporated with Mg materials.

4.2.1 PLA-containing composites

It is generally believed that PLA orthopedic devices suffer from low degradation rate and inadequate osteoconductivity, and often lose efficacy in the late stage of implantation because of inflammatory response of acid products and inability in its integration to bone [27]. PLA was reinforced with 2 and 5 wt% magnesium particles using solvent casting and in vitro degradation and biomineralization were studied [27]. It was reported that (i) the pH value and variations in mass analysis during the in vitro degradation showed that the Mg incorporation could effectively neutralize the acidic products of PLA as well as induce more apatite deposition; (ii) great decrease in molecular weight of 2 and 5 wt% Mg/PLA composites as compared to the PLA after 8-week immersion made it possible to modulate the degradation rate of the PLA by controlling the proportion of Mg content and other key factors such as size and shape of the Mg reinforcements; (iii) in vitro cell culture revealed good biocompatibility of Mg/PLA and the favorable characteristic for osteoblastic cells to adhere and spread; (iv) the cellular biomineralization results demonstrated significantly higher bone-like nodules deposition (both in number and area) achieved on the composite surfaces than that on PLA surface after 14 and 28 days culture; and (v) the promoting bone-forming ability derives from the degradation of Mg particles, suggesting the positive effects of Mg incorporated to PLA matrix on the degradation and osteogenesis, and the composite can provide an alternative for the currently used PLA implants. Li et al. [28] investigated the effects of dynamic compressive loading on the in vitro degradation behavior of pure PLA and PLA-based composite unidirectionally reinforced with microarc-oxidized magnesium alloy wires (MAWs) (Mg/PLA). It was mentioned that (i) dynamic compressive loading is shown to accelerate degradation of pure PLA and Mg/PLA; (ii) as the applied stress is increased from 0.1 to 0.9 MPa or frequency from 0.5 to 2.5 Hz, the overall degradation rate goes up; (iii) after immersion for 21 days at 0.9 MPa and 2.5 Hz, the bending strength retention of the composite and pure PLA is 60.1% and 50%, respectively; and (iv) the synergistic reaction between MAWs and PLA in the composite is further clarified by electrochemical tests. Cai et al. [29, 30] prepared the biodegradable composite rod with Mg–2Zn wires reinforced PLA for potential application in orthopedic internal fixation hot-press method. The used Mg–2Zn wires were subjected to surface modifications including microarc oxidation (MAO) and chemical conversion using dopamine, hydrogen fluoride acid and γ-amino-propyl-triethoxysilane (KH550). It was reported that (i) in contrast, MAO treatment significantly improved the interfacial bonding between wires and PLA matrix due to the strong electrostatic interaction and the microanchoring interaction according to single-wire pull-out experiments and molecular dynamic simulation; (ii) the surface roughness of wires after MAO is 192.0 ± 5.0 nm, most of pore size are in the range of 0.5–1.5 μm and the average interface thickness is about 1.5 μm; and (iii) the essential reason leading to the differences of interfacial bonding is revealed from atomic level, which is useful for optimizing the preparation technology of Mg–2Zn wires/PLA composite rod. Similarly, Cai et al. [31] prepared Mg wire/PLA composite rods by hot-pressing (HP) and hot-drawing (HD) processes, which show desirable application potential as a biodegradable implant in orthopedics.

The influences of the volume content of Mg wires and processing steps on the degradation behavior of composite rods as well as the mutual influence between Mg and PLA during degradation were investigated. During degradation, the improved interface bonding between Mg and PLA by MAO can effectively inhibit the diffusion of the medium from the ends to the central part, supported by XR-CT (X-ray computed tomography) results, which show the degradation cracks in PLA, initiated and propagated along the radial direction of the rod rather than the axial direction. When compared with the hot-pressed rod, the three passes hot-drawn rod had lower degradation rate and better strength retention during long-time immersion. This is ascribed to the higher crystallinity of the PLA matrix by HD. It was mentioned that the 3D morphology of cracks in composite rods enlightened us a clear understanding about the emergence and evolution of cracks, which revealed the reason for the failure of composite rods. Li et al. [32] examined biodegradable composites of unidirectionally reinforced 50-Mg/PLA (50% Mg wire by volume) to replace conventional nondegradable metallic implants for fixing long-bone fractures. The samples were also evaluated for degradation over a duration of 56 days by immersion in phosphate-buffered saline solution at the human body temperature of 37 °C; variations in wet mass and dry mass, and pH was used as indicators for degradation. It was mentioned that (i) the 50C–Mg/PLA composite (with coated wires) suppressed mass loss, controlled the pH and promoted the deposition of Ca and P compounds and (ii) the retention of tensile and flexural properties significantly improved for the immersion period as the interface was better protected by the coating; indicating that the 50C–Mg/PLA composite has good potential as a biodegradable implant for load-bearing bone fractures. Li et al. [33] prepared degradable PLA-based composite reinforced with 20 vol.% MAWs for weight-bearing bone fracture healing. It was found that (i) the dynamic loading would overall accelerate the degradation of the composite; (ii) as the loading magnitude increases from 0.2 to 1 MPa or frequency from 0.5 to 2.5 Hz, the degradation rate goes up; (iii) under the staged dynamic loading condition, the degradation behaviors of the composite would show staged change determined by the dynamic loading condition at each stage; and (iv) the composite could theoretically provide sufficient stabilization for >8 weeks in a feasible dynamic environment to achieve successful bone fracture healing.

4.2.2 PLLA-containing composites

The polymeric matrix will benefit from the higher strength and modulus of the Mg particles, whereas Mg will benefit from the surrounded protective polymeric matrix that will control its degradation rate. Cifuentes et al. [34] developed PLLA/Mg composites as new biodegradable and bioresorbable materials for osteosynthesis implants by combining solvent casting of PLLA loaded with 30 wt% of Mg particles and further molding by compression. It was mentioned that (i) reinforcing the polymer matrix with Mg particles improves its mechanical properties (hardness up to 340 MPa and yield strength up to 100 MPa) and (ii) the modulus of elasticity increases up to 8 GPa. Cifuentes et al. [35] further examined the suitability of processing PLLA/Mg (Mg particles up to 7 wt%) composites by hot extrusion. It was reported that (i) the extrusion causes a reduction of almost 20% in the viscosity average molecular weight of PLLA, which further decreases with increasing Mg content; (ii) extrusion gave always rise to a homogeneous distribution of Mg particles within the PLLA matrix; (iii) the composite processing was not compromised by the degradation of the polymeric matrix because the processing temperature was always below the onset degradation temperature; (iv) degradation of the composite slightly increases as more Mg is added up to 5 wt%, but is very high at 7 wt%; (v) Mg particles improved the stiffness and compression strength of neat PLLA until 5 wt% of Mg content, which dropped drastically when the material had 7 wt% of Mg; and (vi) the filler-strengthening factor decreases with the increment in Mg content. Recently, Cifuentes et al. [36] investigated the effect of the type and crystalline degree of the polymeric matrix on in vitro degradation kinetics of PLA/Mg composites. The effect of the nature of the matrix has been studied by comparing a composite with a PLLA matrix with another with a poly-L, D-lactic (PLDA) matrix. It was mentioned that (i) a PLDA matrix is more effective in lowering the degradation rate of Mg particles than PLLA, (ii) the crystalline degree plays a major role in PLA/Mg composites degradation, (iii) the composite with the near-amorphous matrix exhibited the lowest degradation rate and the highest cell viability, whereas, cell viability decreases markedly on the high-crystalline composites, which is likely related to the accelerated release of degradation products and (iv) it was indicated that these findings highlight the importance of matrix crystallinity on the degradation kinetics and cytocompatibility of PLA/Mg composites.

Although biodegradable polymers, such as PLLA, are very useful in many biomedical applications, their degradation by-products have been much of a concern as they are the sources of inflammatory reactions in the body [37]. To test the hypothesis that a novel composite system composed of PLLA and oligolactide-grafted magnesium hydroxide (Mg-OLA) can overcome drawbacks caused by poor mechanical properties and inflammatory response of PLLA for biomedical applications, Kum et al. [37] prepared Mg-OLAs by the ring-opening polymerization. It was reported that (i) the tensile strength and modulus of PLLA/Mg80-OLA20 (0–20 wt%) were higher than those of PLLA/magnesium hydroxide, (ii) the PLLA/Mg80-OLA20 composite was also very effective in neutralizing the acidic environment caused by the degradable by-product of the PLLA matrix, (iii) in vitro cell viability increased to around 100% with increasing the amount of Mg80-OLA20 from 0 to 20 wt% and (iv) the expression levels of IL-6 and COX-2 were reduced dramatically when increasing the proportion of Mg80-OLA20 from 0 to 50 wt%. Based on these findings, it was concluded that the incorporation of Mg-OLAs into the PLLA matrix could reinforce the mechanical properties as well as reduce the inflammatory response of the hybrid PLLA, so that the hybrid composite system blending Mg-OLA in biodegradable polymers would be a promising strategy for avoiding current fatal problems in biomedical applications. Yu et al. [38] synthesized silane-coated Mg/PLLA composites containing 1%, 2%, 3%, 4% and 5% Mg microparticles. It was found that (i) the bending and tensile strength of PLLA matrix was reduced by incorporation of Mg microparticles, (ii) Mg/PLLA composites with higher Mg microparticles ratio showed higher Mg^{2+} leaching rate and pH value in immersion solutions, (iii) MC3T3-E1 preosteoblasts incubated with Mg/PLLA composites containing higher ratio of Mg microparticles showed higher cytocompatibility, cell viability, osteogenesis differentiation and migration, (iv) in vitro cellular responses showed that MC3T3-E1 preosteoblasts had the highest cell viability at 50 ppm Mg^{2+} and (v) in vivo animal studies showed that there was no change in serum Mg^{2+} concentration after implanting Mg/PLLA composites comparing with control and the implants of silane-coated Mg/PLLA composites accelerated bone formation; summarizing that the silane-coated Mg/PLLA composites with Mg microparticles ratio of 3–5% were optimal substitutes for bone regeneration.

4.2.3 PLGA-containing composites

Wu et al. [39] prepared AZ31 magnesium alloy fiber-reinforced PLGA composites. It was reported that (i) with the addition of AZ31 fibers, the composites had a significant increment in tensile strength and elongation; (ii) for the direct cell attachment test, all the cells showed a healthy morphology and spread well on the experimental sample surfaces; and (iii) the immersion results indicated that pH values of the immersion medium increased with increasing AZ31 fiber contents; indicating that the new kind of magnesium alloy fibers reinforced PLGA composites show a potential for future biomedical applications. Brown et al. [40] developed a metallic magnesium particle/PLGA composite scaffold to overcome the limitations of currently used dental bone grafting materials, being synthesized using a solvent-casting, salt-leaching method. It was reported that (i) incorporation of varying amounts of magnesium into the PLGA scaffolds increased the compressive strength and modulus, as well as provided a porous structure suitable for cell infiltration, as measured by mercury intrusion porosimetry, (ii) combining basic-degrading magnesium with acidic-degrading PLGA led to an overall pH-buffering effect and long-term release of magnesium over the course of a 10-week degradation assay, as measured with inductively coupled plasma-atomic emission spectroscopy; (iii) using an indirect proliferation assay adapted from ISO 10993:5, it was found that extracts of medium from degrading magnesium/PLGA scaffolds increased the bone marrow stromal cell proliferation in vitro, a phenomenon observed by other groups investigating magnesium impact on cells; and (iv) magnesium/PLGA scaffold biocompatibility was assessed in a canine socket preservation model and microcomputed tomography and histological analysis showed the magnesium/PLGA scaffolds to be safer and more effective at preserving bone height than empty controls.

4.2.4 CFRP-containing composites

Pan research group had extensively developed lamellae composite materials of CFRP/Mg alloys [41–43]. Mg sheet was subjected to the grit blasting [41], electrochemical treating in Na_2SiO_3–KOH–KF and KOH–KF electrolytes [42] or the MAO in KOH electrolyte [43]. It was then reported that the rougher surface significantly improves the peel strength of laminates, while the shear strength of laminates increases only slightly with increasing surface roughness; hence, the rougher surface exhibits a good overall interlaminar strength under peel and shear loading when compared to the smoother surfaces [41]. Removal of silicate in the Na_2SiO_3–KOH–KF electrolyte can cause the transition of conversion film from ceramic-like oxide film to pitted oxide film. The pitted oxide film can effectively enhance the peel strength of CFRP/Mg laminates compared with the ceramic-like oxide film, and an average enhancement of 6.5 times was observed. The pitted oxide film on magnesium can provide an excellent protection against the galvanic corrosion in CFRP/Mg laminates as the ceramic-like oxide film [42]. With the increase of KOH in electrolytes solutions, mode I (peel) strength of the lamellae composite sharply decreases due to the decrease of roughness in local regions and the emergence of interspace between magnesium and epoxy. With the rise of KF in electrolyte solutions, mode I strength of lamellae composite declines rapidly on account of the sharply weakening of electrochemical reactions, which causes the decrease of surface roughness. The specimen exhibits the optimal mode I interlaminar strength of 2.04 N/mm when the KOH and KF concentration is 7.28 and 2.9 g/L, respectively [43].

4.3 Mg-based composites with ceramic materials

Hydroxyapatite (HA) can be found in teeth and bones within the human body. Bone is the structural component of our body and can be considered as a natural biocomposite comprising of biopolymers (collagen and noncollagenous proteins) and minerals (HA), together with void spaces (porosity); more precisely, bone is a specialized form of mineralized connective tissue consisting by weight of 33% organic matrix (of which 28% are type I collagen (COL I) and the other 5% are noncollagenous glycoproteins, including osteonectin, osteocalcin (OCN), bone morphogenetic proteins, bone protepglycan and bone sialoprotein) and the other 67% inorganic portion of the bone is made up of HA, which permeates the organic matrix [44]. Composites made up of various Mg alloys as matrix and various ceramics as reinforcements with different fabrication routes have been extensively investigated to assess their viability in biomedical applications. A group of biomaterials which have similar characteristics with the mineral parts of bone seems very promising for hard-tissue engineering applications [4]. This group includes calcium phosphates, especially HA, beta-tricalcium phosphate (β-TCP) and bicalcium phosphate which is the combination of HA and β-TCP [1, 4]. In this section, we will discuss Mg-based biocomposites which are incorporated with various calcium phosphate groups (HA, β-TCP, Ca-P, etc.), carbon and carbides, nitrides and borides.

4.3.1 Mg–HA biocomposites

Gu et al. [45] prepared pure Mg/HA (10, 20 and 30 wt%) composites by powder metallurgy method. It was reported that (i) the main constitutional phases of Mg/HA composites were simply α-Mg and HA; (ii) the HA particulates distributed uniformly in Mg matrix for Mg/10HA composite, and few HA clustering occasionally spread over the Mg/20HA composite, whereas severe agglomeration of HA particulates could be seen for Mg/30HA composite; (iii) the yield tensile strength of Mg/10HA composite increased compared with that of the as-extruded bulk pure magnesium, yet the yield tensile strength, UTS and ductility of Mg/HA composites decreased with the further increase of HA content; (iv) the corrosion rate of Mg/HA composites increased with the increment of HA content; and (v) the cytotoxicity tests indicated that Mg/10HA extract showed no toxicity to L-929 cells, whereas Mg/20HA and Mg/30HA composite extracts induced significantly reduced cell viability. Sunil et al. [46] fabricated nano-HA (nHA)-reinforced magnesium composite by friction stir processing. It was mentioned that (i) grain refinement from 1,500 to ca. 3.5 μm was observed after the process, (ii) in vitro bioactivity studies by immersing the samples in supersaturated simulated body fluid (SBF) indicate that the increased hydrophilicity and pronounced biomineralization are due to grain refinement and the presence of nHA in the composite, respectively; (iii) electrochemical test to assess the corrosion behavior also clearly showed the improved corrosion resistance due to grain refinement and enhanced biomineralization; and (iv) using MTT (3-(4,5-dimethylthiazol-2-yl)-2,5-diphenyltetrazolium bromide) colorimetric assay, cytotoxicity study of the samples with rat skeletal muscle (L6) cells indicate marginal increase in cell viability of the FSP–Mg–nHA sample, accompanied with good cell adhesion.

Mg–Zn alloy was reinforced as Cui et al. [47] fabricated nHA incorporated in Mg–5.5Zn alloy by spark plasma sintering. It was found that (i) with the increasing of the nHA content (from 0 wt% to 10 wt%), the compressive yield strength is improved remarkably, (ii) comparing with Mg–5.5Zn alloy, of the nHA (10 wt%) can improve the compressive yield strength by 43% and bending strength by 14%, (iii) the in vitro immersion tests revealed the positive and negative effects of nHA content on the corrosion behavior of Mg–5.5Zn/HA composite, (iv) the nHA can improve the degradation resistance of the Mg–5.5Zn matrix, (v) addition of 10 wt% HA can decrease the corrosion rate by 49% and (vi) the composite exhibits acceptable cytotoxicity to L-929 cells, and impressive potential to be used as an orthopedic implant material. Liu et al. [48] prepared HA/Mg–Zn composites, using the thermal-treated HA particles, by means of powder metallurgy technology. It was mentioned that (i) no evident reaction happened between HA particles and Mg matrix during sintering process, and Zn atoms diffused into Mg matrix to form a single phase Mg–Zn alloy matrix, (ii) the addition of HA particles changed the corrosion mechanism of Mg matrix, (iii) during the corrosion process, HA particles would adsorb $(PO_4)^{3-}$ and Ca^{2+} ions efficiently and induce the deposition of Ca–P compounds on the surface of composites, so that HA could improve the corrosion resistance of magnesium matrix composites in SBF and restrain the increase of its pH value and (iv) the addition of Zn was favorable to improve the corrosion resistance of HA/Mg composites due to the densification of composites and the formation of Mg–Zn alloy matrix.

Witte et al. [49] investigated MMC comprised of a magnesium alloy AZ91D as a matrix and HA particles as reinforcements. It was reported that (i) the mechanical properties of the composites were adjustable by the choice of HA particle size and distribution, (ii) corrosion tests revealed that HA particles stabilized the corrosion rate and exhibited more uniform corrosion attack in artificial sea water and cell solutions, (iii) the phase identification showed that all samples contained hcp-Mg, $Mg_{17}Al_{12}$ and HA before and after immersion, (iv) after immersion in artificial sea water $CaCO_3$ was found on the composite surfaces, while no formation of $CaCO_3$ was found after immersion in cell solutions with and without proteins and (v) cocultivation of the composite with human bone-derived cells (HBDC), cells of an osteoblasts lineage (MG-63) and cells of a macrophage lineage (RAW264.7) revealed that RAW264.7, MG-63 and HBDC adhere, proliferate and survive on the corroding surfaces of MMC-HA. Based on these findings, it was concluded that biodegradable HA/AZ91D composites are cytocompatible biomaterials with adjustable mechanical and corrosive properties. Chen et al. [50] prepared AZ91/HA composite using squeeze-casting method. It was reported that (i) the molten AZ91 alloy completely infiltrated the preform without destroying the porous structure of the HA preform, (ii) the compressive strength of AZ91/HA composite increased significantly compared with that of the porous HA and (iii) the immersion test indicated that AZ91 alloy shows a lower corrosion resistance and is easier to be corroded in comparison with HA. Razavi et al. [51, 52] reinforced AZ91 alloy with fluorapatite nanoparticles as reinforcement. It was reported that (i) the addition of fluorapatite nanoparticle reinforcements to magnesium alloys can improve the mechanical properties, reduce the corrosion rate and accelerate the formation of an apatite layer on the surface, which provides improved protection for the AZ91 matrix; and (ii) the formation of an apatite layer on the surface of magnesium alloys can contribute to the improved osteoconductivity of magnesium alloys for biomedical applications.

Mg–Zn–Zr alloy was composited with nHA particles. Ye et al. [53] fabricated biocomposites using Mg–2.9Zn–0.7Zr alloy as the matrix and 1 wt% nHA particles as reinforcements. It was found that (i) the average corrosion rate of MMC is 0.75 mm/year after immersion in SBF for 20 days, and the surface of the composite is covered with white Ca–P precipitates, (ii) the electrochemical test results show that the corrosion potential (E_{CORR}) of the composite increases to –1.615 V and its polarization resistance (R_P) is 2.56 KΩ with the addition of nHA particles, (iii) the cocultivation of the composite with osteoblasts results in the adhesion and proliferation of cells on the surface of the composite and the maximum cell density is calculated to be $(1.85 \pm 0.15) \times 10^4$/L after 5 days of coculture with osteoblasts and (iv) the average cell numbers for two groups after culturing for 3 and 5 days are significantly different; suggesting that the Mg–Zn–Zr/nHA composite can be potentially used as biodegradable bone fixation material. Liu et al. [54] studied the hot deformation behavior of HA/Mg–3Zn–0.8Zr composites. It was reported that (i) the flow stress increases increasing strain rates at a constant temperature, and decreases with increasing deforming temperatures at a constant strain rate, (ii) under the same processing conditions, the flow stresses of the 1HA/Mg–3Zn–0.8Zr specimens are higher than those of the Mg–3Zn–0.8Zr alloy specimens, and the difference is getting closer with increasing deformation temperature, (iii) the optimum process conditions of 1HA/Mg–3Zn–0.8Zr composite is concluded as between the temperature window of 300 °C–350 °C with a strain rate range of 0.001–0.1/s and (iv) a higher volume fraction and smaller grain size of dynamic recrystallization grains was observed in 1HA/ Mg–3Zn–0.8Zr specimens after the hot compression deformation compared with Mg–3Zn–0.8Zr alloy, which was ascribed to the presence of the HA particles that play an important role in particle-stimulated nucleation mechanism and can effectively hinder the migration of interfaces.

Wang et al. [55] fabricated a complicated composite consisted of HA + β-TCP/ Mg–5Sn with interpenetrating networks by infiltrating Mg–5Sn alloy into porous HA + β-TCP using suction-casting technique. It was found that (i) the molten Mg–5Sn alloy has infiltrated not only into the pores but also into the struts of the HA + β-TCP scaffold to forming a compact composite, (ii) the microstructure observation also shows that the Mg alloy contacts to the HA + β-TCP closely, and no reaction layer can be found between Mg–5Sn alloy and scaffold, (iii) the ultimate compressive strength of the composite is as high as 176 MPa, which is about four fifths of the strength of the Mg–5Sn bulk alloy, (iv) the electrochemical and immersion tests indicate that the corrosion resistance of the composite is better than that of the Mg–5Sn bulk alloy and (v) the corrosion products on the composite surface are mainly $Mg(OH)_2$, $Ca_3(PO_4)_2$ and HA; indicating that appropriate mechanical and corrosion properties of the (HA + β-TCP)/Mg–5Sn composite indicate its possibility for new bone tissue implant materials.

There are several reports on Ca-containing Mg-based alloys reinforced with HA particles. Gu et al. [56] fabricated Mg–Ca alloy/HA–TCP composite using the liquid alloy infiltration technique. It was reported that (i) the composite had a strength about 200-fold higher than that of the original porous HA–TCP scaffold but retained half of the strength of the bulk Mg–Ca alloy, (ii) the corrosion test indicated that the resulting composite exhibited an average corrosion rate of 0.029 $mL/cm^2/h$ in the Hank's solution at 37 °C, which was slower than that of the bulk Mg–Ca alloy alone, (iii) the indirect cytotoxicity evaluation revealed that 100% concentrated (i.e., undiluted or as-collected) extract of the Mg–Ca/HA–TCP composite showed significant toxicity to L-929 and MG63 cells and (iv) in contrast, the diluted extracts with 50% and 10% concentrations of the Mg–Ca/HA–TCP composite exhibited a similar degree of cell viability, equivalent to the grade I cytotoxicity of the standard ISO 10993-5. Lim et al. [57] produced Mg–1Ca/HA composites by blending Mg–1Ca alloys with 5, 10 and 15 wt% of HA. Biocompatibility assessments were performed using an indirect contact method by culturing human adipose mesenchymal stem cells (hASCs) in the extracts of Mg–1Ca alloy, Mg–1Ca/HA composites and Dulbecco's modified eagle's medium. It was mentioned that (i) Mg–1Ca/HA composites could promote cell proliferation, and at the same time, enhanced COL I and OCN expressions of hASCs and (ii) among the Mg–1Ca/HA composites, 10 wt% of HA is the optimum amount to be added into Mg–1Ca alloy for enhanced bioactivity, thus emerging as a potential biomaterial for orthopedic fixation. Liu et al. [58] fabricated a biodegradable HA-particle-reinforced magnesium-matrix composite Mg-3Zn-0.2Ca-1HA (wt%) by a combination of high shear solidification (HSS) and hot extrusion technology. It was reported that (i) in comparison with the matrix alloy, the as-cast Mg-3Zn-0.2Ca-1HA composite obtained by HSS technology exhibited a uniform and fine-grained structure, further refined after a hot extrusion ratio of 36:1, (ii) the yield strength, UTS and elongation of the extruded composite were 322 MPa, 341 MPa and 7.6%, respectively, (iii) the corrosion rate of the as-extruded Mg-3Zn-0.2Ca-1HA composite was measured to be 1.52 mm/year and (iv) electrochemical and immersion tests showed that the corrosion resistance of the composite is slightly improved comparing to that of the matrix alloy.

A mixture of HA and TiO_2 was used as a reinforcement element to fabricate biocomposites of pure Mg using a milling–pressing–sintering technique to evaluate the effect of addition TiO_2 powder on the corrosion behavior and mechanical properties of Mg/HA-based composites [59, 60]. It was reported that the corrosion resistance of Mg/HA-based composites was significantly improved by addition of 15 wt% of TiO_2 and decreasing HA amount to 5 wt%, and this was inferred from the lower corrosion current; 4.8 $\mu A/cm^2$ versus 285.3 $\mu A/cm^2$ for the 27.5 wt% HA addition, the higher corrosion potential; −1,255.7 versus −1,487.3 mV_{SCE}, the larger polarization resistance; 11.86 versus 0.25 $k\Omega \cdot cm^2$ and the significantly lower corrosion rate; 0.1 versus 4.28 mm/year. Compressive failure strain significantly increased from 1.7% in Mg/27.5HA to 8.1% in Mg/5HA/15TiO_2 which exhibited high corrosion resistance, cytocompatibility and mechanical properties and can be considered as a promising material for implant applications [59]. By sintering the Mg/HA/TiO_2 nanocomposites, $MgTiO_3$ nanoflakes were formed with a hierarchical microstructure on the surface of the samples. The compression and electrochemical tests indicated that the ternary Mg/12.5HA/10TiO_2 nanocomposite had a good combination of mechanical properties and corrosion resistance of 12.17 $k\Omega \cdot cm^2$ in the SBF solution. The cell culture results indicated that the Mg/HA/TiO_2 nanocomposite was biocompatible with osteoblasts [60].

4.3.2 Mg–β-TCP biocomposites

β-TCP – $Ca_3(PO_4)_2$ – exhibits excellent biocompatibility, bioactivity and bioabsorbable characters in physiological conditions and possesses high dissolution rate as compared with HA, which helps to achieve complete degradation of implant material after healing of fractured tissue. When a calcium phosphate is incorporated with Mg materials, it has been pointed out that in vivo corrosion rate becomes controllable along with required mechanical properties [61]. Yu et al. [62] prepared composites with 5%, 10% and 15% β-$Ca_3(PO_4)_2$ with Mg–6Zn alloy through powder metallurgy methods, and studied their corrosion behavior and mechanical properties in SBF at 37 °C. It was reported that (i) the α-Mg, MgZn and β-$Ca_3(PO_4)_2$ phases in these sintered composites, (ii) the density and elastic modulus of the β-$Ca_3(PO_4)_2$/Mg–6% Zn composite match those of natural bone, and the strength is approximately double that of natural bone, (iii) the 10% β-$Ca_3(PO_4)_2$/Mg–6% Zn composites exhibit good corrosion resistance, as determined by a 30-day immersion test and electrochemical measurements in SBF at 37 °C, (iv) the 10% β-$Ca_3(PO_4)_2$/Mg–6% Zn composite is safe for cellular applications, with a cytotoxicity grade of ~0–1 against L-929 cells in in vitro testing, (v) the β-$Ca_3(PO_4)_2$/Mg–6% Zn composite also exhibits good biocompatibility with the tissue and the important visceral organs the heart, kidney and liver of experimental rabbits and (vi) the corrosion products, such as $Mg(OH)_2$ and $Ca_5(PO_4)_6(OH)_2$, can improve the biocompatibility of the β-$Ca_3(PO_4)_2$/Mg–Zn composite. Furthermore, Yu et al. [63], using a Mg–6%Zn–15%$Ca_3(PO_4)_2$ composite, investigated in vivo biocompatibility and biodegradation in Zelanian rabbits. It was reported that (i) the Mg^{2+}, Zn^{2+} and Ca^{2+} ions are in the normal range in the animal's blood during the whole experiment period; (ii) all the tissues are normal during the composite degradation process, which indicates that the composite exhibits good biocompatibility to these visceral organs; and (iii) the biodegradation of composite benefits in stimulating the bone formation around the prefracture.

There are some studies on Mg–Zn–Zr alloy composited with β-TCP. He et al. [64] added nano-β-TCP particles (0.5%, 1.0% and 1.5%) into Mg–3Zn–0.8Zr alloy to improve its microstructure and the properties. It was mentioned that (i) the grains of Mg–Zn–Zr/β-TCP composites were significantly refined and the tensile tests indicate that the UTS and the elongation of composites were improved with the addition of β-TCP and (ii) the electrochemical test result in simulation body fluid shows that the corrosion resistance of the composites was strongly enhanced comparing with that of the alloy and the corrosion potential of Mg–3Zn0.8–Zr/1.0β-TCP composite is −1.547 V and its corrosion current density is 1.20×10^{-6} A/cm^2. Feng et al. [65] fabricated ZK60A matrix composites reinforced with 2.5, 5, 7.5and 10 wt% calcium polyphosphate particles, which were sphere-like in shape with average size of about 750 nm, by powder metallurgy. It was found that ultrafine calcium polyphosphate particles uniformly distribute in the ZK60A matrices without voids for the composites containing 2.5 and 5 wt% calcium polyphosphate. For the composites containing 7.5 and 10 wt% calcium polyphosphate, however, calcium polyphosphate particles agglomerate in the ZK60A matrices, and some obvious voids appear. The UTSs, yield strengths and elastic moduli of the composites tend to increase when the calcium polyphosphate contents increase from 0 to 5 wt%; however, they appear to decrease with the further increase of calcium polyphosphate from 5 to 10 wt%. The weight losses of the composites, pH values and Mg ion concentrations of the solutions immersing the composites gradually decrease with increase of calcium polyphosphate content, which indicates that the addition of more calcium polyphosphate into ZK60A alloy results in significant degradation slow-up of the composites, which might be attributed to the formation of dense corrosion product layers on the composites. The composites have good mechanical properties and controllable degradation rates and thereby have potential to be used as load-bearing bone implants. Zheng et al. [66] produced Mg–3Zn–0.8Zr composites with unmodified (MZZT) and modified (MZZMT) nanoparticles of β-TCP by high-shear mixing technology. It was reported that after hot extrusion deformation and dynamic recrystallization, the grain size of MZZMT was the half size of MZZT and the distribution of β-TCP particles in the matrix was more uniform than β-TCP particles. The yield tensile strength, UTS and corrosion potential of MZZMT were higher than MZZT, and the corrosion current density of MZZMT was lower than MZZT. Cell proliferation of cocultured MZZMT and MZZT composite samples were roughly the same and the cell number at each time point is higher for MZZMT than for MZZT samples.

Wang et al. [67] fabricated a novel interpenetrating β-TCP/Mg–Zn–Mn composite by infiltrating Mg–Zn–Mn alloy into porous β-TCP using suction-casting technique. It was mentioned that (i) the composite had a compact structure and the interfacial bonding between Mg–Zn–Mn alloy and β-TCP scaffold was very well, (ii) the composite had an ultimate compressive strength of 140 ± 20 MPa, which is near with the natural bone (2–180 MPa) and about 1,000-fold higher than that of the original porous β-TCP scaffold, and it still retained about two-fifths of the strength of the bulk Mg–Zn–Mn alloy and (iii) the electrochemical and immersion tests indicated that the corrosion resistance of the composite was better than that of the Mg–Zn–Mn matrix alloy, and the corrosion products on the composite surface were mainly $Mg(OH)_2$, $Ca_3(PO_4)_2$ and HA. Yuan et al. [68] investigated the effect of cooling rate on the microstructure and corrosion behavior of a biodegradable β-TCP/Mg–Zn–Ca composite under a series of cooling rates using a wedge-shaped casting mold. It was reported that (i) faster cooling rates were shown to refine the secondary phase and grain size, and produce a more homogenous microstructure and (ii) the refined microstructure resulted in a more uniform distribution of β-TCP particles, which is believed to be beneficial in the formation of a stable and compact corrosion product layer, leading to improved corrosion resistance for the composite. Wang et al. [69] fabricated the biomedical cocontinuous (β-TCP + MgO)/Zn–Mg composite by infiltrating Zn–Mg alloy into porous β-TCP + MgO using suction exsorption technique. It was reported that the molten Zn–Mg alloy had infiltrated not only into the pores but also into the struts of the porous β-TCP + MgO scaffold to form a compact composite. The Zn–Mg alloy contacted to the β-TCP + MgO scaffold closely, and no reaction layer can be found between the alloy and the scaffold. The compressive strength of the composite was as high as 244 MPa, which was about 1,000 times higher than that of the original porous β-TCP + MgO scaffold and two-thirds of the strength of the Zn–Mg bulk alloy. The electrochemical and immersion tests in SBF solution indicated that the corrosion resistance of the composite was better than that of the Zn–Mg bulk alloy and the corrosion products on the composite surface were mainly $Zn(OH)_2$, indicating that the (β-TCP + MgO)/Zn–Mg composite fabricated by suction exsorption would be a very promising candidate for bone substitute.

TCP has three polymorphs: the rhombohedral β-TCP and two high temperature forms, monoclinic α-TCP and hexagonal α'-TCP. It was reported that β-TCP has a crystallographic density of 3.066 g/cm^3 while the high temperature forms are less dense, α-TCP has a density of 2.866 g/cm^3 and α'-TCP has a density of 2.702 g/cm^3 [70, 71]. There are differences in chemical and biological properties between the beta and alpha forms, the alpha form is more soluble and biodegradable [72]. There are some studies to differentiate between α-TCP and β-TCP. Grandi et al. [73] conducted comparative histomorphometric analysis and conclude that (i) both materials are osteoconductive and biocompatible and (ii) perhaps the larger rate of new bone formation observed in the α-TCP group and it also occurs in the β-TCP/HA group within a longer time period. Merten et al. [74] conducted intraindividual comparison of these two TCPs in animal model and concluded that defined degradation of these ceramics allows early functional bone regeneration with an additional undisturbed biofunctional unisotropic orientation of new trabeculae. Ikeo et al. [75] prepared Mg–Ca alloy composited with α-TCP by powder metallurgical method. It was reported that (i) refinement of the α-TCP particle size caused more uniform distribution and microstructure; (ii) consequently, the composite with finer α-TCP particle size had better ductility to the alloy lacking α-TCP; and (iii) the biodegradation properties were improved by the addition of α-TCP, and the refinement of the α-TCP particles led to a slower degradation rate in electrochemical and immersion tests.

4.3.3 Mg–carbon/carbides biocomposites

Mg materials are incorporated with carbon fiber filament, carbon nanotube (CNT), silicon carbide and other types of carbides. These Mg matrix composites are fabricated usually through stirring casting, powder forming, injecting deposition, liquid metal infiltration or die casting.

4.3.3.1 Carbon fiber

Qi et al. [76] fabricated C_{sf}/Mg composites via infiltration of porous short carbon fiber by liquid magnesium under pressurized nitrogen. It was reported that (i) the preform was infiltrated thoroughly by melt magnesium and the fabricated C_{sf}/Mg composites have excellent mechanical properties compared with the magnesium alloys and (ii) C_{sf}/Mg composites should be very promising candidates for automobile parts and portable electronic appliance parts in the future. Tian et al. [77] characterized the fiber orientation in the extruded C_{sf}/Mg composites. It was mentioned that (i) the fiber orientation variation factor V of the finite element simulations and of the extrusion experiments match well such that the fiber orientation variation factor V is valid and convenient to characterize the fiber orientation variation in the extruded C_{sf}/Mg composites and (ii) the distribution of the fiber orientation variation factors illustrates that the fibers in the extruded C_{sf}/Mg composites are reoriented toward the direction of the maximum principal strain and deviated from the directions of the medium and minimum principal strains. Zhang et al. studied the effect of admixing of Gd element [78] and Y element [79] in C_f/Mg composite. It was reported that (i) the RE Gd tended to segregate at interface area to form Gd_2O_3 layer and particle phase Mg_7Gd, and both the interfacial products enhanced the interfacial bonding strength which can be identified by the increase of interlaminar shear strength, (ii) the Gd addition promoted the shear strength and bending strength greatly, with an increase by 60.4% and 25.3% compared with C_f/Mg composite, respectively [78], (iii) the RE element Y added to C_f/Mg composite improved the interfacial bonding strength, (iv) the interfacial products were identified to be MgO, Mg_2Y and $Mg_{24}Y_5$, (v) the interfacial products enhanced the interfacial bonding strength, which could be confirmed by the increase of interlaminar shear strength and (vi) the C_f/Mg composite with 5.7 wt% Y addition increases the shear strength by about 120.9% from 46.2 to 102.3 MPa [79]. Qi et al. [80] investigated the mechanical properties of magnesium matrix composites reinforced by pyrolytic carbon-coated short carbon fiber at temperatures close to and above the solidus temperature. It was reported that (i) tensile strength of the composites decreased monotonously with temperature, an exponential equation relating the tensile strength to temperature and liquid fraction was derived; (ii) the elongation increases monotonously with temperatures from 400 to 428 °C (solidus temperature), and then decreases gradually with increasing fraction of liquid except a trough at 432 °C; (iii) the composites almost have no ductility and cannot sustain tensile stress when the fraction of liquid reaches 8%; and (iv) the amount and distribution of liquid phase in the composites directly determines their mechanical properties and damage behavior. Qi et al. [81], using two types of device design, namely, internal localization and external localization, studied the mechanical behavior of C_f/Mg composite and reported that (i) the internal localization forming device produced good surface quality and compact C_f/Mg composite components, (ii) the longitudinal microstructures are uniform and conductive to the excellent properties of C_f/Mg composites and (iii) the measured bending strength and elastic modulus are 367 MPa and 59 GPa, respectively, or a 45.6% and 31.1% improvement in comparison to those of the casting AZ91D magnesium alloy.

4.3.3.2 Carbon nanotube

Gupta et al. [82] synthesized CNT-reinforced magnesium using the powder metallurgy technique followed by hot extrusion with up to 0.3 wt% addition of CNTs as reinforcements. It was mentioned that (i) the thermomechanical property results show an increase in thermal stability with increasing amount of CNTs in the Mg nanocomposites and (ii) mechanical property characterizations reveal an improvement of yield strength, ductility and work of fracture with higher weight percentages of CNTs incorporated. Liang et al. [83] developed a process for preparing CNT-reinforced magnesium nanocomposites, which combined friction stir processing and ultrasonic-assisted extrusion. It was reported that (i) a very good dispersion of CNTs in AZ91D alloy could be observed; (ii) the strength of Mg nanocomposites was remarkably enhanced, which might be contributed to dislocation strengthening mechanism and stress transfer mechanism, not concerned with the grain refinement; and (iii) the composites maintained good ductility. The interfaces between CNTs and Mg matrix were well bonded, and the interfacial reaction product formation of Al_2MgC_2 was confirmed. Kumar et al. [84] added the multiwalled CNTs of 20 mm diameter to the highly reactive magnesium alloys in various combinations to produce a lightweight high-strength composites for aerospace and terrain applications by a stir-casting technique under desired conditions in order to overcome defects since the base metal is highly affinitive to volatile oxygen. Furthermore, Kumar et al. [85] produced the MgAZ91D/CNT composites by the emerging stir-casting method.

4.3.3.3 SiC

Roy et al. [86] hot extruded the cast Mg/SiCp and AZ91/SiCp composites up to low ($R = 15:1$) and high ($R = 54:1$) extrusion ratios at 350 °C. It was reported that (i) significant matrix grain refinement was noticed after extrusion due to dynamic recrystallization, the degree of refinement being relatively higher for the two composites; (ii) the AZ91-based materials (AZ91 and AZ91/SiCp) exhibited comparatively finer grain size both in cast condition and after extrusion due to strong pinning effect from alloying elements as well as $Mg_{17}Al_{12}$ intermetallic phase; (iii) compositional analyses eliminated the possibility of any interfacial reaction between matrix (Mg/AZ91) and second-phase reinforcement (SiCp) in case of the composites; (iv) microhardness did not significantly increase on extrusion in comparison to the respective cast materials for both composites and unreinforced alloys; and (v) dynamic mechanical analysis, however, confirmed that the damping properties were affected by the extrusion ratio and to a lesser extent, due to the presence of second phase at room temperature as well as at higher temperature (300 °C). Eamaily et al. [87] investigated the capability of the developed rheocasting technique in combination with the RheoMetal process for producing SiC particulate-reinforced AM50 and AZ91D matrix composites. It was mentioned that (i) solid fraction, particle size and oxidation of SiC particles had strong impacts on the overall quality of the composites; (ii) the composites produced by 40% solid fraction and oxidized micron-sized SiC particles exhibited an excellent casting quality; (iii) a low-quality composite was obtained when nonoxidized submicron-sized SiC particles were employed, showing the formation of various types of intermetallic particles and carbides such as MgO, Mg_2Si, Al_2MgC_2, Mg_2C_3 and Al_4C_3 as the interfacial reaction products of SiC/Mg alloy's melts; and (iv) Mg hydride (α-MgH_2) was also identified in interdendritic regions of the MMCs. Wang et al. [88] fabricated 1 wt% SiC nanoparticles reinforced Mg–9Al–1Zn magnesium matrix composite by stir casting and hot extrusion. It was reported that (i) the grains of the matrix in the as-cast SiCp/Mg–9Al–1Zn nanocomposite stirring for 30 min are mainly refined; however, the mechanical properties of nanocomposite decline due to the increase of agglomerated SiC nanoparticles and $Mg_{17}Al_{12}$ phases with network morphology along the grain boundaries, (ii) after hot extrusion, a bimodal microstructure composed of alternate arrays of fine recrystallized grains and relatively coarse recrystallized grains forms and (iii) particularly, for extruded nanocomposites stirring for 30 min, the fine recrystallized region increases and the distribution of SiC nanoparticles is more homogenous, which exhibits superior mechanical properties compared with as-extruded SiCp/Mg–9Al–1Zn nanocomposite stirring for 10 min. He et al. [89] synthesized Mg-based nanocomposite with hierarchical structure via mechanical alloying followed by spark plasma sintering, which was reinforced by 15 vol% nanometer-sized SiC particles. It was shown that the hierarchical microstructure consists of an isolated soft pure Mg phase, with flake-like morphology, uniformly distributed in the Mg/SiC nanocomposite. The quasistatic compression test demonstrates that the hierarchical nanocomposite shows significantly higher ductility than that of counterpart with homogeneous microstructure while the result of dynamic test suggests that the ductility of the hierarchical nanocomposite has not improved significantly at high strain rate. The fracture morphology shows both brittle and ductile features partially resulting from the flake-like soft phase, as well as the hierarchical microstructure.

Chang et al. [90] reinforced Mg–5Al–2Ca alloys with 2, 5 and 10 vol% 5 μm SiCp by stir casting, followed by the hot extrusion. It was found that (i) in the cast composites, addition of SiCp disturbs the network distribution of Al_2Ca phase along grain boundaries; (ii) after extrusion, grains of the matrix are refined further and the Al_2Ca phase break into particulates and the Al_2Ca phase and grain size can be further refined by the addition of SiCp; (iii) compared with Mg–5Al–2Ca alloy, the addition of SiCp introduces obvious improvement of tensile yield strength and work-hardening rate, however, at the expense of elongation; (iv) unlike the tensile yield strength, the UTS of SiCp/Mg–5Al–2Ca composite does not change monotonously with increasing SiCp's content, and the highest UTS appears when the SiCp's volume fraction is 5%; and (v) the interfacial debonding between SiCp and Al_2Ca phase and cracked particles are considered as the main crack source for SiCp/Mg–5Al–2Ca composite. Based on the fact that a production of fully dense Mg–SiC nanocomposites with a homogeneous distribution of SiC nanoparticles through powder metallurgy techniques is still a challenging issue, Penther et al. [91] proposed to combine sintering and hot extrusion of mechanically milled composite powders to encompass the known difficulties of conventional processing. Cold-isostatic pressing, sintering and indirect hot extrusion were used for compaction and consolidation. It was reported that (i) near-dense Mg–SiC nanocomposites with 1 and 10 vol% SiC nanoparticles were successfully produced with a homogeneous distribution of the nanoparticles; (ii) the nanoparticles pin the grain boundaries and foster dynamic recrystallization, so that a nanograined Mg matrix develops and is preserved even after the final consolidation step; and (iii) very good interface adherence between nanoparticles and matrix contributing to the high hardness of the nanocomposites was noticed. Kamrani et al. [92] employed the high-energy ball milling to produce magnesium matrix nanocomposites reinforced with SiC nanoparticles. It was shown that (i) with increasing volume fraction of SiC nanoparticles, a finer nanocomposite powder with more uniform particle size distribution is obtained, (ii) a homogeneous distribution of SiC nanoparticles, even up to 10% volume fraction, in magnesium matrix after 25 h milling was confirmed by elemental mapping and TEM results, (iii) the analysis of the XRD patterns accompanied by dark-field TEM images revealed that magnesium crystallites refine to fine nanocrystalline sizes after the mechanical milling and (iv) the crystallite size of the magnesium matrix reduced with increasing SiC nanoparticle content in addition to the induced lattice strain. Ghasemi et al. [93] mechanically mixed mixtures of magnesium powder and SiC nanoparticles at various volume fractions to produce nanocrystalline Mg–SiC nanocomposites. It was reported that (i) mechanical milling is a proper method to achieve a uniform distribution of the SiC nanoparticles, even up to 10% in the Mg matrix, (ii) higher volume fraction of the SiC nanoparticles raise the value of measured microstrain and reduce the crystallite size of the Mg matrix and (iii) the SiC nanoparticles (even up to 10 vol%), well distributed in the magnesium matrix, remarkably improve the reduced elastic modulus and nanohardness of the nanocomposite powders. Shen et al. [94] investigated the microstructure evolution and fracture behavior of Mg–2.7Al–0.8Zn (AZ31B) reinforced with 1 vol% nanosilicon carbide particle (nn-SiCp) and 4 vol% submicron SiCp (sm-SiCp) during room temperature tensile test. It was mentioned that (i) the addition of double-sized SiCp resulted in the extensive accumulation of dislocation near the interface between SiCp and matrix, and the dislocation density is increased as the increase of strain, (ii) the formation of high-density dislocation zone was identified as one of the main causes of strength enhancement, (iii) some microcracks can be found in the interface between sm-SiCp and matrix, which show that the high stress concentration exists in the sm-SiCp/Mg interface due to the particle size and polygonal morphology; however, the bonding interfaces of nn-SiCp/Mg were still continuous, and no microcracks were present around nn-SiCp and (iv) as a result of nondeforming sm-SiCp resisting the crack propagation, an appreciable crack-blunting effect is generated, which contributes to the overall strengthening effect of double-sized SiCp/Mg composite.

4.3.4 Magnesium nitride biocomposites

Chen et al. [95] developed a new process for the preparation of ultrafine AlN particles reinforced Mg–Al matrix composites to control the agglomeration of ultrafine AlN particles. It was mentioned that (i) for AlN–Mg mixture, AlN particles were separately cladded in Mg coating and homogeneously distributed in the mixture after milling for 15 h and (ii) Mg–Al matrix alloy particles were significantly refined after milling for 20 h, and the strip-type Al was fragmented and uniformly distributed in Mg matrix. Yang et al. [96] synthesized AlN particles reinforced Mg-9 wt% Al matrix composites by bubbling nitrogen gas method. It was reported that (i) nanosized AlN particles were uniformly distributed in the matrix, which resulted in grain refinement of a-Mg from 90 to 100 μm to 30–40 μm after solutionizing, and then $Mg_{17}Al_{12}$ phase was dispersed and decreased and (ii) subsequently, significant improvements of tensile strength (~226 MPa) and elongation (~21%) were obtained in the as-cast AlN/Mg–9Al composites. Moreover Yang et al. mentioned that the higher UTSs (200–230 MPa) and the higher fracture elongations (16–47%) were obtained in the AlN/Mg–9Al permanent mold-casting composites [97]. Gao et al. [98] fabricated $ZrAl_3$ and AlN-reinforced Mg–Al composite. By inserting Al–10ZrN master alloy into Mg matrix and reheating the cooled ingot to 550 °C, Al and Mg atoms diffuse to the opposite side. It was mentioned that (i) as a result, liquid melt occurs once the interface areas reach to proper compositions, then dissolved Al atoms react with ZrN, leading to the in-situ formation of $ZrAl_3$ and AlN particles, while the Al matrix is finally replaced by Mg and (ii) this new method is claimed as matric exchange synthesization.

The effect of boron nitride BN nanoparticles reinforcement (0%, 0.5%, 1.5% and 2.5%) on dry sliding wear behavior of pure Mg and magnesium nanocomposites was investigated, using powder metallurgy, followed by a hot extrusion [99]. It was mentioned that Mg reinforced with 0.5% boron nitride shows lower wear rates and low friction coefficient values compared with magnesium reinforced with 1.5% boron nitride and 2.5% boron nitride nanocomposites.

4.3.5 Magnesium borides biocomposites

Xiao research group have extensively studied effect of TiB_2 admixed to Mg-based AZ91 alloy [100–103]. The submicron TiB_2 particles (2.5 wt%)-reinforced AZ91 matrix composites are processed by the master alloy method combined with an optimized self-propagating high-temperature synthesis [100]. It was found that (i) only TiB_2 phase is in situ formed in the Al–TiB_2 master alloy and exhibits the size distribution of 100–700 nm, (ii) compared with the unreinforced AZ91 alloy, the grain size and morphology of $Mg_{17}Al_{12}$ phase in as-cast composites are much refined, (iii) the ageing process of composites is accelerated and the peak-aged time of composites decreases from 42 to 22 h significantly with the introduction of TiB_2 particles, (iv) large numbers of fine $Mg_{17}Al_{12}$ in composites preferentially precipitate at grain boundaries and near TiB_2 particles regions. In addition, the hardness, yield strength, UTS and elongation of as-cast composites are improved by 16.1%, 53.0%, 26.3% and 25.6%, respectively, and after T6 heat treatment, the strength of composites is increased further due to large amounts of submicron $Mg_{17}Al_{12}$ phase, and the age-hardening efficiency of composites is higher than that of AZ91 alloy [100]. The hot deformation behavior of in-situ nanosized TiB_2/AZ91 composite was studied by analyzing the constitutive equation, hot processing maps and microstructure evolutions, under hot compression tests at different temperatures (250–400 °C) and strain rates range from 0.001 to 1/s with a constant strain of 0.69. It was reported that (i) deformation temperatures and strain rates have a strong influence on the flow behavior of the composite, exhibiting typical work hardening, softening and steady stages; (ii) the stress exponent (*n*) is calculated as 5.4, suggesting that the hot deformation mechanism of TiB_2/AZ91 composite is dominated by the dislocation climb; (iii) by observing microstructures, full dynamic recrystallization occurs in the safe regions, while the mechanism of instability region is dominated by mechanical twining and high-density dislocation [101]. Furthermore, Mg matrix composites reinforced with 2.5 wt% nanosized TiB_2 particles were fabricated by adding Al–TiB_2 master alloy prepared by the chemical reaction of Al–K_2TiF_6–KBF_4 system into molten magnesium. It was mentioned that (i) the TiB_2 particles display a dominant number of particles less than 100 nm and a uniform distribution in the composites; (ii) the grain size of composites is decreased compared with AZ91 alloy; (iii) the yield strength, UTS and elongation to fracture of composites are improved by 49.4%, 25.5% and 51.1%, respectively; and (iv) among the strengthening mechanisms of nanosized particles reinforced Mg matrix composites, dislocation strengthening and Orowan strengthening play a more important role in increasing the strength [102].

4.3.6 Mg-based biocomposites with other ceramic materials

4.3.6.1 Glass

Bioglass (which will be discussed in the next section) is admixed to Mg-based materials to improve surface biocompatibility and bioactivity. Huan et al. [103, 104] added bioactive glass (BG, 45S5) particles to a biodegradable magnesium alloy (ZK30) through a semisolid high-pressure casting process. It was reported that (i) homogeneous dispersion of BG particles in the matrix. SEM, EDX and EPMA showed the retention of the morphological characteristics and composition of BG particles in the as-cast composite materials, (ii) in vitro tests in a cell culture medium confirmed that the composites indeed possessed an enhanced ability to induce the deposition of a bone-like apatite layer on the surface, indicating an improved surface biocompatibility as compared with the matrix alloy [103], (iii) immersion tests in the minimum essential medium with Earle's balanced salts at 37 °C showed that the composites with 5% and 10% bioglass had lower rates of degradation and hydrogen evolution than the matrix alloy, (iv) the composites possessed an enhanced ability to induce calcium and phosphate ion deposition on sample surfaces during degradation, suggesting accelerated surface mineralization that would lead to improved bioactivity when compared with the matrix alloy, (v) in vitro cytotoxicity tests showed that the ionic products of the composites formed during degradation possessed a superior ability to support the survival, proliferation and osteoblastic differentiation of bone marrow stromal cells to those of the ZK30 alloy and (vi) the ZK30-BG composites with enhanced bioactivity and reduced degradation rate could be promising biodegradable materials for orthopedic implants [104]. Ashuri et al. [105] prepared a bioceramic-based composite by sintering compacts made up of mixtures of HA and sol–gel-derived bioactive glass ($64SiO_2$-26CaO-5MgO-5ZnO) (by mol %) powders (up to 30 wt%). It was reported that (i) compressive strength of the specimen was decreased 65% after maintaining in the SBF for 14 days, (ii) the study of degradation behavior revealed Si release capability of this composite and (iii) biological evaluations in vitro confirmed that the composite studied could induce osteoblast-like cells' activities.

4.3.6.2 Oxides

There are several studies on metallic oxides such as titania, alumina or magnesia to enhance Mg-based materials.

As mentioned previously, the effect of addition of TiO_2 nanopowders on the corrosion behavior and mechanical properties of Mg/HA-based nanocomposites fabricated using a milling–pressing–sintering technique for medical applications was investigated [59]. Ong et al. [106], conducted Young's modulus measurements and indirect cytotoxicity tests on Mg (0.97, 1.98, 2.5) vol% TiO_2, Mg (0.58, 0.97, 1.98) vol % TiC and Mg (0.58, 0.97, 1.98) vol% TiN, synthesized using the disintegrated melt-deposition technique to determine the cytotoxicity of low-volume nanoparticulate reinforcement on magnesium. It was mentioned that (i) the results of the indirect MTT assay on day 3 and day 5 indicate that 2.5 vol% TiO_2, TiC and TiN has little effect on the cytotoxicity when added as low-volume fraction reinforcement to magnesium, (ii) while (0.97, 1.98) vol% TiO_2 negatively affected the cytotoxicity when added to Mg and (iii) the Young's modulus of the materials was found to remain close to that of cortical bone which would suggest that the stress-shielding effect would be reduced as the increase in Young's modulus was mitigated by the low-volume addition of reinforcements. Mg–Ca–TiO_2 (MCT) composite scaffolds loaded with different concentrations of doxycycline (DC) with a network of interconnected pores with good compressive strength (5 ± 0.1 MPa) were fabricated via space holder method [107]. It was reported that (i) MCT-DC scaffolds possess a porosity and pore size in the range of 65–67% and 600–800 µm, respectively, (ii) the bioactivity results exhibited the apatite formation on the MCT-DC scaffold surface, indicating that DC did not obstruct the bioactivity of MCT, (iii) the MCT-DC scaffolds drug release profiles show the initial burst and sustained drug release (55–75%) and the release rate could be adjusted via altering the DC concentration, (iv) the MCT loaded with 1% and 5% DC did not indicate cytotoxic behavior against MG63 cells while further DC loading resulted in toxicity and (v) antimicrobial properties of MCT-DC scaffolds against *Staphylococcus aureus* (*S. aureus*) and *Escherichia coli* (*E. coli*) bacteria were examined and the results reveal oblivious inhibition zone around each MCT-DC scaffold, whereas no obvious inhibition is observed around the MCT scaffold; hence, MCT-DC composite scaffolds with low concentration of DC could be alternative candidates for infection prevention and bone tissue engineering.

In order to improve the corrosion resistance and mechanical properties of magnesium alloys for biomedical implant applications, Lin et al. [108] fabricated biodegradable Mg–3Zn–0.2Ca (wt%) matrix composites, reinforced by adding various contents of MgO nanoparticles (0.1, 0.2, 0.3 and 0.5 wt%) using high-shear melt conditioning. An optimum solution treatment (450 °C, 48 h) and subsequent hot extrusion was carried out to produce the Mg–3Zn–0.2Ca/MgO composites. It was mentioned that (i) the as-extruded composite exhibited a fine-grain structure with relatively uniformly distributed MgO particles, (ii) a substantial reduction in the secondary phase content was found in the solution-treated sample, (iii) in vitro immersion, electrochemical and mechanical tensile tests were used to characterize the corrosion behavior and mechanical properties, (iv) the UTS increased to 329.03 ± 2.01 MPa and the yield tensile strength increased by 22.81% with 0.5 wt% MgO loading, while the ductility did not substantially deteriorate, (v) the polarization resistance of the composite was shown to increase from 0.95 to 2.02 $k\Omega \cdot cm^2$ with the addition of 0.2 wt% MgO and (vi) with increasing MgO content, agglomeration of the MgO particles was detected in the analyzed composite, resulting in decreased ductility and the occurrence of pitting corrosion. Kimiyama et al. [109] fabricated corrosion-resistant films on Mg alloy AZ31 substrates by steam coating method using $Al(NO_3)_3 \cdot 9H_2O$ aqueous solution as a steam source under treatment temperature of was maintained at 160 °C for 3, 5, 7 and 9 h. It was found that (i) XRD analysis demonstrated that the coated films were composed of a mixed structure of $Mg(OH)_2$ and Mg–Al layered double hydroxide (Mg-Al LDH) phases, (ii) the potentiodynamic polarization curves of the film coated for 7 h exhibited the lowest corrosion current density, which was almost four orders of magnitude lower than that of bare AZ31 and (iii) the enhanced corrosion resistance was well consistent with the increase of Mg-Al LDH content in the films.

Liu et al. [110] synthesized Mg–Al_2O_3 nanocomposite powders, with Al_2O_3 particles of 50 nm size, by mechanical alloying starting from a mixture of 70 vol.% pure Mg and 30 vol.% Al_2O_3 powders. It was shown that (i) a mixture of Mg, Al_2O_3 and MgO phases were obtained on mechanical alloying, (ii) on annealing the milled powders at 600 °C for 30 min, a displacement reaction occurred between the Mg and Al_2O_3 phases, when the formation of a mixture of pure Al and MgO phases was observed, (iii) a reaction occurred between the initial Mg powder and Al formed as a result of the displacement reaction, leading to the formation of $Mg_{17}Al_{12}$, $Al_{0.58}Mg_{0.42}$ and Al_3Mg_2 phases and (iv) the powder annealed after milling the Mg + Al_2O_3 powder mix for 25 h consisted of Al, MgO and Al_3Mg_2 phases. Alaneme et al. [111] investigated the fabrication characteristics and mechanical behavior of Al–Mg–Si alloy matrix composites reinforced with alumina (Al_2O_3) and rice husk ash (RHA, an agrowaste) to assess the viability of developing high-performance Al-matrix composites at reduced cost. Al_2O_3 particulates added with 0, 2, 3 and 4 wt% RHA were utilized to prepare 10 wt% of the reinforcing phase with Al–Mg–Si alloy as matrix using two-step stir-casting method. It was reported that (i) the less dense Al–Mg–Si/RHA/Al_2O_3 hybrid composites have estimated percent porosity levels as low as the single Al_2O_3-reinforced grade (<2.3% porosity), (ii) the hardness of the hybrid composites decreases slightly with increase in RHA content with a maximum reduction of less than 11% observed for the Al-4 wt% RHA-6 wt% Al_2O_3 composition (in comparison with the Al-10 wt% Al_2O_3 single reinforced composition), (iii) the tensile strength reductions of 8% and 13%, and specific strengths which were 3.56% and 7.7% lower were respectively observed for the 3 and 4 wt% RHA containing hybrid composites, (iv) the specific strength, percent elongation and fracture toughness of the 2 wt% RHA-containing hybrid composite was however, higher than that of the single Al_2O_3 reinforced and other hybrid composite compositions worked on. RHA, thus, has great promise to serve as a complementing reinforcement for the development of low-cost high-performance aluminum-hybrid composites.

4.3.6.3 Minerals

Dezfuli et al. [112] determined the mechanical properties of Mg–bredigite – $Ca_7Mg(SiO_4)_4$, prior to and during degradation. It was reported that (i) by optimizing the process parameters of pressure-assisted sintering, low-porosity Mg–bredigite composites with strong interfaces between homogeneously distributed bredigite particles and the Mg matrix could be fabricated, (ii) by reinforcing Mg with 20 vol% bredigite particles, the ultimate compressive strength and ductility of Mg increased by 67% and 111%, respectively, (iii) the in vitro degradation rate of the Mg–20% bredigite composite in a cell culture medium was 24 times lower than that of monolithic Mg and (iv) as a result of retarded degradation, the mechanical properties of the composite after 12 days of immersion in the cell culture medium were comparable to those of cortical bone. Voronkova et al. [113] prepared both undoped and Mg-doped Nd_2MoO_6 oxymolybdate single crystals and polycrystalline samples by flux growth and solid-state reactions. It was mentioned that (i) the $(MgO)_x(Nd_2MoO_6)_{(1-x)/2}$ solid solution series has been shown to extend to $x = 0.20$, (ii) doping of Nd_2MoO_6 single crystals with Mg leads to splitting of the Mo, Nd_1 and O_2 sites, (iii) a structural model in which the Mg atoms partially substitute for Mo atoms and reside near the Mo site, 0.28 Å from it, ensures the best agreement with the observed diffraction pattern and (iv) the conductivity of the undoped and doped polycrystalline samples approaches 10^{-4} S/cm at 800 °C and is assumed to have an anionic nature.

4.3.6.4 Compounds

Huang et al. [114] admixed small amounts (up to 1 wt%) of WS_2 nanotubes with AZ31 alloy using melt-stirring process above 700 °C. It was mentioned that (i) the MMC nanocomposites exhibit much superior mechanical properties over the undoped alloy, (ii) metallographic investigation demonstrates that the average grain size has been reduced in inverse proportion to the added amounts of nanotubes up to 1 wt% and (iii) physical considerations suggest that the main mechanism responsible for the reinforcement effect lies in the mismatch between the thermal expansion coefficients of the metal and the nanotubes and this mismatch induced large density of dislocations in the grain boundaries in the vicinity of the nanotube-matrix interface, which obstruct the crack propagation. Zhong et al. [115] investigated the hydrolysis properties and air stability of Mg–Ca hydride (MCH)-based material improved by ball milling with NH_4Cl. It was reported that (i) the addition of NH_4Cl by ball milling significantly enhances the hydrolysis performance, (ii) the MCH–5% NH_4Cl composite (powder) milled for 0.5 h displays the highest hydrogen yield of 1,006 mL/$g_{(com)}$ at 25 °C without stirring, and has the fastest hydrogen generation rate (872 mL/$g_{(com)}$/min in the initial 1 min), (iii) the hydrogen yield of the MCH–5% NH_4Cl composite plate still reaches 726 mL/$g_{(com)}$ at 25 °C without stirring when being exposed to the air for 5 h with 80% humidity at 30 °C and (iv) these characteristics demonstrate that the MCH–NH_4Cl composites in plate can be a promising and practicable hydrogen generation material on portable power supplies. Liu et al. [116] prepared the composites of Mg–$x$wt% $CaNi_5$ ($x = 20$, 30 and 50) by hydriding combustion synthesis (HCS) and investigated the phase evolution during HCS as well as the hydriding properties of the products. It was found that (i) Mg reacted with $CaNi_5$ forming Mg_2Ni and Ca during the heating period of HCS, (ii) afterward, the resultant Mg_2Ni and Ca as well as the remnant Mg reacted with hydrogen during the cooling period, (iii) the lower platform in the P–C isotherms corresponds to the hydriding of Mg, and the higher one corresponds to Mg_2Ni, (iv) with the increase of the content of $CaNi_5$ from 20 to 50 wt%, the hydrogen content of the HCS products increases at first and then decreases and (v) the Mg-30 wt% $CaNi_5$ composite has the maximum hydrogen capacity of 4.74 wt%, and it can absorb 3.51 wt% of hydrogen in the first hydriding process without activation.

Li et al. [117] catalyzed the magnesium hydrolyzing reaction in situ using a layered Mg_2Ni compound, rapidly producing hydrogen in NaCl solution. The post-H_2 generation residue (mixture of $Mg(OH)_2$ and Mg_2Ni catalyst) was recycled to recover pure Ni powder from the waste mixture. It was mentioned that (i) pure Mg (153 g) and pure Ni (47 g) in a eutectic composition were easily melted to form a molten alloy by a super-high-frequency (35 kHz) induction furnace, (ii) the lamellar material had an $Mg/Mg_2Ni/Mg/Mg_2Ni$ layered structure, in which each layer was ~0.8 μm thick; Mg was an anodic phase and Mg_2Ni was a cathodic phase (the catalyst), (iii) bulk Mg/Mg_2Ni composite alloy contains many microgalvanic cells. Owing to the lamellar microstructure, no dense hydrated oxide film that might have caused surface passivation was found, allowing continuous H_2 generation until no magnesium remained to participate in the hydrolysis and (iv) the activation energy of the hydrolysis reaction in simulated seawater was ~36.35 kJ/mol. Fang et al. [118] developed a $Mg–Mg_2Sn$ composite. The Mg_2Sn reinforcement was synthesized effectively by milling microsized Mg and nanosized Sn powders. It was shown that (i) high surface activation of raw nanosized Sn powder would be greatly beneficial to accelerate transformation efficiency of Mg_2Sn nanophase from Mg–Sn mixture; (ii) after sintering, Mg_2Sn cluster consisting of Mg_2Sn nanophase was uniformly distributed in the matrix; and (iii) the $Mg–Mg_2Sn$ composite exhibited an appreciable benefit in terms of hardness and compressive strength, while ductility remained quite high. Jiang et al. [119] produced an Mg_2Si/Mg gradient composite by electromagnetic directional solidification. It was reported that (i) the microstructure of the composite changed longitudinally along with a primary Mg_2Si-rich layer at the bottom and a Mg-rich eutectic layer at the top, respectively, (ii) both layers exhibited a much higher biocorrosion resistance than pure Mg, especially, the primary Mg_2Si-rich phase revealed the greatest biocorrosion resistance due to the corrosion blocking effect and (iii) all the components originated from the gradient composite showed an excellent biocompatibility without toxicity to osteoblasts; indicating a new insight into the designing of gradient Mg_2Si/Mg composite as a promising candidate for orthopedic implants. Cai et al. [120] fabricated an $Mg–MgF_2$ nanocomposite by reactive milling. It was mentioned that the thermal stability is largely enhanced from ~100 °C for nanocrystalline Mg to ~450 °C for $Mg-MgF_2$. The bulk $Mg–MgF_2$ nanocomposite consolidated at a high temperature of 500 °C under 6 GPa exhibits a high compressive yield strength of 582 MPa; meanwhile, the MgF_2 nanoparticles significantly improve the high-temperature hardness of nanocrystalline Mg. The fine, dispersed and thermally stable MgF_2 nanoparticles with a strong interfacial bonding with the matrix are the microstructural features that dominate the superior properties – high thermal stability and high strength at room and elevated temperatures. Yu et al. [121] fabricated AZ91D-based composites reinforced by Ti_2AlC phases particles by the stir-casting technology. It was mentioned that (i) the Ti_2AlC particles were generally distributed along α Mg grain boundaries and strongly impeded the dendritic growth of α-Mg; (ii) the yield strength, Vickers hardness, ultimate compressive strength and Young's moduli increased with increasing Ti_2AlC fraction in composites, while the optimized UTS was found for 10 vol% of Ti_2AlC; (ii) the theoretical calculation on tensile yield strength reveals that individual strengthening contribution was mainly from Hall–Petch strengthening and Forest strengthening, followed by Orowan strengthening effect;

(iii) in situ tensile test revealed that the cracks were initiated in Ti_2AlC particles and propagated along α-Mg grain boundaries; and (iv) during this process, no decohesion occurred at the Ti_2AlC and AZ91D interfaces.

4.4 Mg-based glassy materials

Nandi et al. [122] mentioned that, during the orthopedic surgery, autograft plays a crucial role for correction of fracture repair or other bone pathologies. However, the autograft and/or allograft materials possess several limitations including immunogenic response to the host, low osteogenicity as well as possibilities of disease transmission. Accordingly, demands for developing of alternatives biomaterials that has a capability to initiate osteogenesis, and the graft should closely mimic the natural bone along with regeneration of fibroblasts. As we have seen previously, a variety of artificial materials such as demineralized bone matrix, coralline HA and calcium phosphate-based ceramics such as HA, β-TCP and bioactive glass have been used over the decades to fill bone defects almost without associated soft tissue development [122]. Since bulk metallic glasses (BMGs), when compared with the conventional crystalline metallic counterparts, have unique amorphous structures, they exhibit higher strength, lower Young's modulus, improved wear resistance, good fatigue endurance and excellent corrosion resistance [123]. Hence, BMGs have recently attracted much attention for biomedical applications. Such BMGs should include Ti-based, Zr-based, Fe-based, Mg-based, Zn-based, Ca-based and Sr-based alloying systems for biomedical applications [123]. BMGs are a relatively new class of metallic materials developed over the past three decades. Whereas conventional alloys have a crystalline structure, BMGs exhibit no long-range atomic order, appearing instead as an atomically frozen liquid. With increasing knowledge of the materials science of BMGs and improvements in their properties and processing, there are numerous researches reported for Mg-based BMGs which are showing promise in bioabsorbable implants [124–127].

In the following section, the glass-forming ability (GFA), macro- and microstructures, mechanical behaviors and corrosion behaviors are reviewed.

4.4.1 Glass formability

The GFA of any alloy refers to the ease with which it can be produced in amorphous form by cooling from the liquid. A high GFA indicates a relatively low required cooling rate and a resultant high maximum or critical diameter when cast into a copper mold [128]. There are several types of substituting element to improve the glass formability. The BMGs of $Mg_{60}Ni_{23.6}Y_xLa_{(16.4-x)}$ and $Mg_{65}Ni_{20}Y_xLaMM_{(15-x)}$ with $0 \le x \le 1$ at% were fabricated by injection casting, where MM represents mischmetal [129]. It was found that (i) for the La-containing alloy, a maximum amorphous diameter of 4 mm for $x = 0.5$ and 0.75 was obtained; (ii) the LaMM-containing alloy showed a maximum amorphous diameter of 2 mm for $x = 0$ and 0.25, but decreased to 1 mm with further Y additions; and (iii) the GFA of the $Mg_{60}Ni_{23.6}La_{16.4}$ alloy decreased when La is partially substituted by small amounts of small atoms (Si or B) or by large atoms (Y and Si). Perrière et al. [129] investigated the substitution of Y by MM ($Ce_{55}La_{25}Nd_{20}$) on the $Mg_{65}Cu_{25}Y_{10}$ metallic glass, in order to reduce pure RE content and improve manufacturing for potential applications. It was mentioned that (i) this substitution is well accommodated by partial substitution of Cu by Ni, (ii) alloys were prepared by planar flow melt spinning, with various amounts of MM (0, 5 or 10 at%) and Ni (0, 5, 12.5, 20 or 25 at%) and (iii) with increasing content of MM and nickel, the GFA, especially the width of the supercooled liquid region tends to decrease; however, an optimal substitution of Cu by Ni (12.5 at.%) in an alloy free from Y has been identified to present an appreciable GFA with a supercooled liquid region of 35 K. Zhang et al. [130] developed a group of pseudo-ternary Mg-(Cu-Ag)-Dy BMGs by copper mold casting. It was reported that (i) the GFA is significantly improved by the coexistence of similar elements of Ag and Cu and (ii) the critical diameter for glass formation increases from 10 mm for ternary $Mg_{56.5}Cu_{32}Dy_{11.5}$ alloy to 18 mm for pseudo-$Mg_{56.5}Cu_{27}Ag_5Dy_{11.5}$ alloy. The solidification procedures of Mg-based amorphous alloys were simulated based on the thermodynamics and obtained the critical cooling rates for the formation of Mg-based amorphous alloy [131]. Zhao et al. [132] synthesized Mg–Zn–Ca powders of $Mg_{63+x}Zn_{32-x}Ca_5$ ($x = 0$, 3, 7 and 10 by at%) with the diameter from 2 to 180 μm by gas atomization. It was reported that (i) fully glass powders with the particle diameter < 150 μm can be atomized for alloys with $x \leq 7$ and these Mg–Zn–Ca metallic glass powders exhibit remarkably superior corrosion resistance and degradation capacity in Direct Blue 6 solution to their crystalline counterparts and Fe powders and (ii) nano-whiskers were formed uniformly and loosely on the reacted surface of the $Mg_{70}Zn_{25}Ca_5$ glassy powder, which is considered as the mechanism of high degrading capacity for these Mg–Zn–Ca glassy alloys.

The glass transition (or glass–liquid transition) phenomenon is one of the most important properties of amorphous and semicrystalline materials, including inorganic glasses, amorphous metals, polymers, pharmaceuticals and others and is the gradual and reversible transition in amorphous materials (or in amorphous regions within semicrystalline materials) from a hard and relatively brittle "glassy" state into a viscous or rubbery state as the temperature is increased. An amorphous solid that exhibits a glass transition is called a glass. The reverse transition, achieved by supercooling a viscous liquid into the glass state, is called vitrification. The glass-transition temperature T_g of a material characterizes the range of temperatures over which this glass transition occurs. It is always lower than the melting temperature, T_m, of the crystalline state of the material. It also describes the temperature region where the mechanical properties of the materials change from hard and brittle to more soft, deformable or rubbery. Sun et al. [133] studied the effect of the Cd addition on the GFA, and mechanical properties was studied in $(Mg_{61}Cu_{28}Gd_{11})_{100-x}Cd_x$ ($x = 0$, 0.5, 1.0, 2.0, 3.0 and 5.0 at%) alloys. It was reported that with increase of Cd addition, glass transition temperature T_g and onset temperature of crystallization T_x both increase gradually from 146 °C and 207 °C for $Mg_{61}Cu_{28}Gd_{11}$ to 153 °C and 223 °C for $(Mg_{61}Cu_{28}Gd_{11})_{97}Cd_2$, but then decrease, resulting in the maximum supercooled liquid region ΔT_x obtained by glassy alloy with 2.0 at% Cd. The slightly increase of y-value and the reduced glass-transformation temperature T_{rg} with the increase of Cd content consistent with the experimental results of GFA. By increasing the Cd content to 2.0 at%, the compressive strength and plastic strain of Mg-Cu-Gd-Cd glassy alloy reaches about 904 MPa and 0.45%, respectively. The fracture morphology is changed from netlike striation to homogeneous dimples and local vein pattern, indicating that the minor addition of Cd clearly improves the plasticity of Mg-based glassy alloys, suggesting that the Cd addition could enhance the strength and plasticity of Mg-based glassy alloys by increasing the structural stability during deformation. Li et al. [134] synthesized Mg-Zn-Ca-Ag metallic glasses by copper mold casting and melt spinning and investigated the effects of Ag addition on the glass formation, thermal stability, microhardness, hydrogen evolution, corrosion resistance and cytocompatibility of the Mg-based glassy alloys. It was mentioned that (i) the corrosion resistance and the capability of suppressing the hydrogen evolution are enhanced for the Ag-containing alloys, in comparison to the Mg–Zn–Ca metallic glasses, though the incorporation of Ag decreases the GFA but influences insignificantly on microhardness and (ii) the higher cellular viability of the Ag-containing alloys than that of the Ag-free alloy was also revealed by direct cell-culture experiments; indicating that Mg-Zn-Ca-Ag metallic glasses possess the potential to be employed as biodegradable materials.

4.4.2 Macro- and microstructure

Wang et al. [135] investigated the effects of Mn substitution for Mg on the microstructure, mechanical properties and corrosion behavior of $Mg_{69-x}Zn_{27}Ca_4Mn_x$ ($x = 0$, 0.5 and 1 at%) alloys using XRD, compressive tests, electrochemical treatments and immersion tests, respectively. It was shown that microstructural observations showed that the $Mg_{69}Zn_{27}Ca_4$ alloy was mainly amorphous. Wang et al. [136] conducted similar tests on the microalloying effects of Y on the microstructure, mechanical properties and biocorrosion behavior of $Mg_{69-x}Zn_{27}Ca_4Y_x$ ($x = 0$, 1 and 2 at %) alloys and found that the $Mg_{69}Zn_{27}Ca_4$ alloy was found to be absolutely amorphous. Baulin et al. [125] developed a new ribbon-metallic glass with two different compositions, $Mg_{(85-x)}Ca_{(8+x)}Au_7$ (with $x = 0$, 2 and 4) and $Mg_{(81-x)}Ca_{10}Au_7Yb_{(2+x)}$ (with $x = 0$ and 8). It was reported that (i) the supercooled liquid region was evaluated to be $\Delta T = T_x - T_g = 22$ °C, where T_x is the temperature of crystallization and T_g is the glass transition temperature and (ii) no crystallization was detected after 30 min at 120 °C, which is of major interest for sterilization processes in the medical field.

Li et al. [137] fabricated Mg–Zn–Ca alloys by copper mold-casting method. The microstructure, amorphous nature and mechanical properties of as-cast samples were investigated by SEM, XRD and compressive tests. It was mentioned that (i) amorphous alloys or amorphous matrix composites can be formed in the composition of 1–6 at% Ca for the samples with 2, 3 or 4 mm in diameters and (ii) the best composition range defined both by strength and plastic deformation should be 3–5 at % Ca for $Mg_{72-x}Zn_{28}Ca_x$ ($x = 0–6$) alloys. Zhang et al. [138] prepared metallic glasses in the composition range of $Ca_4Mg_{72-x}Zn_{24+x}$ ($x = 0–12$, $\Delta x = 2$) using the melt-spinning technique. It was reported that the crystallization was initiated at lower temperatures by the precipitation of $Mg_{51}Zn_{20}$ crystals. Mg-hcp and $Ca_{16.7}Mg_{38.2}Zn_{45.1}$ (IM1) ternary compound precipitated from the retained amorphous phase during the second crystallization event. Then, the ternary compound $Ca_{1.5}Mg_{55.3}Zn_{43.2}$ (IM4) was formed at higher temperatures and the crystallization event terminated via IM4 transforming to $Ca_2Mg_5Zn_{13}$ (IM3) before melting. All crystallization reactions were found to be in qualitative agreement with the equilibrium phase diagram. Wu et al. [139] fabricated a novel multilayer structure of metallic glass film deposited Mg alloy by combining surface mechanical attrition treatment and magnetron sputtering. It was mentioned that (i) the multilayer structure consists of amorphous layer and gradient structure sequentially from surface, following with the coarse grains inside; (ii) gradient structure significantly decreases hardness mismatch between the amorphous layer and the matrix of Mg alloy; and (iii) wear resistance is increased by two orders for this novel multilayer structure with the simultaneous improvement of corrosion resistance. Tsarkov et al. [140] fabricated a Mg–Cu–Yb system-based metallic glassy alloys using induction melting and further injection on a spinning copper wheel and investigated the effect of alloying by Ag and Ca on the GFA and the kinetics of crystallization of Mg–Cu–Yb system-based alloys. It was reported that (i) an increase of the Ca and Ag content has a positive effect on the GFA, the effective activation energy of crystallization, and the enthalpy of mixing, (ii) the highest indicators of the GFA and the thermal stability were found for alloys that contain both alloying elements, (iii) the Ag addition suppresses precipitation of the Mg_2Cu phase during crystallization, (iv) a dual-phase glassy-nanocrystalline Mg structure was obtained in $Mg_{65}Cu_{25}Yb_{10}$ and $Mg_{59.5}Cu_{22.9}Yb_{11}Ag_{6.6}$ alloys after annealing, (v) bulk samples with a composite glassy-crystalline structure were obtained in $Mg_{59.5}Cu_{22.9}Yb_{11}Ag_{6.6}$ and $Mg_{64}Cu_{21}Yb_{9.5}Ag_{5.5}$ alloys and (vi) a thermodynamic database for the Mg-Cu-Yb-Ca-Ag system was created to compare the process of crystallization of alloys with polythermal sections of the Mg-Cu-Yb-Ca-Ag phase diagram. Cheng et al. [141] studied the glass formation and microstructure evolution of $Mg_{61}Cu_{28}Gd_{11}$ and alloys laying on the line linking this composition to pure magnesium, that is, alloys with fixed Cu:Gd ratio but increasing Mg content. It was mentioned that the alloys located in the

Mg_2Cu-Mg_2CuGd-Mg_6CuGd ternary phase region have higher GFA than alloys with increased magnesium content.

Babilas research group conducted extensive works on structural characterization on $Mg_{60}Cu_{30}Y_{10}$ [142], $Mg_{65}Cu_{20}Y_{10}Ni_5$ [143] and $Mg_{65}Cu_{20}Y_{10}Zn_5$ [144]. It was reported that (i) glassy alloys were annealed to become nanocomposite containing 200 nm crystallites in an amorphous matrix; (ii) the microstructure of bulk glassy alloy and nanocomposite obtained during heat treatment; (iii) the composite material contained very small particles in the amorphous matrix [142]; (iv) the amorphous structure was described by peak values of partial pair correlation functions and coordination numbers, which illustrated some types of cluster packing; (v) the interplanar spacing identified for the orthorhombic Mg_2Cu crystalline phase is similar to the value of the first coordination shell radius from the short-range order [143]; (vi) the structure of the melt-spun glass is homogeneous, but some medium-range order regions as small as 1–2 nm were observed; (vii) an average coordination number for Mg–Mg and Mg–Cu atoms is 8.1 and 2.5, adequately; (viii) the formation of nanocrystalline structure after annealing was observed containing very small particles in the amorphous matrix with size of 4–10 nm; and (ix) hexagonal Mg and orthorhombic Mg_2Cu phases were identified [144].

4.4.3 Mechanical behaviors

Due to the nature of glassy state, there are several characteristics associated with the BMGs: (1) BMGs inherently lack dislocations and hence slip planes lead to exceptionally high strength and elasticity, approaching the theoretical limit; (2) BMGs can display toughness comparable to crystalline metals while oxide glasses and ceramics exhibit low toughness and brittle failure; (3) because of lack of the grain boundaries, BMGs are homogeneous and exhibit isotropic behavior, even at submicrometer length scales; and (4) without grain boundaries or precipitates as oxidation sites, corrosion rates are significantly reduced compared to conventional metals. Although many BMGs exhibit high strength and show substantial fracture toughness, as Hofmann et al. [145] and Rao et al. [146] pointed out, they lack ductility and fail in an apparently brittle manner in unconstrained loading geometries. For instance, some BMGs exhibit significant plastic deformation in compression or bending tests, but all exhibit negligible plasticity (<0.5% strain) in uniaxial tension. In order to overcome brittle failure in tension, BMG–matrix composites have been introduced [147, 148]. Hays et al. [147] fabricated a ductile metal-reinforced BMG-matrix composite based on glass-forming compositions in the Zr-Ti-Cu-Ni-Be system with a ductile crystalline Ti–Zr–Nb β-phase, with bcc structure and mentioned that under unconstrained mechanical loading organized shear band patterns develop throughout the sample, leading to a dramatic increase in the plastic strain to failure, impact resistance and toughness of the metallic glass. Szuecs et al. [148] fabricated BMG composites with ductile phase by rapid quenching of a homogenous $Zr_{56.2}Ti_{13.8}Nb_{5.0}Cu_{6.9}Ni_{5.6}Be_{12.5}$ melt. It was reported that (i) the composite material demonstrates strongly improved Charpy impact toughness and ductility (average fracture strain up to 8.3% in compression and 5.5% in tension); indicating that these remarkable improvements are attributed to the effect of the mechanically soft and ductile second phase, which acts stabilizing against shear localization and critical crack propagation.

Li et al. [137] studied mechanical properties of bulk Mg–Zn–Ca amorphous alloys and amorphous matrix composites and reported that (i) the highest strength up to 828 MPa and plastic deformation of 1.28% were obtained for Mg–28Zn–$4Ca_4$ alloy with a monolithic amorphous structure; (ii) the best composition range defined both by strength and plastic deformation should be 3–5 at% Ca for $Mg_{72-x}Zn_{28}Ca_x$ ($x = 0$–6) alloys; (iii) at least over 400 MPa of fracture strength was obtained for the samples with an amorphous matrix, indicating that Mg–Zn–Ca alloys can be good candidates for amorphous matrix composites fabrication; and (iv) in order to further consider the amorphous matrix effect on mechanical properties, $Mg_{95-x}Zn_xCa_5$ ($x = 15$–33) alloys were investigated and Mg–15Zn–5Ca alloy with no obviously amorphous structure exhibits a lower yielding strength of 307 MPa, but it shows excellent plastic strain over 3.5%. Wang et al. [135] investigated mechanical properties of Mn-doped Mg–Zn–Ca BMG composites and reported that the addition of Mn decreases the GFA, which results in a decreased strength from 545 to 364 MPa; however, this strength is still suitable for implant application. Wang et al. [149] synthesized Mg–27Zn–4Ca with a spot of Fe particle-reinforced alloys by Cu mold-injection casting and reported that with Fe particle addition, ductile α-Mg and Mg–Zn dendrites were embedded in the amorphous matrix, which enhanced the compressive strength and fracture strain. Wang et al. [136] also studied mechanical properties of Mg–Zn–Ca BMG and reported that the Mg-27Zn-4Ca-1Y alloy exhibited an ultrahigh compressive strength above 1,010 MPa as well as high capacity for plastic strain above 3.1%. Laws et al. [150] investigated magnesium-precious metal-based BMGs from the ternary Mg–Ag–Ca, Mg–Ag–Yb, Mg–Pd–Ca and Mg–Pd–Yb alloy systems with Mg content greater than 67 at%. It was reported that (i) BMGs from the Mg–Pd–Ca alloy system exhibit high GFA with critical casting sizes of up to 3 mm in dimeter, the highest glass-transition temperatures (>200 °C) of any reported Mg-based BMG to date, and sustained compressive ductility and (ii) alloys from the Mg–Pd–Yb family exhibit critical casting sizes of up to 4 mm in diameter, and the highest compressive plastic (1.59%) and total (3.78%) strain to failure of any so far reported Mg-based glass. Erkartal et al. [151] investigated mechanical properties of Mg–20Zn–5Ca and Mg–35Zn–5Ca BMGs and reported that (i) an increase of Zn (≥30%) content in the alloy yields embrittlement in the alloys, (ii) under uniaxial compressions, both compositions undergo structural failure between 6 and 8 GPa and (iii) under hydrostatic pressure, a diminishing in fcc/hcp ordering and an enlargement of the ideal icosahedral ordering may indicate a more disordered structure.

Song et al. [152] studied the effects of amorphous thickness and crystal orientation on the plastic deformation mechanism of dual-phase crystalline/amorphous Mg/Mg–Al nanolaminates under tensile loading by using molecular dynamics simulation method. It was mentioned that (i) the uniform plastic deformation is achieved by combining complete basal–prismatic transformation in crystal phase and uniformly distributed shear transformation zones in amorphous phase and (ii) for the large amorphous thickness model, there is an obvious secondary hardening stage in the plastic deformation process, and the large amorphous phase is conducive to the formation of basal–prismatic interface.

4.4.4 Corrosion behaviors

It is well stated that the original requirement of biocompatible materials was bioinertness and Ti-based as well as CoCr-based alloys are in this category [153]. Less-inert metals including Mg-based materials were, therefore, not deemed suitable, although the ions released on dissolution are generally not harmful to the human body. However, current design requirements for biomaterials induce an appropriate host response and this can include the need to biodegrade and resorb [154]. There are potential advantages for BMGs that span applications of first-generation bioinert biometals through to third-generation materials that seek a controlled degradation profile and interaction with the host [155, 156].

Mg-based biomaterials are considered as attractive biodegradable materials, but their corrosion is accompanied by hydrogen evolution, which is sometimes uncontrollable and problematic in many biomedical applications. Zberg et al. [156] reported, on a distinct reduction in hydrogen evolution in Zn-rich MgZnCa glasses, that (i) above a particular Zn-alloying threshold (≈28 at.%), a Zn- and oxygen-rich passivating layer forms on the alloy surface, which we explain by a model based on the calculated Pourbaix diagram of Zn in SBF, and (ii) animal studies confirmed the great reduction in hydrogen evolution and revealed good tissue compatibility as seen for crystalline Mg implants; indicating that the glassy $Mg_{60+x}Zn_{35-x}Ca_5$ ($0 \leq x \leq 7$) alloys show great potential for deployment in a new generation of biodegradable implants. Wang et al. [136] tested biocorrosion properties of Mg–Zn–Ca BMG and reported that (i) the Y-doped Mg–Zn–Ca alloys had good biocorrosion resistance in SBF at 37 °C and (ii) the results of the cytotoxicity test showed high cell viabilities for these alloys, which means good biocompatibility. Wang et al. [149] conducted similar studies on Mg–27Zn–4Ca with a spot of Fe particle-reinforced alloys and reported that the $Mg_{69}Zn_{27}Ca_4$ glassy alloy and Mg–27Zn–4Ca/Fe alloy remarkably improved the corrosion resistance in 3.5 wt% NaCl solution compared with AZ31 and pure Mg. Zhao et al. [132] tested on Mg–Zn–Ca powders of $Mg_{63+x}Zn_{32-x}Ca_5$ and reported that these Mg–Zn–Ca metallic glass powders exhibit remarkably superior corrosion resistance and degradation capacity in Direct Blue 6 solution to their crystalline counterparts and Fe powders. Wang et al. [135] tested the effects of Mn substitution for Mg on the corrosion behavior of $Mg_{69-x}Zn_{27}Ca_4Mn_x$ ($x = 0$, 0.5 and 1 at%) alloys and reported that polarization and immersion tests in the SBF at 37 °C revealed that (i) the Mn-doped Mg–Zn–Ca alloys have significantly higher corrosion resistance than traditional ZK60 and pure Mg alloys, (ii) cytotoxicity test showed that cell viabilities of osteoblasts cultured with Mn-doped Mg–Zn–Ca alloys' extracts were higher than that of pure Mg, (iii) Mg-27Zn-4Ca-0.5Mn exhibits the highest biocorrosion resistance, biocompatibility and has desirable mechanical properties. Wang et al. [149] tested corrosion behavior of Mg–27Zn–4Ca with a spot of Fe particle-reinforced alloys and reported that the Mg–27Zn–4Ca glassy alloy and Mg–27Zn–4Ca/Fe alloy remarkably improved the corrosion resistance in 3.5 wt% NaCl solution compared with AZ31 and pure Mg. Li et al. [134] tested the effect of Ag on Mg-Zn-Ca-Ag BMGs in terms of its corrosion behavior and reported that the corrosion resistance and the capability of suppressing the hydrogen evolution are enhanced for the Ag-containing alloys, in comparison to the Mg–Zn–Ca, though the incorporation of Ag decreases the GFA but influences insignificantly on microhardness and (ii) the higher cellular viability of the Ag-containing alloys than that of the Ag-free alloy was also revealed by direct cell-culture experiments; suggesting that Mg-Zn-Ca-Ag BMGs possess the potential to be employed as biodegradable materials.

4.5 Mg-based intermetallic compounds

4.5.1 In general

An intermetallic (which are also called an intermetallic compound, intermetallic alloy, ordered intermetallic alloy or a long-range ordered alloy) is a type of metallic alloy that forms a solid-state compound exhibiting defined stoichiometry and ordered crystal structure. Generally, there are three typical types of intermetallic compounds found in the phase diagrams. They are type I: stoichiometric ordered intermetallics, like CuAu or Cu_3Au, possess compositional width on its both sides and ordered lattice arrangement will distort at a certain temperature (below the melting point), characterized by metallic bonding nature and sometimes called as Kurnakov type [157]. Type II: stoichiometric-ordered intermetallics, like Ni_2Al_3 or Ni_3Al, possess compositional width on both sides but the ordered lattice arrangements are stable until the decomposition at a certain temperature, characterized by ionic or covalent bonding nature and sometimes called as Berthollide type [158]. Type III: stoichiometric-ordered intermetallics, like Pt_2Si or PtSi, are not accompanied with compositional width on both sides, characterized by ionic or covalent bonding nature and sometimes called as Daltonide type [159]. There are several methods to fabricate intermetallics, including (1) melting using variety of heat sources such as electroresistance heating, high-induction heating, electrobeam heating, plasma arc heating; (2) solid-state diffusion technique; (3) chemical or physical vapor deposition method; (4) mechanical alloying technique; or (5) friction stir processing. Hort et al. [160] mentioned that (i) intermetallic phases can be found in almost every magnesium alloy and (ii) these intermetallic compounds play a very important role in optimizing the microstructure and mechanical properties and on their stabilities such as dissolvable intermetallics at low temperatures and thermally stable intermetallics at elevated temperatures.

4.5.2 Characterizations

The intermetallics of two AJ62 Mg alloys with low- and high-Sr content were characterized [161]. It was mentioned that (i) the high-Sr version contained a ternary intermetallic, in addition to Al4Sr eutectic present in all AJ62 Mg alloys, (ii) the chemical composition of the ternary phase corresponded to a stoichiometry of Mg_9Al_3Sr, (iii) in order to study the stability of the intermetallics, the heat treatment was done and an increased Al/Sr ratio of Al_4Sr, while its Mg content in solid solution decreased was observed and (iv) after an initial change of the Al/Sr ratio, the ternary intermetallic decomposed during heat treatment into α-Mg and Al_4Sr. Huang et al. [162] investigated phase compositions, lattice structures and phase equilibria of Mg–Zn–La system in Mg-rich corner at 345 °C by equilibrated alloy method and diffusion couple technique. It was reported that (i) a binary solid solution of Mg12La is confirmed as $(Mg,Zn)_{12}La$ with 0–4.96 at% Zn; (ii) it has a body-centered tetragonal lattice structure with giant unit cell of $a = b \approx 1.032$ nm and $c \approx 7.748$ nm; (iii) another linear ternary intermetallic $(Mg,Zn)_{11}La$ (Zn ≈ 8.66–43.39 at%) has been identified and also $(Mg,Zn)_{11}La$ has a C-centered orthorhombic structure, and the unit cell of which becomes smaller with the increase of Zn content; (iv) the smallest lattice parameters of it are a ≈ 1.1191 nm, b ≈ 0.9701 nm and $c \approx 0.9498$ nm; (v) both $(Mg,Zn)_{12}La$ and $(Mg,Zn)_{11}La$ are in equilibrium with Mg solid solution in their composition range; (vi) in addition, MgZn phase containing about 1.53 at% La is confirmed, which is in equilibrium with Mg solid solution and $(Mg,Zn)_{11}La$ at 345 °C; and (vii) it was indicated that it is impossible for $Mg_{17}Zn_{21}La_2$ reported in literature to be in equilibrium with Mg solid solution as a stable phase at this temperature. Gil-Santos et al. [163] studied the ternary Mg–Si–Sr system which has twelve compositions located in the Mg rich corner of the ternary system. It was shown that (i) apart from the Mg matrix, various intermetallic phases are observed, (ii) the binary compounds, Mg_2Si and $Mg_{17}Sr_2$, are identified, as well as, two ternary phases, MgSiSr and $MgSi_2Sr$, (iii) the Mg-rich side of the Mg–Si–Sr phase diagram is constructed based on descriptions of the binary phase diagrams Mg–Si, Mg–Ca and Ca–Si from literature and assuming complete solubility (i.e., a line compound) between the ternary phase MgSiSr and the binary phase Sr_2Si and (iv) it is also assumed that $MgSi_2Sr$ is a stoichiometric compound and these assumptions were made based on the chemical similarities between Ca and Sr and between Si and Sn, and the similarity in crystal structures between the two studied ternary compounds of the Mg–Si–Sr diagram and the ternary compounds present in the Ca–Mg–Si and Mg–Sn–Sr system. Verissimo et al. [164] investigated on the Mg–12 wt% Zn alloy which was directionally solidified (DS) under an extensive range of cooling rates. It was mentioned that (i) the volume fraction of rod-like eutectic is shown to increase with the decrease in cooling rate during solidification; (ii) the DS Mg–12 wt% Zn samples was characterized and found that two different nonequilibrium IMCs (intermetallic compounds), $MgZn_2$ and Mg_4Zn_7 were identified, which are distributed as nanoparticles throughout the a-Mg matrix; (iii) the Mg–Zn eutectic morphologies (lamellar and rod-like) are found to be constituted by a-Mg/$Mg_{21}Zn_{25}$ phases, the latter being formed by the decomposition of the eutectic IMC $Mg_{51}Zn_{20}$ through a eutectoid reaction. Hagihara et al. [165] investigated Mg- or Ca-based intermetallic compounds of Mg_2Ca, Mg_2Si, Ca_2Si and CaMgSi as possible new candidates for biodegradable implant materials, attempting to improve the degradation behavior compared to Mg and Ca alloys. It was reported that the reactivity of Ca can be indeed reduced by the formation of compounds with Mg and Si, but its reactivity is still high for applications as an implant material. In contrast, Mg_2Si shows higher corrosion resistance than conventional Mg alloys while retaining biodegradability. In cytotoxicity tests, under the severe condition conducted in this study, both pure Mg and Mg_2Si showed relatively high cytotoxicity on preosteoblast MC3T3-E1; however, the cell viability cultured in the Mg_2Si extract medium was confirmed to be better than that in a pure Mg extract medium in all the conditions investigated with the exception of the 10% extract medium, because of the lower corrosion rate of Mg_2Si. The cytotoxicity derived from the Si ion was not significantly detected in the Mg_2Si extract medium in the concentration level of ~70 mg/L measured in the present study.

4.5.3 Mechanical properties

Li et al. [166] studied the effect of the RE element Er on the microstructures and properties of Mg–Al intermetallic. It was found that (i) metallographic and XRD results showed that the microstructures of Mg–Al–Er alloys varied with Er content, (ii) the Mg–44Al–0.5Er and Mg–43.8Al–1.0Er alloys were both composed of $Mg_{17}Al_{12}$ matrix and Al_3Er phase, whereas Mg–43Al–3.0Er and Mg–42Al–5.0Er were composed of $Mg_{17}Al_{12}$ matrix, Al_3Er phase, and Mg–$Mg_{17}Al_{12}$ eutectic, (iii) the Mg–42Al–5.0Er alloy showed the highest microhardness, and the values remained nearly stable as Er content increased from 1.0 wt% to 5.0 wt% and (iv) the dispersed second-phase Al_3Er caused the grain refinement of the Mg–Al–Er alloy, which was the main reason for the improvement in microhardness. Nelson et al. [167] fabricated Mg and Mg-alloy MMCs reinforced with the MAX phases,

Ti_3SiC_2 and Cr_2AlC. Pure Mg and Al-containing Mg-alloys with varying Al content (AZ31, AZ61 and AZ91) were pressureless melt-infiltrated into 55 ± 1 vol% porous MAX preforms. It was reported that (i) similar to Ti_2AlC/Mg composites increasing the Al content in the matrix enhanced the mechanical properties of the Mg/Ti_3SiC_2 composites but had little effect on the properties of the Mg/Cr_2AlC composite system; the latter were inferior to those reinforced with the other MAX phases. The Ti_3SiC_2/AZ91 composite achieved the highest Vickers hardness (1.9 ± 0.1 GPa), yield strength (346 ± 4 MPa) and ultimate compressive strength (617 ± 10 MPa) obtained in this study, (ii) all composites exhibited fully and spontaneously reversible hysteresis loops, evidence of energy dissipation, during compression cycling and (iii) having an elastic modulus of ≈160 GPa, the Ti_3SiC_2/AZ91 composite may be suited for high specific strength and high damping applications. Zhao et al. [168] fabricated the bimetal composite rods composed of a softer AZ31 sleeve and a harder WE43 core via a special process by combining hot-pressing diffusion with coextrusion. It was shown that (i) a well-bonded interface with a diffusion layer of ~20 μm in thickness was achieved, (ii) the texture in the interfacial region adjacent to the WE43 core changed with the basal poles largely perpendicular to the extrusion direction and (iii) compared with the monolithic Mg billet, the coextruded AZ31/WE43 bimetal composite rods could achieve a gradient of both composition and microstructure; such gradients along with the superior interfacial bonding led to a higher compressive and tensile yield strength of AZ31/WE43 bimetal composite rods compared with the AZ31 sleeve: indicating that combining hot-pressing diffusion with coextrusion is an effective method to fabricate the bimetal composites with superior mechanical properties.

4.5.4 Corrosion behaviors

Zhang et al. [169] produced $Mg_{17}Al_{12}$ (β-phase) and Mg_2Al_3 (γ-phase) intermetallic layers by cold spraying of pure Al powder on a pure Mg substrate together with subsequent postspray annealing treatment. It was mentioned that these layers showed significantly better nanomechanical properties, including the reduced elastic modulus and nanohardness, which were determined using nanoindentation, than commercial-purity Mg and AZ91 alloys; (ii) combined with their improved corrosion resistance, it is believed that both the γ-phase and the β-phase layers can provide effective protection of Mg alloys from wear and corrosion; and (iii) the effect of postspray annealing process on the formation of thick, uniform and dense intermetallic layers on pure Mg substrate was also investigated. Yang et al. [170] fabricated continuous intermetallic compounds coatings on AZ91D Mg alloy by diffusion reaction of Mg–Al couples at relatively low temperature of 300 °C to improve its wear and corrosion resistance. It was shown that (i) SEM/EDXS and XRD analysis showed the coatings consisted of β-phase ($Mg_{17}Al_{12}$) layer and γ-phase (Mg_2Al_3) layer, (ii) the thickness range of the coatings was 16–110 μm, depending on the treatment time, (iii) the hardness and the corrosion resistance of the AZ91D Mg alloy were greatly improved due to the formation of the continuous intermetallic compounds layers and (iv) the continuous intermetallic compounds layers exhibited passive behavior and no appreciable hydrogen evolved during immersion in 3.5% NaCl solution for 72 h. Li [168] examined the effect of Er element to Mg–Al intermetallic on the corrosion behavior and reported that the Er-containing alloys had the ability to suppress hydrogen evolution, which was the main reason for the higher corrosion resistance of the modified alloys than that of the Mg–44.3Al alloy. Han et al. [171] fabricated a novel Mg–RE (Nd,Ce) coating containing intermetallic compound on the surface of the AZ91D magnesium alloy by bathing the sample in a NaCl-KCl-LiCl-$NdCl_3$-$CeCl_3$ molten salt. It was reported that (i) the SEM observation indicated that a continuous and compact diffusion coating was obtained on the surface of AZ91D magnesium alloy and the XRD and TEM investigations revealed that the new phases were Al_2Ce and Al_2Nd intermetallic and (ii) the potentiodynamic polarization curves showed that the Mg-RE coating improved the corrosion resistance of the AZ91D magnesium alloy, and the corrosion current density of the coated sample was about 1,510 mA/cm^2 lower than the uncoated sample.

References

[1] Oshida Y, Guven Y, Aktoren O. Hydroxyapatite-based biocomposites. In: Oshida Y ed., Hydroxyapatite – Synthesis and Applications. Momentum Press, New York NY 2015, 213–262.

[2] Hull D. An Introduction to Composite Materials. Cambridge University Press, UK, 1982.

[3] Kuśnierczyk K, Basista M. Recent advances in research on magnesium alloys and magnesium-calcium phosphate composites as biodegradable implant materials. Journal of Biomaterials Applications. 2017, 31, 878–900.

[4] Bommala VK, Krishna MG, Rao CT. Magnesium matrix composites for biomedical applications: A review. Journal of Magnesium and Alloys. 2019, 7, 72–9.

[5] Sezer N, Evis Z, Kayhan SM, Tahmasebifar A, Koç M. Review of magnesium-based biomaterials and their applications. Journal of Magnesium and Alloys. 2018, 6, 23–43.

[6] Feng B, Xin Y, Yu H, Hong R, Liu Q. Mechanical behavior of a Mg/Al composite rod containing a soft Mg sleeve and an ultra hard Al core. Materials Science and Engineering: A. 2016, 675, 204–11.

[7] Wu Y, Feng B, Xin Y, Hong R, Liu Q. Microstructure and mechanical behavior of a Mg AZ31/Al 7050 laminate composite fabricated by extrusion. Materials Science and Engineering: A. 2015, 640, 454–9.

[8] Hai C, Mingyi Z. Effect of intermetallic compounds on the fracture behavior of Mg/Al laminated composite fabricated by accumulative roll bonding. Rare Metal Materials and Engineering. 2016, 45, 2242–5.

[9] Ham B, Zhang X. High strength Mg/Nb nanolayer composites. Materials Science and Engineering: A. 2011, 528, 2028–33.

[10] Sadeghi A, Inoue J, Kyokuta N, Koseki T. In situ deformation analysis of Mg in multilayer Mg-steel structures. Materials & Design. 2017, 119, 326–37.

[11] Nie H, Liang W, Chen H, Zheng L, Li X. Effect of annealing on the microstructures and mechanical properties of Al/Mg/Al laminates. Materials Science and Engineering: A. 2018, 732, 6–13.
[12] Nie H, Liang W, Chen H, Wang F, Li X. A coupled EBSD/TEM study on the interfacial structure of Al/Mg/Al laminates. Journal of Alloys and Compounds. 2019, 781, 696–701.
[13] Habila W, Azzeddine H, Mehdi B, Tirsatine K, Bradai D. Investigation of microstructure and texture evolution of a Mg/Al laminated composite elaborated by accumulative roll bonding. Materials Characterization. 2019, 147, 242–52.
[14] Chen L, Tang J, Zhao G, Zhang C, Chu X. Fabrication of Al/Mg/Al laminate by a porthole die co-extrusion process. Journal of Materials Processing Technology. 2018, 258, 165–73.
[15] Liu CY, Wang Q, Jia YZ, Jing R, Liu RP. Microstructures and mechanical properties of Mg/Mg and Mg/Al/Mg laminated composites prepared via warm roll bonding. Materials Science and Engineering: A. 2012, 556, 1–8.
[16] Nie H, Hao X, Chen H, Kang X, Liang W. Effect of twins and dynamic recrystallization on the microstructures and mechanical properties of Ti/Al/Mg laminates. Materials & Design. 2019, 181, https://doi.org/10.1016/j.matdes.2019.107948.
[17] Wang Q, Shen Y, Jiang B, Tang A, Pan F. Enhanced stretch formability at room temperature for Mg-Al-Zn/Mg-Y laminated composite via porthole die extrusion. Materials Science and Engineering: A. 2018, 731, 184–94.
[18] Anne G, Ramesh MR, Nayaka HS, Arya SB, Sahu S. Development and characteristics of accumulative roll bonded Mg-Zn/Ce/Al hybrid composite. Journal of Alloys and Compounds. 2017, 724, 146–54.
[19] Braszczyńska-Malik KN, Przełożyńska E. The influence of Ti particles on microstructure and mechanical properties of Mg-5Al-5RE matrix alloy composite. Journal of Alloys and Compounds. 2017, 728, 600–6.
[20] Li DS, Zhang XP, Xiong ZP, Mai Y-W. Lightweight NiTi shape memory alloy based composites with high damping capacity and high strength. Journal of Alloys and Compounds. 2010, 490, L15–9.
[21] Guo W, Kato H. Development of a high-damping NiTi shape-memory-alloy-based composite. Materials Letters. 2015, 158, 1–4.
[22] Wakeel S, Manakari V, Parande G, Kujur MS, Gupta M. Synthesis and Mechanical Response of NiTi SMA Nanoparticle Reinforced Mg Composites Synthesized through Microwave Sintering Process. Materials Today: Proceedings. 2018, 5, 28203–10.
[23] Aydogmus T. Processing of interpenetrating Mg–TiNi composites by spark plasma sintering. Materials Science and Engineering: A. 2015, 624, 261–70.
[24] Vahid A, Hodgson P, Li Y. New porous Mg composites for bone implants. Journal of Alloys and Compounds. 2017, 724, 176–86.
[25] Tian B, Cheng ZG, Tong YX, Li L, Li QZ. Effect of enhanced interfacial reaction on the microstructure, phase transformation and mechanical property of Ni–Mn–Ga particles/Mg composites. Materials & Design. 2015, 82, 77–83.
[26] Jayalakshmi S, Sahu S, Sankaranarayanan S, Gupta S, Gupta M. Development of novel Mg–Ni60Nb40 amorphous particle reinforced composites with enhanced hardness and compressive response. Materials & Design. 2014, 53, 849–55.
[27] Zhao C, Wu H, Ni J, Zhang S, Zhang X. Development of PLA/Mg composite for orthopedic implant: Tunable degradation and enhanced mineralization. Composites Science and Technology. 2017, 147, 8–15.
[28] Li X, Qi C, Han L, Chu C, Chu PK. Influence of dynamic compressive loading on the in vitro degradation behavior of pure PLA and Mg/PLA composite. Acta Biomaterialia. 2017, 64, 269–78.

[29] Cai H, Zhang Y, Meng J, Li X, Bai J. Enhanced fully-biodegradable Mg/PLA composite rod: Effect of surface modification of Mg-2Zn wire on the interfacial bonding. Surface & Coatings Technology. 2018, 350, 722–31.

[30] Cai H, Zhang Y, Li X, Meng, Bai J. Self-reinforced biodegradable Mg-2Zn alloy wires/polylactic acid composite for orthopedic implants. Composites Science and Technology. 2018, 162, 198–205.

[31] Cai H, Meng J, Li X, Xue F, Bai J. In vitro degradation behavior of Mg wire/poly(lactic acid) composite rods prepared by hot pressing and hot drawing. Acta Biomaterialia. 2019, 98, 125–41.

[32] Li W, Mehboob A, Han M-G, Chang S-H. Effect of fluoride coating on degradation behaviour of unidirectional Mg/PLA biodegradable composite for load-bearing bone implant application. Composites. Part A, Applied Science and Manufacturing. 2019, 124, https://doi.org/10.1016/j.compositesa.2019.05.032.

[33] Li X, Yu W, Han L, Chu C, Xue F. Degradation behaviors of Mg alloy wires/PLA composite in the consistent and staged dynamic environments. Materials Science and Engineering: C. 2019, 103, https://doi.org/10.1016/j.msec.2019.109765.

[34] Cifuentes SC, Frutos E, González-Carrasco JL, Muñoz M, Multigner M, Chao J, Benavente R, Lieblich M. Materials Letters. 2012, 74, 239–42.

[35] Cifuentes SC, Lieblich M, López FA, Benavente R, González-Carrasco JL. Effect of Mg content on the thermal stability and mechanical behaviour of PLLA/Mg composites processed by hot extrusion. Materials Science and Engineering: C. 2017, 72, 18–25.

[36] Cifuentes SC, Lieblich M, Saldaña L, González-Carrasco JL. Benavente R. In vitro degradation of biodegradable polylactic acid/Mg composites: Influence of nature and crystalline degree of the polymeric matrix. Materialia. 2019, 6, https://doi.org/10.1016/j.mtla.2019.100270.

[37] Kum CH, Cho Y, Joung YK, Choi J, Park K, Seo SH, Park YS, Ahn DJ, Han DK. Biodegradable poly (L-lactide) composites by oligolactide-grafted magnesium hydroxide for mechanical reinforcement and reduced inflammation. Journal of Materials Chemistry B. 2013, 1, 2764–72.

[38] Yu X, Huang W, Zhao D, Yang K, Yuan Y. Study of engineered low-modulus Mg/PLLA composites as potential orthopaedic implants: An in vitro and in vivo study. Colloids and Surfaces. B, Biointerfaces. 2019, 174, 280–90.

[39] Wu YH, Li N, Cheng Y, Zheng YF, Han Y. *In vitro* study on biodegradable AZ31 magnesium alloy fibers reinforced PLGA composite. Journal of Material Science and Technology 2013, 29, 545–50.

[40] Brown A, Zaky S, Ray H, Sfeir C. Porous magnesium/PLGA composite scaffolds for enhanced bone regeneration following tooth extraction. Acta Biomater C. 2015, 11, 543–53.

[41] Pan Y, Wu G, Huang Z, Li M, Zhang Z. Effect of surface roughness on interlaminar peel and shear strength of CFRP/Mg laminates. International Journal of Adhesion and Adhesives. 2017, 79, 1–7.

[42] Pan Y, Wu X, Huang Z, Wu G, Zhang Z. A new approach to enhancing interlaminar strength and galvanic corrosion resistance of CFRP/Mg laminates. Composites. Part A, Applied Science and Manufacturing. 2018, 105, 78–86.

[43] Sun S, Pan Y, Wu G, Lin X. Effect of electrolyte composition ratio of micro-arc oxidation on interlaminar strength of CFRP/M laminates. International Journal of Adhesion and Adhesives. 2018, 87, 98–104.

[44] Oshida Y, Wang C-S, Ou K-L. Introduction to Hydroxyapatite. In: Oshida Y. ed., Hydroxyapatite – Synthesis and Applications. Momentum Press, New York NY 2015, 1–6.

[45] Gu X, Zhou W, Zheng Y, Dong L, Xi Y, Chai D. Microstructure, mechanical property, bio-corrosion and cytotoxicity evaluations of Mg/HA composites. Materials Science & Engineering C. 2010, 30, 827–32.

[46] Sunil BR, Sampath Kumar TS, Chakkingal U, Nandakumar V, Doble M. Friction stir processing of magnesium–nanohydroxyapatite composites with controlled *in vitro* degradation behavior. Materials Science & Engineering C. 2014, 39, 315–24.

[47] Cui Z, Li W, Cheng L, Gong D, Wang W. Effect of nano-HA content on the mechanical properties, degradation and biocompatible behavior of Mg-Zn/HA composite prepared by spark plasma sintering. Materials Characterization. 2019, 151, 620–31.

[48] Liu DB, Chen MF, Ye XY. Fabrication and corrosion behavior of HA/Mg-Zn biocomposites. Frontiers of Materials Science in China 2010, 4, 139–44.

[49] Witte F, Feyerabend F, Maier P, Fischer J, Störmer M, Blawert C, Dietzel W, Hort N. Biodegradable magnesium–hydroxyapatite metal matrix composites. Biomaterials. 2007, 28, 2163–74.

[50] Chen B, Yin KY, Lu TF, Sun BY, Dong Q, Zheng JX, Lu C, Li ZC. AZ91 magnesium alloy/porous hydroxyapatite composite for potential application in bone repair. Journal of Material Science and Technology 2016, 32, 858–64.

[51] Razavi M, Fathi MH, Meratian M. Fabrication and characterization of magnesium–fluorapatite nanocomposite for biomedical applications. Materials Characterization. 2010, 61, 1363–70.

[52] Razavi M, Fathi MH, Meratian M. Bio-corrosion behavior of magnesium-fluorapatite nanocomposite for biomedical applications. Materials Letters. 2010, 64, 2487–90.

[53] Ye X, Chen M, Yang M, Wei J, Liu D. In vitro corrosion resistance and cytocompatibility of nano-hydroxyapatite reinforced Mg–Zn–Zr composites. Journal of Material Science and Material Medicines 2010, 21, 1321–8.

[54] Liu D, Liu Y, Zhao Y, Huang Y, Chen M. The hot deformation behavior and microstructure evolution of HA/Mg-3Zn-0.8Zr composites for biomedical application. Materials Science and Engineering: C. 2017, 77, 690–7.

[55] Wang X, Li JT, Xie MY, Qu LJ, Li XL. Structure, mechanical property and corrosion behaviors of (HA+β-TCP)/Mg–5Sn composite with interpenetrating networks. Materials Science and Engineering: C. 2015, 56, 386–92.

[56] Gu XN, Wang X, Li N, Li L, Zheng YF, Miao X. Microstructure and characteristics of the metal–ceramic composite (MgCa-HA/TCP) fabricated by liquid metal infiltration. Journal of Biomedicine Materials and Research – Part B Applied Biomaterials 2011, 99, 127–34.

[57] Lim PN, Lam RN, Zheng YF, Thian ES. Magnesium-calcium/hydroxyapatite (Mg-Ca/HA) composites with enhanced bone differentiation properties for orthopedic applications. Materials Letters. 2016, 172, 193–7.

[58] Liu D, Xu G, Jamali SS, Zhao Y, Jurak T. Fabrication of biodegradable HA/Mg-Zn-Ca composites and the impact of heterogeneous microstructure on mechanical properties, in vitro degradation and cytocompatibility. Bioelectrochemistry. 2019, 129, 106–15.

[59] Khalajabadi SZ, Ahmad N, Yahya A, Yajid MAM, Kadir MRA. The role of titania on the microstructure, biocorrosion and mechanical properties of Mg/HA-based nanocomposites for potential application in bone repair. Ceramics International. 2016, 42, 18223–37.

[60] Khalajabadi SZ, Ahmad N, Izman S, Abu ABH, Kadir MRA. In vitro biodegradation, electrochemical corrosion evaluations and mechanical properties of an Mg/HA/TiO2 nanocomposite for biomedical applications. Journal of Alloys and Compounds. 2017, 696, 768–81.

[61] Kuśnierczyk K, Basista M. Recent advances in research on magnesium alloys and magnesium-calcium phosphate composites as biodegradable implant materials. Journal of Biomaterials Applications 2016, 31, 1–23.

[62] Yu K, Chen L, Zhao J, Li S, Dai Y, Huang Q, Yu Z. In vitro corrosion behavior and in vivo biodegradation of biomedical β-$Ca_3(PO_4)_2$/Mg–Zn composites. Acta Biomaterialia. 2012, 8, 2845–55.

[63] Yu K, Chen L, Zhao J, Wang R, Dai Y, Huang Q. *In vivo* biocompatibility and biodegradation of a Mg-15%$Ca_3(PO_4)_2$ composite as an implant material. Materials Letters. 2013, 98, 22–5.
[64] He SY, Sun Y, Chen MF, Liu DB, Ye XY. Microstructure and properties of biodegradable *β*-TCP reinforced Mg-Zn-Zr composites. Transactions of Nonferrous Metals Soceity of China. 2011, 21, 814–9.
[65] Feng A, Han Y. Mechanical and in vitro degradation behavior of ultrafine calcium polyphosphate reinforced magnesium-alloy composites. Materials & Design. 2011, 32, 2813–20.
[66] Zheng HR, Li Z, You C, Liu DB, Chen MF. Effects of MgO modified b-TCP nanoparticles on the microstructure and properties of b-TCP/Mg-Zn-Zr composites. Bioactive Materials. 2017, 2, 1–9.
[67] Wang X, Zhang P, Dong LH, Ma XL, Li JT, Zheng YF. Microstructure and characteristics of interpenetrating β-TCP/Mg–Zn–Mn composite fabricated by suction casting. Materials & Design. 2014, 54, 995–1001.
[68] Yuan Q, Huang Y, Liu D, Chen M. Effects of solidification cooling rate on the corrosion resistance of a biodegradable β-TCP/Mg-Zn-Ca composite. Bioelectrochemistry. 2018, 124, 93–104.
[69] Wang X, Nie Q-D, Ma X-L, Fan J-L, Li X-L. Microstructure and properties of co-continuous (β-TCP+MgO)/Zn-Mg composite fabricated by suction exsorption for biomedical applications. Transactions of Nonferrous Metals Society of China. 2017, 27, 1996–2006.
[70] Yashima M, Sakai A, Kamiyama T, Hoshikawa A. Crystal structure analysis of beta-tricalcium phosphate $Ca_3(PO_4)_2$ by neutron powder diffraction. Journal of Solid State Chemistry. 2003, 175, 272–7.
[71] Frasnelli M, Sglavo VM. Alpha-Beta Phase Transformation in Tricalcium Phosphate (TCP) Ceramics: Effect of Mg^{2+} Doping. In: Narayan RJ ed., Ceramic Engineering and Science Proceedings, The American Ceramic Society. 2015.
[72] Carrodeguas RG, De Aza, S. α-Tricalcium phosphate: Synthesis, properties and biomedical applications. Acta Biomaterialia. 2011, 7, 3536–46.
[73] Grandi G, Heitz C, Dos Santos LA, Silva ML, Sant'Ana Filho M, Pagnocelli RM, Silva DS. Comparative histomorphometric analysis between α-Tcp cement and β-Tcp/Ha granules in the bone repair of rat calvaria. Advanced Materials Research. 2011, 4, https://doi.org/10.1590/S1516-14392011005000020.
[74] Merten HA, Wiltfang J, Hönig JF, Funke M, Luhr HG. Intra-individual comparison of alpha- and beta-TCP ceramics in an animal experiment. Mund-, Kiefer- Und Gesichtschirurgie : MKG. 2000, 2, S509–15.
[75] Ikeo N, Kawasaki H, Watanabe H, Mukai T. Fabrication and characterization of Mg–0.2 at% Ca/α-tricalcium phosphate composites. Materials Letters. 2019, 241, 96–9.
[76] Qi LH, Zhou JM, Su LZ, Quang HB, Li HJ. Fabrication of C_{sf}/Mg composites using extrusion directly following vacuum infiltration – part 2: forming process study. Solid State Phenomena. 2008, 141/143, 91–6.
[77] Tian W, Qi L, Zhou J. Quantitative characterization of the fiber orientation variation in the Csf/Mg composites. Computational Materials Science. 2015, 98, 56–63.
[78] Zhang S, Chen G, Pei R, Hussain M, Wu G. Effect of Gd content on interfacial microstructures and mechanical properties of Cf/Mg composite. Materials & Design. 2015, 65, 567–74.
[79] Zhang S, Chen G, Pei R, Wang Y, Li D, Wang P, Wu G. Effect of Y content on interfacial microstructures and mechanical properties of C_f/Mg composite. Materials Science and Engineering: A. 2015, 647, 105–12.
[80] Qi L, Liu J, Guan J, Zhou J, Li H. Tensile properties and damage behaviors of C_{sf}/Mg composite at elevated temperature and containing a small fraction of liquid. Composites Science and Technology. 2012, 72, 1774–80.

[81] Qi L, Wei X, Ju L, Ma Y, Deng W, Li H. Design and application of forming device for the thin-walled Cf/Mg composite component. Journal of Materials Processing Technology. 2016, 238, 459–65.
[82] Gupta M, Goh CS, Wei J, Lee LC. Development of novel carbon nanotube reinforced magnesium nanocomposites using the powder metallurgy technique. Nanotechnology. 2006, 17, 7–12.
[83] Liang J, Li H, Qi L, Tian W, Wei J. Fabrication and mechanical properties of CNTs/Mg composites prepared by combining friction stir processing and ultrasonic assisted extrusion. Journal of Alloys and Compounds. 2017, 728, 282–8.
[84] Kumar SP, Selvamani ST, Vigneshwar M, Hariharan SJ. Tensile, microhardness, and microstructural analysis on Mg-CNT nano composites. Materials Today: Proceedings. 2018, 5, 7882–8.
[85] Kumar SP, Selvamani ST, Vigneshwar M, Palanikumar K. Developing an empirical relationship to predict maximum strength on friction stir welded (Mg+ CNT) nanocomposites. Materials Today: Proceedings. 2019, 16, 1152–7.
[86] Roy S, Kannan G, Suwas S, Surappa MK. Effect of extrusion ratio on the microstructure, texture and mechanical properties of (Mg/AZ91)m–SiCp composite. Materials Science and Engineering: A. 2015, 624, 279–90.
[87] Eamaily M, Mortazavi N, Svensson JE, Halvarsson M, Jarfors AEW. A new semi-solid casting technique for fabricating SiC-reinforced Mg alloys matrix composites. Composites Part B: Engineering. 2016, 94, 176–89.
[88] Wang W, Wang H, Ren G, Cheng W, Zhang S. Effect of hot extrusion on the microstructure and mechanical properties of the SiCp/Mg-9Al-1Zn nanocomposite fabricated by different stir time. Rare Metal Materials and Engineering. 2017, 46, 2847–51.
[89] He X, Liu J, An L. The mechanical behavior of hierarchical Mg matrix nanocomposite with high volume fraction reinforcement. Materials Science and Engineering: A. 2017, 699, 114–7.
[90] Chang H, Wang C, Deng K, Nire K, Ting L. Effects of SiCp content on the microstructure and mechanical properties of SiCp/Mg-5Al-2Ca composites. Rare Metal Materials and Engineering. 2018, 47, 1377–84.
[91] Penther D, Ghasemi A, Riedel A, Fleck C, Kamrani S. Effect of SiC nanoparticles on manufacturing process, microstructure and hardness of Mg-SiC nanocomposites produced by mechanical milling and hot extrusion. Materials Science and Engineering: A. 2018, 738, 264–72.
[92] Kamrani S, Penther D, Ghasemi A, Riedel R, Fleck C. Microstructural characterization of Mg-SiC nanocomposite synthesized by high energy ball milling. Advanced Powder Technology. 2018, 29, 1742–8.
[93] Ghasemi A, Penther D, Kamrani S. Microstructure and nanoindentation analysis of Mg-SiC nanocomposite powders synthesized by mechanical milling. Materials Characterization. 2018, 142, 137–43.
[94] Shen M, Jia J, Ying T, He N. Fracture mechanism of nano- and submicron-SiCp/Mg composite during room temperature tensile test: Interaction between double sized particles and dislocations. Journal of Alloys and Compounds. 2019, 791, 452–60.
[95] Chen J, Bao C, Ma Y, Chen Z. Distribution control of AlN particles in Mg-Al/AlN composites. Journal of Alloys and Compounds. 2017, 695, 162–70.
[96] Yang C, Zhang B, Zhao D, Lü H, Liu F. Microstructure and mechanical properties of AlN particles in situ reinforced Mg matrix composites. Materials Science and Engineering: A. 2016, 674, 158–63.
[97] Yang C, Zhang B, Zhao D, Li X, Liu F. In-situ synthesis of AlN/Mg-Al composites with high strength and high plasticity. Journal of Alloys and Compounds. 2017, 699, 627–32.

[98] Gao T, Li Z, Hu K, Han M, Liu X. Synthesizing (ZrAl3 + AlN)/Mg–Al composites by a 'matrix exchange' method. Results in Physics. 2018, 9, 166–70.
[99] Vara Prasad Kaviti R, Jeyasimman D, Parande G, Gupta M, Narayanasamy R. Investigation on dry sliding wear behavior of Mg/BN nanocomposites. Journal of Magnesium and Alloys. 2018, 6, 263–76.
[100] Xiao P, Gao Y, Yang X, Xu F, Zheng Q. Processing, microstructure and ageing behavior of in-situ submicron TiB2 particles reinforced AZ91 Mg matrix composites. Journal of Alloys and Compounds. 2018, 764, 96–106.
[101] Xiao P, Gao Y, Xu F, Yang S, Zhao S. Hot deformation behavior of in-situ nanosized TiB2 particulate reinforced AZ91 Mg matrix composite. Journal of Alloys and Compounds. 2019, 798, 1–11.
[102] Xiao P, Gao Y, Yang C, Liu Z, Xu F. Microstructure, mechanical properties and strengthening mechanisms of Mg matrix composites reinforced with in situ nanosized TiB2 particles. Materials Science and Engineering: A. 2018, 710, 251–9.
[103] Huan Z, Zhou J, Duszczyk J. Magnesium-based composites with improved in vitro surface biocompatibility. Journal of Material Science and Material Medicines 2010, 21, 3163–9.
[104] Huan Z, Leeflang S, Zhou J, Zhai W, Chang J, Duszczyk J. *In vitro* degradation behavior and bioactivity of magnesium-Bioglass® composites for orthopedic applications. Journal of Biomedicine Materials and Research – Part B Applied Biomaterials B. 2012, 100, 437–46.
[105] Ashuri M, Moztarzadeh F, Nezafati N, Ansari Hamedani A, Tahriri M. Development of a composite based on hydroxyapatite and magnesium and zinc-containing sol–gel-derived bioactive glass for bone substitute applications. Materials Science and Engineering C. 2012, 32, 2330–9.
[106] Ong THD, Yu N, Meenashisundaram GK, Schaller B, Gupta M. Insight into cytotoxicity of Mg nanocomposites using MTT assay technique. Materials Science and Engineering: C. 2017, 78, 647–52.
[107] Bakhsheshi-Rad HR, Hamzah E, Staiger MP, Dias GJ, Kashefian M. Drug release, cytocompatibility, bioactivity, and antibacterial activity of doxycycline loaded Mg-Ca-TiO2 composite scaffold. Materials & Design. 2018, 139, 212–21.
[108] Lin G, Liu D, Chen M, You C, Li W. Preparation and characterization of biodegradable Mg-Zn-Ca/MgO nanocomposites for biomedical applications. Materials Characterization. 2018, 144, 120–30.
[109] Kamiyama N, Panomsuwan G, Yamamoto E, Sudare T, Ishizaki T. Effect of treatment time in the Mg(OH)2/Mg–Al LDH composite film formed on Mg alloy AZ31 by steam coating on the corrosion resistance. Surface & Coatings Technology. 2016, 286, 172–7.
[110] Liu J, Suryanarayana C, Ghosh D, Subhash G, An L. Synthesis of Mg–Al2O3 nanocomposites by mechanical alloying. Journal of Alloys and Compounds. 2013, 563, 165–70.
[111] Alaneme KK, Akintunde IB, Olubambi PA, Adewale TM. Fabrication characteristics and mechanical behaviour of rice husk ash – Alumina reinforced Al-Mg-Si alloy matrix hybrid composites. Journal of Materials Research and Technology. 2013, 2, 60–7.
[112] Dezfuli SN, Leeflang S, Huan Z, Chang J, Zhou J. Fabrication of novel magnesium-matrix composites and their mechanical properties prior to and during in vitro degradation. Journal of the Mechanical Behavior of Biomedical Materials 2016, 67, 74–86.
[113] Voronkova VI, Kharitonova EP, Orlova EI, Sorokina NI, Grebenev VV. Synthesis, structure, and physical properties of layered tetragonal Mg-doped Nd2MoO6 compounds. Journal of Alloys and Compounds. 2019, 803, 1045–53.
[114] Huang S-J, Ho C-H, Feldman Y, Tenne R. Advanced AZ31 Mg alloy composites reinforced by WS2 nanotubes. Journal of Alloys and Compounds. 2016, 654, 15–22.

[115] Zhong S, Wu C, Chen Y, Feng Z, Xia Y. Enhanced hydrolysis performance and the air-stability of Mg-Ca hydride-chloride composites. Journal of Alloys and Compounds. 2019, 792, 869–77.

[116] Liu D, Liu X, Zhu Y, Li L. Hydriding combustion synthesis of Mg–CaNi5 composites. Journal of Alloys and Compounds. 2008, 458, 394–7.

[117] Li S-L, Lin H-M, Uan J-Y. Production of an Mg/Mg2Ni lamellar composite for generating H2 and the recycling of the post-H2 generation residue to nickel powder. International Journal of Hydrogen Energy. 2013, 38, 13520–8.

[118] Fang C, Wen Z, Liu X, Hao H, Zhang X. Microstructures and mechanical properties of Mg2Sn-nanophase reinforced Mg–Mg2Sn composite. Materials Science and Engineering: A. 2017, 684, 229–32.

[119] Jiang W, Wang J, Yu W, Ma Y, Guo S. In-situ formation of a gradient Mg2Si/Mg composite with good biocompatibility. Surface & Coatings Technology. 2019, 361, 255–62.

[120] Cai XC, Yang TT, Yu H, Sun BR, Shen TD. A thermally stable and strong Mg-MgF2 nanocomposite. Materials Letters. 2017, 209, 476–8.

[121] Yu W, Wang X, Zhao H, Ding C, Ziong S. Microstructure, mechanical properties and fracture mechanism of Ti_2AlC reinforced AZ91D composites fabricated by stir casting. Journal of Alloys Compounds 2017, 702, 199–208.

[122] Nandi SK, Mahato A, Kundu B, Mukherjee P. Doped Bioactive Glass Materials in Bone Regeneration. In: Zorzi AR et al. ed., Advanced Techniques in Bone Regeneration, Croatia 2016.

[123] Li HF, Zheng YF. Recent advances in bulk metallic glasses for biomedical applications. Acta Biomaterialia. 2016, 36, 1–20.

[124] Meagher P, O'Cearbhaill ED, Byrne JH, Browne DJ. Bulk metallic glasses for implantable medical devices and surgical tools. Advanced Materials (Deerfield Beach, Fla.). 2016, 28, 5755–62.

[125] Baulin O, Fabrègue D, Kato H, Liens A, Pelletier J-M. A new, toxic element-free Mg-based metallic glass for biomedical applications. Journal of Non-crystalline Solids. 2018, 481, 397–402.

[126] Li H, He W, Pang S, Liaw PK, Zhang T. In vitro responses of bone-forming MC3T3-E1 pre-osteoblasts to biodegradable Mg-based bulk metallic glasses. Materials Science and Engineering: C. 2016, 68, 632–41.

[127] Dambatta MS, Izman S, Yahya B, Lim JY, Kurniawan D. Mg-based bulk metallic glasses for biodegradable implant materials: A review on glass forming ability, mechanical properties, and biocompatibility. Journal of Non-crystalline Solids. 2015, 426, 110–5.

[128] González S, Figueroa IA, Todd I. Influence of minor alloying additions on the glass-forming ability of Mg–Ni–La bulk metallic glasses. Journal of Alloys and Compounds. 2009, 484, 612–8.

[129] Perrière L, Béucia B, Ochin P, Champion Y. Nickel improves glass-forming ability of mischmetal substituted yttrium in the Mg–Cu based alloys. Journal of Non-crystalline Solids. 2013, 371/372, 37–40.

[130] Zhang L, Li R, Wang J, Zhang H, Zhang T. The influence of Ag substitution for Cu on glass-forming ability and thermal properties of Mg-based bulk metallic glasses. Journal of Non-crystalline Solids. 2012, 358, 1425–9.

[131] Cai AH, Ziong X, Liu Y, An WK, Li XS. Estimation of glass forming ability of Mg-based alloys based on thermodynamics. Journal of Non-crystalline Solids. 2013, 376, 68–75.

[132] Zhao YF, Si JJ, Song JG, Yang Q, Hui XD. Synthesis of Mg–Zn–Ca metallic glasses by gas-atomization and their excellent capability in degrading azo dyes. Materials Science and Engineering: B. 2014, 181, 46–55.

[133] Sun YD, Chen QR, Li GZ. Enhanced glass forming ability and plasticity of Mg-based bulk metallic glass by minor addition of Cd. Journal of Alloys and Compounds. 2014, 584, 273–8.

[134] Li H, Pang S, Liu Y, Liaw PK, Zhang T. In vitro investigation of Mg–Zn–Ca–Ag bulk metallic glasses for biomedical applications. Journal of Non-crystalline Solids. 2015, 427, 134–8.
[135] Wang J, Huang S, Li Y, Wei Y, Cai K. Microstructure, mechanical and bio-corrosion properties of Mn-doped Mg–Zn–Ca bulk metallic glass composites. Materials Science and Engineering: C. 2013, 33, 3832–8.
[136] Wang J, Li Y, Huang S, Wei Y, Pan F. Effects of Y on the microstructure, mechanical and bio-corrosion properties of Mg–Zn–Ca bulk metallic glass. Journal of Materials Science & Technology. 2014, 30, 1255–61.
[137] Li Q-F, Weng H-R, Suo Z-Y, Ren Y-L, Qiu K-Q. Microstructure and mechanical properties of bulk Mg–Zn–Ca amorphous alloys and amorphous matrix composites. Materials Science and Engineering: A. 2008, 487, 301–8.
[138] Zhang YN, Rocher GJ, Briccoli B, Kevorkov D, Medraj M. Crystallization characteristics of the Mg-rich metallic glasses in the Ca–Mg–Zn system. Journal of Alloys and Compounds. 2013, 552, 88–97.
[139] Wu G, Liu Y, Liu C, Tang Q-H, Lu J. Novel multilayer structure design of metallic glass film deposited Mg alloy with superior mechanical properties and corrosion resistance. Intermetallics. 2015, 62, 22–6.
[140] Tsarkov AA, Zanaeva EN, Churyumov AY, Ketov SV, Louzguine-Luzgin DV. Crystallization kinetics of Mg–Cu–Yb–Ca–Ag metallic glasses. Materials Characterization. 2016, 111, 75–80.
[141] Cheng JL, Chen G, Zhao W, Wang ZZ, Zhang ZW. Correlation of the glass formation and phase selection of the Mg-Cu-Gd bulk metallic glass forming alloys. Journal of Non-crystalline Solids. 2017, 472, 61–4.
[142] Babilas R, Nowosielski R, Pawlyta M, Fitch A, Burian A. Microstructural characterization of Mg-based bulk metallic glass and nanocomposite. Materials Characterization. 2015, 102, 156–64.
[143] Babilas R, Łukowiec D, Temleitner L. Atomic structure of Mg-based metallic glass investigated with neutron diffraction, reverse Monte Carlo modeling and electron microscopy. Journal of Nanotechnolgy. 2017, 8, 1174–82.
[144] Babilas R, Bajorek A, Temleitner L. Structural study of amorphous and nanocrystalline Mg-based metallic glass examined by neutron diffraction, X-ray photoelectron spectroscopy, Reverse Monte Carlo calculations and high-resolution electron microscopy. Journal of Non-crystalline Solids. 2019, 505, 421–30.
[145] Hofmann DC, Suh J-Y, Wiest A, Duan G, Lind M-L, Demetriou MD, Johnson WL. Designing metallic glass matrix composites with high toughness and tensile ductility. Nature. 2008, 451, 1085–9.
[146] Rao X, Si PC, Wang JN, Xu Z, Xu S, Wang WM, Hwang W. Preparation and mechanical properties of a new Zr-Al-Ti-Cu-Ni-Be bulk metallic glass. Material Letters. 2001, 50, 279–83.
[147] Hays CC, Kim CP. Johnson WL. Microstructure controlled shear band pattern formation and enhanced plasticity of bulk metallic glasses containing in situ formed ductile phase dendrite dispersions. Physical Review Letters. 2000, 84, 2901–4.
[148] Szuecs F, Kim CP, Johnson WL. Mechanical properties of Zr56. 2Ti13. 8Nb5. 0Cu6. 9Ni5. 6Be12. 5 ductile phase reinforced bulk metallic glass composite. Acta Materialia. 2001, 49, 1507–13.
[149] Wang J, Huang S, Wei Y, Guo S, Pan F. Enhanced mechanical properties and corrosion resistance of a Mg–Zn–Ca bulk metallic glass composite by Fe particle addition. Materials Letters. 2013, 91, 311–4.
[150] Laws KJ, Shamlaye KF, Granata D, Koloadin LS, Löffler JF. Electron-band theory inspired design of magnesium-precious metal bulk metallic glasses with high thermal stability and extended ductility. Scientific Reports. 2017, 7, doi: 10.1038/s41598-017-03643-7.
[151] Erkartal M, Durandurdu M. An in-depth investigation of Mg-Zn-Ca metallic glasses: A first principles study. Computational Materials Science. 2018, 153, 326–37.

[152] Song HY, Dai JL, An MR, Xial MX, Li YL. Atomic simulation of deformation behavior of dual-phase crystalline/amorphous Mg/Mg-Al nanolaminates. Computational Materials Science. 2019, 165, 88–95.

[153] Demetriou MD, Wiest A, Hofmann DC, Johnson WL, Han B, Wolfson N, Wang PK, Liaw G. Amorphous metals for hard-tissue prosthesis. JOM. 2010. 62, 83–91.

[154] Morgan NB. Medical shape memory alloy applications – the market and its products. Material Sciemce and Engineering A. 2004, 378, 16–23.

[155] Hench LL, Polak JM. Third-generation biomedical materials. Science. 2002, 295, 1014–17.

[156] Zberg B, Uggowitzer PJ, Löffler JF. MgZnCa glasses without clinically observable hydrogen evolution for biodegradable implants. Nature Materials. 2009, 8, 887–91.

[157] Suzuki A, Takeyama M. Formation and morphology of Kurnakov type $D0_{22}$ compound in disordered face-centered cubic γ–(Ni, Fe) matrix alloys. Journal of Materials and Research. 2006, 21, 21–6.

[158] Sugimura H, Kaneko Y, Takasugi T. Alloying Behavior of Ni3Nb. Materials Transactions. 2010, 51, 72–7.

[159] Russel AM. Ductility in intermetallic compounds. Advanced Engineering Materials. 2003, 5, 629–39.

[160] Hort N, Huang Y, Kainer KU. Intermetallics in Magnesium Alloys. Advanced Engineering Materials. 2006, 8, 235–40.

[161] L'Espérance G, Plamondon P, Kunst M, Fischersworring-Bunk A. Characterization of intermetallics in Mg–Al–Sr AJ62 alloys. Intermetallics. 2010, 18, 1–7.

[162] Huang ML, Li HX, Ding H, Zhao JW, Hao SM. Study of intermetallics and phase equilibria of Mg–Zn–La system in Mg-rich corner at 345°C. Journal of Alloys and Compounds. 2014, 612, 479–85.

[163] Gil-Santos A, Moelans N, Hort N, Van der Biest O. Identification and description of intermetallic compounds in Mg–Si–Sr cast and heat-treated alloys. Journal of Alloys and Compounds. 2016, 669, 123–33.

[164] Verissimo NC, Brito C, Afonso CR, Spinelli JE, Garcia A. Microstructure characterization of a directionally solidified Mg-12wt.%Zn alloy: Equiaxed dendrites, eutectic mixture and type/morphology of intermetallics. Materials Chemistry and Physics. 2018, 204, 105–31.

[165] Hagihara K, Fujii K, Matsugaki A, Nakano T. Possibility of Mg- and Ca-based intermetallic compounds as new biodegradable implant materials. Materials Science Engineering C: Materials for Biological Applications. 2013, 33, 4101–11.

[166] Li Y, Wei Y, Hou L, Guo C, Han P. Effect of erbium on microstructures and properties of Mg-Al intermetallic. Journal of Rare Earths. 2014, 32, 1064–72.

[167] Nelson M, Agne Mt, Anasori B, Yang J, Barsoum MW. Synthesis and characterization of the mechanical properties of Ti3SiC2/Mg and Cr2AlC/Mg alloy composites. Materials Science and Engineering: A. 2017, 705, 182–8.

[168] Zhao KN, Xu DX, Li HX, Zhang JS, Chen DL. Microstructure and mechanical properties of Mg/Mg bimetal composites fabricated by hot-pressing diffusion and co-extrusion. Materials Science and Engineering: A. 2019, 764, https://doi.org/10.1016/j.msea.2019.138194.

[169] Zhang M-X, Huang H, Spencer K, Shi Y-N. Nanomechanics of Mg–Al intermetallic compounds. Surface & Coatings Technology. 2010, 204, 2118–22.

[170] Yang HY, Guo XW, Wu GH, Wang S, Ding W. Continuous intermetallic compounds coatings on AZ91D Mg alloy fabricated by diffusion reaction of Mg-Al couples. Surface & Coatings Technology. 2011, 205, 2907–13.

[171] Han B, Gu D, He Q, Zhang X, Yang C. Fabrication of a novel Mg-RE (Nd,Ce) intermetallic compound coating by molten salt diffusion and its effect on corrosion resistance of magnesium alloys. Journal of Rare Earths. 2016, 34, 731–5.

Chapter 5
Physical metallurgy

When pure Mg is alloyed with other elements, for example, Ca, the underlying microstructures and phases define the mechanical properties of the alloy and control other important properties including chemical (in particular, corrosion) behavior. Some of the most important commercial Mg-based binary systems including alloying elements to form binary Mg-based alloys are Al, Zn, Mn, Ca, Sr, Y, Ni, Ce, Nd, Cu and/or Sn. There are also more complicated ternary alloys and some of the most common commercial Mg-based ternary alloys should include AZ series (Mg–Al–Zn), AM series (Mg–Al–Mn), AE series (Mg–Al–RE), EZ series (Mg–RE–Zn), ZK series (Mg–Zn–Zr), AX or AXJ series (Mg–Al–Ca) and AJ series (Mg–Al–Sr) [1–3]. Essential microstructural features should be understood for developing optimum alloying designs with aimed properties which could be varied from mechanical properties, physical properties to chemical or electrochemical properties, regardless of such alloys employed as structural materials or functional materials [4–9]. The microstructural parameters such as the grain size, grain boundary (GB) and phase distribution, grain refinements, precipitates, thermal stabilities of various phases, static and dynamic recrystallization (DRX), dislocation and its interaction with various phases are essential and will be discussed in this chapter.

5.1 Phases

5.1.1 Long-period stacking ordered phase

Among many practical structural metallic materials, Mg is recognized to show lightweight (1/4 of specific density of Fe, 1/3 of Ti and 2/3 of Al) and versatile applications. Although high strength, ductility and toughness are required to produce promising structural materials; the formability is constrained at the basal plane due to a strong anisotropy in plastic deformation because of characteristic hexagonal closed-packed (HCP) crystalline structure of Mg, resulting in reducing the ductility. It is well recognized that Al-based alloys (particularly, 6000 and 7000 series alloys) are precipitation-strengthened by the presence of Guinier–Preston (GP) zone associated with the age hardening and bursting into further industrial applications. Similar remarkable revolution took placed with Mg materials. In early 2000, $Mg_{97}Zn_1Y_2$ (by at.%) alloy prepared by rapidly solidified powder metallurgy and hot extrusion processes was developed to exhibit ultimate tensile strength (UTS) of 610 MPa with 5% of tensile elongation [10] and the principle mechanism for this strengthening is the appearance of strengthening phase of the long-period stacking ordered (LPSO) phase [11]. Following the development of Mg-based complicated

https://doi.org/10.1515/9783110676945-005

alloys accompanied by the LPSO phase, there are numerous researches conducted on further developing new Mg alloys and characterizing them. Among them, there are reports on polytypes of LPSO structures. Magnesium exhibits the HCP stacking order of constituent atoms in which the stacking order is disturbed not to follow the stacking sequence (called stacking fault). If the stacking fault takes place along the *c*-axis at every 18 periods (6 periods × 3 times), such structure is designed as 18R-type LPSO structure; while it occurs at every 14 periods (7 periods × 2 times) as 14H-type LPSO structure and at every 10 periods (5 periods × 2 times) as 10H-type LPSO structure as well [12, 13]. In general, these polytypes of LPSO structures can be found in Mg–TM–RE (TM: transition element = Zn, Cu and Ni; RE: rare earth element = Y, La, Ce, Pr, Sm, Nd, Dy, Ho, Er, Gd and Tm) alloys. Recently, Kishida et al. [14] classified the RE elements that form LPSO phases in the Mg–Zn–RE systems into two types: (i) type I includes Y, Dy, Ho and Er, and the LPSO phase is reported to form during solidification in these ternary systems and the LPSO phase formed during solidification is generally based on the 18R-type stacking and it transforms into that based on the 14H-type stacking upon annealing, (ii) type II includes Gd, Tb and Tm, and the LPSO phase of the 14H-type is reported to form during annealing while it is absent immediately after solidification.

There are just a few to list the Mg-based alloys showing LPSO. In Table 5.1, marks are made for identifying either 14H-type or 18R-type structure.

Table 5.1: Typical Mg-based alloys exhibiting LPSO structures.

	Gd	RE	Y	Cu	Ni	Zn	Yb	14H	18R	15R
Mg–Al	[15]	[16]						[16]	[16]	[15]
Mg–Zn			[17]							
Mg–MM				[18]						
Mg–Dy					[19]			[19]	[19]	
Mg–Ho						[20]				
Mg–Co			[21]							
Mg–Y						[22–24]		[23, 24]	[23, 24]	
Mg–Gd							[25]	[25]		

Note: MM, misch metal; RE, rare earth.

It was mentioned that the LPSO phase can strengthen the alloys without sacrificing the ductility. Meanwhile, the existence of the LPSO phase can retain the strength of Mg alloys during the hot deformation, and then enhance their creep resistance. In addition, LPSO containing Mg-alloys exhibit a better corrosion resistance when compared to the conventional Mg alloys such as AZ31, WE43, ZK60 and ZX60 [26].

5.1.2 Precipitation

The precipitation-hardening (or age-hardening) process is a heat-treatment process by producing uniformly dispersed particles within grain structures, so that displacement is hindered, resulting in strengthening materials. Although magnesium alloys are generally not age hardenable due to low age-hardening response, microalloying may be a path to develop high-strength precipitation-hardening magnesium alloys [27]. Precipitation hardening is typically composed of three steps: (1) solution treatment at a relatively high temperature within the α-Mg single-phase region, (2) water quenching to obtain a supersaturated solid solution of alloying elements in magnesium and (3) subsequent aging at a relatively low temperature to achieve a controlled decomposition of the supersaturated solid solution into a fine distribution of precipitates in the magnesium grain matrices [28]. The decomposition of the supersaturated solid solution often involves the formation of a series of metastable or equilibrium precipitate phases that have a different resistance to dislocation shearing. Therefore, the control of precipitation is important if the maximum precipitation strengthening effect needs to be achieved. Additionally, it should be carefully controlled during the aging process not to overage the material, which could result in large and ineffective precipitates. The typical Mg-based binary or ternary alloys which are considered as age hardenable should include the following along with intermetallic compounds as precipitates listed within parentheses: Mg–Al-based alloys ($Mg_{17}Al_{12}$, Mg_2Al_3), Mg–Zn-based alloys (Mg_7Zn_3, Mg_9Zn, Mg_2Zn_3), Mg–Ca-based alloys (Mg_2Ca), Mg–Sn-based alloys (Mg_2Sn), Mg–Nd-based alloys (Mg_4Nd_5, Mg_3Nd, Mg_2Nd), Mg–Ce-based alloys ($Mg_{12}Ce$, $Mg_{41}Ce_5$, Mg_3Ce, Mg_2Ce), Mg–Y-based alloys (Mg_2Y, MgY), Mg–Ni-based alloys (Mg_2Ni, $MgNi_2$) and Mg–Gd-based alloys (Mg_xGd with $x = 5, 3, 2$ and 1) [28–45].

Precipitation can be promoted not only by static thermal treatment as mentioned earlier, but also by strain-induced dynamic precipitation; for example, by hot deformation (from 300 to 450 °C) in Mg–Al–Ca alloy [29], high strain-rate rolling in a temperature range (from 250 to 400 °C) in Mg–Zn–Mn [30], strain hot rolling in Mg–Al alloys [31], high-pressure torsion processing in Mg–Zn alloy [34]. The precipitation sequence has been identified as (in basic scheme) supersaturated solid solution → clusters → nucleation → equilibrium precipitate [38–41].

5.1.3 GP zone and Laves phase

It is generally believed that a GP zone is a fine-scale metallurgical phenomenon, involving early-stage precipitation and is associated with the phenomenon of age hardening, whereby room-temperature reactions continue to occur within a material through time, resulting in changing physical properties. This phenomenon occurs in several Al-based alloy series (such as the Al–Mg–Si 6000 and Al–Zn 7000 series alloys). Physically, GP zones are extremely fine-scaled (on the order of 3–10 nm in size) solute-enriched regions of the material, which offer physical obstructions to the motion of dislocations, above that of the solid solution strengthening of the solute components [46]. Normally, these GP zone phases do not appear in the equilibrium phase diagram. Besides, strictly speaking, because this phase is a small-scale segregation of the solute atom(s) within the supersaturated solid solution, there should not be any crystallographic alterations. Therefore, this phase should not be considered as a precipitate. In several works, the GP zones are identified in Mg–Ag–RE [47], Mg–Ca [48], Mg–Sn [49], Mg-Gd-Y-Zn-Ni-Mn [50], Al-Zn-Mg-Cu [51] and Mg-Al-Ca-Mn [52, 53].

In an equilibrium phase diagram, we can find various types of intermetallic compounds with different compositions, in which the generalized formula of AB_2 is particularly called as Laves phase. The Laves phases are classified, on the basis of geometry, into three different classes: cubic $MgCu_2$ (C15), hexagonal $MgZn_2$ (C14) and hexagonal $MgNi_2$ (C36). Suzuki et al. [54] identified C36 – $(Mg,Al)_2Ca$ – in Mg-5Al-3Ca-0.15Sr alloy, which is transformed to C15 (Al_2Ca) during annealing at 300 °C. Zhong et al. [55] found C14 (Mg_2Ca) and C15 (Al_2Ca) in Mg–Al–Ca alloy. For the same alloy system, Zubair et al. [56] mentioned that the volume fraction, type and morphology of Laves phases can be controlled through the Ca/Al ratio, so that the Ca/Al ratio can be used to manipulate the mechanical properties of this alloy system in order to achieve optimum creep resistance. $MgZn_2$ C14 Laves phase was identified in Mg–Zn alloy [57].

5.1.4 Other phases

In Mg-based alloys, there are other types of phases that contribute to strengthen the matrices, which should include the quasicrystal icosahedral phase (I-phase) and W-phase.

5.1.4.1 I-phase

In 1993, Luo et al. [58] first discovered this phase in the Mg–Zn–(Y, RE) alloy system. Mg-25.7Zn-1.5Y-0.8Ce alloy was added into molten AZ91 and remelted. In the subsequent metal mold cooling process, the I-phases nucleated. Since I-phases are heat-stable phases [31], they remain in the alloys and will not be broken down into other phases even in high-temperature heating process. Thus, they can play significant roles for the matrix after heat treatment [59]. Since then, various Mg-based complicated alloy systems have been subjected to the investigation on evolution of the I-phase. I-phase was identified in Mg–Zn–Y alloy [60, 61], in Mg-Zn-Y-Zr alloy [62, 63], in Mg–Zn–Nd alloy [64, 65], in Mg–Zn–Gd alloy [66], in Mg–Zn–Er [67], in Mg-Li-Zn-Y alloy [68], in Mg-Li-Zn-Gd alloy [69], in Mg–Li–Y alloy [70, 71] and in Mg–Sn–Zn and Mg-Sn-Zn-Al alloys [72].

5.1.4.2 W-phase

Padezhnova et al. [73] first determined the W-phase with face-centered cubic structure in Ma–Zn–Y alloy. W-phase would transform into another compound under certain condition by the diffusion and rearrangement [74, 75]. Luo et al. [74] mentioned that the occurrence of W-phase in Mg–Zn–Gd alloy indirectly reveals that W-phase would transform under some condition. It was further reported that the existence of W-phase was unfavorable to the mechanical properties of as-extruded alloys; accordingly, the formation range of the W-phase should be avoided during the design of I-phase strengthening Mg–Zn–Gd as-extruded alloys [76–79]. W-phase was also found in Mg–Zn–Er alloy [80] and in Mg-Zn-Y-Zr alloy [62, 63]. There are other types of phases reported. Chen et al. [81] found numerous phases in Mg–Zn–RE alloys; Z ($Mg_{12}ZnRE$), Z + W ($Mg_3Zn_3RE_2$) and a mixture of W and W + I (Mg_3Zn_6RE) ternary phases. Zhang et al. [82] reported the X-phase ($Mg_{12}YZn$) and W-phase (MgY_2Zn_3) in Mg-Y-Zn-Zr alloy.

5.2 Grain refining

Pure Mg (as a form of α-Mg) normally possesses an equiaxed coarser grains that are observed in as-cast pure Mg. As discussed in previous chapters, various alloying element(s) are added to α-Mg to produce more practical and useful materials. In this chapter, grain refining will be reviewed. The strengthening method for Mg is based on the structure design, such as grain refinement, surface modification and with other reinforcement.

5.2.1 Metallurgical routes

Grain refinement via metallurgical routes has been exploited in magnesium alloys to achieve desired microstructures, mechanical properties and improved corrosion resistance.

Table 5.2 lists typical grain refiners to various Mg-based alloys, which also includes several types of master alloys. A master alloy is a base metal, such as Al, Cu or Ni, combined with a relatively high percentage of one or two other elements and is a semifinished product. Among various reasons for adding master alloys to a melt, it should be pointed out that master alloy plays an important role for adjusting the composition of the liquid metal to meet the desired chemical specification and controlling microstructure to influence the mechanical, physical and chemical properties. Depending on its effects on final outcomes, the master alloy is called as hardener, grain refiner or grain modifier.

Table 5.2: Grain refiners to various Mg-based alloys.

	Mg	Mg–Al	Mg–Al–Zn	Mg–Al–RE	Mg–Al–Ca	Mg–Al–Si	Mg–Zn	Mg–Zn–Zr	Mg–Li–Al	Mg–Sn	Mg–Sn–Zn	Mg–Sm	Mg–Gd	Mg–Mn	Mg–Ce	Mg–Nd
Cd	[83]															
Mn	[84]												[85]			
Zn	[84]									[86]						
Al											[87]	[88]			[89]	[90]
Ce		[91]					[92]	[93–95]						[96]		
Sm		[97]						[98]								
Sc											[99]					
C		[100, 101]														
Ca		[101, 102]	[103]				[92]		[104]	[86]						
Sr		[105]														
Mn			[106, 107]							[108]						
Gd				[109]			[110]									
Sn					[111]	[112]			[113]							
Y								[93]	[114]		[115]					

Nd			[116]		
Dy			[116]		
Ag					[117]
Zr					[85]
Sc					[85]
C1					
C2	[118]	[119]			
C3	[120]				
C4	[121–123]				
M1		[124, 125]			
M2		[126]			
M3		[127]			
M4				[128, 129]	
M5				[130]	

Note: C1, NiC; C2, SiC; C3, HfC; C4, Al_4C_3; M1, Mg–Sr master alloy; M2, Mg–Al_4C_3 master alloy; M3, Al–4B master alloy; M4, Al–5Ti–1B master alloy; M5, TiB_2 + Al_3Ti compound.

5.2.2 Mechanical routes

Severe plastic deformation processes have been adopted to improve the mechanical properties and plastic deformation of Mg materials [131]. Table 5.3 lists typical severe plastic deformation methods for grain refining to Mg-based alloys, mainly including single, multiple pass or reciprocating extrusion, forging or rolling.

5.2.3 Hall–Petch relationship

There is an empirical equation between grain size and mechanical strength (yield strength), known as the Hall–Petch equation; $\sigma_y = \sigma_o + k_y\, d^{-1/2}$, where σ_y is the resultant yield strength, σ_o is a material's constant for the starting stress for dislocation movement (or the resistance of the lattice to dislocation motion), k_y is the strengthening coefficient (a material's constant based in solid-solution properties) and d is the average grain diameter, which can be regulated by previously discussed metallurgical routes, mechanical routes or appropriate heat treatment. The basic concept for the GB strengthening (or Hall–Petch strengthening) is based on the fact that GBs are normally behave like strong borders for dislocations and that the number of dislocations within a grain have an effect on how stress builds up in the adjacent grain, which will eventually activate dislocation sources and thus enable deformation in the neighboring grain, resulting in piling up of the number of dislocations at the GB and yield strength [163–166]. This strengthening mechanism works till d approaches approximately 10 nm, as shown in Figure 5.1 [163]. Strengthening is limited by the size of dislocations. Once the grain size reaches about 10 nm, GBs start to slide and deformations within each grain are not obstructed at GBs.

About the Hall–Petch behavior in Mg materials, it was mentioned that (i) the value of k_y in Mg alloys varies with texture, grain size, temperature and strain, and (ii) the influence of texture and grain size on k_y is found to be an essential result of the variation of deformation mode on k_y value [167, 168]. Studying the rolled Mg–1.02Zn alloys with strong basal textures and Mg–0.76Y alloys with weakened basal textures which were subjected to annealing in order to obtain different grain structures with keeping the textures nearly unchanged, Shi et al. [169] reported that (i) the Mg–1.02Zn specimens exhibit two slopes (k_y) of Hall–Petch relationships, that is, the coarse-grained (>49 μm) specimens reveal an abnormally enhanced tendency of k_y (~472 MPa $\mu m^{1/2}$) with increased strains, while fine-grained (≤49 μm) specimens exhibit a slightly decreased tendency of k_y with increased strains and (ii) the Mg–0.76Y specimens follow a single slope of Hall–Petch relationship well in the grain regime with slightly declined k_y with increased strains; attributing to the distinguished twinning responses and/or twinning–slipping interactions dependence of grain size with different initial textures.

Table 5.3: Grain refining by mechanical routes to various Mg-based alloys.

	Mg	Mg–Al	Mg–Al–Zn	Mg–Al–Sn	Mg–Zn	Mg–Zn–Ca	Mg–Zn–Zr	Mg–Zn–Y	Mg–Zn–Nd	Mg–Zn–Mn	Mg–Zn–Gd	Mg–Y	Mg–Li	Mg–Bi	Mg–Ca	Mg–Gd	Mg–Gd–Y
HPT	[132]				[133]	[134]											[135, 136]
SSE	[137]	[137]			[138]											2	
PM		[139]															
ECAP			[140, 141]							[142]							[143]
ECASD			[144]														
ETD			[145]														
LSP			[146]														
DHC			[147, 148]														
HPR				[149]													
BDR					[150]												
HE							[151]	[152]	[153]								

(continued)

Table 5.3 (continued)

	Mg	Mg–Al	Mg–Al–Zn	Mg–Al–Sn	Mg–Zn	Mg–Zn–Ca	Mg–Zn–Zr	Mg–Zn–Y	Mg–Zn–Nd	Mg–Zn–Mn	Mg–Zn–Gd	Mg–Y	Mg–Li	Mg–Bi	Mg–Ca	Mg–Gd	Mg–Gd–Y
RE							[154]	[155]									
MAF											[156]						
FSP												[157]					
DR												[158]					
OSE													[159]	[160]	[161]		
HF																	[162]

Note: HPT, high-pressure torsion; SSE, simple shear extrusion PM, planetary milling; ECAP, equal-channel angular pressing; ECASD, equal-channel angular sheet drawing; ETD, extrusion and torsion deformation; LSP, laser shock peening; DHC, dynamic hot compression; HPR, hard-plate rolling; BDR, bidirectional rolling; HE, hot extrusion; RE, reciprocating extrusion; MAF, multiaxial forging; FSP, friction stir processing; DR, dynamic rolling; OSE, one-step extrusion; HF, hot forging.

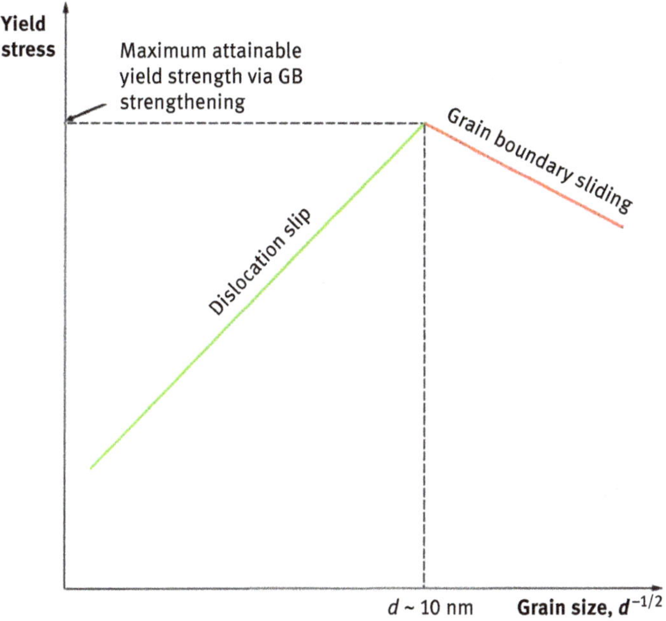

Figure 5.1: Limitation of the Hall–Petch strengthening [163].

5.3 Recrystallization

In general, there are two processes for the recrystallization phenomenon: DRX and static recrystallization (SRX). There are distinct differences between DRX (dynamic) and SRX [170–175]. In DRX, as opposed to SRX, (i) the nucleation and growth of new equiaxial grains occurs in a plastically deformed metallic material, rather than afterward as part of a separate heat treatment, (ii) DRX begins when a critical strain value is reached during deformation, (iii) the reduction of grain size increases the risk of GB sliding at elevated temperatures, while also decreasing dislocation mobil ity within the material, (iv) the new grains are less strained, causing a decrease in the hardening of a material, (v) recrystallization is much faster than creep, which is typically occurring under much lower stresses and (vi) after DRX, the ductility of the material increases. In SRX, the recrystallization process is slow and occurs between subsequent rolling and a plastic deformation where the majority of the grain refinement takes place. Both SRX and DRX are unaffected by the temperature of deformation.

According to Huang et al. [175], referring to Figure 5.2, there are three different processes for DRX occurrence. Discontinuous recrystallization (caused by the interplay

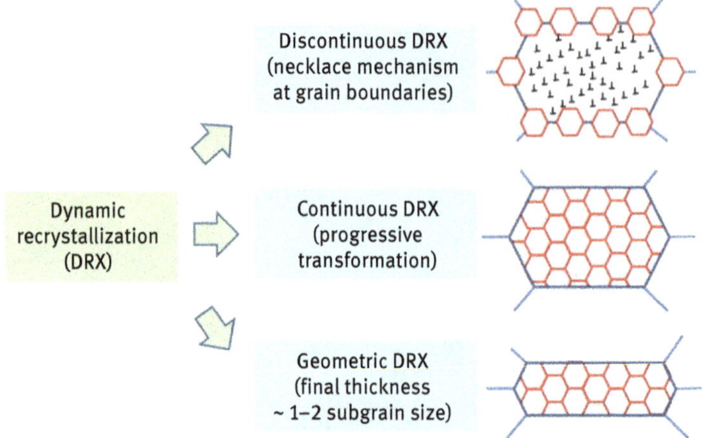

Figure 5.2: Three typical processes for dynamic recrystallization occurrence [175].

of work hardening and recovery) is heterogeneous; there are distinct nucleation and growth stages characterized by (i) recrystallization, which does not occur until the threshold strain has been reached, and (ii) nucleation, which generally occurs along preexisting GBs. Continuous DRX typified materials with high stacking fault energies characterized by the following: as strain increases, subgrain boundary misorientation increases; as low-angle GBs evolve into high-angle GBs, and as deformation increases, crystallite size decreases. Geometric DRX occurs in grains with local serrations and is characterized by the fact that it generally occurs with deformation at elevated temperatures in materials with high stacking fault energy; stress increases and then declines to a steady state; and pinning of GBs causes an increase in the required strain.

5.3.1 Dynamic recrystallization

It is important to mention here that the Zener–Hollomon (Z) parameter [176], which is known as the temperature-compensated strain rate, is used to describe the high-temperature creep strain of a material. There are several reports on DRX kinetics in Mg-based alloys that have been expressed as a function of the Zener–Hollomon parameter which is a function of the microstructure evolution, the DRX fraction, the DRX rate and the DRX sensitive rate and others [176–184].

Figure 5.3 shows the relationship between Z parameter and DRXed grain size [177], indicating that (i) the larger the Z parameter, DRXed grain gets refiner and (ii) elements for solid solution controls this relationship and the higher the solid solution, the finer the grain size.

Table 5.4–5.7 lists the various types of severe deformation methods employed during the DRX process.

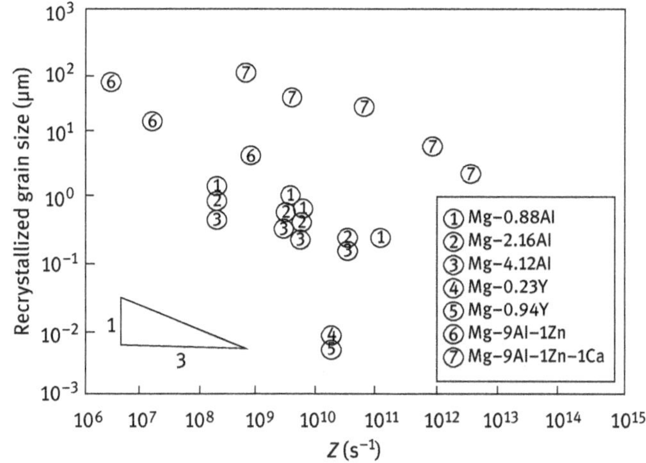

Figure 5.3: Relationship between Z parameter and DRXed grain size [177].

Table 5.4: DRX for Mg–Zn-based alloys.

	Mg–Zn	Mg–Zn–Zr	Mg–Zn–Ca	Mg–Zn–MM	Mg–Zn–Mn	Mg–Zn–RE	Mg–Zn–Y	Mg–Zn–Sn	Mg–Zn–Er
ECAP	[185]								
HEX	[186]	[187–189]	[190, 191]		[192]			[193, 194]	[195]
HDF	[196]								
HCP		[197]			[198]		[199, 200]	[201]	
HSRR		[202]			[203]				
HRL		[204]				[205]	[206]		
HPT		[207]					[208]		
UCP			[209]				[210]		
IDEX			[211]						

Table 5.4 (continued)

	Mg–Zn	Mg–Zn–Zr	Mg–Zn–Ca	Mg–Zn–MM	Mg–Zn–Mn	Mg–Zn–RE	Mg–Zn–Y	Mg–Zn–Sn	Mg–Zn–Er
WRL				[212]					
HSRCP					[213]				

Note: MM, misch metal (55Ce–25La–25Nd); RE, rare earth elements; ECAP, equal-channel angular pressing (with backpressure); HEX, hot extrusion; HDF, hot deformation; HCP, hot compression; HSRR, high strain rate rolling; HRL, hot rolling; HPT, high-pressure torsion; UCP, uniaxial compression; IDEX, indirect extrusion; WRL, warm rolling; HSCP, high strain rate compression.

Table 5.5: DRX for Mg–Al-based and Mg–Li-based alloys.

	Mg–Al–Zn	Mg–Al–Y	Mg–Al–Sn	Mg–Al–Ca	Mg–Li–Zn	Mg–Li–Al
ECAP	[214]					
HEX	[215, 216]	[217]	[218]	[219]	[220]	[221–223]
HDF	[224]		[225]	[226]	[227]	
HCP	[228, 229]				[230]	[231]
HSRR		[232–234]				
HRL	[235]		[236]			
HPT						
UCP						
IDEX						
WRL						
HSRCP						
EPT	[237, 238]					

Table 5.5 (continued)

	Mg–Al–Zn	Mg–Al–Y	Mg–Al–Sn	Mg–Al–Ca	Mg–Li–Zn	Mg–Li–Al
ERL	[239]					
SFT	[240]					
MDIF	[241]					
BEX	[242]					
DCCAP						[243]

Note: ECAP, equal-channel angular pressing (with backpressure); HEX, hot extrusion; HDF, hot deformation; HCP, hot compression; HSRR, high strain rate rolling; HRL, hot rolling; HPT, high-pressure torsion; UCP, uniaxial compression; IDEX, indirect extrusion; WRL, warm rolling; HSCP, high strain rate compression; EPT, electropulsing tension; ERL, electrostatic rolling; SF, sliding friction treatment; MDIF, multidirectional impact forging; BEX, backward extrusion; DCCAP, double change channel pressing.

Table 5.6: DRX for Mg–Gd-based and Mg–Y-based alloys.

	Mg–Gd	Mg–Gd–Y	Mg–Gd–Zn	Mg–Y	Mg–Y–Mg	Mg–Y–RE
ECAP		[244]				
HEX		[245]		[246]		
HDF			[247]			[248]
HCP		[249–252]		[253]		
HSRR						
HRL					[206]	
HPT						
UCP		[254]				
IDEX		[255]				

Table 5.6 (continued)

	Mg–Gd	Mg–Gd–Y	Mg–Gd–Zn	Mg–Y	Mg–Y–Mg	Mg–Y–RE
WRL						
HSRCP						
EPT						
ERL		[239]				
SFT						
MDIF						
BEX						
DCCAP						
SMAT		[256]				

Note: RE, rare earth elements; ECAP, equal-channel angular pressing (with backpressure); HEX, hot extrusion; HDF: hot deformation; HCP, hot compression; HSRR, high strain rate rolling; HRL, hot rolling; HPT, high-pressure torsion; UCP, uniaxial compression; IDEX, indirect extrusion; WRL, warm rolling; HSCP, high strain rate compression; EPT, electropulsing tension; ERL, electrostatic rolling; SF, sliding friction treatment; MDIF, multidirectional impact forging; BEX, backward extrusion; DCCAP, double change channel pressing; SMAT, surface mechanical attrition treatment.

Table 5.7: DRX for other types of Mg-based alloys.

	Mg–Sn–Al	Mg–Sn–Zn	Mg–Sm–Zn	Mg–Bi–Al	Mg–Mn	Mg–Mn–Sr	Mg–Nd–Zn
HEX		[257]	[258]	[259]	[160]	[260]	[260]
HDF							[261]

Note: HEX, hot extrusion; HDF, hot deformation.

5.3.2 Static recrystallization

The majority of the SRXs are related to hardening mechanism which should be affected by a certain type of heat treatment. Here, for the purpose of comparing this to DRX, several works are reviewed and the detailed discussions on interrelated between heat treatment and hardening phenomena will be done in Chapter 8.

SRX plays a key role in the fabrication of thin Mg wires as well as the mechanical properties of the final wires. Meng et al. [262] studied the effect of annealing parameters on the evolution of the microstructures, textures and mechanical properties of cold-drawn pure Mg wire and reported that (i) the mechanical properties of as-annealed pure thin Mg wire is affected not only by the average grain size but also by the uniformity of the recrystallization grains, including the uniformity of grain size and crystal orientation distribution (more random texture component); (ii) with increasing annealing temperature and time, the uniformity of recrystallization grain size first improved and then declined after obvious grain growth; (iii) at the same time, the randomness of the basal texture component declined with the development of recrystallization; and (iv) annealing at 300 °C for 30 min caused the most uniform grain size and orientation distribution in the microstructures, thus contributing to the best plasticity among all experimental wires, concluding that more uniform and regular recrystallized grains and a more randomly distributed crystal orientation would benefit the mechanical properties of Mg wires.

A comparative study between Mg–3Al–1Zn (AZ31) and Mg–3Zn–0.5Ca (ZX31) was conducted to investigate the texture evolution during annealing of hot-rolled sheets [263]. It was mentioned that (i) ZX31 shows faster recrystallization kinetics than AZ31, (ii) during SRX of as-rolled sheet, no significant change in texture takes place in AZ31, while much weaker basal texture develops in ZX31, indicating that discontinuous recrystallization occurs during annealing of ZX31 sheet, (iii) such a development of weaker basal texture in the ZX31 sheet is related to the mode of twins generated during rolling process, that is, the deformation bands consisted of compression, and secondary twins induce accelerated nucleation of recrystallized grains during annealing. ZX31 exhibits significantly enhanced room temperature formability than AZ31 and (iv) the enhanced formability would be closely related with different texture evolution mode during annealing as well as typical strain hardening behavior in ZX31. Ce element containing Mg alloy (Mg–1.5Zn–0.2Ce) was subjected to investigate its SRX at 480 °C annealing [264] and it was reported that (i) double twins mostly exist in deformed grains with basal orientations, and statically recrystallized grains mainly nucleate at the intersections of double twins and preexisting GBs, (ii) statically recrystallized grains tend to exhibit transverse direction (TD)-tilted orientations and grow along double twins to consume adjacent basal-oriented grains; due to inducing the change from a rolling direction-split texture to a well-weakened TD-split texture during annealing and (iii) the residual unrecrystallized grains with TD-tilted orientations and the growth advantage of TD-tilted grains also enhance the formation of TD-split texture. Liu et al. [265] investigated the effect of Gd, Ce and Y elements on texture, recrystallization and mechanical properties of Mg–1.5Zn alloys. It was found that (i) the addition of Gd, Ce and Y elements in Mg–1.5Zn alloy, which rolled at 450 °C and subsequently annealed at 350 °C for 1 h, can effectively weaken and modify the basal texture, characterized by the splitting basal pole toward TD, leading to the yield and tensile strength, the highest along the rolling direction and the lowest along the TD; (ii) the unique basal texture contributes to the significant improvement of elongation at room temperature; (iii) the nonbasal texture in Mg–1.5Zn–0.2RE alloys can be attributed to the obstructive effect of SRX and the nonbasal orientation grains nucleation near preexisting GBs during annealing; and (iv) the Mg–1.5Zn–0.2Gd sheet exhibits much excellent plasticity with the elongation of 27% than Mg–1.5Zn–0.2Ce and Mg–1.5Zn–0.2Y alloys, resulting from the less and smaller second phase of MgZnGd. Yang et al. [266] studied the SRX of hot-deformed magnesium alloy AZ31 during isothermal annealing at temperature of 300 °C. It was reported that the grain size change during isothermal annealing is categorized into three regions, that is, an incubation period for grain growth, rapid grain coarsening and normal grain growth. The number of fine grains per unit area, however, decreases remarkably even in incubation period, leading to grain coarsening that takes place continuously in the whole period of annealing. In contrast, the deformation texture scarcely changes even after full annealing at high temperatures, indicating that the annealing processes operating in hot-deformed magnesium alloy with continuous dynamic recrystallized grain structures can be mainly controlled by grain coarsening without texture change, that is, continuous SRX.

Zhang et al. [267] investigated the effects of Er addition and its existing form on the SRX and grain growth during annealing of an extruded Mg–1.5Zn–0.6Zr alloy. It was mentioned that (i) microstructure stability was much improved by Er addition and the best thermal ability was obtained in 2 wt% Er-containing alloy, (ii) for the incomplete DRX microstructures extruded at a lower temperature of 350 °C, Er addition increased the resistance of SRX; and for the complete DRX microstructures extruded at a relatively high temperature of 420 °C and (iii) Er addition suppressed grain growth. Examining the microstructure and texture evolution during the recrystallization annealing of cold-rolled Mg–1Y and Mg–0.2Zn–1Y alloys, it was reported that (i) at the early annealing stage, new grains are nucleated on subunits with 200–300 nm surrounded by dislocation walls within shear bands and (ii) Zn and Y addition reduced the stacking fault energy which results in the high activity of nonbasal deformation mechanisms and formation of segregation zones along the stacking faults; causing the orientation of recrystallization nuclei to be effectively retained so that the texture weakens during the recrystallization without reducing the basal pole split into the sheet TD.

Based on the fact that the recrystallization process has been reported to be responsible for the formation of nonbasal texture in Mg–RE and Mg–Zn–RE alloy,

Zhao et al. [268] characterized the microstructure, macrotexture, grain orientation and misorientation evolution during annealing of Mg–Zn–Gd alloy at 150–480 °C to understand the evolution of nonbasal texture from a cold-rolled elliptical annular texture to a TD-split texture with double peaks tilting away from normal direction (ND) to TD. It was reported that (i) SRX begins to take place at 200 °C, and an almost fully recrystallized microstructure is obtained at 300 °C and obvious grain growth from 300 to 400 °C and (ii) the texture evolution during SRX is mostly related to preferred grain growth which may be caused by the special misorientation or/and the segregation of Zn and Gd solute atoms on special GBs. Shah et al. [269] studied the SRX behavior of a Mg-9.02Gd-4.21Y-0.48Zr (GW94) alloy during annealing treatment in the temperature range of 350–500 °C and mentioned that, after multidirectional impact forging process, (i) coarse grains containing parallel and intersected twins while small grains containing only parallel twins were observed and (ii) TBs/GBs are stable at 350 °C, but SRX governed by the increased TB/GB mobilities begins at 400–450 °C temperature range.

5.4 Thermal stability

Many of practical alloys are strengthened by solid-state precipitates that are produced by an age-hardening process. Although the basic physical strengthening phenomena of both precipitation hardening and age hardening are the same, that is, hardening via second-phase precipitation, strictly speaking there should be a slight difference there between, namely, precipitation hardening is strengthened by precipitates of a second phase during cooling of homogeneous solid solution, while age hardening is strengthened by precipitates of a second phase during annealing of a supersaturated solid solution and can result in the release of built-in stresses or permit phases locked in (due to quenching) to transform. Both these treatments are very time/temperature sensitive since incorrect temperatures or times can result in developing negative artifacts rather than positive artifacts in the microstructure of the materials being considered. Many magnesium casting and wrought alloys achieve their useful mechanical properties via age hardening, which involves (i) solution treatment at a relatively high temperature within the α-Mg single-phase region, (ii) water quenching to obtain a supersaturated solid solution of alloying elements in magnesium, and (iii) subsequent aging at a relatively low temperature to achieve a controlled decomposition of the supersaturated solid solution into a fine distribution of precipitates in the magnesium matrix [28]. Thermal stability of microstructure, particularly, precipitates play a significant role in mechanical properties.

Various alloying elements have been studied in terms of their influences on thermal stability of microstructures. Xu et al. [270] studied the effects of Nd and Yb on the microstructures, their thermal stability and tensile properties of Mg–5.5Zn–0.6Zr alloy. It was mentioned that (i) an addition of Nd or Yb both brings about the precipitation of a new γ (Mg, Nd) Zn_2 or γ (Mg, Yb) Zn_2 eutectic phase and results in a refinement in dendritics, (ii) however, the combination addition of Nd and Yb has an opposite effect on dendritics and leads to the formation of γ (Mg, Nd + Yb) Zn_2 eutectic phases in the shape of network-like, even the lamellar eutectics are somehow thickened, (iii) the tensile strength, yield strength and the elongation are about 255.6 MPa, 163.6 MPa and 17.4%, respectively, at room temperature; mainly being attributed to combined strengthening factors induced by Yb addition and (iv) at the elevated temperature, the Mg–5.5Zn–0.6Zr alloy with addition combination of Nd and Yb has a good performance in thermal stability, but inferiority in elongation. Hradilová [271] studied the as-cast, T4 heat-treated and equal-channel angular pressing (ECAP) Mg–4Zn and Mg–4Zn–0.4Ca alloys, which consisted of α-Mg dendrites, MgZn and $Ca_2Mg_6Zn_3$ phases. It was reported that (i) the ECAP process resulted in significant structural refinement, fragmentation and the precipitation of intermetallic phases, (ii) the maximum UTS of the ECAPed Mg–4Zn–0.4Ca alloy was 250 MPa and (iii) mechanical tests at elevated temperatures and after heat treatments revealed that the ternary Mg–4Zn–0.4Ca alloy exhibited better thermal stability than the binary Mg–4Zn alloy. Hou et al. [272] prepared the Mg-8Gd-2Y-1Nd-0.3Zn-0.6Zr alloy sheet by hot extrusion technique and studied the structure and mechanical properties of the extruded alloy. It was found that (i) the alloy in different states is mainly composed of α-Mg solid solution and secondary phases of Mg_5RE and $Mg_{24}RE_5$ (RE = Gd, Y and Nd); (ii) at aging temperatures from 200 to 300 °C the alloy exhibits obvious age-hardening response and the great improvement of mechanical properties is observed in the peak-aged state alloy (aged at 200 °C for 60 h); (iii) the UTS, tensile yield strength and elongation are 376 MPa, 270 MPa and 14.2% at room temperature, and 206 MPa, 153 MPa and 25.4% at 300 °C, respectively, suggesting an excellent thermal stability. Kubásek et al. [273] investigated structure and mechanical properties of the as-cast AJ62 (Mg–6Al–2Sr) alloy which was developed for elevated temperature applications and these properties were compared to commercial casting AZ91 (Mg–9Al–1Zn) and WE43 (Mg–4Y–3RE) alloys. The structure of the AJ62 alloy consisted of primary α-Mg dendrites and interdendritic network of the Al_4Sr and massive $Al_3Mg_{13}Sr$ phases. Comparing hardness and compressive strengths among three alloys, it was indicated that AJ62 alloy is inferior to AZ91 but superior to WE43 in terms of thermal stabilities at a temperature of 250 °C.

Lin et al. [274] investigated the microstructure of a new Mg-4Zn-2Al-0.5Ca alloy, which was aged at 120 or 160 °C. It was reported that (i) the microstructure of alloy aged at 120 °C for 230 h consists of cellular textures, ordered zone, elongated precipitates and disc-like precipitates, while the microstructure of the alloy aged at 160 °C for 32 h consists of edge dislocations, ordered zones and moiré fringe and (ii) no MgZn precipitates are found in the peak aged microstructures of alloys aged at 120 and 160 °C; suggesting that Ca is a particularly effective trace addition in improving the thermal stability of precipitation in Mg–4Zn–2Al alloy aged at 120 and 160 °C. Liu et al. [275] added Sr to Mg–5 wt% Sn alloy, resulting in grain refinement and the formation of a rod-shaped and a bone-shaped MgSnSr intermetallic phase which are mainly straddle on the GBs. It was also mentioned that (i) the yield strength is improved, while the tensile strength and elongation first increased, and then decreased with a large addition of Sr, (ii) optimum mechanical properties at ambient temperature are obtained at a content of 2.14 wt% Sr and (iii) tensile properties of the alloys at elevated temperatures are improved, and the decrease of strength at elevated temperature slowed down with increasing Sr addition, indicating that Sr can improve the thermal stability of Mg–Sn alloys. The investigations of microstructure and mechanical properties of AME503 (Mg-5Al-0.4Mn-3RE) and AME505 (Mg-5Al-0.4Mn-5RE) experimental alloys were performed along with the microstructures of α-Mg, $Al_{11}RE_3$ and $Al_{10}RE_2Mn_7$ intermetallic phases [276]. Based on results of a significant influence of RE elements on the Brinell hardness, tensile and compression properties at ambient temperature and especially on creep properties at 200 °C, it was mentioned that improved alloy properties with a rise in RE elements mass fraction results from an increase in $Al_{11}RE_3$ phase volume fraction and suppression of $\alpha + \gamma$ eutectic volume fraction in the alloy microstructure, indicating the improvement of the thermal stability of the intermetallic phases during creep testing. Hanna et al. [277] processed an Mg–0.41Dy (wt%) alloy by high-pressure tension (HPT) through five turns at room temperature. The evolution of the recrystallization microstructure and the texture and mechanical properties of the deformed alloy were investigated after annealing at 200 and 400 °C for 1 h. It was reported that the HPT processing led to significant grain refinement with an average grain size of ~0.5 ± 0.1 µm which increased to ~1.2 ± 0.8 µm after annealing at 400 °C, demonstrating that this slow increase in grain size at a high temperature demonstrates a good thermal stability of the microstructure.

Cheng et al. [278] studied the thermal stability and crystallization kinetics of the $Mg_{65}Cu_{25}Y_{10}$ and $Mg_{65}Cu_{25-x}Y_{10}B_x$ ($x = 1$–10 in at.%) amorphous alloys and compared in terms of nonisothermal and isothermal differential scanning calorimetry measurements. It is mentioned that (i) with the minor addition of 1–5 at% B, the incubation time for crystallization is prolonged and the activation energy is increased, suggesting an improvement of the thermal stability, (ii) nevertheless, the overall nucleation and growth characteristics of the parent and B-additive alloys are similar, (iii) the minor B element appears to impose resistance to the crystallization of the major Mg_2Cu phase, possibly by blocking the path of Mg and Cu diffusion and (iv) with further addition of B up to 10 at%, secondary crystallization phases such as MgB_4 or YB would be induced and thus lower the thermal stability. Minárik et al. [279] processed as-cast WE43 (containing yttrium and RE elements) by ECAP, leading to a significant grain refinement together with a massive precipitation of the secondary phase particles and investigated the thermal stability of the ultrafine grain structure together with microstructural changes due to exposure to elevated temperatures range of 160–500 °C. It was reported that (i) ultrafine grain structure consisting of grains with size of ~340 nm and high density of Mg_5RE particles is stable up to 280 °C for 1 h of annealing; (ii) only negligible change of the microstructure occurred after annealing for 16 h at 250 °C; (iii) excellent thermal stability of ultrafine grain structure was caused by fine Mg_5RE particles, which suppressed the grain growth; (iv) exceeding the limit of thermal stability of these particles above 280 °C resulted in material softening; (v) statistically significant hardening of the ultrafine grain material occurred in the temperature range of 200–280 °C; and (vi) segregation of yttrium and RE elements and eventually precipitation at GBs was proved to be responsible for observed hardening.

When deformation twins and creation of TBs occur, they act as obstacles for dislocation movement and become impermeable for the dislocation to pass through. When dislocations pile up around TB and a larger stress is required for piled dislocation to overcome this energy barrier, resulting in the increase of the strength and ductility of crystal. Hence, the thermal stability of twins is important. Hence, the thermal stability of twins is also important. Zhang et al. [280] pretwinned AZ31 rods which were subjected to different annealing treatments, for studying the effect of annealing temperature, annealing time and preannealing on the thermal stability of the {10–12} twins. It was reported that although the mobility of {10–12} TBs at 250 °C is quite limited, an annealing for 12 h can remove a part of twins. Enhancing annealing temperature greatly increases mobility of TBs and a longer annealing duration further reduces the amount of twins; however, a temperature higher than 375 °C is necessary to completely remove all the twins. The initial grain size in a range of 15–32 μm does not pose a great influence on the thermal stability of {10–12} twins. Recovery process by a preannealing at 200 °C for 6 h is not effective to enhance the thermal stability at higher temperature. During annealing, both the consumption of twins by matrix and that of matrix by twins take place, leading to hardly changed texture components in the annealed samples. Liu et al. [281] discussed the stability of twins, especially {10–12} twins, in Mg alloys. Liu et al. [281] mentioned that (i) the pretwinning is considered to be an effective method for adjusting the microstructure and properties of wrought Mg alloys, (ii) especially, formation of twin texture can remarkably improve formability of rolled-Mg alloys, (iii) the initial {10–12} twins may either grow or shrink under further deformation, and may be removed by SRX under thermal effect and (iv) improving the stability of twin structure could enhance the contribution of twin texture on subsequent plastic formability.

5.5 Twinning and dislocation engineering

5.5.1 Twinning

It is generally believed that (i) twinning is an important mode in plastic deformation of the hexagonal close-packed Mg-based alloys that are promising lightweight structural metals, (ii) the hardness, strength and stretch formability of Mg alloys can be improved by pretwinning, (iii) the most usually detected twin types in Mg alloys are {10–12} extension twins and {10–11} contraction twins and (iv) the most common twin modes in Mg alloys are tension twinning and compression twinning and both are single twins [282–286]. In Mg–Al-based alloys, $Mg_{17}Al_{12}$ is the principle precipitate and it was reported that twinning becomes difficult to occur when the size and number density of this precipitate increases [287]. Studying the precipitate–twin interactions in the Mg–Al alloys and effects of precipitate shape on twinning in Mg–7.7Al alloy, Gharghouri et al. [288] mentioned that (i) the nature of the interaction between the twins and the second phase was found to be dependent on the relative thickness of the twin and the precipitate and (ii) twins were observed to engulf, bypass or impinge upon the precipitates, but the precipitates themselves were not twinned. Similarly, Mg–Zn-based alloys, there are mainly precipitate of MgZn and/or Mg_7Zn_3. Dobroň et al. [289] investigated Mg–1Zn alloy and mentioned that the proper thermomechanical treatment can improve mechanical properties of extruded Mg alloys through a solute segregation and precipitation along TBs. Robson et al. [290], studying the twin behavior of compressed Mg–5Zn alloy, reported that (i) the number of {1012} twins formed in the alloy increased when precipitate particles were present, reaching a maximum in the peak-aged condition, and (ii) particles were observed to promote twin nucleation, but inhibit twin growth.

There are several researches on twin and dislocation interactions in practical Mg–Al–Zn alloys (AZ31 and AZ91). Wang et al. [291] investigated the effect of twinning–detwinning on the mechanical properties of AZ31-extruded magnesium alloy which was subjected to precompression and prestretch deformation along extrusion direction at 1%, 3% and 5% strain levels. It was reported that (i) the detwinning behavior occurred during the inverse tension after the precompression, (ii) although due to the aforementioned effect the tensile yield strength decreased, by increasing the precompressive levels both fracture elongation and peak strength improved and (iii) in the inverse compressive tests after prestretch the {10–12} twinning was restrained and the volume fraction of twins decreased, leading to the improvement of yield strength by increasing in prestretching levels. Xu et al. [292] studied the influence of solute atoms together with dislocations at {1012} TB on mechanical behavior of a detwinning predominant deformation in an Mg alloy AZ31 plate. It was found that (i) a large number of {1012} twins disappear during recompression along the ND, (ii) both the TB–dislocation interaction and TB–solute–dislocation interaction can greatly enhance the yield stress of the recompression along the ND, (iii) the samples with TB–dislocation interaction show a similar working hardening performance with that subjected to a TB–solute–dislocation interaction and (iv) both the TB–dislocation interaction and TB–solute–dislocation interaction greatly reduce the value of work-hardening peaks during a detwinning predominant deformation. Based on the fact that the reaction of lattice dislocation with TB plays a crucial role in the plastic deformation of magnesium alloys, Zhang et al. [293] studied the basal dislocation–twin interaction in a hot-rolled AZ31 sheet through precompression along rolling direction and subsequent compression along 45° of rolling direction and ND, with focus on the TB structure evolution and nucleation structure characterization. It was reported that (i) basal dislocation slip dominates the compression deformation when the strain along 45° of rolling direction and ND is less than 14%; when the strain reaches 14%, new deformation modes are initiated and (ii) when the strain is in the range of 5–14%, basal–prismatic boundaries are created by dislocation–twin interaction. Meantime, the number of the basal–prismatic boundaries increase linearly with strain, leading to an extremely incoherent TB. Mao et al. [294] investigated the twinning-stress correlation of a basal textured Mg–Al–Zn alloy after impact test and found that (i) both the tension and compression region of the sample were dominated by high density deformation twins and (ii) various twinning modes and variant selections were determined by trace method and misorientation analysis. Mao et al. [295] introduced a gradient twin microstructure in which the density of twins decreases with depth when inserted into an AZ31B Mg alloy plate by laser shock peening, followed by the sliding tests performed on surfaces with varying twin volume fraction under dry condition. It was reported that (i) both the coefficient of friction and wear rate decrease with the increase of twin volume fraction, (ii) a possible mechanism responsible for the effect of surface pretwinning on the triboperformance of Mg alloys is proposed and (iii) the improved triboperformance of Mg alloys by pretwinning are attributed to the twinning-induced hardening effect, twin growth and saturation phenomenon, and twinning-induced surface crystallographic texture change during sliding.

There are still studies on different Mg-based alloys, including Mg–Zn–Zr alloy [296], Mg-8Gd-2Y-1Nd-0.3Zn-0.6Zr alloy [297], Mg–Y alloys [298], Mg–Li–Al [299], Mg-Zn-Y-Nd-Zr alloy [300] or Mg–Gd–Mn alloy [301].

5.5.2 Dislocation engineering

High strength and good ductility are mutually exclusive demands for materials for structural applications and these properties appear to exhibit the strength–ductility trade-off nature in metallic materials. Huang et al. [302] described that (i) current alloy design strategies for improving the ductility of ultrahigh strength alloys mainly focus on the selection of alloy composition (atomic length scale) or manipulating ultrafine and nanograined microstructure (grain length scale) and (ii) the intermediate length scale between atomic and grain scales is the dislocation length scale; suggesting that the new alloy design concept be called the dislocation engineering. In fact, the transformation-induced plasticity effect is a sort of the hindsight of the dislocation engineering, by which high dislocation density is mainly responsible for the improved yield strength through dislocation forest hardening, while the improved ductility is achieved by the glide of intensive mobile dislocations [302]. Liu et al. [303] employed the one-step thermal mechanical treatment, that is, hot rolling, can effectively enhance the yielding strength of the metastable austenitic steel from 322 ± 18 MPa to 675 ± 15 MPa, while retaining both the formability and hardenability. Naraparaju et al. [304] applied the dislocation engineering and studied its effects on oxidation behavior of steel, by shot peening of the surface of steel. It was reported that severer microforging action by the shot peening resulted in an increase of the dislocation density, which can act in Cr-containing steels as fast diffusion paths for Cr promoting the formation of protective Cr oxides. Wang et al. [305] applied the dislocation engineering for developing strong and ductile Mg alloys. It was reported that (i) high density of <*c* + *a*> dislocations could be generated at appropriate temperature and retained in the Mg alloy after quenching to room temperature; (ii) those <*c* + *a*> dislocations inherited from the warm deformation could provide <*c* + *a*> dislocation sources when the Mg alloy is deformed at room temperature, resulting in good ductility; and (iii) the high dislocation density generated at warm deformation provides dislocation forest hardening, leading to improved yield strength of Mg alloy.

References

[1] Uddin MS, Hall C, Murphy P. Surface treatments for controlling corrosion rate of biodegradable Mg and Mg-based alloy implants. Science and Technology of Advanced Materials. 2015, 16: DOI: 10.1088/1468-6996/16/5/053501

[2] Mezbahul-Islam M, Mostafa AO, Medraj M. Essential magnesium alloys binary phase diagrams and their thermochemical data. Journal of Materials. 2014; 2014: https://doi.org/10.1155/2014/704283.

[3] Boby A, Pillai U, Pillai B, Pai B. Developments in magnesium alloys for transport applications – an overview. Indian Foundry Journal. 2011, 57, 29–37.

[4] Sezer N, Evis Z, Kayhan SM, Tahmasebifar A, Koç M. Review of magnesium-based biomaterials and their applications. Journal of Magnesium and Alloys. 2018, 6, 23–43.

[5] Cheng W, Ma S, Bai Y, Cui Z, Wang H. Corrosion behavior of Mg-6Bi-2Sn alloy in the simulated body fluid solution: The influence of microstructural characteristics. Journal of Alloys and Compounds. 2017, 731, 945–54.

[6] Lu Y, Bradshaw AR, Chiu YL, Jones IP. Effects of secondary phase and grain size on the corrosion of biodegradable Mg–Zn–Ca alloys. Materials Science and Engineering: C. 2015, 48, 480–6.

[7] Zhang X, Yuan G, Mao L, Niu J, Fu P, Ding W. Effects of extrusion and heat treatment on the mechanical properties and biocorrosion behaviors of a Mg-Nd-Zn-Zr alloy. Journal of the Mechanical Behavior of Biomedical Materials. 2012, 7, 77–86.

[8] Li X, Liu X, Wu S, Yeung KWK, Zheng Y, Chu PK. Design of magnesium alloys with controllable degradation for biomedical implants: From bulk to surface. Acta Biomaterialia. 2016, 45, 2–30.

[9] Kumar N, Choudhuri D, Banerjee R, Mishra RS. Strength and ductility optimization of Mg–Y–Nd–Zr alloy by microstructural design. International Journal of Plasticity. 2015, 68, 77–97.

[10] Kawamura Y, Hayashi K, Inoue A, Masumoto T. Rapidly solidified powder metallurgy $Mg_{97}Zn_1Y_2$alloys with excellent tensile yield strength above 600 MPa. Material Transactions. 2001, 42, 1172–6.

[11] Abe E, Kawamura Y, Hayashi K, Inoue A. Long-period ordered structure in a high-strength nanocrystalline Mg-1 at% Zn-2 at% Y alloy studied by atomic-resolution *Z*-contrast STEM. Acta Materialia. 2002, 50, 3845–57.
[12] Yokobayashi H, Kishida K, Inui H, Yamasaki M, Kawamura K. Enrichment of Gd and Al atoms in the quadruple close packed planes and their in-plane long-range ordering in the long period stacking-ordered phase in the Mg–Al–Gd system. Acta Materialia. 2011, 59, 7287–99.
[13] Abe E, Ono A, Itoi T, Yamasaki M, Kawamura Y. Polytypes of long-period stacking structures synchronized with chemical order in a dilute Mg-Zn-Y alloy. Journal of Philosophical Magazine Letter. 2011, 91, 690–6.
[14] Kishida K, Yokobayashi H, Unui H. A formation criterion for Order-Disorder (OD) phases of the Long-Period Stacking Order (LPSO)-type in Mg-Al-RE (Rare Earth) Ternary Systems. Scientific Reports. 2017, 7; DOI: 10.1038/s41598-017-12506-0.
[15] Cai Q et al. Effects of magnetic field on the microstructure and mechanical property of Mg-Al-Gd alloys. Materials Characterization. 2019, 154, 233–40.
[16] Yang Q et al. Coexistence of 14H and 18R-type long-period stacking ordered (LPSO) phases following a novel orientation relationship in a cast Mg–Al–RE–Zn alloy. Journal of Alloys and Compounds. 201, 766, 902–7.
[17] Ma Y et al. Effect of TiB2-doping on the microstructure and mechanical properties of Mg-Zn-Y-Mn alloy. Materials Science and Engineering: A. 2018, 724, 529–35.
[18] Leng Z et al. Microstructure and mechanical properties of Mg–9RY–4Cu alloy with long period stacking ordered phase. Materials Science and Engineering: A. 2013, 580, 196–201.
[19] Bi G et al. Microstructure and mechanical properties of an extruded Mg-Dy-Ni alloy. Materials Science and Engineering: A. 2019, 760, 246–57.
[20] Liu J et al. Effects of Ho content on microstructures and mechanical properties of Mg-Ho-Zn alloys. Materials Characterization. 2019, 149, 198–205.
[21] Gao S et al. Effect of different Co contents on the microstructure and tensile strength of Mg-Co-Y alloys. Materials Science and Engineering: A. 2019, 750, 91–7.
[22] Horváth K et al. Effect of Extrusion Ratio on Microstructure and Resulting Mechanical Properties of Mg Alloys with LPSO Phase. In: Solanki K. et al., ed., Magnesium Technology 2017. The Minerals, Metals & Materials Series. Springer, 2017, 29–34.
[23] Liu H et al. Formation behavior of 14H long period stacking ordered structure in Mg–Y–Zn cast alloys with different α-Mg fractions. Journal of Materials Science & Technology. 2016, 32, 1267–73.
[24] Gao J et al. Structural features and mechanical properties of Mg-Y-Zn-Sn alloys with varied LPSO phases. Journal of Alloys and Compounds. 2018, 768, 1029–38.
[25] Li B et al. Influence of various Yb additions on microstructures of a casting Mg–8Gd–1.2Zn–0.5Zr alloy. Journal of Alloys and Compounds. 2019, 789, 720–9.
[26] Xu D, Han E-H, Xu Y. Effect of long-period stacking ordered phase on microstructure, mechanical property and corrosion resistance of Mg alloys: A review. Progress in Natural Science: Materials International. 2016, 26, 117–28.
[27] Mendis CL, Kainer KU, Hort N. High strength magnesium alloys through precipitation hardening and micro alloying: considerations for alloy design. JOM 2015, 67, 2427–32.
[28] Nie J-F. Precipitation and hardening in magnesium alloys. Metallurgical and Materials Transactions A. 2012, 43, 3891–939.
[29] Su J, Kaboli S, Kabir ASH, Jung I-H, Yue S. Effect of dynamic precipitation and twinning on dynamic recrystallization of micro-alloyed Mg–Al–Ca alloys. Materials Science and Engineering: A. 2013, 587, 27–35.

[30] Chen C, Chen J, Yan H, Su B, Zhu S. Dynamic precipitation, microstructure and mechanical properties of Mg-5Zn-1Mn alloy sheets prepared by high strain-rate rolling. Materials & Design. 2016, 100, 58–66.
[31] Guo F, Zhang D, Yang X, Jiang L, Pan F. Strain-induced dynamic precipitation of Mg17Al12 phases in Mg–8Al alloys sheets rolled at 748K. Materials Science and Engineering: A. 2015, 636, 516–21.
[32] Guo Y, Li Y, Liu B, Liu W, Li Q. Precipitation mechanism of Mg2Ni in Mg-Ni-Y studied by STEM, 3DAP and first-principles calculations. Journal of Alloys and Compounds. 2018, 750, 117–23.
[33] Kim S-H, Lee JU, Kim YJ, Bae JH, Park SH. Accelerated precipitation behavior of cast Mg-Al-Zn alloy by grain refinement. Journal of Materials Science & Technology. 2018, 34, 265–76.
[34] Meng F, Rosalie JM, Singh A, Tsuchiya K. Precipitation behavior of an ultra-fine grained Mg–Zn alloy processed by high-pressure torsion. Materials Science and Engineering: A. 2015, 644, 386–91.
[35] Son H-T, Lee J-B, Jeong H-G, Konno TJ. Effects of Al and Zn additions on mechanical properties and precipitation behaviors of Mg–Sn alloy system. Materials Letters. 2011, 65, 1966–9.
[36] Jo SM, Kim SD, Kim T-H, Go Y, Kim YM. Sequential precipitation behavior of Mg17Al12 and Mg2Sn in Mg-8Al-2Sn-1Zn alloys. Journal of Alloys and Compounds. 2018, 749, 794–802.
[37] Chen Y, Wang Y, Gao J. Microstructure and mechanical properties of as-cast Mg-Sn-Zn-Y alloys. Journal of Alloys and Compounds. 2018, 740, 727–34.
[38] Dai J, Zhu S, Easton MA, Xu W, Ding W. Precipitation process in a Mg–Gd–Y alloy grain-refined by Al addition. Materials Characterization. 2014, 88, 7–14.
[39] Zheng J-X, Li Z, Tan L-D, Xu X-S, Chen B. Precipitation in Mg-Gd-Y-Zr Alloy: Atomic-scale insights into structures and transformations. Materials Characterization. 2016, 117, 76–83.
[40] Zhang X-M, Tang C-P, Deng Y-L, Yang L, Liu W-J. Phase transformation in Mg–8Gd–4Y–Nd–Zr alloy. Journal of Alloys and Compounds. 2011, 509, 6170–4.
[41] Xu WC, Han XZ, Shan DB. Precipitates formed in the as-forged Mg–Zn–RE alloy during ageing process at 250°C. Materials Characterization. 2013, 75, 176–83.
[42] Chen J, Chen Z, Yan H, Zhang F. Microstructural characterization and mechanical properties of a Mg–6Zn–3Sn–2Al alloy. Journal of Alloys and Compounds. 2009, 467, l1–7.
[43] Devaraj A, Wang W, Vemuri R, Kovarik L, Rohatgi A. Grain boundary segregation and intermetallic precipitation in coarsening resistant nanocrystalline aluminum alloys. Acta Materialia. 2019, 165, 698–708.
[44] Zindal A, Jain J, Prasad R, Singh SS. Effect of pre-strain and grain size on the evolution of precipitate free zones (PFZs) in a Mg-8Al-0.5Zn Alloy. Materials Letters. 2017, 201, 207–10.
[45] Zhang Y, Rong W, Wu Y, Peng L, Birbilis N. A comparative study of the role of Ag in microstructures and mechanical properties of Mg-Gd and Mg-Y alloys. Materials Science and Engineering: A. 2018, 731, 609–22.
[46] Duparc OH. The preston of the Guinier-Preston zones. Guinier. Metallurgical and Mater Trans. 2010, 41, 925–34.
[47] Barucca G, Ferragut R, Lussana D, Mengucci P, Riontino G. Phase transformations in QE22 Mg alloy. Acta Materialia. 2009, 57, 4416–25.
[48] Pan H, Qin G, Ren Y, Wang L, Meng X. Achieving high strength in indirectly-extruded binary Mg–Ca alloy containing Guinier–Preston zones. Journal of Alloys and Compounds. 2015, 630, 272–6.
[49] Liu CQ, Chen HW, Liu H, Zhao XJ, Nie JF. Metastable precipitate phases in Mg–9.8 wt%Sn Alloy. Acta Materialia. 2018, 144, 590–600.
[50] Liu Z, Pei Z, Chen B, Ding W, Zeng X. Unexpected capture of Guinier-Preston zone and γ″ phase in as-cast Mg-Gd-Y-Zn-Ni-Mn alloy: Atomic-scale insights. Materials Characterization. 2019, 153, 103–7.

[51] Hou X, Li J, Liu F, Yan L, Bai P. Coherent strain of Guinier–Preston II zone in an Al–Zn–Mg–Cu alloy. Micron. 2019, 124; https://doi.org/10.1016/j.micron.2019.102711.
[52] Bhattacharyya JJ, Nakata T, Kamado S, Agnew SR. Origins of high strength and ductility combination in a Guinier-Preston zone containing Mg-Al-Ca-Mn alloy. Scripta Materialia. 2019, 163, 121–4.
[53] Bhattacharyya JJ, Sasaki TT, Nakata T, Hono K, Kamado S, Agnew SR. Determining the strength of GP zones in Mg alloy AXM10304, both parallel and perpendicular to the zone. Acta Materialia. 2019, 171, 231–9.
[54] Suzuki A, Saddock ND, Jones JW, Pollock TM. Structure and transition of eutectic $(Mg,Al)_2Ca$ Laves phase in a die-cast Mg–Al–Ca base alloy. Scripta Materialia. 2004, 51, 1005–10.
[55] Zhong Y, Luo A, Sofo J, Liu Z-K. Laves phases in Mg-Al-Ca alloys. Minerals, Metals and Materials Soc. 2004, 317–23.
[56] Zubair M, Sandlöbes S, Wollenweber MA, Kusche CF, Korte-Kerzel S. On the role of Laves phases on the mechanical properties of Mg-Al-Ca alloys. Materials Science and Engineering: A. 2019, 756, 272–83.
[57] Kawano S, Iikubo S, Ohtani H. Thermodynamic stability of Mg-based laves phases. Material Transactions. 2018, 59, 890–6.
[58] Luo ZP, Zhang SQ, Tang YL, Zhao DS. Quasicrystals in As-cast Mg-Zn-RE Alloys. Scripta Metallurgica Et Materialia, 1993, 28, 1513–8.
[59] Wang Z, Zhao W. Mg-Based Quasicrystals. InTech. 2012; http://dx.doi.org/10.5772/481633.
[60] Li KN, Zhang YB, Zeng Q, Huang GH, Yin DD. Effects of semisolid treatment and ECAP on the microstructure and mechanical properties of Mg-6.52Zn-0.95Y alloy with icosahedral phase. Materials Science and Engineering: A. 2019, 751, 283–91.
[61] Lee JY, Lim HK, Kim DH, Kim WT, Kim DH. Effect of icosahedral phase particles on the texture evolution in Mg–Zn–Y alloys. Materials Science and Engineering: A. 2008, 491, 349–55.
[62] Xu DK, Tang WN, Liu L, Xu YB, Han EH. Effect of Y concentration on the microstructure and mechanical properties of as-cast Mg–Zn–Y–Zr alloys. Journal of Alloys and Compounds. 2007, 432, 129–34.
[63] Xu DK, Han EH. Effects of icosahedral phase formation on the microstructure and mechanical improvement of Mg alloys: A review. Progress in Natural Science: Materials International. 2012, 22, 364–85.
[64] Zhang JS, Yan J, Liang W, Xu CX, Zhou CL. Icosahedral quasicrystal phase in Mg–Zn–Nd ternary system. Materials Letters. 2008, 62, 4489–91.
[65] Zhang JS, Yan J, Liang W, Du EL, Xu CX. Microstructures of Mg–Zn–Nd alloy including small quasicrystalline grains. Journal of Non-crystalline Solids. 2009, 355, 836–9.
[66] Liu Y, Yuan G, Lu C, Ding W. Stable icosahedral phase in Mg–Zn–Gd alloy. Scripta Materialia. 2006, 55, 919–22.
[67] Wang Q, Du W, Liu K, Wang Z, Wen K. Microstructure, texture and mechanical properties of as-extruded Mg–Zn–Er alloys. Materials Science and Engineering: A. 2013, 581, 31–8.
[68] Wei G-B, Peng X-D, Zhang B, Hadadzadeh A, Xie W-D. Influence of I-phase and W-phase on microstructure and mechanical properties of Mg–8Li–3Zn alloy, Transactions of Nonferrous Metals Society of China. 2015, 25, 713–20.
[69] Zhang Y, Zhang J, Wu G, Liu W, Ding W. Microstructure and tensile properties of as-extruded Mg–Li–Zn–Gd alloys reinforced with icosahedral quasicrystal phase. Materials & Design. 2015, 66, 162–8.
[70] Xu DK, Zu TT, Yin M, Xu YB, Han EH. Mechanical properties of the icosahedral phase reinforced duplex Mg–Li alloy both at room and elevated temperatures. Journal of Alloys and Compounds. 2014, 582, 161–6.

[71] Li CQ, Xu DK, Yu S, Sheng LY, Han EH. Effect of icosahedral phase on crystallographic texture and mechanical anisotropy of Mg–4%Li based alloys. Journal of Materials Science & Technology. 2017, 33, 475–80.
[72] Kim YK, Sohn SW, Kim DH, Kim WT, Kim DH. Role of icosahedral phase in enhancing the strength of Mg–Sn–Zn–Al alloy. Journal of Alloys and Compounds. 2013, 549, 46–50.
[73] Padezhnova EM, Melnik EV, Miliyevskiy RA, Dobatkina TV, Kinzhibalo VV. Investigation of the Mg-Zn-Y System. Russ. Metall. 1982, 4, 185–8.
[74] Luo L, Liu Y, Duan M. Phase formation of Mg-Zn-Gd alloys on the Mg-rich corner. Materials. 2018, 11, 1351; DOI:10.3390/ma11081351.
[75] Yamasaki M, Anan T, Yoshimoto S, Kawamura Y. Mechanical properties of warm-extruded Mg-Zn-Gd alloy with coherent 14H long periodic stacking ordered structure precipitate. Scripta Materilia. 2005, 53, 799–803.
[76] Xu DK, Liu L, Xu YB, Han EH. The influence of element Y on the mechanical properties of the as-extruded Mg-Zn-Y-Zr alloys. Journal of Alloys Compounds 2006, 426, 155–61.
[77] Geng, JW, Teng XY, Zhou GR, Zhao DG. Microstructure transformations in the heat-treated Mg-Zn-Y alloy. Journal of Alloys Compounds 2013, 577, 498–506.
[78] Feng H, Yang Y, Chang HX. Influence of W-phase on mechanical properties and damping capacity of Mg-Zn-Y-Nd-Zr alloys. Material Science and Engineering A. 2014, 609, 7–15.
[79] Liu JF, Yang ZQ, Ye HQ. Solid-state formation of icosahedral quasicrystals at Zn3Mg3Y2/Mg interfaces in a Mg-Zn-Y alloy. Journal of Alloys Compounds 2015, 650, 65–9.
[80] Liu K, Sun C, Wang Z, Li S, Du W. Microstructure, texture and mechanical properties of Mg–Zn–Er alloys containing I-phase and W-phase simultaneously. Journal of Alloys and Compounds. 2016, 665, 76–85.
[81] Chen TJ, Zhang DH, Wang W, Ma Y, Hao Y. Effects of Zn content on microstructures and mechanical properties of Mg–Zn–RE–Sn–Zr–Ca alloys. Materials Science and Engineering: A. 2014, 607, 17–27.
[82] Zhang Z, Liu X, Hu W, Li J, Cui J. Microstructures, mechanical properties and corrosion behaviors of Mg–Y–Zn–Zr alloys with specific Y/Zn mole ratios. Journal of Alloys and Compounds. 2015, 624, 116–25.
[83] Gao S et al. Effect of Cd addition on microstructure and properties of Mg-Cd binary magnesium alloy. Rare Metal Materials and Engineering. 2015, 44, 2401–4.
[84] Gu J et al. Effects of Mn and Zn Solutes on Grain Refinement of Commercial Pure Magnesium. In: Solanki K. et al., ed., Magnesium Technology 2017. The Minerals, Metals & Materials Series. Springer, 2017, 191–198.
[85] Fang XY et al. Effect of Zr, Mn and Sc additions on the grain size of Mg–Gd alloy. Journal of Alloys and Compounds. 2009, 470, 311–6.
[86] Chai Y et al. Effects of Zn and Ca addition on microstructure and mechanical properties of as-extruded Mg-1.0Sn alloy sheet. Materials Science and Engineering: A. 2019, 746, 82–93.
[87] Kim B et al. Grain refinement and reduced yield asymmetry of extruded Mg–5Sn–1Zn alloy by Al addition. Journal of Alloys and Compounds. 2016, 660, 304–9.
[88] Wang C et al. Effect of Al additions on grain refinement and mechanical properties of Mg–Sm alloys. Journal of Alloys and Compounds. 2015, 620, 172–9.
[89] Jiang Z et al. Role of Al modification on the microstructure and mechanical properties of as-cast Mg–6Ce alloys. Materials Science and Engineering: A. 2015, 645, 57–64.
[90] Liu D et al. Effect of Al content on microstructure and mechanical properties of as-cast Mg-5Nd alloys. Journal of Alloys and Compounds. 2018, 737, 263–70.
[91] Chaubey AK et al. Microstructure and mechanical properties of Mg–Al-based alloy modified with cerium. Materials Science and Engineering: A. 2015, 625, 46–9.

[92] Langelier B et al. Improving microstructure and ductility in the Mg–Zn alloy system by combinational Ce–Ca microalloying. Materials Science and Engineering: A. 2015, 620, 76–84.
[93] Liu L et al. Effect of Y and Ce additions on microstructure and mechanical properties of Mg–Zn–Zr alloys. Materials Science and Engineering: A. 2015, 644, 247–53.
[94] Jeong HY et al. Effect of Ce addition on the microstructure and tensile properties of extruded Mg–Zn–Zr alloys. Materials Science and Engineering: A. 2014, 612, 217–2.
[95] He ML et al. Effects of Cu and Ce co-addition on the microstructure and mechanical properties of Mg-6Zn-0.5Zr Alloy. Journal of Alloys and Compounds. 2018, 767, 1216–24.
[96] Ma N et al. Effects of cerium on microstructures, recovery behavior and mechanical properties of backward extruded Mg–0.5Mn alloys. Materials Science and Engineering: A. 2013, 564, 310–6.
[97] Hu X et al. On grain coarsening and refining of the Mg–3Al alloy by Sm. Journal of Alloys and Compounds. 2016, 663, 387–94.
[98] Zhang Y et al. Effects of samarium addition on as-cast microstructure, grain refinement and mechanical properties of Mg-6Zn-0.4Zr magnesium alloy. Journal of Rare Earths. 2017, 35, 494–502.
[99] Wang P et al. The influence of Sc addition on microstructure and tensile mechanical properties of Mg–4.5Sn–5Zn alloys. Journal of Magnesium and Alloys. 2019, 7, 456–65.
[100] Kim YM et al. Grain refining mechanism in Mg–Al base alloys with carbon addition. Scripta Materialia. 2007, 57, 691–4.
[101] Du J et al. Improvement of grain refining efficiency for Mg–Al alloy modified by the combination of carbon and calcium. Journal of Alloys and Compounds. 2009, 470, 134–40.
[102] Nagasivamuni B et al. An analytical approach to elucidate the mechanism of grain refinement in calcium added Mg–Al alloys. Journal of Alloys and Compounds. 2015, 622, 789–95.
[103] Jiang B et al. Grain refinement of Ca addition in a twin-roll-cast Mg–3Al–1Zn alloy. Materials Chemistry and Physics. 2012, 133, 611–6.
[104] Zeng Y et al. Effect of Ca addition on grain refinement of Mg–9Li–1Al alloy. Journal of Magnesium and Alloys. 2013, 1, 297–302.
[105] Du J et al. Effect of strontium on the grain refining efficiency of Mg–3Al alloy refined by carbon inoculation. Journal of Alloys and Compounds. 2009, 470, 228–32.
[106] Qin GW et al. Grain refining mechanism of Al-containing Mg alloys with the addition of Mn–Al alloys. Journal of Alloys and Compounds. 2010, 507, 410–3.
[107] Peng C et al. Effect of manganese on grain refinement of Mg–Al based alloys. Scripta Materialia. 2006, 54, 1853–8.
[108] Liao H et al. Effects of Mn addition on the microstructures, mechanical properties and work-hardening of Mg-1Sn alloy. Materials Science and Engineering: A. 2109, 754, 778–85.
[109] Wei J et al. Microstructure refinement of Mg-Al-RE alloy by Gd addition. Materials Letters. 2019, 246, 125–8.
[110] Yang J et al. Influences of Gd on the microstructure and strength of Mg–4.5Zn alloy. Materials Characterization 2008, 59, 1667–74.
[111] Wu H et al. Effects of Sn on Microstructures and Mechanical Properties of As-Extruded Mg–6Al–1Ca–0.5Mn Magnesium Alloy. In: Joshi V. et al., ed., Magnesium Technology 2019. The Minerals, Metals & Materials Series. Springer, 2019, 111–117.
[112] Hu T et al. Effects of B and Sn additions on the microstructure and mechanical property of Mg-3Al-1Si alloy. Journal of Alloys and Compounds. 2019, 796, 1–8.
[113] Xiang Q et al. Influence of Sn on microstructure and mechanical properties of Mg–5Li–3Al–2Zn alloys. Journal of Alloys and Compounds. 2009, 477, 832–5.
[114] Cui C et al. Influence of yttrium on microstructure and mechanical properties of as-cast Mg–5Li–3Al–2Zn alloy. Journal of Alloys and Compounds. 2011, 509, 9045–9.

[115] Chen Y et al. Microstructure and mechanical properties of as-cast Mg-Sn-Zn-Y alloys. Journal of Alloys and Compounds. 2018, 740, 727–34.
[116] Wan YC et al. Effect of Nd and Dy on the microstructure and mechanical property of the as extruded Mg–1Zn–0.6Zr alloy. Materials Science and Engineering: A. 2015, 625, 158–63.
[117] Li RG et al. Effect of Ag addition on microstructure and mechanical properties of Mg–14Gd–0.5Zr Alloy. Materials Characterization. 2015, 109, 43–9.
[118] Hung Y et al. Mechanism of grain refinement of Mg–Al alloys by SiC inoculation. Scripta Materialia. 2011, 64, 793–6.
[119] Bae JH et al. Investigation of Grain Refinement Method for AZ91 Alloy Using Carbide Inoculation. In: Orlov D. et al., ed., Magnesium Technology 2018. TMS 2018. The Minerals, Metals & Materials Series. Springer, 2018, 71–77.
[120] Wang L et al. Effect of hafnium carbide on the grain refinement of Mg-3wt.% Al alloy. Journal of Alloys and Compounds. 2010, 500, 12–5.
[121] Suresh M et al. Microstructural refinement and tensile properties enhancement of Mg–3Al alloy using charcoal additions. Materials Science and Engineering: A. 2011, 528, 2502–8.
[122] Liu Y et al. Grain refinement of Mg–Al alloys with Al4C3–SiC/Al master alloy. Materials Letters. 2004, 58, 1282–7.
[123] Nimityongskul S et al. Grain refining mechanisms in Mg–Al alloys with Al4C3 microparticles. Materials Science and Engineering: A. 2010, 527, 2104–11.
[124] Peng X et al. Effects of Different State Mg-5Sr-10Y Master Alloys on the Microstructure Refinement of AZ31 Magnesium Alloy. Rare Metal Materials and Engineering. 2013, 42, 2421–6.
[125] Yang M et al. Effect of Mg–10Sr master alloy on grain refinement of AZ31 magnesium alloy. Materials Science and Engineering: A. 2008, 491, 440–5.
[126] Liu S et al. Grain refinement of AZ91D magnesium alloy by a new Mg–50%Al4C3 master alloy. Journal of Alloys and Compounds. 2015, 624, 266–9.
[127] Suresh M et al. Influence of boron addition on the grain refinement and mechanical properties of AZ91 Mg alloy. Materials Science and Engineering: A. 2009, 525, 207–10.
[128] Jiang B et al. Grain refinement of Mg-Li-Al cast alloys by adding typical master alloys. Progress in Natural Science: Materials International 2011, 21, 236–9.
[129] Zhang Q et al. Grain refinement and mechanical properties of Mg–5Li–3Al alloy inoculated by Al–5Ti–1B master alloy. Materials Science and Engineering: A. 2014, 619, 152–7.
[130] Jiang B et al. A new approach to grain refinement of an Mg–Li–Al cast alloy. Journal of Alloys and Compounds. 2010, 492, 95–8.
[131] Radha R, Sreekanth D. Insight of magnesium alloys and composites for orthopedic implant applications – a review. Journal of Magnesium and Alloys 2017, 5, 286–312.
[132] Qiao XG et al. Hardening mechanism of commercially pure Mg processed by high pressure torsion at room temperature. Materials Science & Engineering. A, Structural Materials 2014, 619, 95–106.
[133] Meng F et al. Ultrafine grain formation in Mg–Zn alloy by in situ precipitation during high-pressure torsion. Scripta Materialia. 2014, 78/79, 57–60.
[134] Gao JH et al. Homogeneous corrosion of high pressure torsion treated Mg–Zn–Ca alloy in simulated body fluid. Materials Letters. 2011, 65, 691–3.
[135] Sun WT et al. Exceptional grain refinement in a Mg alloy during high pressure torsion due to rare earth containing nanosized precipitates. Materials Science and Engineering: A. 2018, 728, 115–23.
[136] Sun WT et al. Evolution of microstructure and mechanical properties of an as-cast Mg-8.2Gd-3.8Y-1.0Zn-0.4Zr alloy processed by high pressure torsion. Materials Science and Engineering: A. 2017, 700, 312–20.

[137] Tork NB et al. Microstructure and texture characterization of Mg–Al and Mg–Gd binary alloys processed by simple shear extrusion. Journal of Materials Research and Technology. 2019, 8, 1288–99.
[138] Das A et al. Investigation on the microstructural refinement of an Mg–6wt.% Zn alloy. Materials Science and Engineering: A. 2006, 419, 349–56.
[139] Diez M et al. Improving the mechanical properties of pure magnesium by three-roll planetary milling. Mater. Sci. Eng. A: Structural Materials. 2014, 612, 287–92.
[140] Kang FJ et al. Equal Channel Angular Pressing of a Mg–3Al–1Zn Alloy with Back Pressure. Advances in Engineering Materials 2010, 12, 730–4.
[141] Zúberová Z et al. Fatigue and tensile behavior of cast, hot-rolled, and severely plastically deformed AZ31 magnesium alloy. Metallurgical and Materials Transactions. A 2007, 38, 1934–40.
[142] Ge Q et al. The processing of ultrafine-grained Mg tubes for biodegradable stents. Acta Biomaterialia. 2013, 9, 8604–10.
[143] Yang HJ et al. Enhancing strength and ductility of Mg–12Gd–3Y–0.5Zr alloy by forming a bi-ultrafine microstructure. Materials Science and Engineering: A. 2011, 528, 4300–11.
[144] Peláez D et al. Mechanical and microstructural evolution of Mg AZ31 alloy using ECASD process. Journal of Materials Research and Technology. 2015, 4, 392–7.
[145] Lu L et al. Modification of grain refinement and texture in AZ31 Mg alloy by a new plastic deformation method. Journal of Alloys and Compounds. 2015, 628, 130–4.
[146] Ge M-Z et al. Effect of laser energy on microstructure of Mg-3Al-1Zn alloy treated by LSP. Journal of Alloys and Compounds. 2018, 734, 266–74.
[147] Zhao F et al. Strength–ductility combination of fine-grained magnesium alloy with high deformation twin density. Journal of Alloys and Compounds. 2019, 798, 350–9.
[148] Miura H et al. Mechanisms of grain refinement in Mg–6Al–1Zn alloy during hot deformation. Materials Science and Engineering: A. 2012, 538, 63–8.
[149] Zhang H et al. The synergy effect of fine and coarse grains on enhanced ductility of bimodal-structured Mg alloys. Journal of Alloys and Compounds. 2019, 780, 312–7.
[150] Nayak S et al. Strengthening of Mg based alloy through grain refinement for orthopaedic application. Journal of the Mechanical Behavior of Biomedical Materials 2016, 59, 57–70.
[151] Wang H-Y et al. Tensile properties, texture evolutions and deformation anisotropy of as-extruded Mg-6Zn-1Zr magnesium alloy at room and elevated temperatures. Materials Science and Engineering: A. 2017, 697, 149–57.
[152] Du BN et al. Optimization of microstructure and mechanical property of a Mg-Zn-Y-Nd alloy by extrusion process. Journal of Alloys and Compounds. 2019, 775, 990–1001.
[153] Cai C et al. Effect of microstructure evolution on tensile fracture behavior of Mg-2Zn-1Nd-0.6Zr alloy for biomedical applications. Materials & Design. 2019, 182; https://doi.org/10.1016/j.matdes.2019.108038.
[154] Li Z et al. The synergistic effect of trace Sr and Zr on the microstructure and properties of a biodegradable Mg-Zn-Zr-Sr alloy. Journal of Alloys and Compounds. 2017, 702, 290–302.
[155] Guo X et al. Reciprocating extrusion of rapidly solidified Mg–6Zn–1Y–0.6Ce–0.6Zr alloy. Journal of Materials Processing Technology 2007, 187, 640–4.
[156] Trivedi P et al. Grain refinement to submicron regime in multiaxial forged Mg-2Zn-2Gd alloy and relationship to mechanical properties. Materials Science and Engineering: A. 2016, 668, 59–65.
[157] Xi W et al. Promotion effect of secondary phase particles on grain refinement of deformed Mg–Y–Nd–Zn alloy. Materials Science and Engineering: A. 2015, 628, 247–51.
[158] Asgari H et al. Effect of grain size on high strain rate deformation of rolled Mg–4Y–3RE alloy in compression. Materials Science and Engineering: A. 2015, 633, 92–102.

[159] Jiang B et al. Effect of Sr on microstructure and aging behavior of Mg–14Li alloys. Progress in Natural Science: Materials International. 2012, 22, 160–8.
[160] Meng S et al. Microstructure and mechanical properties of an extruded Mg-8Bi-1Al-1Zn (wt%) alloy. Materials Science and Engineering: A. 2017, 690, 80–7.
[161] Pan H et al. Ultra-fine grain size and exceptionally high strength in dilute Mg–Ca alloys achieved by conventional one-step extrusion. Materials Letters. 2019, 237, 65–8.
[162] Xiao Z et al. Microstructural development under interrupted hot deformation and the mechanical properties of a cast Mg–Gd–Y–Zr alloy. Materials Science and Engineering: A. 2016, 652, 377–83.
[163] Callister WD. Fundamentals of Materials Science and Engineering, 2nd ed. John Wiley & Sons. 2004.
[164] Naik SN, Walley SM. The Hall–Petch and inverse Hall–Petch relations and the hardness of nanocrystalline metals. Journal of Material Science. 2020, 55, 2661–81.
[165] Ryou H, Drazin JW, Wahl KJ, Qadri SB, Gorzkowski EP, Feigelson BN, Wollmershauser JA. Below the Hall–Petch limit in nanocrystalline ceramics. ACS Nano. 2018, 12, 3083–94.
[166] Whang SH. Nanostructured Metals and Alloys: Processing, Microstructure, Mechanical Properties and Applications. Woodhead Pub. 2011.
[167] Yu H, Xin Y, Wang M, Liu Q. Hall-Petch relationship in Mg alloys: A review. Journal of Materials Science & Technology. 2018, 34, 248–56.
[168] Wang Y, Choo H. Influence of texture on Hall–Petch relationships in an Mg alloy. Acta Materialia. 2014, 81, 83–97.
[169] Shi BQ, Cheng YQ, Shang XL, Yan W, Ke W. Hall-Petch relationship, twinning responses and their dependences on grain size in the rolled Mg-Zn and Mg-Y alloys. Materials Science and Engineering: A. 2019, 743, 558–66.
[170] Lenard JG. Dynamic recrystallization. Comprehensive Materials Processing. 2014; https://www.sciencedirect.com/topics/engineering/dynamic-recrystallization
[171] Laughlin DE, Hono K. Static recrystallization. Physical Metallurgy. 2015: https://www.sciencedirect.com/topics/engineering/static-recrystallization
[172] Shkatove V, Mazur I. Modeling the dynamic recrystallization and flow curves using the kinetics of static recrystallization. Materials. 2019, 12, 3024–33.
[173] Guo-Zheng Q. Characterization for Dynamic Recrystallization Kinetics Based on Stress-Strain Curves, Recent Developments in the Study of Recrystallization, Peter Wilson, IntechOpen. 2013; https://www.intechopen.com/books/recent-developments-in-the-study-of-recrystallization/characterization-for-dynamic-recrystallization-kinetics-based-on-stress-strain-curves.
[174] McQueen HJ. Development of dynamic recrystallization theory. Materials Science and Engineering: A. 2004, 387/389, 203–8.
[175] Huang K, Logé RE. A review of dynamic recrystallization phenomena in metallic materials. Materials & Design. 2016, 111, 548–74.
[176] Zener C, Hollomon JH. Effect of strain rate upon plastic flow of steel. Journal of Applied Physics 1944, 15, 22–32.
[177] Watanabe H, Tsutsui H, Mukai T, Ishikawa H, Okanda Y, Kohzu M, Higashi K. Grain size control of commercial wrought Mg-Al-Zn alloys utilizing dynamic recrystallization. Materials Transactions. 2001, 42, 1200–5.
[178] Takigawa Y, Honda M, Uesugi T, Higashi K. Effect of initial grain size on dynamically recrystallized grain size in AZ31 magnesium alloy. Materials Transactions. 2008, 49, 1979–82.
[179] Hirai K, Smekawa H, Takigawa Y, Higashi K. Superplastic forging with dynamic recrystallization of Mg–Al–Zn alloys cast by thixo-molding. Scripta Mater. 2007, 56, 237–40.

[180] Kaibyshev RO, Galiev AM, Sokolov BK. Phys. Effect of grain size on the plastic deformation and dynamic recrystallization of a magnesium alloy. The Physics of Metals and Metallography. 1994, 78, 209–17.

[181] Yang X, Miura H, Sakai T. Dynamic Evolution of New Grains in Magnesium Alloy AZ31 during Hot Deformation. Materials Transactions. 2003, 44, 197–203.

[182] Duygulu Ö. Production and development of wrought Magnesium alloys. PhD Dissertation, Istanbul Technical University, 2009.

[183] Li L, Wang Y, Li H, Jiang W, Garmestani H. Effect of the Zener-Hollomon parameter on the dynamic recrystallization kinetics of Mg–Zn–Zr–Yb magnesium alloy. Computational Materials Science. 2019, 166, 221–9.

[184] Yu S, Liu C, Gao Y, Jiang S, Bao Z. Dynamic recrystallization mechanism of Mg-8.5Gd-2.5Y-0.4Zr alloy during hot ring rolling. Materials Characterization. 2017, 131, 135–9.

[185] Němec M et al. Influence of alloying element Zn on the microstructural, mechanical and corrosion properties of binary Mg-Zn alloys after severe plastic deformation. Materials Characterization. 2017, 134, 69–75.

[186] Du YZ et al. The microstructure, texture and mechanical properties of extruded Mg–5.3Zn–0.2Ca–0.5Ce (wt%) alloy. Materials Science and Engineering: A. 2015, 620, 164–71.

[187] Guan K et al. Effects of samarium content on microstructure and mechanical properties of Mg–0.5Zn–0.5Zr alloy. Journal of Materials Science & Technology. 2019, 35, 1368–77.

[188] Lv S et al. Influence of Nd addition on microstructures and mechanical properties of a hot-extruded Mg–6.0Zn–0.5Zr (wt.%) alloy. Journal of Alloys and Compounds. 2019, 806, 1166–79.

[189] Shahzad M et al. The roles of Zn distribution and eutectic particles on microstructure development during extrusion and anisotropic mechanical properties in a Mg–Zn–Zr alloy. Materials Science and Engineering: A. 2015, 620, 50–7.

[190] Geng L et al. Microstructure and mechanical properties of Mg–4.0Zn–0.5Ca Alloy. Materials Letters. 2009, 63, 557–9.

[191] Sun H-F et al. Evolution of microstructure and mechanical properties of Mg–3.0Zn–0.2Ca–0.5Y alloy by extrusion at various temperatures. Journal of Materials Processing Technology. 2016, 229, 633–40.

[192] Hu G-S et al. Microstructures and mechanical properties of as-extruded and heat treated Mg–6Zn–1Mn–4Sn–1.5Nd alloy. Transactions of Nonferrous Metals Society of China. 2015, 25, 1439–45.

[193] Wang C et al. Microstructure and mechanical properties of Mg-5Zn-3.5Sn-1Mn-0.5Ca-0.5Cualloy. Materials Characterization. 2019, 147, 406–13.

[194] Lu X et al. Microstructure and mechanical properties of Mg-3.0Zn-1.0Sn-0.3Mn-0.3Ca alloy extruded at different temperatures. Journal of Alloys and Compounds. 2018, 732, 257–69.

[195] Zheng X et al. Effect of trace addition of al on microstructure, texture and tensile ductility of Mg-6Zn-0.5Er Alloy. Journal of Magnesium and Alloys. 2016, 4, 135–9.

[196] Du Y et al. Effects of precipitates on microstructure evolution and texture in Mg-Zn alloy during hot deformation. Vacuum. 2018, 148, 27–32.

[197] Hadadzadeh A et al. Modeling dynamic recrystallization during hot deformation of a cast-homogenized Mg-Zn-Zr alloy. Materials Science and Engineering: A. 2018, 720, 180–8.

[198] Wu Q et al. Dynamic precipitation behavior before dynamic recrystallization in a Mg-Zn-Mn alloy during hot compression. Materials Characterization. 2019, 153, 14–23.

[199] Zhang Y et al. Deformation behavior and dynamic recrystallization of a Mg–Zn–Y–Zr alloy. Materials Science and Engineering: A. 2006, 428, 91–7.

[200] Fan Z et al. Dynamic recrystallization kinetic of fine grained Mg-Zn-Y-Zr alloy solidified under high pressure. Journal of Rare Earths. 2017, 35, 920–6.

[201] Zhao D-Q et al. Constitutive modeling for dynamic recrystallization kinetics of Mg–4Zn–2Al–2Sn alloy. Transactions of Nonferrous Metals Society of China. 2018, 28, 340–7.
[202] Yu H et al. Effects of minor Gd addition on microstructures and mechanical properties of the high strain-rate rolled Mg–Zn–Zr alloys. Journal of Alloys and Compounds. 2014, 586, 757–65.
[203] Chen C et al. Dynamic precipitation, microstructure and mechanical properties of Mg-5Zn-1Mn alloy sheets prepared by high strain-rate rolling. Materials & Design. 2016, 100, 58–66.
[204] Fang X et al. Effects of yttrium on recrystallization and grain growth of Mg4.9Zn-0.7Zr Alloy. Journal of Rare Earths. 2008, 26, 392–7.
[205] Ha C et al. Deformation and Recrystallization Mechanisms and Their Influence on the Microstructure Development of Rare Earth Containing Magnesium Sheets. In: Orlov D. et al., ed., Magnesium Technology 2018. TMS 2018. The Minerals, Metals & Materials Series. Springer, 2018, 209–216.
[206] Farzadfar SA et al. On the deformation, recrystallization and texture of hot-rolled Mg–2.9Y and Mg–2.9Zn solid solution alloys – A comparative study. Materials Science and Engineering: A. 2012, 534, 209–19.
[207] Zheng R et al. Simultaneously enhanced strength and ductility of Mg-Zn-Zr-Ca alloy with fully recrystallized ultrafine grained structures. Scripta Materialia. 2017, 131, 1–5.
[208] Singh A et al. Nucleation of recrystallized magnesium grains over quasicrystalline phase during severe plastic deformation of a Mg-Zn-Y alloy at room temperature. Scripta Materialia. 2017, 134, 80–4.
[209] Hradilová M et al. Effect of Ca-addition on dynamic recrystallization of Mg–Zn alloy during hot deformation. Materials Science and Engineering: A. 2013, 580, 217–26.
[210] Farzadfar SA et al. Role of yttrium in the microstructure and texture evolution of Mg. Materials Science and Engineering: A 2011, 528, 6742–53.
[211] Tong LB et al. Influence of deformation rate on microstructure, texture and mechanical properties of indirect-extruded Mg–Zn–Ca alloy. Materials Characterization. 2015, 104, 66–72.
[212] Kang H et al. Deformation behavior of a statically recrystallized Mg–Zn–MM alloy sheet. Materials Science and Engineering: A. 2013, 582, 203–10.
[213] Zou J et al. Effects of Sn addition on dynamic recrystallization of Mg-5Zn-1Mn alloy during high strain rate deformation. Materials Science and Engineering: A. 2018, 735, 49–60.
[214] Dogan E et al. Dynamic precipitation in Mg-3Al-1Zn alloy during different plastic deformation modes. Acta Materialia. 2016, 116, 1–13.
[215] Razzaghi M et al. Unraveling the effects of Zn addition and hot extrusion process on the microstructure and mechanical properties of as-cast Mg–2Al magnesium alloy. Vacuum. 2019, 167, 214–22.
[216] Park SH et al. Influence of Sn addition on the microstructure and mechanical properties of extruded Mg–8Al–2Zn alloy. Materials Science and Engineering: A. 2015, 626, 128–35.
[217] Wang J et al. The effect of Y content on microstructure and tensile properties of the extruded Mg–1Al-xY alloy. Materials Science and Engineering: A 2019, 765; https://doi.org/10.1016/j.msea.2019.138288.
[218] She J et al. Microstructure and mechanical properties of Mg–Al–Sn extruded alloys. Journal of Alloys and Compounds 2016, 657, 893–905.
[219] Li ZT et al. Effect of Ca/Al ratio on microstructure and mechanical properties of Mg-Al-Ca-Mn alloys. Materials Science and Engineering: A. 2017, 682, 423–32.
[220] Li S et al. Microstructure and mechanical properties of hot extruded Mg-8.89Li-0.96Zn alloy. Results in Physics 2019, 13; https://doi.org/10.1016/j.rinp.2019.02.084.
[221] Sun Y et al. Microstructure, texture, and mechanical properties of as-extruded Mg-xLi-3Al-2Zn-0.2Zr alloys (x = 5, 7, 8, 9, 11 wt%). Materials Science and Engineering: A. 2019, 755, 201–10.

[222] Yang Y et al. Microstructure and Mechanical Behavior of a New α+β-Type Mg-9Li-3Al-2.5Sr Alloy. Rare Metal Materials and Engineering. 2014, 43, 1281–5.
[223] Li J et al. Microstructure, mechanical properties and aging behaviors of as-extruded Mg–5Li–3Al–2Zn–1.5Cu alloy. Materials Science and Engineering: A. 2011, 528, 3915–20.
[224] Ahn K et al. Material model for dynamic recrystallization of Mg–8Al–0.5Zn alloy under uni-axial compressive deformation with variation of forming temperatures. Materials Science and Engineering: A. 2016, 651, 1010–7.
[225] Kabir ASH et al. Effect of strain-induced precipitation on dynamic recrystallization in Mg–Al–Sn alloys. Materials Science and Engineering: A. 2014, 616, 252–9.
[226] Su J et al. Effect of dynamic precipitation and twinning on dynamic recrystallization of micro-alloyed Mg–Al–Ca alloys. Materials Science and Engineering: A. 2013, 587, 27–35.
[227] Junwei L et al. Microstructure evolution and constitutive equation for the hot deformation of LZ91 Mg alloy. Catalysis Today. 2018, 318, 119–25.
[228] Xie C et al. Transition of dynamic recrystallization mechanisms of as-cast AZ31 Mg alloys during hot compression. International Journal of Plasticity. 2018, 111, 211–33.
[229] Prakash P et al. Microstructure and Texture Evolution During Hot Compression of Cast and Extruded AZ80 Magnesium Alloy. In: Joshi V. et al., ed., Magnesium Technology 2019. The Minerals, Metals & Materials Series. Springer, 2019, 89–94.
[230] Zhou Y et al. Effects of second phases on deformation behavior and dynamic recrystallization of as-cast Mg-4.3Li-4.1Zn-1.4Y alloy during hot compression. Journal of Alloys and Compounds. 2019, 770, 540–8.
[231] Xu TC et al. Dynamic recrystallization behavior of Mg–Li–Al–Nd duplex alloy during hot compression. Journal of Alloys and Compounds. 2015, 639, 79–88.
[232] Su J et al. Dynamic recrystallization mechanisms during high speed rolling of Mg–3Al–1Zn alloy sheets. Scripta Materialia 2016, 113, 198–201.
[233] Lee JH et al. Dynamic recrystallization behavior and microstructural evolution of Mg alloy AZ31 through high-speed rolling. Journal of Materials Science & Technology. 2018, 34, 1747–55.
[234] Guo F et al. Deformation behavior of AZ31 Mg alloys sheet during large strain hot rolling process: A study on microstructure and texture evolutions of an intermediate-rolled sheet. Journal of Alloys and Compounds. 2016, 663, 140–7.
[235] Jin Z-Z et al. Effects of Mg17Al12 second phase particles on twinning-induced recrystallization behavior in Mg–Al–Zn alloys during gradient hot rolling. Journal of Materials Science & Technology 2019, 35, 2017–26.
[236] Luo D et al. Microstructure evolution and tensile properties of hot rolled Mg–6Al–3Sn alloy sheet at elevated temperatures. Materials Science and Engineering: A. 2015, 643, 149–55.
[237] Liu Y et al. Recrystallization and microstructure evolution of the rolled Mg–3Al–1Zn alloy strips under electropulsing treatment. Journal of Alloys and Compounds. 2015, 622, 229–35.
[238] Xu Q et al. Thermal and electromigration effects of electropulsing on dynamic recrystallization in Mg–3Al–1Zn alloy. Materials Science and Engineering: A. 2011, 528, 4431–6.
[239] Li X et al. Deformation mechanisms and recrystallization behavior of Mg-3Al-1Zn and Mg-1Gd alloys deformed by electroplastic-asymmetric rolling. Materials Science and Engineering: A. 2019, 742, 722–33.
[240] Zhang W et al. Dynamic recrystallization in nanocrystalline AZ31 Ma-alloy. Vacuum. 2017, 143, 236–40.
[241] Jiang MG et al. Microstructure, texture and mechanical properties in an as-cast AZ61 Mg alloy during multi-directional impact forging and subsequent heat treatment. Materials & Design. 2015, 87, 891–900.
[242] Chen Y et al. Effects of extrusion ratio on the microstructure and mechanical properties of AZ31 Mg alloy. Journal of Materials Processing Technology. 2007, 182, 281–5.

[243] Yang Y et al. Microstructure and mechanical behavior of Mg–10Li–3Al–2.5Sr alloy. Materials Science and Engineering: A. 2014, 611, 1–8.
[244] Liu H et al. Microstructure and mechanical property of a high-strength Mg–10Gd–6Y–1.5Zn–0.5Zr alloy prepared by multi-pass equal channel angular pressing. Journal of Magnesium and Alloys. 2017, 5, 231–7.
[245] Zhou X et al. Microstructure and mechanical properties of extruded Mg-Gd-Y-Zn-Zr alloys filled with intragranular LPSO phases. Materials Characterization. 2018, 135, 76–83.
[246] Tong LB et al. Dynamic recrystallization and texture evolution of Mg–Y–Zn alloy during hot extrusion process. Materials Characterization. 2014, 92, 77–83.
[247] Hoseini-Athar MM et al. Effect of Zn addition on dynamic recrystallization behavior of Mg-2Gd alloy during high-temperature deformation. Journal of Alloys and Compounds. 2019, 806, 1200–6.
[248] Fatemi SM et al. Dynamic precipitation and dynamic recrystallization during hot deformation of a solutionized WE43 magnesium alloy. Materials Science and Engineering: A. 2019, 762; https://doi.org/10.1016/j.msea.2019.138076.
[249] Zhang D et al. Dynamic recrystallization behaviors of Mg-Gd-Y-Zn-Zr alloy with different morphologies and distributions of LPSO phases. Materials Science and Engineering: A. 2018, 715, 389–403.
[250] Yang Z et al. Effect of homogenization on the hot-deformation ability and dynamic recrystallization of Mg–9Gd–3Y–0.5Zr alloy. Materials Science and Engineering: A. 2009, 515, 102–7.
[251] Lu SH et al. The effect of twinning on dynamic recrystallization behavior of Mg-Gd-Y alloy during hot compression. Journal of Alloys and Compounds. 2019, 803, 277–90.
[252] Wu WX et al. Effect of initial microstructure on the dynamic recrystallization behavior of Mg–Gd–Y–Zr alloy. Materials Science and Engineering: A. 2012, 556, 519–25.
[253] Cottam R et al. Dynamic recrystallization of Mg and Mg–Y alloys: Crystallographic texture development. Materials Science and Engineering: A. 2008, 485, 375–82.
[254] Xiao HC et al. Hot deformation and dynamic recrystallization behaviors of Mg–Gd–Y–Zr alloy. Materials Science and Engineering: A. 2015, 628, 311–8.
[255] Chi YQ et al. Effect of trace zinc on the microstructure and mechanical properties of extruded Mg-Gd-Y-Zr alloy. Journal of Alloys and Compounds. 2019, 789, 416–27.
[256] Shi XY et al. Microstructure evolution and mechanical properties of an Mg–Gd alloy subjected to surface mechanical attrition treatment. Materials Science and Engineering: A. 2015, 630, 146–54.
[257] Kim S-H et al. Effect of Ce addition on the microstructure and mechanical properties of extruded Mg-Sn-Al-Zn alloy. Materials Science and Engineering: A. 2016, 657, 406–12.
[258] Kim S-H et al. Controlling the microstructure and improving the tensile properties of extruded Mg-Sn-Zn alloy through Al addition. Journal of Alloys and Compounds. 2018, 751, 1–11.
[259] Guan K et al. Microstructures and mechanical properties of a high-strength Mg-3.5Sm-0.6Zn-0.5Zr alloy. Materials Science and Engineering: A. 2017, 703, 97–107
[260] Borkar H et al. Effect of extrusion temperature on texture evolution and recrystallization in extruded Mg–1% Mn and Mg–1% Mn–1.6%Sr alloys. Journal of Alloys and Compounds. 2013, 555, 219–24.
[261] Zhang D et al. Effect of heat treatment on dynamic recrystallization behaviors and mechanical properties of Mg–2.7Nd–0.5Zn–0.8Zr alloy. Materials Science and Engineering: A. 2016, 675, 128–37.
[262] Meng J, Sun L, Zhang Y, Xue F, Chu C, Bai J. Evolution of recrystallized grain and texture of cold-drawn pure Mg wire and their effect on mechanical properties. Materials. 2020, 13, 427; DOI:10.3390/ma13020427.

[263] Lee J-Y, Yun Y-S, Suh B-C, Kim N-J, Kim D-H. Comparison of static recrystallization behavior in hot rolled Mg–3Al–1Zn and Mg–3Zn–0.5Ca Sheets. Journal of Alloys and Compounds. 2014, 589, 240–6.
[264] Huang X, Suzuki K, Chino Y. Static recrystallization behavior of hot-rolled Mg-Zn-Ce magnesium alloy sheet. Journal of Alloys and Compounds. 2017, 724, 981–90.
[265] Liu P, Jiang H, Cai Z, Kang Q, Zhang Y. The effect of Y, Ce and Gd on texture, recrystallization and mechanical property of Mg–Zn alloys. Journal of Magnesium and Alloys. 2016, 4, 188–96.
[266] Yang X-Y, Zhu Y-K, Miura H, Sakai T. Static recrystallization behavior of hot-deformed magnesium alloy AZ31 during isothermal annealing. Transactions of Nonferrous Metals Society of China. 2010, 20, 1269–74.
[267] Zhang J, Li W, Guo Z. Static recrystallization and grain growth during annealing of an extruded Mg–Zn–Zr–Er magnesium alloy. Journal of Magnesium and Alloys. 2013, 1, 31–8.
[268] Zhao LY, Yan H, Chen RS, Han E-H. Study on the evolution pattern of grain orientation and misorientation during the static recrystallization of cold-rolled Mg-Zn-Gd alloy. Materials Characterization. 2019, 150, 252–66.
[269] Shah SSA, Wu D, Chen RS, Song GS. Static recrystallization behavior of multi-directional impact forged Mg-Gd-Y-Zr alloy. Journal of Alloys and Compounds. 2019, 805, 189–97.
[270] Xu C, Wang X, Zhang J, Zhang Z. Effect of Nd and Yb on the Microstructure and Mechanical Properties of Mg-Zn-Zr Alloy. Rare Metal Materials and Engineering. 2014, 43, 1809–14.
[271] Hradilová M, Vojtěch D, Kubásek J, Čapek J, Vlach M. Structural and mechanical characteristics of Mg–4Zn and Mg–4Zn–0.4Ca alloys after different thermal and mechanical processing routes. Materials Science and Engineering: A. 2013, 586, 284–91.
[272] Hou X, Peng Q, Cao Z, Xu S, Wang L. Structure and mechanical properties of extruded Mg–Gd based alloy sheet. Materials Science and Engineering: A. 2009, 520, 162–7.
[273] Kubásek J, Vojtěch D, Martínek M. Structural characteristics and elevated temperature mechanical properties of AJ62 Mg alloy. Materials Characterization. 2013, 86, 270–82.
[274] Lin X, Dong Y, Ye J, Song B. The microstructure of Mg–4Zn–2Al–0.5Ca aged alloy. Materials Science and Engineering: A. 2012, 538, 231–5.
[275] Liu H, Chen Y, Zhao H, Wei S, Gao W. Effects of strontium on microstructure and mechanical properties of as-cast Mg–5wt.%Sn Alloy. Journal of Alloys and Compounds. 2010, 504, 345–50.
[276] Braszczyńska-Malik KN, Grzybowska A. Influence of phase composition on microstructure and properties of Mg-5Al-0.4Mn-xRE (x=0, 3 and 5wt.%) alloys. Materials Characterization. 2016, 115, 14–22.
[277] Hanna A, Azzeddine H, Huang Y, Bradai D, Langdon TG. An investigation of the thermal stability of an MgDy alloy after processing by high-pressure torsion. Materials Characterization. 2019, 151, 519–29.
[278] Cheng YT, Hung TH, Huang JC, Hsieh PJ, Jang JSC. Thermal stability and crystallization kinetics of Mg–Cu–Y–B quaternary alloys. Materials Science and Engineering: A. 2007, 449/451, 501–5.
[279] Minárik P, Veselý J, Čížek J, Zemková M, Stráská J. Effect of secondary phase particles on thermal stability of ultra-fine grained Mg-4Y-3RE alloy prepared by equal channel angular pressing. Materials Characterization. 2018, 140, 207–16.
[280] Zhang H, Yan C, Li C, Xin Y, Liu Q. Thermal stability of extension twins in Mg-3Al-1Zn rods. Journal of Alloys and Compounds. 2017, 696, 428–34.
[281] Liu T, Yang Q, Guo N, Lu Y, Song B. Stability of twins in Mg alloys – A short review. Journal of Magnesium and Alloys. 2020, 8, 66–77.
[282] Shi D, Liu T, Wang T, Hou D, Zhao S, Hussain S. {10–12} Twins across twin boundaries traced by *in situ* EBSD. Journal of Alloys and Compounds. 2017, 690, 699–706.

[283] Zhu B, Li X, Xie C, Wu Y, Zhang J. {10–12} extension twin variant selection under a high train rate in AZ31 magnesium alloy during the plane strain compression. Vacuum. 2019, 160, 279–85.
[284] Gu X-F, Wang M, Shi Z-Z, Chen L, Yang P. Asymmetrical Precipitation on the {10-12} Twin Boundary in the Magnesium Alloy. Metallurgical and Materials Transactions A. 2018, 49, 4446–51.
[285] Kumar MA, Clausen B, Capolungo L, McCabe RJ, Liu W, Tischler JZ, Tomé CN. Deformation twinning and grain partitioning in a hexagonal close-packed magnesium alloy. Nature Communications. 2018, 9; DOI:10.1038/s41467-018-07028-w.
[286] Wan X, Zhang J, Mo X, Pan F. 3D atomic-scale growth characteristics of {10–12} twin in magnesium. Journal of Magnesium and Alloys. 2019, 7, 474–86.
[287] Clark JB. Age hardening in a Mg-9 wt.% Al alloy. Acta Metall 1968, 16, 141–52.
[288] Gharghouri MA, Weatherly GC, Embury JD. The interaction of twins and precipitates in a Mg-7.7 At.% Al Alloy. Phil. Mag. A. 1998, 8, 1137–49.
[289] Dobroň P, Drozdenko D, Hegedűs M, Olejňák J, Horváth K, Bohlen J. Thermo-Mechanical Treatment of Extruded Mg–1Zn Alloy: Cluster Analysis of AE Signals. In: Orlov D. et al., ed., Magnesium Technology 2018. TMS 2018. The Minerals, Metals & Materials Series. Springer, 2018, 217–221.
[290] Robson JD, Stanford N, Barrnet MR. Effect of particles in promoting twin nucleation in a Mg–5 wt.% Zn alloy. Scripta Materialia. 2010, 63, 823–26.
[291] Wang L, Huang G, Quan Q, Bassani P, Mostaed E, Vedani M, Pan F. The effect of twinning and detwinning on the mechanical property of AZ31 extruded magnesium alloy during strain-path changes. Materials & Design. 2014, 63, 177–84.
[292] Xu J, Guan B, Yu H, Cao X, Liu Q. Effect of Twin Boundary–Dislocation–Solute Interaction on Detwinning in a Mg–3Al–1Zn Alloy. Journal of Materials Science & Technology. 2016, 32, 1239–44.
[293] Zhang J, Xi G, Wan X, Fang C. The dislocation-twin interaction and evolution of twin boundary in AZ31 Mg alloy. Acta Materialia. 2017, 133, 208–16.
[294] Mao L, Liu C, Chen T, Gao Y, Wang R. Twinning behavior in a rolled Mg-Al-Zn alloy under dynamic impact loading. Scripta Materialia. 2018, 150, 87–91.
[295] Mao B, Siddaiah A, Zhang X, Li B, Liao Y. The influence of surface pre-twinning on the friction and wear performance of an AZ31B Mg alloy. Applied Surface Science. 2019, 480, 998–1007.
[296] Qiao H, Agnew SR, Wu PD. Modeling twinning and detwinning behavior of Mg alloy ZK60A during monotonic and cyclic loading. International Journal of Plasticity. 2015, 65, 61–84.
[297] Hou X, Cao Z, Sun X, Wang L-d, Wang L-m. Twinning and dynamic precipitation upon hot compression of a Mg–Gd–Y–Nd–Zr alloy. Journal of Alloys and Compounds. 2012, 525, 103–9.
[298] Sandlöbes S, Friák M, Neugebauer J, Raabe D. Basal and non-basal dislocation slip in Mg–Y. Materials Science and Engineering: A. 2013, 576, 61–8.
[299] Pugazhendhi BS, Kar A, Sinnaeruvadi K, Suwas S. Effect of aluminium on microstructure, mechanical property and texture evolution of dual phase Mg-8Li alloy in different processing conditions. Archives of Civil and Mechanical Engineering. 2018, 18, 1332–44.
[300] Wang J, Zhou H, Wang L, Zhu S, Guan S. Microstructure, mechanical properties and deformation mechanisms of an as-cast Mg–Zn–Y–Nd–Zr alloy for stent applications. Journal of Materials Science & Technology. 2019, 35, 1211–7.
[301] Zhao T, Hu Y, He B, Zhang C, Pan F. Effect of manganese on microstructure and properties of Mg-2Gd magnesium alloy. Materials Science and Engineering: A. 2019, 765; https://doi.org/10.1016/j.msea.2019.138292.
[302] Huang MX, He BB. Alloy design by dislocation engineering. Journal of Materials Science & Technology. 2018, 34, 417–20.

[303] Liu J, Jin Y, Fang X, Chen C, Feng Q, Liu X, Chen Y, Suo T, Zhao F, Huang T, Wang H, Wang X, Fang Y, Wei Y, Meng L, Lu J, Yang W. Dislocation strengthening without ductility trade-off in metastable austenitic steels. Scientific Reports. 2016, 6; https://doi.org/10.1038/srep35345.
[304] Naraparaju R, Christ H-J, Renner FU, Kostka A. Dislocation engineering and its effect on the oxidation behaviour. Journal of Materials at High Temperatures. 2012, 29, 116–22.
[305] Wang M, He BB, Hunag MX. Strong and ductile Mg alloys developed by dislocation engineering. Journal of Materials Science & Technology. 2019, 35, 394–5.

Chapter 6
Synthesis and casting

Magnesium casting technology was well developed during and after World War II, both in gravity sand and permanent mold casting as well as high-pressure die casting, for aerospace, defense and automotive applications. In the last 20 years, most of the development has been focused on thin-wall die casting applications in the automotive industry, taking advantages of the good castability due to excellent fluidity of modern magnesium alloys. Recently, the continued expansion of magnesium casting applications in automotive, defense, aerospace, electronics, power tools and even implants and other medical applications has led to the diversification of casting processes into vacuum die casting, low-pressure die casting, squeeze casting, lost foam casting and ablation casting as well as semisolid casting [1–4]. Secondary products in various forms (like foil, film, sheet, pipe, tube or closer to final shapes) can be fabricated and processed using the primary products which are synthesized by various methods, including fully liquid state methods (e.g., casting) or solid-state techniques (e.g., mechanical alloying (MA) or powder metallurgy) [5]. Our discussion will start with characterizing solidification phenomenon and its effect on subsequent properties which are directly related to casting methods and will continue to various types of casting technologies. Then, we will proceed to elucidate solid-state methods as well as advanced additive manufacturing (AM).

6.1 Casting

6.1.1 Solidification behaviors

During solidification process from the melt, metal crystal (or crystal aggregates) can take different forms. The description of the structure of growing crystals is performed by morphology of solidification, whose relationship with casting properties have been worked out so that reliable conclusions regarding its casting behavior in practice can be drawn if the solidification behavior of an alloy is known [6]. Wang et al. [7] studied the effects of Zn and rare earth (RE) element additions on the solidification behavior of Mg–9Al alloy and reported that (i) Zn additions decreased the end-solidifying temperature, promoted the precipitation of $Mg_{17}Al_{12}$ in grain boundaries and increased the hot tearing susceptibility coefficient, (ii) Al_4RE phase precipitation slowed down the temperature decrease at the initial stage of solidification and (iii) RE additions had little effect on hot tearing susceptibility of Mg–9Al with low or no Zn content, while when Zn content exceeded 0.8 wt%, RE additions decreased the hot tearing susceptibility of Mg–9Al alloys distinctly. Javaid et al. [8] investigated the

https://doi.org/10.1515/9783110676945-006

solidification behavior of dilute Mg–Zn–Nd alloys and the commercial grade ZEK100 (Mg-Zn-RE-Zr). It was found that (i) for a constant Zn content of 2% and 4%, an increase in Nd content in the range of 1–2% caused a reduction in liquidus temperature but increase in solidus and eutectic temperatures; (ii) as verified by controlled solidification experiments, the cooling rate during solidification affected the refinement of alloy microstructure, a volume fraction of intermetallic precipitates and their distribution; (iii) there was no obvious influence of Nd content on the value of secondary dendrite arm spacing for all cooling rates examined; however, there was an influence of Zn where an increase of its content from 1% to 4% halved the average secondary dendrite arm spacing; and (iv) the beneficial role of Zr is confirmed and a presence of 0.25% Zr in ZEK100 caused a dendrite refinement comparable to that achieved through an increase in a cooling rate from 30 to 110 °C/s. Fu et al. [9] investigated the effect of calcium addition on nesting fluidity of Mg-4.2Zn-1.7Ce-0.5Zr alloy and reported that (i) the as-cast alloys consisted of α-Mg matrix, Ca-contained T-phase and $Mg_{51}Zn_{20}$ phase, (ii) addition of 0.2–0.6 wt% Ca led to effective grain refinement and enhanced the fluidity of the alloys, (iii) when the content of Ca was 0.2 wt%, the alloy exhibited the finest grain size of 35.9 μm, and the filling length was increased by approximately 55.4% compared with that of quaternary alloy, (iv) the improvement of the fluidity was attributed to the grain refinement, less energy dissipation and the oxidation resistance of Ce and Ca and (v) with an increase in Ca content, the yield strength (YS) increased gradually, whereas the ultimate tensile strength (UTS) and elongation (EL) showed a decreasing tendency.

6.1.2 Cooling rate during solidification

Cooling rate during the solidification should play an important role and exhibit crucial influence on subsequent microstructure (accordingly, directly or indirectly following mechanical and other) properties. Zhou et al. [10] studied the effect of cooling rate on the microstructure of Mg-Gd-Y-Zr alloy and reported that (i) the increase of cooling rate can refine the solidified microstructure obviously, (ii) the grains are refined and the morphology of the primary phases is changed from coarse to thin, (iii) with the increase of cooling rate, the eutectic distributes more homogeneously and its volume fraction decreases and (iv) higher cooling rate can increase the solid solubility, which contributes to the reduction of dendritic segregation of solutes of Gd and Y in Mg-Gd-Y-Zr alloy. Zhang et al. [11] studied the effect of cooling rate of 10^4 K/s or slow solidification at different cooling rates (0.5, 0.1, 0.01 and 0.005 K/s) on microstructure of Mg-10Gd-3Y-1.8Zn-0.5Zr (wt%) (GWZ1032K) alloys. It was shown that (i) there is no long-period stacking order (LPSO) structure in the alloy prepared by melt spinning at cooling rate of 10^4 K/s, (ii) in the alloy prepared by permanent mold casting at cooling rate of 5 K/s, fine lamellar 14 H-LPSO structure appears in the matrix nearby grain boundaries, (iii) with the cooling rates slowing down from 0.5 to 0.005 K/s, $(Mg,Zn)_3RE$ phase is gradually replaced by 14 H-LPSO phase at grain boundaries, and lamellar 14 H-LPSO structure also propagates in α-Mg matrix, (iv) both $(Mg,Zn)_3RE$ phase and 14 H-LPSO phase are present at grain boundaries in the alloys solidified at cooling rates of 0.5 and 0.1 K/s and (v) when the cooling rate is very slow (0.005 K/s), lamellar 14 H-LPSO structure penetrates throughout the matrix grain. Wang et al. [12], studying on Mg–27Zn–4Ca alloys fabricated using copper mold injection casting, indicated that (i) microstructural analysis reveals that the alloy with a diameter of 1.5 mm is almost completely composed of amorphous phase; however, with the cooling rate decline, a little α-Mg and MgZn dendrites can be found in the amorphous matrix, (ii) the ductile dendrites are conceived to be highly responsible for the enhanced compressive strain from 1.3% to 3.1% by increasing the sample diameter from 1.5 to 3 mm and (iii) the Mg-based alloys show much better corrosion resistance than the traditionally commercial wrought magnesium alloy ZK60 in simulated seawater. Liu et al. [13] investigated the effect of solidification cooling rate on the corrosion resistance of an Mg–Zn–Ca alloy developed for biomedical applications. It was found that (i) increasing cooling rate resulted in a significant improvement in the corrosion resistance of the Mg–Zn–Ca alloy and (ii) this can be attributed to solidification behavior in association with the change in solubility of the alloying elements, microstructural homogeneity and refinement and chemical homogeneity as well as the increased cooling rates. Yuan et al. [14] studied the effect of cooling rate on the microstructure and corrosion behavior of a biodegradable β-TCP/Mg–Zn–Ca composite. The composite was fabricated under a series of cooling rates using a wedge-shaped casting mold. It was mentioned that (i) faster cooling rates were shown to refine the secondary phase and grain size and produce a more homogenous microstructure and (ii) the refined microstructure resulted in a more uniform distribution of β-TCP particles, which is believed to be beneficial in the formation of a stable and compact corrosion product layer, leading to improved corrosion resistance for the composite.

A systematic study was conducted on the structure, phase composition, strength and hardness of the rapidly solidified $Mg_{100-2x}Cu_xY_x$ alloys [15]. It was reported that (i) the structure mostly consists of relatively large dendritic grains of hexagonal close-packed Mg phase and smaller grains of $CuMg_2$ phase, (ii) nanoparticles of $CuMg_2$ phase were also observed as a result of decomposition of the supersaturated Mg-solid solution, (iii) as in the $Mg_{98}Cu_1Y_1$ alloy studied earlier, some fraction of the glassy phase was observed and the volume fraction of the glassy phase increases with increase in Cu and Y content and (iv) yield stress and Vickers microhardness values in general increase with increase in solute content and reach a saturation at $x = 4–5$. Zhou et al. [16] studied microstructure characterization, phase compositions and thermal stability of the Mg–6Zn–5Ca alloy melt and subsequent splat quenching on the water-cooled copper twin rollers in the form of flakes. It was found that (i) with adding RE (Ce and La), the stable intermetallic compounds, namely, the $Mg_xZn_yRE_z$ phase with a few Ca (about 3 at%), shortened as the T′ phase, were formed at the expense of the binary

Mg–Zn and $Ca_2Mg_6Zn_3$ phases, which was possibly beneficial to the enhanced thermal stability of the alloy, (ii) in the Mg-6Zn-5Ca-3Ce-0.5La alloy, the composition of the T′ phase in the grain interior was different from that at the grain boundaries, in which the segregation of the La elements was found, and the atomic percentage ratio of Zn to Ce in the T′ phase within the grains was close to two and (iii) the stable Mg_2Ca phases were detected around the T′ phases at the grain boundaries in the alloy. Zhao et al. [17] investigated microstructure, corrosion behavior and cytotoxicity of biodegradable Mg–Sn alloys fabricated by subrapid solidification. It was reported that the microstructure of Mg–1Sn alloy was almost a equiaxed grain, while the Mg–Sn alloys with higher Sn content (Sn ≥ 3 wt%) displayed α-Mg dendrites, and the secondary dendrite arm spacing of the primary α-Mg decreased significantly with increasing Sn content, (ii) the Mg–Sn alloys consisted of primary α-Mg matrix, Sn-rich segregation and Mg_2Sn phase, and the amount of Mg_2Sn phases increased with increasing Sn content, (iii) the corrosion rates of Mg–Sn alloys increased with increasing Sn content and (iv) cytotoxicity test showed that Mg–1Sn and Mg–3Sn alloys were harmless to MG63 cells, indicating that Mg–1Sn and Mg–3Sn alloys were promising to be used as biodegradable implants. Ye et al. [18] fabricated ribbons of an Mg–9.76 wt% Sn alloy rapid solidification technology and reported that (i) X-ray diffraction (XRD) and transmission electron microscopy confirm that the rapidly solidified ribbons consist of α-Mg, β-Mg_2Sn and β″-Mg_3Sn phases, (ii) the predominant fraction of the β-Mg_2Sn phase distributes at the grain boundaries of the α-Mg grains and (iii) the minor fraction of the β-Mg_2Sn phase reveals a spherical morphology with a typical grain size of 170 nm.

6.1.3 Directional solidification

Directional solidification is solidification that occurs from farthest end of the casting and works its way toward the sprue, having greatest importance in the field of metallurgical casting. Wang et al. [19] investigated the effects of the solidification parameters (growth rate v from 10–200 μm/s and temperature gradient δT of 20, 25 and 30 K/mm) on microstructure and room-temperature mechanical properties of Mg–2.35Gd (mass fraction, %) magnesium alloy under the controlled solidification conditions. It was reported that (i) the cellular spacing λ decreases with increasing v for constant δT or with increasing δT for constant v, (ii) an improved tensile strength and a corresponding decreased EL are achieved in the directionally solidified experimental alloy with increasing growth rate and temperature gradient and (iii) the directionally solidified experimental alloy exhibits higher room-temperature tensile strength than the nondirectionally solidified alloy. Furthermore, Wang et al. [20] studied the effects of the growth rate on the microstructures of Mg–1.5Gd (wt%) magnesium alloy under controlled directional solidification conditions: a constant temperature gradient (40 K/mm) at a wide range of growth rate (10–200 μm/s). It was mentioned that (i) the microstructures are cellular, and the relationship between cellular spacing (λ) and growth rate (V) is established in the form: $\lambda = 130.2827\ V^{-0.2228}$ by a linear regression analysis, which is in good agreement with the calculated values by Trivedi model, (ii) the thermodynamics solidification path calculations by Scheil model and experimental observations confirm that the solidification microstructure in the alloy consists of primary α(Mg) phase and binary eutectic α(Mg) + Mg_5Gd phase and (iii) the microsegregation of the alloying element predicted by the Scheil model agrees reasonably with the electron probe microanalysis measurements. Yang et al. [21] investigated the microstructural evolution, phase constitution and mechanical properties of directionally solidified Mg–5.5Zn–xGd (x = 0.8, 2.0 and 4.0) alloys under $\delta T = 30$ K/mm at a wide range of V (10–100 μm/s). It was reported that (i) a mixture of α(Mg) and I (Mg_3Zn_6Gd) are found in Mg–5.5Zn–0.8Gd alloy, and a mixture of α(Mg), I (Mg_3Zn_6Gd) and W($Mg_3Zn_3Gd_2$) in Mg–5.5Zn–(2.0, 4.0)Gd alloys, respectively, (ii) the criterion growth rate for cellular–columnar dendrite transition for Mg–5.5Zn–xGd alloys decreased with the increase of Gd content, (iii) the tensile test showed that the room-temperature UTS increased and the EL decreased with the increase of the growth rate for a certain composition of Mg–5.5Zn–xGd alloy, (iv) for a certain growth rate, UTS first increased from 0 to 2.0 wt% of Gd content, and then decreased with the further increase of Gd content and (v) the directionally solidified Mg–5.5Zn–2.0Gd experimental alloy showed the maximum UTS. Liu et al. [22] mentioned that the Mg–Li alloy is a unique system with a narrow dual-phase region and superstructure transformation, and these characteristics might exhibit significant influence on the solidification behavior. The directional solidification experiments were performed on alloys with different Li contents (6.3–7.8 wt%) at varied growth rates (3–21 μm/s) and it as reported that (i) as the Li content increases, the microstructures transform from divorced eutectic structure to lamellar structure, then to lamellae/α-Mg rod mixed structure, and finally to α-Mg rod-like structure, (ii) fully eutectic structure is produced at a wide range of off-eutectic compositions (iii) the effect of growth rate on the α-Mg rod-like structure is mainly to diminish the interrod spacing as growth rate increases, while additionally to affect the morphology of lamellar structure and (iv) high growth rate is found to be beneficial for producing straight and uniform lamellar structure. Muto et al. [23] conducted compression tests of directionally solidified Mg–6Zn–9Y alloys from surface observations and acoustic emission (AE) measurements. It was fund that (i) in the compression tests, deformation bands were generated in the early deformation stage, (ii) the number of microcracks started to increase from approximately 100 MPa and rapidly increased around the yielding point, (iii) there are two clusters in AE events: one cluster was considered to be AE events generated by kink deformation and the other was considered to be AE events generated by microcracks and (iv) AE analysis is an effective method to evaluate the dynamic deformation behavior of directionally solidified Mg–Zn alloys containing LPSO phases.

6.1.4 Pressurized solidification

Dong et al. [24] analyzed the microstructure of Mg–8Zn–1Y alloy solidified under super-high pressure. It was reported that (i) the microstructure of Mg–8Zn–1Y alloy solidified under ambient pressure and super-high pressure was both mainly composed of α-Mg and quasicrystal I-Mg_3Zn_6Y, (ii) solidification under super-high pressure contributed to refining solidified microstructure and changing morphology of the intergranular second phase, (iii) the morphology of intergranular second phase (quasicrystal I–Mg_3Zn_6Y) was transformed from continuous network (ambient pressure) to long island (high pressure) and finally to granular (super-high pressure) with the increase in pressure, (iv) the compressive strength, YS and rupture strain of the samples solidified under ambient pressure were significantly improved from 262.6 MPa, 244.4 MPa and 13.3% to 437.3 MPa, 368.9 MPa and 24.7% under the pressure of 6 GPa, respectively, and (v) when it was solidified under the pressure ranging from 4 to 6 GPa, cleavage plane on compressive fracture was small and coarse. Similarly, Zhou et al. [25] studied the effect of high pressure during solidification on the microstructure and mechanical property of Mg–6Zn–1Y and Mg–6Zn–3Y. It was found that (i) under atmospheric-pressure solidification, Mg–6Zn–1Y consisted of α-Mg, Mg_7Zn_3 and Mg_3YZn_6; whilst Mg–6Zn–3Y consisted of α-Mg, $Mg_3Y_2Zn_3$ and Mg_3YZn_6, (ii) under 6 GPa high-pressure solidification, both alloy consisted of α-Mg, MgZn and $Mg_{12}YZn$, (iii) the shape of the main second phase changed from a lamellar structure formed for atmospheric-pressure solidification to small particles formed for solidification at 6 GPa pressure, (iv) the dendrite microstructure was refined and was more regular, and the length of the primary dendrite arm increased under 6 GPa high-pressure solidification, which was attributed to increasing thermal undercooling, compositional undercooling and kinetics undercooling and (v) after solidification at 6 GPa pressure, the solid solubility of Y in the second phase and the Vickers hardness increased from 15 wt% and 69 MPa for Mg–6Zn–1Y to 49 wt% and 97 MPa and from 19 wt% and 71 MPa for Mg–6Zn–3Y alloy to 20 wt% and 92 MPa, respectively. Pan et al. [26] studied the dendritic growth in pressurized solidification of Mg–Al alloy during squeeze casting and reported that (i) the grains are refined, the dendritic growth rate tends to increase and the secondary dendrite arms are more developed as the pressure is increased from 0.1 to 100 MPa, which showed a good agreement with the experimental results of direct squeeze casting of Mg–Al alloy and (ii) as the pressure increases, the largest dendritic growth rate can be obtained under the pressure between 200 and 250 MPa, while the growth rate decreases with a further increase of pressure.

6.1.5 Gravity casting and centrifugal casting

Gravity casting is among the oldest known processes for fabricating metals and metal alloys, involving the pouring of molten metal from a crucible into a mold under only the force of gravity, without the use of pressurized gases, vacuums or centrifugal force. Fu et al. [27] investigated the microstructure and mechanical properties of gravity cast Mg-2.75Nd-*x*Zn-Zr ($x = 0–2.0$ wt%) and Mg-*y*Nd-0.2Zn-Zr ($y = 1.25–3.25$ wt%) alloys in as-cast, solution-treated and 200 °C peak-aged conditions and reported that when Zn addition was 0.2 wt% and Nd addition was 3.0 wt%, the alloy revealed the best combination of strength and EL and was chosen as optimal chemical composition. Lee et al. [28] studied the effect of alloying elements on microstructure and properties of Mg-Sn-Al-Si alloy. It was mentioned that (i) the microstructures of the alloys were mainly consisted of α-Mg, $Mg_{17}Al_{12}$, Mg_2Si and Mg_2Sn phases, (ii) Sr and Zn addition improved tensile strength and (iii) for the corrosion resistance of the TAS652 alloy, the addition of small amount of Sr was beneficial but the Zn addition was detrimental. Wang et al. [29] studied the microstructures and mechanical properties of Mg-*x*Zn-1.25RE-Zr ($x = 3.5$, 4.2, 5.0 wt%) and Mg-4.2Zn-*y*RE-Zr ($y = 1.0$, 1.25, 1.5 wt%) alloys in as-cast and 325 °C peak-aged condition. It was reported that (i) the as-cast Mg-*x*Zn-*y*RE-Zr alloys consist of α-Mg matrix, T-phase and $Mg_{51}Zn_{20}$ phase, (ii) for Mg-*x*Zn-1.25RE-Zr alloys, 4.2 wt% Zn addition led to smallest average grain size and better eutectics morphology of discontinuous network, short bar and island shape, (iii) for Mg-4.2Zn-*y*RE-Zr alloy, increase in RE content gradually refined the microstructure and contributed to more triangular particles and networks, (iv) after peak aged at 325 °C, the strengthening of Mg-*x*Zn-*y*RE-Zr alloys occurred through the precipitations of rod-like β'_1 phases, (v) with Zn content from 3.5 to 5.0 wt%, the strengthening effect first increased and then decreased, with a turning point of 4.2 wt% Zn, due to the formation of plate-like β'_2 phases and reduced number density of β'_1 phases, (vi) with RE addition from 1.0 to 1.5 wt%, the strengthening effect increased because of the denser and finer β'_1 phases and (vii) when $x = 4.2$ and $y = 1.25–1.5$ wt%, the Mg-*x*Zn-*y*RE-Zr alloy reveals good combination of strength and EL in 325 °C peak-aged condition and was chosen as optimal chemical composition.

Centrifugal casting is a casting technique that is typically used to cast thin-walled cylinders, typically used to cast materials such as metals, glass and concrete. Luo et al. [30] fabricated Mg–5Sn alloy by a horizontal centrifugal casting method. It was mentioned that (i) the developed columnar dendritic crystals under the gravity casting condition can be mostly transformed into fine equiaxed grains by the centrifugal casting, (ii) compared with the gravity casting, compression strength, YS and EL to failure are significantly improved by the centrifugal casting, which increase from 181.6 to 257.5 MPa, 38.7 to 52.3 MPa and 14.9% to 21.2% on position r_1 (centrifugal radius $r_1 = 0.05$ m), respectively, (iii) the centrifugal casting also enhances work-hardening ability of the alloy and (iv) the transformation of crystals results in the enhancement of the compression properties and work-hardening ability. Liu et al. [31]

fabricated AZ31B magnesium alloy ring with a large diameter and a thick wall using a centrifugal casting technique and studied the microstructures and tensile properties of the ring were compared with conventional casting. It was found that (i) in the case of dendritic growth, both the primary and secondary arms were broken by the cyclical centrifugal force field and the flow shear of the semisolid slurry, and the primary phase with dendritic morphology in the centrifugal casting of AZ31B magnesium alloy has readily transformed into a spherical nucleus, (ii) the microstructures of the ring by centrifugal casting are formed in equiaxed grains and their size significantly refined and (iii) there is a semisolid slurry preparation process within the solidification process of centrifugal casting.

6.1.6 Suction casting

Suction casting represents an economic and promising process route and improves mechanical properties [32]. Wang et al. [33] fabricated a novel interpenetrating C/Mg–Zn–Mn composite by infiltrating Mg–Zn–Mn alloy into porous carbon using suction casting technique and reported that (i) the composite had a compact structure and the interfacial bonding between Mg–Zn–Mn alloy and carbon scaffold was very well, (ii) the composite had an ultimate compressive strength of (195 ± 15) MPa, which is near with the natural bone (2–180 MPa) and about 150-fold higher than that of the original porous carbon scaffold, and it still retained half of the strength of the bulk Mg–Zn–Mn alloy, (iii) the corrosion test indicated that the mass loss percentage of the composite was 52.9% after 30 days immersion in simulated body fluid at 37 °C, and the corrosion rates were 0.043 and 0.028 mg/cm^{2}h after 3 and 7 days of immersion, respectively, and (iv) the corrosion products on the composite surface were mainly $Mg(OH)_2$ and HA. Similarly, Wang et al. [34] fabricated an interpenetrating β-TCP/Mg–Zn–Mn composite by infiltrating Mg–Zn–Mn alloy into porous β-TCP using suction casting technique. It was reported that (i) the composite had a compact structure and the interfacial bonding between Mg–Zn–Mn alloy and β-TCP scaffold was very well, (ii) the composite had an ultimate compressive strength of 140 ± 20 MPa, which is near with the natural bone (2–180 MPa) and about 1,000-fold higher than that of the original porous β-TCP scaffold, and it still retained about two fifths of the strength of the bulk Mg–Zn–Mn alloy and (iii) the electrochemical and immersion tests indicated that the corrosion resistance of the composite was better than that of the Mg–Zn–Mn matrix alloy, and the corrosion products on the composite surface were mainly $Mg(OH)_2$, $Ca_3(PO_4)_2$ and HA. Zhou et al. [35] investigated the influence of small amount of Ca addition on the microstructures and mechanical properties of three near-eutectic Mg–*x*Li ($x = 6.8, 7.5, 8.4$ wt%) binary alloys under rapid solidification condition by using Cu-mold suction casting technique. It was mentioned that (i) the microstructures were very distinct from those by conventional gravity casting technique in the morphology, grain size and the volume fraction of α-Mg phase; (ii) mechanical properties of the Ca-modified Mg–*x*Li binary alloys were significantly enhanced; (iii) a eutectic growth mode transition from their regular divorced eutectic growth to regular coupled eutectic structure was induced in Mg–8.4Li alloy via Ca addition; and (iv) the eutectic transition mechanisms in three Mg–*x*Li alloys by Ca addition were discussed in terms of the freezing rate, Mg_2Ca particle segregation, the relative volume fraction of α-Mg phase.

6.1.7 Solidification pathways

Various casting parameters including dendritic growth, solid diffusion on primary solidification, a continuation of the solidification involving multiphase reactions and resulting microsegregation are affecting the solidification pathways. Liang et al. [36] investigated the solidification behavior of AZ91 and AM50 with Ca addition (AZC91*x* and AMC50*x* alloys) by a computer-aided cooling curve analysis system. It was reported that (i) the Ca-containing phase formation mainly depends on Ca content and Ca/Al ratio, (ii) with increasing the Ca/Al ratio, these phases transform from Al_2Ca to $(Mg, Al)_2Ca$ and Mg_2Ca, (iii) Ca addition decreases the liquidus temperature of Mg–Al alloys, but influences the solidus temperature in a more complex way and (iv) increasing the Ca content also decreases the solid fraction at which dendrite coherency occurs. Huang et al. [37] investigated the microstructure evolution with composition variation during solidification process in Mg-Zn-Y-Zr alloys (ZW alloys). It was shown that (i) two pseudobinary eutectic reactions appear one after another during solidification due to the different Zn/Y ratio (ranged from 0.35 to 3.33), (ii) in ZW62 alloy, a peritectic reaction happens before I-phase formation through pseudobinary eutectic reaction distinguishing it from other alloys, (iii) the changes of characteristic temperature points for phase transformation are studied in detail, (iv) microstructure observation shows dominating secondary phases in the alloys that differ from one another according to various Zn/Y ratios and (v) divorced massive eutectic Z-phase is formed during solidification in a low Zn/Y ratio; W-phase comes out when Zn/Y ratio grows to 0.85; if the Zn/Y ratio increases further to a certain level, I-phase forms by a peritectic reaction through W-phase and the liquid. Wong et al. [38] studied the solidification path and microstructure evolution in Mg–3Al–14La alloy and reported that (i) the solidification sequence begins with the precipitation of primary Al_5La_2, followed by a eutectic with the products α-Mg + Al_5La_2, then a monovariant binary eutectic with the products α-Mg + $Mg_{12}La$ and lastly a ternary eutectic with the products α-Mg + $Mg_{12}La$ + $(Al,Mg)_3La$, (ii) this solidification sequence is found to be significantly different from the current Mg–Al–La thermodynamic description and (iii) the two main discrepancies are as follows: (a) with Al_5La_2 being the primary phase, the Mg–3Al–14La alloy is a hypereutectic alloy rather than a hypoeutectic alloy as currently described and (b) the

$(Al,Mg)_3La$ phase, which was recently identified as a new phase in the Mg–Al–La system, is also present in the Mg–3Al–14La alloy. Zhang et al. [39] studied the influence of Al addition on solidification oath and hot tearing susceptibility of Mg-2Zn-(3 + 0.5*x*)Y-*x*Al ($x = 0$, 2 and 3 at%) alloys. It was shown that (i) minimum grain size, optimal dendritic coherency and minimum hot tearing susceptibility are exhibited by Mg-2Zn-(3 + 0.5*x*)Y-*x*Al alloy ($x = 2$) and (ii) when Al content was increased to 3 at %, Al_2Y phase exhibited a peritectic reaction and transformed into a mixed structure of Al_2Y and Al + Al_3Y phases, which increased the HTS (hot tearing susceptibility) of the alloy due to reduced fine-grained Al_2Y content.

6.1.8 Hot tearing

Hot tearing is often a major casting defect in magnesium alloys and is a complicated solidification phenomenon showing a significant impact on the quality of their casting products. Hot tearing (or hot cracking) is one of the most severe solidification defects commonly encountered during casting and is identified as cracks, either on the casting surface or in the casting interior. In general, two major factors contribute to hot tearing: (1) when casting regions with mushy alloy are separated from incoming liquid metal and, (2) when the mush zone is under uniaxial tensile loading [40]. Wang et al. [41] studied the hot tearing susceptibility of Mg–9Al–*x*Zn alloys using the crack-ring molds to assess the hot tearing susceptibility. It was found that (i) hot tearing originates along the grains at the end of solidification, (ii) with Zn additions, the quantity of phase with low melting point in grain boundaries is increased, its melting point is decreased and the hot tearing susceptibility is increased and (iii) the segregation of Zn element in grain boundaries is the main contribution to the high hot tearing susceptibility of Mg–9Al–*x*Zn alloys. Cao et al. [42] investigated hot cracking of binary Mg–Al (0.25–8 wt%) alloys in permanent mold casting. It was mentioned that (i) the curve of the crack susceptibility versus the Al content showed a peak near 1 wt% Al, (ii) the onset of hot cracking during casting was detected by connecting a load cell to a rod solidifying in a similar steel mold and recording the temperature at the end of the rod where cracking occurred and (iii) a cracking susceptibility coefficient based on the time at the onset of cracking was found to correlate well with the crack susceptibility curve. Kierzek et al. [43] mentioned that the main criteria of magnesium alloys weldability assessment is their susceptibility to hot cracking, which constitute the greatest difficulty during welding, and their overlay welding capacity. Bichler et al. [44] mentioned that although there were extensive studies on hot tearing in magnesium and aluminum alloys so far, the interactions between the solidification parameters, microstructural development, and stress and strain at the onset of hot tearing in magnesium alloys remain unclear; in particular, the stress and strain conditions required to nucleate hot tears are unknown. Based on this background, the ex situ neutron-diffraction residual strain mapping was carried out on AZ91D magnesium alloy castings at the onset of hot tearing and the results indicated that (i) tensile strain alone was not sufficient to nucleate a hot tear, (ii) a minimum threshold tensile stress of ~12 MPa was necessary to open interdendritic shrinkage pores into hot tears and enable their propagation and (iii) deformation along a certain crystallographic planes played a dominant role on the high-temperature deformation and hot tearing in the AZ91D alloy [44]. Easton et al. [45] studied a series of Mg-based binary alloys with Res (such as La, Ce, Nd, Y and Gd) and found that Mg–La based alloys are least susceptible to hot tearing whilst alloys containing Nd, Y or Gd tend to have very high hot tearing susceptibility. It is a well-known practical observation that hot tearing can be reduced or eliminated in controlled casting conditions that prevent formation of large temperature and stress gradients, so that preheating permanent molds could alleviate or eliminate hot tearing.

6.2 Casting types

6.2.1 Sand casting

Sand (molded) casting produces over 60% of all metal castings and is characterized using sand as the mold material. Cao et al. [46] investigated the microstructure, mechanical properties and fracture behavior of sand-cast Mg-10Gd-3Y-0.5Zr alloy under T6 condition (air cooling after solid solution and then aging heat treatment) and reported that (i) the optimum T6 heat treatments for sand-cast Mg-10Gd-3Y-0.5Zr alloy are (525 °C, 12 h + 225 °C, 14 h) and (525 °C, 12 h + 250 °C, 12 h) according to age-hardening curve and mechanical properties, respectively, (ii) the UTS, YS and EL of the Mg-10Gd-3Y-0.5Zr alloy treated by the two optimum T6 processes are 339.9 MPa, 251.6 MPa, 1.5% and 359.6 MPa, 247.3 MPa, 2.7%, respectively, and (iii) the tensile fracture mode of peak-aged Mg-10Gd-3Y-0.5Zr alloy is transgranular quasicleavage fracture. Pang et al. [47] studied the influence of the pouring temperature ranging from 680°C to 780 °C on the solidification behavior, the microstructure and mechanical properties of the sand-cast Mg-10Gd-3Y-0.4Zr alloy. It was mentioned that (i) the nucleation undercooling of the α-Mg phase increased from 2.3 to 6.3 °C, (ii) the average α-Mg grain size increased from 44 to 71 μm, but then decreased to 46 μm, (iii) the volume fraction of β-$Mg_{24}RE_5$ phase increased and its morphology transformed from particle into rod-like, (iv) YS increased from 138 to 151 MPa, and UTS increased from 186 to 197 MPa, (v) the alloy poured at 750 °C had optimal combining strength and ductility and (vi) the average α-Mg grain size played a main role in the YS of sand-cast Mg-10Gd-3Y-0.4Zr alloy, besides other factors, that is, microporosity, morphology of eutectic compounds, reoxidation inclusion and solute concentration. Liu et al. [48] studied microstructure and mechanical properties of sand mold cast Mg-4.58Zn-2.6Gd-0.18Zr magnesium alloy after different heat treatments. It was reported that (i) as-cast alloy was composed of α(Mg) matrix, interdendritic α(Mg) + W($Mg_3Zn_3Gd_2$) eutectic, icosahedral quasicrystalline I(Mg_3Zn_6Gd) phase and Mg_3Gd particles within α(Mg) matrix, (ii) after solution treatment at 505 °C for 16 h, most of the α(Mg) + W($Mg_3Zn_3Gd_2$) eutectic dissolved into α(Mg) matrix, but a new phase, Zn_2Zr_3, precipitated within α(Mg) matrix, (iii) the appropriate aging treatment was done at 220 °C for 16 h, after which some dispersive fine eutectics reprecipitated along the grain boundary and (v) the UTS, YS and EL of the experimental alloy in the T6 state at room temperature were 280 MPa, 175 MPa and 7.5%, respectively. Zhang et al. [49] investigated microstructure, mechanical properties and fracture behaviors of sand-cast Mg-4Y-3Nd-1Gd-0.2Zn-0.5Zr (wt%) alloy in different thermal conditions. It was mentioned that (i) the as-cast alloy was comprised of α-Mg matrix, $Mg_{24}Y_5$, $Mg_{41}Nd_5$ and β_1 phases, (ii) after solution treatment at 525 °C for 6 h, the eutectics dissolved into α-Mg matrix, leading to a huge improvement of plasticity, (iii) alloys peak aged at 200 and 225 °C exhibit high strength due to fine dense β″ and β′ precipitates, (iv) aged at 250 °C for 10 h, the precipitates in the alloy are coarse sparse coupled β_1/β′ phases, (v) a desirable combination of strength and ductility was obtained with 198 MPa in YS, 276 MPa in UTS and 7.6% in EL when overaged at 250 °C for 10 h and (vi) alloys under different thermal conditions show different fracture behaviors, which are closely linked to the structures of both inner grains and grain boundaries. The microstructures and mechanical properties of a series of sand-cast Mg-Sm-Zn-Zr alloys under as-cast, solution-treated and peak-aged states were investigated [50], reporting that (i) substitution Nd in the conventional Mg-2.5Nd-0.6Zn-0.5Zr alloy with different contents of Sm has comparative grain refinement effect and will fully change the dominant intermetallic phase and (ii) the substituted alloys have clearly higher strength with comparative ductility at both as-cast and peak-aged conditions and much greater age-hardening response than the referential alloy. Li et al. [51] studied the effects of processing parameters (pouring temperature and mold preheating temperature) and flame-retardant content on the microstructure and fluidity of sand-cast Mg-10Gd-3Y-0.5Zr (GW103K). It was reported that (i) the increase of pouring temperature leads to coarsened microstructure and decreased fluidity of sand-cast GW103K alloy, (ii) increase of mold preheating temperature incurs coarsening of as-cast microstructure and increase of fluidity, (iii) the addition of flame retardant into molding sand has a negligible influence on the microstructure of sand-cast GW103K alloy, (iv) with the increase in flame-retardant content, fluidity of the alloy initially increases and then decreases and (v) the optimized process parameters and flame-retardant addition were obtained to have pouring temperature of 750 °C, mold temperature of 110 °C and flame-retardant addition of 1%.

6.2.2 Die casting

Many studies have been reported on Mg–Al-based die cast alloys. These should include Mg–9Al–1Zn with conclusion that the improvement was ascribed to the refinement of the primary α-Mg grains formed in both shot sleeve and die cavity and to the reduction of porosity as well as refinement of $Mg_{17}Al_{12}$ phases [52], AZ91D–2Ca with conclusion that with the melting conditioning, the melt-conditioned high-pressure die casting samples not only have considerably refined size of externally solidified crystals but also have significantly reduced cast defects, thus provide superior mechanical properties to conventional high-pressure die castings [53] and Mg–Al–RE [54, 55] concluding that changing the RE content of the alloy from Ce-rich mischmetal to lanthanum gives a further improvement in the tensile and creep properties, and the later could be attributed to the better thermal stability of $Al_{11}La_3$ phase in Mg-4Al-4La-0.4Mn alloy than that of $Al_{11}RE_3$ phase in Mg-4Al-4RE-0.4Mn alloy and Mg-4Al-4RE-0.3Mn [56]. Furthermore, there are studies on Mg-Al-La-Y [57] with a conclusion that (i) the alloy exhibits significantly improved tensile and compressive YS at room temperature and 200 °C and (ii) the outstanding mechanical properties are mainly attributed to the formation of $Al_{11}La_3$ intermetallics, which is present in a high volume fraction, and possesses fine morphology and relatively good thermal stability, mentioning that small amount of RE element addition enhanced the mechanical properties.

Besides Mg–Al-based alloys, there are still a variety of Mg-based alloys that are subjected to investigations. There are Mg-Al-Ce-Mn [58], Mg-Al-Ce-Y [59], Mg-Al-Sm=Mn [60], Mg-Al-Gd-Mn [61], Mg-Al-Zn (AZ91D) [62] and Mg-Zn-Al-RE [63]. Re element addition imporve mechanical properties. Mg–Zr [64 and Mg–Sn–Ce [65, 66] indicate that Ce addition improved both mechanical and corrosion resistance properties, whilst Mg–La–RE [65] and Mg-Gd-Y-Zr [66, 67] show significant improvements of mechanical properties and ductility.

6.2.3 Continuous casting

Both continuous casting (or strand casting) and semicontinuous casting are processes to solidify molten metal into a semifinished billet, bloom or slab for subsequent rolling in the finishing mills; hence molten metal enter from one end and exit as solid metal on the other end [68]. Zhang et al. [69] examined directionally solidified binary Mg–Al eutectic alloy wires of approximately 5 mm in diameter produced by the continuous casting process. It was reported that (i) the wires possess obvious unidirectional growth characteristic along its axial direction, (ii) the microstructure consists of parallel columnar grains that resulted from the competitive growth of equiaxed grains solidified on the head of dummy bar (iii) each columnar grain comprises regular eutectic αa-Mg and β-$Mg_{17}Al_{12}$ phases, which grew along the axial direction of the wires and (iv) the morphology of the eutectic is mainly lamellar, meanwhile rod eutectic exists. Kido et al. [70], using the semisolid casting method, fabricated magnesium alloy slurry with an inclined cooling plate instead of electromagnetic or mechanical stirring during solidification. It was mentioned that (i) the microstructures of the sheets contained refined and globular primary crystals and (ii) the most important factors are casting temperature and twin-roll speed that influences sheet casting.

Zhao et al. [71] prepared Mg-1.5Zn-0.2Zr-xCe ($x = 0$, 0.1, 0.3, 0.5, mass fraction, %) alloys by conventional semicontinuous casting. It was mentioned that (i) Ce element exists in the form of $Mg_{12}Ce$ phase and has an obvious refining effect on the microstructure of test alloys, (ii) as the Ce content increases, the grain size reduces, the grain boundaries turn thinner and the distribution of $Mg_{12}Ce$ precipitates becomes more and more dispersed and (iii) the Mg–1.5Zn–0.2Zr alloy with 0.3% Ce has the best refinement effect. Du et al. [72] investigated the microstructures and mechanical properties of Mg–5.3Zn–0.2Ca–0.5Ce (wt%) alloy fabricated by semicontinuous casting and reported that (i) the as-cast alloy consists of α-Mg, $Ca_2Mg_6Zn_3$ and T'_1 phase with orthorhombic structure, (ii) T'_1 phase mainly distributes at the triple conjunctions while the $Ca_2Mg_6Zn_3$ at the grain boundaries and (iii) the as-cast alloy exhibits high strength retention due to the stable $Ca_2Mg_6Zn_3$ and T'_1 phase at the grain boundaries. Chen et al. [73] prepared a large sheet made of Mg-1.2Zn-3.4Y-4.7Gd-0.5Zr alloy by semicontinuous casting, followed by homogenization and hot extrusion. It was reported that (i) during homogenization, the generation of 14 H LPSO phase was mainly achieved by two phase transition processes of Mg_5(Gd,Y,Zn) phase → 14 H LPSO phase and 18 R LPSO phase → 14 H LPSO phase, (ii) during extrusion, the evolution of LPSO phases with various morphologies was driven by severe deformation and dynamic recrystallization, (iii) due to the decreased solubility of Zn, Y and Gd in the extruded alloy matrix, the solution elements of Zn, Y and Gd were impelled to precipitate at the scattering arranged stacking faults and formed the needle-like LPSO phase and (iv) the gliding of Shockley partial dislocation(s) on basal plane was structurally needed during the precipitation of needle-like LPSO phase.

6.2.4 Twin-roll casting

Twin-roll casting has been developed for aluminum, which turns liquid aluminum into strip directly, and is a combination integrated process: on the one hand, completes continuous cooling and solidification, on the other hand, produces plastic deformation [74–76]. Twin-roll strip casting process is a near-net-shape casting technology, for the production of thin strips having thickness of about 0.1 to 6.0 mm. This process produces thin strips directly from the liquid metal by combining casting and rolling in a single step. This process provides better control over the microstructure and mechanical properties of the cast strip [76].

Bae et al. [77] cladded Mg alloy with Al by simultaneous casting, cladding and rolling using twin-roll casting process and reported that (i) the as-cast microstructure shows the presence of $Mg_{17}Al_{12}$ in the reaction zone with good interfacial bonding between the Al and the base Mg alloy, (ii) annealing of the clad sheet results in the additional formation of Mg_2Al_3 along the Mg/Al interface and (iii) subsequent rolling of the as-annealed sheet reduces the thickness of the reaction zone with a resultant improvement in the formability of the clad sheet. Jiang et al. [78] found that addition of 0.08 wt% Ca into AZ31 melts significantly reduces the average grain size of thin strips produced by twin-roll cast to 30 μm from 100 μm. It was further mentioned that like Zr, due to the high chemical activity, the Ca added into the melts reacts with Al and forms Al_2Ca intermetallic compound and Al_2Ca is a potential and effective grain refiner for Mg alloys and the grain refinement through addition of Ca in the AZ31 alloy is attributed to the inoculation effect of Al_2Ca particles formed in the melts. Bhattacharjee et al. [79] mentioned that (i) the twin roll cast and hot rolled Mg–6.2 wt%Zn alloys microalloyed with Zr, Ca and Ag show tensile yield strength (TYS) exceeding 300 MPa in the T6 (peak aged) condition with reasonable formability in the T4 condition and (ii) the addition of Zr and Ca plays a critical role in the development of weak textured recrystallized microstructure in Mg–6.2 wt%Zn alloys so Mg-6.2Zn-0.5Zr-0.2Ca (wt%) alloy shows equivalent mechanical properties with Mg-6.2Zn-0.5Zr-0.2Ca-0.4Ag (wt%) alloy even without expensive Ag.

AZ31 Mg alloys produced by twin-roll casting were coated by plasma electrolytic oxidation in solution of potassium hydroxide (KOH) and different concentration of sodium metasilicate pentahydrate ($Na_2SiO_3 \cdot 5H_2O$) electrolytes at 0.140 A/cm^2 current density for 60 min [80]. It was reported that (i) forsterite (Mg_2SiO_4) and periclase (MgO) phases were formed on the surface of the coated magnesium alloys, (ii) the surface of the coatings is very porous and rough due to the presence of microdischarges through plasma electrolytic oxidation process and (iii) the wear rate, hardness and surface roughness of the coatings were increased when the concentration of $Na_2SiO_3 \cdot 5H_2O$ electrolyte was increased [80]. Park et al. [81] analyzed two types of cladding process by vertical twin-roll casting. Mg–AZ31 sheet was cladded with molten AA3003 in type I while molten Mg–AZ31 was cladded with two AA1100 sheets in type II. It was mentioned that (i) the Mg–AZ31 sheet was found to be pulled in tension under roll pressure and thinned with a risk of fracture in type I and (ii) however, the Mg–AZ31 melt was found to be incompletely solidified because of low interfacial heat transfer coefficient vale at the interface between the roll and the AA1100 sheet in type II. Bian et al. [82] produced sheet of Mg-1.3Al-0.8Zn-0.7Mn-0.5Ca (wt%) (AZMX1110) alloy produced by low-cost twin-roll casting process that exhibits excellent room-temperature formability with a large index Erichsen value of 7.8 mm at room temperature in a solution-treated condition (T4). It was indicated that (i) the alloy exhibited rapid age-hardening response at 170 °C, resulting in a significant increase of the flow stress from 198 to 238 MPa within 20 min; such bake hardenability has never been explored in magnesium sheet alloys before and (ii) the microstructure of the bake-hardened sample revealed that Al, Zn and Ca atoms are segregated to basal dislocations and contribute to the strengthening by pinning dislocation motions, along with the co-clustering of these atoms.

6.2.5 Squeeze casting

Squeeze casting technology is a combination of casting and forging process, resulting in the highest mechanical properties attainable in a cast product. Goh et al. [83] prepared AZ91–(1–3 wt%) Ca alloys by direct squeeze casting in which the melt was solidified under applied pressure and studied the effects of processing parameters (such as applied pressure and pouring temperature) and Ca content on microstructure and mechanical properties of squeeze-casting AZ91–Ca alloys. It was found that (i) the microstructure was refined with the increase of applied pressure, and the mechanical properties were improved; (ii) when the pouring temperature was lowered down to near the liquidus, the microstructure was further refined and α-Mg grains turned rosette-like; (iii) the negative effect on ambient-temperature mechanical properties caused by the addition of Ca into AZ91 alloy was inhibited by squeeze casting; and (iv) compared to conventional casting, squeeze-casting process can offer AZ91–Ca alloys better mechanical properties, especially in EL to failure. Kurnaz et al. [84] investigated the effect of titanium and chromium (0, 0.1, 0.2, 0.3 and 0.4 wt%) on the microstructure, mechanical and wear properties of a magnesium-based alloy (Mg–Al 6 wt%) which was produced under a controlled atmosphere by a squeeze-casting process. It was reported that (i) the addition of Ti element modified the structure and decreased the grain size; (ii) a similar trend is also observed in the alloys containing Cr; (iii) the results of hardness, tensile and impact testing indicate that the hardness, tensile and impact strength of Mg–6Al alloy increased by adding Ti up to 0.2 wt% and then is relatively constant with increasing Ti; (iv) a similar result is also observed in the alloys containing Cr; (v) the wear rate of Mg–6Al alloy decreased with increasing alloying elements up to 0.2 wt %, then the wear rate is relatively constant with the addition of more alloying elements; and (vi) while the friction coefficient value of Mg–6Al alloy gradually increased with increasing Cr, the friction coefficient value of Mg–6Al alloy decreased with increasing Ti up to 0.2 wt%, then the friction coefficient value is constant with increasing Ti. The effect of Ag (0, 0.2, 0.5 and 1 wt%) on the microstructure and mechanical properties of Mg-based alloy (Mg-6Al-1Sn-0.3Mn-0.3Ti by wt%) produced under a controlled atmosphere by a squeeze-casting process was investigated [85]. It was mentioned that (i) X-ray diffractometry revealed that the main phases are α-Mg, α-Ti, β-$Mg_{17}Al_{12}$ and Al_8Mn_5 in the all of alloys; (ii) $Al_{81}Mn_{19}$ phase was found with Ag additive; (iii) the amount of β-$Mg_{17}Al_{12}$ phase was decreased with increasing amount of Ag; (iv) the strength of the base alloy was increased by solid solution mechanism and decreasing the amount of β-$Mg_{17}Al_{12}$ phase with addition of Ag; and (v) existence of $Al_{81}Mn_{19}$ phase plays an important role in increasing the mechanical properties of the alloys [85].

Mo et al. [86] prepared a new magnesium alloy Mg-12Zn-4Al-0.5Ca (ZAX12405) by squeeze casting and studied the effects of processing parameters including applied pressure, pouring temperature and dwell time on the microstructure and mechanical properties of squeeze-cast ZAX12405 alloy. It was shown that (i) squeeze-cast ZAX12405 alloy exhibited finer microstructure and much better mechanical properties than gravity casting alloy; (ii) increasing the applied pressure led to significant cast densification and a certain extent of grain refinement in the microstructure, along with obvious promotion in mechanical properties; (iii) lowering the pouring temperature refined the microstructure of ZAX12405 alloy, but deteriorated the cast densification, resulting in that the mechanical properties first increased and then decreased; (iv) a combination of highest applied pressure (120 MPa), medium pouring temperature (650 °C) and dwell time (30 s) brought the highest mechanical properties, under which the UTS is 211 MPa, YS is 113 MPa and EL to failure is 5.2%; and (v) for squeeze-cast Mg-12Zn-4Al-0.5Ca alloy, cast densification was considered more important than microstructure refinement for the promotion of mechanical properties. Zhu et al. [87] fabricated a new high-strength Mg-6Zn-4Al-0.5Cu alloy by direct squeeze casting and studied the effects of applied pressure on the microstructure and mechanical properties of the squeeze-cast alloy. It was reported that (i) the squeeze-cast Mg-6Zn-4Al-0.5Cu alloy exhibits finer and much more uniform microstructure compared with gravity cast one, but increasing the applied pressure does not result in further grain refinement; (ii) the porosities are decreased markedly with increasing applied pressure and eventually disappear when the applied pressure is 90 MPa; (iii) the UTS and EL of the alloy are obviously improved with the application of pressure, which is mainly attributed to the full density of the samples; and (iv) when the applied pressure is 60 MPa, the heat-treated Mg-6Zn-4Al-0.5Cu alloy exhibits the optimal tensile properties with the YS, the UTS and EL of 216 MPa, 337 MPa and 12%, which are improved by 66%, 20% and 13%, respectively, as compared with that of the as-cast sample. Kumar et al. [88] investigated the effects of individual and combined additions of Sb and Sr on microstructure and creep properties of the squeeze-cast AZ91D alloy. It was mentioned that (i) individual and combined additions refine the grain size and β-$Mg_{17}Al_{12}$ phase, which is more pronounced with combined addition, (ii) besides α-Mg and β-$Mg_{17}Al_{12}$ phases, a new rod-shaped Mg_3Sb_2 and an irregular shaped Al_4Sr phases are formed following individual additions of Sb and Sr in the AZ91D alloy, (iii) with combined additions, both Mg_3Sb_2 and Al_4Sr phases are formed in the AZ91D alloy, (iv) all the alloys have been creep tested at a temperature of 175 °C and at an initial stress of 70 MPa, (v) all the modified AZ91D alloys exhibit superior creep resistance as compared to the base AZ91D alloy, (vi) individual addition of Sb is more effective as compared to the individual addition of Sr in improving creep resistance of the AZ91D alloy owing to the higher thermal stability of the Mg_3Sb_2 phase and (vii) among the modified alloys, the best creep resistance is obtained in the AZ91D alloy pertaining combined addition of both Sb and Sr, owing to the reduced amount of β-$Mg_{17}Al_{12}$ phase and increased amount of high melting point Mg_3Sb_2 and Al_4Sr intermetallic phases. Zhao et al. [89] studied microstructural evolution of Mg-15Gd-1Zn-0.4Zr (GZ151K, wt%) alloys, cast under 0 MPa (gravity cast) and 6 MPa (squeeze cast). It was reported that (i) the grain size of squeeze-cast GZ151K alloy with applied stress 6 MPa is much smaller than that of the gravity cast counterpart, (ii) the squeezing pressure hinders the transition from β' precipitates to $β_1$ precipitates during subsequent aging process, leading to reduced volume fraction of $β_1$ precipitates in the squeeze-cast alloy and (ii) the relatively lower volume fraction of $β_1$ precipitates in the squeeze-cast GZ151K results in higher hardness increment and stronger precipitation hardening effect.

6.2.6 Direct chill casting

Direct chill (DC) casting is a method for the fabrication of cylindrical or rectangular solid ingots from nonferrous metals, especially Al, Cu, Mg and their alloys. The casting method reduces the internal stress in the cooled material by allowing contractions on all side, as opposed to only on the top of the ingot in a traditional trough mold [90]. Figure 6.1 compares vertical DC casting for both conventional design and hot top cold design with the electromagnetic casting mold [90]. DC casting is a vertical semicontinuous casting process used for fabrication of cylindrical billets or rectangular ingots/blooms from nonferrous metals such as Al-based, Cu-based and Mg-based alloys. DC cast ingots are further processed by either extrusion, rolling or forging technologies. The most popular application of the DC process is casting aluminum billets for the extrusion and more than a half of aluminum in the world is cast by the DC process. There are two principal designs for the DC casting molds: float-controlled melt flow (conventional design) and hot top design and the latter possesses advantages such as (i) flow control is not required, (ii) the melt is protected from oxidation and (iii) reduces heat losses. Electromagnetic mold uses an alternating electromagnetic field generated by the mold itself for repealing the liquid metal from the mold wall. The alternating current flowing through the inductor induces eddy currents in the melt. The eddy currents interact with the magnetic field generated by the inductor and the Lorenz forces produced as a result of such interaction hold the melt apart from the mold wall, resulting in that the mold forms the ingot shape but does not remove the heat. The entire heat is extracted by the water jets flowing from the mold onto the ingot surface. The main advantages of the DC casting in electromagnetic

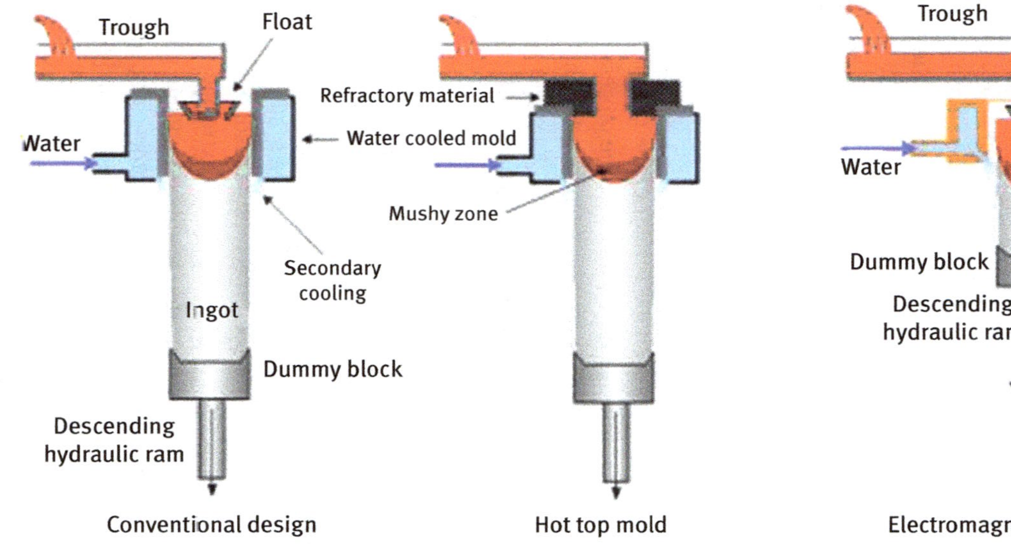

Figure 6.1: Different mold designs in direct chill casting [90].

mold are (i) good surface quality due to the absence of direct contact and friction between the ingot and mold surfaces and (ii) fine grain structure due to the fast cooling provided by the DC only (without heat transfer through the mold wall) and the melt agitation produced by the electromagnetic forces [90].

Zheng et al. [91] prepared high-quality Mg-Nd-Zn-Zr magnesium alloy billets with diameter of 200 mm by DC casting. It was reported that (i) microstructures of the as-cast billet prepared by DC casting are mainly composed of equiaxed a-Mg and $Mg_{12}Nd$ eutectic compound distributing along the grain boundaries, (ii) the average grain size decreases along the radius of the billet, (iii) the alloying elements of Nd and Zn distribute homogeneously across the large billet and (iv) the optimum process parameters for DC casting of the Mg-Nd-Zn-Zr magnesium alloy billet with diameter of 200 mm have been experimentally determined as follows: casting temperature 710 °C, and casting speed 80 mm/min.

6.2.7 Semisolid metal casting

Semisolid metal casting (SSM) is a near-net shape variant of die casting. The process is used with nonferrous metals, such as Al, Cu and Mg. The process combines the advantages of casting and forging. SSM is done at a temperature that puts the metal between its liquidus and solidus temperature [92, 93]. Among a number of different techniques to produce semisolid castings, thixocasting and rheocasting are popular [94–96].

6.2.7.1 Thixocasting

Thixocasting utilizes a precast billet with a nondendritic microstructure that is normally produced by vigorously stirring of the melt as the bar is being cast. Induction heating is normally used to reheat the billets to the semisolid temperature range and die casting machines are used to inject the semisolid material into hardened steel dies. Thixocasting has the ability to produce extremely high-quality components due to the product consistency that results from using precast billet that is manufactured under the same ideal continuous processing conditions that are employed to make forging or rolling stock [94–96]. Amira et al. [97] studied the microstructure and phase composition of die cast and thixocast ZAEX10430 (Mg-10Zn-4Al-3Ce-0.3Ca) alloy. It was mentioned that (i) two intermetallic phases were identified in both the die cast and the thixocast specimens: the τ-phase doped with calcium $(Mg,Ca)_{32}(Al,Zn)_{49}$ (or τ′-phase) and the $(Al,Zn)_xCe$ isomorphous phase with Al_2CeZn_2 and Al_4Ce, (ii) in all of the specimens, the τ′-phase crystallized mostly as fine elongated particles and within a lamellar constituent, (iii) needle-like $(Al,Zn)_xCe$ phase particles were visible in the die cast specimens, whereas coarse particles of various cross-sectional shapes (polygonal, elliptical, rod-like, etc.) were observed in the thixocast specimens and (iv) the difference in morphology of the intermetallic $(Al,Zn)_xCe$ particles in the matrix and the presence of large primary α-Mg grains in the thixocast specimens was used to explain the different creep behavior of diecast and thixocast ZAEX10430 alloy reported previously.

6.2.7.2 Rheocasting

Unlike thixocasting, which reheats a billet, rheocasting develops the semisolid slurry from the molten metal produced in a typical die casting furnace. This is a big advantage over thixocasting because it results in less expensive feedstock, in the form of typical die casting alloys, and allows for direct recycling [94–96]. Fang et al. [98] fabricated a novel Mg-3RE-6Zn-1.4Y alloy by rheo-squeeze casting. It was reported that (i) the increase of the pressure not only contributes to the refinement of α-Mg grains but also results in the increasing solid solubility in the matrix and uniform distribution of RE-rich intermetallic compounds along the grain boundary, (ii) the tensile properties increase continuously with the increase of applied pressure and (iii) the YS, UTS and EL of rheo-squeeze cast sample under 200 MPa pressure are 110 MPa, 180 MPa and 8.6%, which are improved by 17.0%, 19.2% and 81.7%, respectively, than the corresponding values of the samples without pressure. Poddar et al. [99] investigated the microstructure and mechanical properties of conventional cast and rheocast Mg–Sn alloy. It was mentioned that (i) the microstructure of conventional cast Mg–5%Sn and Mg–8%Sn alloys showed different phases, such as primary α-Mg, β-Mg_2Sn phase that precipitates at the grain boundary, and eutectic α-Mg, a dark area surrounding the precipitate phase; (ii) with the addition of mischmetal in Mg–5%Sn alloy, the refinement of microstructure was observed and also the interdendritic second phase changed from rod/irregular shaped to rod and feathery shaped; (iii) in Mg-8%Sn-3%Al-1%Si alloy, α-Mg, Mg_2Sn, $Mg_{17}Al_{12}$ and Mg_2Si phases were observed; (iv) with the addition of Al–Sc master alloy in Mg–8%Sn alloy, the matrix grain size became finer; (v) the rheocast microstructures showed that the primary α-Mg phase is nondendritic and globular shaped; (vi) solution heat treatment at 520 °C for 48–72 h leads to complete dissolution of Mg_2Sn intermetallic in Mg–Sn alloys; (vii) during aging at 200 °C, discontinuous precipitates were formed at the grain boundaries in the initial stage and later continuous precipitates occurred in the remaining regions; and (viii) hardness values were significantly improved after 100 h of aging for all the alloys compared to as-cast alloys. Bartex et al. [100] investigated morphological evolution of microstructures and tensile properties in Mg–Al alloy containing La and Ca (Mg-6Al-3La-1Ca) processed by rheocasting with different solid fractions (f_S) with conducting isothermal mechanical stirring experiments with f_S = 0.30, 0.49 and 0.61 at 950 rpm for 10 min. It was reported that (i) microstructure in conventional casting is composed by α-Mg dendritic matrix and $Al_{11}La_3$, $(Al,Mg)_2Ca$ and Mg_2Ca compounds, (ii) nondendritic and globular microstructures were observed in the rheocasting, (iii) for f_S = 0.30 the acicular $Al_{11}La_3$ phase precipitated at globule boundaries, while for the f_s = 0.49 and f_s = 0.61 the acicular phase precipitated both inside and at globule boundaries, (iv) the ideal rheocasting condition was achieved f_s = 0.30 due to the improvement of 76% for the UTS and 80% in the strain to fracture when compared to the conventional casting and (v) fracture surface analysis pointed to a mixed ductile–brittle fracture mode containing dimples and quasicleavage facets for the lowest solid fraction (f_s = 0.3), and a fully brittle fracture mode consisting exclusively of cleavage planes for the highest solid fraction (f_s = 0.61).

6.3 Sol–gel method and other chemical/electrochemical methods

The name sol–gel derived from the fact that micro particles or molecules in a solution (sols) agglomerate and under controlled conditions eventually link together to form a coherent network (gel). The process of the settling of (nm sized) particles from a colloidal suspension onto a preexisting surface results in ceramic materials. The desired solid particles (e.g., metal alkoxides) are suspended in a liquid, forming the sol, which is deposited on a substrate by spinning, dipping or coating or transferred to a mold. The particles in the sol are polymerized by partial evaporation of the solvent, or addition of an initiator, forming the gel, which is then heated at high temperature to give the final solid product [101, 102].

Tailoring optical bandgap of ZnO nanostructured thin films are doped with different elements that facilitate potential material for photonic applications. Different methods of fabrication process result in different optical and structural properties for the same amount of Mg content. Therefore, detailed investigation of structural and optical parameters and their correlation need to be revealed to utilize the fabricated thin films. Mia et al. [103] fabricated Mg-doped ZnO thin film of 200 nm thickness by sol–gel spin coating method on a glass substrate for four different Mg content levels. It was mentioned that (i) the spectroscopic analysis showed a uniform crystalline nanostructured surface with less structural defects, enhanced transmittance and higher optical bandgap than that of pure ZnO nanostructured thin film and (ii) changing trend of structural and optical parameters with Mg content showed nonlinear, nonmonotonic relation. Shi et al. [104] prepared thin films of ZnO, K-doped ZnO (KZO) and (Mg, K) codoped ZnO (MKZO) thin films using sol–gel method and reported that (i) all the films have a preferential c-axis orientation and an average transmittance of over 93% in the visible range, (ii) the optical band gap decreases by K doping, but gradually increases by Mg doping at a given K doping concentration and (iii) photoluminescence (PL) spectra show that the visible emission was enhanced, which indicates that the number of defects should be changed at Mg doping concentration of 8 mol%. Nadumane et al. [105] synthesized new nickel ferrite and Mg-doped nickel ferrite photocatalysts under modified green sol–gel route and reported that (i) the PL analysis indicates that the present nanoparticles (NPs) are an effective white component in display applications, (ii) these synthesized NPs were used for photocatalytic decomposition of recalcitrant pollutants in aqueous media under sunlight irradiation, (iii) among investigated samples, the $NiFe_2O_4$: Mg^{2+} (1 mol%) exhibits the highest photocatalytic efficiency for the decomposition of recalcitrant pollutants, which is higher than that of the commercial P25 and (iv) this enhancement in photocatalytic performance can be mainly attributed to the balance between the parameters, crystallanity, band gap, morphology, crystallite size, defects, dopant amount and combined facets of photocatalysis. Luo et al. [106] synthesized magnesium oxide (MgO) nanopowders by a sol–gel method with different amounts of ammonium hydroxide ($NH_3 \cdot H_2O$). It was reported that (i) the structure and morphology of MgO nanopowders can be regulated by the addition of $NH_3 \cdot H_2O$, (ii) when an appropriate amount of $NH_3 \cdot H_2O$ was added into the reaction system, plate-like nano-MgO was obtained, (iii) the antibacterial activity test of MgO revealed that the MgO nanoplates have great antibacterial effect with an minimum inhibitory concentration (MIC) value of 600 mg/L and the bactericidal rate was about 99.8% at a concentration of 500 mg/L, (iv) the effect of $NH_3 \cdot H_2O$ on the structure and morphology of MgO nanopowders and on the growth mechanism are briefly discussed and (v) the hydroxide ion of $NH_3 \cdot H_2O$, in favor of $Mg(OH)_2$ generation in the precursors, is essential for the formation of MgO nanoplates.

There are still variety of synthesis methods including electrochemical or chemical method. Zhang et al. [107] prepared Mg–Li alloys by electrolysis in a molten salt electrolyte of 50% LiCl–50% KCl (mass%) at low temperature of 420–510 °C and studied the effects of electrolytic temperature and cathodic current density on alloy formation rate and current efficiency. It was reported that (i) for the deposition of metallic lithium on the cathode consisting of solid Mg and liquid Mg–Li, both electrolytic temperature and cathodic current density have no obvious influence on current efficiency; while for the deposition of metallic lithium on the solid magnesium cathode, both electrolytic temperature and cathodic current density greatly affect alloy formation rate and current efficiency, (ii) the optimum electrolysis condition is molten salt mixture, LiCl:KCl = 1:1 (mass%), electrolytic temperature: 480 °C, cathode current density: 1.13 A/cm^2 and (iii) Mg–Li alloys with low lithium content (about 25 wt% Li) were prepared via electrolysis at low temperature followed by thermal treatment at higher temperature. Yan et al. [108] investigated the electrochemical codeposition of Mg, Li, and Zn on a molybdenum electrode in LiCl-KCl-$MgCl_2$-$ZnCl_2$ melts at 670 °C to form Mg–Li–Zn alloys. It was reported that (i) cyclic voltammograms showed that the potential of Li metal deposition, after the addition of $MgCl_2$ and $ZnCl_2$, is more positive than the Li metal deposition before the addition, (ii) the analysis of energy dispersive spectrometry showed that the elements of Mg and Zn distribute homogeneously in the Mg–Li–

Zn alloy and (iii) the plasma analysis showed that the chemical compositions of Mg–Li–Zn alloys are consistent with the phase structures of the XRD patterns, and the lithium and zirconium contents of Mg–Li–Zn alloys depend on the concentrations of $MgCl_2$ and $ZnCl_2$. Chen et al. [109] investigated the electrochemical behavior of Yb^{3+} and electrodeposition of Mg–Yb alloy film at solid magnesium cathode in the molten LiCl–KCl–$YbCl_3$ (2 wt%) system at 500 °C. It was mentioned that (i) the reduction process of Yb^{3+} is stepwise reactions which are single-electron and double-electron reversible charge transfer reactions, (ii) a very thin Mg_2Yb alloy film (~200 nm) was formed by potentiostatic electrolysis at −1.85 V (vs Ag/AgCl) for 12 h, (iii) a much thicker Mg_2Yb alloy film (~450 μm) was obtained at −2.50 V (vs Ag/AgCl) for 2.5 h and (iv) the corrosion resistance of magnesium can be enhanced by electrochemical formation of Mg–Yb alloy film on its surface. Cao et al. [110] studied the electrodeposition of erbium on molybdenum electrodes and the formation of Mg–Li–Er alloys in LiCl–KCl molten salts. It was mentioned that (i) cyclic voltammograms showed that the underpotential deposition of lithium on predeposited Mg–Er alloy led to the formation of a Mg–Li–Er alloy, (ii) XRD identified Er_5Mg_{24} phase formed via potentiostatic electrolysis and (iii) scanning electron microscopy revealed that Er atoms mainly concentrated at the grain boundaries while Mg element evenly located in the alloy. Li et al. [111] prepared films of Mg-Mn-Fe-Co-Ni-Gd alloy films by electrodeposition and reported that (i) the surface morphology can be controlled by deposition potential and solution composition, (ii) hollow microspheres and core–shell microspheres can be obtained, (iii) the as-deposited alloy is amorphous and (iv) the ferromagnetism to diamagnetism transition can be observed when the contents of Mg is lower than 20%. Li et al. [112] fabricated a three-dimensional (3D) nanoporous bimetallic Ag–Cu alloy with uniform chemical composition by dealloying Mg-12.5Ag-12.5Cu-10Y metallic glass in dilute (0.04 M) H_2SO_4 aqueous solution under free-corrosion conditions. It was reported that the nanoporous Ag–Cu evolves through two distinct stages: first, ligaments of the nanoporous structure, consisting of supersaturated Ag(Cu) solid solution with a constant Ag/Cu mole ratio of 1:1, are yielded and second, with excessive immersion, some Cu atoms separate from the metastable nanoporous matrix and form spherical Cu particles on the sample surface.

Zhao et al. [113] developed a new Mg–Cu system to fabricate monolithic nanoporous copper ribbons and bulk nanoporous Cu through chemical dealloying in a 5 wt% HCl solution. It was mentioned that (i) the compositions of the melt-spun Mg–Cu alloys have an important effect on the dealloying process and microstructures of the nanoporous Cu ribbons and (ii) the synergetic dealloying of Mg_2Cu and $MgCu_2$ in two-phase Mg–Cu alloys results in the formation of nanoporous Cu with a uniform porous structure.

Wang et al. [114] fabricated the biomedical cocontinuous (β-TCP + MgO)/Zn–Mg composite by infiltrating Zn–Mg alloy into porous β-TCP + MgO using suction exsorption technique. It was mentioned that (i) the molten Zn–Mg alloy had infiltrated not only into the pores but also into the struts of the porous β-TCP + MgO scaffold to form a compact composite, (ii) the Zn–Mg alloy is in contact with the β-TCP + MgO scaffold closely, and no reaction layer can be found between the alloy and the scaffold, (iii) the compressive strength of the composite was as high as 244 MPa, which was about 1,000 times higher than that of the original porous β-TCP + MgO scaffold and two-thirds of the strength of the Zn–Mg bulk alloy, (iv) the electrochemical and immersion tests in simulated body fluid solution indicated that the corrosion resistance of the composite was better than that of the Zn–Mg bulk alloy and the corrosion products on the composite surface were mainly $Zn(OH)_2$ and (v) appropriate mechanical and corrosion properties indicated that the (β-TCP + MgO)/Zn–Mg composite fabricated by suction exsorption would be a very promising candidate for bone substitute.

Rong et al. [115] developed a high-strength Mg-Gd-Zn-Zr alloy by a novel extrusion method (differential-thermal extrusion: DTE). It was reported that (i) different from traditional isothermal extrusion (ITE) with the same billet and mold temperature, the billet temperature for the DTE is remarkably higher than the mold temperature, (ii) the finer grains and less LPSO structure in the DTE sample resulted from its higher cooling speed after deformation, (iii) the stronger precipitation strengthening effect was caused by the higher billet preheat temperature which reserved the precipitation ability before extrusion; as a result, the finer grains and stronger precipitation strengthening led to the strong TYS (380 MPa) and UTS (461 MPa) of the aged DTE sample, while those of the aged ITE sample are only 338 MPa and 420 MPa, respectively, and (iv) the higher strengths indicate that the DTE is a better extrusion process for producing high-strength Mg alloys than the traditional ITE.

Zheng et al. [116] investigated a preparation of Mg–Li alloys by vacuum silicothermic reduction process. It was mentioned that (i) the main phase of the product is Mg and that of slag is Ca_2SiO_4, (ii) the product successively presents lamellar, short rod-like and flocculent shape along with the condensation, (iii) when no fluorite was added, the impacts of extraction conditions, including ferrosilicon addition, temperature, compacting pressure and holding time, on Mg and Li recoveries were evaluated and (iii) under the conditions of temperature of 1,250 °C, ferrosilicon addition of 110%, compacting pressure of 15 MPa and holding time of 150 min, Mg and Li recoveries are 81.38% and 99.58%, respectively.

6.4 Mechanical alloying and microalloying

6.4.1 Mechanical alloying

MA is a solid-state powder processing technique involving repeated welding, fracturing and rewelding of powder particles in a high-energy ball mill. MA has now been shown to be capable of synthesizing a variety of equilibrium and nonequilibrium alloy phases starting from blended elemental or prealloyed powders. The nonequilibrium phases synthesized include supersaturated solid solutions, metastable crystalline and quasicrystalline phases, nanostructures and amorphous alloys [117, 118].

Lu et al. [119] synthesized a quaternary Mg-5Al-10.3Ti-4.7B (by wt%) alloy using mechanical milling and reported that (i) extremely large EL at room temperature of 43% in the binary Mg–10.3 wt%Ti alloy has been obtained and (ii) the quarternary alloy gives the highest YS and UTS via the formation of titanium boride particulates. Gennari et al. [120] investigated the MA of the 2 Mg–0.5Ni–0.5Ge mixture at room temperature under argon atmosphere and reported that (i) a new alloy in the Mg–Ni–Ge system was synthesized by MA of the 2 Mg–0.5Ni–0.5Ge mixture and by the combination of MA and subsequent thermal treatment, (ii) no evidence of the formation of Ni–Ge compounds was observed, (iii) the new ternary alloy can be considered isostructural with Mg_3Ni_2M-type compound, with a F cubic cell and a lattice parameter $a = 11.521$ Å and (iv) thermal studies show that the Mg–Ge–Ni alloy is stable upon heating up to 500 °C. Rojas et al. [121] studied the microstructural evolution during MA of Mg and Ni. It was reported that (i) a large number of defects were produced during the first hours of milling and these defects led to the amorphization of part of the system and promoted an extensive refinement of the microstructure as well, but later on, the formation of the Mg_2Ni compound due to the crystallization of the amorphous phase was observed and (ii) subsequent heat treatments of the milled powder showed that the amorphous phase could also be transformed into Mg_2Ni by heating. Al–Mg and Al–Mg–Zr alloys were processed by MA [122]. It was mentioned that (i) in as-milled powders, an Al(Mg) solid solution was formed with up to 40 at% Al, which after annealing transformed to the equilibrium β-Al_3Mg_2 phase, (ii) for high Mg concentrations (60–90 at%), the dominant phase was γ-$Al_{12}Mg_{17}$ in accordance with the equilibrium phase diagram, (iii) the addition of Zr led to the appearance of Zr–Al intermetallics causing Mg to precipitate out of the Al(Mg) solution and (iv) the effect of zirconium was also to refine the structure and to retard grain growth. Brett et al. [123], using electrochemical impedance spectroscopy, studied the electrochemical behavior (in 0.1 M Na_2SO_4 and 0.01 M NaCl electrolyte solutions) of ternary $Mg_{60}Ti_{10}Si_{30}$ and $Mg_{88}Ti_5Si_7$ alloy by MA of the elemental powders in an argon atmosphere. It was shown that (i) corrosion is greater for $Mg_{88}Ti_5Si_7$ which contains free magnesium; however, in sulfate solution a protective oxide layer formed can reduce the corrosion rate and (ii) in $Mg_{60}Ti_{10}Si_{30}$, heat treatment increases corrosion, which is explained through a greater tendency for pitting corrosion. Lee et al. [124] synthesized amorphous and composite Mg–Ni–Ca metal hydrides by MA. It was reported that (i) $(Mg_{0.5}Ca_{0.5})Ni_2$ yielded the composite of Mg_2Ni and $CaNi_5$, while $MgNi_{0.95}$ $Ca_{0.05}$ produced the amorphous phase, (ii) the initial discharge capacities of the amorphous $MgNi_{0.95}$ $Ca_{0.05}$ alloy and the composite $(Mg_{0.5}Ca_{0.5})Ni_2$ alloy were 460 and 210 mAh/g, respectively, (iii) after 20 cycles, the amorphous electrode retained 11% of the initial discharge capacity while the composite electrode maintained 64% of the initial discharge capacity and (iv) after 10 cycles, the X-ray photoelectron spectroscopic analysis showed that Mg spectra of the amorphous $MgNi_{0.95}$ $Ca_{0.05}$ alloy was shifted to a lower binding energy because Mg reacted with OH^- of the electrolyte; however, Mg spectra of the composite $(Mg_{0.5}Ca_{0.5})Ni_2$ alloy showed that the binding energy did not change during the cycle test, indicating that the amorphous phase had the highest discharge capacity, and the composite formation improved the cyclic stability. Zhang et al. [125] prepared $Mg_{2-x}Zr_xNi$ ($x = 0$, 0.15, 0.3, 0.45 and 0.6) electrode alloys by MA. It was found that (i) the substitution of Zr for Mg is favorable for the formation of an amorphous phase, (ii) for a fixed milling time, the amorphous phase in the alloy increases with increasing Zr content and (iii) the electrochemical measurements indicate that the substitution of Zr can dramatically enhance the discharge capacity with preferable cycle stability and markedly improve the discharge voltage characteristics of the alloys.

Datta et al. [126] studied room-temperature solid-state diffusion reaction induced by MA of elemental blends of Mg, Zn and Ca of nominal composition of 60 Mg–35Zn–5Ca by at%. It was mentioned that (i) the amorphous powder consolidated using cold isostatic pressing showed an envelope density ~80% of absolute density, which increased to an envelope density ~84% of absolute density after sintering at an optimized temperature of ~250 °C for 9 h, (ii) electrochemical biocorrosion testing of the cold isostatic pressing compacted amorphous pellet as well as the sintered pellet performed in Dulbecco's modified Eagle's medium, showed improved corrosion resistance in comparison to the as-cast pure Mg and (iii) cytotoxicity testing of the cold isostatic pressing compacted amorphous pellet, performed using the MTT (3-(4,5-dimethylthiazol-2yl)-2,5-diphenyltetrazolium bromide) assay with MC3T3 osteoblastic cells, showed low cytotoxicity in comparison to the as-cast pure Mg. Phase evolution during MA of elemental Mg and Cu powders and their subsequent heat treatment was investigated [127]. Elemental Mg and Cu powders in a 2:1 atomic ratio was mechanically alloyed in a SPEX 8000D mill using a 10:1 ball-to-powder ratio. It was reported that (i) the combination of differential scanning calorimetry, heat treatment and XRD has shown a sequence of phase transformations resulting in the intermetallic Mg_2Cu from an amorphous precursor; and (ii) the amorphous phase is converted into Mg_2Cu by heating at low temperature (134 °C) and short MA times, and the formation of the amorphous precursor, together with its subsequent transformation into Mg_2Cu at low temperatures, represents an advantageous alternative route for its preparation. Khalajabadi et al. [128] synthesized a magnesium matrix nanocomposite comprising bioactive ceramics of Mg-substituted hydroxyapatite (HA), farringtonite ($Mg_3(PO_4)_2$), perovskite ($CaTiO_3$), geikielite ($MgTiO_3$) and brucite ($Mg(OH)_2$) through MA and annealing of a Mg-HA-TiO_2-MgO mixture by mechanically induced self-propagating reactions. It was reported that (i) after 16 h of milling, the powder mixture exhibited a homogenous distribution of fine agglomerates composed of spherical particles with an average size of 83 nm, (ii) the crystallinity and thermal stability of the HA phase decreased with increasing milling time because of the substitution of Mg atoms in the HA structure, (iii) the mean crystallite size of the product phases was approximately 75 nm after 8 h of MA, and these values increased slightly to 82 and 88 nm after 1 h of annealing at 500°C and 630 °C, respectively, (iv) the biocorrosion test of the nanocomposites revealed that the corrosion potential of the as-blended samples shifted toward a nobler direction from – 1,565 to –1,457 mV_{SCE} by increasing the amount of HA from 12.5 to 25 wt%, (v) after 16 h of milling, the corrosion resistance of the milled samples comprising 12.5 and 25 wt% HA increased to 4.63 and 4.97 $k\Omega \cdot cm^2$, respectively, and (vi) the milled samples annealed at 63 0 °C exhibited lower corrosion rates compared with those annealed at 500 °C, suggesting that the high-energy ball milling of the Mg-HA-TiO_2-MgO mixture accompanied with post annealing is a promising option for controlling the rapid corrosion rate. Chaubey et al. [129] produced high-dense ultrafine grain Mg–7.4%Al bulk samples with grain size of about 300 nm by powder metallurgy through hot consolidation of mechanically alloyed powders. It was mentioned that room-temperature compression tests of the consolidated bulk material reveal remarkable mechanical properties: high compressive strength of about 690 MPa combined with a plastic strain exceeding 9%, being attributed to the combination of three different strengthening mechanisms, namely, grain size refinement, dispersion strengthening and solid solution strengthening. The fracture surface shows transgranular quasicleavage fracture in nature. The MgO-rich regions often acted as the microcrack initiation source and thereby stop the main crack. The uniformly distributed intermetallic (γ-$Al_{12}Mg_{17}$) particles in the matrix-deflected main crack resulted in a tortuous crack path, demonstrating that powder metallurgy, MA combined with hot consolidation, is a suitable method for the production of nanostructured Mg-based materials characterized by high strength and considerable plastic deformation.

Kursun et al. [130] synthesized nanocrystalline $Mg_{55}Cu_{40}Ni_5$ alloy from the elemental powders by MA. It was shown that (i) after 50 h of milling time, nanostructured α-Cu(Mg,Ni) solid solution, MgO and $Mg_{0.85}Cu_{0.15}$ phases whose crystallite sizes are below 20 nm were obtained and (ii) the elemental powder particles which were initially of different size, shape and distribution became uniform, confirming the compositional homogeneity of the $Mg_{55}Cu_{40}Ni_5$ alloy, and particle size decreased rapidly with increasing milling time. Salleh research group had extensive investigation on biodegradable MAed Mg–Zn alloy on density and hardness [131], effect of milling duration [132] and elastic modulus [133]. It was reported that (i) density of sintered Mg–Zn alloy was between 1.80 and 1.99 g/cm^3 which is close to the density of human bone and hardness of pure Mg increased from 27 HV to 54 HV to 94 HV with the addition of 3–10 wt% Zn [131], (ii) a prolonged milling time has increased the density and microhardness of the sintered Mg–Zn alloy [132] and (iii) the elastic modulus of biodegradable Mg–Zn alloy was between 40.18 and 47.88 GPa, which was improved and resembled that of natural bone (30–57 GPa) and corrosion resistance (mass loss of pure Mg, 33.74 mg) was enhanced with addition of 3–10% Zn (between 9.32 and 15.38 mg) [133].

The method of mechanical milling was applied to synthesize nanocrystalline Mg_xTi_{100-x} ($x = 95, 90, 85$) composite powders [134]. It was mentioned that (i) mechanical milling is an effective method for preparing Mg–Ti composite powders, which consist of nanocrystalline Mg matrix and fine dispersed Ti particles; (ii) the microstructure evolution and morphology of the as-milled powders were observed, and the corresponding mechanisms were also discussed; (iii) after milling for 60 h, the crystallite size of the matrix Mg in Mg_xTi_{100-x} composite powders was refined to 105, 84 and 76 nm, respectively; (iv) the average size of the dispersed Ti particles in Mg_xTi_{100-x} ($x = 90$) composite powders was refined to about 1 μm; (v) for all these Mg–Ti composite powders, the solid solubility of Ti in Mg seemed to be closely related with the milling time and the content of Ti and (vi) in the 60 h milled Mg_xTi_{100-x} ($x = 95, 90, 85$) composite powders, the solid solubility of Ti in Mg was estimated to be 0.56 at%, 1.32 at% and 2.35 at%, respectively. Asano et al. [135] studied the synthesis process of Mg–Ti alloys by ball milling and reported that (i) the $Mg_{50}Ti_{50}$ body-centered cubic (BCC) phase with the lattice parameter of $a = 0.342(1)$ nm and the grain size of 3 nm was formed, (ii) during milling of Mg and Ti to synthesize the BCC alloy, Mg and Ti were deformed mainly by the basal plane slip and the twinning deformation, respectively, (iii) Ti acted as abrasives for Mg which had stuck on the surface of the milling pot and balls and (iv) the BCC phase was found after Mg dissolved in Ti. Khan et al. [136] produced nanocrystalline Mg–xAl ($x = 0$, 5, 10 and 20 wt%) alloys via high-energy ball milling followed by compaction under uniaxial pressure of 3 GPa at room temperature, followed by heat treatment for 1 h at various temperatures ranging from room temperature to 425 °C. It was found that (i) hardness of the ball milled Mg–xAl alloys was higher than many commercial Mg alloys, (ii) hardness of the alloys was influenced by the Al addition and heat treatment and it was correlated with the crystallite size and microstructure and (iii) high hardness of Mg–xAl alloys was attributed to the grain refinement and Al addition. Cryomilling is a broadly applied technique to synthesize nanostructured alloys and composites through powder metallurgy processing. Nezafati et al. [137] studied the interaction of nitrogen and Mg lattice in Mg alloys synthesized by the cryomilling process. It was reported that the diffusion of N atoms is much easier than that of N_2 molecule in the Mg matrix. Habila et al. [138] investigated the microstructure and texture of an Al1050/AZ31/Al1050 laminated composite fabricated by accumulative roll bonding (ARB) at 400 °C up to five cycles. It was reported that (i) ARB processing led to microstructural refinement with equiaxed grain microstructure in AZ31 layers and to the development of elongated grains parallel to the rolling direction in Al 1050 layers, (ii) no new phases formed at the bond interface after the first ARB cycle while $Mg_{17}Al_{12}$ and Mg_2Al_3 phases appeared after subsequent cycles, (iii) the microhardness of Al1050/AZ31/Al1050 laminated composite increased with increasing ARB cycles and almost saturated after five ARB cycles, (iv) the YS and ultimate strength increased gradually between one and three ARB cycles due to the strain hardening and grain refinement and decreased with further increasing of the ARB cycles because of crack and failure of the Mg_xAl_y intermetallic compounds which developed during fourth and fifth ARB cycles and (v) the deformation behavior of the laminated composite becomes rather similar to the behavior of AZ31 alloy that underwent a dynamic recrystallization during processing.

6.4.2 Microalloying

Chen et al. [139] prepared Mg–Nd coatings by high-energy microarc alloying on AZ31 magnesium alloy and the coatings were treated with Ar shielding gas in ambient atmosphere. It was shown that (i) the phases formed of Mg–Nd coatings were similar to that of Mg–Nd electrode, (ii) the corrosion behavior of the coated AZ31 in 3.5 wt% NaCl solutions indicate that the corrosion resistance of coated alloy was higher than that of AZ31 substrate, and the corrosion potential of Mg–Nd coatings was much positive to that of AZ31 substrate and (iii) the corrosion resistance is bad due to the presence of defects when treated with undesired processing parameters. Langelier et al. [140] enhanced the microstructure and mechanical properties of Mg–Zn alloys by combining microalloying additions of the RE element Ce and the non-RE element Ca. It was reported that (i) the double additions of Ce–Ca are found to significantly increase tensile EL compared to binary Mg–Zn, or single additions of either Ce or Ca, (ii) microstructure analysis reveals that the Ce–Ca additions increase ductility by modifying texture and refining grain size, (iii) texture modification is attributed to solute effects from the microalloying elements, particularly Ca, while grain refinement is additionally influenced by a fine dispersion of $Mg_6Ca_2Zn_3$ precipitates that form during rolling and pin grain boundaries, (iv) the microalloying element additions also lead to large secondary phase particles in the alloys, which can limit ductility enhancement by promoting early fracture and (v) by scaling Zn content in the Mg-Zn-Ce-Ca alloys, the $Mg_6Ca_2Zn_3$ phase fraction and Zn solute content can be controlled for optimum ductility or strengthening potential. Macchi et al. [141] studied effects of microalloying with Ag on the precipitation process in an Al–Cu–Mg alloy with high Mg:Cu ratio during artificial aging of the ternary and quaternary compositions Al–1.5Cu–4 Mg(–0.5Ag) by wt% at 175 °C. It was mentioned that (i) data obtained for the silver-free alloy immediately after quenching from the solution treatment temperature, vacancy v–Cu–Mg clusters are formed in the supersaturated solid solution, (ii) during the early stages of aging these clusters become richer in Cu and Mg and laths of the *S* phase (Al_2CuMg) nucleate preferentially on dislocation lines, (iii) for the silver-containing Al–Cu–Mg alloy, vacancy v-Cu-Mg-Ag aggregates also form immediately after quenching and the solute transport mechanisms are the same, (iv) for both alloys, no evidence was found that the Z phase is preceded by any preprecipitate or Guinier–Preston zones and (v) additional aging experiments at 240 °C showed that neither the Z phase or T phase are formed in the ternary alloy, but only precipitates of the S phase, while in the quaternary alloy the *S* phase is strongly suppressed and mainly Z phase precipitates are formed. Candan et al. [142] investigated micro-Ti-alloyed AZ91 Mg alloys (AZ91 + 0.5 wt%Ti) in order to clarify effectiveness of microalloying and/or cooling rate on their corrosion properties. It was reported that (i) the $Mg_{17}Al_{12}$ (β) intermetallic phase in the microstructure of AZ91 Mg alloy formed as a net-like structure, (ii) the Ti addition has reduced the distribution and continuity of β intermetallic phase and its morphology has emerged as fully divorced eutectic, (iii) compared to AZ91 alloy, the effect of the cooling rate in Ti-added alloy on the grain size was less pronounced and (iv) electrochemical test results showed that while I_{corr} values of AZ91 decrease with the increase in the cooling rate, the effect of the cooling rate on I_{corr} values was much lower in the Ti-added alloy.

et al. research group conducted an extensive work on Mg–Zn alloy systems in terms of the effect of microalloyed Ca and La on mechanical properties [143], microstructures and mechanical properties [144] and effects of Ce and La on mechanical properties [145]. It was reported that (i) YS, UTS and EL to failure of the alloy are 325 MPa, 341 MPa and 15%, respectively; being attributed to grain refinement, dense precipitation and high density of dislocations [143], (ii) the second phase in the as-cast Mg–6Zn alloy is Mg_4Zn_7, which is replaced by $Ca_2Mg_6Zn_3$ with an increase of Ca addition, and microalloying by Ca affects the grain size, dynamic recrystallization and dynamic precipitation of Mg–6Zn alloys during extrusion and inhibits dynamic recrystallization and grain growth due to the pinning effect of fine precipitates, giving rise to fine dynamic recrystallized grains [144] and (iii) Ce or Ca refined the microstructure and affected the texture obviously and (iv) compared with Ca, Ce was more effective to modify the texture and improve the plasticity [145]. Gao et al. [146] investigated in vitro and in vivo antibacterial functionality of Mg alloys through microalloying with Sr and Ga (0.1 wt%). It was reported that (i) a small amount additions of Ga and/or Sr reduce the degradation kinetics of Mg matrix, and the release of Ga^{3+} ions plays a crucial role in disabling the viability of all selected bacterial strains, (ii) the histological tests confirm that the growth of fibrous tissue has been accelerated in the vicinity of Mg-based implants, in comparison to that of blank and commercially pure Ti controls and (iii) the smallest number density of *Staphylococcus aureus* bacteria was found on the surface of the retrieved Ga-containing Mg rod implants.

6.5 Powder metallurgy

6.5.1 Powder metallurgy

A powder metallurgy route has been used to fabricate Mg–Zn–Y alloys reinforced by quasicrystalline particles, using rapidly solidified powders of Mg–2.1Zn–0.6Y and Mg–3.3Zn–0.43Y which were extruded in the temperature range 260–400 °C and it was mentioned that (i) as the extrusion temperature decreases, the yield stress increases due to grain size refinement and (ii) the Mg–3.3Zn–0.43Y alloy showed a yield stress of 410 MPa with a 12% EL [147]. Zhou et al. investigated microstructure and mechanical properties of PMed Mg-6Zn-5Ce-1.5Ca (wt%) alloy [148] and Mg–6Zn and Mg–6Zn–5Ca (wt%) alloys [149] and reported that (i) Mg-6Zn-5Ce-1.5Ca alloy was the characteristics of very fine grains with the size ranging from 200 to 650 nm and was composed of α-Mg, $Mg_xZn_yCe_z$ phase with a few Ca (about 1 at%) shortened as the $Mg_xZn_yCe_z$–(Ca) phase, and a small quantity of $Mg_{51}Zn_{20}$ phases and (ii) the atomic percentage ratio of Zn to Ce in the $Mg_xZn_yCe_z$–(Ca) phase around the grain boundary was close to 1.5 [148], (iii) with an addition of 5 wt% Ca to the Mg–6Zn alloy, the microstructure of the alloy was refined significantly, in which the grain size ranged from 500 nm to 1 µm and the number of finely dispersed particles increased substantially, resulting in an increase in the compressive strength of alloy up to 408 MPa at room temperature, (iv) although the strength of both the alloys decreased with an increase in test temperature, the Mg–6Zn–5Ca alloy exhibited a high strength of 202 MPa at 200 °C, which resulted mainly from the formation of particles of the stable intermetallic phase $Ca_2Mg_6Zn_3$, which were effective in pinning dislocations and grain boundaries at elevated temperatures and (v) the formation of deformation twins and their intersections, and the interaction between the twins and the $Ca_2Mg_6Zn_3$ particles during compressive deformation at 200 °C contributed to the strengthening of the alloy; however, the Mg–6Zn alloy exhibited a very low strength of 41 MPa at 200 °C, which resulted from dynamic recrystallization softening [149]. Fang et al. [150] fabricated Mg–3Al–Zn alloys with ultrafine grain size by consolidation of ball milling nanocrystalline powders. It was mentioned that (i) the bulk alloys with an average grain size of 180 nm showed a yield stress of 379MPa, which was 2 times higher than that of the coarse-grained AZ31, and their ultimate strength was 417MPa with a 5% EL, being attributed to three strengthening mechanism: the fine grain strengthening, dispersion strengthening and solid solution strengthening and (ii) low strain hardening was observed in the ultrafine grain alloy, which may be caused by room-temperature dynamic recovery during plastic deformation. A bulk Mg–Zn–Y alloy reinforced by quasicrystalline particles was produced by hot extrusion of rapidly solidified powders of $MgZn_{4.3}Y_{0.7}$ powders with different particle sizes which were prepared by an inert gas atomizer and then extruded at 380 °C with extrusion ratios of 10:1, 15:1 and 20:1 [151]. It was mentioned that (i) the mechanical strength and hardness of the extruded materials were enhanced by employing finer Mg alloy powders, (ii) more uniform deformation of powders in extruded billets with good tensile properties was achieved at higher extrusion ratios, especially for finer powders and (iii) the high strength of the $MgZn_{4.3}Y_{0.7}$ alloy was preserved at elevated temperatures due to the presence of icosahedral phase nanoparticles (NPs) [151]. Rashad et al. [152] fabricated PMed Mg–1Cu–xAl ($x = 1, 3, 6, 9$ wt%)

alloys to study the influence of copper and aluminum on mechanical behavior of pure magnesium. It was found that (i) microstructural evaluation revealed the presence of $Mg_{17}Al_{12}$ and Mg_2Cu intermetallic phases in synthesized alloys, (ii) the increase in aluminum content lead to increase in Vickers hardness, 0.2% YS and ultimate strength (both in tension and compression), (iii) the tensile failure strain of alloys increases till the threshold of 3 wt% Al is reached and (iv) the decline in failure strain for the alloys containing higher wt% Al contents (i.e., 6 and 9 wt% Al) might be attributed to the formation of brittle intermetallic phase $Mg_{17}Al_{12}$. Yang yet al. [153] produced PMed Mg–(15–50)Al (at%) foams with closed cells, where $CaCO_3$ is selected as the blowing agent. It was reported that (i) the key point of successful foaming is Al addition and the proper sintering treatment, which lead to the formation of intermetallic compounds and can make the gas release reaction between Mg melt and $CaCO_3$ happen during the foaming process and (ii) the high precursor compact degree, proper foaming temperature (~620 °C) and foaming time (~150 s) are required to fabricate Mg–Al alloy foam with good cellular structure.

Yu et al. [154] prepared Mg–Zn alloys by a powder metallurgy method using Mg powder and Zn powder as starting materials. It was reported that (i) the sintered compacts have finer grain size and higher sintered density upon Zn addition, (ii) the density of the sintered products increases with the increase of Zn content, (iii) the Mg–3 wt%Zn alloy is mainly composed of α-Mg phase, (iv) when the content of Zn is 4 wt%, the Mg–Zn alloys is composed of α-Mg and $MgZn_2$ phases, (v) with the increase of the Zn content, the bending strength of the Mg–Zn alloys first increases and then decreases, but the microhardness HV of Mg–Zn alloys always increases, (vi) the bending strength and microhardness of Mg–3 wt%Zn alloys are 123.6 MPa and 1,017 MPa, respectively, which are 58% and 45% higher than those of pure Mg samples and (vii) corrosion resistance measurements show that the corrosion rate of the Mg–Zn alloys decreases with the addition of Zn element, and the Mg–3 wt%Zn alloy shows the lowest corrosion rate and the best corrosion resistance. Hou et al. [155] prepared Mg–Al–Ni alloys by powder metallurgy and investigated their microstructure and elevated temperature mechanical properties. It was mentioned that (i) in addition to α-Mg matrix, both coarse Al_3Ni_2 particles and fine AlNi nanoparticles exist in the Mg–Al–Ni alloys, (ii) the strength at 150 °C is improved with the increase in Ni content, (iii) Mg–18.3Al–8Ni alloy possesses a compressive strength of 234.7 MPa and a YS of 146.5 MPa, (iv) plasticity is also improved with a low concentration of Ni, (v) Mg–11.3Al–2Ni alloy possesses a compression ratio of 17.3%, (vi) the phases of Al_3Ni_2 and AlNi in the alloys block the movements of grain boundaries and dislocations during the deformation at elevated temperature, (vii) the existence of AlNi phase provides a nonbasal slip system, leading to the improvement in plasticity and (viii) the formation mechanism of Al–Ni phases in the process is discussed with thermodynamics and kinetics. Kubásek et al. [156] prepared Mg-4Y-3RE-Zr (WE43) alloy by the powder metallurgy technique and mentioned that there was a partial improvement in the mechanical properties and superior corrosion resistance of PWed WE43, but the texture strength of PMed WE43 was low, and therefore, anisotropy of mechanical properties was suppressed. Kekule et al. [157] studied response to isochronal annealing up to 440 °C of squeeze-cast Mg–Y–Zn alloy and of the same alloy prepared by powder metallurgy and extruded at 280 °C. It was reported that (i) relatively high density of planar defects was found in grain interiors of the cast alloy with the grain size approximately 50 µm; (ii) secondary phase particles decorate grain boundaries in this alloy; (iii) three precipitation processes were detected in the cast alloy during repeated isochronal annealing up to 440 °C, whereas only one significant process was revealed in the PMed alloy and these processes were identified as embedding of stacking faults by solutes, development and rearrangement (18 R → 14 H) of LPSO phase and development of grain boundary particles; (iv) a coarsening of grain boundary particles rich in Y and Zn only proceeds in the PMed alloy; and (v) activation energies of the precipitation processes were determined. Microhardness exhibits good thermal stability against annealing up to 360 °C in the powder metallurgy alloy. Medina et al. [158] synthesized a high-strength Mg-6Zn-1Y-1Ca (wt%) alloy by powder metallurgy route. Rapidly solidified powders with a particle size below 100 µm were used as a way for preventing formation of ternary MgZnCa compounds during subsequent extrusion at 250 °C. It was reported that (i) the microstructure of the extruded alloy consists of an ultrafine-grain magnesium matrix, with an average grain size of 444 nm, embedding a high volume fraction of fine I-phase particles aligned along the extrusion direction, (ii) the alloy combines an excellent ductility (14% of EL to failure) with a high strength (ultimate strength of 469 MPa and yield stress of 461 MPa) at room temperature, mainly due to grain size refinement (around 70% of the yield stress) and (iii) the strength is kept high up to 150 °C (yield stress of 279 MPa) and above this temperature, the mechanical strength decreases to very low values but the ability to deform plastically is considerably enhanced, exhibiting superplastic behavior from 200 to 350 °C, with a maximum EL of 477% at 350 °C.

Schaper et al. [159] developed conventional AZ81 alloy by the metal injection molding and reported that (i) a YS of approximately 120 MPa and an UTS of approximately 255 MPa with EL at fracture of approximately 7% was achieved and (ii) T4 heat treatment at 420 °C for 10 h does not reveal a positive influence on the mechanical properties; this could be caused by an observed grain growth effect; this is in contrast to conventional material, for example, as cast, where T4 heat treatment is known to improve the mechanical properties especially EL at fracture. Zhou et al. [160] employed the hot isostatic pressing (HIP) to Mg-6Gd-3Y-0.5Zr (GW63) alloy to reduce shrinkage porosity, thus, to enhance the integrity and reliability of castings. It was mentioned that (i) during HIP process, shrinkage porosity was closed by grain compatible deformation and subsequent diffusion across the bonding interface, (ii) HIP was testified to be effective on shrinkage porosity reduction in GW63 alloy due to its relatively narrow solidification range and resultant low content of initial shrinkage porosity in most sections, leading to higher tensile properties both in as-cast and cast-T6 condition and (iii) the improvement in tensile properties was mainly because of shrinkage porosity reduction and resultant effective rare-earth elements homogenization and precipitation strengthening. Zhao et al. [161] fabricated ultrafine Mg-5.1Zn-0.18Zr-3Y alloys (by wt%) via powder metallurgy. It was reported that (i) RE element Y-containing alloys with uniformly equiaxed fine grains exhibited weaker texture intensity and (ii) deformation twinning in compression was hardly activated and replaced by dislocation and prismatic slips, (iii) the combined effect of the added Y and grain refinement resulted in the simultaneous enhancement of strength and ductility, especially for the compressive YS of the extruded alloy and (iv) the tension/compression asymmetry of the material was significantly reduced due to the changed deformation mechanism.

6.5.2 Plasma arc sintering

There are several works utilizing the spark plasma sintering method. Aydogmus et al. [162] fabricated Mg/$Ti_{49.4}Ni_{50.6}$ interpenetrating composites via spark plasma sintering technique. It was mentioned that (i) the microstructure of TiNi shape-memory alloy (SMA) reinforcement material is highly sensitive to processing conditions especially to sintering time, (ii) different sintering times resulted in different phase formations and accordingly different phase transformation temperatures due to the overlap of sintering temperature with aging temperature, (iii) room-temperature yield and compressive strength of the composite samples were in the range of 53–113 MPa and 226–315 MPa, respectively, depending on the reinforcement content (10–30 vol%) and the texture formation during processing, (iv) ductility of the composites on the other hand was in the range of 9.6–20%, (v) 30% TiNi addition resulted in minimum ductility, whereas composite samples with 20% TiNi reinforcement exhibited maximum ductility values, (vi) Mg/TiNi composites displayed extraordinary mechanical properties at high temperatures, (vii) YS and elastic modulus of the composites increased with increasing temperature up to 150 °C due to the increase of transformation stress and the elastic modulus of TiNi shape memory reinforcements with increasing temperature and beyond 150 °C, both properties decreased with further temperature increase, (viii) TiNi alloys seem to be promising candidates for reinforcement of pure Mg and Mg alloys to be used in automotive powertrain applications and (ix) composites produced with 20% and 30% TiNi content meet the high strength and elastic modulus requirements at the service conditions of 150–200 °C and the stress levels of 50–70 MPa. Zhang et al. [163] admixed Mg powders, Al and nano SiC particles by mechanical stirring assisted with ultrasonic vibration method, followed by spark plasma sintering to fabricate reinforced Mg–1Al–xSiC (x = 0.3, 0.6, 1.2, 2.4 wt%) composites. It was reported that (i) there was a nearly uniform distribution and good dispersion of nano-SiC particles within the Mg matrix, although some of localized agglomerates were found in the matrix, (ii) mechanical properties tests indicated that the addition of nano-SiC particles along with 1.0 wt% Al particles to pure Mg resulted in a significant enhancement in tensile and compressive properties of the Mg–1Al–*x*SiC composites and (iii) compared to monolithic Mg, Mg–1Al–1.2SiC composite exhibited higher 0.2% TYS (176 MPa vs 98 MPa, increased by ~80%), UTS(246 MPa vs 188 MPa, increased by ~31%), 0.2% compressive YS (140 MPa vs 81 MPa, increased by ~73%) and ultimate compressive strength (338 MPa vs 255 MPa, increased by ~33%) without much reduction on failure strain. Similarly, Prakash et al. [164] synthesized Mg-Zn-Mn-HA composite by spark plasma sintering process for orthopedic applications. It was mentioned that (i) HA compound-induced composite not only refined the grain but also enhanced porosity, which favored osseointergation, (ii) the microstructure examination of the composite reveals the formation of high degree of structural porosity (15–25%), witnessed at low alloying time and high temperature, (iii) XRD pattern analysis confirmed the formation of MgCaO, β-TCP, Mn–CaO and Ca–Mg–Zn phases, enhanced mechanical properties and corrosion characteristics and (iv) the degradation rate of Mg-Zn-Mn-HA alloy was reduced from 1.98 to 0.97 mm/year by the alloying of HA elements. Singh et al. [165] synthesized a bioinspired biodegradable Mg-Zn-Mn-Si alloy by MA and spark plasma technique. It was found that (i) the microstructure examination of the compact revealed that Si not only refined the gain structure but also formed Mg_2Si in the structure and (ii) XRD pattern analysis confirmed the formation of Mg_2Si, Mg–Zn, Mn–Si, SiO_2 and ZnO_2 due to heat developed during the process, which enhanced the mechanical properties and corrosion characteristics. Soderlind et al. [166] characterized the microstructural evolution as a function of sintering temperature from 250 to 450 °C for the alloy WE43. It was reported that (i) the gas-atomized powder microstructure consists of Mg-rich dendrites and a percolating interdendritic Mg–Nd–Y ternary phase with structure $Mg_{14}Nd_2Y$, surrounded by a high Nd and Y content in solid solution, (ii) this microstructure is maintained up to a sintering temperature of 350 °C, while with higher sintering temperatures, segregation of Nd and Y dominates, (iii) the percolating ternary phase breaks up into faceted globular precipitates with structure Mg_5Nd, which is isomorphous to $Mg_{14}Nd_2Y$, (iv) Y comes out of solution and migrates to previous powder-particle surfaces, possibly forming Y_2O_3 and (v) sample densities ranged from 64% to 100% for sintering temperatures of 250 to 450 °C, respectively, and the grain size remained constant at about 10 µm.

Wakeel et al. [167] synthesized NiTi SMA NP-reinforced Mg composites through microwave sintering process and investigated mechanical responses. Mg is reinforced with 2 wt% NiTi SMA NPs and the SMA particle effect on the mechanical properties and microstructural evolution of monolithic magnesium were studied. It was reported that (i) a near dense Mg–2 wt% NiTi nanocomposite was obtained during the study, (ii) the addition of NiTi NP resulted in a ~29% and ~73% enhancement in the microhardness and grain size of pure Mg, (iii) damping capacity and loss rate of pure Mg also had a superior enhancement of ~119% and ~2.6 times, respectively, due to the presence of NiTi NP and (iv) the compressive strength properties also exhibited a visible enhancement due to the presence of NiTi nanoparticle without compromising the fracture strain of the material.

6.6 Additive manufacturing

AM refers to a process by which digital 3D design data is used to build up a component in layers by depositing material. The AM technologies can be broadly divided into three types. The first type is sintering by which the material is heated without being liquefied to create complex objects. Direct metal laser sintering uses metal powder whereas selective laser sintering uses a laser on thermoplastic powders so that the particles stick together. The second AM technology melts the materials, including direct laser metal sintering which uses a laser to melt layers of metal powder and electron beam melting, which uses electron beams to melt the powders. The third type of AM technology is stereolithography, which uses a process called photopolymerization, whereby an ultraviolet laser is fired into a vat of photopolymer resin to create torque-resistant ceramic parts that are able to endure extreme temperatures [168, 169].

Liu et al. [170] fabricated porous Mg–Ca alloys by the laser additive manufacturing (LAM) and investigated effect of laser processing parameters on porosity, surface morphology, microstructure, microhardness and compression performance. It was reported that (i) the porosity and surface morphology of the LAMed samples depend on the laser energy input, (ii) when energy density is between 875 and 1,000 J/mm^3, the porosity of porous magnesium alloy is between 18.48% and 24.60%, and the samples with better surface quality can be obtained, (iii) the LAMed porous Mg–Ca alloy shows overlapped cladding lines and periodic morphological features, (iv) all the LAMed samples only consist of α-Mg phase and a lesser degree of MgO phase, (v) the microhardness of LAMed samples is between 60 HV and 68 HV and the microhardness is superior to that of as-cast pure magnesium, which is mainly attributed to the grain refinement and solid solution strengthening and (vi) as laser energy input increases, the porosity decreases and the compression performance enhances; indicating that the LAMed porous Mg–Ca alloy is a promising biodegradable material for future clinical application. Guo et al. [171] fabricated AZ80M by wire arc additive manufacturing (WAAM) with high deposition efficiencies and studied the microstructure and mechanical properties of the WAAMed AZ80M. It was reported that (i) the WAAMed AZ80M was mainly composed of α-Mg, β-$Mg_{17}Al_{12}$ and Al_2Y phases and had obvious inhomogeneous characteristics along the deposition direction and (ii) because of the microstructure inhomogeneity and micro defects in the interlayer region of the WAAMed AZ80M, its average tensile strength at the horizontal and vertical directions was different with the values of 308.7 and 237.3 MPa, respectively.

References

[1] Luo AA. Magnesium casting technology for structural applications. Journal of Magnesium and Alloys. 2013, 1, 2–22.

[2] Sahoo M. Technology for Magnesium Castings: Design, Products & Applications. American Foundry Society, 2011.

[3] New Casting Technology of Magnesium Alloys in the Automotive Industry: Part One, 2011. https://www.totalmateria.com/page.aspx?ID=CheckArticle&site=KTN&NM=273.

[4] New Casting Technology of Magnesium Alloys in the Automotive Industry: Part Two, 2011. https://www.totalmateria.com/page.aspx?ID=CheckArticle&site=KTN&NM=275.

[5] Vahidgolpayegani A, Wen C, Hodgson P, Li Y. Production methods and characterization of porous Mg and Mg alloys for biomedical applications. Metallic Foam Bone. 2017, 25–82; https://doi.org/10.1016/B978-0-08-101289-5.00002-0.

[6] Liu Y, Liu M, Luo L, Wang J, Liu C. The Solidification Behavior of AA2618 Aluminum Alloy and the Influence of Cooling Rate. Materials (Basel). 2014, 7, 7875–90.

[7] Wang Y, Wang Q, Ma C, Ding W, Zhu Y. Effects of Zn and RE additions on the solidification behavior of Mg–9Al magnesium alloy. Materials Science and Engineering: A. 2003, 342, 178–82.

[8] Javaid A, Hadadzadeh A, Czerwinski F. Solidification behavior of dilute Mg-Zn-Nd alloys. Journal of Alloys and Compounds. 2019, 782, 132–48.

[9] Fu Y, Wang H, Liu X, Hao H. Effect of calcium addition on microstructure, casting fluidity and mechanical properties of Mg-Zn-Ce-Zr magnesium alloy. Journal of Rare Earths. 2017, 35, 503–9.

[10] Zhou J, Yang Y, Tong W, Wang J, Wang B. Effect of Cooling Rate on the Solidified Microstructure of Mg-Gd-Y-Zr Alloy. Rare Metal Materials and Engineering. 2010, 39, 1899–902.

[11] Zhang S, Yuan GY, Lu C, Ding WJ. The relationship between (Mg,Zn)3RE phase and 14H-LPSO phase in Mg–Gd–Y–Zn–Zr alloys solidified at different cooling rates. Journal of Alloys and Compounds. 2011, 509, 3515–21.

[12] Wang J-F, Huang S, Guo S-F, Wei Y-Y, Pan F-S. Effects of cooling rate on microstructure, mechanical and corrosion properties of Mg–Zn–Ca alloy. Transactions of Nonferrous Metals Society of China. 2013, 23, 1930–5.

[13] Liu D, Liu Y, Huang Y, Song R, Chen M. Effects of solidification cooling rate on the corrosion resistance of Mg–Zn–Ca alloy. Progress in Natural Science: Materials International. 2014, 24, 452–7.

[14] Yuan Q, Huang Y, Liu D, Chen M. Effects of solidification cooling rate on the corrosion resistance of a biodegradable β-TCP/Mg-Zn-Ca composite. Bioelectrochemistry. 2018, 124, 93–104.

[15] Méar FO, Louzguine-Luzgin DV, Inoue A. Structural investigations of rapidly solidified Mg–Cu–Y alloys. Journal of Alloys and Compounds. 2010, 496, 149–54.

[16] Zhou T, Chen Z, Yang M, Hu J, Xia H. Investigation on microstructure characterization and property of rapidly solidified Mg–Zn–Ca–Ce–La alloys. Materials Characterization. 2012, 63, 77–82.

[17] Zhao C, Pan F, Zhao S, Pan H, Tang A. Microstructure, corrosion behavior and cytotoxicity of biodegradable Mg–Sn implant alloys prepared by sub-rapid solidification. Materials Science and Engineering: C. 2015, 54, 245–51.

[18] Ye L, Zhuang Y Zhao D, Jia S, Wang J. Transmission electron microscopy investigations of the microstructures in rapidly solidified Mg-Sn ribbons. Micron. 2018, 115, 1–6.

[19] Wang J-H, Yang G-Y, Liu S-J, Jie W-Q. Microstructure and room temperature mechanical properties of directionally solidified Mg–2.35Gd magnesium alloy. Transactions of Nonferrous Metals Society of China. 2016, 26, 1294–1300.

[20] Wang J, Wang J, Song Z. Microstructures and Microsegregation of Directionally Solidified Mg-1.5Gd Magnesium Alloy with Different Growth Rates. Rare Metal Materials and Engineering. 2017, 46, 12–6.

[21] Yang G, Luo S, Liu S, Xiao L, Jie W. Microstructural evolution, phase constitution and mechanical properties of directionally solidified Mg-5.5Zn-xGd (x = 0.8, 2.0, and 4.0) alloys. Journal of Alloys and Compounds. 2017, 725, 145–54.

[22] Liu D, Zhang H, Li Y, Chen X, Liu Y. Effects of composition and growth rate on the microstructure transformation of β-rods/lamellae/α-rods in directionally solidified Mg-Li alloy. Materials & Design. 2017, 119, 199–207.

[23] Muto Y, Shiraiwa T, Enoki M. Evaluation of the deformation behavior in directionally solidified Mg–Y–Zn alloys containing LPSO phases by AE analysis. Materials Science and Engineering: A. 2017, 689, 157–65.

[24] Dong Y, Lin X, Xu R, Zheng R, Wang Z. Microstructure and compression deformation behavior in the quasicrystal-reinforced M-8Zn-1Y alloy solidified under super-high pressure. Journal of Rare Earths. 2014, 32, 1048–55.

[25] Zhou H, Liu K, Zhang L, Lu L, Lu D. Influence of high pressure during solidification on the microstructure and strength of Mg-Zn-Y alloys. Journal of Rare Earths. 2016, 34, 435–40.

[26] Pan H, Han Z, Liu B. Study on Dendritic Growth in Pressurized Solidification of Mg–Al Alloy Using Phase Field Simulation. Journal of Materials Science & Technology. 2016, 32, 68–75.

[27] Fu P, Pemg L, Jiang H, Ma L, Zhai C. Chemical composition optimization of gravity cast Mg–yNd–xZn–Zr alloy. Materials Science and Engineering: A. 2008, 496, 177–88.

[28] Lee SG, Jeon JJ, Park KC, Park YH, Park IM. The effects of alloying elements on microstructure and properties of gravity casting Mg–Sn–Al–Si alloy. Materials Chemistry and Physics. 2011, 128, 208–13.

[29] Wang Y, Wu G, Liu W, Pang S, Ding W. Effects of chemical composition on the microstructure and mechanical properties of gravity cast Mg–xZn–yRE–Zr alloy. Materials Science and Engineering: A. 2014, 594, 52–61.

[30] Luo D, Wan H-Y, Ou-Yang Z-T, Chen L, Jiang Q-C. Microstructure and mechanical properties of Mg–5Sn alloy fabricated by a centrifugal casting method. Materials Letters. 2014, 116, 108–11.

[31] Liu JW, Peng XD, Chen DS, Yi Y, Yu YQ. Microstructure and mechanical properties of centrifugal casting of AZ31B magnesium alloy ring. Mater Res Innovations. 2014, 18, 169–72.

[32] Zeng X, Ma Y, Liu W, Huang Y, Tang S, Chen B. Effect of suction casting process on microstructure and mechanical properties of Au80Sn20 alloy flake. Materials Research Express. 2019, 6; DOI: 10.1088/2053-1591/ab15e7.

[33] Wang X, Dong LH, Ma XL, Zheng YF. Microstructure, mechanical property and corrosion behaviors of interpenetrating C/Mg-Zn-Mn composite fabricated by suction casting. Materials Science and Engineering: C. 2013, 33, 618–25.

[34] Wang X, Zhang P, Dong LH, Ma XL, Zheng YF. Microstructure and characteristics of interpenetrating β-TCP/Mg–Zn–Mn composite fabricated by suction casting. Materials & Design. 2014, 54, 995–1001.

[35] Zhou Y, Bian L, Chen G, Wang L, Liang W. Influence of Ca addition on microstructural evolution and mechanical properties of near-eutectic Mg–Li alloys by copper-mold suction casting. Journal of Alloys and Compounds. 2016, 664, 85–91.

[36] Liang SM, Chen RS, Blandin JJ, Suery M, Han EH. Thermal analysis and solidification pathways of Mg–Al–Ca system alloys. Materials Science and Engineering: A. 2008, 480, 365–72.

[37] Huang ZH, Liang SM, Chen RS, Han EH. Solidification pathways and constituent phases of Mg–Zn–Y–Zr alloys. Journal of Alloys and Compounds. 2009, 468, 170–8.

[38] Wong C, Nogita K, Styles MJ, Zhu S, Easton MA. Solidification path and microstructure evolution of Mg-3Al-14La alloy: Implications for the Mg-rich corner of the Mg-Al-La phase diagram. Journal of Alloys and Compounds. 2019, 784, 527–34.

[39] Zhang G, Wang Y, Liu Z, Liu S. Influence of Al addition on solidification path and hot tearing susceptibility of Mg–2Zn–(3 + 0.5x)Y–xAl alloys. Journal of Magnesium and Alloys. 2019, 7, 272–82.

[40] Song J, Pan F, Jiang B, Atrens A, Ming-Zhang M-X, Lu Y. A review on hot tearing of magnesium alloys. Journal of Magnesium and Alloys. 2016, 4, 151–72.

[41] Wang Y, Wang Q, Wu G, Zhu Y, Ding W. Hot-tearing susceptibility of Mg–9Al–xZn alloy. Materials Letters. 2002, 57, 929–34.

[42] Cao G, Kou S. Hot cracking of binary Mg–Al alloy castings. Materials Science and Engineering: A. 2006, 417, 230–8.

[43] Kierzek A, Adamiec J. Evaluation of susceptibility to hot cracking of magnesium alloy joints in variable stiffness condition. Archives of Metallurgy and Materials. 2011, 56; DOI: 10.2478/v10172-011-0084-y.

[44] Bichler L, Ravindran CRR. Investigations on the Stress and Strain Evolution in AZ91D Magnesium Alloy Castings During Hot Tearing. Journal of Materials Engineering and Performance. 2015, 24, 2208–18.

[45] Easton M, Gavras S, Gibson M, Zhu S, Nie J-F, Abbott T. Hot Tearing in Magnesium-Rare Earth Alloys. In: Singh A. et al. ed., Magnesium Technology 2016. Springer, Cham, 123–128.

[46] Cao L, Liu W-C, Li Z-Q, Wu G-H, Ding W-J. Effect of heat treatment on microstructures and mechanical properties of sand-cast Mg-10Gd-3Y-0.5Zr magnesium alloy. Transactions of Nonferrous Metals Society of China. 2014, 24, 611–8.

[47] Pang S, Wu G-H, Liu W-C, Zhang L, Ding W-J. Influence of pouring temperature on solidification behavior, microstructure and mechanical properties of sand-cast Mg-10Gd-3Y-0.4Zr alloy. Transactions of Nonferrous Metals Society of China. 2015, 25, 363–74.

[48] Liu SJ, Yang GY, Luo SF, Jie WQ. Microstructure and mechanical properties of sand mold cast Mg–4.58Zn–2.6Gd–0.18Zr magnesium alloy after different heat treatments. Journal of Alloys and Compounds. 2015, 644, 846–53.

[49] Zhang H, Fan J, Zhang L, Wu G, Feng S. Effect of heat treatment on microstructure, mechanical properties and fracture behaviors of sand-cast Mg-4Y-3Nd-1Gd-0.2Zn-0.5Zr alloy. Materials Science and Engineering: A 2016, 677, 411–20.

[50] Zhang D, Yang Q, Zhang D, Guan K, Meng J. Effects of substitution of Nd in a sand-cast Mg-2.5Nd-0.6Zn-0.5Zr alloy with x wt.% Sm (x = 2.5, 4, and 6). Journal of Rare Earths. 2017, 35, 1261–7.

[51] Li Y, Wu G, Chen A, Liu W, Zhang L. Effects of processing parameters and addition of flame-retardant into moulding sand on the microstructure and fluidity of sand-cast magnesium alloy Mg-10Gd-3Y-0.5Zr. Journal of Materials Science & Technology. 2017, 33, 558–66.

[52] Zhang Y, Patel JB, Wang Y, Fan Z. Variation improvement of mechanical properties of Mg-9Al-1Zn alloy with melt conditioned high pressure die casting. Materials Characterization. 2018, 144, 498–504.

[53] Liang S-M, Zhang H-W, Xia M-X, Chen R-S, Fan Z-Y. Microstructure and mechanical properties of melt-conditioned high-pressure die-cast Mg-Al-**Ca** alloy. Transactions of Nonferrous Metals Society of China. 2010, 20, 1205–11.

[54] Zhang J, Yu P, Liu K, Fang D, Meng J. Effect of substituting cerium-rich mischmetal with lanthanum on microstructure and mechanical properties of die-cast Mg–Al–RE alloys. Materials & Design. 2009, 30, 2372–8.
[55] Meng F, Lv S, Yang Q, Qin P, Meng J. Developing a die casting magnesium alloy with excellent mechanical performance by controlling intermetallic phase. Journal of Alloys and Compounds. 2019, 795, 436–45.
[56] Yang Q, Guan K, Li B, Lv S, Meng J. Microstructural characterizations on Mn-containing intermetallic phases in a high-pressure die-casting Mg–4Al–4RE–0.3Mn alloy. Materials Characterization. 2017, 132, 381–7.
[57] Zhang J, Liu S, Leng Z, Liu X, Wu R. Structure stability and mechanical properties of high-pressure die-cast Mg–Al–La–Y-based alloy. Materials Science and Engineering: A. 2012, 531, 70–5.
[58] Zhang J, Leng Z, Zhang M, Meng J, Wu R. Effect of Ce on microstructure, mechanical properties and corrosion behavior of high-pressure die-cast Mg–4Al-based alloy. Journal of Alloys and Compounds. 2011, 509, 1069–78.
[59] Zhang J-H, Liu S-J, Leng Z, Zhang M-L, Wu R-Z. Structure stability and mechanical properties of high-pressure die-cast Mg–Al–Ce–Y-based alloy. Transactions of Nonferrous Metals Society of China. 2012, 22, 262–7.
[60] Yang Q, Guan K, Qiu X, Zhang D, Meng J. Structures of Al2Sm phase in a high-pressure die-cast Mg–4Al–4Sm–0.3Mn alloy. Materials Science and Engineering: A 2016, 675, 396–402.
[61] Qin P, Yang Q, Guan K, Meng F, Meng J. Microstructures and mechanical properties of a high pressure die-cast Mg–4Al–4Gd–0.3Mn alloy. Materials Science and Engineering: A. 2019, 764; https://doi.org/10.1016/j.msea.2019.138254.
[62] Xu N, Bao Y, Shen J. Enhanced strength and ductility of high pressure die casting AZ91D Mg alloy by using cold source assistant friction stir processing. Materials Letters. 2017, 190, 24–7.
[63] Xiao W, Zhu S, Easton MA, Dargusch MS, Nie J-F. Microstructural characterization of high pressure die cast Mg-Zn-Al-RE alloys. Materials Characterization 2012, 65, 28–36.
[64] Yang W, Liu L, Zhang J, Ji S, Fan Z. Heterogeneous nucleation in Mg–Zr alloy under die casting condition. Materials Letters. 2015, 160, 263–7.
[65] Yarkadaş G, Kumruoğlu LC, Şevik H. The effect of Cerium addition on microstructure and mechanical properties of high pressure die cast Mg-5Sn alloy. Materials Characterization. 2018, 136, 152–6.
[66] Özarslan S, Şevik H, Sorar I. Microstructure, mechanical and corrosion properties of novel Mg-Sn-Ce alloys produced by high pressure die casting. Materials Science and Engineering: C. 2019, 105; https://doi.org/10.1016/j.msec.2019.110064.
[65] Gavras S, Easton MA, Gibson MA, Zhu S, Nie J-F. Microstructure and property evaluation of high-pressure die-cast Mg–La–rare earth (Nd, Y or Gd) alloys. Journal of Alloys and Compounds. 2014, 597, 21–9.
[66] Li S-Y, Li D-J, Zeng X-Q, Ding W-J. Microstructure and mechanical properties of Mg–6Gd–3Y–0.5Zr alloy processed by high-vacuum die-casting. Transactions of Nonferrous Metals Society of China. 2014, 24, 3769–76.
[67] Wang Z-Q, Zhang B, Li D-J, Fritzsch R, Ding W-J. Effect of heat treatment on microstructures and mechanical properties of high vacuum die casting Mg–8Gd–3Y–0.4Zr magnesium alloy. Transactions of Nonferrous Metals Society of China. 2014, 24, 3762–8.
[68] Jung HC, Shin KS. Continuous Casting of Magnesium Billets for Semi-Solid Processing. Materials Science Forum. 2005, 475/479, 517–20.
[69] Zhang ZM, Lii T, XU CJ, Guo XF. Microstructure of binary Mg-Al eutectic alloy wires produced by the Ohno continuous casting process. Acta Metallurgica Sinica (English Letters). 2008, 21, 275–81.

[70] Kido F, Motegi T. Continuous Casting of Magnesium Alloy Sheet Using Semisolid Slurry. Materials Transactions. 2012, 53, 495–9.
[71] Zhao K-Y, Peng X-D, Xie W-D, Wei Q-Y, Wei G-B. Effects of Ce on microstructure of semi-continuously cast Mg-1.5Zn-0.2Zr magnesium alloy ingots. Transactions of Nonferrous Metals Society of China. 2010, 20, s324-30.
[72] Du YZ, Zheng MY, Qiao XG, Lv WX. Microstructure and mechanical properties of Mg–Zn–Ca–Ce alloy processed by semi-continuous casting. Materials Science and Engineering: A. 2013, 582, 134–9.
[73] Chen T, Shao J, Wang R, Liu C. Evolution of LPSO phases in a Mg-Zn-Y-Gd-Zr alloy during semi-continuous casting, homogenization and hot extrusion. Materials & Design. 2018, 152, 1–9.
[74] Lokyer S, Yun M, Hunt J. Twin roll casting of aluminium alloys. Materials Science and Engineering: A. 2000, 280, 116–23.
[75] Westengen H, Nes K. Twin Roll Casting of Aluminium: The Occurrence of Structure Inhomogeneities and Defects in as Cast Strip. The Minerals, Metals & Materials Society. 2016, 972–80.
[76] Sahoo S. Review on Vertical Twin-Roll Strip Casting: A Key Technology for Quality Strips. Journal of Metallurgy. 2016: https://doi.org/10.1155/2016/1038950.
[77] Bae JH, Pasada Rao AK, Kim KH, Kim NJ. Cladding of Mg alloy with Al by twin-roll casting. Scripta Materialia. 2011, 64, 836–9.
[78] Jiang B, Liu W, Qiu D, Zhang M-X, Pan F. Grain refinement of Ca addition in a twin-roll-cast Mg–3Al–1Zn alloy. Materials Chemistry and Physics. 2012, 133, 611–6.
[79] Bhattacharjee T, Suh B-C, Sasaki TT, Ohkubo T, Hono K. High strength and formable Mg–6.2Zn–0.5Zr–0.2Ca alloy sheet processed by twin roll casting. Materials Science and Engineering: A. 2014, 609, 154–60.
[80] Aktuğ SL, Durdu S, Kutbay I, Usta M. Effect of Na2SiO3·5H2O concentration on microstructure and mechanical properties of plasma electrolytic oxide coatings on AZ31 Mg alloy produced by twin roll casting. Ceramics International. 2016, 42, 1246–53.
[81] Park J-J. Numerical analyses of cladding processes by twin-roll casting: Mg-AZ31 with aluminum alloys. International Journal of Heat and Mass Transfer. 2016, 93, 491–9.
[82] Bian MZ, Sasaki TT, Makata T, Yoshida Y. Hono K. Bake-hardenable Mg–Al–Zn–Mn–Ca sheet alloy processed by twin-roll casting. Acta Materialia. 2018, 158, 278–88.
[83] Goh CS, Soh KS, Oon PH, Chua BW. Effect of squeeze casting parameters on the mechanical properties of AZ91–Ca Mg alloys. Materials & Design. 2010, 31, s50–3.
[84] Kurnaz SC, Sevik H, Açıkgöz S, Özel A. Influence of titanium and chromium addition on the microstructure and mechanical properties of squeeze cast Mg–6Al alloy. Journal of Alloys and Compounds. 2011, 509, 3190–6.
[85] Açıkgöz Ş, Şevik H, Kurnaz SC. Influence of silver addition on the microstructure and mechanical properties of squeeze cast Mg–6Al–1Sn–0.3Mn–0.3Ti. Journal of Alloys and Compounds. 2011, 509, 7368–72.
[86] Mo W, Zhang L, WU G, Zhang Y, Wang C. Effects of processing parameters on microstructure and mechanical properties of squeeze-cast Mg–12Zn–4Al–0.5Ca alloy. Materials & Design. 2014, 63, 729–37.
[87] Zhu S, Luo T, Li Y, Yang Y. Characterization the role of squeezing pressure on microstructure, tensile properties and failure mode of a new Mg-6Zn-4Al-0.5Cu magnesium alloy. Journal of Alloys and Compounds. 2017, 718, 188–96.
[88] Kumar P, Mondal AK, Chowdhury SG, Krishna G, Kumar Ray A. Influence of additions of Sb and/or Sr on microstructure and tensile creep behaviour of squeeze-cast AZ91D Mg alloy. Materials Science and Engineering: A. 2017, 683, 37–45.

[89] Zhao Q, Wu Y, Rong W, Wang K, Peng L. Effect of applied pressure on microstructures of squeeze cast Mg–15Gd–1Zn–0.4Zr alloy. Journal of Magnesium and Alloys 2018, 6, 197–204.
[90] Kopeliovich D. Direct Chill (DC) Casting. Substances & Technologies; http://www.substech.com/dokuwiki/doku.php?id=direct_chill_dc_casting.
[91] Zheng X, Dong J, Wang S. Microstructure and mechanical properties of Mg-Nd-Zn-Zr billet prepared by direct chill casting. Journal of Magnesium and Alloys. 2018, 6, 95–9.
[92] Lowe A, Ridgway K, Atkinson H. Thixoforming. Materials World. 1999, 7, 541–3.
[93] Mohammed MN, Omar MZ, Salleh MS, Alhawari KS, Kapranos P. Semisolid Metal Processing Techniques for Nondendritic Feedstock Production. The Scientific World Journal. 2013; https://doi.org/10.1155/2013/752175.
[94] Husain NH, Ahmad AH, Rashidi MM. An overview of thixoforming process. Material Science and Engineering. 2017, 257: DOI: 10.1088/1757-899X/257/1/012053.
[95] Aziz AM, Omar MZ, Sajuri Z, Salleh MS. Microstructural morphology of rheocast A319 aluminium alloy. Advances in Mechanical Engineering. 2016, 8; https://doi.org/10.1177/1687814016649354.
[96] Rosso M. Thixocasting and rheocasting technologies, improvements going on. Journal of Achievement in Materials and Manufacturing Engineering. 2012, 54, 110–9.
[97] Amira S, Dubé D, Tremblay R, Ghali E. Microstructure of die cast and thixocast ZAEX10430 (Mg–10Zn–4Al–3Ce–0.3Ca) alloy. Materials Characterization. 2013, 76, 48–54.
[98] Fang X, Lü S, Zhao L, Wang J, Wu S. Microstructure and mechanical properties of a novel Mg–RE–Zn–Y alloy fabricated by rheo-squeeze casting. Materials & Design. 2016, 94, 353–9.
[99] Poddar P, Sahoo KL. Microstructure and mechanical properties of conventional cast and rheocast Mg–Sn based alloys. Materials Science and Engineering: A. 2012, 556, 891–905.
[100] Bartex SLT, Dos Santos CA, de BArcellos VK, Schaeffer L. Effect of solid fraction on microstructures and mechanical properties of a Mg-Al-La-Ca alloy processed by rheocasting. Journal of Alloys and Compounds. 2019, 776, 297–305.
[101] Dulay MT, Quirino JP, Bennett BD, Kato M, Zare RN. Photopolymerized sol–gel monoliths for capillary electrochromatography. Analytical Chemistry 2001, 73, 3921–6.
[102] Roman GT, Hiaus T, Bass KJ, Seelhammer TG, Culbertson CT. Sol–gel modified poly (dimethylsiloxane) microfluidic devices with high electroosmotic mobilities and hydrophilic channel wall characteristics. Analytical Chemistry. 2005, 77, 1414–22.
[103] Mia MNH, Pervez MF, Hossain MK, Rahman R, Hoq M. Influence of Mg content on tailoring optical bandgap of Mg-doped ZnO thin film prepared by sol-gel method. Results in Physics. 2017, 7, 2683–91.
[104] Shi S, Xu J, Li L. Effect of Mg concentration on morphological, structural and optical properties of Mg-K co-doped ZnO thin films prepared by sol-gel method. Materials Letters. 2018, 229, 178–81.
[105] Nadumane A, Shetty K, Anantharaju KS, Nagaswarupa HP, Prashantha SC. Sunlight photocatalytic performance of Mg-doped nickel ferrite synthesized by a green sol-gel route. Journal of Science: Advanced Materials and Devices. 2019, 4, 89–100.
[106] Luo F, Lu J, Wang W, Tan F, Qiao X. Preparation and antibacterial activity of magnesium oxide nanoplates via sol-gel process. Micro & Nano Letters. 2013, 8, 479–82.
[107] Zhang ML, Yan YD, Hou ZY, Fan LA, Tang DX. An electrochemical method for the preparation of Mg–Li alloys at low temperature molten salt system. Journal of Alloys and Compounds. 2007, 440, 362–6.
[108] Yan YD, Zhang ML, Xue Y, Han W, Cao DX, Wei SQ. Study on the preparation of M–Li–Zn alloys by electrochemical codeposition from LiCl–KCl–MgCl2–ZnCl2 melts. Electrochimica Acta. 2009, 54, 3387–93.

[109] Chen Y, Ye K, Zhang M. Preparation of Mg-Yb alloy film by electrolysis in the molten LiCl-KCl-YbCl3 system at low temperature. Journal of Rare Earths. 2010, 28, 128–33.
[110] Cao P, Zhang M, Han W, Yan Y, Zheng T. Electrochemical behaviour of erbium and preparation of Mg-Li-Er alloys by codeposition. Journal of Rare Earths. 2011, 29, 763–7.
[111] Li H, Sun H, Wang C, Wei B, Ma H. Controllable electrochemical synthesis and magnetic behaviors of Mg–Mn–Fe–Co–Ni–Gd alloy films. Journal of Alloys and Compounds. 2014, 598, 161–5.
[112] Li R, Wu N, Liu J, Jin Y, Zhang T. Formation and evolution of nanoporous bimetallic Ag-Cu alloy by electrochemically dealloying Mg-(Ag-Cu)-Y metallic glass. Corrosion Science. 2017, 119, 23–32.
[113] Zhao C, Qi Z, Wang X, Zhang Z. Fabrication and characterization of monolithic nanoporous copper through chemical dealloying of Mg–Cu alloys. Corrosion Science. 2009, 51, 2120–5.
[114] Wang X, Nie Q-D, Ma X-L, Fan J-L, Li X-L. Microstructure and properties of co-continuous (β-TCP+MgO)/Zn-Mg composite fabricated by suction exsorption for biomedical applications. Transactions of Nonferrous Metals Society of China. 2017, 27, 1996–2006.
[115] Rong W, Zhang Y, Wu Y, Chen Y, Li D. Fabrication of high-strength Mg-Gd-Zn-Zr alloys via differential-thermal extrusion. Materials Characterization. 2017, 131, 380–7.
[116] Zheng X, Peng X, Li J, Wei Q. Preparation of Mg-Li Alloys via Vacuum Silicothermic Reduction Process. Rare Metal Materials and Engineering. 2014, 43, 2079–82.
[117] Suryanarayana C. Mechanical alloying and milling. Progress in Materials Science 2001, 46, 1–184.
[118] Suryanarayana C, Ivanov E, Boldyrev VV. The science and technology of mechanical alloying. Materials Science and Engineering. 2001, A304/A306, 151–8.
[119] Lu L, Lai MO, Toh YH, Froyen L. Structure and properties of Mg–Al–Ti–B alloys synthesized via mechanical alloying. Materials Science and Engineering: A. 2002, 334, 163–72.
[120] Gennari FC, Urretavizcaya G, Andrade Gamboa JJ, Meyer G. New Mg-based alloy obtained by mechanical alloying in the Mg–Ni–Ge system. Journal of Alloys and Compounds. 2003, 354, 187–92.
[121] Rojas P, Ordoñez S, Serafini D, Zúñiga A, Lavernia E. Microstructural evolution during mechanical alloying of Mg and Ni. Journal of Alloys and Compounds. 2005, 391, 267–76.
[122] Al-Aqeeli N, Mendoza-Suarez G, Labrie A, Drew RAL. Phase evolution of Mg–Al–Zr nanophase alloys prepared by mechanical alloying. Journal of Alloys and Compounds. 2005, 400, 96–9.
[123] Brett CMA, Dias L, Trindade B, Fischer R, Mies S. Characterisation by EIS of ternary Mg alloys synthesised by mechanical alloying. Electrochimica Acta. 2006, 51, 1752–60.
[124] Lee EY, Jung KS, Lee KS. Synthesis of composite Mg–Ni–Ca metal hydride by mechanical alloying. Journal of Alloys and Compounds. 2007, 446/447, 129–33.
[125] Zhang Y-H, Han X-Y, Li B-W, Ren H-P, Wan X-L. Effects of substituting Mg with Zr on the electrochemical characteristics of Mg2Ni-type electrode alloys prepared by mechanical alloying. Materials Characterization. 2008, 59, 390–6.
[126] Datta MK, Chou D-T, Hong D, Saha P, Kumta PN. Structure and thermal stability of biodegradable Mg–Zn–Ca based amorphous alloys synthesized by mechanical alloying. Materials Science and Engineering: B. 2011, 176, 1637–43.
[127] Martínez C, Ordoñez S, Guzmán D, Serafini D, Bustos O. Phase evolution and thermal stability of 2 Mg–Cu alloys processed by mechanical alloying. Journal of Alloys and Compounds. 2013, 581, 241–5.
[128] Khalajabadi SZ, Kadir MRA, Izman S, Bakhsheshi-Rad HR, Farahany S. Effect of mechanical alloying on the phase evolution, microstructure and bio-corrosion properties of a Mg/HA/TiO2/MgO nanocomposite. Ceramics International. 2014, 40, 16743–59.

[129] Chaubey AK, Scudino S, Khoshkhoo MS, Prashanth KG, Eckert J. High-strength ultrafine grain Mg–7.4%Al alloy synthesized by consolidation of mechanically alloyed powders. Journal of Alloys and Compounds. 2014, 610, 456–61.
[130] Kursun C, Gogebakan M. Characterization of nanostructured Mg–Cu–Ni powders prepared by mechanical alloying. Journal of Alloys and Compounds. 2015, 619, 138–44.
[131] Salleh EM, Zuhailawati H, Ramakrishnan S, Abdel-Hady Gepreel M. A statistical prediction of density and hardness of biodegradable mechanically alloyed Mg–Zn alloy using fractional factorial design. Journal of Alloys and Compounds. 2015, 644, 476–84.
[132] Salleh EM, Ramakrishnan S, Hussain Z. Synthesis of Biodegradable Mg-Zn Alloy by Mechanical Alloying: Effect of Milling Time. Procedia Chemistry. 2016, 19, 525–30.
[133] Salleh EM, Zuhailawati H, Ramakrishnan S. Synthesis of biodegradable Mg-Zn alloy by mechanical alloying: Statistical prediction of elastic modulus and mass loss using fractional factorial design. Transactions of Nonferrous Metals Society of China. 2018, 28, 687–99.
[134] Zhou H, Hu L, Sun Y, Zhang H, Yu H. Synthesis of nanocrystalline AZ31 magnesium alloy with titanium addition by mechanical milling. Materials Characterization. 2016, 113, 108–16.
[135] Asano K, Enoki H, Akiba E. Synthesis process of Mg–Ti BCC alloys by means of ball milling. Journal of Alloys and Compounds. 2009, 486, 115–23.
[136] Khan MUF, Mirza F, Gupta RK. High hardness and thermal stability of nanocrystalline Mg–Al alloys synthesized by the high-energy ball milling. Materialia. 2018, 4, 406–16.
[137] Nezafati M, Giri A, Hofmeister C, Cho K, Kim C-S. Atomistic study on the interaction of nitrogen and Mg lattice and the nitride formation in nanocrystalline Mg alloys synthesized using cryomilling process. Acta Materialia. 2016, 115, 295–307.
[138] Habila W, Azzeddine H, Mehdi B, Tirsatine K, Bradai D. Investigation of microstructure and texture evolution of a Mg/Al laminated composite elaborated by accumulative roll bonding. Materials Characterization. 2019, 147, 242–52.
[139] Chen C, Wang M, Wang D, Jin R, Liu Y. Microstructure and corrosion behavior of Mg–Nd coatings on AZ31 magnesium alloy produced by high-energy micro-arc alloying process. Journal of Alloys and Compounds. 2007, 438, 321–6.
[140] Langelier B, Nasiri AM, Lee SY, Gharghouri MA, Esmaeili S. Improving microstructure and ductility in the Mg–Zn alloy system by combinational Ce–Ca microalloying. Materials Science and Engineering: A. 2015, 620, 76–84.
[141] Macchi C, Tolley A, Giovachini R, Polmear IJ, Somoza A. Influence of a microalloying addition of Ag on the precipitation kinetics of an Al–Cu–Mg alloy with high Mg:Cu ratio. Acta Materialia. 2015, 98, 275–87.
[142] Candan S, Celik M, Candan E. Effectiveness of Ti-micro alloying in relation to cooling rate on corrosion of AZ91 Mg alloy. Journal of Alloys and Compounds. 2016, 672, 197–203.
[143] Du YZ, Qiao XG, Zheng MY, Wu K, Xu SW . Development of high-strength, low-cost wrought Mg–2.5mass% Zn alloy through micro-alloying with Ca and La. Materials & Design. 2015, 85, 549–57.
[144] Du YZ, Qiao XG, Zheng MY, Wang DB, Golovin IS. Effect of microalloying with Ca on the microstructure and mechanical properties of Mg-6 mass%Zn alloys. Materials & Design. 2016, 98, 285–93.
[145] Du Y, Zheng M, Jiang B. Comparison of microstructure and mechanical properties of Mg-Zn microalloyed with Ca or Ce. Vacuum. 2018, 151, 221–5.
[146] Gao Z, Song M, Liu R-L, Shen Y, Liu X. Improving in vitro and in vivo antibacterial functionality of Mg alloys through micro-alloying with Sr and Ga. Materials Science and Engineering: C. 2019, 104; https://doi.org/10.1016/j.msec.2019.109926.
[147] Mora E, Garcés G, Oñorbe E, Pérez P, Adeva P. High-strength Mg–Zn–Y alloys produced by powder metallurgy. Scripta Materialia. 2009, 60, 776–9.

[148] Zhou T, Xia H, Yang M, Zhou Z, Chen Z. Investigation on microstructure characterizations and phase compositions of rapidly solidification/powder metallurgy Mg–6wt.% Zn–5wt.% Ce–1.5wt.% Ca alloy. Journal of Alloys and Compounds. 2011, 509, L145–9.
[149] Zhou T, Yang M, Zhou Z, Hu J, Chen Z. Microstructure and mechanical properties of rapidly solidified/powder metallurgy Mg–6Zn and Mg–6Zn–5Ca at room and elevated temperatures. Journal of Alloys and Compounds. 2013, 560, 161–6.
[150] Fang W-B, Fang W, Sun H-F. Preparation of high-strength Mg–3Al–Zn alloy with ultrafine-grained microstructure by powder metallurgy. Powder Technology. 2011, 212, 161–5.
[151] Asgharzadeh H, Yoon EY, Chae HJ, Kim TS, Kim HS. Microstructure and mechanical properties of a Mg–Zn–Y alloy produced by a powder metallurgy route. Journal of Alloys and Compounds. 2014, 586, s95–s100.
[152] Rashad M, Pan F, Asif M. Room temperature mechanical properties of Mg–Cu–Al alloys synthesized using powder metallurgy method. Materials Science and Engineering: A. 2015, 644, 129–36.
[153] Yang D, Hu Z, Chen W, Lu J, Ma A. Fabrication of Mg-Al alloy foam with close-cell structure by powder metallurgy approach and its mechanical properties. Journal of Manufacturing Processes. 2016, 22, 290–6.
[154] Yu J, Wang J. Li Q, Shang J, Cao J, Sun X. Effect of Zn on Microstructures and Properties of Mg-Zn Alloys Prepared by Powder Metallurgy Method. Rare Metal Materials and Engineering. 2016, 45, 2757–62.
[155] Hou L, Li B, Wu R, Cui L, Sun B. Microstructure and mechanical properties at elevated temperature of Mg-Al-Ni alloys prepared through powder metallurgy. Journal of Materials Science & Technology. 2017, 33, 947–53.
[156] Kubásek J, Dvorský D, Čavojský M, Vojtěch D, Fousová M. Superior Properties of Mg–4Y–3RE–Zr Alloy Prepared by Powder Metallurgy. Journal of Materials Science & Technology. 2017, 33, 652–60.
[157] Kekule T, Smola B, Vlach M, Kudrnova H, Stulikova I. Thermal stability and microstructure development of cast and powder metallurgy produced Mg–Y–Zn alloy during heat treatment. Journal of Magnesium and Alloys. 2017, 5, 173–80.
[158] Medina J, Pérez P, Garcés G, Stark A, Adeva P. High-strength Mg-6Zn-1Y-1Ca (wt%) alloy containing quasicrystalline I-phase processed by a powder metallurgy route. Materials Science and Engineering: A. 2018, 715, 92–100.
[159] Schaper JG, Wolff M, Wiese B, Ebel T, Willumeit-Römer R. Powder metal injection moulding and heat treatment of AZ81 Mg alloy. Journal of Materials Processing Technology. 2019, 267, 241–6.
[160] Zhou B, Wu D, Chen RS, Han E-H. Enhanced tensile properties in a Mg-6Gd-3Y-0.5Zr alloy due to hot isostatic pressing (HIP). Journal of Materials Science & Technology. 2019, 35, 1860–8.
[161] Zhao L, Ma G, Jin P, Yu Z. Role of Y on the microstructure, texture and mechanical properties of Mg–Zn–Zr alloys by powder metallurgy. Journal of Alloys and Compounds. 2019, 810; https://doi.org/10.1016/j.jallcom.2019.151843.
[162] Aydogmus T. Processing of interpenetrating Mg–TiNi composites by spark plasma sintering. Materials Science and Engineering: A. 2015, 624, 261–70.
[163] Zhang H, Zhao Y, Yan Y, Fan J, Xu B. Microstructure evolution and mechanical properties of Mg matrix composites reinforced with Al and nano SiC particles using spark plasma sintering followed by hot extrusion. Journal of Alloys and Compounds. 2017, 725, 652–64.
[164] Prakash C, Singh S, Verma K, Sidhu SS, Singh S. Synthesis and characterization of Mg-Zn-Mn-HA composite by spark plasma sintering process for orthopedic applications. Vacuum. 2018, 155, 578–84.

[165] Singh B, Singh R, Mehta JS, Gupta A, Prakash C. Nano-mechanical Characterization of Mg-Zn-Mn-Si Alloy Fabricated by Spark Plasma Sintering for Biomedical Applications. Materials Today: Proceedings. 2018, 5, 27742–8.
[166] Soderlind J, Cihova M, Schäublin R, Risbud S, Löffler JF. Towards refining microstructures of biodegradable magnesium alloy WE43 by spark plasma sintering. Acta Biomaterialia. 2019, 98, 67–80.
[167] Wakeel S, Manakari V, Parande G, Kujur MS, Gupta M. Synthesis and Mechanical Response of NiTi SMA Nanoparticle Reinforced Mg Composites Synthesized through Microwave Sintering Process. Materials Today: Proceedings. 2018, 5, 28203–10.
[168] Jahangir MN, Mamun MAH, Sealy MP. A review of additive manufacturing of magnesium alloys. AIP Conference Proceedings 2018: https://doi.org/10.1063/1.5044305
[169] Karunakaran R, Ortgies S, Tamayol A, Michael FB, Sealy P. Additive manufacturing of magnesium alloys. Bioactive Materials. 2020, 5, 44–54.
[170] Liu C, Zhang M, Chen C. Effect of laser processing parameters on porosity, microstructure and mechanical properties of porous Mg-Ca alloys produced by laser additive manufacturing. Materials Science and Engineering: A. 2017, 703, 359–71.
[171] Guo Y, Pan H, Ren L, Quan G. Microstructure and mechanical properties of wire arc additively manufactured AZ80M magnesium alloy. Materials Letters. 2019, 247, 4–6.

Chapter 7
Thixotechnology

The rheological behavior of flow-induced structural changes is a variable viscosity. If the changes are reversible and time-dependent shear thinning, the effect is called thixotropy [1]. The thixotropy is originally combined with two Greek words "thixis" (meaning stirring or shaking) and "trepo" (turning or changing). It is believed that certain gels or fluids (that are normally thick or viscous under static conditions) will flow (become thinner, less viscous) over time when they are shaken, agitated, shear stressed or otherwise stressed (time-dependent viscosity). They then take a fixed time to return to a more viscous state [2]. There are several unique fabrication methods and forming using the thixotropy behavior of magnesium materials such as thixocasting, thixoforming or thixomolding.

7.1 Thixocasting

Thixomolding is known for its effective process control, microstructural engineering and property enhancement. The potential benefits from its application for net-shape forming of magnesium alloys have been described [3, 4]. The benefits are associated with (i) the semisolid state of the alloy, having a high and controllable viscosity which promotes the nonturbulent filling of the mold, and (ii) the molding effectively combines the slurry-making and part-forming operations into a one-step process and the facility is freed from having to deal with the transport of the liquid metal [5]. Czerwinski et al. [4] discussed the importance of selection of proper manufacturing process in injection molding for different components made up of magnesium alloys. It was indicated that (i) there are many factors that affect the processing route selection; (ii) the component size, its geometry and wall thicknesses define requirements regarding mold-filling conditions; (iii) since there is a factor of energy economy pointing toward lower temperatures, an optimum between these factors is a key for the selection of the appropriate method of manufacturing components with a minimum porosity and satisfactory properties; and (iv) the ultimate goal is the same as that for semisolid processing in general – to manufacture components with sound structural integrity and properties comparable to wrought products at a low cost similar to castings.

The thixocasting process is a semisolid metal processing route (SSM), which involves forming of alloys in the semisolid state to near-net-shaped products. The process of thixocasting offers a number of advantages, such as improved mechanical properties, good surface finish and near-net shape. However, the thixocasting process has also a number of disadvantages, such as the need for special feedstock with near spherical primary crystals. In order to cast such special billets for thixocasting one has to pay a more expensive premium than normal. Eliminating this additional

https://doi.org/10.1515/9783110676945-007

specialized casting step leads to savings in both costs and time. Compared with the conventional casting technologies, thixocasting has a lower forming temperature, significantly longer die life, high part precision, production efficiency and comprehensive mechanical properties. As compared with hot forging technologies, thixocasting has quite a low yield strength, high fluidity, low forming load and low surface roughness. Especially in the thixocasting process, a complex geometry product can be obtained by only one-step forming. This technology has been widely applied in nonferrous metal forming and satisfactory results were derived, but not with ferrous metal [6]. Kim et al. [7] conducted the feasibility study of producing high-strength Mg–Cu–Y alloys by the thixocasting process. It was mentioned that a microstructure, consisting of globular primary Mg particles surrounded by quenched liquid (partly amorphized), could be obtained and gave significantly high tensile strength compared to conventional Mg castings. Amira et al. [8] studied the microstructure and phase composition of die cast and thixocast ZAEX10430 (Mg-10Zn-4Al-3Ce-0.3Ca) alloy. It was reported that (i) two intermetallic phases were identified in both the die cast and the thixocast specimens: the τ-phase doped with calcium $(Mg,Ca)_{32}(Al,Zn)_{49}$ (or τ′-phase) and the $(Al,Zn)_xCe$ isomorphous phase with Al_2CeZn_2 and Al_4Ce; (ii) in all of the specimens, the τ′-phase crystallized mostly as fine elongated particles and within a lamellar constituent; (iii) needle-like $(Al,Zn)_xCe$ phase particles were visible in the die cast specimens, whereas coarse particles of various cross-sectional shapes (polygonal, elliptical, rod-like, etc.) were observed in the thixocast specimens; and (iv) the difference in morphology of the intermetallic $(Al,Zn)_xCe$ particles in the matrix and the presence of large primary α-Mg grains in the thixocast specimens was used to explain the different creep behavior of die cast and thixocast ZAEX10430 alloy reported previously. Szklarz et al. [9] investigated the influence of SSM (called also as thixoforming) of thixocast ZE41A T6 Mg alloy on the electrochemical behavior in 0.1 M NaCl solution. It was reported that (i) the heat treatment and thixoforming significantly improved mechanical properties of ZE41A alloy; (ii) the global corrosion potential is slightly higher for treated sample which is related to the presence of Zr–Zn nanoparticles distributed in solid solution; (iii) the corrosion behavior differences between feedstock and thixocast after T6 samples are also visible in local scale; however there is no improvement in corrosion behavior after treatment; and (iv) corrosion morphology of the treated sample indicates higher susceptibility to pitting and filiform corrosion.

7.2 Thixoforming

Thixoforming is a forming process that exploits metal rheological behavior during solidus and liquidus range temperature. Numerous investigations on thixoforming are currently focusing on the raw material used to produce superior mechanical properties and excellent formability components, especially in automotive industries.

Furthermore, the thixoforming process [10–15] also produced less casting defect component such as macrosegregation, shrinkage and porosity. The thixoforming methods that widely used are thixocasting, thixoforging, thixorolling, thixoextrusion and thixomolding [10, 11].

Meng et al. [12] selected cast and extruded Mg-5.15Y-3.75Gd-3.05Zn-0.75Zr alloys as starting materials in a series of reheating experiments and thixocompression tests. It was reported that (i) homogenous spherical semisolid slurries were obtained when the reheating temperature and isothermal holding time were 560 °C and 20 s, respectively; however, the different grain sizes and different distributions of eutectic compounds in the starting materials resulted in different morphologies of the semisolid slurries; (ii) the thixoforming properties of the semisolid slurry were affected by the forming temperature, strain rate and its morphology; (iii) the dependency of thixoforming properties on the stain rate and morphology of semisolid slurry decreased at higher forming temperature; and (iv) when the extruded alloy was formed at 560 °C with a strain rate of 0.1/s, a sample with a smooth surface was formed by a lower forming load. Meng et al. [13] examined the feasibility of the semisolid forming in manufacturing of Mg-Gd-Y-Zn-Zr alloy products, partial melting and backward thixoextrusion experiments of Mg-8.20Gd-4.48Y-3.34Zn-0.36Zr alloy in semisolid temperature range of it (520–580 °C) and studied the microstructural evolution of this alloy during partial melting and backward thixoextrusion. It was mentioned that (i) the alloy exhibited different microstructural morphologies and formability at different extrusion temperature; (ii) at lower semisolid temperature (520–560 °C), liquid phase with lower volume fraction cannot improve the ductility of this alloy effectively, while at higher semisolid temperature (580–620 °C), handling and transferring of semisolid slurry became quite difficult, owing to the liquid phase with higher volume fraction; and (iii) the occurrence of liquid segregation and plastic deformation of solid particles during thixoextrusion at higher semisolid temperature resulted in inhomogeneous distribution of microstructure and mechanical properties of the sample.

Chen et al. [13] conducted thixoforming of equal-channel angular extrusion formed AM50 alloy and investigated the mechanical properties of thixoformed components. It was found that (i) the tensile properties of thixoformed from equal channel extrusion state are much higher than those from as-cast state and (ii) magnesium alloy semisolid billet with fine and spheroidal grains, which is suitable for semisolid processing, could be obtained by the combination of the equal channel extrusion and partial remelting. Magnesium is particularly challenging material, when formed from liquid phase because of high flammability risk. An alternative process for casting is thixoforming, which involves a lower temperature of process and operation in the partially solidified state. Rogal et al. [14] studied the influence of SSM on EZ33A magnesium alloy (Mg-Zn-RE-Zr) microstructure and mechanical properties. It was reported that (i) ingot microstructure revealed globular grains with coarse eutectic mixture consisting of Mg_7Zn_3RE, T-phase – $RE(Mg,Zn)_{11}$ and α(Mg); (ii) heterogeneous nucleation of magnesium solid solution allowed to obtain the structure appropriate for thixoforming; (iii) using differential scanning calorimetry, temperature of process was determined to be 622 °C, which corresponded to about 30% of the liquid phase; (iv) thixocast microstructure consisted of α(Mg) globular grains with a size of 76 ± 1.1 surrounded by fine eutectic mixture in a volume of 35%; and (v) T6 heat treatment (solution at 500 °C for 6 h and aging at 190 °C for 33 h) caused an increase of grain size to 92 μm and the precipitation of two kinds of phases within the α(Mg): β′1 and β′2 are responsible for the increase of yield strength to 135 MPa, compression strength to 383 MPa and hardness to 73 HV.

References

[1] Mewis J, Wagner NJ. Thixotropy. Advances in Colloid and Interface Science. 2009, 147/148, 214–27.

[2] Morrison I. Dispersions. Kirk-Othmer encyclopedia of chemical technology. Kirk-Othmer Encyclopedia of Chemical Technology. 2003; https://doi.org/10.1002/0471238961.0409191613151818.a01.

[3] Carnahan RD. Magnesium and Magnesium Alloys. In: Avedesian MM et al, ed., ASM Specialty Handbook, Inter., Materials Park, Ohio, 1999, 90–97.2.

[4] Czerwinski F. Processing features of thixomolding magnesium alloys. Die Casting Engineer. 2004, 48, 52–8.

[5] Czerwinski F. The oxidation behavior of AZ91D magnesium alloy at high temperatures, Acta Materialia. 2002, 50, 2639–54.

[6] https://www.totalmateria.com/page.aspx?ID=CheckArticle&site=ktn&NM=318.

[7] Kim J-M, Shin K, Kim K-T, Jung W-J. Microstructure and mechanical properties of a thixocast Mg–Cu–Y alloy. Scripta Materialia. 2003, 49, 687–91.

[8] Amira S, Dubé D, Tremblay R, Ghali E. Microstructure of die cast and thixocast ZAEX10430 (Mg–10Zn–4Al–3Ce–0.3Ca) alloy. Materials Characterization. 2013, 76, 48–54.

[9] Szklarz Z, Bisztyga M, Krawiec H, Lityńska-Dobrzyńska L, Rogal Ł. Global and local investigations of the electrochemical behavior the T6 heat treated Mg–Zn–RE magnesium alloy thixo-cast. Applied Surface Science. 2017, 405, 529–39.

[10] Husain NH, Ahmad AH, Rashidi MM. An overview of thixoforming process. License 2017; DOI: 10.1088/1757-899X/257/1/012053.

[11] Haga T, Kapranos P. Billetless simple thixoforming process. Journal of Materials Processing Technology. 2002, 130/131, 581–6.

[12] Meng Y, Li Q, Tang Y, Sugiyama S. Partial melting behaviors and thixoforming properties of cast and extruded Mg-5.15Y-3.75Gd-3.05Zn-0.75Zr alloys. Vacuum. 2018, 150, 173–85.

[13] Meng Y, Zhou J-C, Peng F, Liu J, Yanagimoto J. Effects of backwards thixo-extrusion on the microstructure and mechanical properties of Mg–8.20Gd–4.48Y–3.34Zn–0.36Zr alloy. Procedia Engineering. 2017, 2–7, 2137–42.

[14] Chen T, Wang L, Yang J, Lu S. Thixoforming of AM50 magnesium alloy. International Journal of Advanced Manufacturing Technology. 2017, 90, 1639–47.

[15] Rogal L, Kania A, Beront K, Janus K, Lityńska-Dobrzyńska L. Microstructure and mechanical properties of Mg–Zn–RE–Zr alloy after thixoforming. Journal of Materials Research and Technology. 2019, 8, 1121–31.

Chapter 8
Heat treatment and strengthening

In general, alloys are subjected to heat treatment to generate other phase(s) of the alloy. If the metallurgical conditions between high temperature and low temperature differ from each other, we can quench the alloy to bring it at a nonequilibrium state, so that any possible changes between high and low temperatures can be prevented. During quenching, three cases occur, depending on the reaction rate due to temperature difference and cooling (quenching) rate. (1) Formation of pseudo-precipitation phase: the high-temperature state S_H can be preserved to bring it at the low temperature; (2) formation of intermediate phase: although S_H cannot be preserved as it is, the final product will be S_I (intermediate state) during the changing process to S_L (low-temperature state); and (3) formation of stable precipitate phase: at even rapid cooling only S_L state is formed. Hence, quenching is meaningless if case (3) takes place. In case (2), the martensite in steels is the typical S_I phase. For case (1), if S_H is mechanically stronger than S_L, as-quenched phase can be used in practical applications. If S_H phase exhibits mechanically soft condition, it can be plastically worked. In other cases, S_H is subjected to further heat treatment to proceed the nonequilibrium state to transform to S_L, resulting in hardening of the alloy, which is referred to as the precipitation-aging process. In the articles cited in this chapter, there are notations like γ-phase, β-phase and α-phase. These three phases are distinct phases in the aging process and are shown in the process sequence as follows: γ-phase (unstable supersaturated solid solution (S.S.S.S.)) → β-phase (intermediate phase) → α-phase (stable solid solution that can be found in the phase diagram).

Mg-based alloys have been subjected to a variety of heat-treatment methods (for both cast and wrought products) in practice to alter metallurgical features, mechanical properties (strength or ductility or both), physical properties (thermal conductivity or electrical conductivity) and chemical behavior (such as corrosion resistance). The type of heat treatment depends on the nature and extent of the changes to be made. By one treatment, the tensile strength and elongation may be substantially raised. By another treatment, the yield strength and hardness may be considerably increased but with appreciable loss of ductility [1]. Although it is recognized that there are three basic types of thermal treating processes commonly applied to magnesium alloys, including solution heat treatment, precipitation or aging and annealing, there are some others that could be used, such as stabilizing, annealing, homogenization, quenching and thermomechanical treatment. As a result of an appropriate heat treatment, Mg-based alloys are hardened and/or strengthened, depending on the outcome of metallurgical features during the heat treatment. In this chapter, we discuss various heat treatment and major strengthening methods.

https://doi.org/10.1515/9783110676945-008

8.1 In general

Although the term "tempering" is basically used for steel as a heat treatment that improves the toughness of hard, brittle steels so that they will hold up during processing, it is also applied to Mg-based alloys, which are previously solution treated or aged, to dress/modify the mechanical properties (in particular to reach a desired hardness/toughness ratio). The designations for temper are used for all forms of magnesium and magnesium alloy products, except ingots. They are based on the sequence of basic treatments that are used to produce various tempers, and basic temper designation consists of letters to add the following materials' designation code. Table 8.1 lists all tempering specifications [2].

Taking an example of this designation system, consider a magnesium alloy AZ81A-T4. AZ81 designates the alloy code, indicating that A for Al, Z for Zn, 8 for rounded-off nominally 8 wt% for Al and 1 for 1 wt% for Zn [3–6]. The third part "A" indicates that it is the fifth alloy standardized with 8% Al and 1% Zn as the principal alloying additions. Then the fourth part, T4, denotes that the alloy is solution heat treated, as listed in Table 8.1.

8.2 Effects of heat treatment

Main effects of having heat treatments on various types of Mg-based alloys are listed in Tables 8.2–8.5.

8.3 Homogenization

In general, almost all metal alloys are suffered from significant intercrystalline segregation of solute elements during solidification. As a result, this elemental partitioning can severely degrade as-cast material properties and lead to difficulties during post-processing, so that many castings are subjected to a homogenization (or diffusion annealing) heat treatment in order to minimize segregation, ensure microstructural homogeneity and improve their performance. On the other hand, since the homogenization heat treatment is conducted at relatively high temperature, causing coarse-grained microstructure; hence, homogenization is normally followed by subsequent heat-treatment process to incorporate the desired set of properties (particularly in the steel castings) and such heat treatments should include conventional full annealing, normalizing or normalizing followed by tempering, depending upon the specified property requirement.

There are several reports on the effects of homogenization or influence of homogenized conditions of Mg–Zn-based alloys. Kang et al. [65] processed Mg–4Zn–0.5Ca alloy by the combination of forging, homogenization and extrusion and mentioned

Table 8.1: Temper designations [2].

F	As fabricated. Applies to products that acquire some temper from shaping processes not having special control over the amount of strain hardening or thermal treatment.
O	Annealed, recrystallized (wrought products only). Applies to the softest temper of wrought products.
H	Strain hardened (wrought products only). Applies to products that have their strength increased by strain hardening with or without supplementary thermal treatment to produce partial softening. The H is always followed by two or more digits.
Subdivisions of the "H" temper	
H1	Strain hardened only. Applies to products that are strain hardened to obtain the desired mechanical properties without supplementary thermal treatment. The number following this designation indicates the final degree of strain hardening.
H2	Strain hardened and then partially annealed. Applies to products that are strain hardened more than the desired and then reduced in strength to the desired final amount by partial annealing. The number following this designation indicates the final degree of strain hardening remaining after the product has been partially annealed.
H3	Strain hardened and then stabilized. Applies to products that are strain hardened and then stabilized by low-temperature heating to slightly lower their strength and increase ductility. This designation applies only to alloys that, unless stabilized, gradually age soften at room temperature. The number following this designation indicates the degree of strain hardening that remains once the product has been strain hardened at a specific amount and then stabilized.
Subdivisions of "H1," "H2" and "H3" tempers	
The digit following the designation H1, H2 and H3 indicates the final degree of strain hardening. Tempers between 0 (annealed) and 8 (full hard) are designated by numerals 1 through 7. A material having a strength about midway between that of the 0 temper and that of the 8 temper is designated by the numeral 4 (half hard), between 0 and 4 by the numeral 2 (quarter hard), between 4 and 8 by the numeral 6 (three-quarter hard) and so on. The third digit, when used, indicates a variation of a two-digit H temper. It is used when the degree of control of temper or the mechanical properties are different from but close to those for the two-digit H temper to which it is added. Numerals 1 through 9 may be arbitrarily assigned to an alloy and its product to indicate a specific degree of control of temper or specified mechanical property limits.	
W	Solution heat treated. An unstable temper applicable only to alloys that spontaneously age at room temperature after solution heat treatment. This designation is specific only when the period of natural aging is indicated, for example, W1/2 hour.
T	Thermally treated to produce stable tempers other than F, O or H. Applies to products that are thermally treated, with or without supplementary strain hardening, to produce stable tempers. The T is always followed by one more digit. Numerals 1 through 10 have been assigned to indicate specific sequence of basic treatments as follows.

Table 8.1 (continued)

Subdivisions of the "T" tempers	
T1	Cooled from an elevated temperature shaping process and naturally aged to a substantially stable condition. Applies to products for which the rate of cooling from an elevated temperature shaping process, such as casting or extrusion, is such that their strength is increased by room-temperature aging.
T2	Annealed (cast products only). Applies to a type of annealing treatment used to improve ductility and increase stability of castings.
T3	Solution heat treated and then cold worked. Applies to products that are cold worked to improve strength, or in which the effect of cold work in flattening and straightening is recognized in applicable mechanical properties.
T4	Solution heat treated and naturally aged to a substantially stable condition. Applies to products that are not cold worked after solution heat treatment, or in which the effect of cold work in flattening or straightening may not be recognized in applicable mechanical properties.
T5	Cold from an elevated temperature shaping process and then artificially aged. Applies to products that are cooled from an elevated temperature shaping process, such as casting or extrusion, and then artificially aged to improve mechanical properties or dimensional stability or both.
T6	Solution heat treated and then artificially aged. Applies to products that are not cold worked after solution heat treatment, or in which the effect of cold work in flattening or straightening may not be recognized in applicable mechanical properties.
T7	Solution heat treated and then stabilized. Applies to products that are stabilized to carry them beyond the point of maximum strength to provide control of some special characteristics.
T8	Solution heat treated, cold worked and then artificially aged. Applies to products that are cold worked to improve strength, or in which the effect of cold work in flattening or straightening is recognized in applicable mechanical properties.
T9	Solution heat treated, artificially aged and then cold worked. Applies to products that are cold worked to improve strength.
T10	Cooled from an elevated temperature shaping process, artificially aged and then cold worked. Applies to products that are artificially aged after cooling from an elevated temperature shaping process, such as casting or extrusion, and then cold worked to further improve strength.

A period of natural aging at room temperature may occur between or after the operations listed for temper T3 through T10. Control of this period is exercised when it is metallurgically important. Additional digits may be added to designations T1 through T10 to indicate a variation in treatment that significantly alters the characteristics of the product.

Table 8.2: Typical effects of heat treatment.

	Mg–Al–Zn	Mg-Al-Zn-Si	Mg-Al-Ca-Mn-Zn	Mg-Al-Sn-Zn	Mg–Y	Mg-Y-Nd-Zr	Mg-Y-Gd-Zn-Zr	Mg-Y-Sm-Zr
Stable precipitate	[7–9]	[10]		[11]	[12]	[13]	[14, 15]	[16]
Strength	[17]		[18]			[13, 19, 20]		[16]
Ductility	[17]					[13, 19, 20]		
Biocompatibility					[21, 22]			
Biodegradation					[21, 22]			
Hardness							[14]	

Table 8.3: Typical effects of heat treatment.

	Mg–Zn	Mg–Zn–Zr	Mg–Zn–Y	Mg-Zn-Y-Zr	Mg-Zn-Mn-Sn-Nd	Mg-Zn-Si-Mn	Mg–Zn–Ca	Mg–Zn–Al	Mg-Zn-Y-Nd	Mg-Zn-Mn-Nd
Stable precipitate		[23]	[24, 25]	[26–28]	[29]	[30]		[31]		
Strength		[23]		[26, 28]		[30]	[32]	[31]	[33]	[34]
Ductility		[23]				[30]		[31]	[33]	[34]
Biocompatibility	[2]								[33]	
Biodegradation										
Corrosion resistance	[35, 36]						[32]			

that (i) homogenization treatment between forging and extrusion process can release stored energy and diminish precipitated $MgZn_2$ phase, both of which result in the finer size and low volume fraction of dynamic recrystallized grains and (ii) when compared with the as-extruded alloy without homogenization treatment, the alloy exhibited high yield strength which is thought to originate from the dislocation strengthening and texture strengthening. Xiao et al. [66] studied the microstructure evolution and

Table 8.4: Typical effects of heat treatment.

	Mg–Sn–Mn	Mg-Sn-Zn-Al-Mn-Na	Mg-Sn-Y-Zr	Mg-Gd-Zn	Mg-Gd-Y	Mg-Gd-Y-Zn-Zr	Mg-Gd-Zr	Mg-Gd-Y-Zr	Mg-Gd-Y-Nd-Zr	Mg-Gd-Nd-Y-Ho-Er-Zn
Stable precipitate			[37]	[38]	[39, 40]	[41]	[42]	[43]	[44]	
Strength	[45, 46]	[47]			[39, 48]	[49]	[42]	[50]		[51]
Ductility	[46]	[47]			[48]					[51]
Biocompatibility										
Biodegradation										
Hardness								[52]		
Creep strength	[45]	[53]								
Fracture						[49]		[50]		

Table 8.5: Typical effects of heat treatment.

	Mg-Nd-Zn-Zr	Mg-Nd-Gd-Zn-Zr	Mg-Li-Al-Zn-Y	Mg-Li-Al-Zn-RE	Mg–Ca	Mg–Sr	Mg–Ni	Mg–Cu
Stable precipitate	[54, 55]	[56]	[57]					
Strength	[58]	[56]	[59, 60]	[61]		[62]		
Ductility	[58]	[56]		[61]		[62]		
Biocompatibility						[62]		
Biodegradation								
Corrosion resistance					[63]	[62]	[64]	[64]
Hardness								
Creep strength								
Fracture	[58]		[57]					
Fatigue strength	[55]							

mechanical properties of Mg–6Zn–2Gd–0.5Zr alloy during homogenization treatment. It was reported that (i) the as-cast alloy was found to be composed of dendritic primary α-Mg matrix, α-Mg + W ($Mg_3Zn_3Gd_2$) eutectic along grain boundaries and icosahedral quasicrystalline I (Mg_3Zn_6Gd) phase within the α-Mg matrix; (ii) during homogenization process, α-Mg + W ($Mg_3Zn_3Gd_2$) eutectic and I phase gradually dissolved into α-Mg matrix, while some rod-like rare earth (RE) hydrides (GdH_2) formed within the α-Mg matrix; (iii) both the tensile yield strength and the elongation showed a similar tendency as a function of homogenization temperature and holding time; and (iv) the optimized homogenization parameter was determined to be 505 °C for 16 h according to the microstructure evolution. Zhang et al. [67] investigated the microstructure evolution during homogenization of a low-alloying Mg–7Zn–3Al magnesium alloy and mentioned that (i) shorter holding time results in the so-called in situ precipitation phenomena, which is attributed to the insufficient diffusion of elements Zn and Al from solute-rich grain boundary region to the inner side of grain during homogenization and (ii) a homogenization treatment at 325 °C for at least 50 h is just enough allowing complete homogenization for such an alloy, in point of both morphology and microchemistry of the microstructure, which is deemed to be a key precondition for the optimum combined properties through proper thermomechanical treatment. Yan et al. [68] studied the microstructure evolution of Mg-5.9Zn-1.6Zr-1.6Nd-0.9Y alloy during homogenization and reported that (i) the microstructure of as-cast Mg-5.9Zn-1.6Zr-1.6Nd-0.9Y alloy consists of α-Mg, $Mg_3(Y,Nd)_2Zn_3$ (W), Zn–Zr, $Mg_{12}(Y,Nd)Zn$ (X) and $Mg_3(Y,Nd)Zn_6$ (I) phases; (ii) the as-cast sample has an endothermic peak at 510 °C, which disappears in the alloy homogenized at 500 °C for 16 h; (iii) a small quantity of W phases dissolve at 470 and 490 °C; however, after homogenization at 500 °C for 16 h, there is only a small number of W, I and X phases, and dendritic segregation is almost eliminated. Hence, the optimum homogenization parameter is 500 °C for 16 h and homogenization can effectively decrease the hardness of the as-cast Mg-5.9Zn-1.6Zr-1.6Nd-0.9Y alloy from 1,852 to 1,442 MPa, so it is beneficial to further deformation of the alloy.

In terms of effects of homogenization on Mg–Gd-based alloys, Yang et al. [69] prepared as-cast and homogenized Mg-9Gd-3Y-0.5Zr alloys, which were subjected to hot compression at strain rate of 0.1 s^{-1} and temperatures ranging from 350 to 450 °C. It was found that (i) flow stresses are sensitive to the compression temperature and pretreatment state and (ii) comparing with the as-cast alloy, homogenized alloy has a higher flow stress and strain-hardening rate. Liu et al. [70] investigated the microstructure and mechanical properties of the Mg-5Y-4Gd-0.5Zn-0.4Zr alloy and reported that (i) the 14 H LPSO (long-period stacking ordered) structure was formed during isothermal homogenization; (ii) the presence of the 14 H LPSO structure resulted in refined microstructure and weak texture while harmful to improve age-hardening response after hot extrusion, (iii) the alloy after homogenization for 16 h at 500 °C followed by subsequent hot extrusion displayed the highest peak hardness value during aging at 220 °C and (iv) the yield tensile strength and the ultimate tensile strength of the peak-aged alloy were about 300 and 370 MPa, respectively. Zhang et al. [71] investigated that the microstructures and mechanical properties of the Mg-7.68Gd-4.88Y-1.32Nd-0.63Al-0.05Zr alloy were investigated both in the as-cast condition and after homogenization heat treatment from 535 to 555 °C in the time range 0–48 h. The as-cast alloy consisted of α-Mg matrix, $Mg_5(Y_{0.5}Gd_{0.5})$ phase which is a eutectic phase, strip of $Al_2(Y_{0.6}Gd_{0.4})$ phase, little Al_3Zr and $Mg(Y_3Gd)$ phase. It was mentioned that (i) with the increasing homogenization temperature and time, the $Mg_5(Y_{0.5}Gd_{0.5})$ phase was completely dissolved into the matrix; (ii) the $Al_2(Y_{0.6}Gd_{0.4})$ phase was almost not dissolved which impeded grain boundaries motion making the grain size almost not changed in the process of homogenization; (iii) the optimum homogenization condition was 545 °C × 16 h; and (iv) the tensile strength increased, yield strength decreased and the plasticity improved obviously after 545 °C × 16 h homogenization treatment. Li et al. [72] conducted a similar research to study the microstructures evolution and mechanical properties of Mg-7Gd-3Y-1Nd-*x*Zn-0.5Zr ($x = 0.5$, 1 and 2 wt%) alloys before and after homogenization and reported that the microstructure of the as-cast alloy with 0.5% Zn consists of α-Mg, $(Mg, Zn)_3RE$ phase, $Mg_5(RE, Zn)$ phase and stacking fault, and the addition of 1% and 2% Zn results in the disappearance of $Mg_5(RE, Zn)$ phase, but a block-like 14H LPSO phase is observed in the alloy with 2% Zn. After homogenization at 520 °C for 32 h, the 14H LPSO phase appear in the alloys with 1% and 2% Zn, but no other phase can be seen in the alloy with 0.5% Zn. The tensile tests at room temperature exhibit that the as-cast alloy containing 1% Zn shows the optimal mechanical properties and the ultimate tensile strength, yield strength and elongation are 187 MPa, 143 MPa and 3.1%, respectively, but the mechanical properties of the as-homogenized alloy containing 2% Zn exhibit the highest mechanical properties and the ultimate tensile strength, yield strength and elongation are 245 MPa, 166 MPa and 12.6%, respectively. Xu et al. [73] utilized different cooling processes (such as quenching in warm water and cooling in furnace) to homogenize Mg-8.2Gd-3.8Y-1.0Zn-0.4Zr alloy. It was mentioned that (i) the as-quenched sample was comprised of α-Mg matrix, Mg5RE phase and 18R LPSO phase distributed at the grain boundaries and a few of RE-rich particles distributed randomly; (ii) during the process of cooling in furnace, Mg_5RE and 18R LPSO phases were transformed into block-shaped 14H LPSO phase and lamellar-shaped 14H LPSO phase, respectively, due to the diffusion of solute atoms into the α-Mg matrix; (iii) the as-quenched sample exhibits tensile yield strength of 130 MPa, ultimate tensile strength of 206 MPa and elongation to failure of 5.5%, while the sample cooled in the furnace exhibits higher tensile yield strength but lower ultimate tensile strength and ductility due to the coarse grains and formation of block-shaped 14H LPSO phase.

There are still some studies on different Mg-based alloys. Bao et al. [74] studied the Mg–3Li–0.4Zr alloys containing RE elements (Gd, La, Nd) to reveal the influence of homogenization treatment on microstructures and distributions of RE, Zr elements and mentioned that (i) 300 °C × 24 h homogenization treatment shows better improvement on the microstructure including the refinement of grain size, the dispersion of cellular dendrite and low melting point particles; (ii) before treatment, La and Nd segregate effectively at grain boundary and Zr segregates in the form of precipitates; and (iii) homogenization treatment induces the reduction of RE segregation; however, the segregation of Zr in precipitates cannot be abated due to the relatively low diffusion rate compared with RE elements. Peng et al. [75] investigated the effects of homogenization treatment of Mg-8Li-3Al-Y alloy and indicated that (i) there existed five phases in the as-cast alloy: α, β, Al_2Y, AlLi and $MgAlLi_2$; (ii) the spheroidized α-phase grew gradually and its microstructure and composition became homogeneous when it was treated at 300 °C for 12 h; and (iii) the alloy has a good comprehensive mechanical property compared with other homogenization schedules, suggesting that a homogenization treatment at 300 °C for 12 h was determined to be the optimal homogenization treatment for Mg-8Li-3Al-Y alloy. Tan et al. [76] studied the effect of homogenization on enhancing the failure strain of a high-strength $MgY_{1.06}Zn_{0.76}Al_{0.42}$ (at%) alloy. It was reported that (i) bulk 14 H LPSO phases (≥10 μm) were progressively broken down into acicular fine platelets (≤2 μm) with increase in homogenization time (1, 2, 4 and 6 h) at 450 °C; (ii) the high density of fine LPSO platelets (≤2 μm interparticle spacing) were experimentally observed to be more effective than the bulk LPSO phases (≥10 μm interphase spacing) for promoting dynamic recrystallization via particle-simulated nucleation during extrusion, which was critical for basal texture weakening to enhance the failure strain of the as-extruded alloy; and (iii) the alloy homogenized for 2 h prior to hot extrusion displayed the highest tensile yield (376 MPa) and ultimate tensile strength (416 MPa) with significant improvement in failure strain (+80%) compared to as-extruded alloy (homogenized for 1 h prior to hot extrusion).

8.4 Solution treatment

Solution heat treatment consists in heating the alloy material to a temperature at which certain constituents go into solution, and then quenching so as to hold these constituents in solution during the cooling. Quenching is done in still or moving air, and liquids are not generally used. For magnesium alloy castings, the solution heat-treating temperature lies in the range of about 340–565 °C, depending upon the composition and details of the operation, for a range of 16–24 h. Solution heat-treated material has the temper designation T4 for castings, which requires high strength and maximum toughness.

Naghdi et al. [77] investigated the effect of solution treatment on the microstructure, mechanical properties and creep resistance of cast Mg–4Zn–0.3Ca (wt%) alloy by the impression creep testing at 175 and 225 °C. It was reported that (i) a semicontinuous network of $Ca_2Mg_6Zn_3$ phase was found to form at grain boundaries after a single-step solution treatment (500 °C × 4 h), which was, however, completely dissolved into the matrix after a double-step solution treatment (350 °C × 20 h + 510 °C × 3 h); (ii) single-step-treated samples exhibited better mechanical properties and creep resistances due to the presence of the thermally stable $Ca_2Mg_6Zn_3$ phase, mainly at grain boundaries, which made the single-step-treated samples more susceptible to brittle fracture by acting as preferred sites for initiation of microcracks that could easily propagate through the intergranular phase network; and (iii) on the other hand, double-step-treated samples had inferior mechanical properties and creep resistances, as compared to the single-step-treated condition due to the elimination of the intergranular phases and activation of twinning during deformation. Miao et al. [78] conducted the in vitro study on the microstructure, mechanical properties and corrosion of Mg–2.4Zn–0.8Gd (wt%) alloy with and without solution treatment before extrusion. It was mentioned that (i) the volume of secondary phases decreased after solution treatment, leading to more homogeneous microstructure distribution of as-extruded samples; (ii) the solution treatment before extrusion contributed to an elongation increase by 24%, and corrosion resistance was improved by about 20% according to hydrogen evolution and weight loss test; and (iii) with solution treatment before extrusion, the corrosion morphology was transformed from localized pitting corrosion to uniform corrosion due to the more homogeneous microstructure. Jia et al. [79] investigated the solution treatment parameters, mechanical properties and corrosion behavior of binary Mg–4Zn alloy and found that (i) after the solution treatment at 335 °C for 16 h, Mg–4Zn alloy had an ultimate tensile strength of 184.13 MPa and elongation of 9.43% and (ii) the corrosion resistance in 3.5% NaCl solution revealed that the corrosion current density of the solution treatment Mg alloy was 11.2 $\mu A/cm^2$. It was lower than 15.8 $\mu A/cm^{-2}$ for the as-cast Mg alloy under the same conditions, which was greatly associated with the microcathode effect of the second phases. Shahri et al. [80] solution treated a binary Mg–6Zn biodegradable alloy to evaluate the effects of resulting microstructure changes on the alloy's degradation rate and mechanisms in vitro, under 350 °C for 6–48 h treatment conditions. It was reported that (i) over 24 h solution treatment dissolves intermetallic phases in matrix and produces an almost single-phase microstructure; (ii) decreasing the intermetallic phases results in lower cathode/anode region ratios and lowers corrosion rates; (iii) solution at 350 °C × 24 h enhances the corrosion resistance (in simulated body fluid at 37 °C) of the as-cast alloy more than 60% and decreasing intermetallic phases in the microstructure accompanied a lower pH rise reduced corrosion rate and (iv) solution treatment is suggested as a corrosion improving process for the application of Mg–Zn alloys as biodegradable implant materials.

Li et al. [81] studied the effect of temperature and strain rate on tensile ductility of a solutionized Mg-Gd-Y-Zr alloy under the uniaxial tensile testing. It was found that (i) with the increment of temperature, this alloy exhibited drop of ductility at 350 °C along with intergranular fracture, due to the local precipitation at grain boundary by holding process before tension was responsible for the grain boundary embrittlement at 350 °C; (ii) plastic deformation preferentially occurred at the softer *solute-depleted zones* concurrent with grain boundary precipitates, whereas dislocation movement would be effectively inhibited at the hard grain boundary precipitates, inducing stress concentration and cracking along the grain boundary as the solute-depleted zone deformed to its plastic limit; (iii) the ductility at 350 °C was closely related to the holding time which significantly determined the size and distribution of precipitates and (iv) the occurrence of local grain boundary precipitation dependent on temperature and time was predominantly attributed to RE elements segregation to grain boundary. Wu et al. [82] mentioned that (i) solid-solution-treated Mg-10.2Li-1.2Al-0.4Zn (LAZ1010) alloy specimens aged at room temperature reach the maximal hardness after ≈20 h of aging, (ii) X-ray diffraction tests show that θ precipitates is much smaller in size than α ones, which may be attributed to the hardening phenomenon observed in the solid-solution-treated and -aged LAZ1010 alloy and (iii) during aging, the decrease in hardness of solid-solution-treated specimens with severe cold rolling at its maximal hardness is slower than that without, because specimens with severe cold rolling have abundant nucleus sites and thus have θ precipitates of smaller size. The microstructure evolution of Mg–9Li–6Al–xLa ($x = 0, 2, 5$) alloy under different solid solution parameters was investigated [83] and it was reported that during solution treatment at 350 °C, the lamellar AlLi is precipitated from α-Mg in Mg–9Li–6Al, while the $MgLi_2Al$ is dissolved into the matrix; however, during solution treatment at 450 °C, the AlLi phase is wholly dissolved into matrix, while the $MgLi_2Al$ is precipitated from β-Li. The addition of La can reduce the size of α-Mg, restrain the formation of AlLi, and make the precipitated $MgLi_2Al$ from β-Li at 450 °C be finer than that in Mg–9Li–6Al. With the addition of La, the decrease of the amount of AlLi and $MgLi_2Al$ leads to a descent of hardness, while the refinement, Al–La phase precipitation, and the solution of Al atoms can improve the hardness of the alloys.

The effect of solution heat treatment at 420 °C on the morphology of Mg_2Si particles in Mg–Al–Si alloys was studied and it was mentioned that the Mg_2Si precipitates tended to be spherodized during the treatment due to the diffusion of Si atoms along the Mg_2Si/Mg interface, which is benefit the mechanical properties of the alloys [84]. Wang et al. [85] investigated the effects of solution heat treatment on the microstructure and mechanical properties of Mg–3Al–1Si–0.3Mn–xSr ($x = 0, 0.2, 0.4$) alloy. It was mentioned that Sr could play a role in the surface refinement and form a new binary or multiple phases with the matrix elements; however, excessive Sr has no metamorphism. After solution treatment, magnesium alloy showed spheroidization and Mg_2Si phase experienced the process from passivation to fusion. The mechanical properties of the alloy had been significantly improved in 420 °C × 10 h (T4) treatment process. After aging treatment, the microstructure of the alloy had no obvious change and the mechanical properties had a slight increase. The tensile properties of the alloy were approximately proportional to the holding time. Zeng et al. [86] studied morphology and microstructure of precipitate phases in a Mg–12Dy–3Nd–0.4Zr (wt%) alloy, before and after extrusion. It was found that (i) the eutectic phase, with composition of $Mg_5(Nd_{0.47}Dy_{0.53})$, has a face-centered cubic (fcc) crystal structure (a_o = 2.24 nm); (ii) the rectangular particles, at or near grain boundaries in the solution-treated state, has an fcc crystal structure (a_o = 0.526 nm) with composition of $Dy_{17}Mg_3$ and (iii) many elliptical particles, distributed almost homogeneously across the matrix in the as-extruded alloy, was identified an fcc crystal structure (a_o = 2.24 nm) with composition of $Mg_5(Nd_{0.50}Dy_{0.50})$, which should be identical to the eutectic phases except the difference in morphology. Zhang et al. [87] investigated the effect of solid-solution treatment on corrosion and electrochemical mechanisms of Mg–15Y alloy in 3.5 wt% NaCl solution and indicated that (i) the corrosion resistance of Mg–15Y sample gradually deteriorated with increase in immersion time, which was consistent with the observation of corrosion morphologies, (ii) the solid-solution treatment decreased the amounts of second phase $Mg_{24}Y_5$ and (iii) the corrosion potential (E_{CORR}) and corrosion rate of as-cast samples were both lower than those of solid-solution-treated samples, and both increased with increase in solid-solution-treated time. Yang et al. [88] identified the NdH_2 precipitates in Mg–2.5%Nd (wt%) alloy in 540 °C × 6 h solution-treated state.

8.5 Quenching

Quenching involves the rapid cooling of a metal to adjust the mechanical properties of its original state by heating the metal to a temperature greater than that of normal conditions (typically above the recrystallization temperature and below its melting temperature), followed by rapid cooling into quenching media (either air, oil, water or brine; as increasing manner in cooling rate). Quenching metals possess two-hold purposes: (1) to prevent cooling process from dramatically changing the metal's microstructure and (2) to preserve the high-temperature metallurgical state in a nonequilibrium condition (e.g., S.S.S.S.).

It is generally believed that the higher the cooling rate during the quenching process, the more amount of the supersaturated solution can exist, so that the subsequent aging treatment can show higher strengthening effect. Hence, quenching sensitivity and cooling rate are important factors to control the resultant age-hardening effect. Wang et al. [89] characterized the quench sensitivity of Mg–12Gd–0.8Zn–0.4Zr (GZ1208K) (by wt%) under the water cooling (WC) and air cooling (AC) conditions. This alloy contains an LPSO phase. It was reported that (i) GZ1208K alloy indicates significant quench sensitivity, that is, the yield strength of GZ1208K-WC alloy is 25.2% and 21.6% higher than GZ1208K-AC alloy, when aged at 225 °C for 8 and 32 h; (ii) the significant quench sensitivity is due to the formation of long basal precipitates during cooling in the air, which probably is a mixture of basal γ′ precipitate and the LPSO phases; and (iii) the strengthening effect of solution atom, fine LPSO precipitate and prismatic precipitate in GZ1208K alloy can be listed in the following order: prismatic precipitate ≫ fine LPSO precipitate > solution atom. Hagihara et al. [90] found that the addition of

5 at% of Al to Mg0Li alloy, combined with rapid quenching, caused an extreme increase in yield stress up to ~470 MPa; this is compared with ~50 MPa in a Mg–Li binary crystal. Increased valence electron to atom ratio and development of chemical modulation in the alloy by Al addition are probable causes of the enhancement of plastic anisotropy and the drastic increase in yield stress, respectively.

Candan et al. [91] investigated micro-Ti-alloyed AZ91 Mg alloys (AZ91 + 0.5 wt%Ti) to determine the effectiveness of microalloying and/or cooling rate on their corrosion properties in 3.5% NaCl solution. It was shown that (i) the $Mg_{17}Al_{12}$ (β) intermetallic phase in the microstructure of AZ91 Mg alloy formed as a net-like structure; (ii) the Ti addition has reduced the distribution and continuity of β-intermetallic phase and its morphology has emerged as fully divorced eutectic; (iii) compared with AZ91 alloy, the effect of the cooling rate in Ti-added alloy on the grain size was less pronounced; (iv) when AZ91 and its Ti-added alloys were compared under the same cooling conditions, the Ti addition showed notably high corrosion resistance; (v) electrochemical test results showed that while I_{CORR} (corrosion current) values of AZ91 decrease with increase in the cooling rate, the effect of the cooling rate on I_{CORR} values was much lower in the Ti-added alloy; and (vi) the corrosion resistance of AZ91 Mg alloy was sensitive toward the cooling rates while Ti-added alloy was not affected much from the cooling conditions. The effect of cooling rate on the transition of dendrite morphology of a Mg–6Gd (wt%) alloy was semiquantitatively analyzed under a constant temperature gradient [92]. It was reported that (i) equiaxed dendrites, including exotic "butterfly-shaped" dendrite morphology, dominate at high cooling rate (>1 K/s); (ii) when the cooling rate decreases in the range of 0.5–1 K/s, the equiaxed-to-columnar transition takes place, and solute segregates at the center of two long dendrite arms of the "butterfly-shaped" dendrite; and (iii) when the cooling rate is lower than 0.3 K/s, directional solidification occurs and the columnar dendritic growth direction gradually rotates from the crystalline axis to the thermal gradient direction with an increase in cooling rate [92]. Meng et al. [93] conducted the reheating and rapid cooling experiments, and semisolid compression tests on extruded Mg-8.20Gd-4.48Y-3.34Zn-0.36Zr alloy using a multistage hot compression test machine. It was mentioned that, depending on reheating temperature, heating rate and isothermal holding time, the dynamic arrangement of alloying elements and phase transformation took place during subsequent rapid cooling. These microstructural behaviors not only changed the anisotropy in microstructural morphology of the extruded alloy but also affected the anisotropy in forming properties of it. When this alloy was reheated to 580 °C with a heating rate of 20 °C/s and held isothermally for 20 s, semisolid slurry without anisotropy in microstructural morphology and forming properties exhibiting a homogeneous spherical microstructure was obtained.

Rapidly quenched amorphous Mg-based alloys were subjected to metallurgical study [94, 95]. In terms of primary crystallization in $Mg_{76}Ni_{19}Y_5$ alloy, the crystallization starts with formation of the equilibrium hexagonal Mg_2Ni phase, obeying a continuous nucleation and parabolic growth kinetics law during the whole transformation;

while $Mg_{78}Ni_{18}Y_4$ alloy forms a nanocrystalline metastable phase during primary crystallization [94]. With Mg-rich near eutectic Mg–Ni amorphous alloys ($Mg_{88}Ni_{12}$ and $Mg_{87}Ni_{12}Y_1$), it was mentioned that (i) the influence of Y substitution for Mg and quenching rate on the crystallization process was noticeable, (ii) the metastable compound decomposes in a large temperature interval with a very broad exothermic effect for both alloys, (iii) due to the very low rate of transformation its differential scanning calorimetry peak and the associated enthalpy change can be detected only at high heating rates (>40 K/min) and (iv) the isothermal crystallization kinetics analysis revealed a three-dimensional linear growth of existing nuclei mechanism for the $Mg_{\sim 6}Ni$ formation in both $Mg_{87}Ni_{12}Y_1$ and $Mg_{88}Ni_{12}$ glasses, appearing as a second crystallization reaction after the primary α-Mg formation.

8.6 Cryogenic treatment

A cryogenic treatment is the process of treating workpieces to cryogenic temperatures (i.e., below −190 °C), usually using liquid nitrogen, in order to remove residual stresses and improve wear resistance (particularly on steels). Although cryogenic treatment has been extensively applied to steels, it should not be limited to steels but can also be applied to Mg-based alloys.

Liu et al. [96] investigated the effect of cryogenic treatment on the microstructure and mechanical properties of Mg–1.5Zn–0.15Gd (at%) alloy and reported that (i) numerous W phase particles precipitated from the Mg matrix after cryogenic treatment, (ii) with increasing cryogenic treatment duration from 1 min to 24 h, the volume fraction of W phase precipitate also increased, (iii) after cryogenic treatment for 24 h, the ductility of alloy was enhanced by 79%, since the homogenous distributed W phase with nanoscale activated the nucleation of twins during deformation and (iv) cryogenic treatment could be efficient only for the formation of precipitate with a much lower atom density than the matrix. Li et al. [97] reported that the tensile tests of Mg–2Zn–0.7Ce (at%) alloys before and after cryogenic treatment show that it can significantly increase the plasticity of the alloy. The yield strength, tensile strength and elongation of the as-extruded alloy were 245 MPa, 197 MPa and 9.6%, respectively; after cryogenic treatment at −196 °C for 24 h, the elongation of the alloy increased to 17.5%, but the tensile strength did not change significantly, whereas the hardness increased slightly and the yield strength decreased slightly. The fracture mechanism of alloy after cryogenic treatment changed from brittle fracture to ductile fracture. Yang et al. [98] investigated the wear behavior of Mg–1.5Zn–0.15Gd alloy before and after cryogenic treatment by dry sliding wear test and mentioned that (i) the wear resistance of the alloys has been significantly improved after cryogenic treatment; (ii) the friction coefficient and wear rate decrease with the increase in cryogenic treatment, which is attributed to the increase of volume fraction of the secondary phase particles and its refinement due to the treatment; and (iii) the alloy after cryogenic treatment exhibits a much smoother worn surface.

There are some studies on AZ series. Jiang et al. [99] studied the effect of cryogenic treatment (−196 °C) on the microstructure and mechanical properties of AZ31 alloy and mentioned that the tensile stress and the hardness of the samples treated in a cryogenic environment are higher than those of the untreated sample, due to the generation of a type of "frame-like" twinning during the cryogenic treatment, which also leads to the evolution of grain orientation. Li et al. [100] investigated the microstructure and mechanical properties of AZ31 alloy, which was cryogenically treated at −196 °C for 1, 5 and 24 h, respectively. It was reported that (i) the grains of AZ31 were initially refined and grew up with increase in cryogenic time, the second phase decreased gradually, and the rigidity and tensile strength decreased drastically and then increased; and (ii) as a result, AZ31 magnesium alloys subjected to 1 h cryogenic treatment were able to obtain the optimal combination properties. The microstructural behavior of a high-pressure die-casting AZ91 alloy, submitted to T6 and T6 with deep cryogenic treatment prior to aging was studied [101]. It was mentioned that (i) the mechanical properties were improved by both treatments though yield strength was higher following T6 treatment and elongation was greater following T6 with deep cryogenic treatment and (ii) continuous precipitation was promoted by cryogenic treatment, resulting in an improvement in elongation by 20%.

8.7 Aging

When a metal is quenched down to room temperature, the alloying elements become supersaturated in nonequilibrium state and have a driving force to form precipitates and different phases. Aging treatment consists in heating the quenched alloy at a moderately elevated temperature to affect the precipitation of the constituents held in solid solution. The temperature of treatment may be in the range of about 150–260 °C, with exposures from 3 to 16 h. The temper designation for solution heat-treated and -aged material is T6. High yield strength and hardness are developed by the T6 treatment. For aging the solution-treated materials, as mentioned in this section, there are two types of aging methods, that is, natural aging and artificial aging. Natural aging is done at room temperature in which the metal is removed from the quench bath and allowed to gain its full strength at room temperature. This natural aging may be good because it allows for an initially softer and easier to machine alloy, which then hardens without extra energy/process steps. Artificial aging is the treatment of a metal alloy at elevated temperatures so as to accelerate the changes in the properties of an alloy as a result of the casting and forging process. Generally, the chemical properties of newly cast and forged metals naturally change and settle very slowly at room temperature. Artificial aging will speed up this change more rapidly at higher temperatures. This process ensures quality and accuracy in close tolerance specifications. It also helps manufacturers make machine-ready parts available much more quickly to machinists and distributors. Although aging possesses benefits like enhancing strength of alloys, restoring the equilibrium in the metal and eliminating any unstable conditions brought upon by a prior operation, a special care should be taken to ensure that the aging process is accomplished below the equilibrium solvus temperature. If the process is continued beyond the specified time, eventually the hardness decreases, which is known as an over-aging phenomenon.

Phenomenologically, there are various ways of appearance of precipitates during the precipitation-aging process. Figure 8.1 illustrates a precipitation sequence [102], where [1] before precipitation (supersaturated solid solution) [2]; localized precipitation (2a shows localized precipitation at twin and/or grain boundary and 2b depicts localized precipitation at grain boundary and slip bands) [3]; full precipitation (agglomeration of grain boundary precipitates takes place, leaving precipitate-deficit zone along the grain boundaries); [4a] final stage when precipitation is completed without onset of the grain boundary reaction, resulting in formation of large sizes of precipitates; [4b] proceeding grain boundary reaction, when new grains created at grain boundaries proceed to precipitate; [5b] final stage when a certain percentage of uncompleted grain boundary reaction occurs; [5a] completion of grain boundary reaction, by which all grains are newly reacted and reformed grains; and [6] final stage when grain boundary reaction takes place during precipitation and precipitates agglomerates to form large particles.

Since the precipitation phenomenon is diffusion controlled, the amount of the precipitates should be a function of time and temperature. And the reaction resultant can be evaluated by mechanical properties such as yield strength, as shown in Figure 8.2 [103] (although this data is for Al-4Cu-1Si-0.5Mn alloy, the phenomena of precipitation of Mg alloys should not be different). As mentioned previously, under certain condition, precipitates tend to agglomerate to form coarse size of aggregated precipitates, exhibiting less strength and a prematurely aged phase also indicating less strength due to inadequate precipitate formation. Accordingly, there should be a peak point in terms of strength during the aging condition (a combination of aging time and temperature), called as peak aging. It is obvious that the higher the aging temperature, the sooner the peak aging time is established, and vice versa.

8.7.1 Mg–Al-based alloys

For Mg–Al-based alloys, Bohlen et al. [104] mentioned that a higher content of Al in Mg alloys leads to the formation of the precipitation-hardened intermetallic compound $Mg_{17}Al_{12}$; however, the rollability and the resulting ductility and formability of sheets of such alloys are reduced with increasing Al content. The higher content of aluminum leads to a decrease of rollability at a given rolling schedule as well as

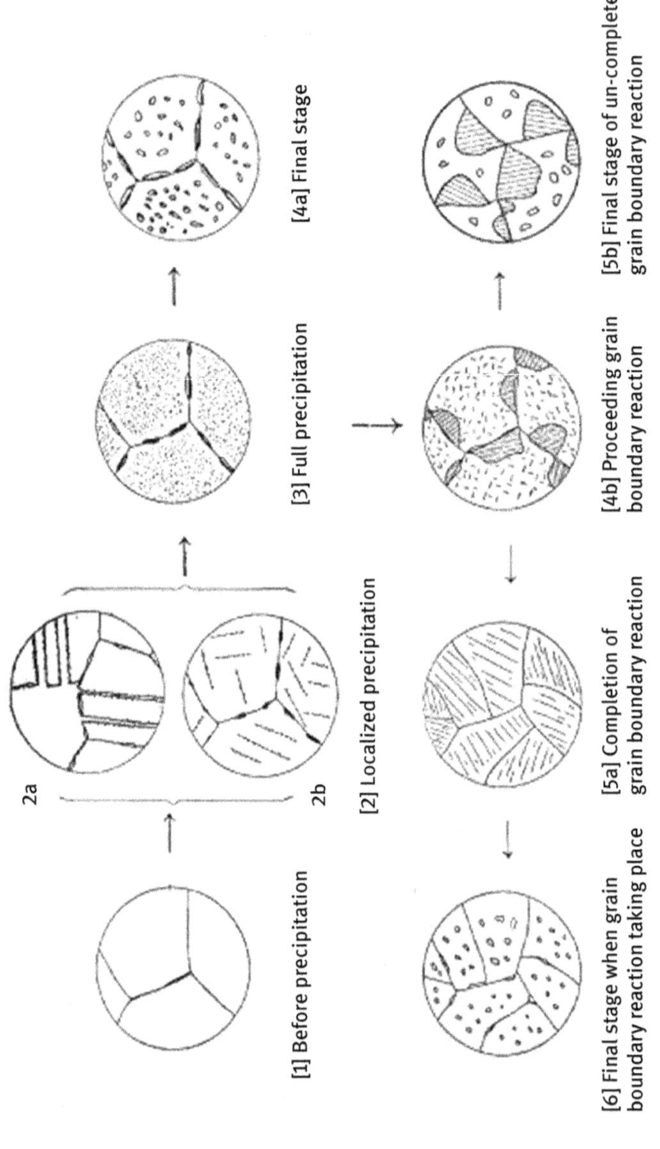

Figure 8.1: Precipitation sequence [102].

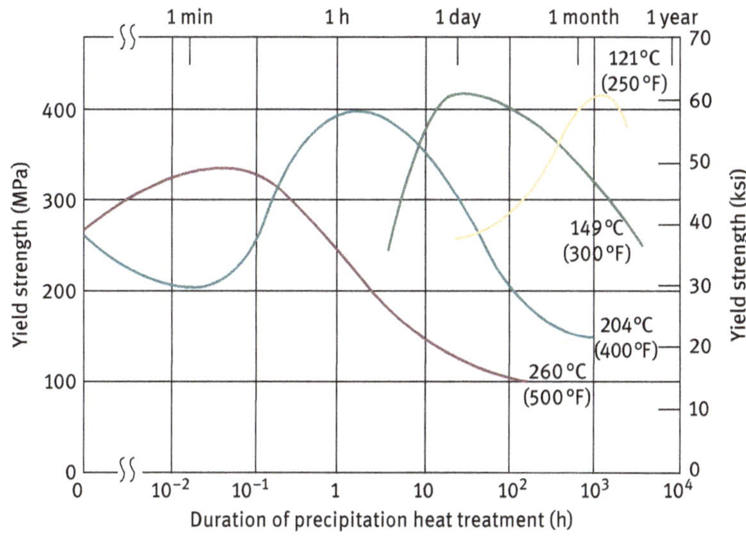

Figure 8.2: Effect of aging condition on yield strength for Al alloy [103].

a decrease of the ductility of the sheets after rolling and annealing. Alloys of the AM (Mg–Al–Mn) series have more advantages compared to AZ (Mg–Al–Zn) series alloys; however, Mn limits the ability to precipitation strengthening. Ge et al. [105] indicated that (i) ultrahigh-pressure technique remarkably extends solid solubility limitation of Al alloying element (~25 at%) in Mg alloys, resulting in unique solid solution strengthening and age-hardening response; and (ii) microhardness, yield strength and ultimate compressive strength are improved simultaneously without degrading plasticity by forming homogeneous and globular-shaped $Mg_{17}Al_{12}$ precipitates of 10–30 nm. Table 8.6 lists the reported Mg–Al-based alloys along with remarkable improvements of various properties.

Table 8.6: Major improvements by aging.

	Aging temperature (°C)	Aging time (h)	Tensile strength (MPa)	Yield strength (MPa)	Elongation (%)	Hardness	Corrosion resistance	Reference
Mg–3Al–1Zn							x	[106]
Mg–6Al–4Zn			x		x			[107]
Mg–8Al–1Zn			x					[108]
Mg–9Al–1Zn			x		x			[109, 110]
Mg–9Al–1Zn	250		366	270	28			[111]
Mg-9Al-1Zn-Ag	175	18	x		x			[112]
Mg-9Al-1Zn-Y			x		x			[113]
Mg-4Al-2Sn-RE	170	8	168	70	14			[114]
Mg-8Al-2Sn-1Zn						x		[115]
Mg-8Al-2Sn-1Zn			408	296	7			[116]
Mg–9Al–6Sn						103 HV		[117]
Mg-9Al-2Sn-Mn	200	8	292	154	5			[118]
Mg-1Al-0.3Ca-0.4Mn			287					[119]
Mg–4Al–4La	200	32	280					[120]

Note: X indicates enhanced or improved.

8.7.2 Mg–Zn-based alloys

Table 8.7 lists major improvements in various properties of Mg–Zn-based alloys.

Table 8.7: Major improvements by aging.

	Aging temperature (°C)	Aging time (h)	Tensile strength (MPa)	Yield strength (MPa)	Elongation (%)	Hardness	Electrical conductivity	Corrosion resistance	Reference
Mg–Zn						70 HV	x		[121]
Mg–3Zn	70					x			[122]
Mg-5Zn-5Sn-2Al	150	70	x	x	x	90 HV			[123]
Mg-5Zn-4Sn-1Mn			401	392	7				[124]
Mg–4Zn–3Sn				129					[125]
Mg-Zn-Cu-Mn						x			[126]
Mg–6Zn–3Cu	200		x (shear)						[127]
Mg-6Zn-1Cu-1Zr	180		x						[128]
Mg–4Zn–1.5Al	150	40	314	236	18				[129]
Mg-4Zn-2Al-0.5Ca	160	30		202		x			[130]
Mg-6Zn-4Al-1Sn			335	175	11				[131]
Mg-6Zn-4Al-0.5Cu			312	202	7				[132]
Mg-8Zn-4Al-1Ca	160	16				x			[133]
Mg–1.2Zn–0.5Ca		2–5	x					x	[32]
Mg–4Zn–0.5Ca	150–200		x						[134]
Mg-4Zn-0.5Ca-Mn	250	6–72	180	175	3–9				[135]
Mg-6Zn-1Mn-4Sn			x	x					[136]
Mg-6Zn-1Mn-4Sn						x			[137]
Mg-6Zn-1Mn-4Sn-Y			376	371	7.7				[138]

Table 8.7 (continued)

	Aging temperature (°C)	Aging time (h)	Tensile strength (MPa)	Yield strength (MPa)	Elongation (%)	Hardness	Electrical conductivity	Corrosion resistance	Reference
Mg–2.4Zn–0.2Ti	70					x			[139]
Mg–2.8Zn–Ba			x						[140]
Mg–8Zn–Co			x						[141]
Mg-2.4Zn-Ag-Ca	160					x			[142]
Mg–2.8Zn–Cr	70					x			[143]
Mg–1Zn–2Gd	227					x			[144]
Mg–8Zn–2Y	200					110 HV			[145]
Mg–4Zn–2Er	200					x			[146]
Mg–2Zn–2Zr	160					x			[147]

Note: X indicates enhanced or improved.

8.7.3 Mg–Gd-based alloys

Table 8.8 lists major enhanced properties of various Mg–Gd-based alloys.

Table 8.8: Major improvements by aging.

	Aging temperature (°C)	Aging time (h)	Tensile strength (MPa)	Yield strength (MPa)	Elongation (%)	Hardness	Thermal conductivity	Electrical resistivity	Corrosion resistance	Creep resistance	Reference
Mg–11.5Gd	230		x								[148]
Mg–12Gd		300					x				[149]
Mg–15Gd	NA	5 years						X			[150]
Mg–6Gd–2Y	175	100				x					[151]
Mg–7Gd–5Y	250		212	140							[152]
Mg–10Gd–3Y						x					[153]
Mg-Gd-Y-Zn-Zr						135 HV					[154]
Mg-1.4Gd-1.2Y-0.4Zn			461	395	6						[155]
Mg-1.5Gd-1.3Y-0.6Zn		100	583		13.1						[156]
Mg-8.2Gd-3.8Y-1.0Zn	225					x					[157]
Mg-8.2Gd-3.8Y-1.0Zn						156 HV					[158]
Mg-8.2Gd-3.8Y-1.0Zn			517	426	4.5						[159]
Mg-10Gd-2Y-0.5Zn	200	60	x	x							[160]
Mg-10Gd-3Y-1.2Zn			315								[161]
Mg-10Gd-6Y-2Zn			432		5						[162]
Mg-12.6Gd-1.3Y-0.9Zn	200		543	475							[163]
Mg-14Gd-3Y-1.8Zn	225	16	366	230	2.8						[164]

Table 8.8 (continued)

	Aging temperature (°C)	Aging time (h)	Tensile strength (MPa)	Yield strength (MPa)	Elongation (%)	Hardness	Thermal conductivity	Electrical resistivity	Corrosion resistance	Creep resistance	Reference
Mg-Gd-Y-Zr						x					[165]
Mg-Gd-Y-Zr	NA	6 years				x					[166]
Mg-7Gd-3Y-0.4Zr	200	120									[167]
Mg-7Gd-3Y-0.4Zr	200	120							x		[168]
Mg-8Gd-2Y-0.2Zr						x					[169]
Mg-10Gd-2Y-0.5Zr	NA,200	3 years	x			x					[170]
Mg-10Gd-3Y-0.5Zr	250		x								[171]
Mg-10Gd-3Y-0.4Zr	225					x					[172]
Mg-10Gd-3Y-0.5Zr			390	245							[173]
Mg-10Gd-5Y-0.6Zr		108							x		[174]
Mg-10Gd-5Y-0.4Zr			302	289							[175]
Mg-Gd-Y-Nd-Zr						x					[176]
Mg-Gd-Y-Nd-Zr			x	x							[177]
Mg-6Gd-3Y-2Nd-0.4Zr	200	92	435	359							[178]
Mg-7Gd-3Y-1Nd-0.5Zr	300		x	x							[179]
Mg-7Gd-5Y-1Nd-0.5Zr	210	180	x	x							[180]

Table 8.8 (continued)

	Aging temperature (°C)	Aging time (h)	Tensile strength (MPa)	Yield strength (MPa)	Elongation (%)	Hardness	Thermal conductivity	Electrical resistivity	Corrosion resistance	Creep resistance	Reference
Mg-8Gd-3.7Y-0.3Ag	200		411	339	3.9						[181]
Mg-2.4Gd-0.4Ag-0.1Zr			X	X							[182]
Mg-3.4Gd-0.5Ag-0.1Zr			410								[183]
Mg-14Gd-2Ag-0.5Zr						X					[184]
Mg–6Gd–0.6Zr						X				X	[185]
Mg-8Gd-0.6Zr-1RE			170	146							[186]
Mg–14Gd–0.5Zr				X							[187]
Mg–15Gd–0.5Zr	250		X	X							[188]
Mg-8Gd-1Er-0.5Zr			560	518	4.8						[189]
Mg–8Gd–2Er	200		308	246							[190]
Mg-8Gd-5Er-0.6Zr			261	173							[191]
Mg-3Gd-3Nd-0.6Zr			X	X							[192]
Mg-8.3Gd-1Dy-0.4Zr			X	X		X					[193]
Mg–Gd–Sm–Zr	225										[194]
Mg-8Gd-3Ho-0.6Zr			279	175							[195]

Note: X indicates enhanced or improved; NA represents natural aging.

8.7.4 Mg–Li-based alloys

Table 8.9 lists major enhanced properties on Mg–Li-based alloy.

Table 8.9: Major improvements by aging.

	Aging temperature (°C)	Aging time (h)	Tensile strength (MPa)	Yield strength (MPa)	Elongation (%)	Hardness	Thermal conductivity	Electrical resistivity	Corrosion resistance	Microstructure	Reference
Mg–4Li–6(Al,Si)			295								[196]
Mg-5Li-3Al-2Zn-2Cu			x	x							[197]
Mg–6Li–6Zn–1.2Y						x				x	[198]
Mg-8Li-3Al-2Zn-0.5Y	125		276	216	11.1						[199]
Mg–9Li–3Sc	200					93 HV					[200]
Mg-9Li-6Al-Y	150									x	[201]
Mg–9Li–6Al	RT	24								x	[202]
Mg-14Li-3Al-3Ce		15	137	196	19.2						[203]
Mg–14Li–Sr (0.15–0.4)										x	[204]

Note: X indicates enhanced or improved; RT represents room temperature.

8.7.5 Mg–Y-based alloy

Table 8.10 lists major enhanced properties of Mg–Y-based alloys.

Table 8.10: Major improvements by aging.

	Aging temperature (°C)	Aging time (h)	Tensile strength (MPa)	Yield strength (MPa)	Elongation (%)	Hardness	Thermal conductivity	Electrical resistivity	Corrosion resistance	Microstructure	Reference
Mg–10Y	220					x					[205]
Mg–12Y						x					[206]
Mg–Y–RE	180	60	388		23						[207]
Mg–4Y–3RE	140, 210	4								x	[208]
Mg-Y-Nd-Zr					18						[209]
Mg–Y–Nd	210									x	[210]
Mg-3.5Y-2.5Nd-0.5Zr	225	34	301	202	6.9						[20]
Mg–4Y–2.4Nd–0.4Zr	200		339	268	4						[211]
Mg-5Y-2.5Nd-1.5Gd										x	[212]
Mg-6Y-3Nd-0.2Ni	200									x	[213]
Mg–5Y–4Nd	250	16								x	[214]
Mg-2Y-3Gd-2Nd	225	10	281.7	198	11.1						[215]
Mg-4Y-2Gd-0.4Zr	220		291	228	28						[216]
Mg-5Y-5Gd-0.3Zr	200	64								x	[217]
Mg-7Y-4Gd-0.5Zr	250					x					[218]
Mg-7Y-5Sm-0.5Zn	200		465	413	6.5						[219]
Mg–10Y–1.5Sm			200								[220]
Mg-6Y-1Zn-0.6Zr						x					[221]
Mg–3Y–1Ni			435		21						[222]

Note: X indicates enhanced or improved.

8.7.6 Mg–Sn-based alloys

Table 8.11 lists improved properties of Mg–Sn-based alloys.

Table 8.11: Major improvements by aging.

	Aging temperature (°C)	Aging time (h)	Tensile strength (MPa)	Yield strength (MPa)	Elongation (%)	Hardness	Thermal conductivity	Electrical resistivity	Corrosion resistance	Microstructure	Reference
Mg–Sn–Hf						x					[223]
Mg–1.3Sn	200					x					[224]
Mg–1.5Sn–0.5Mn	200	100				77 HV					[225]
Mg–2.0Sn–0.4Mn			x	x							[226]
Mg–2.2Sn–0.5Mn	160					95 HV					[227]
Mg-2.2Sn–3Al–0.5Zn	200					72 HV					[228]
Mg–5.0Sn–0.4Sb			x	x							[229]
Mg–5.0Sn							x	x			[230]
Mg–5.0Sn– (0–2)Ag										x	[231]
Mg–5.0Sn–2Zn	150	48	x	x							[232]
Mg-6.0Sn-5Al-2Si										x	[233]
Mg-7.0Sn-1Al-1Zn										x	[234]
Mg–7.0Sn–1Ca–1Ag			482-c			95 HV					[235]
Mg-7.0Sn-1Ca-1Ag	200					80 HV					[236]
Mg-7.0Sn-2Ag-1Zn	160					78 HV					[237]
Mg-8.0Sn-6Zn-2Al			x	x							[238]
Mg-9.0Sn-1.5Y-0.4Zr	250	60	262	218	10.4						[37]

Note: X indicates enhanced or improved; -c represents ultimate compressive strength.

8.7.7 Mg–Nd-based alloys

Table 8.12 lists improvements in major properties of Mg–Nd-based alloys.

Table 8.12: Major improvements by aging.

	Aging temperature (°C)	Aging time (h)	Tensile strength (MPa)	Yield strength (MPa)	Elongation (%)	Hardness	Thermal conductivity	Electrical resistivity	Corrosion resistance	Microstructure	Reference
Mg–Nd										x	[239]
Mg–2.2Nd	295	3								x	[240]
Mg–3.0Nd										x	[241]
Mg-3.0Nd-0.2Zn-Zr	200	14	x	x							[242]
Mg-3.4Sn-0.1Zn-Zr			280	165							[243]

Note: X indicates enhanced or improved.

8.7.8 Other important Mg-based alloys

Table 8.13 lists noticeable improvements on various properties of other types of Mg-based alloys, which include mainly RE element(s) as an effective alloying element.

Table 8.13: Major improvements by aging.

	Aging temperature (°C)	Aging time (h)	Tensile strength (MPa)	Yield strength (MPa)	Elongation (%)	Hardness	Thermal conductivity	Electrical resistivity	Corrosion resistance	Microstructure	Reference
Mg–0.3Ca– (0–2) Zn						69 HV					[244]
Mg–0.3Ca–0.3Zn						x				x	[245]
Mg–0.5Ca– (1–5) Zn	200		x	x		x			x		[246]
Mg–1Ca–1Zn						x					[247]
Mg–2Dy–0.5Zn	180	36–80				x					[248]
Mg–2.2Dy–1Cu	535	4	x	x							[249]
Mg–(10–20)Dy	200		x	x					x		[250]
Mg–4Sm										x	[251]
Mg-4Sm-3Nd-1Zn-1Gd			213		8.6						[252]
Mg-5Sm-1.4Nd-Zn-Zr	200									x	[253]
Mg–Sc										x	[254]
Mg–5Sc	190	8	x	x							[255]
Mg–25Sc	200	5	x	x		232 HV					[256]
Mg–32Sc	200		357		12	143 HV					[257]
Mg–8.8Hg–8Ga									x	x	[258]
Mg–5Ce	180–250									x	[259]
Mg–2Ag–2Re			x	x							[260]
Mg–(1–3) Yb–0.5Zn	200									x	[261]
Mg–Cd–Yb	200					67 HV					[262]

Note: X indicates enhanced or improved.

8.8 Precipitation

The precipitation is a phenomenon that usually follows solution heat treatment. However, a precipitation treatment may be applied to material that has not received definitive solution treatment. Certain manufacturing processes for wrought products (like extruding and forging) result in retaining alloy constituents in solid solution in concentrations substantially greater than the equilibrium solubility at room temperature, leading to air-quenching during hot extrusion or forging from the press. There are various important factors controlling the nucleation and growth of precipitates, including the structure, morphology [263], orientation of precipitates [264], effects of precipitate morphology, and orientation of the strengthening and microstructural factors [265]. As a result of evolution of precipitates, the material is hardened and/or strengthened. Precipitation hardening (also called age-hardening or particle hardening) is a heat-treatment technique employed to enhance the yield strength of materials of most structural alloys such as Al, Mg, Ni, Ti and steels and stainless steels. Although both solution heat treatment and precipitation heat treatment involve precipitates, there should be a definite difference in between; that is, the solid solution strengthening involves formation of a single-phase solid solution via quenching, while the precipitation heat treatment involves the addition of impure particles to increase a material's strength. Precipitation hardening relies on changes in solid solubility with temperature to produce fine particles of an impurity phase, which impede the movement of dislocations, or defects in a crystal's lattice, since dislocations (as a dominant plasticity carrier) lead to hardening of the material [266–268].

Wang et al. [269], using the minima hopping method, calculated the formation energies, constructed the respective zero temperature convex hulls and analyzed their stabilities to predict suitable crystal structures. It was mentioned that the bulk formation energies per solute atom (essentially, the solute chemical potentials) decrease along the observed sequences of precipitation, validating our calculations in Mg–(Nd, Gd, Y, Y–Nd, Nd–Zn, Gd–Zn, Y–Zn, Al, Zn, Sn, Al–Ca, Ca–Zn) alloy systems. Magnesium has been alloyed with other metal elements for engineering applications. The most popular commercial magnesium alloys should include AZ series (Mg–Al–Zn), AM series (Mg–Al–Mn), AE (Mg–Al–RE), EZ (Mg–RE–Zn), ZK (Mg–Al–Zr) and WE (Mg–RE–Zr). Among the various magnesium alloys developed, AZ91, containing about 9 wt% Al and 1 wt% Zn, is the most widely used, not only for making automotive components but also for other structural components because of its combination of excellent castability and reasonable mechanical properties at room temperature with good corrosion resistance. About 90% of the magnesium cast products currently used are made of AZ91 [270–273].

8.8.1 Mg–Al-based alloys

To overcome the metallurgical issues of coursing of grain size during the conventional thermal aging for precipitate evolution, Ma et al. [274] performed dynamic precipitation during low-temperature deformation processing on a coarse-grained, fully solutionized Mg–9Al (wt%) alloy as a starting material, following low-temperature equal channel angular extrusion (ECAE) technique. It was reported that (i) nanoscale $Mg_{17}Al_{12}$ particles within grain interiors (or intergranular) were formed with a high number density and a low aspect ratio due to strain-induced and defect-assisted nucleation, (ii) the dislocation-accelerated nucleation rate and the excess vacancy concentration in Ma intergranular $Mg_{17}Al_{12}$ particles grows as the number of ECAE passes increases and (iii) the results suggest to provide key insights into the evolution of microstructure during dynamic precipitation and recrystallization, and thus provide guidance for the design of improved microstructures in Mg alloys. Wong et al. [275] investigated the solidification path and microstructure evolution in Mg–3Al–14La alloy and mentioned that the solidification sequence begins with the precipitation of primary Al_5La_2, followed by a eutectic with the products α-Mg + Al_5La_2, then a monovariant binary eutectic with the products α-Mg + $Mg_{12}La$ and lastly a ternary eutectic with the products α-Mg + $Mg_{12}La$ +$(Al,Mg)_3La$. Hu et al. [276] modified the commercially used Mg–3Al–1Si (AS31) alloy with B and Sn for grain-refining purpose, and subjected to hot rolling. It was reported that (i) simultaneous addition of B and Sn resulted in large grains and coarse Mg_2Si phase in the as-cast alloy and (ii) the AS31–2Sn sheet exhibited the best yield strength of ~260 MPa with desirable ductility of ~15%, being attributed to a solid solution strengthening, grain boundary strengthening, texture strengthening and dislocation strengthening. Park et al. [277] rapidly solidified Mg–Al–Si–Ca and Mg–Zn–Ca-based alloys by melt spinning at the cooling rate of about a million K/s, followed by aging in the range 100–400 °C for 1 h. It was mentioned that (i) age hardening occurred after aging at 200 °C in the Mg-Al-Si-Ca alloys mainly due to the formation of Al_2Ca and Mg_2Ca phases, whereas in the Mg–Zn–Ca alloys mostly due to the distribution of Mg_2Ca and (ii) spherical Al_2Ca precipitate has the coherent interface with the matrix.

8.8.2 Mg–Zn-based alloys

Gao et al. [278] characterized the strengthening precipitate phases in a Mg–8Zn (et%) alloy, aged isothermally at 200 °C and reported that (i) precipitation at 200 °C involves formation of β1′ and β2′ transition phases, (ii) the β1′ phase is found to have a monoclinic structure similar to that of Mg_4Zn_7 and (iii) the β2′ phase is confirmed to have a hexagonal structure similar to that of $MgZn_2$. Wang et al. [279] studied the mechanical properties of Mg–1Zn–2 MM (mischmetal) alloy, where a typical mischmetal is mainly composed of approximately 55% cerium, 25% lanthanum and 15–

18% neodymium with other RE metals. It was reported that (i) the microstructure identified in the second phase is (La,Ce)$(Mg,Zn)_{12}$, which disperse them uniformly and (ii) hot rolling of Mg–1Zn–2 MM alloy at 500 °C provided a yield strength of 300 MPa, being attributed to a strong second phase. Luo et al. [280] investigated the effects of combined addition of 0.6 wt% Nd and 0.4 wt% Y on the microstructure and mechanical properties of Mg–7Zn–3Al alloy. It was indicated that (i) the Nd and Y addition led to obvious dendrite coarsening, while it could modify the morphology and distribution of τ-$Mg_{32}(Al, Zn)_{49}$ intermetallics; (ii) Al_2REZn_2 phase could be introduced into the alloy with the Nd and Y addition; (iii) with the effective second-phase strengthening, the ultimate tensile strength and elongation in as-cast state can be improved by the Nd and Y addition; and (iv) after aging treatment, the alloy with the Nd and Y addition exhibited better precipitation strengthening effects by forming finer $MgZn_2$ and $Mg_{32}(Al,Zn)_{49}$ precipitates into the α-Mg matrix, resulting that the yield and ultimate strength of Mg-7Zn-3Al-0.6Nd-0.4Y alloy could be increased to 182 and 300 MPa by peak-aging treatment.

8.8.3 Mg–Li-based alloys

Guo et al. [281] prepared Mg–9Li–3Al (wt%) alloys with addition of Sn and Y by vacuum melting followed by hot extrusion process. It was reported that (i) $MgLi_2Sn$ and $MgLi_2Al$ particles were observed in Mg-9Li-3Al-2Sn alloys and significant strength improvement was achieved due to precipitation hardening; (ii) the ultimate tensile strength of Mg-9Li-3Al-2Sn is 251 MPa, which is the highest among all the studied Mg–9Li–3Al alloys; and (iii) on the other hand, the highest elongation (43.8%) at room temperature is obtained in Mg-9Li-3Al-2Y. Zhao et al. [282] fabricated Mg–12Li, Mg–12Li–3 (Al–Si), Mg–12Li–7(Al–Si) and Mg–12Li–9(Al–Si) alloys (wt%) by high-frequency vacuum induction melting in a water-cooled copper crucible, followed by hot rolling and annealing. It was shown that (i) mechanical properties of Mg–12Li alloy were significantly improved by the addition of Al–Si eutectic alloy; (ii) Mg–12Li–7(Al–Si) alloy showed the highest strength of 196 MPa of the investigated alloys, which is about 1.8 times the strength of Mg–12Li alloy, and maintains high elongation of 27%; and (iii) the improved mechanical property with addition of Al and Si in the eutectic proportion into Mg–12Li alloy was attributed to the solution strengthening effect of Al and precipitation-hardening effect from AlLi and Mg_2Si precipitates. Feng et al. [283] evaluated the effect of extrusion ratio on the microstructure and mechanical properties of Mg–8Li-3Al-2Zn-0.5Y (wt%) alloy, which was prepared by casting and then deformed by hot extrusion at 200 °C with four different ratios of 4:1, 9:1, 16:1 and 25:1, respectively. It was reported that (i) the as-cast Mg-8Li-3Al-2Zn-0.5Y alloy is composed of α-Mg, β-Li, AlLi, $MgLi_2Al$ and Al_2Y phases; (ii) after hot extrusion with all four ratios, the microstructure was significantly refined; and (iii) the mechanical properties of Mg-8Li-3Al-

2Zn-0.5Y alloy at room temperature were improved, mainly caused by grain refinement and precipitation strengthening.

8.8.4 Mg–Ca-based alloys

Lalpoor et al. [284] investigated the effect of predeformation on precipitation-hardening response as well as the work-hardening behavior of a binary Mg–Ca alloy. It was mentioned that (i) application of 5% predeformation increases the precipitation-hardening response of the material and decreases the annealing time by 50%; (ii) the dislocations introduced during the predeformation process act as predominant nucleation sites and result in a higher number of precipitates of smaller size; (iii) during the thermomechanical treatments, the work-hardening behavior is altered by the state of the precipitates, namely, under-aged, peak-aged and over-aged; and (iv) the absolute values of the work-hardening rate are far less sensitive to the precipitation stage compared to aluminum alloys, a fact that explains the low work-hardening capacity of magnesium compared to aluminum. Nie et al. [285] identified Mg_2Ca precipitate in Mg–1Ca–1Zn alloy. Jardim [286], studying on the melt-spun Mg–1.5Ca–6Zn (wt%) alloy, mentioned that (i) the as-solidified alloy exhibited both spherical matrix precipitates and elongated precipitates at the grain boundaries; (ii) after heat treatment, the alloy showed faceted precipitates (cuboidal shape), mostly on dislocations; and (iii) the observed precipitate is $Ca_2Mg_6Zn_3$. Moreover, similar studies were carried out on Mg–Ca–Zn alloy [287, 288] and it was reported that (i) the precipitates were two types of equilibrium phases (i.e., Mg_2Ca and $Mg_6Ca_2Zn_3$) and (ii) early stage decomposition of the solid solution had no observable effect on hardness, but was followed by the formation of hardening GP zones [288]. Jayaraji et al. [289] and Chai et al. [290] investigated the precipitation behavior of Mg–Ca–Al alloy. The precipitate of Al_2Ca was identified in Ma–0.5Ca–0.3Al alloy [289]. Chai et al. [290] investigated effects of Al addition (0.0, 0.5, 3.0, 7.2 wt%) on microstructure, texture and mechanical properties of Mg–3.5Ca-based alloys. It was reported that (i) the addition of Al to the as-cast Mg–3.5Ca alloy resulted in the transformation of precipitated secondary phase from Mg_2Ca to $(Mg, Al)_2Ca$, Al_2Ca and even $Mg_{17}Al_{12}$ phase and (ii) the as-cast microstructure evolution influenced dynamic recrystallization and texture formation in the subsequent extrusion process.

8.8.5 Mg–Gd-based alloys

Mg–Gd-based alloys have an excellent aging precipitation strengthening effect; their precipitation sequence and precipitate phases are also very typical in magnesium alloys containing RE elements. Zhang et al., studying the evolution of precipitates in a Mg–16.2Gd–0.4Zr (wt%) alloy [291] and Mg–2.8Gd–0.1Zr (at%), Mg–2.4Gd–0.4Ag–

0.1Zr (at%), Mg–2.8Y–0.1Zr (at%) and Mg–2.4Y–0.4Ag–0.1Zr (at%) [292] during isothermal aging, mentioned that the widely accepted four-stage precipitation sequence of the Mg–Gd(–Zr) alloy system has been accordingly updated to S.S.S.S. → ordered solute clusters → GP zones → β′ → βF′ + tail-like hybrid structures → β_1 → β [291–293]. Zheng et al. [294] studied the precipitation evolution in Mg–Gd–Ag alloy aged at 200 °C and mentioned that (i) basal γ″ precipitates serve as the key strengthening structures in the under-aged sample; (ii) under the peak-aged condition, the alloy is strengthened by basal γ″ and prismatic β′; (iii) at the over-age stage, coarse particles, which are enriched with Ag and Gd, and highly stacked γ″ form within the alloy; and (iv) no γ′ is observed through the aging of this Mg–Gd–Ag alloy. Zhang et al. [295] and Dai et al. [296] investigated precipitation behaviors of Mg–Gd–Y-based alloys. Zhang et al. [295] studied the precipitation processes during the peak-aged and over-aged stages of the as-extruded Mg-11.9Gd-1Y-0.44Zr (wt%) alloy and mentioned that (i) in addition to the dominant precipitate β′, both β_T and β_F' precipitates were also found from the peak-aged stage; (ii) the transformation from β_T to β_F' gives rise to the formation of neck morphology that connects different β-phases; (iii) the age hardening of this alloy strongly depends on the formation of the size of the near-continuous network composed of prismatic precipitates; and (iv) the near-continuous precipitate network was formed in the peak-aged condition while the breakdown of the near-continuous precipitate network results in the significant decrease of hardness. Dai et al. [296] investigated the effect of additions of 0.5–1 wt% Al on grain refinement, heat treatment and mechanical properties of Mg–10Gd–3Y (wt%) alloy and reported that (i) the additions of 0.6–1 wt% Al showed a dramatic grain refinement effect, which is associated with the formation of the $Al_2(Gd_{0.5}Y_{0.5})$ particles that act as nucleants for α-Mg grains; (ii) subsequent aging at low temperatures led to pronounced precipitation hardening and consequently a large improvement in strength; and (iii) in the peak-aged condition, the strength of the Al-refined alloy is comparable to that of the Zr-refined counterpart. Xu et al. [297] studied the effect of LPSO phase and γ′ precipitates on the aging behavior and mechanical properties of the extruded Mg-8.2Gd-3.8Y-1.0Zn-0.4Zr (wt%) alloy. It was indicated that (i) more β′-phases precipitate during aging treatment in the LPSO phase-containing alloy so that it exhibits a higher age-hardening response than the γ′-precipitate-containing alloy; (ii) the precipitation strengthening induced by β′-precipitates is the greatest contributor to the strength of the peak-aged LPSO-containing alloys; (iii) higher strength is achieved in γ′-precipitate-containing alloy due to the more effective strengthening induced by dense nanoscale γ′-precipitates than LPSO phases as well as the higher volume fraction of coarse unrecrystallized grains with strong basal texture; and (iv) the extruded alloy containing γ′-precipitates after T5 peak-aging treatment shows ultra-high tensile yield strength of 462 MPa, high ultimate tensile strength of 520 MPa and superior elongation to failure of 10.6%.

8.8.6 Mg–Sn-based alloys

Fu et al. [298], studying Mg–9Sn (wt%) alloy, mentioned that a hexagonal Mg_2Sn strengthening precipitate has been achieved by high-pressure aging (2 GPa, 400 °C) method. The particle is ellipsoid shaped with an average diameter of 25 nm. Differing from the conventional coarse plate-like or rod-like Mg_2Sn strengthening particles with fcc structure after artificial aging at ~200 °C, the formation of the fine hexagonal Mg_2Sn particles significantly improves the strength of Mg–Sn alloys together with the ductility. The high strength and ductility are mainly associated with the presence of fine strengthening precipitates and the low lattice misfit (0.025) of hexagon-on-hexagon crystallographic orientation, respectively. As the melting point of the precipitate of Mg_2Sn in Mg–Sn alloy (770.5 °C) is much higher than the melting point of the typical precipitate of $Mg_{17}Al_{12}$ in Mg–Al alloy (462 °C), Mg–Sn alloys have attracted much attention, in particular for the high-temperature applications. The precipitate also exhibits excellent oxidation resistance; Chen et al. [299] mentioned that Mg–5Sn (wt%) alloy processed by ECAE showed improved wear resistance due to the grain size refinement and the precipitate of the second phase, Mg_2Sn. Although Mg–Sn binary alloys can be precipitation hardened, their age-hardening response is moderate. Hence, Liu et al. [300] alloyed Mg–Sn alloy with Zn to improve the age-hardening response by refining the distribution of Mg_2Sn precipitates and investigated Mg_2Sn precipitates with different morphologies and orientations in under-, peak- and over-aged samples of a Mg–9.8Sn–1.2Zn (wt%) alloy. It was mentioned that Zn atoms always segregate to the precipitate–matrix interface, irrespective of the interfacial structures and orientation relationships of the Mg_2Sn precipitates. Chen et al. [301] investigated the effects of Y addition on the microstructure and mechanical properties of the as-cast Mg–5Sn–3Zn. It was reported that (i) the addition of Y to Mg–5Sn–3Zn not only refines the grains but also promotes the precipitation of MgSnY phase with high stability; (ii) an increase in the addition of Y from 0.2 to 0.8 wt% increases the amount and size of MgSnY, which would influence the mechanical properties of the as-cast alloys; (iii) the precipitate $MgZn_2$ phase tends to attach to the Mg_2Sn phase because the mismatch degree between them is relatively low, which have some guiding role in increasing the amount of $MgZn_2$ by Sn addition to enhance the performance of Mg–Sn–Zn alloys; (iv) Y to the Mg-5Sn-3Zn alloy generally improves the mechanical properties, but overdose of Y would make it decrease, especially the elongation, which is affected by the grains and precipitates, improved significantly; and (v) the addition of 0.5 wt% Y gives the alloy favorable properties that the ultimate tensile strength reaches to 229 MPa and the elongation peaks at 19.2% at room temperature. Zhang et al. [302] studied the microstructures of a Mg–Sn-based alloy with trace additions of Mn and Si after various aging heat treatments. It was found that the alloy was found to contain mostly $Mg_2Sn(\beta)$ precipitates, which exhibit three shapes: lath, polygon and plate. Huang et al. [303] added Cu and Al to Mg–6Sn–1Mn alloy to study the hardening effect. It was reported that (i) a eutectic structure consists of strong intermetallic phases, that is, Mg_2Cu in the Mg-6Sn-1Mn-2Cu alloy and $Al_{0.93}Cu_{1.07}Mg$ in the Mg-6Sn-1Mn-2Cu-2Al alloy remains stable along the grain boundaries after solution and aging heat treatments; (ii) the precipitate density has been increased significantly and the precipitate size has been refined remarkably during aging at 200 ° C; and (iii) the growth of the precipitates is inhibited remarkably during the over-aging period, indicating that the age-hardening response and over-aging resistance are notably improved.

8.8.7 Mg–Y-based alloys

Precipitation process and microstructures of both Mg–5%Y and Mg–10%Y (mass%) alloys were investigated [304]. It was mentioned that (i) the hardness of Mg–5Y increased slightly by about HV 10 with aging time at temperatures between 150 and 250 °C; (ii) in a Mg–10Y alloy the hardness increased markedly after certain incubation periods for 38.7 ks at aging temperatures between 150 and 225 °C; (iii) the time–temperature–transformation diagram for the precipitation of the β″-phase was determined from the hardness curves of a Mg–10%Y alloy and the nose temperature was 225 °C; (iv) the hardness increase in a Mg–10%Y alloy at 150–225 °C was found to be caused by the homogeneous precipitation of the fine coherent metastable β″-phase; (v) the metastable β′- and stable β-phases precipitated and coarsened in a Mg–10%Y alloy at 250–300 °C; (vi) both the β″- and β′-phases were found to have a base-centered orthorhombic structure; and (vii) the atom configurations in their unit cells, however, were assumed to be different from each other in the β″- and β′-phases because of the existence of weak reflection spots at the forbidden positions. Zhao et al. [305] studied the precipitation behavior of Mg–10Y (wt%) and reported that (i) a Mg–10 wt% Y alloy exhibited age-hardening response by both artificial aging at 220°C (T6) and superhigh-pressure aging (6 GPa) at 300 °C (SHP-300); (ii) a spherical strengthening precipitate ($Mg_{24}Y_5$) was achieved after SHP-300 heat treatment, which was different from conventional plate-shaped strengthening precipitate (β′) after T6 treatment; (iii) compared with the T6 state sample, the peak hardness, strength and ductility were improved by means of SHP-300 treatment and the improved hardness and strength were associated with the nanoscale precipitate ($Mg_{24}Y_5$) and strain hardening; and (iv) the large elongation was ascribed to the formation of spherical precipitate, which can effectively reduce the stress concentration during the deformation process.

It is known that Mg–RE alloys exhibit excellent age-hardening property due to higher solubility for Mg matrix [306], the precipitation sequence in Mg–RE alloys is as S.S.S.S. → β″ → β′ → β [291–293] and stable β-phase in Mg–Sc alloy [307]. Hiragi et al. [308], using three Mg–RE alloys (Mg–Y, Mg–Sc, Mg–Y–Sc) containing the same total amount of solute elements, investigated the effect of Sc on age hardening and precipitation and metastable phase (i.e., GP zones, β″, β′) under high-resolution transmission electron microscopy (HRTEM), selected area electron diffraction

(SAED) technique. It was reported that (i) in HRTEM observation, zig-zag structure and pre-β″ were observed, and both precipitates were confirmed in SAED pattern as diffuse spot in the early stage of aging, (ii) in peak-aged and over-aged conditions, β′-phase was observed in Mg–Y and Mg–Y–Sc alloys and (iii) in the case of Mg–Y–Sc alloy, β′ showed different lattice parameter with close inspection of SAED pattern and HRTEM images. Fu et al. [309] studied the strengthening behavior of Mg–Y–B alloy and reported that (i) the formation of nanoscale YB_{12} particles (~9 nm) with a high melting point improves the strength of the Mg–Y alloy significantly and this is coupled with its thermal stability and (ii) the age-hardening response is weakened because of the decrease in yttrium supersaturation in the Mg matrix. Barucca et al. [310] investigated the formation and evolution of hardening precipitates in a Mg–Y–Nd (WE43) alloy during artificial aging at 150 and 210 °C. It was mentioned that (i) the β″-phase was identified by the small-angle X-ray scattering measurements and (ii) transmission electron microscopy and microhardness results indicate that the hardening mechanism is based on β″ transformation of pre-precipitates and their growth at 150 °C, while at 210 °C hardening is mainly associated with β″ → β′ transformation. Although wrought Mg alloys, especially precipitation-hardened RE alloys, have promising potential for structural applications, wrought Mg alloys usually possess deformation texture leading to strong mechanical anisotropy, providing an obstacle to the application of wrought Mg alloys. Xin et al. [311] investigated the effect of aging precipitation on extruded Mg–Y–Nd alloy. It was reported that (i) the extruded alloy presented a weak basal fiber texture and after peak aging at 210 °C for 59 h, β′ precipitates were primarily formed, (ii) the extruded alloy exhibited obvious anisotropies of yield strength and strain hardening and (iii) after precipitation of β′ precipitates the yield strength anisotropy of the peak-aged alloy was effectively reduced.

8.9 Annealing

Annealing consists of heating the alloy material at a moderate temperature to affect recrystallization, agglomerate precipitate or remove internal strains and can be applied for both heat-treatable and non–heat-treatable alloys to increase ductility with a slight reduction in strength. A typical annealing cycle for wrought magnesium alloys is to heat them to 290–455 °C for at least 1 h. Since most forming operations are done at elevated temperature, most of the wrought material is already fully annealed.

8.9.1 Mg–Al-based alloys

Table 8.14 lists typical improvements by annealing on Mg–Al-based alloys.

Table 8.14: Major improvements by annealing Mg–Al-based alloys.

	Annealing temperature (°C)	Annealing time (h)	Anisotropy	Microstructure	Ductility	Formability/plasticity	Strength	Reference
Mg–3Al–1Zn			X					[312]
	350			X	X			[313]
	RTA			X				[314]
						X		[315]
	175	6				X	X	[316]
	250			X		X		[317]
	250				X		X	[318]
	330	4				X	X	[319]
	275			X				[320]
	200	20		X				[321]
	300	4		X		X	X	[317]
	450	72				X		[322]
						X		[323]
Mg–6Al–1Zn	250/450					X		[324]
				X				[325]
	350	2				X		[326]
				X		X		[327]
					X	X		[328]
	200	12		X			X	[329]
Mg–Al–Mn	420			X				[330]
	200	1,000		X				[331]

Note: X indicates enhanced or improved; RTA indicates rapid thermal annealing.

8.9.2 Mg–Zn-based alloys

Table 8.15 lists typical improvements by annealing on Mg–Zn-based alloys.

Table 8.15: Major improvements by annealing Mg–Zn-based alloys.

	Annealing temperature (°C)	Annealing time (h)	Anisotropy	Microstructure	Ductility	Formability/Plasticity	Strength	Reference
Mg–Zn–Gd				x				[332]
Mg–0.3Zn–0.1Ca	80/200			x			x	[333]
Mg–1.5Zn–0.25Gd	200/400			x				[334]
Mg-1Zn-RE-Zr						x		[335]
Mg–4Zn–3Sn				x			x	[336]
Mg-1.5Zn-0.6Zr-Er	350/420			x				[337]

Note: X indicates enhanced or improved.

8.9.3 Other Mg-based alloy series

Table 8.16 lists typical improvements by annealing on other types of Mg-based alloys.

Table 8.16: Major improvements by annealing other Mg-based alloys.

	Annealing temperature (°C)	Annealing time (h)	Anisotropy	Microstructure	Ductility	Formability/plasticity	Strength	Reference
Mg–3Li–1Sc				x			x	[338]
Mg–5Li–1Al	300						x	[339]
Mg-5Li-3Al-2Zn-Y	220/320	12		x				[340]

Table 8.16 (continued)

	Annealing temperature (°C)	Annealing time (h)	Anisotropy	Microstructure	Ductility	Formability/plasticity	Strength	Reference
Mg–8Li–4Al				x			x	[341]
Mg-11Li-3Al-2Zn-Y				x			x	[342]
Mg–Ni–Nd	150/300			x				[343]
Mg–Mn–Ce	475/550			x				[344]
Mg–1Gd				x				[345]
Mg-Gd-Y-Zr	420	3,000		x				[346]
Mg-8Gd-4Y-1Nd-Zr	470				x		x	[347]
Mg-8.1Gd-1.8Y-Zr				x				[169]
Mg-9Gd-4Y-0.6Zr				x				[348]
Mg-10Gd-3Y-0.3Zr				x			x	[349]
Mg-11.5Gd-4.5Y-Zn				x			x	[350]
Mg–(1,5)Y	300/400			x			x	[351]
Mg–Y–Zn	500	100		x				[352]
Mg–RE–Zn	400/425			x		x		[353]
Mg–Sc				x				[354]
Mg–0.57Nd				x				[355]

Note: X indicates enhanced or improved.

8.10 Thermomechanical treatment

Thermomechanical treatment involves the simultaneous application of mechanical or severe plastic deformation process like compression, forging, rolling, drawing or extrusion and thermal processes like heat treatment, water quenching, heating and cooling at various rates in order to refine microstructure and crystallographic orientation (which is referred to grain boundary engineering), to enhance strength and ductility or improve fatigue strength as well as resistances against the tribological action (e.g., wear) and corrosion. It is known that, although Mg materials are considered for their high specific strength, the conventional mechanical processing is difficult due to their anisotropic material properties. A severe plastic deformation method called equal-channel angular pressing (ECAP) is an effective tool for producing ultra-fine-grained materials. The applied route has a strong influence on the texture, microstructure and mechanical behavior of ECAPed metals [356].

Munitz et al. [357] investigated the influence of thermomechanical treatment on the complex modulus of AZ31 alloy. It was reported that (i) the real component or storage modulus (E') in the elastic modulus ($E^* = E' + iE''$) determined for this alloy was 42.0 ± 2.5 GPa at 25 °C and it was independent of rolling direction (RD) and cold work up to 20% reduction in thickness; (ii) a broad peak was observed in the imaginary component or loss modulus (E'') around 175 °C (for a 1.0 Hz loading frequency) and it was determined that this peak is a superposition of at least four different relaxation mechanisms: a thermally activated mechanism related to precipitate phases near 153 °C and three peaks related to mechanical deformation at 165, 188 and 235 °C; (iii) the latter three peaks were also thermally activated with the activation energy determined to be 1.68 ± 0.04 eV; and (iv) these mechanical relaxation peaks are attributed to microstructural features produced by cold work, and it is demonstrated that the stresses generated by cooling from heat-treatment temperatures influence these peaks, concluding that the grain boundary relaxation peak is above 350 °C. Chang et al. [358] mentioned about the application of ECAP to Mg materials that pure Mg was susceptible to shear localization during ECAP; surface cracking occurred along the direction of shear localization at lower temperatures than 300 °C. Uniform flow occurred at 300 °C, resulting in the successful four repetitive ECAPs. The ECAP of AZ series alloys was unsuccessful at even higher temperature than 300 °C; however, the ECAP temperature of AZ series alloys hot-rolled before ECAP was lowered, and the temperature for successful ECAP decreased with decreasing Al content; in particular, the hot-rolled AZ31 alloy could be ECAPed at 220 °C. The ECAPed AZ31 alloy revealed the microstructure of dynamically recrystallized grains with a grain size in the range of 1–10 μm. The deformation during ECAP was analyzed by dislocation characteristics. Mukai et al. [359] described the possibility of drastic ductility enhancement in a commercial AZ31 alloy without refining its grain structure. It was reported that simple shear was applied by ECAE for the development of a different texture. X-ray diffraction spectra examined for the parallel and perpendicular section to the extrusion direction suggested that the fraction of basal plane was possibly similar to each other for ECAE/annealed alloy, while it was obviously different for the conventionally extruded alloy. From the tensile test it was demonstrated that the elongation to failure of the ECAE/annealed alloy exhibited ~50%, which was twice larger than for the conventionally extruded alloy. Kim et al. [360] investigated microstructure and texture development of an AZ61 Mg alloy during ECAP and correlated with the mechanical properties. It was mentioned that (i) the microstructure was effectively refined by ECAP, and the original fiber texture of the extruded AZ61 alloy was disintegrated and a new texture was gradually developed by repetitive ECAP; (ii) after eight ECAP passes, the yield stress is lower than for the as-extruded AZ61 alloy, indicating that the texture softening is dominant over the strengthening due to grain refinement; (iii) when route A was used, on the other hand, the yield stress slightly increased after eight passes; and (iv) tensile ductility increased after ECAP and the effect of ECAP on ductility is more remarkable when the initial grain size is large. Jafari et al. [361] investigated the microstructure and hardness of commercial AZ63 alloy specimens subjected to two different thermomechanical treatments: (i) after solution treated at the temperature of 380 °C for 20 h, AZ63 alloy specimens were 5% cold worked by rolling process followed by aging at the temperatures of 150 and 250 °C for 3, 9 and 25 h; (ii) the specimens were solution treated at the temperature of 380 °C for 20 h, underwent 2% cold worked and quenched in water of 0 °C. Half of the specimens were then 2% cold worked while the rest were rolled to 8% cold worked. All the specimens were then aged at the temperatures of 150 and 250 °C for 3, 9 and 25 h. It was mentioned that (i) two-step aging enhances the hardness of the specimens due to the distribution of fine β-phase ($Mg_{17}Al_{12}$) in the alloy matrix and (ii) the best hardness from the first thermomechanical treatment was produced by specimen that was preaged at 150 °C, whereas, in the second treatment, aging at 250 °C exhibited the best hardness values. It is well known that the high-cycle fatigue (HCF) performance of severe plastically deformed wrought magnesium alloys is not as good as one might expect from the significant grain size refinement. Although enhanced HCF strength after ECAP as compared to as-cast material was observed, its value was significantly lower than that after conventional extruding. Based on this background, Müller et al. [362] determined whether the relatively poor HCF strength of the ECAPed wrought magnesium alloy AZ80 is associated with the ECAP-induced unfavorable crystallographic textures. It was reported that (i) post-ECAP thermomechanical treatment was found to result in favorable texture modifications as well as in markedly improved HCF performance and (ii) the resulting combination of both ultrafine grain-sized material and beneficial crystallographic texture results in superior HCF performance not achievable by ECAP processing alone.

Thermomechanical treatment consisting of precompression and a subsequent isothermal aging was used to improve the compressive properties of extruded Mg–Zn–Ca (ZX10) alloy [363]. Isothermal aging at 150 and 200 °C was performed on as-extruded samples for various times to find peak aged conditions. To achieve a different twin volume fraction in the alloy, samples were precompressed up to 2%, 3% and 4% along the extrusion direction. Afterward, the peak-aged conditions were applied to the precompressed samples to enhance their mechanical properties. It was mentioned that (i) after 150 °C × 4 h thermomechanical treatment, deformation curves exhibit a distinctive yield plateau independently on the prestrain level, (ii) using the 200 °C × 2 h condition, the yield plateau occurs only after prestrain of 3% and (iii) higher compressive yield strength values were observed for the thermomechanically treated samples at the lower temperature. Furthermore, Dobroň et al. [364], using the same ZX10 alloy, conducted the thermomechanical treatment consisting of precompression and isothermal aging at 150 °C for 16 h in order to reduce tension–compression yield asymmetry and improve mechanical properties via strengthening mechanism. It was reported that (i) with respect to the initial texture of the alloy, precompression leads to the formation of extension twins; (ii) a solute segregation and precipitation along twin boundaries are realized during a subsequent isothermal aging; (iii) after thermomechanical treatment, a solute solution and precipitation hardening contribute to the strengthening of the alloy; and (iv) active deformation mechanisms were monitored during compression or tension using the acoustic emission technique.

Mingler et al. [365] mentioned that (i) the mechanical properties of the AM60 can be improved significantly by severe plastic deformation, (ii) the lower the temperature (down to 150 °C) of ECAP the higher is the resulting strength (up to 310 MPa), which can be ascribed to the concomitant decrease of grain size (down to 1 μm), (iii) after ECAP processing at temperatures 150–210 °C the ductility remains at about the same high level (~15%) as in the initial material, due to the presence of $Al_{12}Mg_{17}$ precipitates with a size of about 500 nm, which reduce the remaining concentration of Al in the solid solution of the matrix, (iv) differential scanning calorimetry revealed four peaks during heating runs and the most remarkable peak occurs at 390 °C in the initial sample, and at 360 °C in the material ECAPed at 150 °C and (v) transmission electron microscopy analyses showed that this peak can be associated with the dissolution of the $Al_{12}Mg_{17}$ precipitates as well as with the annealing of dislocations and possibly vacancy clusters and that ECAP has the potential to induce a shift of a phase boundary to lower temperatures because of ECAP-induced lattice defects.

Tang et al. [366] investigated the effect of thermomechanical processing on the microstructure, texture and mechanical properties of a Mg-5.5Gd-3.0Y-1.0Nd-1.0Zr (wt%) alloy. An overaging treatment before extrusion was introduced to affect the dynamic recrystallization process of the alloy. It was found that (i) a substantial amount of β-equilibrium phases with the composition of $Mg_{5.05}RE$ precipitated from the matrix during the aging process prior to extrusion; (ii) compared to the counterpart with no precipitates, the dynamic recrystallization process was promoted by the mechanism of particle-stimulated nucleation, which led to the formation of uniform fine grains and weakened texture in the extruded rod; (iii) samples with an ultimate tensile strength of 324 MPa and a good elongation of 20.5% were obtained; and (iv) the good ductility was attributed to the uniform fine grains and the modified texture. Li et al. [367] processed an as-solution-treated Mg-6Gd-1Y-0.4Zr alloy by low-temperature thermomechanical treatments, including cold tension with various strains followed by aging at 200 °C to peak hardness. It was shown that (i) the precipitation kinetics of the treated is greatly accelerated and the aging time to peak hardness is greatly decreased with increasing tensile strain and (ii) the tensile yield strength, ultimate tensile strength and elongation at room temperature of the alloy after cold tension with strain of 10% and peak aging at 200 °C are 251 MPa, 296 MPa and 8%, respectively, which are superior to the commercial heat-resistant WE54 alloy, although the latter has a higher RE element content. Zhang et al. [368] studied the microstructural evolution of a thermomechanical-treated Mg–10Gd–3Y–1Sn–0.5Zr (wt%) alloy and its effect on mechanical properties. It was reported that (i) a cuboid-shaped $Mg_2(Sn,Y)_3Gd_2$ was observed in a homogenized/hot-extruded condition; (ii) precipitations involving $Mg_5(Gd,Y)$ particles, $Mg_3(Gd,Y)$-$\beta''(DO_{19})$, $Mg_5(Gd,Y)$-β'(bco) and β_1(fcc) were identified during isothermal aging; (iii) the metastable β'-phase is the key factor for the enhancement in both the Vickers hardness and the tensile strength; and (iv) the highest ultimate tensile strength up to 352 MPa was achieved when aged at 200 °C for 100 h postextrusion. Yu et al. [369] fabricated a high-strength Mg-11Gd-4.5Y-1Nd-1.5Zn-0.5Zr (wt%) alloy via hot extrusion, cold rolling and aging treatment. It was mentioned that (i) the alloy exhibits an average 0.2% proof stress of 481.6 ± 19.9 MPa, an average ultimate tensile strength of 517.4 ± 27.5 MPa and an average elongation to failure of 2.0 ± 0.4% at room temperature, (ii) the best mechanical property obtained in the present study has the 0.2% proof stress of 502.0 MPa, the ultimate tensile strength of 546.8 MPa and an elongation to failure of 2.6%, (iii) the high strength of this alloy is attributed to the fine grains, stacking faults, LPSO phase and precipitates of Mg_5RE phase at grain boundaries and of β'-phase inside the grains, (iv) cold rolling improves the mechanical properties and enhances the age-hardening response but decreases the ductility and (v) two texture components are found simultaneously in the deformed alloy; the typical Mg–RE texture and the unusual prismatic texture.

Kumar et al. [370] studied the influence of alloying and thermomechanical processing on the microstructure and texture evolution on the two Mg–Li–Al-based alloys, namely Mg–9Li–7Al–1Sn (LAT971) and Mg-9Li-5Al-3Sn-1Zn (LATZ9531) (wt%). These Mg–Li–Al-based alloys were cast (induction melting under protective atmosphere) followed by hot rolling at ~300 °C with a cumulative reduction of five. It was reported that (i) a contrary dual-phase dendritic microstructure rich in α-Mg, instead of β-Li phase predicted by equilibrium phase diagram of Mg Li binary alloy was observed; (ii) preferential presence of Mg–Li–Sn primary precipitates (size 4–10 μm) within α-Mg phase and Mg–Li–Al secondary precipitates (<3 μm) interspersed in β-Li indicated their degree of dissolution during hot rolling and homogenization in the dual-phase matrix, (iii) presence of Al, Sn and Zn alloying elements in the Mg–Li-based alloy has resulted in an unusual dual-phase microstructure, change in the lattice parameter and intriguing texture evolution after hot rolling of cast LAT 971 and LATZ9531 alloy and

(iv) role of alloying in rendering distribution of dual-phase structure has strongly influenced dynamic recrystallization and grain growth in the hot-rolled Mg–Li–Al-based alloys. Ding et al. [371] investigated the effect of thermomechanical processing on the microstructure and mechanical properties of the duplex phase Mg-8Li-3Al-0.4Y alloy. It was found that (i) the as-cast alloy was composed of α-Mg, β-Li, AlLi, Al_2Y and $MgAlLi_2$ phases; (ii) annealing of the cold-rolled alloy at 350 °C for 60 min was considered to be optimum, due to full static recrystallization and spheroidization; (iii) a significant β-Li loss occurred when the annealing time was increased to 90 min; (iv) the optimized annealing treatment produced the following values of the yield strength, ultimate strength and elongation: 148 MPa, 184 MPa and 35%, respectively; and (v) the texture evolution of the α-phase and the β-phase changed remarkably during thermomechanical processing.

The microstructure and mechanical properties of an as-cast Mg–4.0Sm–1.0Ca alloy were investigated during thermome chanical treatments consisting of hot extrusion, rolling and aging at 200 °C [372]. It was reported that (i) $Mg_{41}Sm_5$ phases containing Ca and needle-like Mg_2Ca phases formed in the Mg matrix, and the average grain size and elongation were 4.2 μm and 27%, respectively, after hot extrusion, which implied an increase in ductility, (ii) after the rolling, the grain size was further refined, and the tensile strength increased to 293 MPa and (iii) a new precipitate Mg_3Sm was found in the peak-aged Mg–4.0Sm–1.0Ca alloy that displayed the best mechanical properties, with a peak hardness of 83 HV and ultimate tensile strength of 313 MPa; these properties being attributed to grain refinement strengthening, solid solution strengthening, work hardening and precipitation strengthening [372].

8.11 Strengthening

We have been discussing strengthening or hardening via thermal routes (various heat treatments, including quenching, solid-solution treatment, precipitation and aging) and thermomechanical way (such as ECAP process). There are still practically important methods to enhance mechanical properties of Mg-based alloys. In this section, grain boundary and/or texture strengthening based on dislocation engineering and strain hardening will be reviewed.

8.11.1 Grain boundary strengthening

Wang et al. [373] prepared Mg–2Al–0.5Mn alloys with 0–0.5% Zn and 0.5–1.0% La–Ce-misch metal (MM) by metal mold casting method to investigate the effect of alloying elements Zn and MM on microstructures. It was reported that (i) Zn and MM additions led to an obvious grain refinement, (ii) addition of 0.5% Zn resulted in about 30% reduction in grain size for Mg–2Al–0.5Mn alloys, while 0.5% MM addition caused about 40% reduction in grain size, (iii) the tensile properties of the as-cast alloys were tested at room temperature, (iv) Mg–2Al–0.5Mn–0.5Zn–1 MM alloy exhibited the best mechanical properties and (v) improvement of mechanical properties was attributed to the grain-refining effect and the formation of $Al_{11}MM_3$ phase, which could inhibit dislocation movement and grain-boundary sliding during deformation. Hu et al. [374] modified the commercially used Mg–3Al–1Si (AS31) alloy with B and Sn and subjected to hot rolling. It was found that (i) for the as-cast alloys, single addition of B or Sn refined the grains of AS31 alloy, (ii) the B addition could modify the network-shaped Mg_2Si phase into fine particles while the modification effect of Sn was not obvious, (iii) simultaneous addition of B and Sn resulted in large grains and coarse Mg_2Si phase in the as-cast alloy, (iv) the as-cast AS31–2Sn alloy showed the highest tensile strength of 231 MPa and ductility of 19.5%, (v) for the hot-rolled alloys, B or Sn addition distinctly refined the grains of AS31 sheet, while their combination severely retarded dynamic recrystallization, leading to much unrecrystallized structure, (vi) the AS31–2Sn sheet exhibited the best yield strength of ~260 MPa with desirable ductility of ~15% and (vii) such desirable strength can be attributed to solid solution strengthening, grain boundary strengthening, texture strengthening and dislocation strengthening. Go et al. [375] fabricated a new Mg alloy with the composition of Mg-8Al-0.3Zn-0.1Mn-0.3Ca-0.2Y by a low-temperature, low-speed indirect extrusion process. It was reported that the extruded alloy showed excellent mechanical properties, that is, a tensile yield strength of 379.3 MPa, ultimate tensile strength of 421.7 MPa, elongation of 11.3%, and yield asymmetry of 0.95, as well as a very high chip ignition temperature of 820 °C, mainly being attributed to the microstructural characteristics of the extruded alloy, that is, (a) grain boundary strengthening by fine recrystallized grains, (b) precipitation hardening by abundant fine $Mg_{17}Al_{12}$ precipitates, and (c) strain hardening by the deformed nonrecrystallized region with a strong basal texture that is unfavorable for basal slip during tension.

Effects of samarium (Sm) content (0, 2.0, 3.5, 5.0, 6.5 wt%) on microstructure and mechanical properties of Mg–0.5Zn–0.5 Zr alloy under as-cast and as-extruded states were investigated [376]. It was indicated that (i) grains of the as-cast alloys are gradually refined as Sm content increases, (ii) the dominant intermetallic phase changes from Mg_3Sm to $Mg_{41}Sm_5$ till Sm content exceeds 5.0 wt%, (iii) the dynamically precipitated intermetallic phase during hot-extrusion in all Sm-containing alloys is Mg_3Sm, (iv) the intermetallic particles induced by Sm addition could act as heterogeneous nucleation sites for dynamic recrystallization during hot extrusion; promoting dynamic recrystallization via the particle stimulated nucleation mechanism, and resulting in weakening the basal texture in the as-extruded alloys, (v) Sm addition can significantly enhance the strength of the as-extruded Mg–0.5Zn–0.5 Zr alloy at room temperature, with the optimal dosage of 3.5 wt%, (vi) the optimal yield strength and ultimate tensile strength are 368 MPa and 383 MPa, which were enhanced by approximately 23.1% and 20.8% compared with the Sm-free alloy, respectively and (vii) based on microstructural analysis, the dominant strengthening mechanisms are revealed to be grain boundary strengthening and dispersion strengthening [376]. Cai et al. [377] fabricated binary Mg–Zn alloys with high-purity raw materials and by a clean melting process to study the effects of Zn on the microstructure, mechanical property and corrosion behavior of the as-cast Mg–Zn alloys. It was found that (i) the microstructure of Mg–Zn alloys typically consists of primary α-Mg matrix and MgZn intermetallic phase mainly distributed along grain boundary and (ii) the improvement in mechanical performances for Mg–Zn alloys with Zn content until 5% of weight is corresponding to fine grain strengthening, solid solution strengthening and second phase strengthening. Du et al. [378] investigated aging treatment on dynamic recrystallization and texture in Mg–6Zn alloy (wt%). It was mentioned that (i) aging treatment prohibited dynamic recrystallization during deformation, which was because the precipitates inhibited dislocation movement and restricted the formation of deformation bands, (ii) the dynamic recrystallized region and deformed region both contained typical basal texture with basal planes oriented perpendicular compression direction, but the recrystallized region showed a much weaker texture and (iii) the peak-aged alloy containing rod-shaped precipitates exhibited stronger texture intensity after dynamic recrystallization compared with the as-solutionized alloy, which was because the precipitates in the peak-aged alloy inhibited the lattice rotation of the newly formed dynamic recrystallized grains or affected the microstructural evolution. Guan et al. [379] studied effects of samarium (Sm) addition on microstructures and tensile properties of Mg–6.0Zn–0.5Zr (ZK60) alloy under both as-cast and as-extruded states. It was indicated that (i) similar to some other RE additions, the grains of the as-cast ZK60 alloy were refined and the dominant intermetallic phase was changed from $MgZn_2$ to $Mg_3Sm_2Zn_3$ (W) phase by Sm addition, (ii) after extrusion, the ZK60 sample with Sm addition owns much finer dynamic recrystallization (DRX) grains due to the widely spaced large particles and the fine particles on DRX grain boundaries, (iii) some other intermetallic phases were examined in the as-extruded samples such as Mg_4Zn_7 and Mg_7Zn_3 in ZK60 sample, $Mg_{22}Zn_{64}Sm_{14}$ (Z) and $Mg_{21}Zn_{62}Sm_{17}$ (W′) in ZK60 + Sm sample, (iv) Sm addition results in much finer, much more and more stable spherical nanoscale precipitates in matrix and (v) Sm addition further improves the strength of ZK60 alloy, with the dominant strengthening mechanisms being revealed as both fine grain strengthening and precipitation strengthening.

The microstructure, texture and mechanical properties of as-extruded Mg–*x*Li–3Al–2Zn–0.2Zr alloys (x = 5, 7, 8, 9, 11 wt%) were investigated [380]. It was mentioned that (i) after hot extrusion, the filamentous AlLi phase in α-Mg is crushed into tiny particles, while the morphology of round-like AlLi phase in β-Li remains unchanged, (ii) the thread-like $MgLi_2Al$ phase precipitated during hot extrusion only distributes along the grain boundaries of β-Li phase, (iii) the grains of as-extruded alloys are refined markedly due to dynamic recrystallization (DRX), and α-Mg phase undergoes discontinuous DRX while β-Li phase undergoes continuous DRX and (iv) compared with as-homogenized alloys, the mechanical properties of as-extruded alloys are significantly improved owing to grain refinement strengthening, texture hardening, strain hardening and second phase strengthening. Nene et al. [381] hot-rolled Mg–4Li–1Ca (LC41) alloy at 300 °C, which resulted in the refinement of the grain size from 100 to 5 µm by recrystallization in the presence of fine uniformly dispersed eutectic (α-Mg + Mg_2Ca). Evidence of profuse deformation twinning in the microstructure suggested twinning to be the important mode of deformation in the present material. It was further mentioned that room-temperature tensile tests of the alloy at a strain rate of 10^{-4}/s exhibited substantially high specific strength of 142 kN m/kg owing to its low density and combined effect of grain boundary strengthening and dispersion strengthening in the presence of Mg_2Ca phase. Sun et al. [382] studied the effects of combined addition of Sn and Y on the microstructure, texture, and mechanical properties of as-extruded Mg–5Li–3Al–2Zn alloy. It was reported that (i) the microstructure of as-extruded Mg–5Li–3Al–2Zn alloy mainly consists of α-Mg and AlLi phases, (ii) with the addition of Sn and Y, Mg_2Sn and Al_2Y compounds form, while AlLi phase gradually disappears with increasing Y content, (iii) the addition of Sn and Y weakens the basal texture of as-extruded alloy and introduces recrystallization texture due to solute drag effect and dynamic recrystallization, (iv) as-extruded Mg–5Li–3Al–2Zn–0.8Sn–1.2Y alloy exhibits a superior combination of tensile properties with ultimate tensile strength and elongation of 328.0 MPa and 25.1%, which are increased by approximately 32.2% and 41.0% compared with those of as-extruded Mg–5Li–3Al–2Zn alloy (248.2 MPa and 17.8%), respectively; being attributed to solution, dispersion and grain refinement strengthening.

8.11.2 Strain hardening

Kim et al. [383] proposed two thermomechanical processing methods involving severe plastic deformation (SPD) for the development of a novel microstructure having nanosized $Mg_{17}Al_{12}$ (β) particles distributed within the interiors of ultrafine grains in Mg–Al-based alloys. It was mentioned that (i) the first method involves deformation-induced breakup of the β-phase during SPD, while the second method involves low-temperature dynamic precipitation during SPD followed by low-temperature aging and (ii) the resulting processed materials exhibited very high yield strengths of over 380 MPa and distinct strain-hardening properties. Ning et al. [384] employed surface mechanical attrition treatment (SMAT) to produce gradient structures in AZ31B Mg alloy samples with two different initial textures. It was mentioned that (i) the structure of both samples can be regarded as an integration of two main layers: the severely deformed layer exhibited dramatic grain refinement to nano- and submicron scale with weakened and randomized textures; the less deformed layer exhibited the inherited coarse grains with increased dislocation density, possessing the similar texture with the sample prior to SMAT, (ii) all the samples containing different layer constituents cut from the SMAT alloys showed remarkable increase of strength compared to the original Mg alloy; however, the two integral SMAT samples with different initial textures exhibited marked difference in uniform elongation during tension, being attributed to the different strain-hardening behaviors influenced by the deformation coordination and strain partitioning between layers with different orientation relationships, (iii) the 0° oriented SMAT sample showed no macroscopic strain transfer or slip transmission across layers, which was hard to cause dislocation accumulation throughout the whole thickness of the layered sample, resulting in a limited strain hardening and uniform elongation; however, the favored orientation relationship between layers of the 45° oriented SMAT sample facilitated the strain transfer and slip continuity across the layers, causing a generation of a dynamically migrating interface during tension, which allowed the dislocations accumulating over the whole sample volume and a pronounced strain hardening and sustained uniform elongation to an appreciable value. Meng et al. [385] studied the deformation behavior of AZ31 Mg alloy with surface mechanical attrition treatment (SMAT). It was reported that (i) a gradient nanostructure could be formed in sample by SMAT, in which the grain size increased gradually from surface to matrix, (ii) a depth-dependent gradient microhardness was also formed due to the corresponding gradient microstructure, (iii) yield strength and ultimate tensile strength of AZ31 Mg alloy with SMAT were significantly improved combining with decrease of fracture elongation and (iv) the plastic anisotropy of the sample increased significantly after SMAT, which was related to the texture variation of rolled sheet and special deformation behavior of gradient nanostructure.

Zhang et al. [386] reported a new single-phase solid solution as-cast Mg–1Zn–0.4Zr–0.2Yb alloy that possesses excellent ductility and strong work-hardening effect ($n = 0.38$) at room temperature. It was further mentioned that (i) the low stacking fault energy in Mg–1Zn–0.4Zr–0.2Yb alloy might be due to the addition of trace Yb, and the low stacking fault energy is conducive to improving the activity of basal dislocation slip, activations of nonbasal dislocations slips and the formation of deformation twins during tensile deformation, eventually leading to the development of the ductility in Mg–1Zn–0.4Zr–0.2Yb alloy, (ii) the strong work-hardening effect of Mg–1Zn–0.4Zr–0.2Yb alloy is due to the formation of stacking faults and deformation twins induced by low SFE, which can remarkably store dislocations, restrict dislocation motions and result in multiplication and storage of dislocations at twin boundaries. Shou et al. [387] investigated the influence of crystallographic texture on deformation mechanism and work-hardening behavior of the Mg–2Zn–0.1Ca alloy sheet via quasi-in-situ slip traces analysis. It was indicated that (i) the sheet displayed a weakened transverse direction (TD) spread texture. The RD sample exhibited the highest yield strength (104.3 MPa), while the TD samples exhibit the lowest (68.6 MPa), implying a high dependency of yield strength on texture, (ii) a deformation mechanism transition were observed in the RD, 45° and TD samples, that is, basal slip ($\varepsilon = 0.5\%$) → basal slip + nonbasal slip ($\varepsilon = 1.5\%$) → basal slip + nonbasal slip + twinning ($\varepsilon = 7.5\%$), and nonbasal slip was activated to accommodate the imposed deformation due to the increment in an applied shear stress for basal slip with deformation processing, (iii) additionally, the anisotropy of deformation modes is pronounced. At $\varepsilon = 0.5\%$, basal slip primarily operated in the grains with high Schmid factor (SF ≥ 0.35) in TD sample, while in the RD sample, the SFs for basal slip exhibited a wider distribution and prismatic slip also operated, (iv) as strain reached to 7.5%, twinning played more important role in the TD sample than the 45° and RD samples, (v) the texture has a substantial influence on work-hardening behavior. At $\varepsilon = 1.5\%$, work-hardening rate was governed by SF distribution for basal slip and (vi) the sample with more grains exhibiting low SF for basal slip shows higher work-hardening rate; however, twinning plays an important role in effecting work-hardening rate at $\varepsilon = 7.5\%$, and consequently the TD sample with the greatest area fraction of twin has the highest work-hardening rate. Zhao et al. [388] studied the influence of Zn on the strain hardening of as-extruded Mg–*x*Zn ($x = 1$, 2, 3 and 4 wt%) magnesium alloys using uniaxial tensile tests at $10^{-3}\ s^{-1}$ at room temperature. It was mentioned that (i) there were almost no second phases in the as-extruded Mg–Zn magnesium alloys, (ii) average grain sizes of the four as-extruded alloys were about 17.8 µm, (iii) with increasing Zn content from 1 to 4 wt%, the strain-hardening rate increased from 2,850 to 6,810 MPa at $(\sigma - \sigma_{0.2}) = 60$ MPa, the strain-hardening exponent n increased from 0.160 to 0.203, and the hardening capacity, Hc increased from 1.17 to 2.34 and (iv) the difference in strain-hardening response of these Mg–Zn alloys might be mainly caused by weaker basal texture and more solute atoms in the α-Mg matrix with higher Zn content. Tahreen et al. [389] identified the effect of Y addition on the phase development and strain-hardening behavior of an extruded Mg–Zn–Mn (ZM31) alloy. It was mentioned that (i) the addition of a small amount (0.3 wt %) of Y in the alloy led to the formation of icosahedral quasicrystalline I (Mg_3YZn_6) phase, (ii) both I-phase and W-phase ($Mg_3Y_2Zn_3$) were present in the extruded ZM31 + 3.2Y alloy, while LPSO X-phase ($Mg_{12}YZn$) and $Mg_{24}Y_5$ were observed in the extruded ZM31 + 6Y alloy, (iii) the Y addition significantly refined grains in the extruded state, (iv) the presence of I-phase in the extruded ZM31 + 0.3Y alloy increased hardness, compressive yield strength, and stage B strain-hardening rate, (v) the extruded ZM31 + 3.2Y alloy exhibited a lower hardness and stage B hardening rate due to the formation of W-phase, (vi) both extruded ZM31 + 0.3Y and ZM31 + 3.2Y alloys showed a yield point phenomenon with an initial negative strain-hardening rate, (vii) the extruded ZM31 + 6Y alloy had a high hardness and compressive yield strength without stage B hardening, suggesting a change of major deformation mode from twinning to slip mainly due to the role of LPSO X-phase and (viii) after solution treatment and aging, the hardness and compressive yield strength gradually increased with increasing Y content, while the strain-hardening exponent and the extent of stage B strain hardening decreased due to the dissolution of I- and W-phases and the presence of LPSO X-phase. Chen et al. [390] investigated strain-hardening behaviors of extruded ZK60 Mg alloy under different heat treatments (T4, T5 and T6). It was found that (i) T5 and T6 treatments decrease strain hardening of extruded ZK60 alloy, and subsequently give rise to an obvious reduction in tensile uniform strain and (ii) while, as-T4-treated specimen shows the strongest strain-hardening ability among these specimens, and its hardening capacity and strain-hardening exponent are nearly twice those of as-T5- and -T6-treated specimens. Shiraishi et al. [391] evaluated the strain-hardening behavior and microstructural development of polycrystalline as-cast Mg–Zn–Y alloys with various volume fractions of the LPSO phase subjected to cyclic loading. For all alloys, cyclic loading tests with a constant strain amplitude of 0.5% for up to 100 cycles showed asymmetric cyclic-hardening behavior, namely, the absolute value of the compressive peak stress significantly increased during cyclic loading while the tensile peak stress slightly decreased. It was reported that (i) with increasing volume fraction of the LPSO phase, the stress amplitude significantly increased, (ii) cyclic loading tests after compressive preloading up to 200 or 250 MPa resulted in a significant increase in the stress amplitude, while a number of kink bands developed during preloading, (iii) for the cyclic-hardening behavior, the contribution of the increase in kinematic hardening was significant in the alloys with a higher volume fraction of the LPSO phase and (iv) transmission electron microscopy observation of the cyclically deformed $Mg_{85}Zn_6Y_9$ alloy indicated the formation of a deformation-induced band, where the crystal structure was transformed from 18R-LPSO to hcp-Mg with the exclusion of solute elements. Kwak et al. [392] investigated the effect of volume fraction and dispersion of icosahedral phase particles on the strength and work hardening of Mg–Zn–Y alloys. It was found that (i) the cast microstructure of a Mg–13Zn–1.55Y alloy (ZW132) with a high volume fraction of I-phase (7.4%) was refined considerably by severe plastic deformation via high-ratio differential speed rolling (HRDSR), (ii) ultrafine grains (0.7–1.3 μm) with high angle boundary fractions of 0.48–0.50 were obtained after HRDSR with speed ratios of 2 or 3, (iii) the alloy processed at a speed ratio of 3 exhibited high strength and high ductility, with a yield stress of 332 MPa and a tensile elongation of 16.3% and (iv) the ductility of the rolled ZW132 alloy was controlled by the work-hardening rate, which increased as the amount of I-phase, the degree of refinement of the eutectic I-phase pockets, the degree of dispersion of the broken I-phase particles over the matrix, and the size of the resultant grains increased.

Huo et al. [393] treated the Mg–0.6at%Y alloy having an average grain size of 180 μm and random texture to cyclic tensile tests at room temperature. Tensile tests were performed at a strain rate of 1×10^{-3}/s for 10 cycles with the peak stress of 40, 70, and 100 MPa with reference to the 0.2% proof stress of 68 MPa. It was mentioned that (i) hysteresis loops and cyclic strain hardening were observed in all peak stress cases, (ii) the observation of slip traces and twin types suggested that the hysteresis behavior was due to synchronous movement of basal slip and anomalous $\{10\bar{1}2\}$ twinning, and that the cyclic strain hardening was due to nonbasal slip and (iii) prismatic slip led to cyclic strain hardening when peak stress was below the proof stress, and both prismatic and pyramidal slip promoted larger cyclic strain hardening when peak stress was increased over the proof stress. Kula et al [394], studied the flow stress and work-hardening behavior of Mg–Y binary alloys under uniaxial tension and compression at 4, 78 and 298 K. It was reported that (i) electron microscopy observations show that yttrium forms multiatomic clusters distributed randomly in Mg matrix, (ii) during thermomechanical processing, Y accumulates at the grain boundaries and controls recrystallization texture, which acquires lower intensity of the basal component and higher degree of randomness in comparison to polycrystalline Mg, (iii) tensile and compressive yield stress of the alloys is temperature dependent and decreases as temperature increases from 4 to 298 K (25 °C), (iii) the grain size and solution strengthening contributions to the yield stress have been analyzed for all alloys and deformation temperatures, (iv) critical resolved shear stress of individual deformation modes has been obtained from the modelling of the flow stress, indicating that Y strengthens most the <c + a> slip system, followed by pyramidal I, prismatic, twinning and basal systems. All slip systems exhibit monotonic increase of critical resolved shear stress with Y concentration, but at different rates and (v) analysis of the solution strengthening component of the yield stress suggests that it is determined by activity of the basal slip participating in yielding. Yang et al. [395] investigated the effects of secondary phases (W, $Mg_3Y_2Zn_3$), long-period stacking-ordered (LPSO, $Mg_{12}ZnY$) and icosahedral (I, Mg_3YZn_6) phases on the tensile properties and work-hardening behavior of Mg–Y–Zn alloys (Mg–1.32Zn–1.79Y, ZW12; Mg–4.4Zn–2.2Y, ZW42; and Mg–5.2Zn–1.1Y, ZW51) prepared after application of differential speed rolling on their cast microstructures at room temperature. It was reported that (i) the volume fractions of LPSO, W- and I-phase in ZW12, ZW42 and ZW51 were 4.7%, 6.3% and 4.8%, respectively; (ii) the rolled alloys exhibited a similar level of yield strength but different work-hardening characteristics and tensile fracture behavior; (iii) the rolled ZW51 with I-phase particles exhibited the highest work-hardening rate and the largest tensile elongation (with ductile fracture); (iv) the ZW42 with W-phase particles exhibited a work-hardening rate slightly lower than that of the rolled ZW51, despite having the larger amount of secondary phase, and premature fracture occurred far before neck formation in ZW42, while fracture took place after neck formation in ZW51; (v) the rolled ZW12 with LPSO phase, forming a coherent interface with the Mg matrix phase, exhibited a considerably lower work-hardening rate than the rolled ZW51, though they had the similar amounts of secondary phase; thus, the uniform strain of the rolled ZW12 was quite small compared with that of the rolled ZW51, though fracture occurred after necking in both alloys; and (vi) the same work-hardening and tensile elongation behaviors were retained after annealing treatment on the rolled alloys.

Zheng et al. [396] investigated the remarkably enhanced mechanical performance of Mg–8Gd–1Er–0.5Zr alloy with lower RE content, which was achieved on the route of extrusion, rolling and aging processes. It was indicated that (i) the ultrahigh ultimate tensile strength of 560 MPa and YTS of 518 MPa as well as elongation of 4.8% at ambient temperature were obtained, (ii) the β-phase with size of 100–200 nm was precipitated during rolling in accompany with refined grains and strong basal texture, and the layer-structured precipitates with nanoscale were formed during aging and (iii) the fine β-phase coordinating with strong basal texture as well as fine grain size controlled the mechanical performance of the rolled alloy, whereas the layer-structured precipitates contributed to the remarkably enhanced mechanical properties of the aged alloy. Peng et al. [397] studied effect of heat treatment and extrusion temperature on the properties of the recycled Mg–10Gd–2Y–0.5Zr, It was mentioned that (i) the aging response in the recycled specimens is similar to that in as-extruded reference samples, (ii) the deformation temperature is increased in order to inhibit $Mg_{24}(Gd,Y)_5$ particles precipitation and realize interfacial bonding between chips, (iii) after peak-aged treatment at 225 °C, the GW102K alloy consolidated at 450 °C exhibits excellent tensile strength and (iv) it is feasible to obtain the desired tensile properties of the recycled alloys by simultaneously promoting the precipitation of the metastable RE-containing phases and retaining the work-hardening effect during heat treatment.

Liao et al. [398] investigated the effect of Mn addition on the microstructure, mechanical properties and work-hardening behavior of Mg–1Sn (wt%) alloys. It was found that (i) the as-extruded alloys are mainly composed of α-Mg and Mn precipitates, which exist in TM11 and TM12, (ii) the average grain size sharply decreases with Mn addition, (iii) with increase in Mn content, the basal texture of the alloys has strengthened, (iv) Mn addition significantly increases the tensile and compressive yield strengths, ultimate tensile strengths and elongation of the as-extruded Mg–Sn–Mn alloys because of the good microstructures, (v) the decrease in the number of tensile twins in compress leads to the yield asymmetry reduces with Mn addition and (vi) with increasing Mn content, the value of work-hardening exponent and capacity decreases, the work-hardening behavior in stage III significantly improved. Zhao et al. [399] studied the effects of Sn content on strain-hardening behavior of as-extruded Mg–xSn (x = 1.3, 2.4, 3.6 and 4.7 wt%) binary alloys by uniaxial tensile tests at room temperature. Strain-hardening rate, strain-hardening exponent and hardening capacity were obtained from the true plastic stress-strain curves. It was indicated that (i) after hot extrusion, the as-extruded Mg–Sn alloys are mainly composed of α-Mg matrix and second phase Mg_2Sn, which only exists in Mg–3Sn and Mg–4Sn; (ii) average grain size decreases from 15.6 to 3.6 μm with Sn content increasing from 1.3 to 4.7 wt%; (iii) Sn content decreases strain-hardening ability of as-extruded Mg–Sn alloys, but gives rise to an obvious elevation in tensile strength, yield strength and elongation of them; (iv) with increasing Sn content, strain-hardening rate decreases from 3,527 to 1,211 MPa at $(\sigma - \sigma_{0.2}) = 50$ MPa, strain-hardening exponent decreases from 0.21 to 0.13 and hardening capacity decreases from 1.66 to 0.63; and (v) the variation in strain-hardening behavior of Mg–Sn alloys with Sn content is discussed in terms of the influences of grain size and distribution of grain orientation. Jiang et al. [400] investigated strain-hardening and warm deformation behaviors of extruded Mg–2Sn–0.5Yb alloy (at%) sheet in uniaxial tensile test at temperatures of 25–250 °C and strain rates of 1×10^{-3}/s to 0.1/s. It was reported that (i) besides III-stage and IV-stage, the absence of the II-stage strain hardening at room temperature should be related to the sufficient dynamic recrystallization during extrusion; (ii) the decrease of strain-hardening ability of the alloy after yielding was attributed to the reduction of dislocation density with increasing testing temperature; (iii) strain rate sensitivity was significantly enhanced with increasing temperature, and the corresponding m-value was calculated as 0.07–0.12, which indicated that the deformation mechanism was dominated by the climb-controlled dislocation creep at 200 °C; (iv) the grain boundary sliding was activated at 250 °C, which contributed to the higher strain rate sensitivity; and (v) the activation energy was calculated as 213.67 kJ/mol, which was higher than that of lattice diffusion or grain boundary self-diffusion. Nonflammability and high production rate are prerequisites for extending application of Mg extrusion products.

References

[1] Practical Heat Treatment of Magnesium Alloys. 2006; https://www.totalmateria.com/page.aspx?ID=CheckArticle&site=ktn&NM=155.

[2] Temper Designations of Magnesium Alloys, Cast and Wrought. 2002; https://www.totalmateria.com/page.aspx?ID=CheckArticle&site=ktn&NM=34

[3] Kopeliovich D. Classification of magnesium alloys. 2012; https://www.substech.com/dokuwiki/doku.php?id=classification_of_magnesium_alloys.

[4] Sillekens WH, Hort N. Magnesium and Magnesium Alloys. In: Lehmhus et al., ed., Structural Materials and Processes in Transportation, 2013, Wiley-VCH; DOI: 10.1002/9783527649846.ch3.

[5] Introduction to Magnesium Alloys. In: Moosbrugger C, ed., Engineering Properties of Magnesium Alloys, 2017 ASM International; https://www.asminternational.org/documents/10192/22833166/05920G_SampleChapter.pdf/d1a641ad-e4e8-789d-c565-c9c690c1931e.

[6] Magnesium Alloys and Temper Designations. 2001; https://www.totalmateria.com/page.aspx?ID=CheckArticle&site=ktn&NM=4.

[7] Chowdary VS et al. Influence of heat treatment on the machinability and corrosion behavior of AZ91 Mg alloy. Journal of Magnesium and Alloys. 2018, 6, 52–8.

[8] Chai S et al. Effect of partial rolling and heat treatment on the microstructure and mechanical properties of AZ80 Mg joint. Materials Science and Engineering: A. 2015, 646, 66–74.

[9] Zindal A et al. Effect of heat treatment variables on the formation of precipitate free zones (PFZs) in Mg-8Al-0.5Zn Alloy. Materials Characterization. 2018, 136, 175–82.

[10] Mingbo Y et al, Effect of semi-solid isothermal heat treatment on the microstructure of Mg–6A1–1Zn–0.7Si alloy. Journal of Materials Processing Technology. 2008, 206, 374–81.

[11] Liu C et al. Heat-treatable Mg-9Al-6Sn-3Zn extrusion alloy. Journal of Materials Science & Technology. 2018, 34, 284–90.

[12] Mengucci P et al. Structure evolution of a WE43 Mg alloy submitted to different thermal treatments. Materials Science and Engineering: A. 2008, 479, 37–44.

[13] Xu L et al. Effects of heat treatments on microstructures and mechanical properties of Mg–4Y–2.5Nd–0.7Zr alloy. Materials Science and Engineering: A. 2012, 558, 1–6.

[14] Liu K et al. The effect of heat treatment on microstructure of the melt-spun Mg–7Y–4Gd–5Zn–0.4Zr alloy. Journal of Magnesium and Alloys. 2016, 4, 99–103.

[15] Wang Q-D et al. Characterization of phases in Mg-10Y-5Gd-2Zn-0.5Zr alloy processed by heat treatment. Transactions of Nonferrous Metals Society of China. 2010, 20, 2076–80.

[16] Li D et al. Characterization of phases in Mg–4Y–4Sm–0.5Zr alloy processed by heat treatment. Materials Science and Engineering: A. 2006, 428, 295–300.
[17] Jiang MG et al. Microstructure, texture and mechanical properties in an as-cast AZ61 Mg alloy during multi-directional impact forging and subsequent heat treatment. Materials & Design. 2015, 87, 891–900.
[18] Bian MZ et al. A heat-treatable Mg–Al–Ca–Mn–Zn sheet alloy with good room temperature formability. Scripta Materialia. 2017, 138, 151–5.
[19] Liu Z-J et al. Effect of heat treatment on microstructures and mechanical properties of sand-cast Mg–4Y–2Nd–1Gd–0.4Zr magnesium alloy. Transactions of Nonferrous Metals Society of China. 2012, 22, 1540–8.
[20] Li H et al. Effect of heat treatment on microstructures and mechanical properties of a cast Mg-Y-Nd-Zr alloy. Materials Science and Engineering: A. 2016, 667, 409–16.
[21] Torroni A et al. Histo-morphologic characteristics of intra-osseous implants of WE43 Mg alloys with and without heat treatment in an in vivo cranial bone sheep model. Journal of Cranio-Maxillofacial Surgery. 2018, 46, 473–78.
[22] Torroni A et al. Biocompatibility and degradation properties of WE43 Mg alloys with and without heat treatment: In vivo evaluation and comparison in a cranial bone sheep model. Journal of Cranio-Maxillofacial Surgery. 2017, 45, 2075–83.
[23] Chen X-H et al. Effects of heat treatment on microstructure and mechanical properties of ZK60 Mg alloy. Transactions of Nonferrous Metals Society of China. 2011, 21, 754–60.
[24] Geng J et al. Microstructure transformations in the heat-treated M–Zn–Y alloy. Journal of Alloys and Compounds 2013, 577, 498–506.
[25] Liu W et al. Microstructure Evolution of Semisolid Mg-2Zn-0.5Y Alloy during Isothermal Heat Treatment. Rare Metal Materials and Engineering. 2016, 45, 1967–72.
[26] Ma R et al. Mechanical and damping properties of thermal treated Mg–Zn–Y–Zr alloys reinforced with quasicrystal phase. Materials Science and Engineering: A. 2014, 602, 11–8.
[27] Wang SD et al. Effect of heat treatment on the corrosion resistance and mechanical properties of an as-forged Mg–Zn–Y–Zr alloy. Corrosion Science. 2015, 92, 228–36.
[28] Lan et al. Effect of substitution of minor Nd for Y on mechanical and damping properties of heat-treated M–Zn–Y–Zr alloy. Materials Science and Engineering: A. 2016, 651, 646–56.
[29] Hu G-S et al. Microstructures and mechanical properties of as-extruded and heat treated Mg–6Zn–1Mn–4Sn–1.5Nd alloy. Transactions of Nonferrous Metals Society of China. 2015, 25, 1439–45.
[30] Mendis CL et al. Microstructures and mechanical properties of extruded and heat treated Mg–6Zn–1Si–0.5Mn alloys. Materials Science and Engineering: A. 2012, 553, 1–9.
[31] Zhu S et al. Effects of Cu addition on the microstructure and mechanical properties of as-cast and heat treated Mg-6Zn-4Al magnesium alloy. Materials Science and Engineering: A. 2107, 689, 203–11.
[32] Ibrahim H et al. Microstructural, mechanical and corrosion characteristics of heat-treated Mg-1.2Zn-0.5Ca (wt%) alloy for use as resorbable bone fixation material. Journal of the Mechanical Behavior of Biomedical Materials. 2017, 69, 203–12.
[33] Kang Y et al. Optimizing mechanical property and cytocompatibility of the biodegradable Mg-Zn-Y-Nd alloy by hot extrusion and heat treatment. Journal of Materials Science & Technology. 2019, 35, 6–18.
[34] Zhang Y et al. Effects of heat treatment on the mechanical properties and corrosion behaviour of the Mg-2Zn-0.2Mn-xNd alloys. Journal of Alloys and Compounds. 2018, 769, 552–65.
[35] Liu X-B et al. Effects of heat treatment on corrosion behaviors of Mg-3Zn magnesium alloy. Transactions of Nonferrous Metals Society of China. 2010, 20, 1345–50.

[36] Yan et al. Effects of Zn concentration and heat treatment on the microstructure, mechanical properties and corrosion behavior of as-extruded Mg-Zn alloys produced by powder metallurgy. Journal of Alloys and Compounds. 2017, 693, 1277–89.
[37] Zhang D et al. Effects of Heat Treatment on Microstructure and Mechanical Properties of as-Extruded Mg-9Sn-1.5Y-0.4Zr Magnesium Alloy. Rare Metal Materials and Engineering. 2016, 45, 2208–13.
[38] Li J et al. Heat treatment and mechanical properties of a high-strength cast Mg–Gd–Zn alloy. Materials Science and Engineering: A. 2016, 651, 745–52.
[39] Dai J et al. Heat treatment, microstructure and mechanical properties of a Mg–Gd–Y alloy grain-refined by Al additions. Materials Science and Engineering: A. 2013, 576, 298–305.
[40] Dong J et al. Influence of heat treatment on fatigue behaviour of high-strength Mg–10Gd–3Y alloy. Materials Science and Engineering: A. 2010, 527, 6053–63.
[41] Wu L-Y et al. Microstructure evolution during heat treatment of Mg–Gd–Y–Zn–Zr alloy and its low-cycle fatigue behavior at 573 K. Transactions of Nonferrous Metals Society of China. 2017, 27, 1026–35.
[42] Wang Q et al. Effect of heat treatment on tensile properties, impact toughness and plane-strain fracture toughness of sand-cast Mg-6Gd-3Y-0.5Zr magnesium alloy. Materials Science and Engineering: A. 2017, 705, 402–10.
[43] Wu G et al. Microstructure evolution of semi-solid Mg–10Gd–3Y–0.5Zr alloy during isothermal heat treatment. Journal of Magnesium and Alloys. 2013, 1, 39–46.
[44] Tang C et al. Effects of thermal treatment on microstructure and mechanical properties of a Mg-Gd-based alloy plate. Materials Science and Engineering: A. 2016, 659, 63–75.
[45] Yang M-B et al. Effects of heat treatment on microstructure and mechanical properties of Mg-3Sn-1Mn magnesium alloy. Transactions of Nonferrous Metals Society of China. 2011, 21, 2168–74.
[46] Zhao Z et al. Microstructural evolution and mechanical strengthening mechanism of Mg-3Sn-1Mn-1La alloy after heat treatments. Materials Science and Engineering: A. 2018, 734, 200–9.
[47] Sasaki TT et al. Strong and ductile heat-treatable Mg–Sn–Zn–Al wrought alloys. Acta Materialia. 2015, 99, 176–86.
[48] Zhang L et al. Microstructure and mechanical properties of as-cast and heat treated Mg-15Gd-3Y alloy. Journal of Rare Earths. 2011, 29, 77–82.
[49] Jin X et al. Influence of heat treatment on the evolution of microstructure and mechanical properties of Mg-7Gd-5Y-0.6Zn-0.8Zr magnesium alloy. Materials Science and Engineering: A. 2018, 729, 219–29.
[50] Wang Z-Q et al. Effect of heat treatment on microstructures and mechanical properties of high vacuum die casting Mg–8Gd–3Y–0.4Zr magnesium alloy. Transactions of Nonferrous Metals Society of China. 2014, 24, 3762–8.
[51] Li G et al. Development of high mechanical properties and moderate thermal conductivity cast Mg alloy with multiple RE via heat treatment. Journal of Materials Science & Technology. 2018, 34, 1076–84.
[52] Gao Y et al. Effects of heat treatments on microstructure and mechanical properties of Mg-15Gd-5Y-0.5Zr alloy. Journal of Rare Earths. 2008, 26, 298–302.
[53] Sasaki TT et al. Heat-treatable Mg–Sn–Zn wrought alloy. Scripta Materialia. 2009, 61, 80–3.
[54] Liang M-J et al. Microstructure characterization on Mg-2Nd-4Zn-1Zr alloy during heat treatment. Transactions of Nonferrous Metals Society of China. 2012, 22, 2327–33.
[55] Li Z et al. Effect of heat treatment on strain–controlled fatigue behavior of cast Mg–Nd–Zn–Zr alloy. Journal of Materials Science & Technology. 2018, 34, 2091–9.
[56] Liu SJ et al. Microstructure evolution during heat treatment and mechanical properties of Mg–2.49Nd–1.82Gd–0.19Zn–0.4Zr cast alloy. Materials Characterization. 2015, 107, 334–42.

[57] Zhao J et al. Influence of heat treatment on microstructure and mechanical properties of as-cast Mg–8Li–3Al–2Zn–xY alloy with duplex structure. Materials Science and Engineering: A. 2016, 669, 87–94.
[58] Zhang D et al. Effect of heat treatment on dynamic recrystallization behaviors and mechanical properties of Mg–2.7Nd–0.5Zn–0.8Zr alloy. Materials Science and Engineering: A. 2016, 675, 128–37.
[59] Tang Y, Le Q, Misra RDK, Su G, Cui J. Influence of extruding temperature and heat treatment process on microstructure and mechanical properties of three structures containing Mg-Li alloy bars. Materials Science and Engineering: A. 2018, 712, 266–80.
[60] Tang Y et al. Microstructure evolution and strengthening mechanism study of Mg-Li alloys during deformation and heat treatment. Materials Science and Engineering: A. 2017, 704, 344–59.
[61] Wu L et al. Effects of Ce-rich RE additions and heat treatment on the microstructure and tensile properties of Mg–Li–Al–Zn-based alloy. Materials Science and Engineering: A. 2011, 528, 2174–9.
[62] Wang Y et al. Microstructures, mechanical properties, and degradation behaviors of heat-treated Mg-Sr alloys as potential biodegradable implant materials. Journal of the Mechanical Behavior of Biomedical Materials. 2018, 77, 47–57.
[63] Gu XN et al. A study on alkaline heat treated Mg–Ca alloy for the control of the biocorrosion rate. Acta Biomaterialia. 2009, 5, 2790–9.
[64] Ong MS et al. The influence of heat treatment on the corrosion behaviour of amorphous melt-spun binary Mg–18 at.% Ni and Mg–21 at.% Cu alloy. Materials Science and Engineering: A. 2001, 304/306, 510–4.
[65] Kang J-W, Wang C-J, Deng K-K, Nie K-B, Li W-J. Microstructure and mechanical properties of Mg-4Zn-0.5Ca alloy fabricated by the combination of forging, homogenization and extrusion process. Journal of Alloys and Compounds. 2017, 720, 196–206.
[66] Xiao L, Yang G, Liu Y, Luo S, Jie W. Microstructure evolution, mechanical properties and diffusion behaviour of Mg-6Zn-2Gd-0.5Zr alloy during homogenization. Journal of Materials Science & Technology. 2018, 34, 2246–55.
[67] Zhang J, Zuo R, Chen Y, Pan F, Luo X. Microstructure evolution during homogenization of a τ-type Mg–Zn–Al alloy. Journal of Alloys and Compounds. 2008, 448, 316–20.
[68] Yan L, Liu Y, Shi G, Sun J, Liu H. Effect of Homogenization on Microstructure and Mechanical Property of Mg-5.9Zn-1.6Zr-1.6Nd-0.9Y Alloy. Rare Metal Materials and Engineering. 2018, 47, 1393–8.
[69] Yang Z, Li JP, Zhang JX, Guo YC, Liang MX. Effect of homogenization on the hot-deformation ability and dynamic recrystallization of Mg–9Gd–3Y–0.5Zr alloy. Materials Science and Engineering: A. 2009, 515, 102–7.
[70] Liu K, Wang X, Wen K. Effect of isothermal homogenization on microstructure and mechanical properties of the Mg–5Y–4Gd–0.5Zn–0.4Zr alloy. Materials & Design. 2013, 52, 1035–42.
[71] Zhang G, Li X, Ma M, Li Y, Zhang K. Homogenization heat treatment of Mg-7.68Gd-4.88Y-1.32Nd-0.63Al-0.05Zr alloy. Journal of Rare Earths. 2014, 32, 445–50.
[72] Li K, Zhang K, Du ZW, Li XG, Liu JB. The effect of homogenization on microstructures and mechanical properties of Mg–7Gd–3Y–1Nd–xZn–0.5Zr (x=0.5, 1 and 2wt.%) alloys. Materials Characterization. 2015, 109, 66–72.
[73] Xu C, Zheng MY, Wu K, Wang ED, Lv XY. Effect of cooling rate on the microstructure evolution and mechanical properties of homogenized Mg–Gd–Y–Zn–Zr alloy. Materials Science and Engineering: A. 2013, 559, 364–70.

[74] Bao L, Le Q, Zhang Z, Cui J, Li Q. Effect of homogenization treatment on microstructure evolution and the distributions of RE and Zr elements in various Mg–Li–RE–Zr alloys. Journal of Magnesium and Alloys. 2013, 1, 139–44.

[75] Peng QZ, Zhou HT, Zhong FH, Ding HB, Peng Y. Effects of homogenization treatment on the microstructure and mechanical properties of Mg–8Li–3Al–Y alloy. Materials & Design. 2015, 66, 566–74.

[76] Tan XH, Chee KHW, Chan KWJ, Kwok WOR, Gupta M. Effect of homogenization on enhancing the failure strain of high strength quaternary LPSO Mg–Y–Zn–Al alloy. Materials Science and Engineering: A. 2015, 644, 405–12.

[77] Naghdi F, Mahmudi R. Effect of solution treatment on the microstructural evolution and mechanical properties of an aged Mg–4Zn–0.3Ca alloy. Materials Science and Engineering: A. 2015, 631, 144–52.

[78] Miao H, Huang H, Shi Y, Zhang H, Yuan G. Effects of solution treatment before extrusion on the microstructure, mechanical properties and corrosion of Mg-Zn-Gd alloy in vitro. Corrosion Science. 2017, 122, 90–9.

[79] Jia H, Feng X, Yang Y. Influence of solution treatment on microstructure, mechanical and corrosion properties of Mg-4Zn alloy. Journal of Magnesium and Alloys. 2015, 3, 247–52.

[80] Shahri SMG, Idris MH, Jafari H, Gholampour B, Assadian M. Effect of solution treatment on corrosion characteristics of biodegradable Mg–6Zn alloy. Transactions of Nonferrous Metals Society of China. 2015, 25, 1490–9.

[81] Li JL, Wang XX, Zhang N, Wu D, Chen RS. Ductility drop of the solutionized Mg-Gd-Y-Zr alloy during tensile deformation at 350 °C. Journal of Alloys and Compounds. 2017, 714, 104–13.

[82] Wu SK, Li YH, Chien KT, Chien C, Yang CS. X-ray diffraction studies on cold-rolled/solid-solution treated α+β Mg–10.2Li–1.2Al–0.4Zn alloy. Journal of Alloys and Compounds. 2013, 563, 234–41.

[83] Fei P, Qu Z, Wu R. Microstructure and hardness of Mg–9Li–6Al–xLa (x=0, 2, 5) alloys during solid solution treatment. Materials Science and Engineering: A. 2015, 625, 169–76.

[84] Lü YZ, Wang QD, Zeng XQ, Zhu YP, Ding WJ. Behavior of Mg–6Al–xSi alloys during solution heat treatment at 420°C. Materials Science and Engineering: A. 2001, 301, 255–8.

[85] Wang B, Wang X, Zhou J, Zhang G, Liu F. Effects of solution heat treatment on microstructure and mechanical properties of Mg–3Al–1Si–0.3Mn–xSr alloy. Materials Science and Engineering: A. 2014, 618, 210–8.

[86] Zeng XQ, Li DH, Dong J, Lu C, Ding WJ. Effect of solution treatment and extrusion on evolution of microstructure in a Mg–12Dy–3Nd–0.4Zr alloy. Journal of Alloys and Compounds. 2008, 456, 419–24.

[87] Zhang X, Zhang K, Li X, Deng X, Shi Y. Effect of solid-solution treatment on corrosion and electrochemical behaviors of Mg-15Y alloy in 3.5 wt.% NaCl solution. Journal of Rare Earths. 2012, 30, 1158–67.

[88] Yang Y, Peng L, Fu P, Hu B, Ding W. Identification of NdH2 particles in solution-treated Mg–2.5%Nd (wt.%) alloy. Journal of Alloys and Compounds. 2009, 485, 245–8.

[89] Wang D, Fu P, Peng L, Wang Y, Ding W. Quench sensitivity characterization of a LPSO-phase containing Mg alloy. Materials Science and Engineering: A. 2019, 749, 291–300.

[90] Hagihara K, Mori K, Nakano T. Enhancement of plastic anisotropy and drastic increase in yield stress of Mg-Li single crystals by Al-addition followed by quenching. Scripta Materialia. 2019, 172, 93–7.

[91] Candan S, Celik M, Candan E. Effectiveness of Ti-micro alloying in relation to cooling rate on corrosion of AZ91 Mg alloy. Journal of Alloys and Compounds. 2016, 672, 197–203.

[92] Wang Y, Peng L, Ji Y, Cheng X, Chen L-Q. Effect of cooling rates on the dendritic morphology transition of Mg–6Gd alloy by in situ X-ray radiography. Journal of Materials Science & Technology. 2018, 34, 1142–8.
[93] Meng Y, Chen Q, Sugiyama S, Yanagimoto J. Effects of reheating and subsequent rapid cooling on microstructural evolution and semisolid forming behaviors of extruded Mg–8.20Gd–4.48Y–3.34Zn–0.36Zr alloy. Journal of Materials Processing Technology. 2017, 247, 192–203.
[94] Rangelova V, Spassov T. Primary crystallization kinetics in rapidly quenched Mg-based Mg–Ni–Y alloys. Journal of Alloys and Compounds. 2002, 345, 148–54.
[95] Todorova St, Spassov T. Mg6Ni formation in rapidly quenched amorphous Mg–Ni alloys. Journal of Alloys and Compounds. 2009, 469, 193–6.
[96] Liu Y, Shao S, Xu C-S, Zeng X-S, Yang X-J. Effect of cryogenic treatment on the microstructure and mechanical properties of Mg–1.5Zn–0.15Gd magnesium alloy. Materials Science and Engineering: A. 2013, 588, 76–81.
[97] Li Q, Yuan Z, Jiang A, Zhu W, She X. Effect of Cryogenic Treatment on Mechanical Properties of Mg-2Zn-0.7Ce Alloy. 2nd International Symposium on Resource Exploration and Environmental Science IOP Publishing IOP Conf. Series: Earth and Environmental Science. 2018, 170; doi:10.1088/1755-1315/170/3/032135
[98] Yong Liu, Shuang Shao, Chunshui Xu, Xiangjie Yang, Deping Lu, Enhancing wear resistance of Mg-Zn-Gd alloy by cryogenic treatment. Materials Letters 2012, 76, 201–4.
[99] Jiang Y, Chen D, Chen Z, Liu J. Effect of Cryogenic Treatment on the Microstructure and Mechanical Properties of AZ31 Magnesium Alloy. Journal of Materials and Manufacturing Processes. 2010, 25, 837–41.
[100] Li J, Jiang XQ. Effect of Cryogenic Treatment on the Microstructure and Mechanical Properties of AZ31 Magnesium Alloy. Materials Science Forum. 2011, 686, 53–56.
[101] Mónica P, Bravo PM, Cárdenas D. Deep cryogenic treatment of HPDC AZ91 magnesium alloys prior to aging and its influence on alloy microstructure and mechanical properties. Journal of Materials Processing Technology. 2017, 239, 297–302.
[102] Mishima T, Mishima R. Theory of Alloying. Kyouritu Pub. 1954, pp.187–190.
[103] Callister WD Jr. Materials Science and Engineering; An Introduction. 7th ed. John Wiley & Sons, 2007, p.406.
[104] Bohlen J, Telleria Iparragirre A, Arruebarrena G, Letzig D. On the Age Hardening Response of Aluminum Containing Magnesium Sheets with Zinc or Manganese (AZ- and AM Series Alloys). In: Solanki K. et al., ed., Magnesium Technology 2017. The Minerals, Metals & Materials Series. Springer, 2017, 113–21.
[105] Ge B, Fu H, Deng K, Zhang Q, Peng Q. Unique strengthening mechanisms of ultrahigh pressure Mg alloys. Bioactive Materials. 2018, 3, 250–4.
[106] Shahar IA et al. Mechanical and Corrosion Properties of AZ31 Mg Alloy Processed by Equal-Channel Angular Pressing and Aging. Procedia Engineering. 2017, 184, 423–31.
[107] Dong X et al. Microstructure and tensile properties of as-cast and as-aged Mg–6Al–4Zn alloys with Sn addition. Materials & Design. 2013, 51, 567–74.
[108] Jung J-G et al. Improved mechanical properties of Mg–7.6Al–0.4Zn alloy through aging prior to extrusion. Scripta Materialia. 2014, 93, 8–11.
[109] Yuan YC et al. Mechanical properties and precipitate behavior of Mg–9Al–1Zn alloy processed by equal-channel angular pressing and aging. Journal of Alloys and Compounds. 2014, 594, 182–8.
[110] Yuan Y et al. Optimizing the strength and ductility of AZ91 Mg alloy by ECAP and subsequent aging. Materials Science and Engineering: A. 2013, 588, 329–34.

[111] Jiang Y et al. Improved mechanical properties of Mg–9Al–1Zn alloy by the combination of aging, cold-rolling and electropulsing treatment. Journal of Alloys and Compounds. 2015, 626, 297–303.

[112] Li Y et al. Evolution of β Mg17Al12 in MgAlZnAg lloy over time. Materials Science and Engineering: A 2019, 754, 470–8.

[113] Ren LB et al. Effect of Y addition on the aging hardening behavior and precipitation evolution of extruded Mg-Al-Zn alloys. Materials Science and Engineering: A. 2017, 690, 195–207.

[114] Majd AM et al. Effect of RE elements on the microstructural and mechanical properties of as-cast and age hardening processed Mg–4Al–2Sn alloy. Journal of Magnesium and Alloys. 2018, 6, 309–17.

[115] Jo SM et al. Precipitation Behavior of Mg–Al–Sn–Zn–(Na) Alloy. In: Solanki K. et al., ed. Magnesium Technology 2017. The Minerals, Metals & Materials Series. Springer, 2017, 203–207.

[116] Jiang L et al. Effects of Zn addition on the aging behavior and mechanical properties of Mg8Al2Sn wrought alloy. Materials Science and Engineering: A. 2019, 752, 145–51.

[117] Liu C et al. Effects of Zn additions on the microstructure and hardness of Mg–9Al–6Sn alloy. Materials Characterization. 2016, 113, 214–21.

[118] Zhu T et al., Effects of Mn addition on the microstructure and mechanical properties of cast Mg–9Al–2Sn (wt.%) alloy. Journal of Magnesium and Alloys. 2014, 2, 27–35.

[119] Nakata et al. Strong and ductile age-hardening Mg-Al-Ca-Mn alloy that can be extruded as fast as aluminum alloy. Acta Materialia. 2017, 130, 261–70.

[120] Zhu SM et al. Age hardening in die-cast Mg–Al–RE alloys due to minor Mn additions. Materials Science and Engineering: A. 2016, 656, 34–8.

[121] Pan H et al. High-conductivity binary Mg–Zn sheet processed by cold rolling and subsequent aging. Journal of Alloys and Compounds. 2013, 578, 493–500.

[122] Buha J. Reduced temperature (22–100°C) ageing of an Mg–Zn alloy. Materials Science and Engineering: A. 2008, 492, 11–9.

[123] Zhang G et al. Effects of artificial aging on microstructure and mechanical properties of the Mg–4.5Zn–4.5Sn–2Al alloy. Journal of Alloys and Compounds. 2014, 592, 250–7.

[124] Wang C et al. Microstructure and mechanical properties of Mg-5Zn-3.5Sn-1Mn-0.5Ca-0.5Cu alloy. Materials Characterization. 2019, 147, 406–13.

[125] Wei S et al. Effects of Pb/Sn additions on the age-hardening behaviour of Mg–4Zn alloys. Materials Science and Engineering: A. 2014, 597, 52–61.

[126] Buha J. Mechanical properties of naturally aged Mg–Zn–Cu–Mn alloy. Materials Science and Engineering: A. 2008, 489, 127–37.

[127] Golmakaniyoon S et al. Effect of aging treatment on the microstructure, creep resistance and high-temperature mechanical properties of Mg–6Zn–3Cu alloy with La- and Ce-rich rare earth additions. Materials Science and Engineering: A. 2015, 620, 301–8.

[128] Zhu HM et al. Microstructure and mechanical properties of Mg–6Zn–xCu–0.6Zr (wt.%) alloys. Journal of Alloys and Compounds. 2011, 509, 3526–31.

[129] Wang B et al. Microstructure and mechanical properties of as-extruded and as-aged Mg–Zn–Al–Sn alloys. Materials Science and Engineering: A. 2016, 656, 165–73.

[130] Lin X et al. The microstructure of Mg–4Zn–2Al–0.5Ca aged alloy. Materials Science and Engineering: A. 2012, 538, 231–5.

[131] Zhu S et al. Improving mechanical properties of age-hardenable Mg–6Zn–4Al–1Sn alloy processed by double-aging treatment. Journal of Materials Science & Technology. 2017, 33, 1249–54.

[132] Zhu S et al. Effects of Cu addition on the microstructure and mechanical properties of as-cast and heat treated Mg-6Zn-4Al magnesium alloy. Materials Science and Engineering: A. 2017, 689, 203–11.
[133] Dong Y et al. Microstructure of Mg–8Zn–4Al–1Ca aged alloy. Transactions of Nonferrous Metals Society of China. 2014, 24, 310–5.
[134] Naghdi F et al. Microstructure and high-temperature mechanical properties of the Mg–4Zn–0.5Ca alloy in the as-cast and aged conditions. Materials Science and Engineering: A. 2016, 649, 441–8.
[135] Duley P et al. Homogenization-induced age-hardening behavior and room temperature mechanical properties of Mg-4Zn-0.5Ca-0.16Mn (wt%) alloy. Materials & Design. 2019, 164; https://doi.org/10.1016/j.matdes.2018.107554.
[136] Hu G-S et al. Microstructures and mechanical properties of extruded and aged Mg–Zn–Mn–Sn–Y alloys. Transactions of Nonferrous Metals Society of China. 2014, 24, 3070–5.
[137] Qi F et al. Effect of Sn addition on the microstructure and mechanical properties of Mg–6Zn–1Mn (wt.%) alloy. Journal of Alloys and Compounds. 2014, 585, 656–66.
[138] Hu G et al. Effect of Y addition on the microstructures and mechanical properties of as-aged Mg-6Zn-1Mn-4Sn (wt%) alloy. Journal of Alloys and Compounds. 2016, 689, 326–32.
[139] Buha J. Characterisation of precipitates in an aged Mg–Zn–Ti alloy. Journal of Alloys and Compounds. 2009, 472, 171–7.
[140] Buha J. The effect of Ba on the microstructure and age hardening of an Mg–Zn alloy. Materials Science and Engineering: A. 2008, 491, 70–9.
[141] Geng J et al. Enhanced age-hardening response of Mg–Zn alloys via Co additions. Scripta Materialia. 2011, 64, 506–9.
[142] Bhattacharjee T et al. The effect of Ag and Ca additions on the age hardening response of Mg–Zn alloys. Materials Science and Engineering: A. 2013, 575, 231–40.
[143] Buha J. The effect of micro-alloying addition of Cr on age hardening of an Mg–Zn alloy. Materials Science and Engineering: A. 2008, 492, 293–9.
[144] Koizumi T et al. Platelet precipitate in an age-hardening Mg-Zn-Gd alloy. Journal of Alloys and Compounds. 2018, 752, 407–11.
[145] Ye J et al. Influence of pre-strain on the aging hardening effect of the Mg-9.02Zn-1.68Y alloy. Materials Science and Engineering: A. 2016, 663, 49–55.
[146] Li J et al. Effect of aging on microstructure of Mg-Zn-Er alloys. Journal of Rare Earths. 2009, 27, 1042–5.
[147] Mendis CL et al. Effect of Li additions on the age hardening response and precipitate microstructures of Mg–2.4Zn–0.16Zr based alloys. Materials Science and Engineering: A. 2012, 535, 122–8.
[148] Xie H et al. Co-existences of the two types of β′ precipitations in peak-aged Mg-Gd binary alloy. Journal of Alloys and Compounds. 2018, 738, 32–6.
[149] Zhong L et al. Effects of precipitates and its interface on thermal conductivity of Mg–12Gd alloy during aging treatment. Materials Characterization. 2018, 138, 284–8.
[150] Stulikova I et al. Natural and artificial aging in Mg-Gd binary alloys. Journal of Alloys and Compounds. 2018, 738, 173–81.
[151] Yang Z et al. Microstructure evolution of Mg–6Gd–2Y alloy during solid solution and aging process. Materials Science and Engineering: A. 2015, 631, 160–5.
[152] Peng QM et al. Microstructures and properties of Mg–7Gd alloy containing Y. Journal of Alloys and Compound. 2007, 430, 252–6.
[153] Liu WC et al. Effect of microstructures and texture development on tensile properties of Mg–10Gd–3Y alloy. Materials Science and Engineering: A. 2011, 528, 2250–8.

[154] Li et al. Effects of friction stir process and subsequent aging treatment on the microstructure evolution and mechanical properties of Mg-Gd-Y-Zn-Zr alloy. Materials Characterization. 2019, 155; https://doi.org/10.1016/j.matchar.2019.109832.
[155] Yao Y et al. High strength Mg-1.4Gd-1.2Y-0.4Zn sheet and its strengthening mechanisms. Materials Science and Engineering: A. 2019, 747, 17–26.
[156] Liu S et al. Ageing behavior and mechanisms of strengthening and toughening of ultrahigh-strength Mg-Gd-Y-Zn-Mn alloy. Materials Science and Engineering: A. 2019, 758, 96–8.
[157] Xu C et al. Effect of ageing treatment on the precipitation behaviour of Mg–Gd–Y–Zn–Zr alloy. Journal of Alloys and Compounds. 2013, 550, 50–6.
[158] Sun WT et al. Achieving ultra-high hardness of nanostructured Mg-8.2Gd-3.2Y-1.0Zn-0.4Zr alloy produced by a combination of high pressure torsion and ageing treatment. Scripta Materialia. 2018, 155, 21–5.
[159] Xu C et al. Ultra high-strength Mg–Gd–Y–Zn–Zr alloy sheets processed by large-strain hot rolling and ageing. Materials Science and Engineering: A. 2012, 547, 93–8.
[160] Han XZ et al. Effect of precipitates on microstructures and properties of forged Mg–10Gd–2Y–0.5Zn–0.3Zr alloy during ageing process. Journal of Alloys and Compounds. 2011, 509, 8625–31.
[161] Jafari HR et al. Microstructure characterization and high-temperature shear strength of the Mg–10Gd–3Y–1.2Zn–0.5Zr alloy in the as-cast and aged conditions. Journal of Alloys and Compounds. 2015, 619, 826–33.
[162] Zheng L et al. Microstructures and mechanical properties of Mg–10Gd–6Y–2Zn–0.6Zr(wt.%) alloy. Journal of Alloys and Compounds. 2011, 509, 8832–9.
[163] Heng X et al. A super high-strength Mg-Gd-Y-Zn-Mn alloy fabricated by hot extrusion and strain aging. Materials & Design. 2019, 169; https://doi.org/10.1016/j.matdes.2019.107666.
[164] Zhang S et al. Effect of solid solution and aging treatments on the microstructures evolution and mechanical properties of Mg–14Gd–3Y–1.8Zn–0.5Zr alloy. Journal of Alloys and Compounds. 2013, 557, 91–7.
[165] Yu S et al. Age-hardening and age-softening in nanocrystalline Mg-Gd-Y-Zr alloy. Materials Characterization. 2019, 156; https://doi.org/10.1016/j.matchar.2019.109841.
[166] Heng J et al. Segregation of rare earth atoms in Mg-Gd-Y-Zr alloy after a 6-year natural ageing at room temperature: Atomic-scale direct imaging. Materials Letters. 2016, 174, 86–90.
[167] Liang S et al. Precipitation and its effect on age-hardening behavior of as-cast Mg–Gd–Y alloy. Materials & Design. 2011, 32, 361–4.
[168] Liang S et al. Effect of isothermal aging on the microstructure and properties of as-cast Mg–Gd–Y–Zr alloy. Materials Science and Engineering: A. 2011, 528, 1589–95.
[169] Yao Y et al. Annealing-induced microstructural evolution and mechanical anisotropy improvement of the Mg-Gd-Y-Zr alloy processed by hot ring rolling. Materials Characterization. 2018, 144, 641–51.
[170] Yang Z et al. Effect of natural ageing on microstructure and mechanical properties of Mg–10Gd–2Y–0.8Zr Alloy. Materials Science and Engineering: A. 2015, 648, 140–5.
[171] Liu XB et al. Effects of ageing treatment on microstructures and properties of Mg–Gd–Y–Zr alloys with and without Zn additions. Journal of Alloys and Compounds. 2008, 465, 232–8.
[172] Wang D et al. HRTEM studies of aging precipitate phases in the Mg-10Gd-3Y-0.4Zr alloy. Journal of Rare Earths. 2016, 34, 441–6.
[173] Jafari HR et al. Effect of Gd content on microstructure and mechanical properties of Mg–Gd–Y–Zr alloys under peak-aged condition. Materials Science and Engineering: A. 2014, 615, 79–86.
[174] Li H-Z et al. Effect of ageing time on corrosion behavior of Mg-10Gd-4.8Y-0.6Zr extruded-alloy. Transactions of Nonferrous Metals Society of China. 2011, 21, 1498–1505.

[175] Wang J et al. Effect of Y for enhanced age hardening response and mechanical properties of Mg–Gd–Y–Zr alloys. Materials Science and Engineering: A. 2007, 456, 78–84.
[176] Liu X et al. Effects of Nd/Gd value on the microstructures and mechanical properties of Mg–Gd–Y–Nd–Zr alloys. Journal of Magnesium and Alloys. 2016, 4, 214–9.
[177] Liu Q et al. Analysis on micro-structure and mechanical properties of Mg-Gd-Y-Nd-Zr alloy and its reinforcement mechanism. Journal of Alloys and Compounds. 2017, 690, 961–5.
[178] Liu X et al. Microstructures and mechanical properties of high performance Mg–6Gd–3Y–2Nd–0.4Zr alloy by indirect extrusion and aging treatment. Materials Science and Engineering: A. 2014, 612, 380–6.
[179] Yuan J et al. Effect of Zn content on the microstructures, mechanical properties, and damping capacities of Mg–7Gd–3Y–1Nd–0.5Zr Based Alloys. Journal of Alloys and Compounds. 2019, 773, 919–26.
[180] Li T et al. Characterisation of precipitates in a Mg–7Gd–5Y–1Nd–0.5Zr alloy aged to peak-ageing plateau. Journal of Alloys and Compounds. 2013, 574, 174–80.
[181] Wang B et al. Microstructure evolution and mechanical properties of Mg-Gd-Y-Ag-Zr alloy fabricated by multidirectional forging and ageing treatment. Materials Science and Engineering: A. 2017, 702, 22–8.
[182] Zhang Y et al. A comparative study of the role of Ag in microstructures and mechanical properties of Mg-Gd and Mg-Y alloys. Materials Science and Engineering: A. 2018, 731, 609–22.
[183] Yamada K et al. Enhanced age-hardening and formation of plate precipitates in Mg–Gd–Ag alloys. Scripta Materialia. 2009, 61, 636–9.
[184] Li RG et al. Cold-working mediated converse age hardening responses in extruded Mg-14Gd-2Ag-0.5Zr alloy with different microstructure. Materials Science and Engineering: A. 2019, 748, 95–9.
[185] Nie JF et al. Enhanced age hardening response and creep resistance of Mg–Gd alloys containing Zn. Scripta Materialia. 2005, 53, 1049–53.
[186] Peng Q et al. The effect of La or Ce on ageing response and mechanical properties of cast Mg–Gd–Zr alloys. Materials Characterization. 2008, 59, 435–9.
[187] Li R et al. Effect of grain size, texture and density of precipitates on the hardness and tensile yield stress of Mg-14Gd-0.5Zr alloys. Materials & Design. 2017, 114, 450–8.
[188] Chen HW et al. Effect of Ca addition on microstructures of aged Mg-15Gd-0.5Zr alloy. Materials Characterization. 2019, 156; https://doi.org/10.1016/j.matchar.2019.109838.
[189] Zheng X et al. Remarkably enhanced mechanical properties of Mg-8Gd-1Er-0.5Zr alloy on the route of extrusion, rolling and aging. Materials Letters. 2018, 212, 155–8.
[190] Wang X et al. Microstructure evolutions of Mg-8Gd-2Er (wt.%) alloy during isothermal ageing at 200°C. Journal of Rare Earths. 2012, 30, 1168–71.
[191] Peng Q et al. Age hardening and mechanical properties of Mg–Gd–Er alloy. Journal of Alloys and Compounds. 2008, 456, 395–9.
[192] Chen Q et al. Equilibrium and metastable phases in a designed precipitation hardenable Mg–3Gd–3Nd–0.6Zr alloy. Materials Science and Engineering: A. 2017, 686, 26–33.
[193] Peng Q et al. Microstructure and mechanical property of Mg–8.31Gd–1.12Dy–0.38Zr alloy. Materials Science and Engineering: A. 2008, 477, 193–7.
[194] Liu N et al. Microstructure evolution and mechanical properties of Mg-Gd-Sm-Zr alloys. Materials Science and Engineering: A. 2015, 627, 223–9.
[195] Peng Q et al. Aging behavior and mechanical properties of Mg–Gd–Ho alloys. Materials Characterization. 2008, 59, 983–6.
[196] Zhao Z et al. Influence of Al and Si additions on the microstructure and mechanical properties of Mg-4Li alloys. Materials Science and Engineering: A. 2017, 702, 206–17.

[197] Li J et al. Microstructure, mechanical properties and aging behaviors of as-extruded Mg–5Li–3Al–2Zn–1.5Cu alloy. Materials Science and Engineering: A. 2011, 528, 3915–20.
[198] Xu DK et al. Effect of icosahedral phase on the thermal stability and ageing response of a duplex structured Mg–Li alloy. Materials & Design. 2015, 69, 124–9.
[199] Ji H et al. Balance of mechanical properties of Mg-8Li-3Al-2Zn-0.5Y alloy by solution and low-temperature aging treatment. Journal of Alloys and Compounds. 2019, 791, 655–64.
[200] Dutkiewicz J et al. Development of new age hardenable Mg-Li-Sc alloys. Journal of Alloys and Compounds. 2019, 784, 686–96.
[201] Wu R et al. Ageing behavior of Mg–9Li–6Al–xY(x=0, 0.5, 2) alloys. Journal of Alloys and Compounds. 2014, 616, 408–12.
[202] Qu Z et al. The solution and room temperature aging behavior of Mg–9Li–xAl(x=3, 6) alloys. Journal of Alloys and Compounds. 2012, 536, 145–9.
[203] Muga CO et al. Effects of aging and fast-cooling on the mechanical properties of Mg-14Li-3Al-3Ce alloy. Materials Science and Engineering: A. 2017, 689, 195–202.
[204] Jian B et al. Effect of Sr on microstructure and aging behavior of Mg–14Li alloys. Progress in Natural Science: Materials International. 2012, 22, 160–8.
[205] Zhao H et al. Spherical strengthening precipitate in a Mg-10wt%Y alloy with superhigh pressure aging. Materials Letters. 2013, 96, 16–9.
[206] Rokhlin LL et al. Recovery after ageing of Mg–Y and Mg–Gd alloys. Journal of Alloys and Compounds. 1998, 279, 166–170.
[207] Panograhi SK et al. A study on the combined effect of forging and aging in Mg–Y–RE alloy. Materials Science and Engineering: A. 2011, 530, 28–35.
[208] Bhattacharyya JJ et al. Deformation and fracture behavior of Mg alloy, WE43, after various aging heat treatments. Materials Science and Engineering: A. 2017, 705, 79–88.
[209] Zhang D et al. Dynamic recrystallization behaviors and the resultant mechanical properties of a Mg–Y–Nd–Zr alloy during hot compression after aging. Materials Science and Engineering: A. 2015, 640, 51–60.
[210] Xin R et al. Effect of aging precipitation on mechanical anisotropy of an extruded Mg–Y–Nd alloy. Materials & Design. 2012, 34, 384–8.
[211] Su Z et al. Microstructures and mechanical properties of high performance Mg–4Y–2.4Nd–0.2Zn–0.4Zr alloy. Materials & Design. 2013, 45, 466–72.
[212] Tian Z et al. Microstructure and mechanical properties of a peak-aged Mg-5Y-2.5Nd-1.5Gd-0.5Zr casting alloy. Journal of Alloys and Compounds. 2018, 731, 704–13.
[213] Xin R et al. Structural examination of aging precipitation in a Mg–Y–Nd alloy at different temperatures. Materials Characterization. 2011, 62, 535–9.
[214] Lentz M et al. Effect of age hardening on the deformation behavior of an Mg–Y–Nd alloy: In-situ X-ray diffraction and crystal plasticity modeling. Materials Science and Engineering: A. 2015, 628, 396–409.
[215] Luo K et al. Effect of Y and Gd content on the microstructure and mechanical properties of Mg–Y–RE alloys. Journal of Magnesium and Alloys. 2019, 7, 345–54.
[216] Liu K et al. Microstructures and mechanical properties of the extruded Mg-4Y-2Gd-xZn-0.4Zr alloys. Journal of Alloys and Compounds. 2011, 509, 3299–3305.
[217] Lukyanova EA et al. Reversion after ageing in an Mg–Y–Gd–Zr alloy. Journal of Alloys and Compounds. 2015, 635, 173–9.
[218] Liu K et al. Precipitates formed in a Mg–7Y–4Gd–0.5Zn–0.4Zr alloy during isothermal ageing at 250°C. Materials Chemistry and Physics. 2009, 117, 107–12.
[219] Lyu S et al. Fabrication of high-strength Mg-Y-Sm-Zn-Zr alloy by conventional hot extrusion and aging. Materials Science and Engineering: A. 2018, 732, 178–85.

[220] Zhang Q et al. Strength stability of aging hardened Mg-10Y-1.5Sm alloy. Rare Metal Materials and Engineering. 2018, 47, 799–802.
[221] Zhu YM et al. Improvement in the age-hardening response of Mg–Y–Zn alloys by Ag additions. Scripta Materialia. 2008, 58, 525–8.
[222] Wu S et al. A high strength and good ductility Mg–Y–NI–TI alloy with long period stacking ordered structure processed by hot rolling and aging treatment. Materials Science and Engineering: A. 2015, 648, 134–9.
[223] Behdad S et al. Improvement of aging kinetics and precipitate size refinement in Mg–Sn alloys by hafnium additions. Materials Science and Engineering: A. 2016, 651, 854–8.
[224] Mendis CL et al. An enhanced age hardening response in Mg–Sn based alloys containing Zn. Materials Science and Engineering: A. 2006, 435/436, 163–71.
[225] Huang X-F et al. Improved age-hardening behavior of Mg–Sn–Mn alloy by addition of Ag and Zn. Materials Science and Engineering: A. 2012, 552, 211–21.
[226] Lee BD et al. Microstructure and mechanical properties on aging behavior of Zn containing Mg–2Sn–0.4Mn alloy. Intermetallics. 2013, 32, 214–8.
[227] Sasaki TT et al. Effect of double aging and microalloying on the age hardening behavior of a Mg–Sn–Zn alloy. Materials Science and Engineering: A. 2011, 530, 1–8.
[228] Elsayed FR et al. Compositional optimization of Mg–Sn–Al alloys for higher age hardening response. Materials Science and Engineering: A. 2013, 566, 22–9.
[229] Nayyeri G et al. The microstructure, creep resistance, and high-temperature mechanical properties of Mg-5Sn alloy with Ca and Sb additions, and aging treatment. Materials Science and Engineering: A. 2010, 527, 5353–9.
[230] Wang C et al. Electrical and thermal conductivity in Mg–5Sn Alloy at different aging status. Materials & Design. 2015, 84, 48–52.
[231] Huang X et al. Effects of Ag content on the solid-solution and age-hardening behavior of a Mg-5Sn alloy. Journal of Alloys and Compounds. 2017, 696, 850–5.
[232] Hu T et al. Improving tensile properties of Mg-Sn-Zn magnesium alloy sheets using pre-tension and ageing treatment. Journal of Alloys and Compounds. 2018, 735, 1494–504.
[233] Lee SG et al. Investigation on microstructure and creep properties of as-cast and aging-treated Mg–6Sn–5Al–2Si alloy. Materials Science and Engineering: A. 2011, 528, 5394–9.
[234] Jung J-G et al. Effect of aging prior to extrusion on the microstructure and mechanical properties of Mg–7Sn–1Al–1Zn alloy. Journal of Alloys and Compounds. 2015, 627, 324–32.
[235] Li W et al. Enhanced age-hardening response and compression property of a Mg-7Sn-1Ca-1Ag (wt.%) alloy by extrusion combined with aging treatment. Journal of Alloys and Compounds. 2018, 766, 584–93.
[236] Li W et al. Effects of Ca, Ag addition on the microstructure and age-hardening behavior of a Mg-7Sn (wt%) alloy. Materials Science and Engineering: A. 2017, 692, 75–80.
[237] Huang X et al. Effects of extrusion and Ag, Zn addition on the age-hardening response and microstructure of a Mg-7Sn alloy. Materials Science and Engineering: A. 2016, 661, 233–9.
[238] Cheng W et al. Improved tensile properties of an equal channel angular pressed (ECAPed) Mg-8Sn-6Zn-2Al alloy by prior aging treatment. Materials Science and Engineering: A. 2017, 87, 148–54.
[239] Tan J et al. A new insight into the beta‴ structure: Three categories of configurations between beta′ precipitates in aged binary Mg-Nd alloy. Scripta Materialia. 2019, 172, 130–4.
[240] Zhou B et al. Study of age hardening in a Mg–2.2wt%Nd alloy by in situ synchrotron X-ray diffraction and mechanical tests. Materials Science and Engineering: A. 2017, 708, 319–28.
[241] Sun BZ et al. Atomic scale investigation of a novel metastable structure in aged Mg–Nd alloys. Scripta Materialia. 2019, 161, 6–12.

[242] Li ZM et al. Effects of grain size and heat treatment on the tensile properties of Mg–3Nd–0.2Zn (wt%) magnesium alloys. Materials Science and Engineering: A. 2013, 564, 450–60.
[243] Li J-H et al. Effect of gadolinium on aged hardening behavior, microstructure and mechanical properties of Mg-Nd-Zn-Zr alloy. Transactions of Nonferrous Metals Society of China. 2008, 18, s27–s32.
[244] Oh-ishi K et al. Age-hardening response of Mg–0.3at.%Ca alloys with different Zn contents. Materials Science and Engineering: A. 2009, 526, 177–84.
[245] Oh JC et al. TEM and 3DAP characterization of an age-hardened Mg–Ca–Zn alloy. Scripta Materialia. 2005, 53, 675–9.
[246] Ibrahim H et al. Effect of Zn content and aging temperature on the in-vitro properties of heat-treated and Ca/P ceramic-coated Mg-0.5%Ca-x%Zn alloys. Materials Science and Engineering: C. 2019, 103; https://doi.org/10.1016/j.msec.2019.04.079.
[247] Ortega Y et al. Tensile fracture behavior of aging hardened Mg–1Ca and Mg–1Ca–1Zn alloys. Materials Letters. 2008, 62, 3893–5.
[248] Bi G et al. Double-peak ageing behavior of Mg–2Dy–0.5Zn alloy. Journal of Alloys and Compounds. 2011, 509, 8268–75.
[249] Zou G et al. Age strengthening behavior and mechanical properties of Mg–Dy based alloys containing LPSO phases. Materials Science and Engineering: A. 2015, 620, 10–5.
[250] Yang L et al. Influence of ageing treatment on microstructure, mechanical and bio-corrosion properties of Mg–Dy alloys. Journal of the Mechanical Behavior of Biomedical Materials. 2012, 13, 36–44.
[251] Li R et al. Effect of cold rolling on microstructure and mechanical property of extruded Mg–4Sm alloy during aging. Materials Characterization. 2016, 112, 81–6.
[252] Che C et al. The effect of Gd and Zn additions on microstructures and mechanical properties of Mg-4Sm-3Nd-Zr alloy. Journal of Alloys and Compounds. 2017, 706, 526–37.
[253] Cao G et al. Evolution of the hardening precipitates with an enclosed structure in pre-deformed Mg-Sm-Nd-Zn-Zr alloy. Materials Letters. 2019, 246, 117–20.
[254] Ogawa Y et al. Aging precipitation kinetics of Mg-Sc alloy with bcc+hcp two-phase. Journal of Alloys and Compounds. 2018, 747, 854–60.
[255] Peng Q et al. Age hardening response of a Mg–5wt.%Sc alloy under an applied stress field. Materials Letters. 2012, 78, 58–61.
[256] Ando D et al. Age-hardening effect by phase transformation of high Sc containing Mg alloy. Materials Letters. 2015, 161, 5–8.
[257] Ogawa Y et al. Aging effect of Mg-Sc alloy with α + β two-phase microstructure. Material Transactions. 2016, 57, 1119–23.
[258] Feng Y et al. Influence of aging treatments on microstructure and electrochemical properties in Mg–8.8Hg–8Ga (wt%) alloy. Intermetallics. 2013, 33, 120–5.
[259] Saito K et al. TEM study of real precipitation behavior of an Mg–0.5at%Ce age-hardened alloy. Journal of Alloys and Compounds. 2013, 574, 283–9.
[260] Khan F et al. Age hardening, fracture behavior and mechanical properties of QE22 Mg alloy. Journal of Magnesium and Alloys. 2015, 3, 210–7.
[261] Zhang D et al. Microstructural evolution of the as-cast and the peak-aged Mg–xYb–0.5Zn–0.4Zr (x = 0.5, 1, 2, and 3 wt.%) alloy. Journal of Alloys and Compounds. 2017, 726, 295–305.
[262] Xie H et al. Atomic-scale HAADF-STEM characterization of an age-hardenable Mg-Cd-Yb alloy. Journal of Alloys and Compounds. 2019, 770, 742–7.
[263] Fan H, El-Awady JA. Hardening Effects of Precipitates with Different Shapes on the Twinning in Magnesium Alloys. In: Joshi V. et al. ed., Magnesium Technology 2019. The Minerals, Metals & Materials Series. Springer, 2019, 257–261.

[264] Liu F, Xin R, Wang C, Song B, Liu Q. Regulating precipitate orientation in Mg-Al alloys by coupling twinning, aging and detwinning processes. Scripta Materialia. 2019, 158, 131–5.
[265] Nie J-F. Precipitation and Hardening in Magnesium Alloys. Metallurgical and Materials Transactions A. 2012, 43, 3891–939.
[266] Barnett MR, Wang H, Guo T. An Orowan precipitate strengthening equation for mechanical twinning in Mg. International Journal of Plasticity. 2019, 112, 108–22.
[267] Tehranchi A, Yin Bm Curtin WA. Solute strengthening of basal slip in Mg alloys. Acta Materialia. 2018, 151, 56–66.
[268] Ghazisaeidi M, Hector LG, Curtin WA. Solute strengthening of twinning dislocations in Mg alloys. Acta Materialia. 2014, 80, 278–87.
[269] Wang D, Amsler M, Hegde VI, Saal JE, Wolverton C. Crystal structure, energetics, and phase stability of strengthening precipitates in Mg alloys: A first-principles study. Acta Materialia. 2018, 158, 65–78.
[270] Paliwal M, Jung I-H. Precipitation kinetic model and its applications to Mg alloys. Calphad. 2019, 64, 196–204.
[271] Mordike B, Ebert T. Magnesium: Properties – Applications – Potential. Materials Science and Engineering: A. 2001, 302, 37–45.
[272] Bamberger M, Dehm G. Trends in the Development of New Mg Alloys. Annual Review of Materials Research. 2008, 38, 505–33.
[273] Yang Z, Li J, Zhang J, Lorimer G, Robson J. Review On Research And Development Of Magnesium Alloys. Acta Metallurgica Sinica (English Letters). 2008, 21, 313–28.
[274] Ma XL, Prameela SE, Yi P, Ferandez M, Weihs TP. Dynamic precipitation and recrystallization in Mg-9wt.%Al during equal-channel angular extrusion: A comparative study to conventional aging. Acta Materialia. 2019, 172, 185–99.
[275] Wong C, Nogita K, Styles MJ, Zhu S, Easton MA. Solidification path and microstructure evolution of Mg-3Al-14La alloy: Implications for the Mg-rich corner of the Mg-Al-La phase diagram. Journal of Alloys and Compounds. 2019, 784, 527–34.
[276] Hu T, Wang F, Zheng R, Xiao W, Ma C. Effects of B and Sn additions on the microstructure and mechanical property of Mg-3Al-1Si alloy. Journal of Alloys and Compounds. 2019, 796, 1–8.
[277] Park W-W, You B-S, Moon B-G, Kim W-C. Microstructural change and precipitation hardening in melt-spun Mg–X–Ca alloys. Science and Technology of Advanced Materials. 2001, 2, 73–8.
[278] Gao X, Nie JF. Characterization of strengthening precipitate phases in a Mg–Zn alloy. Scripta Materialia. 2007, 56, 645–8.
[279] Wang J-Y, Saufan A, Lin PH, Bor HY, Kawamura Y. Mechanical properties and strengthening behavior of M–Zn–MM alloy. Materials Chemistry and Physics. 2014, 148, 28–31.
[280] Luo J, Qiu K, Wang J, Dong X, Li F. Microstructure and mechanical properties of Mg-7Zn-3Al alloy with Nd and Y additions. Journal of Rare Earths. 2012, 30, 486–91.
[281] Guo J, Chang LL, Zhao YR, Jin YP. Effect of Sn and Y addition on the microstructural evolution and mechanical properties of hot-extruded Mg-9Li-3Al alloy. Materials Characterization. 2019, 148, 35–42.
[282] Zhao Z, Xing X, Ma J, Bian L, Wang Y. Effect of addition of Al-Si eutectic alloy on microstructure and mechanical properties of Mg-12wt%Li alloy. Journal of Materials Science & Technology. 2018, 34, 1564–9.
[283] Feng S, Liu W, Zhao J, Wu G, Ding W. Effect of extrusion ratio on microstructure and mechanical properties of Mg–8Li–3Al–2Zn–0.5Y alloy with duplex structure. Materials Science and Engineering: A. 2017, 692, 9–16.
[284] Lalpoor M, Miroux A, Mendis CL, Hort N, Offerman SE. The interaction of precipitation and deformation in a binary Mg–Ca alloy at elevated temperatures. Materials Science and Engineering: A. 2014, 609, 116–24.

[285] Nie JF, Muddle BC. Precipitation hardening of Mg-Ca(-Zn) alloys. Scripta Materialia. 1997, 37, 1475–81.

[286] Jardim PM, Solórzano G, Vander Sande JB. Precipitate Crystal Structure Determination in Melt Spun Mg-1.5wt%Ca-6wt%Zn Alloy. Microscopy and Microanalysis. 2002, 8, 487–96.

[287] Somekawa H, Mukai T. High strength and fracture toughness balance on the extruded Mg–Ca–Zn alloy. Materials Science and Engineering: A. 2007, 459, 366–70.

[288] Langelier B, Wang X, Esmaeili S. Evolution of precipitation during non-isothermal ageing of an Mg–Ca–Zn alloy with high Ca content. Materials Science and Engineering: A. 2012, 538, 246–51.

[289] Jayaraj J, Mendis CL, Ohkubo T, Oh-ishi K, Hono K. Enhanced precipitation hardening of Mg–Ca alloy by Al addition. Scripta Materialia. 2010, 63, 831–4.

[290] Chai Y, Jiang B, Song J, Wang Q, Pan F. Role of Al content on the microstructure, texture and mechanical properties of Mg-3.5Ca based alloys. Materials Science and Engineering: A. 2018, 730, 303–16.

[291] Zhang Y, Rong W, Wu Y, Peng L, Birbilis N. A detailed HAADF-STEM study of precipitate evolution in Mg–Gd alloy. Journal of Alloys and Compounds. 2019, 777, 531–43.

[292] Zhang Y, Rong W, Wu Y, Peng L, Birbilis N. A comparative study of the role of Ag in microstructures and mechanical properties of Mg-Gd and Mg-Y alloys. Materials Science and Engineering: A. 2018, 731, 609–22.

[293] Tang Y-J, Zhang Z-Y, Jin L, Jie D, Ding W-J. Research progress on ageing precipitation of Mg-Gd alloys. Chinese Journal of Nonferrous Metals. 2013, 24, 8–24.

[294] Zheng JK, Zhu C, Li Z, Luo R, Chen B. On the strengthening precipitate structures in Mg-Gd-Ag alloy: An atomic-resolution investigation using Cs-corrected STEM. Materials Letters. 2019, 238, 66–9.

[295] Zhang F, Wang Y, Duan Y, Wang K. Precipitation processes during the peak-aged and over-aged stages in an Mg-Gd-Y-Zr alloy. Journal of Alloys and Compounds. 2019, 788, 541–8.

[296] Dai J, Zhu S, Easton MA, Zhang M, Ding W. Heat treatment, microstructure and mechanical properties of a Mg–Gd–Y alloy grain-refined by Al additions. Materials Science and Engineering: A. 2013, 576, 298–305.

[297] Xu C, Nakata T, Qiao XG, Zheng MY, Wu K, Kamado S. Ageing behavior of extruded Mg–8.2Gd–3.8Y–1.0Zn–0.4Zr (wt.%) alloy containing LPSO phase and γ′ precipitates. Scientific Reports. 2017, 7; https://doi.org/10.1038/srep43391.

[298] Fu H, Guo J, Wu W, Liu B, Peng Q. High pressure aging synthesis of a hexagonal Mg2Sn strengthening precipitate in Mg–Sn alloys. Materials Letters. 2015, 157, 172–5.

[299] Chen J-H, Shen Y-C, Caho C-G, Liu T-F. Wear Behavior and Microstructure of Mg-Sn Alloy Processed by Equal Channel Angular Extrusion. Materials (Basel). 2017,10; https://doi.org/10.3390/ma10111315.

[300] Liu C, Chen H, Nie JF. Zn Segregation at Precipitate/Matrix Interface in Mg–Sn–Zn Alloys. In: Solanki K. et al., ed., Magnesium Technology 2017. The Minerals, Metals & Materials Series. Springer, 2017, 53–59.

[301] Chen Y, Wang Y, Gao J. Microstructure and mechanical properties of as-cast Mg-Sn-Zn-Y alloys. Journal of Alloys and Compounds. 2018, 740, 727–34.

[302] Zhang M, Zhang W-Z, Zhu G-Z, Yu K. Crystallography of Mg_2Sn precipitates in Mg-Sn-Mn-Si alloy. Transactions of Nonferrous Metals Society of China. 2007, 17, 1428–32.

[303] Huang X, Zhang W, Ma Y, Yin M. Enhancement of hardening and thermal resistance of Mg–Sn-based alloys by addition of Cu and Al. Philosophical Mag Letters. 2014, 94, 460–9.

[304] Sato T, Takahashi I, Tezuka H, Kamio A. Precipitation structures of Mg-Y alloys. Journal of Japan Institute of Light Metals. 1992, 42, 804–9.

[305] Zhao H, Pan J, Li H, Tian Y, Peng Q. Spherical strengthening precipitate in a Mg-10wt%Y alloy with superhigh pressure aging. Materials Letters. 2013, 96, 16–9.
[306] Rokhlin LL. Magnesium Alloys Containing Rare Earth Metals: Structure and Properties. Taylor & Francis, London, 2003, pp. 97–99.
[307] Ogawa Y, Sutou Y, Ando D, Koike J. Aging precipitation kinetics of Mg-Sc alloy with bcc+hcp two-phase. Journal of Alloys and Compounds. 2018, 747, 853–60.
[308] Hiragi T, Tsuchiya T, Lee S, Ikeno S, Matsuda K. Precipitates structure analysis of Mg-Y-Sc alloy by HRTEM. Microscopy 2018, 67; https://doi.org/10.1093/jmicro/dfy108.
[309] Fu H, Peng Q, Guo J, Liu B, Wu W. High-pressure synthesis of a nanoscale YB12 strengthening precipitate in Mg–Y alloys. Scripta Materialia. 2014, 76, 33–6.
[310] Barucca G, Ferragut R, Fiori F, Lussana D, Riontiono G. Formation and evolution of the hardening precipitates in a Mg–Y–Nd alloy. Acta Materialia. 2011, 59, 4151–8.
[311] Xin R, Song B, Zeng K, Huang G, Liu Q. Effect of aging precipitation on mechanical anisotropy of an extruded Mg–Y–Nd alloy. Materials & Design. 2012, 34, 384–8.
[312] Long Z et al. Improving the anisotropy of rolled Mg–3Al–1Zn alloy by pre-strain and annealing. Materials Science and Engineering: A. 2014, 616, 240–5.
[313] Mishra SK et al. Texture evolution during annealing of AZ31 Mg alloy rolled sheet and its effect on ductility. Materials Science and Engineering: A. 2014, 599, 1–8.
[314] Jiang Y et al. Recrystallization and texture evolution of cold-rolled AZ31 Mg alloy treated by rapid thermal annealing. Journal of Alloys and Compounds. 2016, 656, 272–7.
[315] Zhang H et al. Improved formability of Mg–3Al–1Zn alloy by pre-stretching and annealing. Scripta Materialia. 2012, 67, 495–8.
[316] Guo F et al. Obtaining high strength and high plasticity in a Mg-3Al-1Zn plate using pre-tension and annealing treatments. Journal of Alloys and Compounds. 2017, 704, 406–12.
[317] Li J et al. Effect of Annealing Process on Microstructure and Properties of Roll-Casting AZ31B Mg Alloy Sheet. Procedia Engineering. 2012, 27, 895–902.
[318] Su CW et al. Mechanical behaviour and texture of annealed AZ31 Mg alloy deformed by ECAP. Journal of Mater Sci and Technology. 2007, 23, 290–6.
[319] Wang B et al. Deformation and fracture mechanisms of an annealing-tailored “bimodal” grain-structured Mg alloy. Journal of Materials Science & Technology. 2019, 35, 2423–9.
[320] Xu X-Y et al. Influences of pre-existing Mg17Al12 particles on static recrystallization behavior of Mg-Al-Zn alloys at different annealing temperatures. Journal of Alloys and Compounds. 2019, 787, 1104–9.
[321] Afifi MA et al. Characterization of precipitates in an Al-Zn-Mg alloy processed by ECAP and subsequent annealing. Materials Science and Engineering: A. 2018, 712, 146–56.
[322] Abouhilou F et al. Microstructure and texture evolution of AZ31 Mg alloy after uniaxial compression and annealing. Journal of Magnesium and Alloys. 2019, 7, 124–33.
[323] Xin Y et al. Annealing hardening in detwinning deformation of Mg–3Al–1Zn alloy. Materials Science and Engineering: A. 2014, 594, 287–91.
[324] Liao C et al. Hot deformation behavior and flow stress modeling of annealed AZ61 Mg alloys. Progress in Natural Science: Materials International. 2014, 24, 253–65.
[325] Pérez-Prado MT et al. Texture evolution during grain growth in annealed Mg AZ61 alloy. Scripta Materialia. 2003, 48, 59–64.
[326] Ramezani M. Influence of heat treatment techniques on hot formability of AZ61 magnesium alloy. AIP Conference Proceedings. 2017, 1846; https://doi.org/10.1063/1.4983605
[327] Sułkowski B. Structure and properties of hot-rolled and annealed AZ61 Magnesium alloy. Metallurgy and Foundry Engineering. 2017, 43; https://doi.org/10.7494/mafe.2017.43.1.21.
[328] Sułkowski C et al. Deformation behavior of AZ61 magnesium alloy systematically rolled and annealed at 450°C. Kovove Materials. 2016, 54, 147–151.

[329] Yang M-B et al. Effects of solution heat treatment on microstructure and mechanical properties of AZ61-0.7Si magnesium alloy. Transactions of Nonferrous Metals Society of China. 2010, 20, s416–s420.
[330] Rusin NM. Effect of high-temperature annealing on the structure of cast magnesium alloy AM60 + 0.3% TiC. Metal Science and Heat Treatment. 2006, 48, 513–7.
[331] Braszczyńska-Malik KN et al. Microstructure of Mg-5Al-0.4Mn-xRE (x = 3 and 5 wt.%) alloys in as-cast conditions and after annealing. Journal of Alloys and Compounds. 2016, 663.
[332] Tian Y et al. Nanoscale icosahedral quasicrystal phase precipitation mechanism during annealing for Mg–Zn–Gd-based alloys. Materials Letters. 2014, 130, 236–9.
[333] Zeng ZR et al. Annealing strengthening in a dilute Mg–Zn–Ca sheet alloy. Scripta Materialia. 2015, 107, 127–30.
[334] Huang H et al. Precipitation of secondary phase in Mg-Zn-Gd alloy after room-temperature deformation and annealing. Journal of Materials Research and Technology. 2018, 7, 135–41.
[335] Min J et al. Forming limits of Mg alloy ZEK100 sheet in preform annealing process. Materials & Design. 2014, 53, 947–53.
[336] Wei S et al. Effects of Sn addition on the microstructure and mechanical properties of as-cast, rolled and annealed Mg–4Zn alloys. Materials Science and Engineering: A. 2013, 585, 139–48.
[337] Zhang J et al. Static recrystallization and grain growth during annealing of an extruded Mg–Zn–Zr–Er magnesium alloy. Journal of Magnesium and Alloys. 2013, 1, 31–8.
[338] Sha G et al. Effects of Sc Addition and Annealing Treatment on the Microstructure and Mechanical Properties of the As-rolled Mg-3Li alloy. Journal of Materials Science & Technology. 2011, 27, 753–8.
[339] Ruihong L et al. Microstructure and Mechanical Property Development in a Hot-rolled and Annealed Mg-5Li-1Al Alloy Sheet. Rare Metal Materials and Engineering. 2018, 47, 3640–4.
[340] Tang Y et al. Precipitation evolution during annealing of Mg-Li alloys. Materials Science and Engineering: A. 2017, 689, 332–44.
[341] Pugazhendhi BS et al. Effect of aluminium on microstructure, mechanical property and texture evolution of dual phase Mg-8Li alloy in different processing conditions. Archives of Civil and Mechanical Engineering. 2018, 18, 1332–44.
[342] Tang Y et al. Influences of warm rolling and annealing processes on microstructure and mechanical properties of three parent structures containing Mg-Li alloys. Materials Science and Engineering: A. 2018, 711, 1–11.
[343] Yin J et al. Hydrogen-Storage Properties and Structure Characterization of Melt-Spun and Annealed Mg-Ni-Nd Alloy. Materials Transactons. 2002, 43, 417–20.
[344] Lentz M et al. Macro- and microtexture evolution of an extruded Mg–Mn–Ce alloy during annealing. Materials Science and Engineering: A. 2016, 655, 17–26.
[345] Wu WX et al. Grain growth and texture evolution during annealing in an indirect-extruded Mg–1Gd alloy. Journal of Alloys and Compounds. 2014, 585, 111–9.
[346] Yang Y et al. Annealing behavior of a cast Mg-Gd-Y-Zr alloy with necklace fine grains developed under hot deformation. Materials Science and Engineering: A. 2017, 688, 280–8.
[347] Wu Y-P et al. Microstructure, texture and mechanical properties of Mg–8Gd–4Y–1Nd–0.5Zr alloy prepared by pre-deformation annealing, hot compression and ageing. Transactions of Nonferrous Metals Society of China. 2019, 29, 976–83.
[348] Li L et al. Effect of Static Annealing on Microstructure and Texture in Extruded Mg-Gd-Y-Zr Alloy. Rare Metal Materials and Engineering. 2016, 45, 2263–8.
[349] Chen J et al. Annealing strengthening of pre-deformed Mg–10Gd–3Y–0.3Zr alloy. Journal of Alloys and Compounds. 2015, 642, 92–7.

[350] Yu Z et al. Effects of pre-annealing on microstructure and mechanical properties of as-extruded Mg-Gd-Y-Zn-Zr alloy. Journal of Alloys and Compounds. 2017, 729, 627–37.
[351] Huang GH et al. Microstructure, texture and mechanical properties evolution of extruded fine-grained Mg-Y sheets during annealing. Materials Science and Engineering: A. 2018, 720, 24–35.
[352] Liu H et al. Comparative studies on evolution behaviors of 14H LPSO precipitates in as-cast and as-extruded Mg–Y–Zn alloys during annealing at 773K. Materials & Design. 2016, 93, 9–18.
[353] Sun L et al. Effect of annealing on the microstructures and properties of cold drawn Mg alloy wires. Materials Science and Engineering: A. 2015, 645, 181–7.
[354] Silva CJ et al. Grain growth kinetics and annealed texture characteristics of Mg-Sc binary alloys. Journal of Alloys and Compounds. 2016, 687, 548–61.
[355] Liu S et al. Effects of intermediate annealing on twin evolution in twin-structured Mg-Nd alloys. Journal of Alloys and Compounds. 2018, 763, 11–7.
[356] Kràllics G, Horváth M, Nyirő J. Forming and machining of the nano-crystalline alloys. Second International Conference on Multi-Material Micro Manufacture 2006, 175–8.
[357] Munitz A, Ricker RE, Pitchure DJ, Kimmel G. The influence of thermomechanical treatment on the complex modulus of Mg alloy AZ31. Metallurgical and Materials Transactions. A 2005, 36, 2403–13.
[358] Chang SY, Lee KS, Lee SH, Hong SK, Park KT, Shin DH. Effect of Al content and pressing temperature on ECAP of cast Mg alloys. Material Sciemce Forum. 2003, 419/422, 491–6.
[359] Mukai T, Yamanoi M, Watanabe H, Higashi K. Ductility enhancement in AZ31 magnesium alloy by controlling its grain structure. Scripta Materialia. 2001, 45, 89–94.
[360] Kim WJ, Hong SI, Kim YS, Min SH, Jeong HT, Lee JD. Texture development and its effect on mechanical properties of an AZ61 Mg alloy fabricated by equal channel angular pressing. Acta Materialia. 2003, 51, 3293–307.
[361] Jafari H, Idris MH, Ourdjini A, Payganeh G. Effect of thermomechanical treatment on microstructure and hardness behavior of AZ63 magnesium alloy. Acta Metallurgica Sinica (English Letters). 2009, 22, 401–7.
[362] Müller J, Janeček M, Wagner L. Influence of post-ECAP TMT on mechanical properties of the wrought magnesium alloy AZ80. Material Science Forum. 2008, 584/586, 858–63.
[363] Dobroň P, Drozdenko D, Olejňák J, Hegedüs M, Letzig D. Compressive yield stress improvement using thermomechanical treatment of extruded Mg-Zn-Ca alloy. Materials Science and Engineering: A. 2018, 730, 401–9.
[364] Dobroň P, Hegedüs M, Olejňák J, Drozdenko D, Horváth K, Bohlen J. Influence of Thermomechanical Treatment on Tension–Compression Yield Asymmetry of Extruded Mg–Zn–Ca Alloy. In: Joshi V. et al., ed., Magnesium Technology 2019. The Minerals, Metals & Materials Series. Springer, 2019, 77–81.
[365] Mingler B, Kulyasova O, Islamgaliev RK, Korb G, Karnthaler HP, Zehetbauer MJ. DSC and TEM analysis of lattice defects governing the mechanical properties of an ECAP-processed magnesium alloy. Journal of Material Science. 2007, 42, 1477–82.
[366] Tang C, Wang X, Liu W, Feng D, Li Q. Effects of thermomechanical processing on the microstructure, texture and mechanical properties of a Mg-Gd-based alloy. Materials Science and Engineering: A. 2019, 759, 172–80.
[367] Li D-J, Zeng X-Q, Xie Y-C, Wu Y-J, Chen B. Mechanical properties of Mg-6Gd-1Y-0.5Zr alloy processed by low temperature thermo-mechanical treatment. Transactions of Nonferrous Metals Society of China. 2012, 22, 2351–6.

[368] Zhang L, Gong M, Peng LM. Microstructure and strengthening mechanism of a thermomechanically treated Mg–10Gd–3Y–1Sn–0.5Zr alloy. Materials Science and Engineering: A. 2013, 565, 262–8.
[369] Yu Z, Huang Y, Qiu X, Wang G, Meng J. Fabrication of a high strength Mg–11Gd–4.5Y–1Nd–1.5Zn–0.5Zr (wt%) alloy by thermomechanical treatments. Materials Science and Engineering: A. 2015, 622, 121–30.
[370] Kumar V, Govind, Shekhar R, Balasubramaniam R, Balani K. Microstructure evolution and texture development in thermomechanically processed Mg–Li–Al based alloy. Materials Science and Engineering: A. 2012, 547, 38–50.
[371] Ding H-B, Liu Q, Zhou H-T, Zhou X, Atrens A. Effect of thermal-mechanical processing on microstructure and mechanical properties of duplex-phase Mg-8Li-3Al-0.4Y alloy. Transactions of Nonferrous Metals Society of China. 2017, 27, 2587–97.
[372] Luo X, Fang D, Li Q, Chai Y. Microstructure and mechanical properties of an Mg-4.0Sm-1.0Ca alloy during thermomechanical treatment. Journal of Rare Earths. 2016, 34, 1134–8.
[373] Wang J, Shi N, Wang L, Cao Z, Li J. Effect of zinc and mischmetal on microstructure and mechanical properties of Mg-Al-Mn alloy. Journal of Rare Earths. 2010, 28, 794–7.
[374] Hu T, Wang FM, Zheng R, Xiao W, Ma C. Effects of B and Sn additions on the microstructure and mechanical property of Mg-3Al-1Si alloy. Journal of Alloys and Compounds. 2019, 796, 1–8.
[375] Go Y, Jo SM, Park SH, Kim HS, Kim YM. Microstructure and mechanical properties of non-flammable Mg-8Al-0.3Zn-0.1Mn-0.3Ca-0.2Y alloy subjected to low-temperature, low-speed extrusion. Journal of Alloys and Compounds. 2018, 739, 69–76.
[376] Guan K, Meng F, Qin P, Yang Q, Meng J. Effects of samarium content on microstructure and mechanical properties of Mg–0.5Zn–0.5Zr alloy. Journal of Materials Science & Technology. 2019, 35, 1368–77.
[377] Cai S, Lei T, Li N, Feng F. Effects of Zn on microstructure, mechanical properties and corrosion behavior of Mg–Zn alloys. Materials Science and Engineering: C. 2012, 32, 2570–7.
[378] Du Y, Jiang B, Ge Y. Effects of precipitates on microstructure evolution and texture in Mg-Zn alloy during hot deformation. Vacuum. 2018, 148, 27–32.
[379] Guan K, Li B, Yang Q, Qiu X, Meng J. Effects of 1.5 wt% samarium (Sm) addition on microstructures and tensile properties of a Mg–6.0Zn–0.5Zr alloy. Journal of Alloys and Compounds. 2018, 735, 1737–49.
[380] Sun Y, Wang R, Ren J, Peng C, Cai Z. Microstructure, texture, and mechanical properties of as-extruded Mg-xLi-3Al-2Zn-0.2Zr alloys (x = 5, 7, 8, 9, 11 wt%). Materials Science and Engineering: A. 2019, 755, 201–10.
[381] Nene SS, Kashyap BP, Prabhu N, Estrin Y, Al-Samman T. Microstructure refinement and its effect on specific strength and bio-corrosion resistance in ultralight Mg–4Li–1Ca (LC41) alloy by hot rolling. Journal of Alloys and Compounds. 2014, 615, 501–6.
[382] Sun Y, Wang R, Peng C, Feng Y. Effects of Sn and Y on the microstructure, texture, and mechanical properties of as-extruded Mg-5Li-3Al-2Zn alloy. Materials Science and Engineering: A. 2018, 733, 429–39.
[383] Kim WJ, Hong SI, Kim YH. Enhancement of the strain hardening ability in ultrafine grained Mg alloys with high strength. Scripta Materialia. 2012, 67, 689–92.
[384] Ning J, Xu B, Sun MS, Zhao C, Tong W. Strain hardening and tensile behaviors of gradient structure Mg alloys with different orientation relationships. Materials Science and Engineering: A. 2018, 735, 275–87.
[385] Meng X, Duan M, Luo L, Zhan D, Lu J. The deformation behavior of AZ31 Mg alloy with surface mechanical attrition treatment. Materials Science and Engineering: A. 2017, 707, 636–46.

[386] Zhang D, Zhang D, Bu F, Li X, Meng J. Excellent ductility and strong work hardening effect of as-cast Mg-Zn-Zr-Yb alloy at room temperature. Journal of Alloys and Compounds. 2017, 728, 404–12.

[387] Shou H, Zheng J, Zhang Y, Long D, Liu Q. Quasi-in-situ analysis of dependency of deformation mechanism and work-hardening behavior on texture in Mg-2Zn-0.1Ca alloy. Journal of Alloys and Compounds. 2019, 784, 1187–97.

[388] Zhao C, Chen X, Pan F, Wang J, Atrens A. Strain hardening of as-extruded Mg-xZn (x = 1, 2, 3 and 4 wt%) alloys. Journal of Materials Science & Technology. 2019, 35, 142–50.

[389] Tahreen N, Zhang DF, Pan FS, Jiang XQ, Chen DL. Influence of yttrium content on phase formation and strain hardening behavior of Mg–Zn–Mn magnesium alloy. Journal of Alloys and Compounds. 2014, 615, 424–32.

[390] Chen X, Pan F, Mao J, Wang J, Peng J. Effect of heat treatment on strain hardening of ZK60 Mg alloy. Materials & Design. 2011, 32, 1526–30.

[391] Shiraishi K, Mayama T, Yamasaki M, Kawamura Y. Strain-hardening behavior and microstructure development in polycrystalline as-cast Mg-Zn-Y alloys with LPSO phase subjected to cyclic loading. Materials Science and Engineering: A. 2016, 672, 49–58.

[392] Kwak TY, Kim WJ. The effect of volume fraction and dispersion of icosahedral phase particles on the strength and work hardening of Mg-Zn-Y alloys. Materials Science and Engineering: A. 2017, 684, 284–91.

[393] Huo Q, Ando D, Sutou Y, Koike J. Stress-strain hysteresis and strain hardening during cyclic tensile test of Mg-0.6at%Y alloy. Materials Science and Engineering: A. 2016, 678, 235–42.

[394] Kula A, Jia X, Mishra RK, Niewczas M. Flow stress and work hardening of Mg-Y alloys. International Journal of Plasticity. 2017, 92, 96–121.

[395] Yang JY, Kim WJ. Effect of I(Mg3YZn6)-, W(Mg3Y2Zn3)- and LPSO(Mg12ZnY)-phases on tensile work-hardening and fracture behaviors of rolled Mg–Y–Zn alloys. Journal of Materials Research and Technology. 2019, 8, 2316–25.

[396] Zheng X, Du W, Wang Z, Li S, Du X. Remarkably enhanced mechanical properties of Mg-8Gd-1Er-0.5Zr alloy on the route of extrusion, rolling and aging. Materials Letters. 2018, 212, 155–8.

[397] Peng T, Wang Q, Han Y, Zheng J, Guo W. Microstructure and high tensile strength of Mg–10Gd–2Y–0.5Zr alloy by solid-state recycling. Materials Science and Engineering: A. 2010, 528, 715–20.

[398] Liao H, Kim J, Liu T, Tang A, Pan F. Effects of Mn addition on the microstructures, mechanical properties and work-hardening of Mg-1Sn alloy. Materials Science and Engineering: A. 2109, 754, 778–85.

[399] Zhao C, Chen X, Pan F, Gao S, Liu X. Effect of Sn content on strain hardening behavior of as-extruded Mg-Sn alloys. Materials Science and Engineering: A. 2018, 713, 244–52.

[400] Jiang J, Bi G, Wang G, Jiang Q, Jiang Z. Strain-hardening and warm deformation behaviors of extruded Mg–Sn–Yb alloy sheet. Journal of Magnesium and Alloys. 2014, 2, 116–23.

Chapter 9
Formability

To facilitate the wider application of wrought Mg alloys as structural materials, there are several obstacles, including (i) Mg is inherently plastically anisotropic due to low symmetry of their hexagonal close-packed structure, (ii) poor formability at low temperatures due to their strong basal texture and a lack of adequate deformation systems and (iii) poor resistance against the strain localization and failure. Hence, there are extensive researches conducted for improving the formability and for reducing the plastic anisotropy.

9.1 Forming limit diagram

The formability can be simply defined as the ability of a given metal workpiece to undergo plastic deforming processes (such as rolling, extrusion, forging, roll forming, stamping or hydroforming) without fracture, and the plastic deformation capacity of metallic materials, however, is limited to a certain extent, at which point, the material could fracture. The formability of different materials varies depending on the stress conditions, which lead to strain forming. The determination of the forming limit can be measured by different methods. In dependence on the stress conditions and the material, Figure 9.1(b) shows the forming limit diagram (FLD) [1], depicting the forming zones of deep drawing, uniaxial tensile, plane strain and stretch forming. The diagram attempts to provide a graphical description of material failure tests. In

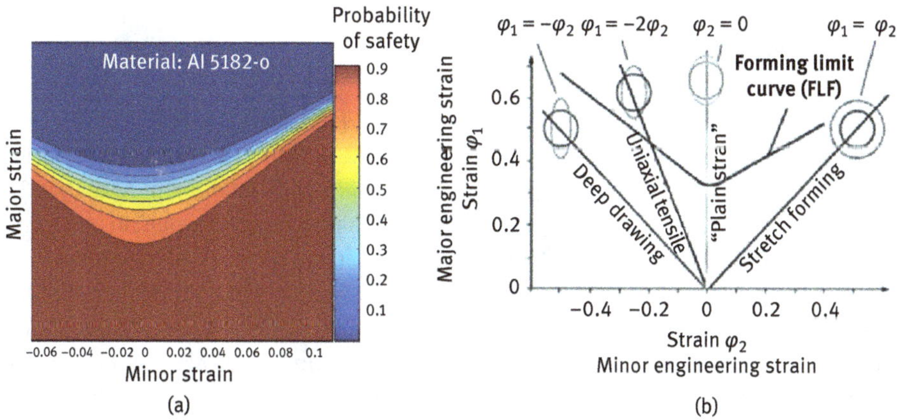

Figure 9.1: Schematic illustration of the forming limit diagram: (a) probability of safety and (b) FLD for various strain conditions.

https://doi.org/10.1515/9783110676945-009

order to determine whether a given region has failed, a mechanical test is performed by placing a circular mark on the work piece prior to deformation, and then measuring the postdeformation ellipse that is generated from the action on this circle. By repeating the mechanical test to generate a range of stress states, the formability limit diagram can be generated as a line at which failure is onset (as a probability of safety or unfractured, shown in Figure 9.1(a) [2]). The lowest formability for sheet metal takes place under plane strain conditions. Figure 9.2 shows FLDs of various materials [3] and Mg–3Al–1Zn (AZ31) alloy [4].

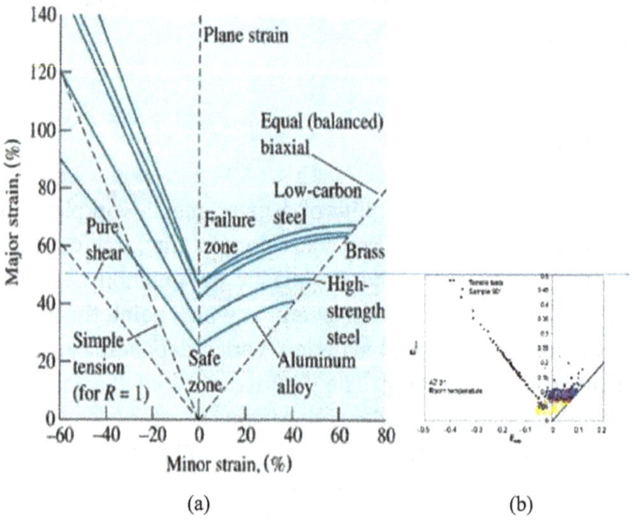

Figure 9.2: Practical FLDs of various materials (a) and AZ31 alloy (b).

9.2 Formability

Formability is affected by metallurgical parameters (such as grain size, alloying elements and heat treatment), physical metallurgy (such as twins) and deformation factor (such as textures) [5]. Lim et al. [6] investigated the effects of addition of Al and/or Zn in Mg–MM (misch metal)–Sn alloy and its effect on microstructural evolution and formability. It was found that Mg-2MM-2Sn-1Zn annealed at 200 °C improves the formability. Studying the influence of Ca and Gd that are microalloyed to hot-rolled Mg–3Al alloy, Jiang et al. [7] found that (i) the combined addition of microalloying Ca and Gd element significantly attenuates basal texture and improves refinement of grain size and room-temperature formability of Mg–3Al alloy (when annealed at 350 °C × 1 h), due to the delayed recrystallization behavior because of the secondary phase, and (ii) combined addition reduces the anisotropy of mechanical property. Zeng et al. [8] found that by adding Sn to pure Mg, (i) the τ_{max} (critical shear strength) in basal slip increased from 114 to 149 MPa, while that in pyramidal slip decreased from 1,571 to 446 MPa and (ii) the decreased τ_{max} ratio of the pyramidal slip to the basal slip might make the pyramidal slip systems more likely to be activated, leading to an improvement in the formability of Mg–Sn alloys. Nie et al. [9] developed a novel TiC_p/Mg–4Zn–0.5Ca nanocomposite by using the ultrasonic-assisted semisolid stirring method, and then extruded at the speed of 0.01 mm/s with low extrusion temperatures of 270, 230 and 190 °C, respectively, and mentioned that the addition of TiC nanoparticles could act as nucleation sites for the recrystallization, and thus coordinating the deformation of matrix, leading to improved low temperature formability. Park et al. [10] investigated formability and viscoplastic self-consistent simulations of Mg-4Zn-X-Ca alloys in an effort to understand the relationship between deformation behaviors and room-temperature formability and reported that (i) Mg-4Zn-X-Ca alloys showed a sound twin-roll cast microstructure without the occurrence of inverse segregation and (ii) among the Mg-4Zn-X-Ca alloys, the ZAX400 alloy exhibited a high yield strength value of 189.3 MPa and excellent formability of 7.5 mm (Erichsen index value) with enhanced yield isotropy, comparable to those of Al alloys. The Erichsen index indicates forming quality of sheet metal. As shown in Figure 9.3 [11], test is conducted by supporting the sheet on a circular ring and deforming it at the center of the

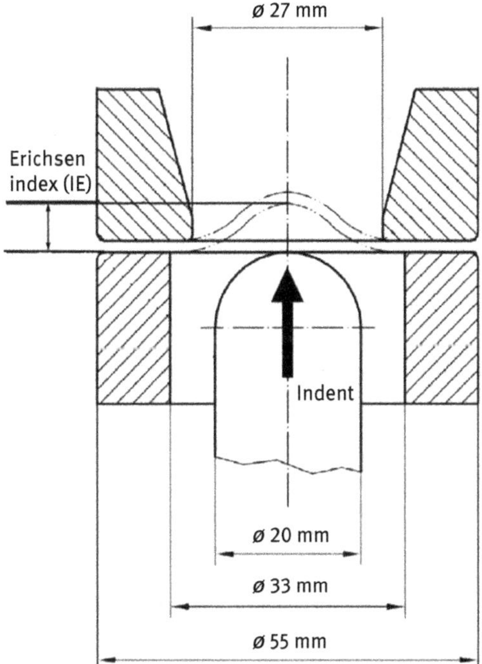

Figure 9.3: Sheet metal forming test to measure the Erichsen index value [11].

ring by a spherical pointed tool and the depth of impression (or cup) in mm required to obtain fracture is defined as the Erichsen index value for the metal. It is obvious that the higher (larger) the value of the Erichsen index the better the (room temperature) formability. Bian et al. [12] mentioned that (i) a newly developed magnesium sheet alloy Mg-1.1Al-0.3Ca-0.2Mn-0.3Zn (at%) shows a large index Erichsen value of 7.7 mm in a solution-treated (T4) condition due to a weak basal texture developed by the trace addition of Zn and (ii) subsequent artificial aging at 200 °C for 1 h (T6) significantly increases the 0.2% proof strength from 144 to 204 MPa, due to a dense distribution of monoatomic layer Guinier–Preston zones on the basal planes of the Mg matrix. Jiang et al. [13] added Al–5Ti–1B master alloy to Mg–14Li–1Al (LA141) alloy, which is later subjected to extrusion and cold rolling to prepare sheets. It was reported that (i) the optimal addition level of Al–5Ti–1B master alloy into LA141 alloy is 1.25% (mass fraction) and LA141 alloy has the finest grains, (ii) with the increase of the total reduction of cold rolling, the grains of the as-rolled LA141 sheets were flattened gradually, (iii) a proper anneal temperature of 200 °C is obtained for the cold-rolled LA141 sheets and (iv) under this condition, microstructure of the LA141 sheets consists of fine and uniform equiaxed grains and has higher Erichsen index value. Chen et al. [14] forward extruded as-cast Mg-Zn-Y-Zr alloy and mentioned that (i) the alloy exhibits an excellent workability at aging temperatures from 250 to 400 °C with a extrusion rate of 10 mm/s and (ii) temperatures higher than 400 °C are not suitable for forming the alloy because of heavy oxidation.

Since extruded or rolled wrought magnesium alloy sheets usually exhibit strong basal texture, which greatly degrades their mechanical performance, He et al. [15] applied a novel texture modification process based on employing in-plane precompression, prestretching and annealing to an extruded Mg–3Al–1Zn (AZ31) sheet to introduce an orthogonal four-peak distribution of basal texture. It was reported that (i) such an orthogonal four-peak texture could provide larger and more balanced Schmid factors for basal slip compared with that of the as-extruded sheet when the sheets were subjected to tension along different directions; (ii) the tensile yield strength was decreased and the ductility was increased effectively, suggesting a considerable improvement in uniaxial deformation ability; (iii) the orthogonal four-peak texture could also provide more balanced mechanical properties along different directions and contribute to reducing the planar anisotropy; and (iv) the Erichsen index value of the sample with orthogonal four-peak texture increased up to ~115% compared with that of the as-extruded sheet, indicating that such a texture modification method was also highly conducive to enhancing the multiaxial stretch formability of the Mg sheets. Zhang et al. [16] conducted the similar technique of prestretching and annealing to modify the microstructure of Mg–3Al–1Zn (AZ31) alloy to enhance its formability and found that the thus-treated specimens exhibited lower basal texture intensities and coarser grain sizes and their Erichsen index values were increased up to 65% compared with the as-received sheet.

Wang et al. [17] investigated residual stress relaxation and the texture evolution of cold-rolled AZ31 Mg alloys using the vibratory stress relief technique with a simple cantilever beam vibration system and found that the vibratory stress relief process for the vibrational aging time of more than 10 min is able to weaken the strong basal textures of AZ31 Mg alloys, leading to the improvement of formability. Gao et al. [18] developed a high-ductility ZME200 (Mg-2.3Zn-0.4Mn-0.2Ce) alloy for vehicle closure and structure applications, based on an earlier ZE20 (Mg–2.0Zn–0.2Ce) alloy for extrusion applications, and mentioned that (i) the hot deformation behavior of as-cast ZME200 alloy varies with processing parameters, namely temperature and strain rate, (ii) the ZME200 alloy sheet exhibits extraordinarily higher ductility (36% in tensile elongation), much superior stretch formability (an Erichsen index value of 9.5 mm), (iii) lower anisotropy, comparable strength and corrosion resistance to AZ31 alloy and (iv) the unique rolling direction–transverse direction (TD) double split texture with remarkably reduced intensity and grain refinement give rise to the significantly improved ductility and formability at room temperature. Nie et al. [19] mentioned that multipass hot rolling can help overcome the poor formability of high-strength Mg–8Gd–3Y alloys at the temperature range of 350–450 °C with a strain rate range of 0.001–0.1/s. It was reported that (i) two kinds of hardening behavior characterized by higher second-pass peak stress than the first-pass unloading stress are discovered; one is caused by precipitation that occurs during holding at a temperature range of 350–400 °C under a strain rate of 0.1/s and the other is grain-growth-induced hardening and takes place at 450 °C with a strain rate range of 0.01–0.1/s and (ii) based on the dynamic material model, three-dimensional power dissipation and instability maps were established, corroborating improved formability under double-pass isothermal compression.

9.3 Stretch formability

Stretch forming is a metal forming process in which a piece of sheet metal is stretched and bent simultaneously over a die in order to form large contoured parts. There are several metallurgical routes for improving the stretch formability of Mg alloys. Somekawa et al. [20] investigated the effect of alloying elements on room-temperature stretch formability and its deformation mechanism using pure magnesium and its binary alloys containing an element of Ag, Al, Ca, Li, Mn, Pb, Sn, Y and Zn. It was found that (i) alloying elements clearly affected stretch formability as measured by Erichsen testing, (ii) the addition of Mn or Y element played a role in improving formability; on the other hand, most of the alloying elements did not improve formability, as exhibited by their limited dome height values, which were similar to or lower than that of pure magnesium, (iii) an intragranular misorientation axis analysis using electron back-scatter diffraction results revealed that the Mg–Y alloy had a high fraction of grains amenable to nonbasal dislocation slips, which is a helpful deformation mode for improving formability; in contrast, pure magnesium and the Mg–Mn alloy, which had a high limited dome height, did not have a high fraction of such grains and (iv) grain boundary sliding compensated for the lack of <**c**>-component, such as activating nonbasal dislocation slips.

Yuasa et al. [21] studied the effects of group II elements (Ca, Sr or Ba) on Mg–Zn-based alloys on tensile and Erichsen behavior tests on cold stretch formability. It was mentioned that (i) the flow stresses of the Mg–Zn–X (Ca, Sr or Ba) alloys were lower than that of the Mg–Zn alloy, (ii) the addition of Ca, Sr or Ba enhanced the stretch formability of Mg–Zn alloys and the effectiveness for this enhanced stretch formability increased in order of decreasing atomic number of the group II elements and (iii) the stretch formability of Mg alloys is suggested to be related not only to thermally activated dislocation processes but also to athermally activated processes. Wang et al. [22] developed a new Mg–0.4Sn–0.7Y (TW00) (wt%) alloy sheet and indicated that the TW00 alloy exhibited a good balance of the ductility and stretch formability at room temperature via extrusion or hot rolling–annealing. Bian et al. [23] rolled Mg-1.2Al-0.3Ca-0.4Mn-0.3Zn (AXMZ1000) (wt%) alloy in three different conditions and studied the effects of the rolling conditions on the microstructure and mechanical properties. It was reported that (i) the sheet subjected to high-temperature reheating at 500 °C for 5 min prior to each 100 °C rolling delivers the highest Erichsen index value of 7.0 mm, (ii) the sheet rolled at 300 °C with 500 °C reheating for 5 min delivers the lowest Erichsen index of 5.4 mm, while the sheet continuously rolled at the same temperature shows a moderate value of 6.0 mm and (iii) systematic observations of the microstructures of T4-treated (with 3mm-streching) samples reveal that the large stretch formability of the sheet rolled at 100 °C with 500 °C reheating is associated the weak basal texture and fine-grained microstructure.

The stretch formability can be improved by mechanical manipulations. For a purpose of tailoring the texture of Mg alloy, He et al. [24] introduced {10-12} tensile twins by in-plane compression in a thin magnesium alloy sheet. It was found that (i) the room-temperature stretch formability of the pretwinned Mg alloy sheet was remarkably improved by 50%, (ii) the activation of the tensile twinning in the pretwinned region, which can effectively accommodate the through-thickness strain during stretch forming, is assumed to be the main reason of stretch formability improvement and (iii) numerical simulation results demonstrate that multidirectional tensile twins induced by multistep compression are more beneficial to improve the formability of Mg alloy sheet, compared with unidirectional twins. Similarly, Song et al. [25] introduced {10-12} twinning for controlling the texture of wrought Mg alloys, particularly in rolled Mg alloy sheets, and mentioned that the micromechanism and impact factors of control in twin orientation, plastic processing techniques of preinducing twins and the application of preinduced twins all influence to an improvement of stretch formability. Mao et al. [26] found that the laser shock peening experiments enhanced the room temperature stretch formability of AZ31B Mg alloy sheet, due to an integrated texture weakening and grain refinement effect induced by the laser shock loading. It is generally believed that weakening or tilting basal texture is an effective way to improve stretch formability of Mg alloy sheets [26, 27]. Song et al. [27] introduced contraction twins (including double twins) in rolled AZ31 sheet by precold rolling to a thickness reduction of 10%. It was reported that (i) the stretch formability of rolled AZ31 sheet can be greatly enhanced by precold rolling and subsequent recrystallization annealing and (ii) the Erichsen index value of rolled AZ31 sheet was increased up to 66% by precold rolling and annealing at 400 °C, mainly due to the formation and growth of recrystallization grains with weak texture nucleated at contraction twins during annealing.

Shi et al. [28] developed a novel final-pass heavy reduction rolling (FHRR) approach and applied it on the as-cast ingots of Mg-1.1Zn-0.76Y-0.56Zr alloy. It was reported that (i) the as-annealed light-reduction rolling sheet exhibits a typical "TD-split" texture, whereas the as-annealed FHRR sheets reveal a unique "oblique-line-split" texture, with the basal poles tilted by about 50° from the normal direction (ND) toward some oblique line with respect to about 40° of TD and (ii) the stretch formability was improved. Meng et al. [29] modified the electromagnetic forming, which can improve the formability of metal sheets without the need for lubricants, combined with the warm forming, which is also believed to be effective to improve the stretch formability. It was reported that (i) the bulging height of Mg sheets increases with moderate discharging energies, (ii) enhancing the discharging voltage is also a more efficient method for increasing bulging height compared to simply increasing the capacity and (iii) when the discharging energy is kept constant, the bulging height first decreases (<150 °C) and then increases (>150 °C) from room temperature to 230 °C and the formability of Mg alloy sheets improves with increasing temperature, while the forming efficiency of the warm and electromagnetic forming decreases under similar conditions.

References

[1] Doege E, Hallfeld T. Doege E, Hallfeld T, Khalfalla Y, Benyounis KY. Metal Working: Stretching of Sheets. Encyclopedia of Materials: Science and Technology (Second Edition), 2001, pp.5518–21.

[2] https://en.wikipedia.org/wiki/Forming_limit_diagram.

[3] Askeland DR, Phulè PP. The Science and Engineering of Materials. 4th Ed., Thompson Brooks, 2003, p.321.

[4] Boissière R, Vacher P, Blandin JJ, Khelil A. Strain Capacities Limits of Wrought Magnesium Alloys: Tension vs. Expansion. Materials Science and Applications: Scientific Research. 2013, 768–72; DOI:10.4236/msa.2013.412097.

[5] Mohmed W, Gollapudi S, Charit I, Murty L. Formability of a wrought Mg alloy evaluated by impression testing. Materials Science and Engineering: A. 2018, 712, 140–5.

[6] Lim HK, Kim DH, Lee JY, Kim WT, Kim DH. Effects of alloying elements on microstructures and mechanical properties of wrought Mg–MM–Sn alloy. Journal of Alloys and Compounds. 2009, 468, 308–14.

[7] Jiang H, Zhang Y, Kang Q, Xu Z, Li H. The influence of Ca and Gd microalloying on microstructure and mechanical property of hot-rolled Mg-3Al alloy. Procedia Engineering. 2017, 207, 932–7.
[8] Zeng Y, Shi OL, Jiang B, Quan GF, Pan FS. Improved formability with theoretical critical shear strength transforming in Mg alloys with Sn addition. Journal of Alloys and Compounds. 2018, 764, 555–64.
[9] Nie K, Guo Y, Deng K, Kang X. High strength TiCp/Mg-Zn-Ca magnesium matrix nanocomposites with improved formability at low temperature. Journal of Alloys and Compounds. 2019, 792, 267–78.
[10] Park SJ, Jung HC, Shin KS. Deformation behaviors of twin roll cast Mg-Zn-X-Ca alloys for enhanced room-temperature formability. Materials Science and Engineering: A. 2017, 679, 329–39.
[11] Source FS, Ngo S, Lowe C, Taylor AC. Quantification of coating surface strains in Erichsen cupping tests. Journal of Materials Science. 2019, 54, 7997–8009.
[12] Bian MZ, Sasaki TT, Suh BC, Nakata T, Hono K. A heat-treatable Mg–Al–Ca–Mn–Zn sheet alloy with good room temperature formability. Scripta Materialia. 2017, 138, 151–5.
[13] Jiang B, Yin H-M, Li R-H, Gao L. Grain refinement and plastic formability of Mg-14Li-1Al alloy. Transactions of Nonferrous Metals Society of China. 2010, 20, s503–7.
[14] Chen Q, Lin J, Shu D, Hu C, Yuan B. Microstructure development, mechanical properties and formability of Mg–Zn–Y–Zr magnesium alloy. Materials Science and Engineering: A. 2012, 554, 129–41.
[15] He J, Mao Y, Fu Y, Jiang B, Pan F. Improving the room-temperature formability of Mg-3Al-1Zn alloy sheet by introducing an orthogonal four-peak texture. Journal of Alloys and Compounds. 2019, 797, 443–55.
[16] Zhang, Huang G, Wang L, Li J. Improved formability of Mg–3Al–1Zn alloy by pre-stretching and annealing. Scripta Materialia. 2012, 67, 495–8.
[17] Wang J-S, Hsieh C-C, Lai H-H, Kuo C-W, Wu W. The relationships between residual stress relaxation and texture development in AZ31 Mg alloys via the vibratory stress relief technique. Materials Characterization. 2015, 99, 248–53.
[18] Gao L, Yan H, Luo J, Luo AA, Chen R. Microstructure and mechanical properties of a high ductility Mg–Zn–Mn–Ce magnesium alloy. Journal of Magnesium and Alloys. 2013, 1, 283–91.
[19] Nie X, Dong S, Wang F, Jin L, Wang Y. Flow behavior and formability of hot-rolled Mg-8Gd-3Y alloy under double-pass isothermal compression. Journal of Materials Processing Technology. 2020, 275; https://doi.org/10.1016/j.jmatprotec.2019.116328.
[20] Somekawa H, Kinoshita A, Kato A. Effect of alloying elements on room temperature stretch formability in Mg alloys. Materials Science and Engineering: A. 2018, 732, 21–8.
[21] Yuasa M, Miyazawa N, Hayashi M, Mabuchi M, Chino Y. Effects of group II elements on the cold stretch formability of Mg–Zn alloys. Acta Materialia. 2015, 83, 294–303.
[22] Wang Q, Shen Y, Jiang B, Tang A, Pan F. A good balance between ductility and stretch formability of dilute M-Sn-Y sheet at room temperature. Materials Science and Engineering: A. 2018, 736, 404–16.
[23] Bian MZ, Sasaki TT, Nakata T, Kamado S, Hono. Effects of rolling conditions on the microstructure and mechanical properties in a Mg–Al–Ca–Mn–Zn alloy sheet. Materials Science and Engineering: A. 2018, 730, 147–54.
[24] He W, Zeng Q, Yu H, Zin Y, Liu Q. Improving the room temperature stretch formability of a Mg alloy thin sheet by pre-twinning. Materials Science and Engineering: A. 2016, 655, 1–8.
[25] Song B, Yang Q, Zhou Tm Chai L, Xin R. Texture control by {10-12} twinning to improve the formability of Mg alloys: A review. Journal of Materials Science & Technology. 2019, 35, 2269–82.

[26] Mao B, Li B, Lin D, Liao Y. Enhanced room temperature stretch formability of AZ31B magnesium alloy sheet by laser shock peening. Materials Science and Engineering: A. 2019, 756, 219–25.

[27] Song B, Xin R, Liao A, Yu, Liu Q. Enhancing stretch formability of rolled Mg sheets by pre-inducing contraction twins and recrystallization annealing. Materials Science and Engineering: A. 2015, 627, 369–73.

[28] Shi BQ, Xiao YH, Shang XL, Cheng YQ, Ke W. Achieving ultra-low planar anisotropy and high stretch formability in a Mg-1.1Zn-0.76Y-0.56Zr sheet by texture tailoring via final-pass heavy reduction rolling. Materials Science and Engineering: A. 2019, 746, 115–26.

[29] Meng Z, Huang S, Hu J, Huang W, Xia Z. Effects of process parameters on warm and electromagnetic hybrid forming of magnesium alloy sheets. Journal of Materials Processing Technology. 2011, 211, 863–7.

Chapter 10
Forming and product forms

There are four basic production processes for producing desired shape of a product: casting, machining, joining and deformation fabrication. For each of these, we discuss in different chapters the casting process (Chapter 6), machining process and machinability (Chapter 9) and joining process (Chapter 11), respectively. In this chapter, we discuss various methods of forming and show different product forms.

10.1 Forming

Deformation processes exploit a remarkable property of metals, which is their ability to flow plastically in the solid state without deterioration of their properties. With the application of suitable stresses, the material is moved to obtain the desired shape with almost no wastage. The required stresses are usually high (depending on the working temperature), and the forming tools and equipment needed are quite expensive. Large production quantities are often necessary to justify the process [1]. For production processes, depending on the type of forming technology, manufacturing engineers select one of five general categorized strategies; repetitive, discrete, job shop, process (batch) and process (continuous) [2] (as shown in Figure 10.1).

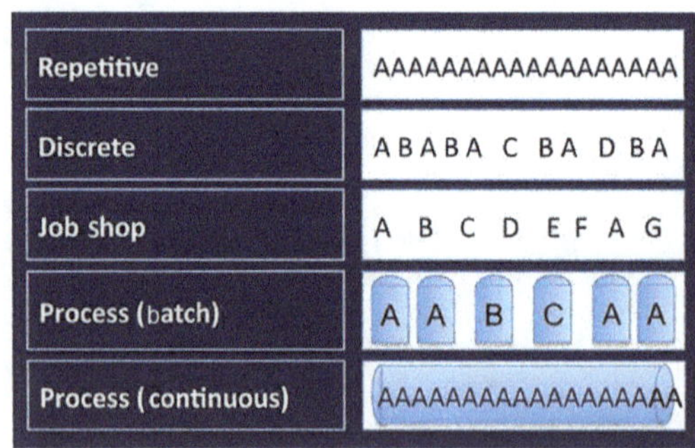

Figure 10.1: Five types of strategies for manufacturing processes [2].

10.1.1 In general

Before the detailed description for individual forming technologies, it will be worthy to look at several important and common parameters. There are normally three temperature-related forming methods, for example, hot rolling, warm rolling and

https://doi.org/10.1515/9783110676945-010

cold rolling. Table 10.1 compares among these three working in terms of major concerns on workpiece nature, working load, tool life and so on along with advantages and disadvantages [3–5].

Table 10.1: Comparison among cold working, warm working and hot working.

Cold working	Warm working	Hot working
In general		
It is generally performed at room temperature. In some cases, slightly elevated temperatures may be used to provide increased ductility and reduced strength. The primary advantage is the material savings achieved through precision shapes that require little finishing. Production rates are very high with exceptional die life	Compared with cold forging, warm forging has the potential advantages of reduced tooling loads, reduced forging press loads, increased metal ductility, elimination of need to anneal prior to forging and favorable as-forged properties that can eliminate heat treatment	Under the action of heat and force, when the atoms of a metal reach a certain higher energy level, the new crystals start forming. This is called recrystallization. When this happens, the old grain structure deformed by previously carried out mechanical working no longer exists, instead new crystals that are strain free are formed
Critical temperature		
Cold working is done at temperatures below the recrystallization temperature of the metal	Warm working is performed at temperature above room temperature but below the recrystallization temperature	Hot working is the process of plastically deforming a metal above the metal's recrystallization temperature
Residual stress buildup		
Internal and residual stresses buildup in the metal	Depending on the operation temperature	No internal and residual stresses buildup in the metal
Work piece		
Directional properties can be imparted and less ductility is available	Greater metal ductility	Greater ductility of material is available, and therefore, more deformation is possible
Recovery of the product		
No considerable metal recovery takes place in cold working	Normally, no considerable metal recovery	Deformation of the metal and its recovery occurs simultaneously in hot working

Table 10.1 (continued)

Cold working	Warm working	Hot working
Cracks		
Cracks propagate, and new cracks are formed in cold working	Depending on the operation temperature	Cracks or pores can be removed in hot working
Uniformity		
The uniformity of the metal is low after cold working	The uniformity is generally close to cold-worked piece	The uniformity of the metal is very high after hot working
Surface finish and dimensional stability		
Better surface finish and better dimensional control is achieved, so that no secondary machining is generally needed	Better dimensional control and surface finish	Poor surface finish of material due to scaling of surface and poor accuracy and dimensional control of parts
Tool loads		
Higher forces are required for deformation	Lesser loads on tooling and equipment	Lesser forces are required for deformation, so equipment of lesser power is needed
Tool life		
Higher tool life	Greater tool life due to lesser thermal shock and fatigue on tooling	Lower tool life
Strengthening effect		
Strain hardening is done without using heat, so that it may require intermediate annealing	Fewer number of annealing operation, due to less strain hardening	No strain hardening

Deformation processes (mostly stress mode, strain rate and operational temperature) exhibit great effects on mechanical and metallurgical properties of workpiece and at the same time deformation-processing parameters are influenced by characteristics of workpiece to be deformed. With the application of suitable pressures, the material is moved to obtain the desired shape with almost no wastage. Depending on final shape of work products and production strategy (see Figure 10.1), manners of stressing (tension, compression and shear) and combination thereof would be complicated. Figure 10.2 illustrates typical stress states for various forming modes [1].

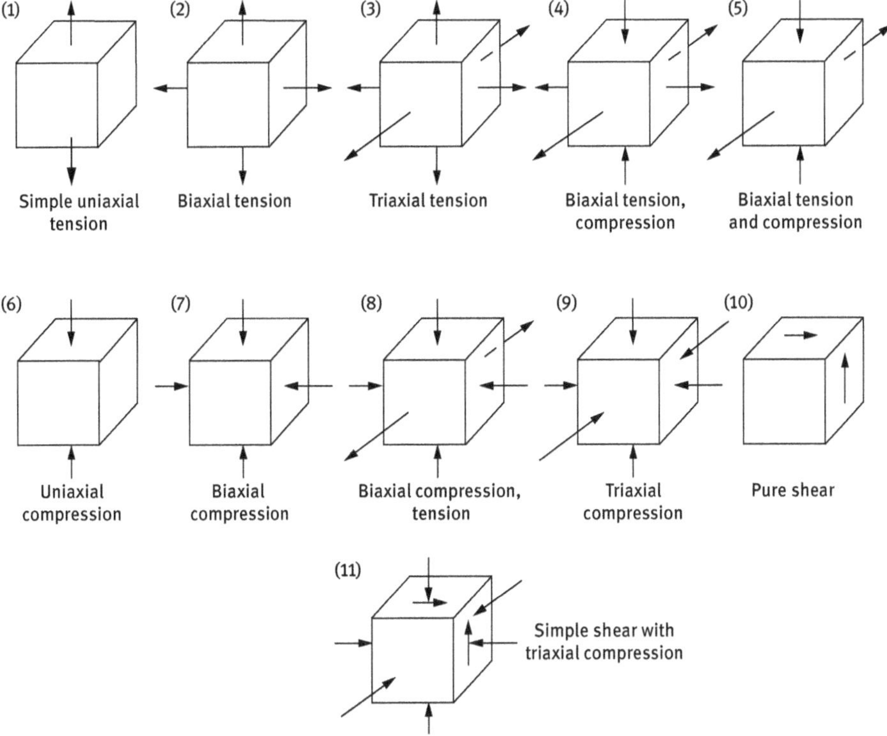

Figure 10.2: Basic state conditions of stressing workpiece during deformation [1].

It is well stated that there is an applicable difficulty associated with wrought magnesium alloys due to the limited low-temperature formability. This poor formability should be attributed to a combination of the limited number of active slip mechanisms (which is characteristic to hexagonal close-packed crystalline structure) and strong basal textures, resulting in strong deformation anisotropy and the brittle nature in mechanical behavior. Although there are several works on the alloying with rare (REs) earth elements that can activate nonbasal slip modes and simultaneously weaken texture, therefore improving the plasticity [6–8], deformation mechanism can be manipulated by rolling variants such as cross-rolling, twin-cast rolling and differential speed rolling to activate the nonbasal deformation mechanisms and weakened or randomized texture to lend magnesium allows more formability [9, 10].

10.1.2 Strain rate sensitivity

As mentioned in subsequent sections of this chapter, there are some studies on strain rate sensitivity of Mg materials that are subjected to various manufacturing methods. The yield criterion is assumed to be independent of the strain rate and can be predicted by von Mises yield criterion theory if the material shows isotropic stress–strain relationship. However, most of materials having variations in grain size and orientation exhibit anisotropic yielding when particularly subjected to a large deformation. For anisotropic yield criterion, there are, for example, Hill's quadratic yield criterion, generalized Hill yield criterion or Hosford yield criterion proposed. At the same time, the plastic flow of materials is sensitive to strain rate, which is known as the strain rate sensitivity (or viscoplasticity). In general, the complete constitutive equation for stress–strain relationship can be expressed by $\sigma = E \times e^n \times \acute{e}^m$, where σ represents stress, E the modulus of elasticity, e the strain, $\acute{e}$ the strain rate, n the strain (work)-hardening exponent and m the strain rate sensitivity exponent, respectively. If the exponent "m" exists, the exponent "n" is not present, and if "m" is unity, the flow is called a viscous flow. When the exponent "m" becomes meaningful during plastic deformation at elevated temperatures, it is characterized to be superplastic flow (see Chapter 15 for details). It is obviously important when the creep deformation is involved [11, 12].

The strain rate sensitivity depends on loading paths (e.g., tension and compression) [12] and operational temperature [13]. Magnesium alloys are strongly rate sensitive at both room and elevated temperatures. Anisotropy is shown to be important in modeling magnesium alloys, and advanced yield criteria with fits to directional variation in strength. Magnesium alloys also exhibit strong tension–compression asymmetry due to twinning under compression, mandating compressive characterization of sheet alloys, which can be difficult. Magnesium alloys also display significant yield surface evolution, which should be captured using advanced constitutive models [14]. Increasing the plastic deformation temperature of Mg alloys results in higher strain rate sensitivity, easier activation of secondary slip modes and impeded twinning [12, 15–20]. When the intergranular deformation becomes dominant, the ductility of an Mg alloy could be evaluated by measuring its average "m" value [21–23].

10.1.3 Bulk deformation processes

In this category, rolling forging and extrusion/drawing are classified (see Figure 10.3 [24]).

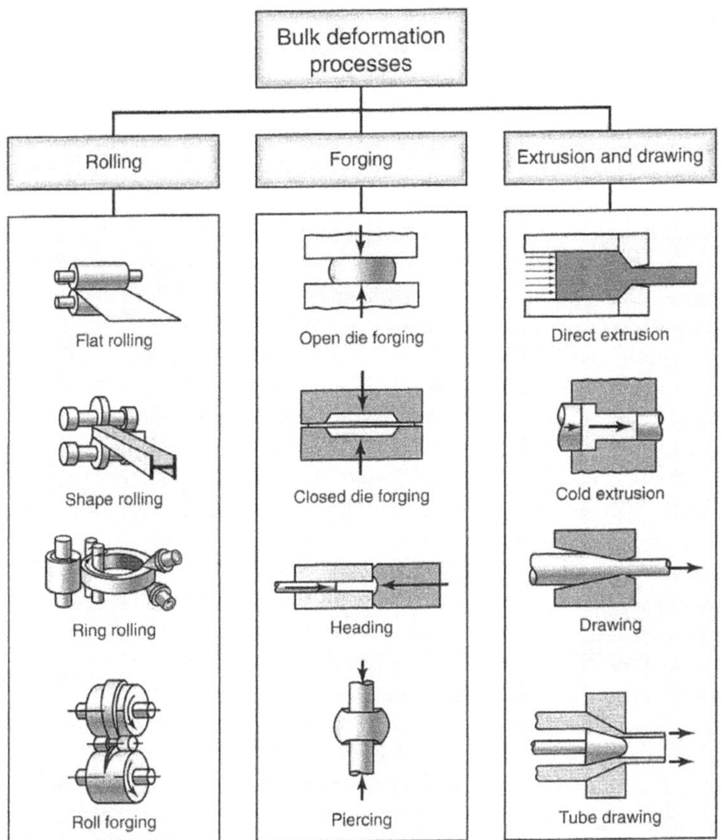

Figure 10.3: Typical bulk forming processes – rolling, forging and extrusion [24].

Table 10.2 lists typical Mg materials that are roll formed at cold, warm and hot temperature zones.

Table 10.2: Roll forming at three operational temperature zones.

	Rolling temperature		
	Cold	**Warm***	**Hot**
Mg–Al			[25, 26]
Mg–Al–Zn: AZ31	[27–45]	[46, 47]	[27, 48–62]
Mg–Al–Zn: AZ61	[63]		

Table 10.2 (continued)

	Rolling temperature		
	Cold	**Warm***	**Hot**
Mg–Al–Zn: AZ91	[64, 65]		[62, 66–68]
Mg–Al–Zn		[69]	
Mg-Al-Zn-Sn	[70]		[70]
Mg-Al-Zn-Mn	[71]		[71]
Mg–Al–Sn	[72, 73]	[74]	[74, 75]
Mg–Al–Ca			[76]
Mg–Al–Mn			[77]
Mg–Zn	[78–81]		[80]
Mg–Zn: ZK60	[82–84]		
Mg–Zn–Y	[85, 86]		[87]
Mg–Zn–Mn	[88]		[89]
Mg–Zn–Gd	[90–92]		[93–95]
Mg–Zn–Ca	[96]	[97]	[98]
Mg–Zn–Ce			[99, 100]
Mg–Zn–Zr			[101, 102]
Mg-Zn-Nd-Zr			[103]
Mg–Li	[104–108]	[109–112]	[109, 113, 114]
Mg–Li–Ca			[115, 116]
Mg-Li-Ca-Zn-Al			[117]
Mg–Ca	[118]		
Mg–Mn	[119]		
Mg–Y			[120, 121]
Mg-Y-Ni-Ti			[122]
Mg–Y–Zn	[123]		
Mg–Y–RE	[124]		
Mg–Gd			[125]
Mg–Gd–Zn	[126]		

Table 10.2 (continued)

	Rolling temperature		
	Cold	**Warm***	**Hot**
Mg–Gd–Y	[127]		[128, 129]
Mg-Gd-Y-Zn-Zr			[130–132]
Mg-Gd-Y-Zr			[133–136]
Mg–Sn–Mn	[137]		[138]
Mg–Sn–Zn			[139]
Mg–Nd			[140]
Mg–Nd–Zn			[141]
Mg–Hg–Ga			[142]

Note: RE, rare earth element; warm*, up to 200 °C.

Table 10.3 lists forged Mg materials at three different temperature zones.

Table 10.3: Forging at three operational temperature zones.

	Forging temperature		
	Cold	**Warm***	**Hot**
Mg–Al–Zn: AZ31	[143]		
Mg–Al–Zn: AZ61	[144]		[144–147]
Mg–Al–Zn: AZ71	[148]		
Mg–Al–Zn: AZ91			
Mg–Al–Zn	[149]		[150]
Mg–Al–Sn			[151]
Mg–Zn–Al			[152]
Mg–Zn: ZK60		[153]	
Mg–Zn–Y			[154]
Mg-Zn-Y-Zr	[155]		[156]

Table 10.3 (continued)

	Forging temperature		
	Cold	**Warm***	**Hot**
Mg–Zn–Gd	[157]		
Mg–Zn–Ca	[158]		
Mg–Y–RE	[159]		
Mg–Gd–Y	[160]		
Mg-Gd-Y-Zr			[134, 161–164]
Mg-Gd-Y-Zr-Ag	[165]		[165]
Mg-Gd-Nd-Zr			[166]
Mg–Si			[167]

Note: RE, rare earth element; warm*, up to 200 °C.

In extrusion processing, there are terms known as direct extrusion versus indirect extrusion or forward extrusion versus backward extrusion. And these terms are used frequently in subsequent cited references. Referring to Figure 10.4 [168], the direct extrusion is the most general extrusion process and is also called forward extrusion. Ram or screw is used to push the billet in the container house through the die. In between the billet and ram, there is a dummy block, which is reusable and is used for keeping them separated. One of the major disadvantages associated with the direct extrusion process is that the force needed for the extrusion of billet is more than what is required in the indirect extrusion process. This is because of the introduction of frictional forces due to the requirement for the billet to move the container's entire length. Hence, greatest force is required at the start of the process, which decreases slowly with the use of billet. On the other hand, in the indirect extrusion (or also called backward extrusion), the die is constant whereas the billet and container move together. To keep the die stationary, a "stem" is used which must be longer than the length of container. The final and maximum extrusion length is decided by the stem's column strength. While the billet movement is along with the container, all the frictional forces are easily eliminated. This results in advantages: (1) 25–30% reduction of friction, allowing extrusion of larger billets, enhanced speed and an increased ability to extrude smaller cross-sections; (2) less tendency for extrusions to crack as no heat formation takes place from friction and (3) container liner lasts longer due to less wear. There are a couple of disadvantages of the indirect or backward extrusion. This process is not as versatile as the process of direct extrusions, as the cross-sectional area is confined by the stem's maximum size. Also, the defects and impurities on the billet's surface affect the extrusion's surface [169].

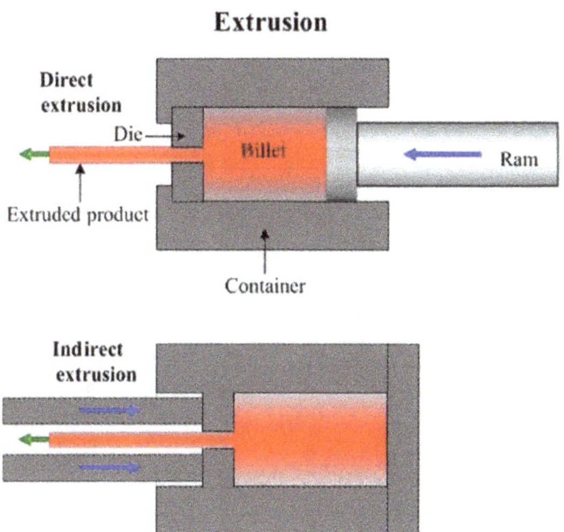

Figure 10.4: Differences between direct (forward) extrusion and indirect (backwards) extrusion [168].

Table 10.4 lists Mg materials that are subjected to extrusion/drawing at three different temperature zones.

Table 10.4: Extrusion/drawing forming at three with operational temperature zones.

	Extrusion temperature		
	Cold	**Warm***	**Hot**
Mg–Al	[170]	[171]	[171–175]
Mg–Al–Zn: AZ31	[42, 176–189]	[190, 191]	[191–194]
Mg–Al–Zn: AZ61			[195–197]
Mg–Al–Zn: AZ63			[198]
Mg–Al–Zn: AZ80	[199, 200]		[199, 201]

Table 10.4 (continued)

	Extrusion temperature		
	Cold	**Warm***	**Hot**
Mg–Al–Zn: AZ81	[202]		[203]
Mg–Al–Zn: AZ82	[203]		
Mg–Al–Zn: AZ91			[204]
Mg–Al–Zn	[173, 205, 206]		[207–212]
Mg-Al-Zn-Sn			
Mg-Al-Zn-Mn			
Mg-Al-Zn-Ca-Mn	[213]		
Mg–Al–Sn	[214]		[214–217]
Mg–Al–Ca	[218–222]		[219, 223–225]
Mg–Al–Mn	[226]		[227]
Mg–Al–Y	[228]		
Mg–Al–Sr			[229]
Mg–Zn	[230–232]	[231]	[233, 234]
Mg–Zn–Zr	[235–237]		[238–241]
Mg–Zn–Zr: ZK60			
Mg–Zn–Y	[242–244]		[245–249]
Mg-Zn-Y-Zr	[250–252]		[252–256]
Mg-Zn-Y-Nd	[257, 258]		[257]
Mg-Zn-Y-Sn			[259]
Mg-Zn-Y-Ca			[260, 261]
Mg–Zn–Mn			[262–265]
Mg-Zn-Mn-Sn	[266, 267]		[266, 267]
Mg–Zn–Gd	[268]		[269–273]
Mg–Zn–Ca	[97, 274–278]	[278]	[158, 279–283]
Mg-Zn-Ca-Mn			[284–287]
Mg-Zn-Ca-Ce			[288, 289]
Mg-Zn-Ca-Y			[290]

Table 10.4 (continued)

	Extrusion temperature		
	Cold	**Warm***	**Hot**
Mg-Zn-Ca-Zr			[291]
Mg–Zn–Ce			
Mg-Zn-Nd-Zr			
Mg–Zn–Al	[292]	[292]	
Mg-Zn-Al-Sn	[293]		
Mg–Zn–Er	[294]		[294–297]
Mg–Zn–Si	[298]		
Mg–Zn–Gd			[299]
Mg–Zn–Sn		[300]	[300]
Mg–Li	[301–305]		[306]
Mg–Li–Ca			
Mg-Li-Ca-Zn-Al			
Mg–Li–Al	[307–313]	[314, 315]	[308, 310, 316–318]
Mg–Li–Zn	[319–321]	[322]	[322–325]
Mg–Ca	[326, 327]		[327]
Mg–Ca–In	[328]		
Mg-Ca-Zn-Zr			[329]
Mg–Y	[330, 331]	[331]	[332–334]
Mg-Y-Ni-Ti			
Mg–Y–Zn	[335]		[336–338]
Mg–Y–RE			
Mg–Y–Nd	[339, 340]		[341]
Mg–Y–Er	[342]		
Mg–Y–Zr	[341]		
Mg–Y–Gd	[343]		[344, 345]
Mg–Y–Sm			[346, 347]
Mg–Y–Mn			[348]

Table 10.4 (continued)

	Extrusion temperature		
	Cold	**Warm***	**Hot**
Mg–Y–Ca			[349]
Mg–Gd	[350, 351]	[171]	[171, 352, 353]
Mg–Gd–Zn			[354–357]
Mg–Gd–Zr	[358]		
Mg–Gd–Y	[359]		
Mg-Gd-Y-Zn-Zr	[356, 360]		[357, 361–365]
Mg-Gd-Y-Zn-Ca			[366]
Mg-Gd-Y-Zr	[367–369]		[367, 368, 370–376]
Mg-Gd-Y-Nd	[377, 378]		[378]
Mg-Gd-Y-Ag			[379]
Mg-Gd-Y-Er	[380]		
Mg-Gd-Er-Zn			[381, 382]
Mg–Sn	[383–387]		[388, 389]
Mg–Sn–Mn			
Mg–Sn–Zn	[384, 390–392]		[391, 393–399]
Mg–Sn–Ca	[400, 401]		
Mg–Sn–Yb	[402, 403]		
Mg–Sn–Al	[404]	[405, 406]	
Mg-Sn-Al-Zn			[405, 407–411]
Mg–Sn–Y	[412]	[413]	[413, 414]
Mg–Nd			
Mg–Nd–Zn			[415]
Mg-Nd-Zn-Zr			[416, 417]
Mg-Nd-Gd-Zn			[418]
Mg–Hg–Ga			
Mg–Dy	[419–421]		
Mg–Dy–Zn			[422, 423]

Table 10.4 (continued)

	Extrusion temperature		
	Cold	**Warm***	**Hot**
Mg–Dy–Ni		[419]	[419]
Mg–Mn	[424]	[424]	[424, 425]
Mg–Mn–Y			[426]
Mg–Mn–Zn			[427]
Mg–Mn–Ce			[428]
Mg–MM	[429]		
Mg–RE	[430]		[431]
Mg–Sm	[432, 433]		
Mg–Er	[434]		
Mg–Er–Zn			[435, 436]
Mg–Sr	[437]		
Mg–Zr	[438]		
Mg–Ce–Zr			[439]
Mg–Ho–Zn			[440]
Mg–Bi–Al			[441]

Note: MM, misch metal; RE, rare earth element; warm*, up to 200 °C.

10.1.4 Equal-channel angular processing

Equal-channel angular processing (ECAP) is one of the most commonly employed severe plastic deformation (SPD) process to drive nano- or ultrafine-grained microstructure at low homologous temperatures. The homologous temperature is the thermodynamic temperature of a material, that is, a fraction of its melting point in Kelvin scale. For ECAP, the common homologous temperature is around 0.3; in other words, the operational temperature for ECAP is about 0.3 of the melting point (in K) of work material. ECAP is most suitable for materials used in industrial-scale application, the process works by introducing a large shear strain by repeated extrusion steps. As a result of multiple-pass ECAP, the microstructure is subjected to SPD and grain refining, so that ECAP is considered as a mechanical hardening treatment for ductile materials [442, 443].

Referring to Figure 10.5 [444], the internal channel is bent through an abrupt angle, Φ, and there is an additional angle, Ψ, which represents the outer arc of curvature where the two channels intersect. The sample, in the form of a rod or bar, is machined to fit within channel, and the die is placed in some form of fuss so that the sample can be pressed through the die using a plunger. The nature of the imposed deformation is simple shear which occurs as the billet passes through the die. The retention of the same cross-sectional area when processing by ECAP, despite the introduction of very large strains, is the important characteristic of SPD processing, and it is this characteristic that distinguishes this type of processing from conventional metal-working operations such as rolling, extrusion and drawing. As the process is capable of maintaining the net dimensions of the workpiece, repetitive extrusion is possible, provided that the material exhibits sufficient ductility to withstand heavy deformations.

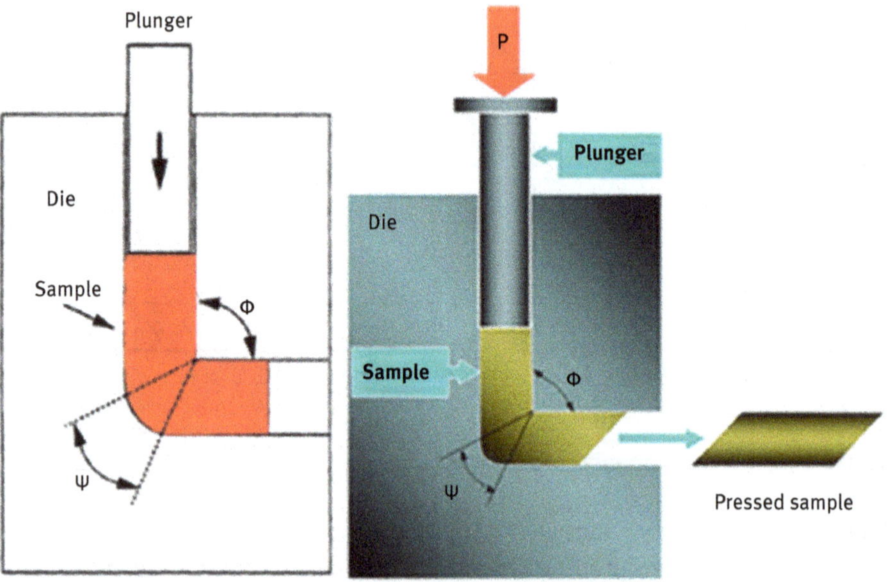

Figure 10.5: Schematic illustration of equal channel angular processing [444].

The ECAPed work possesses several characteristics, including (1) hardened structure with ultrafine grain and subgrain structures; (2) enhanced mechanical properties in terms of tensile strength, stress-controlled fatigue strength and fatigue crack growth resistance and (3) strongly influenced anisotropy of the structure in achieving good ductility [442, 443]. Among various Mg–based alloy, Mg–Al-based alloys are frequently subjected to SPD process such as ECAP. These include Mg–10Al [445], Mg–15Al [446, 447], AZ31 [448–452], AZ91[453], Mg–Al–Y [454] and Mg–Al–Si [455]. Mg–Zn alloy systems are also frequently studied on effects of ECAP on mechanical improvements: Mg–4Zn [456], Mg–6Zn [457, 458], ZA62 [459], ZK60 [460], Mg–Zn–Y [461, 462] and Mg–Zn–Ca [463–465]. ECAPed Mg–Gd alloy systems are investigated: Mg–Gd–Zn [466, 467], Mg–Gd–Y [468, 469] and Mg–Gd–Nd [470]. There are still numerous studies on ECAPed Mg-based alloys, including Mg–Y alloys [471–474], Mg–Li alloys [475, 476], Mg–Sn alloys [477] and Mg–Nd alloys [478, 479].

10.1.5 Friction stir processing

Friction stir processing (FSP) is a sort of the spin-off technology from its precursor – friction stir welding – and is a unique method for altering properties of a metal through intense, localized SPD. This deformation is produced by inserting a nonconsumable tool into the work and revolving the tool in a stirring motion as it is pushed laterally through the workpiece. Figure 10.6 illustrates schematic of FSP [480] along with typical microstructural features [481] observed at the cross section of FSPed work [482], where BM represents the base metal, SZ the stir zone, HAZ the heat-affected zone and TMAZ the thermomechanical affected zone. The underlying material is subjected to high strain during FSP resulting in fragmentation and homogeneous distribution of the dendrites. The inset shows the actual image of the nugget zone of friction stir-processed metallic glass. The highly strained material in the nugget zone comprises fine dendrites compared to elongated ones in the undeformed region [480].

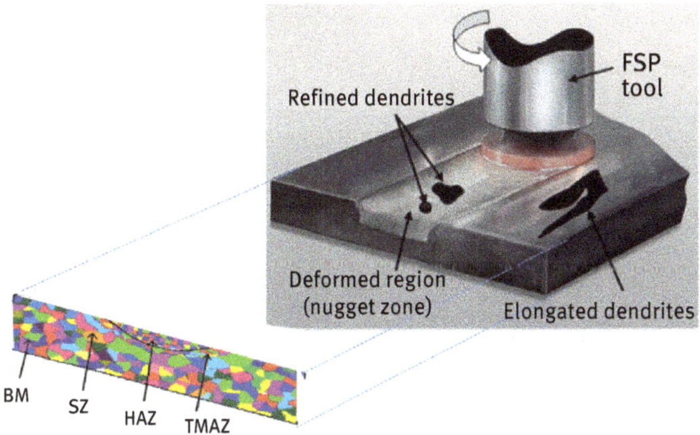

Figure 10.6: FSP schematic and typical changes in microstructures along the FSP line.

When ideally implemented, this process mixes the material without changing the phase (by melting or otherwise) and creates a microstructure with fine, equiaxed grains. FSP also enhances the microhardness, tensile strength and fatigue strength of the metal. Friction between the tool and workpieces results in localized heating that softens and plasticizes the workpiece. A volume of processed material is produced by movement of materials from the front of the pin to the back of the pin. During this process, the material undergoes SPD and results in significant grain refinement [480, 481, 483–485].

Ahmadkhaniha et al. [486] modified pure magnesium by FSP and reported significant improvements in mechanical and biocorrosion resistance. Similar results were mentioned on Mg–Al-based AXM541 alloy [487]. There are more studies on different Mg-based alloys, including AZ31 [488, 489], Mg–Zn alloy [490, 491], Mg–Zn–Ca [492], Mg–Gd alloy [493] and Mg–Nd-based alloys [494–496].

10.2 Product forms

There are basically three types of product shapes as shown in Figure 10.7 [497]. To make final shape of products, in addition to the various technologies mentioned earlier, we have sheet metal processes as shown in Figure 10.8 [24]. Employing single technique or a combination of processing(s), we can produce various shapes of products.

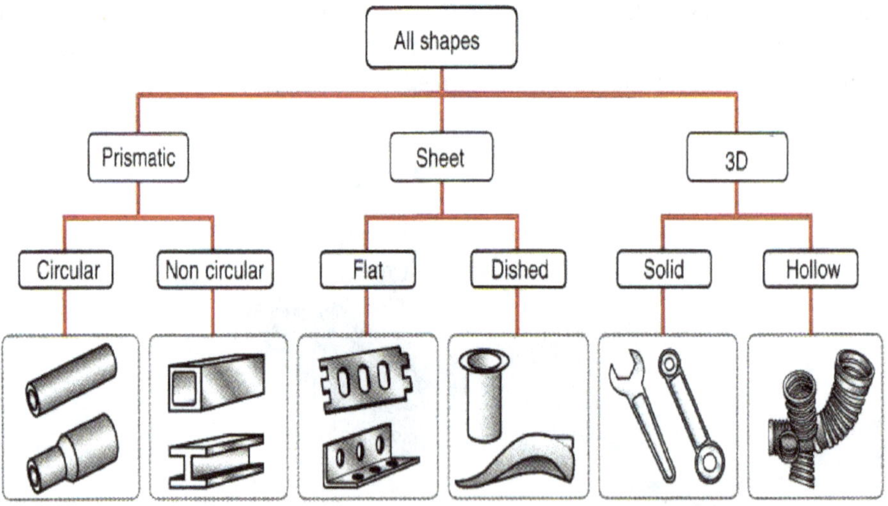

Figure 10.7: Typical shapes of product [497].

10.2.1 Film

To improve the corrosion resistance and mechanical properties of Mg–Gd–Zn alloy, Ba et al. [498] plated the substrate surface with Mg–Al hydrotalcite film by arc ion plating. The similar Mg–Al hydrotalcite film was prepared by cerium-based sealing

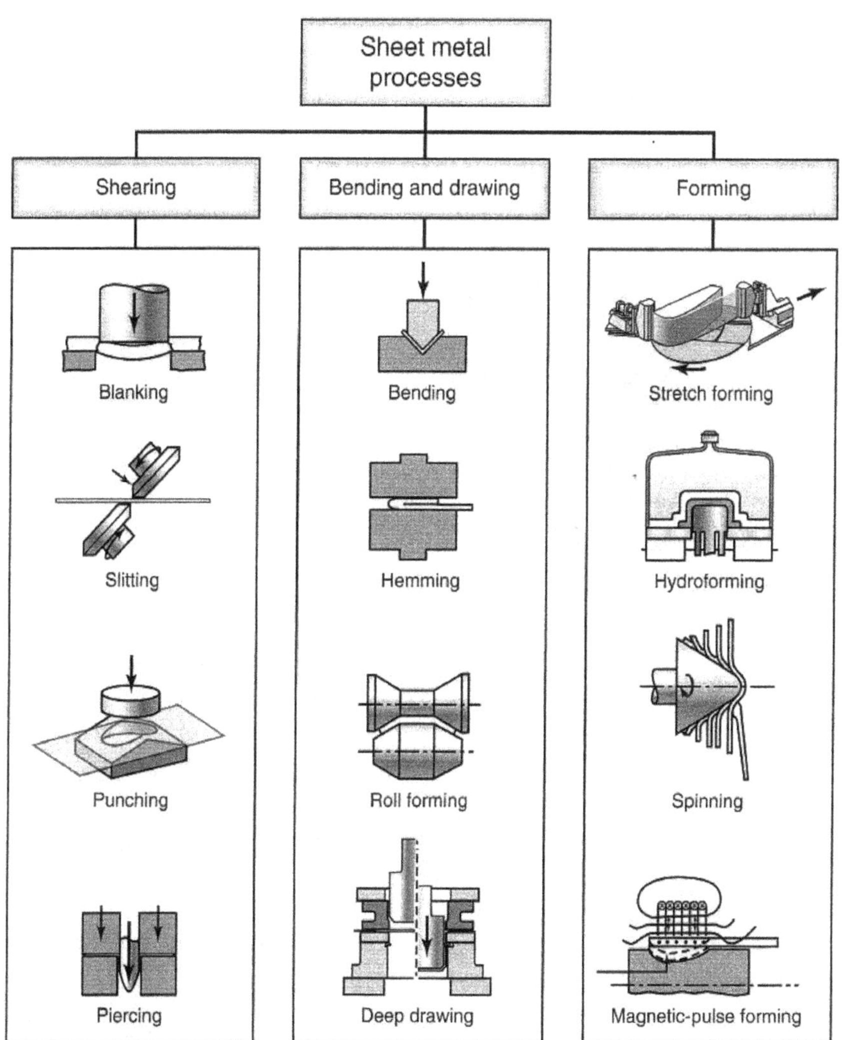

Figure 10.8: Sheet metal fabrication methods [24].

treatment to apply the AZ91 to improve the corrosion resistance [499, 500]. Mg–Zn thin film was prepared by various methods; by thermionic vacuum arc deposition [501], chemically in Kokubo's solution [502] or scattering deposition of Mg–Zn–Ca film [503, 504]. For switchable mirror, Mg–Zr–H thin film was fabricated by cosputtering of Mg and Zr [505] and Mg–Zr–Ni thin film was prepared [506]. There are other types of Mg-based thin films for different purposes; magnetic property of Mg-Mn-Fe-Co-Ni-Gd thin film by electrochemical synthesis [507], for optical application of Mg–Y thin film [508] and biomedical application of Mg–Nb alloy thin film by the magnetron sputtering technique [509].

10.2.2 Sheet

The majority of sheet products are produced via rolling at elevated temperatures. Typical Mg sheet [510] is shown in Figure 10.9.

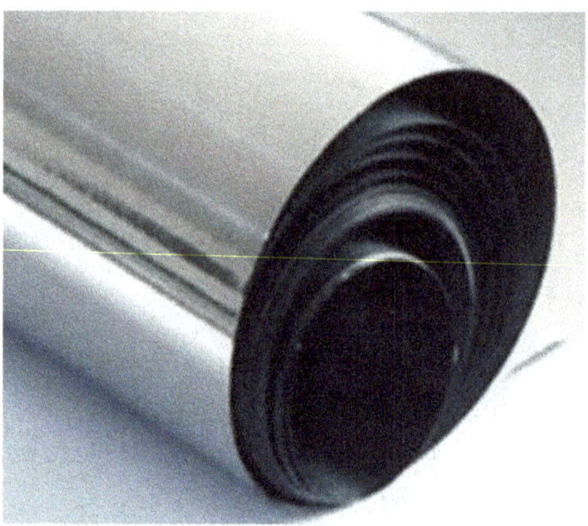

Figure 10.9: Typical Mg sheet [510].

Sheet materials from Mg-based alloys are varied. They should include Mg–Al-based alloys such as Mg–Al–Sn [511], Mg–Al–Zn–Mn [512], Mg–Al–Zn–Ca [513] and Mg–Al–Mn [514].

There are numerous studies on sheet production using AZ31 alloys [515–521] as well as AZ31B [522–525].

There are also many investigations for sheet fabrication using Mg–Zn-based alloys. They should include Mg–Zn–Ca alloys [503, 504, 514, 526–528], Mg–Zn–MM (misch metal) [529], Mg–Zn–Gd [530, 531] and Mg–Zn–RE [519, 532–534].

There are still a variety of Mg materials which are subjected to the rolling to produce sheets such as Mg–Li–Zn [535], Mg–Mn–Ce [536], Mg–Mn–Fe [507], Mg–Y [508], Mg–Gd–Y [537–539], Mg–Zr–H [505], Mg–Zr–Ni [506], Mg–Sn–Yb [540] and Mg–Dy–Zn [541].

10.2.3 Ribbon and wire

Figure 10.10 shows typical wire-shaped products of (a) Mg sound ribbon [542], (b) Mg wires [543] and (c) Mg audio cable [544].

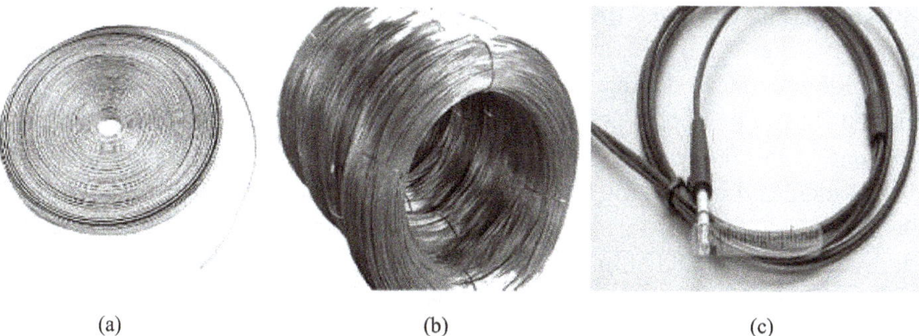

(a) (b) (c)

Figure 10.10: Typical Mg wire-shaped products: (a) ribbon, (b) wire and (c) cable.

There are wire products formed via variously modified rolling processes, including hot rolling and annealing of Mg–Zn [545], twin-roll casting of Mg–Al [546], electroplastic rolling of AZ31 [547] and semisolid rheorolling of Mg–Sn–Mn [548].

Several studies were performed to develop wire-shaped products for medical applications. They are Mg–Ca alloys for surgical applications [549], Mg–Zn–Ca for surgical tack [550], Mg–Zn–Ca for nerve regeneration [551] and Mg–Y for stent self-assembly [552].

10.2.4 Rod and bar

Figure 10.11 shows typical Mg rod (a) [553] and bars (b) [554].

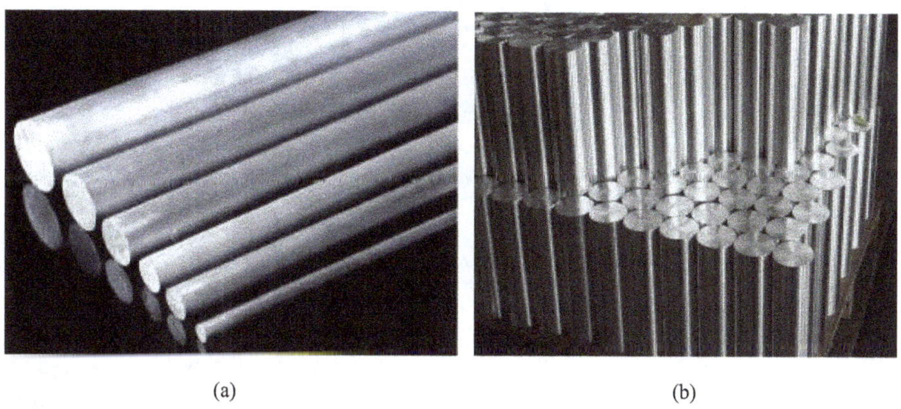

(a) (b)

Figure 10.11: (a) Magnesium rods and (b) bars.

Mroz et al. [555] employed the explosive cladding method to fabricate Mg–Al bimetallic bars. Butt et al. [556] treated AZ31 rod with the fluoride conversion coatings formed porous MgF_2 ceramic layer to adjust the biodegradation and reported that (i) AZ31 Mg rod-reinforced polylactic acid (PLA) plays a crucial role in the degradation rate of PLA/Mg composite, treated with hydrofluoric acid promoting a lower degradation rate than untreated sample, which is attributed only to the microanchoring effect, leading to better mechanical properties and degradation performance in simulated body fluid solution; (ii) untreated promote a faster formation of cracks and, therefore, an increasingly faster degradation of the polymeric matrix; and (iii) with prolonging immersion time in the simulated body liquid until 8 weeks, the MgF_2 porous coatings were corroded gradually, along with the disappearance of original pores and the formation of a relatively smooth surface, resulting in a rapid reduction in mechanical properties for corresponding composite rods owing to the weakening of interfacial binding capacity between PLA and inner layer.

10.2.5 Tube and pipe

Figure 10.12 shows Mg tubes and pipes with different cross-sectional features [557].

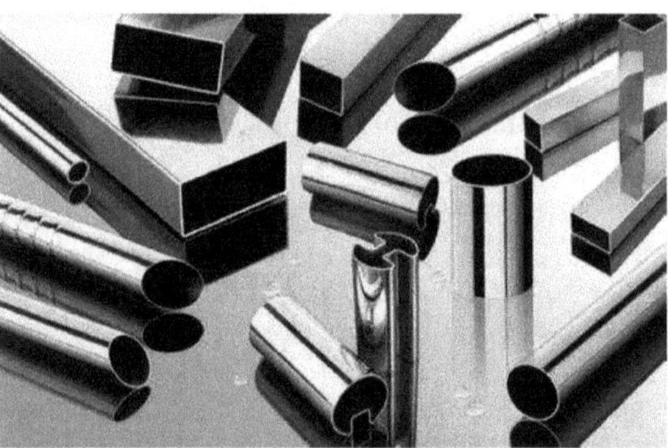

Figure 10.12: Various cross sections of Mg tubes and pipes [557].

Sun et al. [558] studied tension and compression behaviors of Mg–3%Al–1%Zn (AZ31) and Mg–8%Gd–3%Y (GW83) extruded tubes and found that (i) there was an asymmetry in strain hardening behavior; (ii) high strain-hardening rate in AZ31 compression test was caused by the growth of large fraction extension twinning to cover the whole matrix grain; and (iii) the weaker texture, lower volume fraction of twins and multiple dislocation slip in GW83 alloy are responsible for the better yield symmetry and lower strain hardening rate compared with AZ31 alloy tube. Guo et al. [559] investigated mechanical property, microstructure and texture of an extruded Mg–1.0Al–1.5Ca–1.0Mn (wt%) flat–oval tube in both the flat and the oval regions. It was reported that (i) there exists a great difference in microstructure and texture between the flat and the oval region; (ii) both the flat and the oval regions have fine dynamic recrystallized grains of 3–4 µm, while more row-stacked grains are observed in the flat region; (iii) a large number of fine particles with a size of about 0.5 µm are dispersed in both the grain boundary and grain interior; and (iv) the particles exhibit a uniform distribution in the oval region, while they tend to aggregate into bands along the extrusion direction in the flat region. Ge et al. [560] conducted the ECAP and extrusion processing of a ZM21 Mg alloy to obtain an improved candidate material for the manufacturing of biodegradable Mg stents. It was mentioned that (i) a significant improvement in the properties of the ECAP-treated samples compared with the starting coarse-grained ZM21 alloy was recognized; (ii) the 0.2% yield strength rose from 180 to 340 MPa after 150 °C ECAP processing, while maintaining a fairly high tensile ductility; (iii) the ultrafine ZM21 alloy billets were then used for the extrusion of stent precursors having the form of small-size tubes; and (iv) the grain size after extrusion remained in the submicrometer range while the hardness was revealed to be significantly higher than that of the coarse-grained ZM21 Mg alloy, indicating that processing of biodegradable Mg stent having an ultrafine-grained microstructure by ECAP and low-temperature extrusion is feasible and that the obtained products feature promising properties.

10.2.6 Foam

A metallic foam is a cellular structure consisting of a solid metal or alloy with pores that occupy a large portion of the volume (typically 75–95%). The pores can be sealed (closed-cell foam) or interconnected (open-cell foam). Figure 10.13 compares closed-cell foam structure and open-cell foam structure [561]. Furthermore, Kränzlin et al. [562] subdivided porous metals into metal foams, metal sponges and nanoporous metals, as shown in Figure 10.14. However, this classification possesses a sort of controversial issue since there are numerous studies, which will be cited later in this section, that utilize the term “open-cell metal foam” for tissue engineering applications. Synthesis are also listed to each of these cellular structures, although in the most cases, a method suitable for a specific shape might not be the best option for controlling the microscopic features. It was further mentioned that the production strategy greatly affects the efficiency and performance of the porous metal structure in its final application and some applications rely on more complex geometries and pore structures than others, which is indicated on the bottom part of Figure 10.14 [562]. Foams are commonly fabricated by injecting a gas or mixing

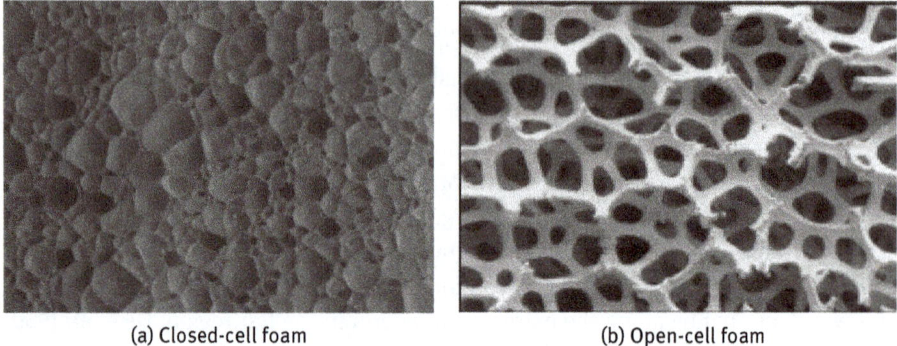

Figure 10.13: Comparison between closed and open cellular foam structures [561].

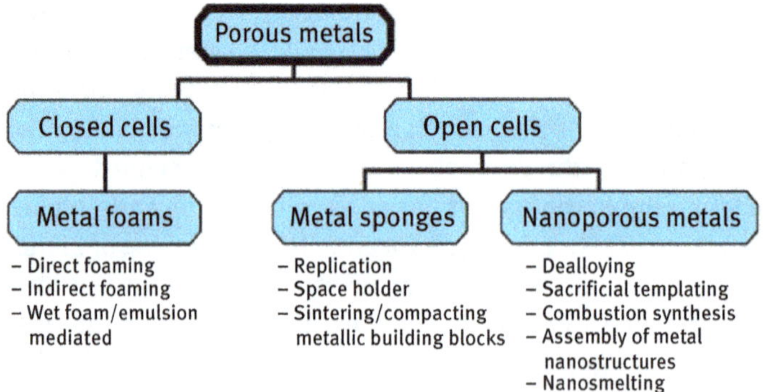

Figure 10.14: Classification of cellular structures and suggested syntheses [562].

foam-making agent into molten metal. Melts can be foamed by creating gas bubbles in the material. Normally, bubbles in molten metal are highly buoyant in the high-density liquid and rise quickly to the surface. This rise can be slowed by increasing the viscosity of the molten metal by adding ceramic powders or alloying elements to form stabilizing particles in the melt, or by other means. Metallic melts can be foamed in one of three ways: (1) by injecting gas into the liquid metal from an external source; (2) by causing gas formation in the liquid by admixing gas-releasing blowing agents with the molten metal; and (3) by causing the precipitation of gas that was previously dissolved in the molten metal [563]. On the other hand, open-cell foams are normally manufactured by foundry or powder metallurgy. In the powder method, the space holders are used to occupy the pore spaces and channels. In casting processes, foam is cast with an open-celled polyurethane foam skeleton.

Practically, there are two different methods for the introduction of the gas phase into the metal: direct foaming processes (see Figure 10.15) and indirect foaming techniques (Figure 10.16).

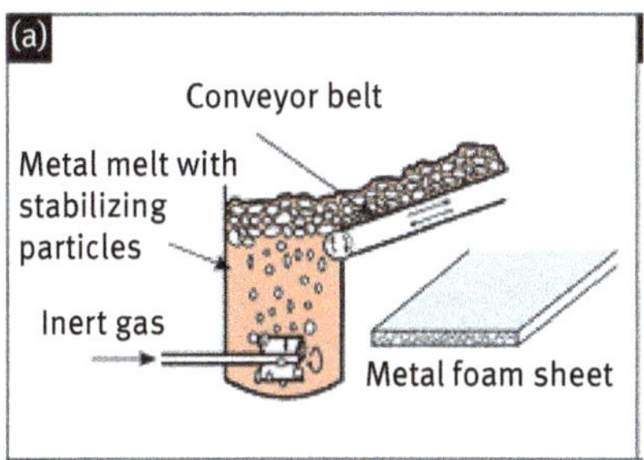

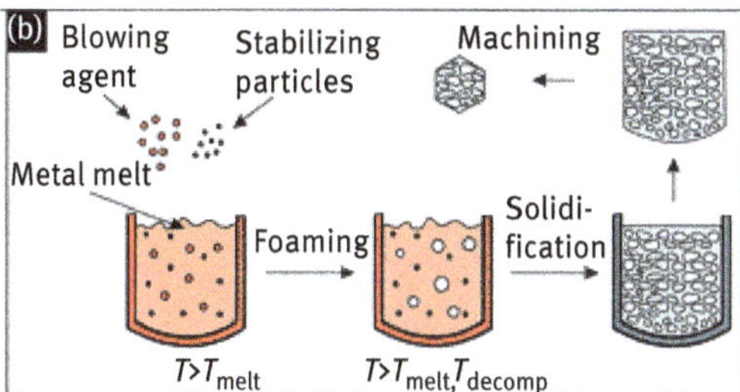

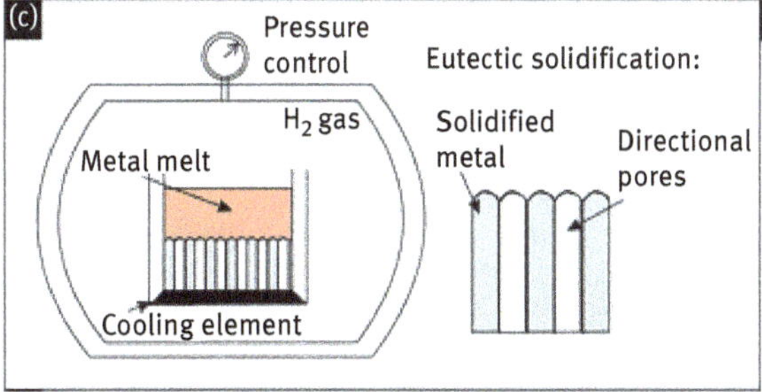

Figure 10.15: Direct foaming processes [562].

Although metal foams typically retain some physical properties of their base material, the strength of the foam structure depends on the density (or porosity). Even if porous metals are divided into closed-cell pores and open-cell pores and these parameters control to some extent basic properties of cellular structures, additional features like relative density, pore structure and macroscopic shape are also critical in determining the functionality of porous metals and thus their application potential beyond structural materials [562, 564].

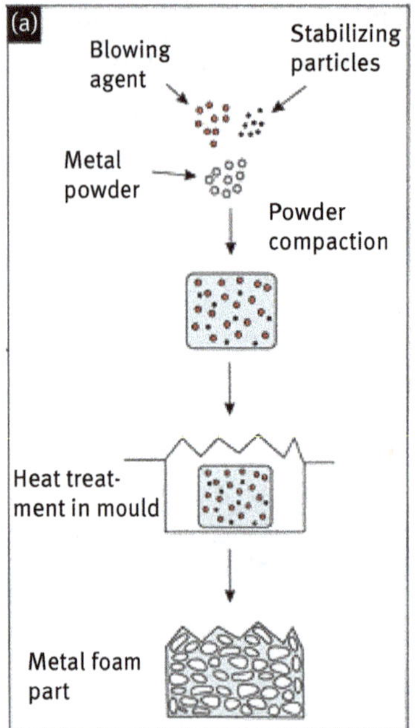

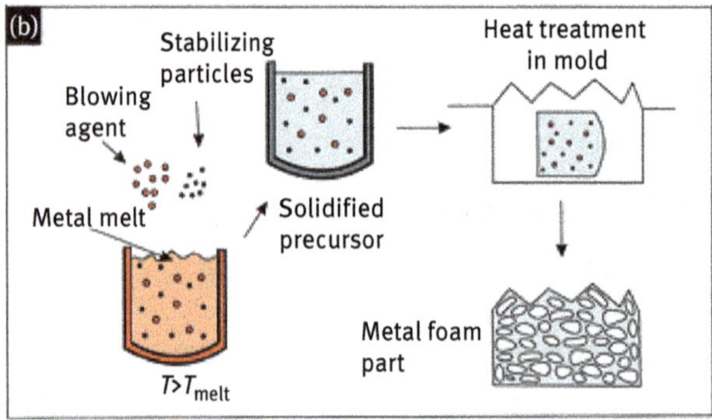

Figure 10.16: Indirect foaming techniques [562].

The applicability of porous metal structure is strongly controlled by three parameters: (1) the composition, (2) the macroscopic shape and (3) the pore structure. The composition determines the intrinsic properties and thus decides on whether or not a specific metal or alloy fulfills the targeted physical (density, electrical/thermal conductivity, strength, elasticity, ductility and machinability) or chemical (oxidation behavior and corrosion stability) requirements. The macroscopic shape is critical for the integration into predesigned devices or for their combination with other materials. The pore structure (relative density, surface area density, mechanical stability, pore size, pore size distribution and connectivity of pores) defines the efficiency of the material during operation. Only when all these three characteristics are carefully engineered, the material can be considered as possible candidate for a given application [13, 565, 566]. Functional applications of metal foam structures are therefore versatile, including medical areas (in which devices for tissue engineering, orthopedic implants and stents should be included); automotive industry (including sound damping and catalytic converters); better heat transfer like heat sinks, energy absorption and electromagnetic shielding; arresting flames and catalytic engineering [567].

Among valuable articles that will be reviewed further, an uncertainty of categorization was reported by Kränzlin et al. [562] and there are numerous reports, in particular, the medical applications in tissue engineering, using the terminology "foam metal" to indicate open-cell metal foam.

10.2.6.1 Closed-cell foam structure

Mg alloy (AZ31) foams with different closed-cell sizes, fixed porosity and uniform structure were prepared by direct foaming method, and it was reported that (i) the pores in the foams were polygon with the porosity of 87%, as shown in Figure 10.17; (ii) decreasing the cell size is beneficial to eliminating the big cell edges in the foams; (iii) decrease of the average cell size improves the strength of the foams by sharing the load with more and smaller cells, however, too small average cell size can impair the strength because no enough metals hold the integrity of the new cell walls; and (iv) the densification strain hardly changes with the varying average cell size and fixed porosity.

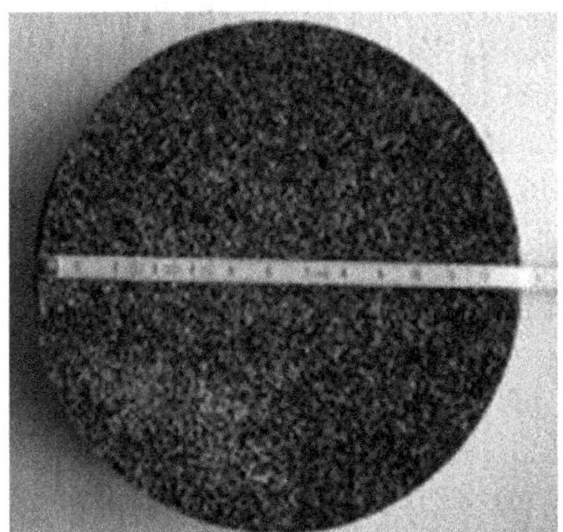

Figure 10.17: Mg alloy closed-cell foam structure [568].

Xia et al. [569] prepared closed-cell AZ31 Mg alloy foams by melt-foaming method and investigated the effects of specimen aspect ratio (the thickness/width ratio) on the compressive properties of closed-cell Mg alloy foams. It was shown that (i) the length of stress–strain plateau stage extended and ideality energy absorption efficiency improved with the specimen thickness/width aspect ratio (AR) increasing and the yield strength decreased and (ii) specimens with the aspect ratio of 1.00 possess good combination of yield strength, plateau stage length and compressive stability when compressed under the experiment conditions. Furthermore, Xia et al. [570], using the same foam structures, studied the effects of homogenizing heat treatment on compressive properties. It was reported that (i) homogenizing heat treatment enhanced the compressive properties in terms of yield strength, mean plateau strength, available energy absorption capacity and ideality energy absorption efficiency of the foams; (ii) homogenizing heat treatment greatly reduced the stress drop rates of the foams; and (iii) specimens homogenized at the temperature of 480 °C for 24 h possessed good combination of yield strength, compressive stability, available energy absorption capacity and ideality energy absorption efficiency under the present experiment conditions. Yang et al. [571] employed Ca particles as thickening agent and $CaCO_3$ powder as blowing agent and fabricated cellular Mg foams with homogeneous closed pore structures by melt-foaming method. It was mentioned that (i) the blowing gas to foam-melted Mg is CO rather than CO_2; (ii) CO is released from the liquid–solid reaction between Mg melt and $CaCO_3$; and (iii) compared to Al/Al alloy foams, the cellular Mg foams possess superior comprehensive mechanical properties, suggesting that the closed cellular Mg foam might have promising future in the practical engineering applications. Lu et al. [572] investigated the compressive behavior of closed-cell Mg alloy foams fabricated by melting method at various temperatures (25, 200, 400 and 500 °C). It was found that the effect of temperature on compressive behavior of the Mg alloy foams is different between high temperature and low temperature and the Mg alloy foams exhibit a brittle compressive behavior at room temperature by the fracture of cell walls; however, the pure brittle fracture mode transforms into a combination of brittle fracture mode and ductile fracture mode at temperature in the range of 200–400 °C; indicating a softening effect of high temperature on the foams matrix and the plasticity of the cell walls at low temperature. Based on these findings, it was concluded that the compressive strength and energy absorption capacity of the closed-cell Mg alloy foams decrease with the increasing temperature.

10.2.6.2 Open-cell foam structure

It is believed that open-cell foams are normally manufactured by foundry or powder metallurgy, in which the space holders are used to occupy the pore spaces and channels. In casting processes, foam is cast with an open-celled polyurethane foam skeleton. However, recently, it was mentioned that the additive manufacturing technology can be applied to manufacture porous materials as a three-dimensional (3D)-printing technology does [573], as shown in Figure 10.18 [574].

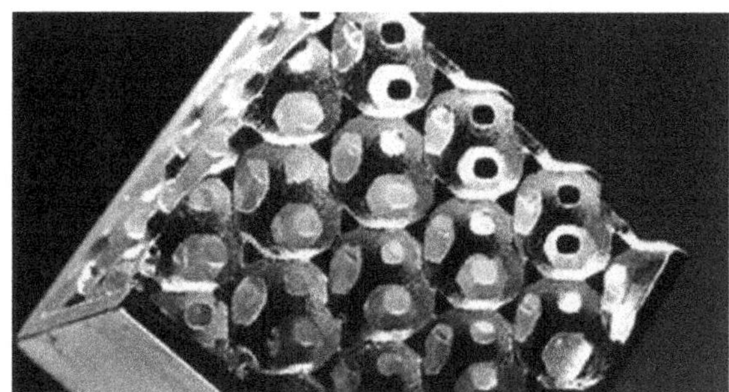

Figure 10.18: Open-cell Al foam by the additive manufacturing.

To manufacture open-cell pure Mg and Mg alloys foams with melting points lower than 950 °C, Lara-Rodriguez et al. [575] developed the replication-casting device, which consisted of three basic parts: a cylindrical reaction chamber, a valve system for controlling the vacuum and the gas injection and a heating system. An example of the thus manufactured open-cell Mg–10 wt% Al alloy foam is shown in Figure 10.19 [575].

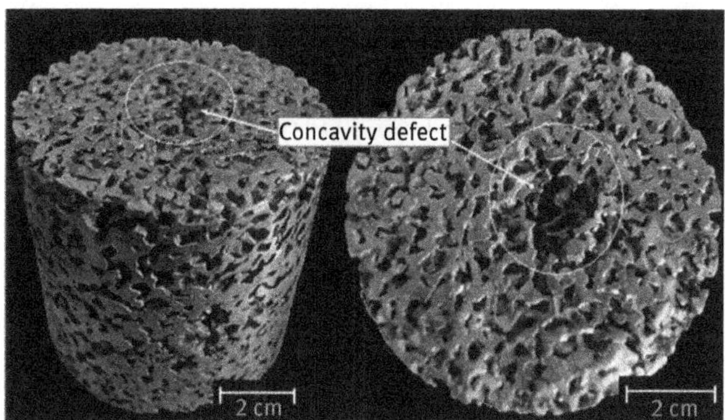

Figure 10.19: Open-cell Mg–Al alloy foam by replication casting [575].

Tissue engineering is a field that aims to regenerate damaged tissues by enhancing tissue growth through the porous architecture of the scaffolds, which is desired to mimic the human cancellous bone. Mg-based scaffolds are gaining importance in the field of tissue engineering owing to its potential application as a biomaterial [576]. There are several reasons for promising applicability of open-cell Mg foam to fabricate scaffold structures: (1) technically, it is not difficult to manufacture open-cell Mg foams, (2) Mg material per se exhibits an excellent biodegradability and (3) Mg shows an excellent osteoinductivity. Porous Mg and Mg alloys can be used as bone substitutes with bone-mimicking characteristics. Since the structures of bone tissue and porous Mg materials are similar, host bone cells can exhibit the bone ingrowth into the pores of an Mg scaffold. Moreover, the gradual biodegradation of porous Mg and Mg alloys after implantation, followed by the absorption of Mg ions in the body, eliminates the necessity of removing the implant via a subsequent surgical procedure, which makes Mg scaffolds more favorable than other porous metallic biomaterials [577]. Singh et al. [576] fabricated a novel Mg-based open-cell porous structure with pore interconnectivity and significant strength via powder metallurgy approach and Ti-woven wire mesh as a space holding material. It was reported that (i) a uniform distribution of pores with porosity varied in range from 50% to 60%; (ii) the measured values of ultimate compressive strength and elastic modulus using quasistatic compression test were found to be 101 MPa and 2 GPa, respectively; and (iii) results of corrosion tests and cytocompatibility studies using L929 cells showed improved corrosion resistance as well as cell viability of more than 90%, suggesting it as a promising development for bone-scaffolding applications in future. Wen et al. [578] investigated mechanical properties of porous magnesium with the porosity of 35–55% and the pore size of about 70–400 μm by compressive tests focusing on the effects of the porosity and pore size on the Young's modulus and strength. It was indicated that (i) the Young's modulus and peak stress increase with decreasing porosity and pore size and (ii) the mechanical properties of the porous magnesium were in a range of those of cancellous bone, suggesting that the porous magnesium is one of promising scaffold materials for hard tissue regeneration. Tan et al. [579] fabricated porous magnesium with a 3D open-cellular structure, potentially employed as bone tissue engineering scaffolds by the mechanical perforation method. The influences of porosity, pore size and pore arrangement on compressive behavior and the anisotropy of new porous Mg were analyzed theoretically using orthogonal arrays and the finite element method. It was found that (i) the parameters of porosity, pore size and pore arrangement had different effects on the compressive properties; (ii) the compressive strength could be improved by optimizing these parameters; and (iii) the theoretical results showed good agreement with the experimental ones before the strain reaches 0.038. Gu et al. [580] prepared the lotus-type porous pure magnesium was prepared using a metal/gas eutectic unidirectional solidification method to evaluate the corrosion behavior, decay of mechanical property and the cytocompatibility. It was found that (i) the porous pure Mg indicates better corrosion resistance than that of compact pure Mg in the simulated body fluid at 37 °C; (ii) the compressive yield strength of compact and porous pure Mg is (110.3 ± 8.5) MPa and (23.9 ± 4.9) MPa before immersion test, and porous pure Mg exhibits slower decay in compressive yield strength with the extension of immersion period than that of compact pure Mg; and (iii) with larger exposed surface area, porous pure Mg shows higher Mg concentration in the extract than that of compact pure Mg, which leads to a higher osmotic pressure to cells and might affect its indirect cytotoxicity assay result.

Highly porous Mg–Ca–Zn–Co alloy scaffolds for tissue engineering applications were produced by powder metallurgy with a space holder (carbamide)-water leaching method, which is potentially applicable as a scaffold material in tissue engineering [581]. It was mentioned that (i) increasing Zn content of the alloy increased the elastic modulus, (ii) Ca addition prevented the oxidation of the specimens during sintering, (iii) corrosion rate decreased with Zn addition from 1.0% up to 3.0% (mass fraction) and then increased and (iv) mass loss of the specimens initially decreased with Zn addition up to about 3% and then increased. Jia et al. [582] produced porous Mg scaffolds, which could be achieved by three steps: (1) defectless NaCl open-porous template with enhanced relative density was prepared with NaCl particles by hot press sintering process; (2) green compact of Mg and the NaCl template was produced by infiltration casting; and (3) open-porous Mg scaffold was achieved after leaching out the template. It was reported that (i) by using spherical NaCl particles and irregular polyhedral NaCl particles, respectively, two different types of templates were prepared, and correspondingly Mg scaffolds with spherical and irregular pores were, respectively, fabricated; and (ii) the irregular pore scaffold (I-scaffold) exhibited higher yield strength, while the spherical pore scaffold (S-scaffold) showed superior interconnectivity and more stable compressive deformability due to the uniform spatial structure (see Figure 10.20) [582].

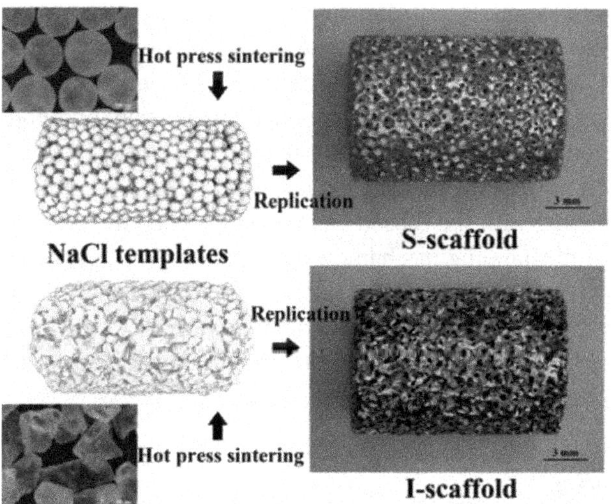

Figure 10.20: Two types of Mg open-cell scaffolds using NaCl templates [582].

Wen et al. [583] employed a new powder process to manufacture Ti and Mg metallic foams and reported that (i) the open-cellular foams (pores: 200–500 μm) have exceptional characteristics (e.g., Ti foam porosity 78%, compressive strength 35 MPa and

Young's modulus 5.3 GPa) and (ii) these show potential applications as biocompatible implant materials. Kang et al. [584] fabricated biodegradable porous Mg with hydroxyapatite (HA) coating suitable for biomedical applications. A blend of Mg and NaCl particles was sintered by spark plasma sintering, followed by dissolving the NaCl to obtain a porous structure. It was reported that (i) different levels of porosity (50%, 60% and 70%) were achieved by adjusting the volume fraction of NaCl, while preserving high pore interconnectivity with a large pore size of ~240 μm, (ii) a dense HA coating layer comprised of needle-shaped HA crystals was formed on the surface of the porous Mg by treatment in an aqueous solution and both bare and HA-coated porous Mg specimens with a porosity of 60% exhibited ductile behavior under compressive loading and similar levels of ultimate compressive strength (~15 MPa); however, HA coating significantly enhanced the corrosion resistance of porous Mg. Wang et al. [585] fabricated Zn-enriched coatings with distinct microstructures and properties on Mg foams by a modified thermal evaporation technique using a tubular resistance furnace. It was mentioned that (i) the Zn coatings brought dramatic improvements in compression strength, but exhibited differently in biodegradation performance; (ii) the diffusion layer accelerated corrosion of Mg foam due to the galvanic effect, while the Zn-based deposition coating displayed excellent anticorrosion performance, showing great potential as bone implant materials; and (iii) this technique provides a novel and convenient approach to tailor the biodegradability of Mg foams for biomedical applications.

There are some nonmedical applications of open-cell Mg foam structures. Hao et al. [586] manufactured open-cellular magnesium foam using powder metallurgy technology basing on space holder fillers. It was mentioned that (i) depending on the volume fraction and the diameter of the carbamide particles, the porosity and pore size can be controlled in the range of 40–80% and 0.5–2.0 mm, respectively, (ii) quasistatic compressive tests indicate that the mechanical behavior of the present magnesium foam is in good agreement with the Gibson–Ashby model when the porosity is over 45% and (iii) the most outstanding mechanical feature, however, may be its long and flat plateau region that is favorable for energy absorbing applications. Yamada et al. [587] developed open-cellular magnesium with a very low density of 0.05 g/cm^3 by the casting method and mentioned that the thus fabricated foam structure shows high potential for usage as energy absorbers.

10.2.6.3 Gradated foam structure

In some applications where both structural integrity and functionality are important, it is not necessary to fabricate the entire structure to be in porous form, rather it should possess gradated porosity from one end to the other. Some authors use the term surface porosity [588, 589], or others call it gradated porosity [29]. Li et al. [27] used an acetic acid (HAc) aqueous solution to dealloy Mg–Al eutectic alloy as an effective electrolyte and found that (i) the corrosion morphologies showed that the Mg–Al eutectic alloy had an obvious selective corrosion character in the HAc solution, (ii) the pore formation mechanism was only governed by the α-Mg dissolution and (iii) with prolonged corrosion time, the dealloying rate was slowed down due to corrosive ion transfer becoming difficult at the corrosion interface. Yang et al. [589] fabricated that surface-porous Mg–Al alloys with different microstructures were fabricated via a new method of electrochemical dealloying in a neutral 0.6 M NaCl solution. It was reported that (i) a bimodal porous structure with 47.57 ± 11.43 μm large pores and 265.60 ± 78.68 nm honeycomb-like fine pores was obtained by direct electrochemical dealloying of as-cast Mg–20Al alloy, (ii) by subsequent annealing, the eutectic structure disappeared and a bicontinuous, single-sized, porous structure with 7.10 ± 1.96 μm ligaments was created by an annealing electrochemical dealloying approach and (iii) the porous formation mechanism is governed by selective dissolution of the α-Mg phase, which leaves the $Mg_{17}Al_{12}$ phase as the porous layer framework. Oshida et al. [590] proposed a concept of gradation of controlled porosity which should correspond to the surrounding anatomical conditions when an implant is placed into bony structure. As shown in Figure 10.21, surface area needs to possess a certain level of porosity to accommodate the bone ingrowth activity, so the biological reaction is high, while the inner portion of the implant should be strong enough to bear an occlusal force (if a case of dental implant) and zones in between should be gradually changing by both increasing the biomechanical strength and decreasing the biological activity. As is well known, the main reason for the HA coating is for establishing the surface roughness to exhibit the morphological compatibility with the receiving hard tissue [591].

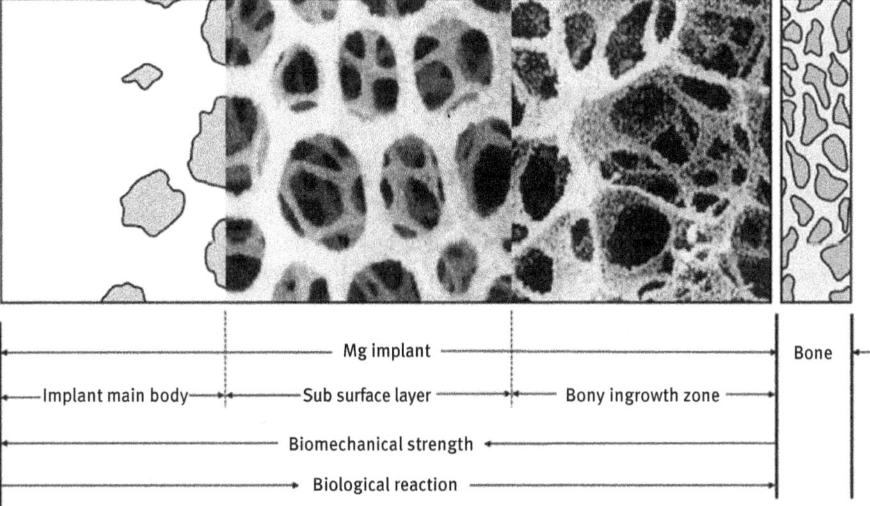

Figure 10.21: Conceptual design of implant with gradated porosity [591].

References

[1] https://nptel.ac.in/content/storage2/courses/112107144/Metal%20Forming%20&%20Powder%20metallurgy/lecture1/lecture1.htm.

[2] https://www.machinedesign.com/community/contributing-technical-experts/article/21831946/the-5-types-of-manufacturing-processes.

[3] https://www.differencebetween.com/wp-content/uploads/2018/02/Difference-Between-Hot-Working-and-Cold-Working.pdf.

[4] https://www.thelibraryofmanufacturing.com/forming_basics.html.

[5] https://www.differencebetween.com/difference-between-hot-working-and-vs-cold-working/.

[6] Luo ZP, Song DY, Zhang SQ. Strengthening effects of rare earths on wrought Mg-Zn-Zr-RE alloys. Journal of Alloys and Compounds. 1995, 230, 109–14.

[7] Hazeli K, Sadeghi A, Pekguleryuz MO, Kontsos A. The effect of strontium in plasticity of magnesium alloys. Materials Science and Engineering: A. 2013, 578, 383–93.

[8] Jiang MG, Xu C, Nakata T, Yan H, Chen RS, Kamado S. Rare earth texture and improved ductility in a Mg-Zn-Gd alloy after high-speed extrusion. Materials Science and Engineering: A. 2016, 667, 233–39.

[9] Mathaudhu SN. The Continued Quest for Low-Temperature Formability in Mg Alloys: Historical Developments and Future Opportunities. In: Solanki K. et al., ed., Magnesium Technology 2017. The Minerals, Metals & Materials Series. Springer, 2017, 9.

[10] Wang H-Y, Feng T-T, Zhang L, Liu C-G, Jiang Q-C. Achieving a weak basal texture in a Mg-6Al-3Sn alloy by wave-shaped die rolling. Materials & Design. 2015, 88, 157–61.

[11] Ghosh AK. On the measurement of strain-rate sensitivity for deformation mechanism in conventional and ultra-fine grain alloys. Materials Science and Engineering: A. 2007, 463, 36–40.

[12] Wang H, Wu P, Kurukuri S, Worswick MJ, Peng Y, Tang D, Li D. Strain rate sensitivities of deformation mechanisms in magnesium alloys. International Journal of Plasticity. 2018, 107, 207–22.

[13] Chapuis A, Liu Q. Modeling strain rate sensitivity and high temperature deformation of Mg-3Al-1Zn alloy. Journal of Magnesium and Alloys. 2019, 7, 433–43.

[14] Bagheriasl R. Tari DG, Kurukuri S, Worswick MJ. Material properties for numerical calculations. Comprehensive Materials Processing. 2014, 1, 227–46.

[15] Korla R, Chokshi AH. Strain-rate sensitivity and microstructural evolution in a Mg–Al–Zn alloy. Scripta Materialia. 2010, 63, 913–16.

[16] Livescu V, Cady CM, Cerreta EK, Henrie BL, Gray GT. The High Strain Rate Deformation Behavior of High Purity Magnesium and AZ31B Magnesium Alloy. In: Mathaudhu SN ed., Essential Readings in Magnesium Technology. The Minerals, Metals, and Materials Society. Springer, Cham. 2016, 375–80.

[17] Matsunaga T, Somekawa H, Hongo H, Tabuchi M. Strain-rate sensitivity enhanced by grain-boundary sliding in creep condition for AZ31 magnesium alloy at room temperature. Materials Science Forum. 2016, 838/839, 106–09.

[18] Hutchinson WB, Barnett MR. Effective values of critical resolved shear stress for slip in polycrystalline magnesium and other hcp metals. Scripta Materialia. 2010, 63, 737–40.

[19] Agnew SR, Mulay RP, Polesak III FJ, Calhoun CA, Bhattacharyya JJ, Clausen B. In situ neutron diffraction and polycrystal plasticity modeling of a Mg-Y-Nd-Zr alloy: Effects of precipitation on individual deformation mechanisms. Acta Materialia. 2013, 61, 3769–80.

[20] Lentz M, Klaus M, Wagner M, Fahrenson C, Beyerlein IJ, Zecevic M, Reimers W, Knezevic M. Effect of age hardening on the deformation behavior of an Mg-Y-Nd alloy: In-situ X-ray

diffraction and crystal plasticity modeling. Materials Science and Engineering A. 2015, 628, 396–409.

[21] Li W, Wang L, Zhou B, Liu C, Zeng X. Grain-scale deformation in a Mg–0.8 wt% Y alloy using crystal plasticity finite element method. Journal of Materials Science & Technology. 2019, 35, 2200–06.

[22] Somekawa H, Basha DA, Singh A. Change in dominant deformation mechanism of Mg alloy via grain boundary control. Materials Science and Engineering: A. 2019, 746, 162–66.

[23] Sun J, Jin L, Dong J, Wang F, Luo AA. Towards high ductility in magnesium alloys – The role of intergranular deformation. International Journal of Plasticity. 2019, 123, 121–32.

[24] Kalpakjian S, Schmid SR. Manufacturing Engineering and Technology. 5th ed., Pearson Prentice Hall, 2006.

[25] Jiang H et al. The influence of Ca and Gd microalloying on microstructure and mechanical property of hot-rolled Mg-3Al alloy. Procedia Engineering. 2017, 207, 932–37.

[26] Guo F et al. Strain-induced dynamic precipitation of Mg17Al12 phases in Mg–8Al alloys sheets rolled at 748K. Materials Science and Engineering: A. 2015, 636, 516–21.

[27] Luo D et al. Effect of differential speed rolling on the room and elevated temperature tensile properties of rolled AZ31 Mg alloy sheets. Materials Characterization. 2017, 124, 223–28.

[28] Ma C et al. Modeling the deformation behavior of a rolled Mg alloy with the EVPSC-TDT model. Materials Science and Engineering: A. 2017, 682, 332–40.

[29] Arab SM et al. On the cold rolling of AZ31 Mg alloy after equal channel angular pressing. Journal of Magnesium and Alloys. 2014, 2, 203–07.

[30] Hua X et al. The anisotropy and diverse mechanical properties of rolled Mg–3% Al–1% Zn alloy. Materials Science and Engineering: A. 2014, 618, 523–32.

[31] Doiphode RL et al. Grain growth in calibre rolled Mg–3Al–1Zn alloy and its effect on hardness. Journal of Magnesium and Alloys. 2015, 3, 322–29.

[32] Xia D et al. Microscopic deformation compatibility during biaxial tension in AZ31 Mg alloy rolled sheet at room temperature. Materials Science and Engineering: A. 2019, 756, 1–10.

[33] Lee JH et al. Improved tensile properties of AZ31 Mg alloy subjected to various caliber-rolling strains. Journal of Magnesium and Alloys. 2019, 7, 381–87.

[34] Ye H et al. Effect of ultrasonic surface rolling process on mechanical properties and corrosion resistance of AZ31B Mg alloy. Surface and Coatings Technology. 2019, 372, 288–98.

[35] Xin R et al. Crystallographic analysis on the activation of multiple twins in rolled AZ31 Mg alloy sheets during uniaxial and plane strain compression. Materials Science and Engineering: A. 2016, 652, 42–50.

[36] Song B et al. Enhancing stretch formability of rolled Mg sheets by pre-inducing contraction twins and recrystallization annealing. Materials Science and Engineering: A. 2015, 627, 369–73.

[37] Li X et al. Improvement of formability of Mg–3Al–1Zn alloy strip by electroplastic-differential speed rolling. Materials Science and Engineering: A. 2014, 618, 500–04.

[38] Zeng Y et al. Effect of Li content on microstructure, texture and mechanical properties of cold rolled Mg–3Al–1Zn alloy. Materials Science and Engineering: A. 2015, 631, 189–95.

[39] He J et al. Texture optimization on Mg sheets by preparing soft orientations of extension twinning for rolling. Materials Science and Engineering: A. 2019, 760, 174–85.

[40] Pan H et al. Mechanical behavior and microstructural evolution in rolled Mg-3Al-1Zn-0.5Mn alloy under large strain simple shear. Materials Science and Engineering: A. 2018, 712, 585–91.

[41] Qian XY et al. Study on mechanical behaviors and theoretical critical shear strength of cold-rolled AZ31 alloy with different Li additions. Materials Science and Engineering: A. 2019, 742, 241–54.

[42] Li X et al. Deformation mechanisms and recrystallization behavior of Mg-3Al-1Zn and Mg-1Gd alloys deformed by electroplastic-asymmetric rolling. Materials Science and Engineering: A. 2019, 742, 722–33.
[43] Jiang Y et al. Recrystallization and texture evolution of cold-rolled AZ31 Mg alloy treated by rapid thermal annealing. Journal of Alloys and Compounds. 2016, 656, 272–77.
[44] Kim S-H et al. Dynamic deformation behavior and microstructural evolution during high-speed rolling of Mg alloy having non-basal texture. Journal of Materials Science & Technology. 2019, 35, 473–82.
[45] Sofinowski K et al. In situ tension-tension strain path changes of cold-rolled Mg AZ31B. Acta Materialia. 2019, 164, 135–52.
[46] Su J et al. Dynamic recrystallization mechanisms during high speed rolling of Mg–3Al–1Zn alloy sheets. Scripta Materialia. 2016, 113, 198–201.
[47] Ko YG et al. Structural features and mechanical properties of AZ31 Mg alloy warm-deformed by differential speed rolling. Journal of Alloys and Compounds. 2018, 744, 96–103.
[48] Kamran J et al. The beneficial effect of AgIn addition on deformation behavior, microstructure and texture in Mg–Al–Zn alloy during single pass warm rolling. Materials & Design. 2015, 81, 11–20.
[49] Mao L et al. Microstructure and mechanical anisotropy of the hot rolled Mg-8.1Al-0.7Zn-0.15Ag alloy. Materials Science and Engineering: A. 2017, 701, 7–15.
[50] Doiphode RL et al. Effects of caliber rolling on microstructure and room temperature tensile properties of Mg–3Al–1Zn alloy. Journal of Magnesium and Alloys. 2013, 1, 169–75.
[51] Lee J-Y et al. Comparison of static recrystallization behavior in hot rolled Mg–3Al–1Zn and Mg–3Zn–0.5Ca sheets. Journal of Alloys and Compounds. 2014, 589, 240–46.
[52] Zheng L et al. Microstructural refinement and improvement of mechanical properties of hot-rolled Mg–3Al–Zn alloy sheets subjected to pre-extrusion and Al-Si alloying. Materials Science and Engineering: A. 2018, 722, 58–68.
[53] Huang W et al. Damage analysis of hot-rolled AZ31 Mg alloy sheet during uniaxial tensile testing under different loading directions. Materials Science and Engineering: A. 2018, 710, 289–99.
[54] Miao Q et al. Grain refining and property improvement of AZ31 Mg alloy by hot rolling. Transactions of Nonferrous Metals Society of China. 2009, 9, s326–s330.
[55] Jia W et al. Heat-transfer analysis of AZ31B Mg alloys during single-pass flat rolling: Experimental verification and mathematical modeling. Materials & Design. 2017, 121, 288–309.
[56] Jia W et al. Role of pre-vertical compression in deformation behavior of Mg alloy AZ31B during super-high reduction hot rolling process. Journal of Materials Science & Technology. 2018, 34, 2069–83.
[57] Gup F et al. Effect of rolling speed on microstructure and mechanical properties of AZ31 Mg alloys rolled with a wide thickness reduction range. Materials Science and Engineering: A. 2014, 619, 66–72.
[58] Gup F et al. Deformation behavior of AZ31 Mg alloys sheet during large strain hot rolling process: A study on microstructure and texture evolutions of an intermediate-rolled sheet. Journal of Alloys and Compounds. 2016, 663, 140–47.
[59] Chai S et al. Effect of partial rolling on the microstructure, mechanical properties and fracture behavior of AZ31 Mg alloy joints. Materials Science and Engineering: A. 2015, 620, 1–9.
[60] Lee JH et al. Dynamic recrystallization behavior and microstructural evolution of Mg alloy AZ31 through high-speed rolling. Journal of Materials Science & Technology. 2018, 34, 1747–55.

[61] Guo F et al. Microstructure, texture and mechanical properties evolution of pre-twinning Mg alloys sheets during large strain hot rolling. Materials Science and Engineering: A. 2016, 655, 92–99.

[62] Guo F et al. The role of Al content on deformation behavior and related texture evolution during hot rolling of Mg-Al-Zn alloys. Journal of Alloys and Compounds. 2017, 695, 396–403.

[63] Yang Q et al. Twinning, grain orientation, and texture variations in Mg alloy processed by pre-rolling. Progress in Natural Science: Materials International. 2019, 29, 231–36.

[64] Jiang Y et al. Mechanism of electropulsing induced recrystallization in a cold-rolled Mg–9Al–1Zn alloy. Journal of Alloys and Compounds. 2012, 536, 94–105.

[65] Jiang Y et al. Improved mechanical properties of Mg–9Al–1Zn alloy by the combination of aging, cold-rolling and electropulsing treatment. Journal of Alloys and Compounds. 2015, 626, 297–303.

[66] Zha M et al. Achieving bimodal microstructure and enhanced tensile properties of Mg–9Al–1Zn alloy by tailoring deformation temperature during hard plate rolling (HPR). Journal of Alloys and Compounds. 2018, 765, 1228–36.

[67] Jin Z-Z et al. Effects of Mg17Al12 second phase particles on twinning-induced recrystallization behavior in Mg–Al–Zn alloys during gradient hot rolling. Journal of Materials Science & Technology. 2019, 35, 2017–26.

[68] Wang H-Y et al. A comparison of microstructure and mechanical properties of Mg–9Al–1Zn sheets rolled from as-cast, cast-rolling and as-extruded alloys. Materials & Design. 2016, 89, 167–72.

[69] Zha M et al. Prominent role of a high volume fraction of Mg17Al12 particles on tensile behaviors of rolled Mg–Al–Zn alloys. Journal of Alloys and Compounds. 2017, 728, 682–93.

[70] Yu Z-P et al. Effect of tensile direction on mechanical properties and microstructural evolutions of rolled Mg-Al-Zn-Sn magnesium alloy sheets at room and elevated temperatures. Journal of Alloys and Compounds. 2018, 744, 211–19.

[71] Cao L et al. Influence of finish rolling temperature on the microstructure and mechanical properties of Mg-8.5Al-0.5Zn-0.2Mn-0.15Ag alloy sheets. Materials Characterization. 2018, 139, 38–48.

[72] Zhang C-C et al. Microstructure and tensile properties of rolled Mg-4Al-2Sn-1Zn alloy with pre-rolling deformation. Materials Science and Engineering: A. 2018, 719, 132–39.

[73] Wang H-Y et al. Achieving a weak basal texture in a Mg–6Al–3Sn alloy by wave-shaped die rolling. Materials & Design. 2015, 88, 157–61.

[74] Luo D et al. Microstructure evolution and tensile properties of hot rolled Mg–6Al–3Sn alloy sheet at elevated temperatures. Materials Science and Engineering: A. 2015, 643, 149–55.

[75] Wang J et al. Microstructure, texture and mechanical properties of hot-rolled Mg–4Al–2Sn–0.5Y–0.4Nd alloy. Journal of Magnesium and Alloys. 2016, 4, 207–13.

[76] Bian MZ et al. Effects of rolling conditions on the microstructure and mechanical properties in a Mg–Al–Ca–Mn–Zn alloy sheet. Materials Science and Engineering: A. 2018, 730, 147–54.

[77] Wang J et al. Effect of hot rolling on the microstructure and mechanical properties of Mg–5Al–0.3Mn–2Nd alloy. Journal of Alloys and Compounds. 2010, 507, 178–83.

[78] Masoumi M et al. The influence of Sr on the microstructure and texture evolution of rolled Mg–1%Zn alloy. Materials Science and Engineering: A. 2011, 529, 207–14.

[79] Wei S et al. Effects of Sn addition on the microstructure and mechanical properties of as-cast, rolled and annealed Mg–4Zn alloys. Materials Science and Engineering: A. 2013, 585, 139–48.

[80] Shi BQ et al. Hall-Petch relationship, twinning responses and their dependences on grain size in the rolled Mg-Zn and Mg-Y alloys. Materials Science and Engineering: A. 2019, 743, 558–66.

[81] Pan H et al. High-conductivity binary Mg–Zn sheet processed by cold rolling and subsequent aging. Journal of Alloys and Compounds. 2013, 578, 493–500.
[82] Yuan Y et al. Superior mechanical properties of ZK60 Mg alloy processed by equal channel angular pressing and rolling. Materials Science and Engineering: A. 2015, 630, 45–50.
[83] Lee T et al. Enhanced yield symmetry and strength-ductility balance of caliber-rolled Mg–6Zn-0.5Zr with ultrafine-grained structure and bulk dimension. Journal of Alloys and Compounds. 2019, 803, 434–41.
[84] Guo H et al. Effect of electropulsing treatment on static recrystallization behavior of cold-rolled magnesium alloy ZK60 with different reductions. Journal of Materials Science & Technology. 2019, 35, 1113–20.
[85] Kim YM et al. Static recrystallization behaviour of cold rolled Mg-Zn-Y alloy and role of solute segregation in microstructure evolution. Scripta Materialia. 2017, 136, 41–45.
[86] Shi BQ et al. Achieving ultra-low planar anisotropy and high stretch formability in a Mg-1.1Zn-0.76Y-0.56Zr sheet by texture tailoring via final-pass heavy reduction rolling. Materials Science and Engineering: A. 2019, 746, 115–26.
[87] Itoi T et al. Microstructure and mechanical properties of Mg-Zn-Y alloy sheet prepared by hot-rolling. Materials Science and Engineering: A. 2013, 560, 216–23.
[88] Jiang J et al. New orientations between β′2 phase and α matrix in a Mg-Zn-Mn alloy processed by high strain rate rolling. Journal of Alloys and Compounds. 2018, 750, 465–70.
[89] Chen C et al. Dynamic precipitation, microstructure and mechanical properties of Mg-5Zn-1Mn alloy sheets prepared by high strain-rate rolling. Materials & Design. 2016, 100, 58–66.
[90] Yan H et al. Room-temperature ductility and anisotropy of two rolled Mg–Zn–Gd alloys. Materials Science and Engineering: A. 2010, 527, 3317–22.
[91] Pan S et al. Tailoring the texture and mechanical anisotropy of a Mg–2Zn–2Gd plate by varying the rolling path. Materials Science and Engineering: A. 2016, 653, 93–98.
[92] Zhao LY et al. Study on the evolution pattern of grain orientation and misorientation during the static recrystallization of cold-rolled Mg-Zn-Gd alloy. Materials Characterization. 2019, 150, 252–66.
[93] Pan S et al. The effect of hot rolling regime on texture and mechanical properties of an as-cast Mg–2Zn–2Gd plate. Materials Science and Engineering: A. 2018, 731, 288–95.
[94] Luo J et al. Effects of Gd concentration on microstructure, texture and tensile properties of Mg–Zn–Gd alloys subjected to large strain hot rolling. Materials Science and Engineering: A. 2104, 614, 88–95.
[95] Verma R et al. Studies on tensile behaviour and microstructural evolution of UFG Mg-4Zn-4Gd alloy processed through hot rolling. Materials Science and Engineering: A. 2017, 704, 412–16.
[96] Zeng ZR et al. Texture evolution during cold rolling of dilute Mg alloys. Scripta Materialia. 2015, 108, 6–10.
[97] Tong LB et al. Effect of warm rolling on the microstructure, texture and mechanical properties of extruded Mg–Zn–Ca–Ce/La alloy. Materials Characterization. 2016, 115, 1–7.
[98] Li Q et al. On the texture evolution of Mg–Zn–Ca alloy with different hot rolling paths. Journal of Magnesium and Alloys. 2017, 5, 166–72.
[99] Huang X et al. Static recrystallization behavior of hot-rolled Mg-Zn-Ce magnesium alloy sheet. Journal of Alloys and Compounds. 2017, 724, 981–90.
[100] Wu T et al. Improved ductility of Mg–Zn–Ce alloy by hot pack-rolling. Materials Science and Engineering: A. 2013, 584, 97–102.
[101] Chen WZ et al. Property improvements in fine–grained Mg–Zn–Zr alloy sheets produced by temperature–step–down multi–pass rolling. Journal of Alloys and Compounds. 2015, 646, 195–203.

[102] Markushev MV et al. Structure, texture and strength of Mg-5.8Zn-0.65Zr alloy after hot-to-warm multi-step isothermal forging and isothermal rolling to large strains. Materials Science and Engineering: A. 2018, 709, 330–38.
[103] Ding W et al. Microstructure and mechanical properties of hot-rolled Mg–Zn–Nd–Zr alloys. Materials Science and Engineering: A. 2008, 483/484, 228–30.
[104] Chiang C-T et al. Rolling route for refining grains of super light Mg-Li alloys containing Sc and Be. Transactions of Nonferrous Metals Society of China. 2010, 20, 1374–79.
[105] Sha G et al. Effects of Sc addition and annealing treatment on the microstructure and mechanical properties of the As-rolled Mg-3Li alloy. Journal of Materials Science & Technology. 2011, 27, 753–58.
[106] Cao F et al. Mechanical properties and microstructural evolution in a superlight Mg-7.28Li-2.19Al-0.091Y alloy fabricated by rolling. Journal of Alloys and Compounds. 2018, 745, 436–45.
[107] Yan H et al. Microstructures and mechanical properties of cold rolled Mg-8Li and Mg-8Li-2Al-2RE alloys. Transactions of Nonferrous Metals Society of China. 2010, 20, s550–s554.
[108] Wu SK et al. X-ray diffraction studies on cold-rolled/solid–solution treated α+β Mg–10.2Li–1.2Al–0.4Zn alloy. Journal of Alloys and Compounds. 2013, 563, 234–41.
[109] Tang Y et al. Influences of warm rolling and annealing processes on microstructure and mechanical properties of three parent structures containing Mg-Li alloys. Materials Science and Engineering: A. 2018, 711, 1–11.
[110] Wang T et al. Influence of rolling directions on microstructure, mechanical properties and anisotropy of Mg-5Li-1Al-0.5Y alloy. Journal of Magnesium and Alloys. 2015, 3, 345–51.
[111] Liu W et al. Effect of rolling strain on microstructure and tensile properties of dual-phase Mg–8Li–3Al–2Zn–0.5Y alloy. Journal of Materials Science & Technology. 2018, 34, 2256–62.
[112] Kim JT et al. Microstructure and mechanical properties of the as-cast and warm rolled Mg-9Li-x(Al-Si)-yTi alloys with x = 1, 3, 5 and y = 0.05 wt.%. Journal of Alloys and Compounds. 2017, 711, 243–49.
[113] Shi Q et al. Effects of adding Al–Si eutectic alloy and hot rolling on microstructures and mechanical behavior of Mg–8Li alloys. Journal of Alloys and Compounds. 2015, 631, 129–32.
[114] Muga C et al. Effects of holmium and hot-rolling on microstructure and mechanical properties of Mg-Li based alloys. Journal of Rare Earths. 2016, 34, 1269–76.
[115] Nene SS et al. Microstructure refinement and its effect on specific strength and bio-corrosion resistance in ultralight Mg–4Li–1Ca (LC41) alloy by hot rolling. Journal of Alloys and Compounds. 2014, 615, 501–06.
[116] Estrin Y et al. New hot rolled Mg-4Li-1Ca alloy: A potential candidate for automotive and biodegradable implant applications. Materials Letters. 2016, 173, 252–56.
[117] Cao F et al. Mechanical properties and microstructural evolution in a superlight Mg-6.4Li-3.6Zn-0.37Al-0.36Y alloy processed by multidirectional forging and rolling. Materials Science and Engineering: A. 2019, 760, 377–93.
[118] Seong JW et al. Development of biodegradable Mg–Ca alloy sheets with enhanced strength and corrosion properties though the refinement and uniform dispersion of the Mg2Ca phase by high-ratio differential speed rolling. Acta Biomaterialia. 2015, 11, 531–42.
[119] Masoumi M et al. The influence of Ce on the microstructure and rolling texture of Mg–1%Mn alloy. Materials Science and Engineering: A. 2011, 528, 3122–29.
[120] Shi Y et al. Enhancing creep properties of a hot-rolled Mg-4Y binary alloy via a new thought of inhibiting cross-slip. Materials Characterization. 2019, 147, 64–71.
[121] Farzadfar SA et al. On the deformation, recrystallization and texture of hot-rolled Mg–2.9Y and Mg–2.9Zn solid solution alloys – A comparative study. Materials Science and Engineering: A. 2012, 534, 209–19.

[122] Wu S et al. A high strength and good ductility Mg–Y–NI–TI alloy with long period stacking ordered structure processed by hot rolling and aging treatment. Materials Science and Engineering: A. 2015, 648, 134–39.
[123] Tong LB et al. Enhanced mechanical properties of extruded Mg–Y–Zn alloy fabricated via low-strain rolling. Materials Science and Engineering: A. 2015, 620, 483–89.
[124] Asgari H et al. Effect of grain size on high strain rate deformation of rolled Mg–4Y–3RE alloy in compression. Materials Science and Engineering: A. 2015, 633, 92–102.
[125] Wu WX et al. Microstructure and texture evolution during hot rolling and subsequent annealing of Mg–1Gd alloy. Materials Science and Engineering: A. 2013, 582, 194–202.
[126] Wu D et al. Strength enhancement of Mg–3Gd–1Zn alloy by cold rolling. Transactions of Nonferrous Metals Society of China. 2013, 23, 301–06.
[127] Wang R et al. Microstructure and mechanical properties of rolled Mg-12Gd-3Y-0.4Zr alloy sheets. Transactions of Nonferrous Metals Society of China. 2008, 18, s189–s193.
[128] Zhang P et al. Mechanical properties of the hot-rolled Mg–12Gd–3Y magnesium alloy. Materials Chemistry and Physics. 2009, 118, 453–58.
[129] Nie X et al. Flow behavior and formability of hot-rolled Mg-8Gd-3Y alloy under double-pass isothermal compression. Journal of Materials Processing Technology. 2020, 275; https://doi.org/10.1016/j.jmatprotec.2019.116328.
[130] Xu C et al. Microstructure and mechanical properties of rolled sheets of Mg–Gd–Y–Zn–Zr alloy: As-cast versus as-homogenized. Journal of Alloys and Compounds. 2012, 528, 40–44.
[131] Xu C et al. Ultra high-strength Mg–Gd–Y–Zn–Zr alloy sheets processed by large-strain hot rolling and ageing. Materials Science and Engineering: A. 2012, 547, 93–98.
[132] Shao J et al. Texture evolution, deformation mechanism and mechanical properties of the hot rolled Mg-Gd-Y-Zn-Zr alloy containing LPSO phase. Materials Science and Engineering: A. 2018, 731, 479–86.
[133] Chen Z-B et al. Effect of rolling passes on the microstructures and mechanical properties of Mg–Gd–Y–Zr alloy sheets. Materials Science and Engineering: A. 2014, 618, 232–37.
[134] Yu S et al. Microstructure, texture and mechanical properties of Mg-Gd-Y-Zr alloy annular forging processed by hot ring rolling. Materials Science and Engineering: A. 2017, 689, 40–47.
[135] Yao Y et al. Annealing-induced microstructural evolution and mechanical anisotropy improvement of the Mg-Gd-Y-Zr alloy processed by hot ring rolling. Materials Characterization. 2018, 144, 641–51.
[136] Yu S et al. Dynamic recrystallization mechanism of Mg-8.5Gd-2.5Y-0.4Zr alloy during hot ring rolling. Materials Characterization. 2017, 131, 135–39.
[137] Guan R-G et al. Microstructure and properties of Mg–3Sn–1Mn (wt%) alloy processed by a novel continuous shearing and rolling and heat treatment. Materials Science and Engineering: A. 2013, 559, 194–200.
[138] Guan RG et al. Microstructure evolution and properties of Mg–3Sn–1Mn (wt%) alloy strip processed by semisolid rheo-rolling. Journal of Materials Processing Technology. 2012, 212, 1430–36.
[139] Shi Z-Z et al. Microstructure and mechanical properties of as-cast and as-hot-rolled novel Mg-xSn-2.5Zn-2Al alloys (x = 2, 4wt%). Materials Science and Engineering: A. 2018, 712, 65–72.
[140] Hadorn JP et al. A new metastable phase in dilute, hot-rolled Mg–Nd alloys. Materials Science and Engineering: A. 2012, 533, 9–16.
[141] Li Z et al. Effect of rolling deformation on microstructure and texture of spray-deposited magnesium alloy containing Mg-Nd-Zn typed LPSO. Journal of Materials Science & Technology. 2017, 33, 630–36.

[142] Wu J et al. Effect of hot rolling on the microstructure and discharge properties of Mg-1.6 wt% Hg-2 wt%Ga alloy anodes. Journal of Alloys and Compounds. 2018, 765, 736–46.
[143] Chen L et al. Effect of ultrasonic cold forging technology as the pretreatment on the corrosion resistance of MAO Ca/P coating on AZ31B Mg alloy. Journal of Alloys and Compounds. 2015, 635, 278–88.
[144] Jiang MG et al. Twinning, recrystallization and texture development during multi-directional impact forging in an AZ61 Mg alloy. Journal of Alloys and Compounds. 2015, 650, 399–409.
[145] Jiang MG et al. Enhanced mechanical properties due to grain refinement and texture modification in an AZ61 Mg alloy processed by small strain impact forging. Materials Science and Engineering: A. 2015, 621, 204–11.
[146] Jiang MG et al. Microstructure, texture and mechanical properties in an as-cast AZ61 Mg alloy during multi-directional impact forging and subsequent heat treatment. Materials & Design. 2015, 87, 891–900.
[147] Xia X-S et al. Microstructure and mechanical properties of isothermal multi-axial forging formed AZ61 Mg alloy. Transactions of Nonferrous Metals Society of China. 2013, 23, 3186–92.
[148] Chen J-K et al. Effects of Nd and rotary forging on mechanical properties of AZ71 Mg alloys. Transactions of Nonferrous Metals Society of China. 2015, 25, 3223–31.
[149] Miura H et al. Microstructure and mechanical properties of multi-directionally forged Mg–Al–Zn alloy. Scripta Materialia. 2012, 66, 49–51.
[150] Yoon J et al. Enhancement of the microstructure and mechanical properties in as-forged Mg–8Al–0.5Zn alloy using T5 heat treatment. Materials Science and Engineering: A. 2013, 586, 306–12.
[151] Jiang MG et al. Microstructural evolution of Mg-7Al-2Sn Mg alloy during multi-directional impact forging. Journal of Magnesium and Alloys. 2015, 3, 180–87.
[152] Sanyal S et al. Influence of hard plate hot forging temperature on the microstructure, texture and mechanical properties in a lean Mg–Zn–Al alloy. Journal of Alloys and Compounds. 2019, 800, 343–54.
[153] Jamali A et al. Evolution of microstructure, texture, and mechanical properties in a multi-directionally forged ZK60 Mg alloy. Materials Science and Engineering: A. 2019, 752, 55–62.
[154] Garcés G et al. Effect of hot forging on the microstructure and mechanical properties of Mg–Zn–Y alloy. Journal of Materials Processing Technology. 2008, 206, 99–105.
[155] Wang SD et al. Effect of heat treatment on the corrosion resistance and mechanical properties of an as-forged Mg–Zn–Y–Zr alloy. Corrosion Science. 2015, 92, 228–36.
[156] Wang D et al. Effects of variable-cavity liquid forging on microstructure and mechanical properties of Mg–Zn–Y–Zr alloy. Materials Characterization. 2019, 151, 96–102.
[157] Li K et al. Nanoscale deformation of multiaxially forged ultrafine-grained Mg-2Zn-2Gd alloy with high strength-high ductility combination and comparison with the coarse-grained counterpart. Journal of Materials Science & Technology. 2018, 34, 311–16.
[158] Kang J-W et al. Microstructure and mechanical properties of Mg-4Zn-0.5Ca alloy fabricated by the combination of forging, homogenization and extrusion process. Journal of Alloys and Compounds. 2017, 720, 196–206.
[159] Panigrahi SK et al. A study on the combined effect of forging and aging in Mg–Y–RE alloy. Materials Science and Engineering: A. 2011, 530, 28–35.
[160] Shah SSA et al. Microstructural evolution and mechanical properties of a Mg-Gd-Y alloy processed by impact forging. Materials Science and Engineering: A. 2017, 702, 153–60.
[161] Liu B et al. Forgeability, microstructure and mechanical properties of a free-forged Mg–8Gd–3Y–0.4Zr alloy. Materials Science and Engineering: A. 2016, 650, 233–39.

[162] Zhou H et al. Finite element simulation and experimental investigation on homogeneity of Mg-9.8Gd-2.7Y-0.4Zr magnesium alloy processed by repeated-upsetting. Journal of Materials Processing Technology. 2015, 225, 310–17.
[163] Zhou H et al. Uniform fine microstructure and random texture of Mg–9.8Gd–2.7Y–0.4Zr magnesium alloy processed by repeated-upsetting deformation. Materials Letters. 2012, 83, 175–78.
[164] Shah SSA et al. Static recrystallization behavior of multi-directional impact forged Mg-Gd-Y-Zr alloy. Journal of Alloys and Compounds. 2019, 805, 189–97.
[165] Wang B et al. Microstructure evolution and mechanical properties of Mg-Gd-Y-Ag-Zr alloy fabricated by multidirectional forging and ageing treatment. Materials Science and Engineering: A. 2017, 702, 22–28.
[166] Xia X et al. Microstructure, texture and mechanical properties of coarse-grained Mg–Gd–Y–Nd–Zr alloy processed by multidirectional forging. Journal of Alloys and Compounds. 2015, 623, 62–68.
[167] Metayer J et al. Microstructure and mechanical properties of Mg–Si alloys processed by cyclic closed-die forging. Transactions of Nonferrous Metals Society of China. 2014, 24, 66–75.
[168] http://aluitaliaco.blogspot.com/2010/08/extrusion-press-directindirect_07.html.
[169] http://www.industrialextrusionmachinery.com/extrusion_process_direct_extrusion_and_indirect_extrusion.html.
[170] Pozuelo M et al. Enhanced compressive strength of an extruded nanostructured Mg–10Al alloy. Materials Science and Engineering: A. 2014, 594, 203–11.
[171] Tork NB et al. Microstructure and texture characterization of Mg–Al and Mg–Gd binary alloys processed by simple shear extrusion. Journal of Materials Research and Technology. 2019, 8, 1288–99.
[172] Park SH et al. Improving mechanical properties of extruded Mg–Al alloy with a bimodal grain structure through alloying addition. Journal of Alloys and Compounds. 2015, 646, 932–36.
[173] Razzaghi M et al. Unraveling the effects of Zn addition and hot extrusion process on the microstructure and mechanical properties of as-cast Mg–2Al magnesium alloy. Vacuum. 2019, 167, 214–22.
[174] Kang J-W et al. High strength Mg-9Al serial alloy processed by slow extrusion. Materials Science and Engineering: A. 2017, 697, 211–16.
[175] Hou J et al. Significantly enhancing the strength + ductility combination of Mg-9Al alloy using multi-walled carbon nanotubes. Journal of Alloys and Compounds. 2019, 790, 974–82.
[176] WU Y et al. Microstructure and mechanical behavior of a Mg AZ31/Al 7050 laminate composite fabricated by extrusion. Materials Science and Engineering: A. 2015, 640, 454–59.
[177] Peláez D et al. Mechanical and microstructural evolution of Mg AZ31 alloy using ECASD process. Journal of Materials Research and Technology. 2015, 4, 392–97.
[178] Xu J et al. Unusual texture formation in Mg–3Al–1Zn alloy sheets processed by slope extrusion. Materials Science and Engineering: A. 2018, 732, 1–5.
[179] Xu J et al. Improved mechanical properties of Mg-3Al-1Zn alloy sheets by optimizing the extrusion die angles: Microstructural and texture evolution. Journal of Alloys and Compounds. 2018, 762, 719–29.
[180] Xu J et al. Effect of effective strain gradient on texture and mechanical properties of Mg–3Al–1Zn alloy sheets produced by asymmetric extrusion. Materials Science and Engineering: A. 2017, 706, 172–80.
[181] Chen H-B et al. Influence of pre-strain and heat treatment on subsequent deformation behavior of extruded AZ31 Mg alloy. Transactions of Nonferrous Metals Society of China. 2015, 25, 3604–10.

[182] Chen C et al. Study on cyclic deformation behavior of extruded Mg–3Al–1Zn alloy. Materials Science and Engineering: A. 2012, 539, 223–29.
[183] Qiao J et al. High temperature tensile behaviors of extruded and rolled AZ31 Mg alloy. Transactions of Nonferrous Metals Society of China, 2010, 20, s540–s544.
[184] Jiang B et al. Mechanical properties and microstructure of as-extruded AZ31 Mg alloy at high temperatures. Materials Science and Engineering: A. 2011, 530, 51–56.
[185] Jiang B et al. Influence of crystallographic texture and grain size on the corrosion behaviour of as-extruded Mg alloy AZ31 sheets. Corrosion Science. 2017, 126, 374–80.
[186] Xu S et al. The interrupted properties of an extruded Mg alloy. Materials & Design. 2013, 45, 166–70.
[187] Kim B et al. Grain refinement and improved tensile properties of Mg–3Al–1Zn alloy processed by low-temperature indirect extrusion. Scripta Materialia. 2014, 76, 21–24.
[188] Xin R et al. Geometrical compatibility factor analysis of paired extension twins in extruded Mg–3Al–1Zn alloys. Materials & Design. 2015, 86, 656–63.
[189] Wang B et al. In-situ investigation on nucleation and propagation of {10-12} twins during uniaxial multi-pass compression in an extruded AZ31 Mg alloy. Materials Science and Engineering: A. 2018, 731, 71–79.
[190] Jin L et al. Microstructure evolution of AZ31 Mg alloy during equal channel angular extrusion. Materials Science and Engineering: A. 2006, 423, 247–52.
[191] Chen Y et al. Effects of extrusion ratio on the microstructure and mechanical properties of AZ31 Mg alloy. Journal of Materials Processing Technology. 2007, 182, 281–85.
[192] Song L et al. The effect of Ca addition on microstructure and mechanical properties of extruded AZ31 alloys. Vacuum. 2019, 168; https://doi.org/10.1016/j.vacuum.2019.108822.
[193] Lu L et al. Microstructure and mechanical property of dual-directional-extruded Mg alloy AZ31. Materials Science and Engineering: A. 2010, 527, 4050–55.
[194] Tian S-G et al. Microstructure and properties of hot extruded AZ31-0.25%Sb Mg-alloy. Transactions of Nonferrous Metals Society of China. 2008, 18, s17–s21.
[195] Hu Z et al. Effects of ultrasonic vibration on microstructure evolution and elevated-temperature mechanical properties of hot-extruded Mg-6Al-0.8Zn-2.0Sm wrought magnesium alloys. Journal of Alloys and Compounds. 2016, 685, 58–64.
[196] Wu H-Y et al. Dynamic behavior of extruded AZ61 Mg alloy during hot compression. Materials Science and Engineering: A. 2012, 535, 68–75.
[197] Gryguć A et al. Multiaxial cyclic behaviour of extruded and forged AZ80 Mg alloy. International Journal of Fatigue. 2019, 127, 324–37.
[198] Kavyani M et al. Texture evaluation in warm deformation of an extruded Mg–6Al–3Zn alloy. Journal of Magnesium and Alloys. 2016, 4, 89–98.
[199] Suh JS et al. Microstructures and Mechanical Properties of Direct-Extruded Novel Mg Alloys. Procedia Engineering 2017, 207, 908–13.
[200] Go Y et al. Microstructure and mechanical properties of non-flammable Mg-8Al-0.3Zn-0.1Mn-0.3Ca-0.2Y alloy subjected to low-temperature, low-speed extrusion. Journal of Alloys and Compounds. 2018, 739, 69–76.
[201] Luo L et al. Enhanced mechanical properties of a hot-extruded AZ80 Mg alloy rod by pre-treatments and post-hot compression. Journal of Alloys and Compounds. 2018, 740, 180–93.
[202] Yu H et al. Development of extraordinary high-strength Mg–8Al–0.5Zn alloy via a low temperature and slow speed extrusion. Materials Science and Engineering: A. 2014, 610, 445–49.
[203] Park SH et al. Influence of Sn addition on the microstructure and mechanical properties of extruded Mg–8Al–2Zn alloy. Materials Science and Engineering: A. 2015, 626, 128–35.

[204] Ying T et al. Recycling of AZ91 Mg alloy through consolidation of machined chips by extrusion and ECAP. Transactions of Nonferrous Metals Society of China. 2010, 20, s604–s607.
[205] He J et al. Improved tension-compression performance of Mg-Al-Zn alloy processed by co-extrusion. Materials Science and Engineering: A. 2016, 675, 76–81.
[206] Peng P et al. Novel continuous forging extrusion in a one-step extrusion process for bulk ultrafine magnesium alloy. Materials Science and Engineering: A. 2019, 764; https://doi.org/10.1016/j.msea.2019.138144.
[207] Chen L et al. Microstructure and mechanical properties of Mg-Al-Zn alloy extruded by porthole die with different initial billets. Materials Science and Engineering: A. 2018, 718, 390–97.
[208] Bu F et al. Study on the assemblage of Y and Gd on microstructure and mechanical properties of hot extruded Mg–Al–Zn alloy. Materials Science and Engineering: A. 2015, 639, 198–207.
[209] Kim S-H et al. Effect of billet diameter on hot extrusion behavior of Mg–Al–Zn alloys and its influence on microstructure and mechanical properties. Journal of Alloys and Compounds. 2017, 690, 417–23.
[210] Bae SW et al. Improvement of mechanical properties and reduction of yield asymmetry of extruded Mg-Al-Zn alloy through Sn addition. Journal of Alloys and Compounds. 2018, 766, 748–58.
[211] Bu F et al. Study on the mutual effect of La and Gd on microstructure and mechanical properties of Mg-Al-Zn extruded alloy. Journal of Alloys and Compounds. 2016, 688, 1241–50.
[212] Chen L et al. Microstructure and texture evolution during porthole die extrusion of Mg-Al-Zn alloy. Journal of Materials Processing Technology. 2018, 259, 346–52.
[213] Wang F et al. Significant improvement in the strength of Mg-Al-Zn-Ca-Mn extruded alloy by tailoring the initial microstructure. Vacuum. 2019, 161, 429–33.
[214] She J et al. Microstructure and mechanical properties of Mg–Al–Sn extruded alloys. Journal of Alloys and Compound. 2016, 657, 893–905.
[215] Wang H-Y et al. Effects of Zn on the microstructure and tensile properties of as-extruded Mg-8Al-2Snalloy. Materials Science and Engineering: A. 2017, 698, 249–55.
[216] Lee S-I et al. Evolution of tension and compression asymmetry of extruded Mg-Al-Sn-Zn alloy with respect to forming temperatures. Materials & Design. 2016, 110, 510–18.
[217] Park SH et al. A new high-strength extruded Mg-8Al-4Sn-2Zn alloy. Materials Letters. 2015, 139, 35–38.
[218] Nakata T et al. Optimization of Mn content for high strengths in high-speed extruded Mg-0.3Al-0.3Ca (wt%) dilute alloy. Materials Science and Engineering: A. 2016, 673, 443–49.
[219] Nakata T et al. Improving mechanical properties and yield asymmetry in high-speed extrudable Mg-1.1Al-0.24Ca (wt%) alloy by high Mn addition. Materials Science and Engineering: A. 2018, 712, 12–19.
[220] Homma T et al. Room and elevated temperature mechanical properties in the as-extruded Mg–Al–Ca–Mn alloys. Materials Science and Engineering: A. 2012, 539, 163–69.
[221] Nakata T et al. High-speed extrusion of heat-treatable Mg–Al–Ca–Mn dilute alloy. Scripta Materialia. 2015, 101, 28–31.
[222] Nakata T et al. Improving tensile properties of dilute Mg-0.27Al-0.13Ca-0.21Mn (at.%) alloy by low temperature high speed extrusion. Journal of Alloys and Compounds. 2015, 648, 428–37.
[223] Li ZT et al. Ultrahigh strength Mg-Al-Ca-Mn extrusion alloys with various aluminum contents. Journal of Alloys and Compounds. 2019, 792, 130–41.
[224] Han G et al. Development of non-flammable high strength extruded Mg-Al-Ca-Mn alloys with high Ca/Al ratio. Journal of Materials Science & Technology. 2018, 34, 2063–68.
[225] Xu SW et al. High-strength extruded Mg–Al–Ca–Mn alloy. Scripta Materialia. 2011, 65, 269–72.

[226] Qiao H et al. Twin-induced hardening in extruded Mg alloy AM30. Materials Science and Engineering: A. 2017, 687, 17–27.
[227] Farbaniec L et al. Spall response and failure mechanisms associated with a hot-extruded AMX602 Mg alloy. Materials Science and Engineering: A. 2017, 707, 725–31.
[228] Wang J et al. The effect of Y content on microstructure and tensile properties of the extruded Mg–1Al-xY alloy. Materials Science and Engineering: A 2019, 765; https://doi.org/10.1016/j.msea.2019.138288.
[229] Bai J et al. Effect of extrusion on microstructures, and mechanical and creep properties of Mg–Al–Sr and Mg–Al–Sr–Ca alloys. Scripta Materialia. 2006, 55, 1163–66.
[230] Zhao C et al. Strain hardening of as-extruded Mg-xZn (x = 1, 2, 3 and 4 wt%) alloys. Journal of Materials Science & Technology. 2019, 35, 142–50.
[231] Ying T et al. Thermal conductivity of as-cast and as-extruded binary Mg–Zn alloys. Journal of Alloys and Compounds. 2015, 621, 250–55.
[232] Drozdenko D et al. Mobility of pinned twin boundaries during mechanical loading of extruded binary Mg-1Zn alloy. Materials Characterization. 2018, 139, 81–88
[233] Ross NG et al. Effect of alloying and extrusion temperature on the microstructure and mechanical properties of Mg–Zn and Mg–Zn–RE alloys. Materials Science and Engineering: A. 2014, 619, 238–46.
[234] Yan K et al. Preparation of a high strength and high ductility Mg-6Zn alloy wire by combination of ECAP and hot drawing. Materials Science and Engineering: A. 2019, 739, 513–18.
[235] Liu W et al. Grain refinement and fatigue strengthening mechanisms in as-extruded Mg–6Zn–0.5Zr and Mg–10Gd–3Y–0.5Zr magnesium alloys by shot peening. International Journal of Plasticity. 2013, 49, 16–35.
[236] Kim B et al. Enhanced strength and plasticity of Mg–6Zn–0.5Zr alloy by low-temperature indirect extrusion. Journal of Alloys and Compounds. 2017, 706, 56–62.
[237] Jeong HY et al. Effect of Ce addition on the microstructure and tensile properties of extruded Mg–Zn–Zr alloys. Materials Science and Engineering: A. 2014, 612, 217–22.
[238] Li X et al. Microstructure, Texture and Mechanical Properties of Extruded Mg-Zn-Zr Mg Alloy Profiles. Rare Metal Materials and Engineering. 2014, 43, 2927–30.
[239] Wang H-Y et al. Tensile properties, texture evolutions and deformation anisotropy of as-extruded Mg-6Zn-1Zr magnesium alloy at room and elevated temperatures. Materials Science and Engineering: A. 2017, 697, 149–57.
[240] Wan YC et al. Effect of Nd and Dy on the microstructure and mechanical property of the as extruded Mg–1Zn–0.6Zr alloy. Materials Science and Engineering: A. 2015, 625, 158–63.
[241] Shazad M et al. The roles of Zn distribution and eutectic particles on microstructure development during extrusion and anisotropic mechanical properties in a Mg–Zn–Zr alloy. Materials Science and Engineering: A. 2015, 620, 50–57.
[242] Medina J et al. Effects of calcium, manganese and cerium-rich misch metal additions on the mechanical properties of extruded Mg-Zn-Y alloy reinforced by quasicrystalline I-phase. Materials Characterization. 2017, 129, 195–206.
[243] Kim T-S. Effect of rapid cooling and extrusion ratio on the mechanical property of Mg alloys. Journal of Alloys and Compounds. 2010, 504, s496–s499.
[244] Li J et al. Evolution of microstructure and tensile properties of extruded Mg-4Zn-1Y alloy. Journal of Rare Earths. 2014, 32, 1189–95.
[245] Hagihara K et al. Strengthening mechanisms acting in extruded Mg-based long-period stacking ordered (LPSO)-phase alloys. Acta Materialia. 2019, 163, 226–39.
[246] Qiao X et al. Influence of hot extrusion and aging treatment on the properties of biodegradable Mg-Zn-Y alloy. Rare Metal Materials and Engineering. 2018, 47, 773–79.

[247] Yamasaki M et al. Effect of multimodal microstructure evolution on mechanical properties of Mg–Zn–Y extruded alloy. Acta Materialia. 2011, 59, 3646–58.
[248] Yang W-P et al. High strength magnesium alloy with α-Mg and W-phase processed by hot extrusion. Transactions of Nonferrous Metals Society of China. 2011, 21, 2358–64.
[249] Singh A et al. Quasicrystal strengthened Mg–Zn–Y alloys by extrusion. Scripta Materialia. 2003, 49, 417–22.
[250] Wang D et al. Effects of Heat Treatment on Microstructure and Mechanical Properties of As-extruded Mg-Zn-Y-Zr Alloy. Rare Metal Materials and Engineering. 2018, 47, 3345–52.
[251] Xu DK et al. The influence of element Y on the mechanical properties of the as-extruded Mg–Zn–Y–Zr alloys. Journal of Alloys and Compounds. 2006, 426, 155–61.
[252] Jiang H et al. Influence of size and distribution of W phase on strength and ductility of high strength Mg-5.1Zn-3.2Y-0.4Zr-0.4Ca alloy processed by indirect extrusion. Journal of Materials Science & Technology. 2018, 34, 277–83.
[253] Du Z et al. Influence of hot extrusion process on microstructure and mechanical properties of Mg-Zn-Y-Zr magnesium alloy. Rare Metal Materials and Engineering. 2018, 47, 1655–61.
[254] Jiang HS et al. The partial substitution of Y with Gd on microstructures and mechanical properties of as-cast and as-extruded Mg-10Zn-6Y-0.5Zr alloy. Materials Characterization. 2018, 135, 96–103.
[255] Jiang HS et al. Ultrahigh strength as-extruded Mg–10.3Zn–6.4Y–0.4Zr–0.5Ca alloy containing W phase. Materials & Design. 2016, 108, 391–99.
[256] Xia X et al. Hot deformation behavior of extruded Mg–Zn–Y–Zr alloy. Journal of Alloys and Compounds. 2015, 644, 308–16.
[257] Wang B et al. Effects of Nd on microstructures and properties of extruded Mg–2Zn–0.46Y–xNd alloys for stent application. Materials Science and Engineering: B. 2011, 176, 1673–78.
[258] Feng Y et al. Fabrication and characterization of biodegradable Mg-Zn-Y-Nd-Ag alloy: Microstructure, mechanical properties, corrosion behavior and antibacterial activities. Bioactive Materials. 2018, 3, 225–35.
[259] Ye L et al. Effects of Sn on the microstructure and mechanical properties of a hot-extruded Mg-Zn-Y-Sn alloy. Materials Science and Engineering: A. 2018, 724, 121–30.
[260] Kang XK et al. Effect of extrusion parameters on microstructure, texture and mechanical properties of Mg-1.38Zn-0.17Y-0.12Ca (at.%) alloy. Materials Characterization. 2019, 151, 137–45.
[261] Mohammadi FD et al. Microstructure characterization and effect of extrusion temperature on biodegradation behavior of Mg-5Zn-1Y-xCa alloy. Transactions of Nonferrous Metals Society of China. 2018, 28, 2199–213.
[262] Peng J et al. Effect of extrusion temperature on the microstructure and thermal conductivity of Mg–2.0Zn–1.0Mn–0.2Ce alloys. Materials & Design. 2015, 87, 914–19.
[263] Tahreen N et al. Characterization of hot deformation behavior of an extruded Mg–Zn–Mn–Y alloy containing LPSO phase. Journal of Alloys and Compounds. 2015, 644, 814–23.
[264] Tahreen N et al. Hot Deformation and Work Hardening Behavior of an Extruded Mg–Zn–Mn–Y Alloy. Journal of Materials Science & Technology. 2015, 31, 1161–70.
[265] Park SH et al. Effects of extrusion parameters on the microstructure and mechanical properties of Mg–Zn–(Mn)–Ce/Gd alloys. Materials Science and Engineering: A. 2014, 598, 396–406.
[266] Hu G-S et al. Microstructures and mechanical properties of as-extruded and heat treated Mg–6Zn–1Mn–4Sn–1.5Nd alloy. Transactions of Nonferrous Metals Society of China. 2015, 25, 1439–45.
[267] Hu G-S et al. Microstructures and mechanical properties of extruded and aged Mg–Zn–Mn–Sn–Y alloys. Transactions of Nonferrous Metals Society of China. 2014, 24, 3070–75.

[268] Jiang MG et al. Rare earth texture and improved ductility in a Mg-Zn-Gd alloy after high-speed extrusion. Materials Science and Engineering: A. 2016, 667, 233–39.
[269] Xiao L et al. Microstructure, texture evolution and tensile properties of extruded Mg-4.58Zn-2.6Gd-0.16Zr alloy. Materials Science and Engineering: A. 2019, 744, 277–89.
[270] Huang H et al. Effects of cyclic extrusion and compression parameters on microstructure and mechanical properties of Mg–1.50Zn–0.25Gd alloy. Materials & Design. 2015, 86, 788–96.
[271] Jiang MG et al. Enhancing strength and ductility of Mg-Zn-Gd alloy via slow-speed extrusion combined with pre-forging. Journal of Alloys and Compounds. 2017, 694, 1214–23.
[272] Chen T et al. The role of long-period stacking ordered phases in the deformation behavior of a strong textured Mg-Zn-Gd-Y-Zr alloy sheet processed by hot extrusion. Materials Science and Engineering: A. 2019, 750, 31–39.
[273] Huang H et al. Microstructure and mechanical properties of double continuously extruded Mg–Zn–Gd-based magnesium alloys. Materials Science and Engineering: A. 2013, 560, 241–48.
[274] Dobroň P et al. Compressive yield stress improvement using thermomechanical treatment of extruded Mg-Zn-Ca alloy. Materials Science and Engineering: A. 2018, 730, 401–09.
[275] Tong LB et al. Microstructures, mechanical properties and corrosion resistances of extruded Mg–Zn–Ca–xCe/La alloys. Journal of the Mechanical Behavior of Biomedical Materials. 2016, 62, 57–70.
[276] Tong LB et al. Reducing the tension–compression yield asymmetry of extruded Mg–Zn–Ca alloy via equal channel angular pressing. Journal of Magnesium and Alloys. 2015, 3, 302–08.
[277] Du YZ et al. Microstructures and mechanical properties of as-cast and as-extruded Mg-4.50Zn-1.13Ca (wt%) alloy. Materials Science and Engineering: A. 2013, 576, 6–13.
[278] Li C-J et al. Microstructure, texture and mechanical properties of Mg-3.0Zn-0.2Ca alloys fabricated by extrusion at various temperatures. Journal of Alloys and Compounds. 2015, 652, 122–31.
[279] Zhang B et al. Effects of calcium on texture and mechanical properties of hot-extruded Mg–Zn–Ca alloys. Materials Science and Engineering: A. 2012, 539, 56–60.
[280] Tong LB et al. Influence of deformation rate on microstructure, texture and mechanical properties of indirect-extruded Mg-Zn-Ca alloy. Materials Characterization. 2015, 104, 66–72.
[281] Tong LB et al. Effect of extrusion ratio on microstructure, texture and mechanical properties of indirectly extruded Mg-Zn-Ca alloy. Materials Science and Engineering: A. 2013, 569, 48–53.
[282] Li W-J et al. Effect of ultra-slow extrusion speed on the microstructure and mechanical properties of Mg-4Zn-0.5Ca alloy. Materials Science and Engineering: A 2016, 677, 367–75.
[283] Du YZ et al. The effect of double extrusion on the microstructure and mechanical properties of Mg-Zn-Ca alloy. Materials Science and Engineering: A. 2013, 583, 69–77.
[284] Jiang MG et al. High-speed extrusion of dilute Mg-Zn-Ca-Mn alloys and its effect on microstructure, texture and mechanical properties. Materials Science and Engineering: A. 2016, 678, 329–38.
[285] Jiang MG et al. Development of dilute Mg–Zn–Ca–Mn alloy with high performance via extrusion. Journal of Alloys and Compounds. 2016, 668, 13–21.
[286] Xu SW et al. Twins, recrystallization and texture evolution of a Mg–5.99Zn–1.76Ca–0.35Mn (wt.%) alloy during indirect extrusion process. Scripta Materialia. 2011, 65, 875–78.
[287] Xu SW et al. Extruded Mg–Zn–Ca–Mn alloys with low yield anisotropy. Materials Science and Engineering: A. 2012, 558, 356–65.
[288] Wang G et al. Effects of Zn addition on the mechanical properties and texture of extruded Mg-Zn-Ca-Ce magnesium alloy sheets. Materials Science and Engineering: A. 2017, 705, 46–54.
[289] Du YZ et al. The microstructure, texture and mechanical properties of extruded Mg–5.3Zn–0.2Ca–0.5Ce (wt%) alloy. Materials Science and Engineering: A. 2015, 620, 164–71.

[290] Sun H-F et al. Evolution of microstructure and mechanical properties of Mg–3.0Zn–0.2Ca–0.5Y alloy by extrusion at various temperatures. Journal of Materials Processing Technology. 2016, 229, 633–40.
[291] Homma T et al. Effect of Zr addition on the mechanical properties of as-extruded Mg–Zn–Ca–Zr alloys. Materials Science and Engineering: A. 2010, 527, 2356–62.
[292] Niu Y et al. Excellent mechanical properties obtained by low temperature extrusion based on Mg-2Zn-1Al alloy. Journal of Alloys and Compounds. 2019, 801, 415–27.
[293] Wang B et al. Microstructure and mechanical properties of as-extruded and as-aged Mg–Zn–Al–Sn alloys. Materials Science and Engineering: A. 2016, 656, 165–73.
[294] Wang Q-F et al. Microstructure evolution and mechanical properties of extruded Mg-12Zn-1.5Er alloy. Transactions of Nonferrous Metals Society of China. 2011, 21, 874–79.
[295] Wang Q et al. Microstructure, texture and mechanical properties of as-extruded Mg–Zn–Er alloys. Materials Science and Engineering: A. 2013, 581, 31–38.
[296] Wang Q et al. Microstructure, texture and mechanical properties of as-extruded Mg–Zn–Er alloys containing W-phase. Journal of Alloys and Compounds. 2014, 602, 32–39.
[297] Liu K et al. Effects of secondary phases on texture and mechanical properties of as-extruded Mg–Zn–Er alloys. Transactions of Nonferrous Metals Society of China. 2018, 28, 890–95.
[298] Mendis CL et al. Microstructures and mechanical properties of extruded and heat treated Mg–6Zn–1Si–0.5Mn alloys. Materials Science and Engineering: A. 2012, 553, 1–9.
[299] Huang H et al. The effect of nanoquasicrystals on mechanical properties of as-extruded Mg-Zn-Gd alloy. Materials Letters. 2012, 79, 281–83.
[300] Lu X et al. Microstructure and mechanical properties of Mg-3.0Zn-1.0Sn-0.3Mn-0.3Ca alloy extruded at different temperatures. Journal of Alloys and Compounds. 2018, 732, 257–69.
[301] Xu DK et al. The strengthening effect of icosahedral phase on as-extruded Mg–Li alloys. Scripta Materialia. 2007, 57, 285–88.
[302] Zeng Y et al. Effect of Li content on microstructure, texture and mechanical behaviors of the as-extruded Mg-Li sheets. Materials Science and Engineering: A. 2017, 700, 59–65.
[303] Li C et al. Effects of icosahedral phase on mechanical anisotropy of as-extruded Mg-14Li (in wt%) based alloys. Journal of Materials Science & Technology. 2019, 35; https://doi.org/10.1016/j.jmst.2019.07.028.
[304] Jiang B et al. Effect of stannum addition on microstructure of as-cast and as-extruded Mg-5Li alloy. Transactions of Nonferrous Metals Society of China. 2011, 21, 2378–83.
[305] Dong H et al. Evolution of microstructure and mechanical properties of a duplex Mg–Li alloy under extrusion with an increasing ratio. Materials & Design. 2014, 57, 121–27.
[306] Jiang B et al. Effects of Sn on microstructure of as-cast and as-extruded Mg–9Li alloys. Transactions of Nonferrous Metals Society of China. 2013, 23, 904–08.
[307] Sun Y et al. Effects of Sn and Y on the microstructure, texture, and mechanical properties of as-extruded Mg-5Li-3Al-2Zn alloy. Materials Science and Engineering: A. 2018, 733, 429–39.
[308] Kim JT et al. Effect of Ca addition on the plastic deformation behavior of extruded Mg-11Li-3Al-1Sn-0.4Mn alloy. Journal of Alloys and Compounds. 2016, 687, 821–26.
[309] Liu J et al. A comparison between DCCAE and conventional extrusion of Mg-9.5Li-3Al-1.6Y alloy. Journal of Rare Earths. 2016, 34, 626–31.
[310] Li J et al. Microstructure, mechanical properties and aging behaviors of as-extruded Mg–5Li–3Al–2Zn–1.5Cu alloy. Materials Science and Engineering: A. 2011, 528, 3915–20.
[311] Sun Y et al. Microstructure, texture, and mechanical properties of as-extruded Mg-xLi-3Al-2Zn-0.2Zr alloys (x = 5, 7, 8, 9, 11 wt%). Materials Science and Engineering: A. 2019, 755, 201–10.
[312] Tang Y et al. Fabrication of high strength α, α+β, β phase containing Mg-Li alloys with 0.2%Y by extruding and annealing process. Materials Science and Engineering: A. 2016, 675, 55–64.

[313] Fu X et al. Microstructure and mechanical properties of as-cast and extruded Mg-8Li-1Al-0.5Sn alloy. Materials Science and Engineering: A. 2108, 709, 247–53.

[314] Qu Z et al. Microstructures and tensile properties of hot extruded Mg-5Li-3Al-2Zn-xRE(Rare Earths) alloys. Materials & Design. 2014, 54, 792–95.

[315] Feng S et al. Effect of extrusion ratio on microstructure and mechanical properties of Mg–8Li–3Al–2Zn–0.5Y alloy with duplex structure. Materials Science and Engineering: A. 2017, 692, 9–16.

[316] Guo J et al. Effect of Sn and Y addition on the microstructural evolution and mechanical properties of hot-extruded Mg-9Li-3Al alloy. Materials Characterization. 2019, 148, 35–42.

[317] Zhang J et al. Microstructure and mechanical properties of as-cast and extruded Mg-8Li-3Al-2Zn-0.5Nd alloy. Materials Science and Engineering: A. 2015, 621, 198–203.

[318] Yang Y et al. Influence of extrusion temperature on microstructure and mechanical behavior of duplex Mg-Li-Al-Sr alloy. Journal of Alloys and Compounds. 2018, 750, 696–705.

[319] Kaami M et al. Hot shear deformation constitutive analysis of an extruded Mg–6Li–1Zn alloy. Materials Letters. 2012, 81, 235–38.

[320] Chen Z et al. Plastic Flow Characteristics of an Extruded Mg-Li-Zn-RE Alloy. Rare Metal Materials and Engineering. 2013, 42, 1779–84.

[321] Zhang Y et al. Microstructure and tensile properties of as-extruded Mg–Li–Zn–Gd alloys reinforced with icosahedral quasicrystal phase. Materials & Design. 2015, 66, 162–68

[322] Karami M et al. Hot shear deformation constitutive analysis of an extruded Mg–6Li–1Zn alloy. Materials Letters. 2012, 81, 235–38.

[323] Shalbafi M et al. Hot deformation of the extruded Mg–10Li–1Zn alloy: Constitutive analysis and processing maps. Journal of Alloys and Compounds. 2017, 96, 1269–77.

[324] Li S et al. Microstructure and mechanical properties of hot extruded Mg-8.89Li-0.96Zn alloy. Results in Physics. 2019, 13; https://doi.org/10.1016/j.rinp.2019.02.084.

[325] Chen Z et al. Hot deformation behavior of an extruded Mg–Li–Zn–RE alloy. Materials Science and Engineering: A. 2011, 528, 961–66.

[326] Pan H et al. Achieving high strength in indirectly-extruded binary Mg–Ca alloy containing Guinier–Preston zones. Journal of Alloys and Compounds. 2015, 630, 272–76.

[327] Pan H et al. Ultra-fine grain size and exceptionally high strength in dilute Mg–Ca alloys achieved by conventional one-step extrusion. Materials Letters. 2019, 237, 65–68.

[328] Nakata T et al. Unexpected influence of prismatic plate-shaped precipitates on strengths and yield anisotropy in an extruded Mg-0.3Ca-1.0In-0.1Al-0.2Mn (at.%) alloy. Scripta Materialia. 2019, 169, 70–75.

[329] Geng J et al. Microstructure and mechanical properties of extruded Mg–1Ca–1Zn–0.6Zr alloy. Materials Science and Engineering: A. 2016, 653, 27–34.

[330] Peng Q et al. Microstructures, aging behaviour and mechanical properties in hydrogen and chloride media of backward extruded Mg–Y based biomaterials. Journal of the Mechanical Behavior of Biomedical Materials. 2013, 17, 176–85.

[331] Fu H et al. High ductility of a bi-modal Mg-7wt.%Y alloy at low temperature prepared by high pressure boriding and semi-solid extrusion. Materials & Design. 2016, 92, 240–45.

[332] Huang GH et al. Microstructure, texture and mechanical properties evolution of extruded fine-grained Mg-Y sheets during annealing. Materials Science and Engineering: A. 2018, 720, 24–35.

[333] Lu JW et al. Plastic anisotropy and deformation behavior of extruded Mg-Y sheets at elevated temperatures. Materials Science and Engineering: A. 2017, 700, 598–608.

[334] Singh A et al. Dislocation structures in a near-isotropic Mg-Y extruded alloy. Materials Science and Engineering: A. 2017, 698, 238–48.

[335] Briffod F et al. Effect of long period stacking ordered phase on the fatigue properties of extruded Mg-Y-Zn alloys. International Journal of Fatigue. 2019, 128; https://doi.org/10.1016/j.ijfatigue.2019.105205.
[336] Tong LB et al. Dynamic recrystallization and texture evolution of Mg–Y–Zn alloy during hot extrusion process. Materials Characterization. 2014, 92, 77–83.
[337] Tong LB et al. Effect of long period stacking ordered phase on the microstructure, texture and mechanical properties of extruded Mg–Y–Zn alloy. Materials Science and Engineering: A. 2013, 563, 177–83.
[338] Leng Z et al. Notch tensile behavior of extruded Mg–Y–Zn alloys containing long period stacking ordered phase. Materials & Design. 2014, 56, 495–99.
[339] Shi G et al. Precipitation behaviors, texture and tensile properties of an extruded Mg-7Y-1Nd-0.5Zr (wt%) alloy bar with large cross-section. Materials Science and Engineering: A. 2017, 685, 300–09.
[340] Xin R et al. Effect of aging precipitation on mechanical anisotropy of an extruded Mg–Y–Nd alloy. Materials & Design. 2012, 34, 384–88.
[341] Xu X et al. Effect of Nd on microstructure and mechanical properties of as-extruded Mg-Y-Zr-Nd alloy. Journal of Materials Science & Technology. 2017, 33, 926–34.
[342] Zhang L et al. Microstructure and mechanical properties of high-performance Mg-Y-Er-Zn extruded alloy. Materials & Design. 2014, 54, 256–63.
[343] Liu K et al. Influence of Zn content on the microstructure and mechanical properties of extruded Mg–5Y–4Gd–0.4Zr alloy. Journal of Alloys and Compounds. 2009, 481, 811–18.
[344] Meng Y et al. Partial melting behaviors and thixoforming properties of cast and extruded Mg-5.15Y-3.75Gd-3.05Zn-0.75Zr alloys. Vacuum. 2018, 150, 173–85.
[345] Liu K et al. Microstructures and mechanical properties of the extruded Mg-4Y-2Gd-xZn-0.4Zr alloys. Journal of Alloys and Compounds. 2011, 509, 3299–305.
[346] Li D-Q et al. Influence of extrusion temperature on microstructure and mechanical properties of Mg-4Y-4Sm-0.5Zr alloy. Transactions of Nonferrous Metals Society of China. 2010, 20, 1311–15.
[347] Lyu S et al. Fabrication of high-strength Mg-Y-Sm-Zn-Zr alloy by conventional hot extrusion and aging. Materials Science and Engineering: A. 2018, 732, 178–85.
[348] Fang D et al. Microstructures and mechanical properties of Mg–2Y–1Mn–1–2Nd alloys fabricated by extrusion. Materials Science and Engineering: A. 2010, 527, 4383–88.
[349] Zhou N et al. High ductility of a Mg–Y–Ca alloy via extrusion. Materials Science and Engineering: A. 2013, 560, 103–10.
[350] Lee SW et al. Twinning and slip behaviors and microstructural evolutions of extruded Mg-1Gd alloy with rare-earth texture during tensile deformation. Journal of Alloys and Compounds. 2019, 791, 700–10.
[351] Peng Q et al. Effect of backward extrusion on microstructure and mechanical properties of Mg–Gd based alloy. Materials Science and Engineering: A. 2012, 532, 443–48.
[352] Hou X et al. Structure and mechanical properties of extruded Mg–Gd based alloy sheet. Materials Science and Engineering: A. 2009, 520, 162–67.
[353] Hadorn JP et al. Solute clustering and grain boundary segregation in extruded dilute Mg–Gd alloys. Scripta Materialia. 2014, 93, 28–31.
[354] Sarebanzadeh M et al. Constitutive analysis and processing map of an extruded Mg–3Gd–1Zn alloy under hot shear deformation. Materials Science and Engineering: A. 2015, 637, 155–61.
[355] Gui Z et al. Mechanical and corrosion properties of Mg-Gd-Zn-Zr-Mn biodegradable alloy by hot extrusion. Journal of Alloys and Compounds. 2016, 685, 222–30.
[356] Li JP et al. Microstructures of extruded Mg–12Gd–1Zn–0.5Zr and Mg–12Gd–4Y–1Zn–0.5Zr alloys. Scripta Materialia. 2007, 56, 137–40.

[357] Zhou X et al. Microstructure and mechanical properties of extruded Mg-Gd-Y-Zn-Zr alloys filled with intragranular LPSO phases. Materials Characterization. 2018, 135, 76–83.
[358] Liu K et al. Microstructures and mechanical properties of extruded Mg–8Gd–0.4Zr alloys containing Zn. Materials Science and Engineering: A. 2009, 505, 13–19.
[359] Zhen R et al. Effect of Zn Content on the Microstructure and Mechanical Properties of the Extruded Mg-6Gd-4Y (wt%) Alloy. Rare Metal Materials and Engineering. 2018, 47, 2957–63.
[360] Liu S et al. On the microstructure and mechanical property of as-extruded Mg-Gd-Y-Zn alloy with Sr addition. Materials Science and Engineering: A. 2017, 679, 183–92.
[361] Xia X et al. Characterization of hot deformation behavior of as-extruded Mg–Gd–Y–Zn–Zr alloy. Journal of Alloys and Compounds. 2014, 610, 203–11.
[362] Du Y et al. Grain Refinement and Texture Evolution of Mg-Gd-Y-Zn-Zr Alloy Processed by Repetitive Usetting-extrusion at Decreasing Temperature. Rare Metal Materials and Engineering. 2018, 47, 1422–28.
[363] Li B et al. Microstructures and mechanical properties of a hot-extruded Mg–8Gd–3Yb–1.2Zn –0.5Zr (wt%) alloy. Journal of Alloys and Compounds. 2019, 776, 666–78.
[364] Yu Z et al. Effects of extrusion ratio and temperature on the mechanical properties and microstructure of as-extruded Mg-Gd-Y-(Nd/Zn)-Zr alloys. Materials Science and Engineering: A. 2019, 762; https://doi.org/10.1016/j.msea.2019.138080.
[365] Zhang G et al. Effects of repetitive upsetting-extrusion parameters on microstructure and texture evolution of Mg–Gd–Y–Zn–Zr alloy. Journal of Alloys and Compounds. 2019, 790, 48–57.
[366] Xu C et al. Effect of extrusion parameters on microstructure and mechanical properties of Mg-7.5Gd-2.5Y-3.5Zn-0.9Ca-0.4Zr (wt%) alloy. Materials Science and Engineering: A. 2017, 685, 159–67.
[367] Wang Q et al. Strengthening and toughening mechanisms of an ultrafine grained Mg-Gd-Y-Zr alloy processed by cyclic extrusion and compression. Materials Science and Engineering: A. 2017, 699, 26–30.
[368] Nam ND et al. Improvement of mechanical properties and saline corrosion resistance of extruded Mg-8Gd-4Y-0.5Zr by alloying with 2 wt.% Zn. Journal of Alloys and Compounds. 2017, 711, 215–21.
[369] Wang H et al. In-situ analysis of the slip activity during tensile deformation of cast and extruded Mg-10Gd-3Y-0.5Zr (wt.%) at 250 °C. Materials Characterization. 2016, 116, 8–17.
[370] Chi YQ et al. Effect of trace zinc on the microstructure and mechanical properties of extruded Mg-Gd-Y-Zr alloy. Journal of Alloys and Compounds. 2019, 789, 416–27.
[371] Chi YQ et al. Tension-compression asymmetry of extruded Mg-Gd-Y-Zr alloy with a bimodal microstructure studied by in-situ synchrotron diffraction. Materials & Design. 2019, 170; https://doi.org/10.1016/j.matdes.2019.107705.
[372] Li X et al. Enhanced strength and ductility of Mg-Gd-Y-Zr alloys by secondary extrusion. Journal of Magnesium and Alloys. 2013, 1, 54–63.
[373] Peng T et al. Microstructure and enhanced mechanical properties of an Mg–10Gd–2Y–0.5Zr alloy processed by cyclic extrusion and compression. Materials Science and Engineering: A. 2011, 528, 1143–48.
[374] Yu Z et al. Microstructure evolution and mechanical properties of as-extruded Mg-Gd-Y-Zr alloy with Zn and Nd additions. Materials Science and Engineering: A. 2018, 713, 234–43.
[375] Zhou H et al. Hot deformation and processing maps of as-extruded Mg–9.8Gd–2.7Y–0.4Zr Mg alloy. Materials Science and Engineering: A. 2013, 576, 101–07.
[376] Yu Z et al. Microstructure evolution and mechanical properties of a high strength Mg-11.7Gd-4.9Y-0.3Zr (wt%) alloy prepared by pre-deformation annealing, hot extrusion and ageing. Materials Science and Engineering: A. 2017, 703, 348–58.

[377] Hou X et al. Microstructure and mechanical properties of extruded Mg–8Gd–2Y–1Nd–0.3Zn–0.6Zr alloy. Materials Science and Engineering: A. 2011, 528, 7805–10.
[378] Liu X et al. Microstructures and mechanical properties of high performance Mg–6Gd–3Y–2Nd–0.4Zr alloy by indirect extrusion and aging treatment. Materials Science and Engineering: A. 2014, 612, 380–86.
[379] Zhou H et al. Microstructure and mechanical properties of extruded Mg–8.5Gd–2.3Y–1.8Ag–0.4Zr alloy. Transactions of Nonferrous Metals Society of China. 2012, 22, 1891–95.
[380] Zheng X et al. Remarkably enhanced mechanical properties of Mg-8Gd-1Er-0.5Zr alloy on the route of extrusion, rolling and aging. Materials Letters. 2018, 212, 155–58.
[381] Liu K et al. Development of extraordinary high-strength-toughness Mg alloy via combined processes of repeated plastic working and hot extrusion. Materials Science and Engineering: A. 2013, 573, 127–31.
[382] Wen K et al. Effect of microstructure evolution on mechanical property of extruded Mg–12Gd–2Er–1Zn–0.6Zr alloys. Journal of Magnesium and Alloys. 2015, 3, 23–28.
[383] Cheng WL et al. Strengthening mechanisms of indirect-extruded Mg–Sn based alloys at room temperature. Journal of Magnesium and Alloys. 2014, 2, 299–304.
[384] Chai Y et al. Effects of Zn and Ca addition on microstructure and mechanical properties of as-extruded Mg-1.0Sn alloy sheet. Materials Science and Engineering: A. 2019, 746, 82–93.
[385] Zhao C et al. Effect of Sn content on strain hardening behavior of as-extruded Mg-Sn alloys. Materials Science and Engineering: A. 2018, 713, 244–52.
[386] Zhao C et al. Preparation and characterization of as-extruded Mg-Sn alloys for orthopedic applications. Materials & Design. 2015, 70, 60–67.
[387] Cheng WL et al. Microstructure and mechanical properties of binary Mg–Sn alloys subjected to indirect extrusion. Materials Science and Engineering: A. 2010, 527, 4650–53.
[388] Cheng W et al. Dependence of Microstructure, Texture and Tensile Properties on Working Conditions in Indirect-Extruded Mg-6Sn Alloys. Rare Metal Materials and Engineering. 2015, 44, 2132–37.
[389] Chen D et al. Microstructures and tensile properties of as-extruded Mg-Sn binary alloys. Transactions of Nonferrous Metals Society of China. 2010, 20, 1321–25.
[390] Kim HJ et al. Influence of alloyed Al on the microstructure and corrosion properties of extruded Mg–8Sn–1Zn alloys. Corrosion Science. 2015, 95, 133–42.
[391] Chai Y et al. Improvement of mechanical properties and reduction of yield asymmetry of extruded Mg-Sn-Zn alloy through Ca addition. Journal of Alloys and Compounds. 2019, 782, 1076–86.
[392] She J et al. Microstructures and mechanical properties of as-extruded Mg-5Sn-1Zn-xAl (x=1, 3 and 5) alloys. Progress in Natural Science: Materials International. 2015, 25, 267–75.
[393] El Mahallawy N et al. Effect of Zn addition on the microstructure and mechanical properties of cast, rolled and extruded Mg-6Sn-xZn alloys. Materials Science and Engineering: A. 2017, 680, 47–53.
[394] Kim B et al. Grain refinement and reduced yield asymmetry of extruded Mg–5Sn–1Zn alloy by Al addition. Journal of Alloys and Compounds. 2016, 660, 304–09.
[395] Luo D et al. Corrosion inhibition of hydrophobic coatings fabricated by micro-arc oxidation on an extruded Mg–5Sn–1Zn alloy substrate. Journal of Alloys and Compounds. 2018, 731, 731–38.
[396] Chang LL et al. Strengthening effect of nano and micro-sized precipitates in the hot-extruded Mg-5Sn-3Zn alloys with Ca addition. Journal of Alloys and Compounds. 2017, 703, 552–59.
[397] Wang Y et al. On the microstructure and mechanical property of as-extruded Mg–Sn–Zn alloy with Cu addition. Journal of Alloys and Compounds. 2018, 744, 234–42.

[398] Kim S-H et al. Underlying mechanisms of drastic reduction in yield asymmetry of extruded Mg-Sn-Zn alloy by Al addition. Materials Science and Engineering: A. 2018, 733, 285–90.
[399] Kim S-H et al. Controlling the microstructure and improving the tensile properties of extruded Mg-Sn-Zn alloy through Al addition. Journal of Alloys and Compounds. 2018, 751, 1–11.
[400] Huang Q et al. On the dynamic mechanical property and deformation mechanism of as-extruded Mg-Sn-Ca alloys under tension. Materials Science and Engineering: A. 2016, 664, 43–48.
[401] Li W et al. Enhanced age-hardening response and compression property of a Mg-7Sn-1Ca-1Ag (wt.%) alloy by extrusion combined with aging treatment. Journal of Alloys and Compounds. 2018, 766, 584–93.
[402] Jiang J et al. Microstructures and mechanical properties of extruded Mg–2Sn–xYb (x=0, 0.1, 0.5 at.%) sheets. Journal of Magnesium and Alloy. 2014, 2, 257–64.
[403] Jiang J et al. Dry sliding wear behavior of extruded Mg-Sn-Yb alloy. Journal of Rare Earths. 2105, 33, 77–85.
[404] Park SS et al. Microstructure and mechanical properties of an indirect-extruded Mg–8Sn–1Al–1Zn alloy. Materials Letters. 2010, 64, 31–34.
[405] Park SH et al. Improving the tensile strength of Mg–7Sn–1Al–1Zn alloy through artificial cooling during extrusion. Materials Science and Engineering: A. 2015, 625, 369–73.
[406] Yoon J et al. Forgeability test of extruded Mg–Sn–Al–Zn alloys under warm forming conditions. Materials & Design. 2014, 55, 300–08.
[407] Kim S-H et al. Effect of Ce addition on the microstructure and mechanical properties of extruded Mg-Sn-Al-Zn alloy. Materials Science and Engineering: A. 2016, 657, 406–12.
[408] Elsayed FR et al. Effect of extrusion conditions on microstructure and mechanical properties of microalloyed Mg–Sn–Al–Zn alloys. Materials Science and Engineering: A. 2013, 588, 318–28.
[409] Park SH et al. Improved strength of Mg alloys extruded at high speed with artificial cooling. Journal of Alloys and Compounds. 2015, 648, 615–21.
[410] Park SH et al. High-speed indirect extrusion of Mg–Sn–Al–Zn alloy and its influence on microstructure and mechanical properties. Journal of Alloys and Compounds. 2016, 667, 170–77.
[411] Park SH et al. Effect of cold pre-forging on the microstructure and mechanical properties of extruded Mg–8Sn–1Al–1Zn alloy. Materials Science and Engineering: A. 2014, 612, 197–201.
[412] Zhang D et al. Effects of Heat Treatment on Microstructure and Mechanical Properties of as-Extruded Mg-9Sn-1.5Y-0.4Zr Magnesium Alloy. Rare Metal Materials and Engineering. 2016, 45, 2208–13.
[413] Jiang J et al. Strain-hardening and warm deformation behaviors of extruded Mg–Sn–Yb alloy sheet. Journal of Magnesium and Alloys. 2014, 2, 116–23.
[414] Zhao H-D et al. Microstructure and tensile properties of as-extruded Mg-Sn-Y alloys. Transactions of Nonferrous Metals Society of China. 2010, 20, s493–s497.
[415] Li J et al. Study on microstructure and properties of extruded Mg–2Nd–0.2Zn alloy as potential biodegradable implant material. Materials Science and Engineering: C. 2015, 49, 422–29.
[416] Zhang X et al. Microstructure, mechanical properties, biocorrosion behavior, and cytotoxicity of as-extruded Mg–Nd–Zn–Zr alloy with different extrusion ratios. Journal of the Mechanical Behavior of Biomedical Materials. 2012, 9, 153–62.
[417] Zhang X et al. Improvement of mechanical properties and corrosion resistance of biodegradable Mg–Nd–Zn–Zr alloys by double extrusion. Materials Science and Engineering: B. 2012, 177, 1113–19.
[418] Xiao L et al. Effects of the Extrusion Temperature on Microstructure, Texture Evolution and Mechanical Properties of Extruded Mg-2.49Nd-1.82Gd-0.19Zn-0.4Zr Alloy. In: Joshi V. et al., ed., Magnesium Technology 2019. The Minerals, Metals & Materials Series. Springer, 2019, 69–75.

[419] Bi G et al. Microstructure and mechanical properties of an extruded Mg-Dy-Ni alloy. Materials Science and Engineering: A. 2019, 760, 246–57.
[420] Zeng XQ et al. Effect of solution treatment and extrusion on evolution of microstructure in a Mg–12Dy–3Nd–0.4Zr alloy. Journal of Alloys and Compounds. 2008, 456, 419–24.
[421] Bi G et al. Microstructure and Mechanical Properties of an Extruded Mg-2Dy-0.5Zn Alloy. Journal of Materials Science & Technology. 2012, 28, 543–51.
[422] Bi G et al. An elevated temperature Mg–Dy–Zn alloy with long period stacking ordered phase by extrusion. Materials Science and Engineering: A. 2011, 528, 3609–14.
[423] Bi G et al. Deformation behavior of an extruded Mg–Dy–Zn alloy with long period stacking ordered phase. Materials Science and Engineering: A. 2015, 622, 52–60.
[424] Ma N et al. Effects of cerium on microstructures, recovery behavior and mechanical properties of backward extruded Mg–0.5Mn alloys. Materials Science and Engineering: A. 2013, 564, 310–16.
[425] Borkar H et al. Effect of extrusion temperature on texture evolution and recrystallization in extruded Mg–1% Mn and Mg–1% Mn–1.6%Sr alloys. Journal of Alloys and Compounds. 2013, 555, 219–24.
[426] Fang D-Q et al. Microstructures and mechanical properties of extruded Mg-1Mn-3.5Y and Mg-1Mn-1Y-2.5Nd alloys. Transactions of Nonferrous Metals Society of China. 2010, 20, s555–s560.
[427] Zhou Y-L et al. Microstructures, mechanical and corrosion properties and biocompatibility of as extruded Mg–Mn–Zn–Nd alloys for biomedical applications. Materials Science and Engineering: C. 2015, 49, 93–100.
[428] Yang Q et al. Evolution of microstructure and mechanical properties of Mg–Mn–Ce alloys under hot extrusion Materials Science and Engineering: A. 2015, 628, 143–48.
[429] Leng Z et al. Microstructure and mechanical properties of Mg–(6,9)RY–4Zn alloys by extrusion and aging. Materials & Design. 2013, 52, 713–19.
[430] Wu YP et al. Effect of secondary extrusion on the microstructure and mechanical properties of a Mg–RE alloy. Materials Science and Engineering: A. 2014, 616, 148–54.
[431] Zhai Y et al. Analysis of Crystallographic Texture and Mechanical Anisotropy of an Extruded Mg-RE Alloy. Rare Metal Materials and Engineering. 2018, 47, 1341–46.
[432] Li R et al. Effect of cold rolling on microstructure and mechanical property of extruded Mg–4Sm alloy during aging. Materials Characterization. 2016, 112, 81–86.
[433] Cai Y et al. Microstructure and mechanical properties of extruded Mg-Sm-Ca alloys. Rare Metal Materials and Engineering. 2016, 45, 287–91.
[434] Wu BL et al. The quasi-static mechanical properties of extruded binary Mg–Er alloys. Materials Science and Engineering: A. 2013, 573, 205–14.
[435] Feng Y et al. Characterization of elevated-temperature high strength and decent thermal conductivity extruded Mg-Er-Y-Zn alloy containing nano-spaced stacking faults. Materials Characterization. 2019, 155; https://doi.org/10.1016/j.matchar.2019.109823.
[436] Zhang M et al. Development of extruded Mg-6Er-3Y-1.5Zn-0.4Mn (wt.%) alloy with high strength at elevated temperature. Journal of Materials Science & Technology. 2019, 35, 2365–74.
[437] Zhao C et al. Microstructure, mechanical properties, bio-corrosion properties and cytotoxicity of as-extruded Mg-Sr alloys. Materials Science and Engineering: C. 2017, 70, 1081–88.
[438] Zhong M et al. Effects of loading conditions on twin characteristics in an extruded Mg-Zr alloy. Materials Science and Engineering: A. 2018, 724, 239–48.
[439] Hu L-F et al. Effect of extrusion temperature on microstructure, thermal conductivity and mechanical properties of a Mg-Ce-Zn-Zr alloy. Journal of Alloys and Compounds. 2018, 741, 1222–28.
[440] Lv S et al. Microstructures and mechanical properties of a hot-extruded Mg–8Ho–0.6Zn–0.5Zr alloy. Journal of Alloys and Compounds, 2019, 774, 926–38.

[441] Meng S et al. Microstructure and mechanical properties of an extruded Mg-8Bi-1Al-1Zn (wt%) alloy. Materials Science and Engineering: A. 2017, 690, 80–87.
[442] Rajmane UC. Review of Eaul Channel Angular Pressing System. Asian Review of Mechanical Engineering. 2016, 5, 11–13.
[443] Aliofkhazraei M. Equal-Channel Angular Pressing (ECAP), In: Ravisankar B ed., Handbook of Mechanical Nanostructuring; Advance Science Series, Wily, 2015; https://doi.org/10.1002/9783527674947.ch13.
[444] http://blog.totalmateria.com/equal-channel-angular-pressing-ecap-part-one/.
[445] Wang H, Zhou K, Xie G, Liang X, Zhao Y. Microstructure and mechanical properties of an Mg–10Al alloy fabricated by Sb-alloying and ECAP processing. Materials Science and Engineering: A. 2013, 560, 787–91.
[446] Wang H, Zhou B, Zhao Y, Zhou K, Liang W. Effect of Si addition on the microstructure and mechanical properties of ECAPed Mg–15Al alloy. Materials Science and Engineering: A. 2014, 589, 119–24.
[447] Cheng W, Wang W, Wang H, Liu Y, Park SH. Improved mechanical properties of ECAPed Mg–15Al alloy through Nd addition. Materials Science and Engineering: A. 2015, 633, 63–68.
[448] Feng X-M, Ai T-T. Microstructure evolution and mechanical behavior of AZ31 Mg alloy processed by equal-channel angular pressing. Transactions of Nonferrous Metals Society of China. 2009, 19, 293–98.
[449] Suh J, Victoria-Hernández J, Letzig D, Golle R, Volk W. Enhanced mechanical behavior and reduced mechanical anisotropy of AZ31 Mg alloy sheet processed by ECAP. Materials Science and Engineering: A. 2016, 650, 523–29.
[450] Suh J, Victoria-Hernandez J, Letzig D, Golle R, Volk W. Improvement of ductility at room temperature of Mg-3Al-1Zn alloy sheets processed by equal channel angular pressing. Procedia Engineering. 2014, 81, 1517–22.
[451] Peláez D, Isaza C, Meza JM, Fernández-Morales P, Mendoza E. Mechanical and microstructural evolution of Mg AZ31 alloy using ECASD process. Journal of Materials Research and Technology. 2015, 4, 392–97.
[452] Shahar IA, Hosaka T, Yoshihara S, MacDonald BJ. Mechanical and corrosion properties of AZ31 Mg alloy processed by equal-channel angular pressing and aging. Procedia Engineering. 2017, 184, 423–31.
[453] Yuan YC, Ma AB, Jiang JH, Sun Y, Song D. Mechanical properties and precipitate behavior of Mg–9Al–1Zn alloy processed by equal-channel angular pressing and aging. Journal of Alloys and Compounds. 2014, 594, 182–88.
[454] Zhao Z, Chen Q, Chao H, Hu C, Huang S. Influence of equal channel angular extrusion processing parameters on the microstructure and mechanical properties of Mg–Al–Y–Zn alloy. Materials & Design. 2011, 32, 575–83.
[455] Gong J, Liang W, Wang H, Zhao X, Bian L. Microstructure and mechanical properties of Mg-12Al-0.7Si magnesium alloy processed by equal channel angular pressing. Rare Metal Materials and Engineering. 2013, 42, 1800–04.
[456] Hradilová M, Vojtěch D, Kubásek J, Čapek J, Vlach M. Structural and mechanical characteristics of Mg–4Zn and Mg–4Zn–0.4Ca alloys after different thermal and mechanical processing routes. Materials Science and Engineering: A. 2013, 586, 284–91.
[457] Yan K, Bai J, Liu H, Jin Z-Y. The precipitation behavior of MgZn2 and Mg4Zn7 phase in Mg-6Zn (wt.%) alloy during equal-channel angular pressing. Journal of Magnesium and Alloys. 2017, 5, 336–39.
[458] Yan K, Sun J, Bai J, Liu H, Wu Y. Preparation of a high strength and high ductility Mg-6Zn alloy wire by combination of ECAP and hot drawing. Materials Science and Engineering: A. 2019, 739, 513–18.

[459] Yan K, Sun YS, Bai J, Xue F. Microstructure and mechanical properties of ZA62 Mg alloy by equal-channel angular pressing. Materials Science and Engineering: A. 2011, 528, 1149–53.
[460] Yuan Y, Ma A, Gou X, Jiang J, Zhu Y. Superior mechanical properties of ZK60 Mg alloy processed by equal channel angular pressing and rolling. Materials Science and Engineering: A. 2015, 630, 45–50.
[461] Wu J, Shi Q, Chiu YL. Fragmentation of Mg24Y5 intermetallic particles in an Mg-Zn-Y alloy during the equal channel angular pressing. Materials Characterization. 2017, 129, 46–52.
[462] Li KN, Zhang YB, Zeng GH, Huang GH, Yin DD. Effects of semisolid treatment and ECAP on the microstructure and mechanical properties of Mg-6.52Zn-0.95Y alloy with icosahedral phase. Materials Science and Engineering: A. 2019, 751, 283–91.
[463] Tong LB, Zheng MY, Chang H, Hu XS, Kojima Y. Microstructure and mechanical properties of Mg–Zn–Ca alloy processed by equal channel angular pressing. Materials Science and Engineering: A. 2009, 523, 289–94.
[464] Tong LB, Zheng MY, Hu XS, Wu K, Kojima Y. Influence of ECAP routes on microstructure and mechanical properties of Mg–Zn–Ca alloy. Materials Science and Engineering: A. 2010, 527, 4250–56.
[465] Tong LB, Zheng MY, Xu SW, Hu XS, Lv XY. Room-temperature compressive deformation behavior of Mg–Zn–Ca alloy processed by equal channel angular pressing. Materials Science and Engineering: A. 2010, 528, 672–79.
[466] Lu FM, Ma AB, Jiang JH, Yang DH, Zhang LY. Formation of profuse long period stacking ordered microcells in Mg–Gd–Zn–Zr alloy during multipass ECAP process. Journal of Alloys and Compounds. 2014, 601, 140–45.
[467] Lu F, Ma A, Jiang J, Chen J, Yang D. Enhanced mechanical properties and rolling formability of fine-grained Mg–Gd–Zn–Zr alloy produced by equal-channel angular pressing. Journal of Alloys and Compounds. 2015, 643, 28–33.
[468] Li B, Teng B, Chen G. Microstructure evolution and mechanical properties of Mg-Gd-Y-Zn-Zr alloy during equal channel angular pressing. Materials Science and Engineering: A. 2019, 744, 396–405.
[469] Liu H, Huang H, Yang X, Li C, Ma A. Microstructure and mechanical property of a high-strength Mg–10Gd–6Y–1.5Zn–0.5Zr alloy prepared by multi-pass equal channel angular pressing. Journal of Magnesium and Alloys. 2017, 5, 231–37.
[470] Zhang J, Kang Z, Zhou L. Microstructure evolution and mechanical properties of Mg–Gd–Nd–Zn–Zr alloy processed by equal channel angular pressing. Materials Science and Engineering: A. 2015, 647, 184–90.
[471] Cabibbo M, Paoletti C, Minárik P, Král R, Zemková M. Secondary phase precipitation and thermally stable microstructure refinement induced by ECAP on Mg-Y-Nd (WN43) alloy. Materials Letters. 2019, 237, 5–8.
[472] Shen J, Gärtnerová V, Kecskes LJ, Kondoh K, Wei Q. Residual stress and its effect on the mechanical properties of Y-doped Mg alloy fabricated via back-pressure assisted equal channel angular pressing (ECAP-BP). Materials Science and Engineering: A. 2016, 669, 110–17.
[473] Minárik P, Veselý J, Čížek J, Zemková M, Stráská J. Effect of secondary phase particles on thermal stability of ultra-fine grained Mg-4Y-3RE alloy prepared by equal channel angular pressing. Materials Characterization. 2018, 140, 207–16.
[474] Minárik P, Veselý J, Král R, Bohlen J, Stráská J. Exceptional mechanical properties of ultra-fine grain Mg-4Y-3RE alloy processed by ECAP. Materials Science and Engineering: A. 2017, 708, 193–98.
[475] Minárik P, Čížek J, Veselý J, Hruška P, Král R. Nanocrystalline aluminium particles inside Mg-4Li-4Al-2RE magnesium alloy after severe plastic deformation. Materials Characterization. 2017, 127, 248–52.

[476] Wei G, Mahmoodkhani Y, Peng X, Hadadzadeh A, Wells MA. Microstructure evolution and simulation study of a duplex Mg–Li alloy during Double Change Channel Angular Pressing. Materials & Design. 2016, 90, 266–75.
[477] Cheng W, Tian L, Wang H, Bian L, Yu H. Improved tensile properties of an equal channel angular pressed (ECAPed) Mg-8Sn-6Zn-2Al alloy by prior aging treatment. Materials Science and Engineering: A. 2017, 687, 148–54.
[478] Zhao S, Guo E, Cao G, Wang L, Feng Y. Microstructure and mechanical properties of Mg-Nd-Zn-Zr alloy processed by integrated extrusion and equal channel angular pressing. Journal of Alloys and Compounds. 2017, 705, 118–25.
[479] Sha G, Li JH, Xu W, Xisa K, Ringer SP. Hardening and microstructural reactions in high-temperature equal-channel angular pressed Mg–Nd–Gd–Zn–Zr alloy. Materials Science and Engineering: A. 2010, 527, 5092–99.
[480] Arora HS, Mridha S, Grewal HS, Singh H, Hofmann DC, Mukherjee S. Controlling the length scale and distribution of the ductile phase in metallic glass composites through friction stir processing. Science and Technology of Advanced Materials. 2014, 15, 1–7.
[481] Mahmoud TS. Effect of friction stir processing on electrical conductivity and corrosion resistance of AA6063-T6 Al alloy. Proceedings of the Institution of Mechanical Engineers, Part C: Journal of Mechanical Engineering Science. 2008, 222, 1117–23.
[482] https://home.iitm.ac.in/rbauri/researchinterest.html.
[483] Du X-H, Wu B-L. Using friction stir processing to produce ultrafine-grained microstructure in AZ61 magnesium alloy. Transactions of Nonferrous Metals Society of China. 2008, 18, 562–65.
[484] Ma ZY. Friction Stir Processing Technology: Review. Metallurgical and Materials Transactions A. 2008, 39, 642–58.
[485] Misha RS. Ma ZY, Charit I. Friction stir processing: a novel technique for fabrication of surface composite. Materials Science and Engineering: A. 2003, 341, 307–10.
[486] Ahmadkhaniha D, Järvenpää A, Jaskari M, Heydarzadeh Sohi M, Karjalainen LP. Microstructural modification of pure Mg for improving mechanical and biocorrosion properties. Journal of the Mechanical Behavior of Biomedical Materials. 2016, 61, 360–70.
[487] Nene SS, Zellner S, Mondal B, Komarasamy M, Cho KC. Friction stir processing of newly-designed Mg-5Al-3.5Ca-1Mn (AXM541) alloy: Microstructure evolution and mechanical properties. Materials Science and Engineering: A. 2018, 729, 294–99.
[488] Peng J, Zhang Z, Huang J, Guo P, Wu Y. The effect of the inhomogeneous microstructure and texture on the mechanical properties of AZ31 Mg alloys processed by friction stir processing. Journal of Alloys and Compounds. 2019, 792, 16–24.
[489] Kondaiah VV, Pananteja P, Khan A, Kumar A, Sunil BR. Microstructure, hardness and wear behavior of AZ31 Mg alloy – fly ash composites produced by friction stir processing. Materials Today: Proceedings. 2017, 4, 6671–77.
[490] Huang Y, Wang Y, Meng X, Wan L, Feng J. Dynamic recrystallization and mechanical properties of friction stir processed Mg-Zn-Y-Zr alloys. Journal of Materials Processing Technology. 2017, 249, 331–38.
[491] Huang Y, Li J, Wan L, Meng X, Xie Y. Strengthening and toughening mechanisms of CNTs/Mg-6Zn composites via friction stir processing. Materials Science and Engineering: A. 2018, 732, 205–11.
[492] Vargas M, Lathabai S, Uggowitzer PJ, Qi Y, Estrin Y. Microstructure, crystallographic texture and mechanical behaviour of friction stir processed Mg-Zn-Ca-Zr alloy ZKX50. Materials Science and Engineering: A. 2017, 685, 253–64.
[493] Xin R, Zheng X, Liu Z, Liu D, Liu Q. Microstructure and texture evolution of an Mg–Gd–Y–Nd–Zr. alloy during friction stir processing. Journal of Alloys and Compounds. 2016, 659, 51–59.

[494] Zheng FY, Wu YJ, Peng LM, Li XW, Ding WJ. Microstructures and mechanical properties of friction stir processed Mg–2.0Nd–0.3Zn–1.0Zr magnesium alloy. Journal of Magnesium and Alloys. 2013, 1, 122–27.
[495] Cao G, Zhang D, Zhang W, Qiu C. Microstructure evolution and mechanical properties of Mg–Nd–Y alloy in different friction stir processing conditions. Journal of Alloys and Compounds. 2015, 636, 12–19.
[496] Han J, Chen J, Peng L, Zheng F, Ding W. Influence of processing parameters on thermal field in Mg–Nd–Zn–Zr alloy during friction stir processing. Materials & Design. 2016, 94, 186–94.
[497] Ashby MF. Materials Selection in Mechanical Design. 3rd edition, Elsevier, New York NY, 2005.
[498] Ba Z, Dong Q, Zhang X, Wang J, Liao Y. Properties of Zr2ON2 film deposited on Mg-Gd-Zn alloy with Mg-Al hydrotalcite film by arc ion plating. Surface and Coatings Technology. 2016, 294, 67–74.
[499] Ba Z, Dong Q, Zhang X, Qiang X, Luo X. Cerium-based modification treatment of Mg-Al hydrotalcite film on AZ91D Mg alloy assisted with alternating electric field. Journal of Alloys and Compounds. 2017, 695, 106–13.
[500] Dong Q, Ba Z, Jia Y, Chen Y, Wang Z. Effect of solution concentration on sealing treatment of Mg-Al hydrotalcite film on AZ91D Mg alloy. Journal of Magnesium and Alloys. 2017, 5, 320–25.
[501] Vladoiu R, Mandes A, Dinca V, Prodan G, Tichý M. Plasma diagnostics and characterization of the Mg and Mg–Zn thin films deposited by thermionic vacuum arc (TVA) method. Vacuum. 2019, 167, 129–35.
[502] Zhang Y, Li J, Li J. Microstructure, mechanical properties, corrosion behavior and film formation mechanism of Mg-Zn-Mn-xNd in Kokubo's solution. Journal of Alloys and Compounds. 2018, 730, 458–70.
[503] Fu Y, Cao QP, Wang XD, Zhang DX, Jiang JZ. Thickness dependent electrical resistivity in amorphous Mg-Zn-Ca thin films. Thin Solid Films. 2019, 672, 182–85.
[504] Fu Y, Cao QP, Liu SY, Wang C, Jiang JZ. Anomalous deformation mode transition in amorphous Mg-Zn-Ca thin films. Scripta Materialia. 2018, 149, 139–43.
[505] Bao S, Yamada Y, Tajima K, Jin P, Yoshimura K. Switchable mirror based on Mg–Zr–H thin films. Journal of Alloys and Compounds. 2012, 513, 495–98.
[506] Tajima K, Yamada Y, Yoshimura K. Switchable mirror glass with a Mg–Zr–Ni ternary alloy thin film. Solar Energy Materials and Solar Cells. 2014, 126, 227–36.
[507] Li H, Sun H, Wang C, Wei B, Ma H. Controllable electrochemical synthesis and magnetic behaviors of Mg–Mn–Fe–Co–Ni–Gd alloy films. Journal of Alloys and Compounds. 2014, 598, 161–65.
[508] Yamada Y, Miura M, Tajima K, Okada M, Yoshimura K. Optical indices of switchable mirrors based on Mg–Y alloy thin films in the transparent state. Thin Solid Films. 2014, 571, 712–14.
[509] Leinartas K, Juzeliūnas E, Staišiūnas L, Grigucevičienė A, Juškėnas R. Mg–Nb alloy films: Structure and stability in a balanced salt solution. Journal of Alloys and Compounds. 2016, 661, 322–30.
[510] https://www.mtixtl.com/Mg-Foil-100w-1000L-0.1th.aspx.
[511] Luo D, Wang H-Y, Zhang L, Liu G-L, Jiang Q-C. Microstructure evolution and tensile properties of hot rolled Mg–6Al–3Sn alloy sheet at elevated temperatures. Materials Science and Engineering: A. 2015, 643, 149–55.
[512] Cao L, Liu C, Gao Y, Jiang S, Liu Y. Influence of finish rolling temperature on the microstructure and mechanical properties of Mg-8.5Al-0.5Zn-0.2Mn-0.15Ag alloy sheets. Materials Characterization. 2018, 139, 38–48.
[513] Nakata T, Xu C, Suzawa K, Yoshida K, Kamado S. Enhancing mechanical properties of rolled Mg-Al-Ca-Mn alloy sheet by Zn addition. Materials Science and Engineering: A. 2018, 737, 223–29.

[514] Ding H-L, Zhang P, Cheng G-P, Kamado S. Effect of calcium addition on microstructure and texture modification of Mg rolled sheets. Transactions of Nonferrous Metals Society of China. 2015, 25, 2875–83.
[515] Guo F, Zhang D, Fan X, Li J, Pan F. Microstructure, texture and mechanical properties evolution of pre-twinning Mg alloys sheets during large strain hot rolling. Materials Science and Engineering: A. 2016, 655, 92–99.
[516] Kim HL, Lee J-H, Lee CS, Bang W, Chnag YW. Shear band formation during hot compression of AZ31 Mg alloy sheets. Materials Science and Engineering: A. 2012, 558, 431–38.
[517] Xia D, Huang G, Liu S, Tang A, Pan F. Microscopic deformation compatibility during biaxial tension in AZ31 Mg alloy rolled sheet at room temperature. Materials Science and Engineering: A. 2019, 756, 1–10.
[518] Han T, Huang G, Ma L, Wang G, Pan F. Evolution of microstructure and mechanical properties of AZ31 Mg alloy sheets processed by accumulated extrusion bonding with different relative orientation. Journal of Alloys and Compounds. 2019, 784, 584–91.
[519] Mekonen MN, Steglich D, Bohlen J, Mosler LJ. Mechanical characterization and constitutive modeling of Mg alloy sheets. Materials Science and Engineering: A. 2012, 540, 174–86.
[520] Wang L, Qiao Q, Liu Y, Song X. Formability of AZ31 Mg alloy sheets within medium temperatures. Journal of Magnesium and Alloys. 2013, 1, 312–17.
[521] Yang X, Patel JB, Huang Y, Mendis CL, Fan Z. Towards directly formable thin gauge AZ31 Mg alloy sheet production by melt conditioned twin roll casting. Materials & Design. 2019, 179; https://doi.org/10.1016/j.matdes.2019.107887.
[522] Nguyen N-T, Lee M-G, Kim JH, Kim HY. A practical constitutive model for AZ31B Mg alloy sheets with unusual stress–strain response. Finite Elements in Analysis and Design. 2013, 76, 39–49.
[523] Wu H-Y, Sun P-H, Zhu F-J, Liu H-C, Chiu C-H. Tensile Properties and Shallow Pan Rapid Gas Blow Forming of Commercial Fine-grained Mg Alloy AZ31B Thin Sheet. Procedia Engineering. 2012, 36, 329–34.
[524] Li J, Li Z, Mao D, Zhang B, Chen S. Effect of Annealing Process on Microstructure and Properties of Roll-Casting AZ31B Mg Alloy Sheet. Procedia Engineering. 2012, 27, 895–902.
[525] Kitahara H, Yada T, Hashiguchi F, Tsushida M, Ando S. Mg alloy sheets with a nanocrystalline surface layer fabricated by wire-brushing. Surface and Coatings Technology. 2014, 243, 28–33.
[526] Zeng ZR, Bian MZ, Xu SW, Davies CHJ, Nie JF. Effects of dilute additions of Zn and Ca on ductility of magnesium alloy sheet. Materials Science and Engineering: A 2016, 674, 459–71.
[527] Zeng ZR, Zhu YM, Bian MZ, Xu SW, Nie JF. Annealing strengthening in a dilute Mg–Zn–Ca sheet alloy. Scripta Materialia. 2015, 107, 127–30.
[528] Ha C, Bohlen J, Yi S, Zhou X, Kainer KU. Influence of Nd or Ca addition on the dislocation activity and texture changes of Mg–Zn alloy sheets under uniaxial tensile loading. Materials Science and Engineering: A. 2019, 761; https://doi.org/10.1016/j.msea.2019.138053.
[529] Kang H, Bae DH. Deformation behavior of a statically recrystallized Mg–Zn–MM alloy sheet. Materials Science and Engineering: A. 2013, 582, 203–10.
[530] Pan S, Huang X, Xin Y, Huang G, Liu Q. The effect of hot rolling regime on texture and mechanical properties of an as cast Mg–2Zn–2Gd plate. Materials Science and Engineering: A. 2018, 731, 288–95.
[531] Luo J, Hu WW, Jin QQ, Yan H, Chen RS. Unusual cold rolled texture in an Mg-2.0Zn-0.8Gd sheet. Scripta Materialia. 2017, 127, 146–50.
[532] Dobroň P, Balík J, Chmelík F, Illková K, Lukáč P. A study of mechanical anisotropy of Mg–Zn–Rare earth alloy sheet. Journal of Alloys and Compounds. 2014, 588, 628–32.
[533] Min J, Lin J, Li J. Forming limits of Mg alloy ZEK100 sheet in preform annealing process. Materials & Design. 2014, 53, 947–53.

[534] Min J, Lin J. An elastic behavior and phenomenological modeling of Mg ZEK100-O alloy sheet under cyclic tensile loading–unloading. Materials Science and Engineering: A. 2013, 561, 174–82.
[535] Lin Y-N, Wu H-Y, Zhou G-H, Chiu C-H, Lee S. Mechanical and anisotropic behaviors of Mg–Li–Zn alloy thin sheets. Materials & Design. 2008, 29, 2061–65.
[536] Yang Q, Jiang B, Li X, Dong H, Pan F. Microstructure and mechanical behavior of the Mg–Mn–Ce magnesium alloy sheets. Journal of Magnesium and Alloys. 2014, 2, 8–12.
[537] Xu C, Zheng MY, Wu K, Wang ED, Liu YT. Effect of final rolling reduction on the microstructure and mechanical properties of Mg–Gd–Y–Zn–Zr alloy sheets. Materials Science and Engineering: A. 2013, 559, 232–40.
[538] Xu C, Zheng MY, Wu K, Wang ED, Lv XY. Influence of rolling temperature on the microstructure and mechanical properties of Mg–Gd–Y–Zn–Zr alloy sheets. Materials Science and Engineering: A. 2013, 559, 615–22.
[539] Wang K, Wang J, Peng X, Gao S, Pan F. Microstructure and mechanical properties of Mg-Gd-Y-Zn-Mn alloy sheets processed by large-strain high-efficiency rolling. Materials Science and Engineering: A. 2019, 748, 100–07.
[540] Jiang J, Bo G, Liu J, Ye CC, Jiang Z. Microstructures and mechanical properties of extruded Mg–2Sn–xYb (x=0, 0.1, 0.5 at.%) sheets. Journal of Magnesium and Alloys. 2014, 2, 257–64.
[541] Luo X-M, Bi G-L, Jiang J, Li M, Hao Y. Compressive anisotropy of extruded Mg–Dy–Zn alloy sheet Transactions of Nonferrous Metals Society of China. 2016, 26, 390–97.
[542] https://www.amazon.com/Wrisky-1Rolls-99-95-Magnesium-Chemicals/dp/B01I9CDW50.
[543] http://mgwiresindustry.com/.
[544] https://www.thephonograph.net/periodic-audio-mg-magnesium-review/.
[545] Du X-H, Hong M, Duan G-S, Wu B-L, Esling C. Preparation of sound ribbons with submicrometer-grained microstructure on a Mg–Zn alloy. Science Bulletin. 2015, 60, 570–73.
[546] Kim M-S, Kim S-H, Kim H-W. Deformation-induced center segregation in twin-roll cast high-Mg Al–Mg strips. Scripta Materialia. 2018, 152, 69–73.
[547] Xu Z, Tang G, Tian S, Ding F, Tian H. Research of electroplastic rolling of AZ31 Mg alloy strip. Journal of Materials Processing Technology. 2007, 182, 128–33.
[548] Guan RG, Zhao ZY, Zhang H, Lian C, Liu CM. Microstructure evolution and properties of Mg–3Sn–1Mn (wt%) alloy strip processed by semisolid rheo-rolling. Journal of Materials Processing Technology. 2012, 212, 1430–36.
[549] Milenin A, Kustra P, Seitz J-M, Bach F-W, Bormann D. Production of thin wires of magnesium alloys for surgical applications. Wire Journal International. 2010, 44, 74–81.
[550] Johnston S, Shi Z, Dargusch MS, Atrens A. Influence of surface condition on the corrosion of ultra-high-purity Mg alloy wire. Corrosion Science. 2016, 108, 66–75.
[551] Monfared A, Ghaee A, Ebrahimi-Barough S. Preparation and characterization of crystallized and relaxed amorphous Mg-Zn-Ca alloy ribbons for nerve regeneration application. Journal of Non-Crystalline Solids. 2018, 489, 71–76.
[552] Peng Q, Fu H, Pang J, Zhang J, Xiao W. Preparation, mechanical and degradation properties of Mg–Y-based microwire. Journal of the Mechanical Behavior of Biomedical Materials. 2014, 29, 375–84.
[553] https://www.aliexpress.com/item/32841630120.html
[554] https://www.pearl-overseas.com/magnesium-products.html
[555] Mroz S, Stradomski G, Dyja H, Galka A. Using the explosive cladding method for production of Mg-Al bimetallic bars. Archives of Civil and Mechanical Engineering. 2015, 15, 317–23.
[556] Butt MS, Bai J, Wan X, Chu C, Zhou G. Mg alloy rod reinforced biodegradable poly-lactic acid composite for load bearing bone replacement. Surface and Coatings Technology. 2017, 309, 471–79.

[557] http://www.winfredint.com/magnesium-metal/magnesium-extrusions/magnesium-alloy-round-square-tube-pipe-been.html.
[558] Sun J, Jin L, Dong S, Zhang Z, Dong J. Asymmetry strain hardening behavior in Mg-3%Al-1%Zn and Mg-8%Gd-3%Y alloy tubes. Materials Letters. 2013, 107, 197–201.
[559] Guo F, Feng B, Fu S, Xin Y, Liu Q. Microstructure and texture in an extruded Mg–Al–Ca–Mn flat-oval tube. Journal of Magnesium and Alloy 2017, 5, 13–19.
[560] Ge Q, Dellasega D, Demir AG, Vedani M. The processing of ultrafine-grained Mg tubes for biodegradable stents. Acta Biomaterialia. 2013, 9, 8604–10.
[561] https://www.slideshare.net/aliaahmeddiaa/foam-by-alia.
[562] Kränzlin N, Niederberger M. Controlled fabrication of porous metals from the nanometer to the macroscopic scale. Materials Horizons. 2015, 2, 59–377.
[563] Banhart J. Manufacturing Routes for Metallic Foams. JOM. Minerals, Metals & Materials Society. 2000, 52, 22–27.
[564] Liu PS, Chen GF. Chapter Three – Application of Porous Metals. Porous Materials; Processing and Applications. 2014, 113–88.
[565] Banhart J. Manufacture, Characterization and application of cellular metals and metal foams. Progress in Materials Science. 2001, 46, 559–632.
[566] DeGroot CT, Straatman AG, Betchen LJ. Modeling forced convection in finned metal foam heat sinks. Journal of Electronic Packaging. 2009, 131; https://doi.org/10.1115/1.3103934.
[567] https://en.wikipedia.org/wiki/Metal_foam.
[568] Xu ZG, Fu JW, Luo TJ, Yang YS. Effects of cell size on quasi-static compressive properties of Mg alloy foams. Materials & Design. 2012, 34, 40–44.
[569] Xia X, Zhao W, Wei Z, Wang Z. Effects of specimen aspect ratio on the compressive properties of Mg alloy foam. Materials & Design. 2012, 42, 32–36.
[570] Xia X, Zhao W, Feng X, Feng H, Zhang X. Effect of homogenizing heat treatment on the compressive properties of closed-cell Mg alloy foams. Materials & Design. 2013, 49, 19–24.
[571] Yang D, Yang S, Ma A, Jiang J, Wang H. Fabrication and compressive properties of cellular Mg foam via melt foaming method. Procedia Engineering. 2012, 27, 1248–56.
[572] Lu X, Zhang Z, Du H, Luo H, Xu J. Compressive behavior of Mg alloy foams at elevated temperature. Journal of Alloys and Compounds. 2019, 797, 727–34.
[573] Guo N, Leu MC. Additive manufacturing: technology, applications and research needs. Frontiers of Mechanical Engineering. 2013, 8, 215–43.
[574] https://www.machinedesign.com/materials/article/21830512/additive-manufacturing-comes-to-metal-foam.
[575] Lara-Rodriguez GA, Figueroa IA, Suarez MA, Novelo-Peralta O, Goodall R. A replication-casting device for manufacturing open-cell Mg foams. Journal of Materials Processing Technology. 2017, 243, 16–22.
[576] Singh S, Vashisth P, Shrivastav A, Bhatnagar N. Synthesis and characterization of a novel open cellular Mg-based scaffold for tissue engineering application. The Journal of the Mechanical Behavior of Biomedical Materials. 2019, 94, 54–62.
[577] Vahidgolpayegni A, Wen C, Hodgson P, Li Y. Production methods and characterization of porous Mg and Mg alloys for biomedical applications. In Wen C ed., Metallic Foam Bone: Processing, Modification and Characterization and Properties. Woodhead Pub, Duxford UK, 2017, pp 25–82; DOI: 10.1016/B978-0-08-101289-5.00002-0.
[578] Wen C, Yamada Y, Shimojima K, Chino Y, Hosokawa H, Mabuchi M. Compressibility of porous magnesium foam: dependency on porosity and pore size. Materials Letters. 2004, 58, 357–60.
[579] Tan L, Gong M, Zheng F, Zhang B, Yang K. Study on compression behavior of porous magnesium used as bone tissue engineering scaffolds. Biomedical Materials. 2009, 4; DOI: 10.1088/1748-6041/4/1/015016.

[580] Gu X, Zhou W, Zheng Y, Liu Y, Li Y. Degradation and cytotoxicity of lotus-type porous pure magnesium as potential tissue engineering scaffold material. Materials Letters. 2000, 64, 1871–74.
[581] Mutlu I. Production and fluoride treatment of Mg-Ca-Zn-Co alloy foam for tissue engineering applications. Transactions of Nonferrous Metals Society of China. 2018, 28, 114–24.
[582] Jia G, Hou Y, Chen C, Niu J, Yuan G. Precise fabrication of open porous Mg scaffolds using NaCl templates: Relationship between space holder particles, pore characteristics and mechanical behavior. Materials & Design. 2018, 140, 106–13.
[583] Wen C, Mabuchi M, Yamada Y, Shimojima K, Chino Y, Asahina T. Processing of biocompatible porous Ti and Mg. Scripta Mater. 2001, 45, 1147–53.
[584] Kang M-H, Jung H-D, Kim S-W, Lee S-M, Kim H-E, Estrin Y, Koh Y-H. Production and bio-corrosion resistance of porous magnesium with hydroxyapatite coating for biomedical applications. Materials Letters. 2013, 108, 122–24.
[585] Wang X, Wang X, Wang D, Zhao M, Han F. A novel approach to fabricate Zn coating on Mg foam through a modified thermal evaporation technique. Journal of Materials Science & Technology. 2018, 34, 1558–63.
[586] Hao GL, Han FS, Li WD. Processing and mechanical properties of magnesium foams. Journal of Porous Materials. 2009, 16, 251–56.
[587] Yamada Y, Shimojima K, Sakaguchi Y, Mabuchi M, Nakamura M, Asahina T, Mukai T, Kanahashi H, Higashi K. Processing of cellular magnesium materials. Advanced Engineering Materials. 2000, 2, 184–87.
[588] Li Y-G, Wei Y-H, Hou L-F, Guo C-L, Han P-J. Fabrication of a surface-porous magnesium–aluminium alloy. Electrochemistry Communications. 2014, 46, 94–98.
[589] Yang F, Yan Z-Y, Wei Y-H, Li Y-G, Hou L-F. Fabrication of surface-porous Mg–Al alloys with different microstructures in a neutral aqueous solution. Corrosion Science. 2018, 130, 138–42.
[590] Oshida Y, Tuna EB, Aktören O, Gençay K. Dental Implant Systems. International Journal of Molecular Sciences. 2010, 11, 1580–678.
[591] Oshida Y. Bioscience and Bioengineering of Titanium Materials. Elsevier, Oxford UK, 2007.

Chapter 11
Joining

11.1 Introduction

Due to the wide application of magnesium alloys in metals manufacturing, it is very important to employ a reliable method of joining these reactive metals together and to other alloys [1]. Along with improved fusion welding techniques, some novel methods and their hybrids were developed, enabling reliable joining of different grades of cast and wrought magnesium alloys [2]. Since interfacial phenomena is crucial and controls the resultant joint strengths and joint characteristics for particularly low-temperature processes (such as soldering and brazing, solid-state diffusion bonding (DB) and even mechanical joining), there are still on-going researches for improvement in joint strength by better control of interface phenomena. In this chapter, we will discuss fusion welding, liquid–solid joining (such as soldering and brazing) and solid-state joining (such as DB).

11.2 Fusion welding

Fusion welding is a generic term for welding processes during which material is melt to join material of similar compositions and melting points. Due to the high-temperature phase transitions involved in the process, a heat-affected zone (HAZ) is created in the materials, although the zone of the HAZ varies depending on the type of heat-input sources. Energy source for the fusion welding varies by thermal sources including arc (gas shielding or flux shielding), resistance, radiation like electron beam welding (operated in vacuum) or conduction like laser beam welding (LBW).

11.2.1 Arc welding

There are two basic methods of arc welding: tungsten inert gas (TIG) and metal inert gas (MIG).

11.2.1.1 Tungsten inert gas

In TIG arc welding, an arc is generated between a nonconsumable tungsten electrode and the welded metal. The electrode and welded metal are shielded with an inert gas, typically argon. In general, weld can be made with or without filler (in a form of wire) [3, 4]. During TIG welding, an arc is produced between a nonconsumable electrode and the workpiece, which melts the base metal (BM) to form a weld/joint. TIG

https://doi.org/10.1515/9783110676945-011

welding is considered as the most preferred industrial welding method for reactive materials such as magnesium; this is attributed to better economy and applicability, which makes it an excellent choice for joining magnesium and its alloys [3].

Peng et al. [5] welded AZ31 and AZ61 plates in 3 mm thick plates with AZ31 and AZ61 welding wires by TIG method and investigated the influence of welding wires on the strength of welded joints of AZ31 and AZ61 magnesium alloy plates. It was reported that (i) the appearance shape was good with whether AZ31 or AZ61 welding wire, (ii) the welded zone was identified to be composed of α-Mg and β-$Mg_{17}Al_{12}$ phases, (iii) HAZs exist both in AZ31 and AZ61 joints, with grains coarser than BM, (iv) relative to AZ61 welding wire, using the AZ31 welding wire tends to get a coarse-grain region of little width, and a fracture point closer to the center line of welding seam, with tensile fracture strength of 161 MPa leading to a 64% strength of the AZ31 BM and (v) with the AZ61 welding wire, a coarse-grain region of more width and a fracture point a little far from the center line occur, the strength of the joints reaches to 210 MPa, 84% of that of its AZ31 BM. Liu et al. [6] employed TIG on superlight Mg–Li alloy plates with a thickness of 2 mm, using argon gas as a protecting atmosphere. It was found that (i) the microstructure in the fusion zone is fine, and the microstructure in the HAZ is coarser than the parent metal, (ii) the tensile strength of the welded joint is about 84% of that of the parent metal, (iii) the fracture occurs in a mixed type of toughness and brittleness in the HAZ and (iv) during the welding process, aluminum and cerium are enriched at grain boundaries in the fusion zone. Song et al. [7] studied cast magnesium alloy AZ80 and wrought magnesium alloy AZ31B subjected to TIG filler wire welding and laser-TIG hybrid filler wire welding. It was obtained that (i) although good welding formation and good tensile strength can be achieved both in two welding methods, hybrid welding possessed wider parameter than TIG welding, which made it more flexible and reliable in industry application; (ii) the weld beads of the two joints both had irregular anchor shapes, and both joints had a sharp angle region on the AZ31B sides; (iii) the microstructure of the joints was composed of α-Mg phases and β-$Mg_{17}Al_{12}$ phases, and α + β divorced eutectic phases were found in the fusion zone, AZ80 BM and AZ80 partially melted zone; (iv) the fusion zone was observed as small equiaxed dendrites and an evident partially melted zone, whose microstructure was a reticular α + β eutectic phase belt and some nongrown α-Mg phases, was observed on the AZ80 sides in both joints; (v) the eutectic phases were tinier and more dispersed in hybrid welding than in TIG welding; (vi) the hardness value of hybrid welding was higher than TIG welding, and the partially melted zone was the hardened zone in both joints; (vii) the tensile test showed that the ultimate tensile strength (UTS) of both joints were over 155 MPa, and the joints fracture at the AZ80 BM; and (viii) the increased hardness and high tensile strength of each joint were attributed to the partially melted zone microstructure.

There are several works on filler materials. For magnesium alloys, filler rods may be of the same chemistry as welded part or lower melting range. The latter allows the weld to remain liquid until other parts of the weld are solid, thus reducing the probability of cracking. Song et al. used TIG hybrid filler [7] and AZ61 filler wires [8] for laser–TIG (LATIG) of AZ31 Mg alloy and steel. Liu et al. [9] used Zn-29-5Al-0.5Ti alloy filler for TIG welding AZ31B and 6061 Al alloy. It was reported that (i) the formation of brittle and hard Mg–Al intermetallic compounds (IMCs) is avoided because of the effects of Zn, Al and Ti, (ii) the average tensile strength of the joint is 148 MPa. Al_3Ti is first precipitated and functions as the nucleus of heterogeneous nucleation during solidification and (iii) the precipitated Al–$MgZn_2$ hypoeutectic phase exhibited a feather-like structure, which enhances the property of the Mg–Al dissimilar joint.

There are some concerns about the IMCs of Mg and Al elements. Welding of Mg and Al alloys is challenging due to the formation of hard and brittle Mg–Al IMCs. Dai et al. [10] designed the gas tungsten arc welding (GTAW)-assisted hybrid ultrasonic seam welding with Sn interlayer to join Mg to Al alloys and investigated effects of Sn interlayer and GTAW current on the microstructure and mechanical properties of the joints. It was reported that (i) Sn interlayer could restrain the formation of Mg–Al IMCs, which were replaced by Mg_2Sn and Sn-based solid solution; (ii) the peak load of the joints increased with the GTAW current increasing and then decreased dramatically at higher GTAW current; (iii) the maximum peak load of the joints with Sn interlayer was approximately 1.3 kN, which was about 30% increase over the joints without Sn interlayer; and (iv) all the joint failures occurred by the interface mode at the Al/Sn interface and the fracture patterns exhibited entirely brittle fracture mode with cleavage facet feature surface. Yang et al. [11] studied the effects of ultrasonic vibration-assisted treatment on the microstructures and mechanical properties of MB3(or AZ80A)/AZ31 dissimilar Mg alloy joints by microstructural characterization, microhardness testing and tensile testing. It was obtained that (i) the welding pores are eliminated and coarse α-Mg grains of fusion zone are refined to 26 μm, owing to the acoustic streaming effect and cavitation effect induced by the ultrasonic vibration-assisted treatment with an optimal ultrasonic power of 1.0 kW; (ii) $Mg_{17}Al_{12}$ precipitation phases are fine and uniformly distributed in the whole fusion zone of weldment; and (iii) microhardness of fusion zone of the Mg alloy joints increases to 53.5 HV after the ultrasonic vibration-assisted process, and the maximum tensile strength with optimized UVA treatment increases to 263 MPa, which leads to fracture occurrence in the Mg alloy base plate; indicating (iv) robust MB3/AZ31 Mg alloy joints can be obtained by ultrasonic vibration-assisted process.

In general, fluxes allow full penetration welding at greater rates using relatively inexpensive gas tungsten arc as the heat source. For transition-metal alloys, chemical fluxes predeposited on the path of gas tungsten electric arcs can significantly increase weld penetration. Several mechanisms for this beneficial contribution of fluxes, including electrical charge redistribution (possibly constriction) and surface-energy-driven flow (Marangoni effect), have been postulated. Using argon shielding and chloride fluxes during the Mg alloy welding, Marya et al. [12] revealed increases in weld penetration as much as 100% were not unusual. It was found that

(i) among all selected chlorides (LiCl, $CaCl_2$, $CdCl_2$, $PbCl_2$ and $CeCl_3$), cadmium chloride was the most effective and (ii) increases in heat input, accompanied by a redistribution of the heat flux, are suggested as the main contribution to the augmented weld penetration with chlorides.

11.2.1.2 Metal inert gas

Similarly, MIG welding has been shown by several researchers to be capable of joining magnesium alloys with greater speed when compared to TIG welding. Unique fast rigging proportions are normally required in the wire feeders since the magnesium terminal wire has a high melt-off rate. The typical wire feeder and power supply utilized for aluminum welding will be appropriate for welding magnesium. The heat input during MIG welding of magnesium alloys, however, results in the formation of a large HAZ containing a coarse-grain structure which lowers the mechanical performance of the weld [13]. Liu et al. [13] developed a novel weld-bonding hybrid process by combining a modified MIG spot welding process with adhesive bonding and applied to join Mg alloy and Al alloy. It was reported that (i) the Mg BM and the fusion zone are metallurgically connected by an Al–Mg transition layer with the thickness of 30–60 μm; (ii) a single nugget of a spot-welded joint can offer high shear strength of 130 MPa, which reaches 81% of that of Mg BM; (iii) the increased strength is due to the intermetallic layer being formed at the region with low stress, so the joint fractures in an Al-rich dendritic region; and (iv) superior mechanical properties can be obtained by weld-bonded joint, benefiting from the advantages of both welding and adhesive bonding.

During an MIG arc welding, the arc is formed between the consumable electrode and the part to be welded. The electrode is continuously provided from the spool. Both the welded area and the arc zone are protected by a gas shield. The solidification microstructure of the weld is controlled by constitutional undercooling depending on the thermal gradient and growth rate. The microstructure of MIG-welded AZ91D alloy with AZ61 as welding wire consisted of solid solution of α-Mg and IMC of $Mg_{17}Al_{12}$ [14]. Sun et al. [14] investigated the microstructure and cracking characteristics of MIG-welded magnesium alloy (AZ91D) joint, and the effect of welding speed on cracking susceptibility. It was reported that (i) the welded joint consists of primary α-Mg and divorced phases (eutectic α-Mg eutectic β-$Mg_{17}Al_{12}$), the latter mainly distributing along the α-Mg grain boundaries; (ii) solidification cracking often occurred in the crater and was also observed at weld center line when welding speed was 300 mm/min, which are associated with segregation of Mn, Al and Zn, and high tensile stresses in the welds; (iii) liquation cracking appeared in HAZ immediately adjacent to the fusion line when low welding speed was used (300 mm/min); (iv) the weld contained roughly 7% of Al; (v) in HAZ near the fusion line, subjected to temperatures between solidus and liquidus, a part of α-Mg solid solution and eutectics, distributed at grain boundaries, experienced melting; thus, after subsequent solidification the boundary regions formed islands of eutectic solid solution of α-Mg surrounded by $Mg_{17}Al_{12}$ precipitates; (vi) it is mainly related to the low welding speed resulting in increasing heat input and tensile stresses in the HAZ; and (vii) it is favorable to decrease heat input for improving the susceptibility of hot cracking during MIG welding of magnesium alloys. Wang et al. [15] investigated AZ31B Mg to Q235 steel (0.2 C-0.35Si-1.4Mn-Fe) joints by MIG arc welding. It was found that (i) the temperature distribution in the joints is uneven, (ii) Mg alloy welds present a fine equiaxed grain structure, (iii) there exists a transition layer consisting mainly of AlFe, $AlFe_3$ and $Mg(Fe, Al)_2O_4$ phases at Mg/steel interface, and it is the weakest link in Mg–steel joints, (iv) the welding heat input and weld Al content have significant effect on the joint strength, (v) the joint strength increases with increasing the heat input from 1,680 to 2,093 J/cm, due to promoting Mg/steel interface reaction, (vi) when weld Al content is increased to 6.20%, the joint strength reaches 192 MPa, 80% of Mg alloy BM strength and (vii) it is favorable to select the suitable welding heat input and weld Al content for improving joint strength. Gaur et al. [16] investigated the physically short- and long-crack growth behavior of Al–5.8%Mg alloy, a special hardened alloy used for welding of Al-5083 plates. It was reported that (i) microstructural analysis on both longitudinal and cross-sectional plane of welded plates showed no crystallographic texture with nearly equiaxed grains of size 85 μm and gas porosities; (ii) during the fatigue tests, it appeared that the physically short cracks initially propagated in closure-free environment and then deviated toward their long-crack growth rates and the physically short-crack growth effect could not be removed completely using the crack-closure concept alone, suggesting the role of other growth-retarding mechanisms; and (iii) a modified empirical model including the effect of other possible growth-retarding mechanisms was proposed to capture the behavior of physically short cracks in this material.

11.2.2 Resistance spot welding

Resistance spot welding (RSW) represents the localized joining of two or more metal parts together by an application of heat and pressure. The weld is formed due to the heat generated by the resistance to the electrical current passage between copper electrodes, being also the source of pressure. As a result, at the interface of welded materials, a liquid pool (weld nugget) is formed. For high electrical conductivity of magnesium and low heat generation in the weld, high welding currents are required. The process is used mainly in assembly lines to weld products made of thin gauge metals and it has potentials for joining sheets of magnesium alloys [17, 18].

11.2.2.1 Mg/Mg similar joint

Xu et al. [19] evaluated microstructures, tensile and fatigue properties of weld-bonded magnesium-to-magnesium (Mg/Mg) similar joints. It was reported that (i) in the weld-bonded Mg/Mg joints, equiaxed dendritic and divorced eutectic structures formed in the fusion zone, (ii) weld-bonded Mg/Mg was significantly stronger than RSWed Mg/steel joints in terms of the maximum tensile shear load and energy absorption, which also increased with increasing strain rate and (iii) fatigue strength was three-fold higher for weld-bonded Mg/Mg than for RSWed- Mg/steel joints. Patel et al. [20] identified failure mode and estimated fatigue life of ultrasonic spot-welded (USWed) lap joints of an AZ31B-H24 magnesium alloy. It was found that (i) the solid-state USWed joints exhibited a superior fatigue life compared with other welding processes, (ii) fatigue failure mode changed from interfacial failure to transverse-through-thickness crack growth with decreasing cyclic load level, depending on the welding energy, (iii) fatigue crack initiation and propagation occurred from both the notch tip inside the faying surface and the edge of sonotrode indentation footprints due to the presence of stress concentration and (iv) the fatigue life estimation, based on the fatigue crack growth model with the global and local stress intensity factors as a function of kink length and the experimentally determined kink angle, agreed well with the obtained experimental results. A series of USW experiments with similar Mg alloy (AZ31B) were performed to determine the process parameters and their effect on weld quality, including weld strength and fracture morphologies [21]. Two dominant welding parameters including vibration amplitude and welding time were evaluated independently to obtain good weld quality. It was reported that the lap joint thinning was significant at higher vibration amplitudes and longer welding times and resulted in the variation of fracture types at the weld interface. Lap shear tests on the USWed Mg alloy lap joints yielded two fracture types: shear and pullout fracture. Metallographic examinations of the fracture surfaces provided insights on the fracture characteristics of the USWed Mg alloys. Variations in the fracture morphologies were the results of the actual weld nugget development and closely related to weld quality. Higher weld strength was obtained at a low welding energy range of 100–140 J.

11.2.2.2 Mg dissimilar joint

The most dissimilar joint cases are reported joining Mg alloy to Al alloy. Penner et al. [22] investigated microstructure and mechanical properties of the dissimilar Al–Mg resistance spot welds made with gold coated and bare nickel interlayers. It was mentioned that (i) welds were made with different welding currents in a range from 16 to 24 kA with a fixed welding time of five cycles. No joints were achieved with a bare nickel interlayer; after welding, specimens were separated without applying any force. Addition of gold coating on nickel surface greatly contributed to the metallurgical bonding at the interfaces and welds easily met requirements of AWS D17·2 standard. Average lap shear strength reached 90% of similar AZ-31B spot weld strength. Similar results were obtained for RSW of AZ31B Mg alloy to Al alloy 5754 using Zn foil and Zn-coated steel interlayers [23]. Patel et al. [24, 25] studied the strength of dissimilar joints of AZ31B-H24 magnesium alloy to 5754-O aluminum alloy by using a tin interlayer inserted in between the faying surfaces during USW. It was reported that (i) the addition of tin interlayer was observed to successfully eliminate the brittle $Al_{12}Mg_{17}$ IMCs, which were replaced by a layer of composite-like tin and Mg_2Sn structure, (ii) failure during the tensile lap shear tests occurred through the interior of the blended interlayer, (iii) the addition of a tin interlayer resulted in a significant improvement in both joint strength and failure energy of magnesium to aluminum dissimilar joints and also led to an energy saving because the optimal welding energy required to achieve the highest strength decreased from ~1,250 to ~1,000 J. Zhang et al. [26] fabricated Mg/Al dissimilar metals joined together utilizing USW with a Zn interlayer. It was shown that (i) four typical regions with different forming morphologies emerged in the interface owing to the uneven distribution of stress and temperature; these four regions were the vortex-like plastic deformation region on the outside of the sonotrode tip teeth, the thinner flat region directly under the sonotrode tip teeth, the network-like diffusion region inside of the sonotrode tip teeth and the thicker flat region between the two sonotrode tip teeth; (ii) the interfacial layer of Mg/Zn/Al USWed joints was mainly composed of a Mg–Zn liquid phase layer of α-Mg + (α-Mg + MgZn) + $MgZn_2$ + (Mg_2Zn_{11} + β-Zn), a residual Zn interlayer and a η-Zn + α-Al solid solution layer; (iii) the addition of Zn interlayer blocked the interdiffusion of Mg and Al atoms successfully and avoided the generation of Mg–Al IMCs; (iv) the formed Mg–Zn system structure and Zn–Al solid solution have relatively good performances and lower brittleness; and (v) in comparison, Mg/Al joints welded with a Zn interlayer in-between displayed the maximum shearing strength about 89.6% greater than those of joints without a Zn interlayer.

Xu et al. [19] also evaluated microstructures, tensile and fatigue properties of weld-bonded magnesium-to-steel (Mg/steel) dissimilar joints, in comparison with resistance spot-welded Mg/steel dissimilar joints. It was mentioned that (i) in the dissimilar joints of RSW and weld-bonded Mg/steel, fusion zone appeared only at Mg side with equiaxed and columnar dendrites; (ii) at steel side, no microstructure changed in the weld-bonded Mg/steel joints, while the microstructure in the RSWed Mg/steel joints consisted of lath martensite, bainite, pearlite and retained austenite leading to an increased microhardness; (iii) the relatively low cooling rate suppressed the formation of shrinkage porosity but promoted the formation of $MgZn_2$ and Mg_7Zn_3 in the weld-bonded Mg/steel joints; (iv) the added adhesive layer diminished stress concentration around the weld nugget; (v) Mg/steel joints were significantly stronger than RSWed Mg/steel joints in terms of the maximum tensile shear load and energy absorption, which also increased with increasing strain rate; (vi) fatigue strength was three-folds higher for weld-bonded Mg/steel joint than for RSWed Mg/steel joints; and (vii) fatigue failure in the RSWed Mg/steel joints occurred from the HAZ near the notch root at lower load levels and in the mode of interfacial fracture at higher load levels, while it occurred in the Mg BM at a maximum cyclic load up to ~10 kN in weld-bonded Mg/steel joint. Effects of insertion of interlayer were recognized by Sn addition for Mg–high strength low-alloy steel joints [25] and Al–Si coating for Mg to 22MnB5 boron steel [27].

11.2.3 Laser beam welding

LBW (also known as conduction welding or radiation welding) is a highly precise form of fusion welding. The laser beam can be split and sent to multiple locations greatly reducing the cost and amount of energy required. LBW finds applications in the automotive industry. Due to a smaller diameter beam and greater control of power input, laser welding permits dissimilar joining of magnesium alloys while limiting the width of the HAZ. Laser welding is usually applied to delicate and thin sheets due to the low penetration of laser beam into the materials.

11.2.3.1 Mg similar joining

Zhou [28] used a 1.5 kW diode laser and a 2 kW CO_2 laser for the welding of AZ31 alloys. It was mentioned that different welding modes exist, that is, keyhole welding with the CO_2 laser and conduction welding with both the CO_2 and the diode lasers. Lei et al. [29] investigated the welding porosity and poor weld formability in the ultrasonic-assisted laser welding process of AZ31B Mg alloy. It was indicated that (i) the cavitation and acoustic streaming of ultrasonic vibration on weld pool can significantly improve weld defect and microstructure morphologies; (ii) with ultrasonic-assisted laser welding technology, the weld appearance becomes smooth and sound; (iii) the weld porosity declines from 4.3% to 0.9% and its average size decreases; (iv) the width of columnar grain zone near fusion line decreases and the equiaxed grains in fusion center zone increase tremendously, the refining effect on the grain is obvious; and (v) the mechanical properties of welds can be significantly improved, the tensile strength and elongation (EL) can be increased to 87% and 64% of the BM. Wahba et al. [30] produced lap joints between AZ91D thixomolded Mg alloy and amorphous polyethylene terephthalate (PET) by direct irradiation of high-power diode laser beam from either plastic or metal side. It was mentioned that (i) the joining mechanism involves the generation of gas bubbles in a narrow region inside PET specimen adjacent to the interface, (ii) the pressure induced by expansion of these bubbles secures tight bonding in the microsize between AZ91D and PET specimens, (iii) discrete bubbles morphology associated with metal-side laser irradiation promoted higher joint strength in comparison with networked wormhole morphology in the case of plastic-side laser irradiation and (iv) the presence of premade pits on the AZ91D specimen surface proved to be effective for the improvement in the performance of plastic-side laser-irradiated joints. Zhao et al. [31] studied the mechanism of pore formation during continuous-wave Nd:YAG LBW of die-cast magnesium alloy AM60B. It was reported that (i) preexisting pores in the BM coalesced and expanded during welding of this alloy and, as a result, large pores were commonly present in the weld metal; (ii) unlike LBW of aluminum alloys, the stability of the keyhole was not a major factor in pore formation during LBW of alloy AM60B; (iii) the porosity in the fusion zone increased with the increase in heat input, that is, increase in the laser power and decrease in the welding speed; and (iv) well-controlled remelting of the fusion zone led to removal of gas bubbles and reduced porosity in the fusion zone. A 3 kW CO_2 laser beam was used to weld the wrought Mg–Al–Mn alloy [32]. It was reported that (i) the wrought Mg–Al–Mn alloy can be joined successfully using optimized welding conditions; (ii) the highest UTS of the joints is up to 94% of that of the BM; (iii) the BM consists of a typical rolled structure, the narrow HAZ has no obvious grain coarsening, and the fusion zone consists of fine grains with a high density of γ-$Mg_{17}Al_{12}$ precipitates; (iv) the hardness test results indicate that the microhardness in the fusion zone is higher than that of the BM; and (v) the elemental analysis reveals that the Mg content in the weld is lower than that of the BM, but the Al content is slightly higher.

Keyhole formation as well as the geometry of weld profiles during Nd:YAG laser welding of ZE41A-T5 were studied through combining various models and concepts [33]. It was reported that (i) weld width and fusion area decrease with increasing welding speed, (ii) in the case of partially penetrated welding, penetration depth decreases with increasing welding speed, (iii) the model predicted that excessive decrease in laser power or increase in defocusing distance decreases surface power density, thereby changing the welding mode from fully penetrated keyhole, to partially penetrated keyhole and then to the conduction mode, (iv) the predicted conditions for keyhole stability and welding modes as well as the weld profiles for various processing conditions were validated by some selected welding experiments and (v) good agreements were found between the model predictions and experimental results indicating the validity of the assumptions made for the development of the model. Dai et al. [34, 35] studied the weldability of a 9.5 mm thick Mg–rare earth (RE) alloy NZ30K using 15 kW high-power CO_2 laser. It was found that (i) when using the right laser welding parameters, good weld forming can be obtained, (ii) the microstructure of the fusion zone is small equiaxed grains, (iii) there was no softening zone to be observed according to the microhardness distribution across the welded joints and (iv) the thick Mg–RE alloy NZ30K plate can be welded by the high power CO_2 laser with good weld quality. Yan et al. [36] investigated the microstructure and mechanical properties of the laser-welded Mg-3Nd-0.2Zn-0.4Zr (NZ30K) magnesium alloy. A fiber optic laser was used to weld 4 mm thick Mg-3Nd-0.2Zn-0.4Zr (NZ30K) and AZ31 magnesium alloy plates. It was found that (i) the NZ30K RE–magnesium alloy showed better properties, especially at a high temperature (200 °C), benefiting from the strengthening phase, compared with the AZ31 joint, such as high-temperature tensile strength, creep resistance at high temperature and corrosion resistance, (ii) the grain of NZ30K in the fusion zone was significantly refined with strengthening-phase distribution on the grain boundary and (iii) the tensile strength of NZ30K laser beam welded joints at a high temperature (200 °C) decreased by 29% compared with that at room temperature, while the tensile strength of AZ31 joint at a high temperature (200 °C) decreased by 53% compared with that at room temperature, which was mainly because of the stable existence of the strengthening phase Mg12Nd in the NZ30K RE–magnesium alloy while the strengthening phase $Mg_{17}Al_{12}$ in AZ31 would soften and coarsen with the rise in temperature.

Fine-grained Mg–5Zn–1Mn–0.6Sn alloy sheets of 2 mm in thickness were welded by fiber laser welding [37]. It was reported that (i) with the lower welding power and higher welding speed, the width and depth of the joints decrease; (ii) some pores are detected at a very high welding speed; (iii) there are two kinds of liquation phenomena in the partially melted zone: one is the liquation network along grain boundaries associated with the liquation of substrate and segregation-induced liquation, the other is the molten pool involved with the liquation of the residual second phases at the boundaries; and (iv) the liquation of substrate and the segregation-induced liquation are the main liquation mechanism in the partially melted zone. Wang et al. [38] investigated the precipitates evolution in the HAZ of laser-welded Mg–Gd–Y–Zr alloy in T6 condition. It was reported that (i) compared with isothermally aged precipitates, the overaged β′-phase presented same morphology and size, while size of needle-shape β became much smaller and (ii) the width of complete dissolution zone of the β′ is smaller than that of partial dissolution and transformation zone.

11.2.3.2 Mg dissimilar joining

Gao et al. [39], using Ti as an interlayer, joined Mg and Al alloys by fiber laser welding. It was mentioned that (i) the formation of Mg–Al IMCs could be totally suppressed and the interfacial layer was composed of Al_3Ti and small amounts of $Al_{18}Ti_2Mg_3$ and (ii) the mechanism of interfacial layer formation was attributed to the thermodynamic behavior of the formation of IMCs in Al–Mg–Ti ternary system and to precise control of the laser power. The immiscible and nonreactive characteristics of Mg/Ti dissimilar metals restrict the metallurgical bonding and reliable joining of them. To solve this problem, the Al interlayer between Mg/Ti was added [40]. It was reported that (i) the Mg/Ti joint without addition of Al interlayer could not be welded. While relatively acceptable appearance was obtained when adding Al interlayer, (ii) the interfacial reaction was improved with the assistance of Al interlayer resulting in metallurgical bonding at the interface, (iii) the $TiAl_3$ phase formed at the direct laser irradiation zone, (iv) the interfacial reaction layer increased little with the increasing thickness of Al interlayer, (v) the interfacial reaction layer was mainly restricted by dissolution of Ti element, (vi) the maximum tensile-shear force could reach 2,230 N/cm (about 81% of that of AZ31B Mg alloy BM) when the laser power was 2,300 W and the thickness of added Al interlayer was 0.05 mm, (vii) the tensile-shear force decreased when network structure of $Mg_{17}Al_{12}$ precipitated in the weld zone and (viii) the fracture path changed from fusion zone/Ti to Mg fusion line when the thickness of Al interlayer exceeded 0.12 mm.

To improve the metallurgical bonding of immiscible and nonreactive Mg/Ti system, Ni electrocoating was employed acting as an intermediate element by reacting with both Mg and Ti in laser heat-conduction welding process [41]. It was found that (i) reliable joints were obtained with suitable laser powers ranging from 1,200 to 1,800 W, (ii) continuous reaction layer of Ti_2Ni and Ti solid solution formed at the interface, (iii) Mg–Al–Ni ternary phase dispersed in fusion zone at Mg side, (iv) diffusion of electroplated Ni was influenced by a bidirectional mechanism to Mg side and Ti side, which resulted in the variation of reaction layer thickness, (v) the maximum tensile-shear load could reach 144 N/mm (about 53.3% of joint efficiency of BM AZ31B Mg alloy) when laser power was 1,500 W and (vi) joint strength and fracture mode were associated with two aspects: interfacial reaction and weld appearance of Mg side.

11.2.3.3 Hybrid laser beam welding

Hybrid laser beam technologies are defined as a combination of a laser beam source with an additional secondary beam source or another joining technique. Lu et al. [42] carried out welding of AZ31B magnesium alloy using hybrid LATIG welding, LBW and TIG welding. It was reported that (i) the welding speed of LATIG was higher than that of TIG, which was caught up with LBW; (ii) the penetration of LATIG doubles that of TIG, and was four times that of LBW; (iii) arc stability was improved in hybrid of LATIG welding compared with using the TIG welding alone, especially at high welding speed and under low TIG current; (iv) the HAZ of joint was only observed in TIG welding; and the size of grains in it was evidently coarse; (v) in fusion zone, the equiaxed grains exist, whose size was the smallest welded by LBW, and was the largest by TIG welding; and (vi) Mg concentration of the fusion zone was lower than that of the base one by Electro-Probe Micro-Analyzer (EPMA) in three welding processes. Joints of Mg alloys and Al alloys were produced by the LATIG hybrid welding process with Ce as an interlayer [43]. It was mentioned that (i) cracks did not occur in the most critical region with Ce as the interlayer, while they did in its absence and (ii) the Ce distributed uniformly in the most critical regions where the major composition changed from Mg to Al. Liu et al. [44], using a laser–GTA hybrid welding technique, studied the weld of the dissimilar alloys of AZ31B Mg alloy and 304 steel. It was reported that (i) a lap joint was formed between the two; (ii) the weld penetration, which determines the mechanical properties of the welded joints, depends on the laser power; (iii) a transition zone formed at the interface of the Mg–Fe during laser–GTA hybrid welding and Mg element diffused into the Fe matrix by forming oxides and reacting in the transition; (iv) during tensile testing, the joints fractured at the interface between the Mg alloy and the steel; and (v) metallic oxides produced at the Mg–Fe interface were the reason for the poor mechanical properties of the weld joints.

Qi et al. [45] investigated the joint interface of Mg alloy to steel with Ni interlayer. It was mentioned that the formation of IMC Mg_2Ni and solid solution of Ni in Fe at the interface altered the bonding mode of joints which contributed to the increase of the tensile shear strength in contrast to the direct joining of Mg alloy to steel. Song et al. [46] joined 1.6 mm AZ31 B Mg alloy 1.0 mm Q235 steel by using laser–GTAW hybrid butt welding with AZ61 filler metal. It was reported that (i) laser–GTAW hybrid welding with filling wire can be used to combine high-performance joints and Mg/steel dissimilar metals during butt assembly; (ii) the maximum average tensile fracture load of the joints can reach up to 3,265 N (the load equal to that of steel BM); (iii) the tensile load of the joints decreases with the decrease in heat input; and (iv) with the decrease in heat input, the Mg/steel butt joints had three fracture modes, including the fracture on the BM of steel, Mg weld seam and Mg/steel interface.

11.2.4 Laser welding–brazing

A laser welding–brazing technology using Mg-based filler has been developed for joining Mg alloy to mild steel and Mg alloy to stainless steel in a lap configuration [47]. It was shown that (i) no distinct reaction layer was observed at the interface of Mg/mild steel and, subsequently, the interface was confirmed as mechanical bonding; (ii) the average tensile-shear strength of Mg/mild steel joint was only 142 N/mm with typical interfacial failure, while that of Mg/stainless steel joint could reach 270 N/mm, representing 82.4% joint efficiency relative to the Mg alloy BM; and (iii) the fracture location of Mg/stainless steel joint was at Mg fusion-welding side, suggesting that the interface was not weak point due to the formation of ultrathin interfacial layer. Li et al. [48] investigated the influence of process variables including heating mode, flux, laser beam offset and travel speed on the weld bead geometry and joint strength was investigated during laser welding–brazing of AZ31B Mg alloy to Zn coated steel. It was reported that (i) dual-beam processing was found to preheat the steel substrate and promote the wettability of molten filler metal on the steel surface, thereby improving the corresponding joint strength; (ii) the joint strength was however found to decrease with increasing travel speed; (iii) the reaction layer thickness varied within a certain range when applying different process parameters, suggesting the growth of interfacial layer was not essentially related to the heat input; (iv) the primary failure mode of the lap specimens was interfacial fracture; (v) cracks propagated along the Mg–Zn reaction layer and steel interface; and (vi) original Fe–Al phase formed during the hot-dip galvanization process hindered the metallurgical bonding of Mg–Zn reaction layer and steel substrate, which was attributed to interfacial-type failure.

Chai et al. [49] studied the evolution of microstructure, porosity and mechanical properties of AZ80 joints during two postweld-processing routes. It was mentioned that (i) during the partial rolling process, the welding area was effectively strengthened and the porosity was largely reduced with increasing rolling reduction, (ii) the $Mg_{17}Al_{12}$ phases in the fusion zone and HAZ were essential on the microstructure evolution during the hot deformation process and subsequent aging process and (iii) by proper processing sequence, the strengthening effect of $Mg_{17}Al_{12}$ phases can be brought into full play, and abnormal grain growth in the HAZ can be reduced. Tan et al. [50] fabricated joints of AZ31B Mg and Ti–6Al–4V alloys with Ni coating by laser welding–brazing process using AZ92 Mg-based filler. It was reported that (i) Ni coating was found to significantly promote good wetting–spreading ability of molten filler on the Ti sheet, (ii) acceptable joints without obvious defects were obtained within a relatively wide processing window, (iii) in the process, metallurgical bonding was achieved by the formation of Ti_3Al phase at direct irradiation zone and Al–Ni phase followed by a layer of Mg–Al–Ni ternary compound adjacent to the fusion zone at the intermediate zone, (iv) the tensile-shear test indicated that joints produced at the laser power of 1,300 W reached 2,387 N fracture load, representing 88.5% joint efficiency with respect to the Mg BM and (v) the corresponding failure occurred in the fusion zone of the Mg BM, while joints fractured at the interface at lower/higher laser power due to the crack or excessive IMC formation along the interface. Laser welding–brazing Mg/Cu-coated Ti in lap configuration using various coating thickness was performed with AZ92 Mg-based filler [51]. It was mentioned that (i) only Ti_3Al interfacial layer was generated at the direct irradiation region and grew obviously when thicker Cu coating was adopted; (ii) the interfacial reaction layer evolved from Ti_3Al to Ti_3Al/Ti_2Cu to $Ti_3Al/Ti_2Cu + AlCu_2Ti$ at the middle region with the increase of Cu coating thickness; (iii) Cu could promote mutual diffusion between Ti and Al. Ti preferred to react with Al than Cu, indicating that Al–Ti compounds were easily produced along the Ti surface; (iv) the maximum fracture load was 2,314N with coating thickness of 10.6 μm, which was 55% higher than that with bare Ti sheet and as high as 85% of Mg parent metal; and (v) the fracture occurred along the Mg/Ti interface at the direct irradiation region while the crack propagated in Mg–Cu eutectic structure near the interfacial layer at the middle region.

Dissimilar AZ31B-Mg and Ni-coated Q235A steel alloys were joined in a lap configuration using a laser welding–brazing process [52]. The effects of the Ni coating thickness on the joint appearance, interfacial reactions and mechanical properties were investigated with the assistance of thermodynamic calculations. It was found that (i) in the direct irradiation region, Ni atoms diffused and were accumulated near the interface due to the driving force of the chemical potential; (ii) Al atoms from the filler were attracted by the concentrated Ni atoms, which resulted in the formation of the FeAl phase; (iii) in the middle region and weld toe region, a Fe(Ni) solid solution formed at the interface; (iv) heterogeneous reaction products were produced at the seam near the interface, varying from only the AlNi phase to the AlNi+(α-Mg + Mg_2Ni) eutectic with the increase of the coating thickness; additionally, a bulky Mg_2Ni phase also formed in the matrix of Mg-Ni eutectic with a coating thickness of 40 μm; (v) strong mutual attraction occurred between the Al and Ni atoms at the seam, resulting in a higher driving force for generating the AlNi phase than for generating the Mg–Ni phase; and (vi) the maximum value of the tensile-shear fracture load approached 230 N/mm with a Ni coating thickness of 20 μm, reaching an 88.5% joint efficiency relative to the Mg BM. Tan et al. [53] conducted dissimilar lap joining of magnesium alloy to titanium alloy using Ni coating by laser welding–brazing process. It was found that (i) in laser irradiation region, Ti_3Al phase formed at fusion zone/Ti interface; (ii) in middle region, Ti_3Al phase still existed at fusion zone/Ti interface, while Mg–Al–Ni ternary IMC generated at fusion zone; (iii) in weld toe region, Ti–Ni binary IMCs were observed at the interface of fusion zone/Ti; (iv) the fracture load first increased and then decreased slightly with increasing coating thickness, the maximum fracture load (2,430 N/cm) represented 90% joint efficiency in relation to the Mg BM; and (v) the fracture mode changed from interfacial failure into fusion zone fracture when the Ni-coating thickness was greater than 4.0 μm. Auwal et al. [54] developed a fiber laser welding–brazing procedure for joining AZ31B magnesium alloy to Cu–Ni coated Ti–6Al–4V titanium sheet using AZ92D filler wire. It was reported that (i) the feasibility of this process depends strongly on the preexisting Cu–Ni layer on the Ti surface that promotes wetting of the AZ92 filler; (ii) depending on the interlayer arrangements chosen, different reactions layers formed inside the joint region; (iii) the tensile-shear fracture load of the joints produced at the optimum laser power reached a maximum value of 2,016.5 N for AZ31B/Ni–Cu/Ti–6Al–4V and 2,014.6 N for AZ31B/Cu–Ni/Ti–6Al–4V, representing an efficiency of 71% compared to AZ31B alloy; (iv) under suitable heat input, the joints failed at the fusion zone of the AZ31B BM; and (v) incomplete brazing or large volume of intermetallics at the brazed interface resulted in interfacial failure at lower/higher heat input.

11.3 Force-assisted joining

There are several ways to apply compressive force to interfaces of faying materials; including mainly, extrusion, rolling or pressing. Xin et al. [55] fabricated successfully Mg/Al multilayer plates with excellent layer–layer bonding by coextrusion of Mg/Al bimetal billets from the as-cast condition. It was reported that (i) a weakened basal texture with a double-peaked basal poles tilting toward the extrusion bonding and a preferred distribution of prismatic planes exist in the inner Mg layer, in comparison to a much stronger peak of basal poles and a random distribution of prismatic planes in the surface Mg layer, (ii) all the Al layers have a strong β-fiber texture and a texture gradient from the surface to the center exists, (iii) both the Mg layer and the Al layer have an inhomogeneous grain structure after the first pass of extrusion, (iv) the inner Mg layer has a similar grain morphology to that of the surface Mg layer, (v) compared to the inner Al layers, the surface Al layer contains more recrystallized grains and (vi) a new cycle of accumulative extrusion bonding at 400 °C does not refine grains, but generates more homogeneous grains, which leads to an improved tension EL. Han et al. [56] applied rolled AZ31 Mg alloy sheets to accumulated extrusion-bonding process at 200 °C with transverse direction parallel (0°), at 45° inclined and perpendicular (90°) to the sizing band. It was found that mechanical properties tests indicated that three accumulated extrusion-bonded samples exhibited similar strength and ductility with higher yield strength (145 vs 169 MPa), UTS (336 vs 392 MPa) and fracture EL (24.9% vs 28.8%) comparing to that of as-received sample along rolling direction. Zhou et al. [57] prepared a new composite made of AZ31B Mg alloy and $Zr_{44}Ti_{11}Cu_{10}Ni_{10}Be_{25}$ (LM1B) bulk metallic glass (BMG) by hot stacking extrusion process based on the thermoplastic forming ability of LM1B BMG within the supercooled liquid range. The stacking extrusion tests were carried out at three different temperatures of 430, 440 and 450 °C, respectively, and the extrusion speed was 5 mm/min. It was reported that (i) the LM1B BMG and AZ31B can be well bonded, and welding defects at the smooth and continuous interface were negligible; (ii) the bonding mode is mainly mechanical bonding, meanwhile, a few of metallurgical bonding does exists; and (iii) significant atomic diffusion was detected in the vicinity of the interface while the nanocrystals and partial crystallization were produced in the LM1B BMG.

Laminated metal composites using Mg and Al have good application potential in the aerospace industry because of their lightweights. Liu et al. [58] prepared two types of composites (Mg/Mg and Mg/Al/Mg) with different reduction ratios by the warm roll-bonding technique. It was indicated that (i) the tensile strengths of the two types of laminated metal composites reached their peak values at 35% reduction ratio and (ii) the delamination mechanism in composites significantly improved the bending properties, although this effect decreases with increasing reduction ratio. Partial rolling processes at different temperatures were conducted on the fusion zone of double-side welded Mg–3Al–1Zn alloy joints with excess weld bead, and Chai et al. [59] studied the effect of rolling reduction and rolling temperature on the microstructure, mechanical properties and fracture behavior of the joints. It was shown that (i) both the strength and EL of the joints increase significantly with rolling reduction owing to the microstructure evolution in the fusion zone, (ii) once rolling reduction exceeds a critical value, tensile fracture location will be transferred from the fusion zone to the substrate and the joints can achieve tensile properties roughly the same as those of the initial substrate and (iii) rolling at a lower temperature is preferred to obtaining a weak basal texture in the fusion zone, for the corresponding critical value is smaller. Anne et al. [60] employed the accumulative roll-bonding process to develop Mg–2%Zn/Ce/Al hybrid composite and investigated microstructure, mechanical and corrosion properties. It was reported that (i) the grains are significantly reduced and reaches up to 1 μm in Mg–2%Zn layer and 1.8 μm in Al layer having high angle misorientation of grain boundaries after subjected to five passes of the accumulative roll-bonding process, (ii) the $Al_{17}Mg_{12}$, $AlMg_4Zn_{11}$ and $Al_{11}Ce_3$ intermetallic phases were observed through the

X-ray diffraction (XRD) analysis, (iii) mechanical properties of the hybrid composite improved with increase in the number of accumulative roll bonding passes which is attributed to work hardening, grain refinement and uniform distribution of Ce particles, (iv) presence of Ce in the hybrid composite restricts the phenomenon of dynamic recrystallization and prevents the grain growth during accumulative roll bonding process and (v) the corrosion rate of Mg–Zn/Ce/Al hybrid composite (0.72 mm/year) improved about 3.3 times as compared to that of Mg–2%Zn alloy (2.37 mm/year).

Song et al. [61] prepared and assembled ZSM-5 (zeolite sconony mobile) layer on Mg–Li alloy by hot pressing, using silane coupling as a bonding agent. It was indicated that (i) the corrosion behavior, assessed by electrochemical measurements, showed that ZSM-5 layer reduced the corrosion activity of Mg–Li alloy; and (ii) the method can potentially provide a general route to synthesize various, uniform layers on other active metals. Arkhurdt et al. [62] investigated the effect of two types of carbon fiber-reinforced plastics (CFRPs) with different matrices, on the strength of a metal alloy–plastic composite joint made by the hot-metal pressing technique. One set of experiments was carried out with a PAN-type CFRP with thermoplastic polyurethane (TPU) matrix, and the other with a PAN-type CFRP with a polyamide 6 (PA6) matrix. Both matrices were joined with either as-received or annealed AZ31 Mg-alloy sheets processed at different annealing durations to produce oxide layers on the alloy sheets. It was mentioned that (i) a reaction between C and MgO was observed at the joint interface for the TPU-CFRP but not for the PA6-CFRP and (ii) the melting/decomposition temperature of the matrix materials and the influence of the oxide layer on the conduction of heat between the materials were the key determinants of the AZ31 Mg alloy–CFRP joint strength.

Chen et al. [63] investigated the effect of multipass rolling and postrolling heat treatment upon the microstructure at interface and mechanical properties of the explosive welding Mg/Al composite plates. The thin explosive welding Mg/Al composite plates with 2.14 mm in thickness and good surface quality were obtained by five passes hot rolling (30% reduction, 400 °C). It was found that (i) the thickness of interfacial diffusion layer increases with the increase of annealing temperature and holding time; (ii) the mechanical properties of composite plates increase first and then decrease with the increase of annealing temperature and holding time; (iii) the tensile strength and EL of the composite plates under 200 °C/2 h annealing condition reach the maximum, which are 285 MPa and 24.5%, respectively; and (v) fractography indicates that the postrolling or annealed composite plates all exhibit mixed mode of ductile and brittle fractures.

Based on the fact that due to their distinct physical and metallurgical properties, using conventional fusion welding to direct join steel and magnesium alloy without interlayer metal faces many challenges, Zhang et al. [64] prepared dissimilar joining of a 304 austenitic stainless steel/AZ31B magnesium alloy (304/AZ31B) cladding plate by explosive welding. It was reported that (i) columnar crystals were found at the bottom of the welded joint while fine equiaxed grains were presented in its center, which is similar to that in a fusion joint, (ii) the transmission electron microscopy (TEM) showed that a thin diffusion layer (80 nm) was formed on the surface of 304 flyer plate and (iii) the diffusion at the surface of the 304 plate and melting–solidification near the AZ31B side showed that the AZ31B and 304 were metallurgically bonded.

11.4 Soldering and brazing

The solid-state welding processes used for bonding these two alloys include: friction welding methods, explosion welding, welding with transient liquid phase (TLP) and diffusion welding [65, 66].

11.4.1 In general

Both soldering and brazing are solid-state joining and the two most common methods used for joining similar or dissimilar metals in which a filler metal is melted and filled into the joints. Both the processes are quite the same, except soldering uses filler alloys with melting temperatures below 450 °C, whereas brazing is to be carried out at temperatures above 450 °C. Typical soldering temperatures may be in the 150–260 °C range, whereas brazing is typically done in the range from 650 to 1,260 °C. Both soldering and brazing use capillary action to distribute the molten filler metal between the unmelted BMs being joined, and those BMs must be very clean prior to joining. The properties of jointed portion should be accordingly different between these two joining methods from metallurgical point of view. It is normally believed that the higher temperatures required for brazing result in very different joint properties in service as compared to soldering; while the lower temperatures of soldering usually allow only minimal interalloying of the filler metal with the BMs being joined, brazing often results in extensive interaction between the filler metal and BM. As a result of these characteristic differences, the way they behave in service will usually be very different, particularly in joint strength and fatigue resistance. At the higher temperatures involved in brazing, the metallurgical reactions and alloying are much more intense than those that occur at the much lower temperatures of soldering, therefore, brazed joints usually approach or exceed the strengths of the BMs being joined. A properly brazed joint (assuming the joint has been properly designed) should always be able to handle the stresses and fatigue placed on the joint by thermal cycling or mechanical shock, whereas solder joints under similar conditions would normally be expected to fail through the solder joint, since the degree of alloying with the BM is usually so much less with soldering than with brazing [67].

11.4.2 Soldering

Due to discrepancies in their thermal expansion coefficients, joining magnesium alloy and aluminum alloys by conventional welding methods is a challenge. Moreover, due to the low melting temperatures of both alloys and the high affinities of magnesium and aluminum to oxygen, fusion welding of both alloys is considered difficult. Spot welding, friction stir welding, TIG welding and laser welding processes result in the formation of brittle MgAl, Mg_2Al_3 and $Mg_{17}Al_{12}$ IMCs in the joint area [68–71], as shown in Figure 11.1. Chang et al. [70] joined AZ31 Mg alloy and 6061 aluminum alloy with Sn–xZn ($x = 5$, 10, 20 and 30 wt%) fillers containing trace RE elements at 250 °C in air without the use of flux or a wetting layer. It was reported that (i) the bond shear strengths of AZ31 magnesium alloy joined to 6061 aluminum alloy with Sn–5Zn–0.1RE, Sn–10Zn–0.1RE, Sn–20Zn–0.1RE and Sn–30Zn–0.1RE fillers were determined to be 14.84, 17.08, 19.39 and 20.86 MPa, respectively; (ii) the shear strengths increased with increasing Zn content; and (iii) the joint strengths of all four alloys significantly decreased with increasing aging time at 150 °C. Based on these findings, it was concluded

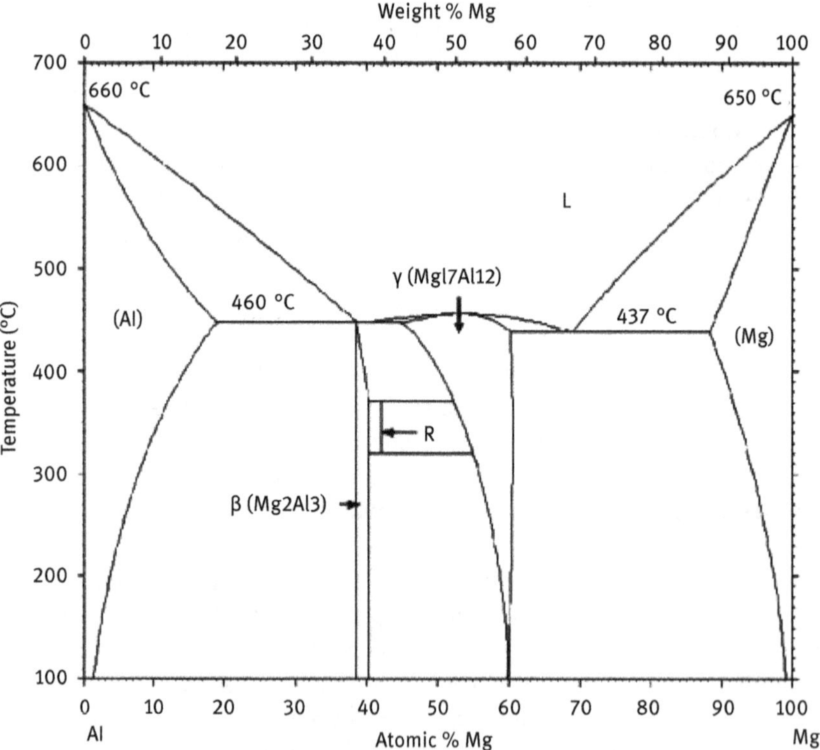

Figure 11.1: Mg–Al phase diagram.

that higher Zn compositions in the solder facilitated the dissolution of aluminum and increased the number of Al-rich clusters in the solder. During the soldering process, Mg dissolved irregularly in the solder and formed Mg_2Sn IMCs, and after aging at 150 °C, irregular blocky Mg_2Sn IMCs formed and led to decreases in joint strength. Similarly, Xu et al. [71] soldered dissimilar Al/Mg alloys by changing the Zn content in Sn-based solders with the assistance of ultrasonic. It was found that (i) the Al/Mg IMCs of Al_3Mg_2 and $Al_{12}Mg_{17}$ were avoided, but a new IMC of Mg_2Sn was formed in the joints; (ii) Mg_2Sn was blocky inside the joints and continuous near the Mg side; (iii) the shear strength of the joints increased with the addition of Zn into the solders; (iv) the maximum shear strength of 49 MPa was obtained when the Sn–16Zn solder was used; (v) the Al content exceeded its ultimate solution in the solder and increased with increasing Zn; and (vi) the floating of Al grains was observed in the joints soldered by Sn, Sn–3Zn and Sn–9Zn because of sound radiation pressure, which was blocked by Zn grains in the joint soldered by Sn–16Zn.

Generally, magnesium is considered "unsolderable" by conventional means [2]. Recently, Ma et al. [72] soldered AZ31 Mg alloy by means of high-frequency induction soldering using a Zn–Al (80.8Zn–19.2Al by wt%) filler metal in argon gas shield condition at a wide temperature range and process time of 120 s. It was mentioned that (i) in the soldering region, the α-Mg solid solution and α-Mg + Mg–Zn eutectoid were formed, (ii) the zinc solid solution and the aluminum solid solution in the original filler metal disappeared completely after the soldering process, (iii) the shear strength of the soldered joint is 19 MPa and (iv) the fracture morphology of the soldered joint exhibits intergranular fracture mode and the crack originates from α-Mg + MgZn eutectoid structure. Li et al. [73] bonded magnesium and aluminum successfully by using Mg–Al eutectic alloy as the solder under different pressures at 450 °C in atmosphere. It was reported that (i) the bond strength of these Mg/Al joints is improved with increasing of holding pressure, while the holding time has not much effect on it; and (ii) to demonstrate the potential application of the Mg–Al eutectic alloy solder, magnesium plate was coated with aluminum foil by this process and its corrosion resistance was evaluated by electrochemical test, showing that the corrosion resistance of the magnesium plate with aluminum coating was remarkably improved, which exhibits a similar corrosion behavior to that of aluminum.

11.4.3 Brazing

When Mg and Al alloys are used in the same products, it is necessary to bond Mg and Al to form a complex structure. However, the different physicochemical properties of these materials make them difficult to join by welding. Brittle Mg–Al IMCs and cracking occur in the joint when Mg/Al is fusion welded, with the result that the strength of the joint is very low [2, 74]. A Zn filler metal was selected as the interlayer for the brazing because Zn does not form IMCs with Al [74, 75]. Furthermore, Zn and Mg have the same crystal lattice, which may somewhat enhance the property of the joints. Liu et al. [74] reported that (i), according to the feature of Mg–Zn eutectic reaction, Al alloy was bonded to Mg alloy by contact-reaction brazing (CRB) using a zinc-based brazing alloy successfully; (ii) Mg–Al IMCs were avoided for the addition of the zinc-based brazing alloy (thickness of up to 30 μm). The Mg substrate and the remanent brazing alloy were bonded with the reaction zone that formed along the zinc-rich- and magnesium-poor interface; (iii) only a few Mg–Zn IMCs ($MgZn_2$) existed homogeneously in the reaction zone; (iv) the substrate and the remanent brazing alloy were bonded with a thin Al–Zn solution; (v) the average tensile-shear strength of the final joints was a little lower than that of the zinc-based brazing alloy owning to some pores at the interface between the reaction zone and the remanent brazing alloy layer; and (vi) the best shear strength was achieved by joints made with a 3 μm thick Zn layer at 360 °C, 5 MPa pressure and bonding times from 10 to 30 min. CRB is a method of brazing, in which the joint is formed by means of a low-melting liquid phase formed by the eutectic reaction of the dissimilar metals. This method is contamination free because the joint can be achieved without the use of flux. Liu et al. [75] studied the microstructure and properties of Mg alloy and Al alloy brazed joints prepared with different thickness of Zn filler metal, ranging from 0 to 30 μm. Mg alloy and Al alloy can be bonded successfully by CRB with and without Zn filler metal in a traditional air furnace. It was reported that (i) the addition of the Zn filler metal can significantly improve the tensile strength, (ii) the reaction layer became thin with the use of thinner Zn filler-metal layers, while the thinner reaction layer brought about higher shear strength and (iii) the best results were associated with a bonding temperature of 360 °C and the use of a 3 μm Zn filler metal to produce bonded joints in times ranging from 10 to 30 min.

Other types of filler materials should include nickel interlay [76], Mg–Al filler [77] and Mg–In–Zn alloy [78]. The differences in physical and metallurgical properties of stainless steels and magnesium alloys make them difficult to join using conventional fusion welding. Therefore, Elthalabawy et al. [76] performed the diffusion brazing of 316 L (Fe-10Cr-10Ni-2Mo with low level of carbon) stainless steel to magnesium alloy (AZ31) using a double stage-bonding process using nickel interlayer. To join these dissimilar alloys, the solid-state DB of 316 L steel to a Ni interlayer was carried out at 900 °C followed by diffusion brazing to AZ31 at 510 °C. It was mentioned that metallographic and compositional analyses show that a metallurgical bond was achieved with a shear strength of 54 MPa; however, during the diffusion brazing stage B_2 IMCs form within the joint and these intermetallics are pushed ahead of the solid/liquid interface during isothermal solidification of the joint; these intermetallics had a detrimental effect on joint strengths when the joint was held at the diffusion brazing temperature for longer than 20 min. Wang et al. [77] developed a Mg–Al filler metal to braze magnesium alloy AZ31B through furnace brazing under the protection of a flux. There are two microstructures in the filler metal: solid solution α-Mg and eutectic structure α-Mg + γ-$Mg_{17}Al_{12}$. It was found that (i) partial BM was dissolved into the brazing seam during the brazing process, where α-Mg solid solution and γ-$Mg_{17}(Al, Zn)_{12}$ compound were formed; (ii) the average shear strength of the brazed joints is 75MPa; (iii) the fracture morphology of the brazed joint exhibits a intergranular brittle feature; and (iv) discontinuous γ-$Mg_{17}(Al, Zn)_{12}$ phase distributed around the α-Mg grains is a main crack source. Watanabe et al. [78] developed filler metal as well as flux for brazing AZ31. It was reported that (i) a flux was successfully developed consisting of $CaCl_2$, LiCl and NaCl with Ca and Li ions, which made the magnesium alloy surface active at around 450 °C; (ii) additionally, brazing filler metals with a melting temperature below 480 °C were successfully developed; magnesium and indium were the main components, along with 0.2–6.4 wt% zinc to lower the melting temperature; (iii) with a small amount of zinc, the flux and filler metals achieved a joint with a high strength equivalent to the BM; and (iv) as the amount of zinc increased, the joint strength decreased.

11.5 Friction stir welding

11.5.1 In general

Friction stir welding (FSW) is a solid-state joining process and is carried out using a nonconsumable rotating pin which travels along the joint to be welded. The combination of tool rotation and localized softening of the material causes movement of the material leading to a weld. The literature shows that weld quality is dependent on the optimization of the welding parameters (tool shape, jig rotational speed, tool speed and joint configuration) [79]. FSW has many advantages when welding magnesium or lightweight alloys. The FSW of magnesium alloy has many potential applications in major industries, that is, land transportation, aerospace, railway, shipbuilding and marine, construction and many other industrial applications. Even magnesium alloys have been used in industrial equipment of nuclear energy as magnesium alloys have low tendency to absorb neutrons, sufficient resistance to carbon dioxide and excellent thermal conductivity [80]. Wang et al. [81] mentioned that the optimal welding condition for realization of the maximum tensile load was predicted: a rotation rate of 20,000 rpm, welding speed of 3 mm/s, plunge depth of 0.85 mm and use of a stepped pin. It was also reported that (i) significant grain refinements and material hardening in the weld zone were observed in multilayer defect-free joints, with a decrease in the bonding length between adjacent layers from the top layer to the bottom layer, and (ii) a more distinct thermomechanically affected zone (TMAZ) was found on the retreating side than on the advancing side. Radj et al. [82] analyzed the effect of tool rotational speed, welding speed and plunging depth with each three levels of magnesium alloy and reported that (i) the UTS, yield strength and percentage EL were evaluated and obtained joint efficiency of 81%, 78% and 85% than that of BM, respectively, and (ii) the microhardness profile obtained on various cross-sectional regions of the welded zone indicates uniform distribution of grains at the nugget zone (NZ). In comparison to the traditional welding zones, the weld produced by FSW was characterized by four distinct zones; stirring zone, TMAZ, HAZ and (BM [81, 82]. Boccarusso et al. [83] mentioned that, on FSWed AA6082 T6 and MgAZ31, all joints are characterized by the presence of three main metallurgical zones: NZ, dynamic recrystallized zone and interpenetrating feature zone. Furthermore, IMCs like $Al_{12}Mg_{17}$ and Al_3Mg_2 have been detected inside the NZ.

11.5.2 Mg/Al dissimilar joints

It is generally believed that the continuous IMCs at the joined zone of dissimilar joints of Mg/Al metals or alloys under FSW easily become crack initiation and propagation path, deteriorating mechanical properties. Hence, it is important to know the formation and properties of IMCs during the dissimilar FSW process. Ji et al. [84] reported that (i) the dissimilar joint of Mg/Al couple was formed with higher tensile shear strength when the Mg alloy was selected as the upper plate, (ii) the Zn-added friction stir lap welding assisted by ultrasound further enlarged the effective lap width and improved the mechanical interlocking and attained the finer disperse Mg–Zn IMCs in the stir zone and (iii) the maximum tensile shear strength of the joint assisted by ultrasound and a Zn interlayer reached 268 N/mm. The effect of joining time on the microstructure and mechanical properties of the dissimilar Mg/Al-welded joints was studied [85], and it was reported that (i) an IMCs layer formed in the joint center after welding and its thickness of approximately 1,100 μm formed at the pin-affected zone and only a 10 μm diffusion layer formed at the sleeve-affected zone, (ii) little liquid eutectic phase formed at 1 s, resulting into a 10 μm IMCs at the pin-affected zone, (iii) thicker IMCs formed with increasing the welding time, (iv) lap shear failure load of the joint first increased and then decreased with increasing the welding time, (v) the maximum failure load of 3.6 kN was obtained at 2 s and (vi) joint fractured through the IMC layer and presented brittle fracture mode. Formation of IMCs during the FSW of dissimilar joint of Mg/Al alloys easily results in the pin adhesion and then deteriorates joint formation. Meng et al. [86] reported that (i) the severe pin adhesion transformed the tapered-and-screwed pin into a tapered pin at a low welding speed of 30 mm/min, (ii) the pin adhesion problem was solved with the help of ultrasonic, (iii) the weldability of Mg/Al alloys was significantly improved due to the good material flow induced by mechanical vibration and the fragments of the IMCs on the surface of a rotating pin caused by acoustic streaming, respectively, (iv) a sound joint with ultrasonic contained long Mg/Al interface joining length and complex mixture of Mg/Al alloys in the stir zone, thereby achieving perfect metallurgical bonding and mechanical interlocking and (v) the ultrasonic could broaden process window and then improve tensile properties, which can reach 115 MPa with ultrasonic assistance.

There are two approaches to reduce the IMCs: one approach is to conduct submerged FSW underwater or under liquid nitrogen, and the other approach is DB, which is a solid-state welding process which is applicable to the similar and dissimilar materials [87, 88].

11.5.3 AZ31 alloy

Combining Mg and Al in one hybrid structure would make possible the use of these alloys for even more applications which will result in desirable weight saving. Given the increasing use of aluminum and magnesium alloys in aviation, aerospace, automotive, electrical and chemical industries, bonding these two alloys together is inevitable. In this regard, fusion welding and solid-state methods are used to join the two alloys. Given the many problems of fusion welding of these alloys, such as thermal cracks, oxidative impurities and formation of brittle IMCs, attention is drawn to bonding the two alloys through solid-state methods [87–90].

There are numerous researches on microstructures and related mechanical properties of dissimilar FSWed AZ31 to other alloys. Chang et al. [91] investigated the improvement in intermetallic layer by using a third material foil between the faying edges of the friction stir-welded and hybrid-welded Al6061-T6/AZ31 alloy plates and compared the difference in microstructural and mechanical characteristics of friction stir-welded and hybrid-welded Al6061-T6/AZ31 joints. It was reported that (i) the hybrid butt welding of aluminum alloy plate to a magnesium alloy plate was successfully achieved with Ni foil as filler material, while defect-free laser-FSW hybrid welding was achieved by using a laser power of 2 kW, and (ii) transverse tensile strength of the joint reached about 66% of the Mg BM tensile strength in the case of hybrid welding with Ni foil and showed higher value than that of the friction stir welded join with and without the third material foil; maybe owing to the presence of less brittle Ni-based intermetallic phases instead of $Al_{12}Mg_{17}$. Liu et al. [92] studied microstructure and mechanical properties of FSWed joints of dissimilar Mg alloys AZ31 with several different welding parameters including the effects of rotation speed and welding speed on the joint quality. It was mentioned that (i) sound joints with good mechanical properties could be easily obtained when AZ31 was at retreating side, but it was difficult to obtain the sound joint with the contrary material arrangement, suggesting that (ii) the material with inferior plastic deformability should be set at the advancing side and the material with superior one should be set at the retreating side in order to get sound FSW joint of dissimilar Mg alloys. Choi et al. [93] evaluated the microstructural and mechanical properties of FSWed AZ31 with CaO Mg alloys under a tool rotation speed of 1,600 rpm and a traveling speed of 80 mm/min. It was reported that (i) an IMC, Al_2Ca, was resulted in the BM;

(ii) in the stir zone, fine grains and IMC particles formed due to dynamic recrystallization and mechanical stirring; and (iii) hardness profiling showed that the stir zone was harder than the BM, likely due to the presence of fine grains and thermally stable IMCs. Friction stir-welded Mg alloys normally exhibit a lower yield strength compared with the base materials, which is a drawback for their application as structure materials. Hence, Xin et al. [94, 95] applied the subsequent tension along the transverse direction and then annealing on FSW AZ31 alloys to modify the microstructure and texture in weld zone and to improve the joint strength. It was obtained that by subsequent tension ~4.5% strain along transverse direction and then annealing, the yield strength could be greatly enhanced for the FSWed AZ31 alloys; specifically, the YS was improved from ~86 to ~177 MPa by subsequent 4.5% tension and then reduced to ~156 MPa after annealing. For the initial joint sample, fracture occurred in the stir-zone side during the transverse tensile test. However, after subsequent tension, all the samples fractured in the base materials whether subjected to annealing or not. Sihuddin et al. [96] performed friction spot welding (or refill friction stir spot welding) to consolidate dissimilar AA5754 Al and AZ31 Mg alloys. It was reported that (i) the IMCs $Al_{12}Mg_{17}$ and Al_3Mg_2 were primarily found in the weld, distributed at the interface between the base materials and in the Al top sheet and (ii) the material flow induced by tool movement plays an important role in both the distribution of the IMCs and the interfacial area between the base materials. Singh et al. [97] studied the effect of FSW parameters on mechanical and metallurgical properties of AZ31B-O Mg alloy joints. The selected material was welded using combination of different parameters, that is, tool rotational speed, welding speed and tool shoulder diameter. The effect of weld pitch, that is, ratio of welding speed to tool rotational speed (0.0020 to 0.05 mm/rev) was examined on the mechanical and microstructural properties of friction stir-welded joints of AZ31B-O Mg alloy. It was reported that (i) the linear relationship between tensile strength and weld pitch was observed, (ii) the maximum value of tensile strength, that is, 187.8 N/mm^2 was obtained at weld pitch of 0.05 mm/rev using 20 mm tool shoulder diameter and (iii) most of the tensile test specimens fractured in the area between stir zone and TMAZ (similar to HAZ in fusion welding) toward the advancing side. The fine and equiaxed grains were observed due to dynamic recrystallization at higher value of weld pitch. One of the major drawbacks associated with Mg alloys is poor weldability, caused by porosity formation during conventional fusion-welding processes. Templeman et al. [98] investigated the microstructure and corrosion properties of FSWed Mg alloys, studying representatives of two commercial families: wrought AZ31-H24 and die-cast AM50. It was found that (i) in both alloys, recrystallization occurred during the FSW; (ii) in AM50, the mechanism of the recrystallization was continuous, manifested by dislocation rearrangement into subgrain boundaries; (iii) in AZ31, discontinuous recrystallization had occurred through grain boundaries migration – twins rotated with respect to the matrix, turning into low-angle grain boundaries; and (iv) in the AZ31 alloy, no change in Al concentration had occurred, and the surface potential measured in the nugget was only slightly higher than in the BM. Kim et al. [99] studied the evolution of the microtexture in the stir-zone portion of AZ31 Mg alloys during FSW via microtexture analysis and polycrystal modeling. It was reported that the electron backscatter diffraction analysis revealed that the FSW process induced the development of strong fiber textures in the stir-zone portion, and that the texture development was strongly dependent on the moving path of the material point with respect to the rotating pin. Shang et al. [100] performed the FSW for a single plate of extruded AZ31 alloy at different tilt angles relative to the extrusion direction, with the aim to investigate the evolution of local texture in the weld as well as its effect on the mechanical behavior of the joint. It was shown that (i) the formation of specific-textured NZ and prevalent twinning activated at low strain brought about the reduction of yield anisotropy in the tensile test, (ii) relatively higher EL of the joints was achieved with the welding direction aligned at 45° to the extrusion direction, (iii) the fracture locations were observed to occur in different regions and shift with the variation of the welding direction, which was mainly attributed to the strain localization induced by incompatible deformation of different subregions, (iv) electron backscatter diffraction analysis indicated that the microstructure and texture evolution in both the NZ and the TMAZ played a vital role in the inconsistent deformation behavior and (v) for the wrought Mg alloys, the strong texture may greatly affect their fracture behavior and mechanical property. Xu et al. [101] conducted the FSW a 2.4 mm thick AZ31 Mg alloy sheet and 1.5 mm Q234 steel sheet with a hot-dipped Al-containing Zn coating using a pinless tool. It was reported that (i) the Al-containing Zn coating played a crucial role in joining the Mg alloy and steel during FSW, (ii) the Zn coating observably improved the Mg-steel interfacial wettability during FSW, and the Al_5Fe_2 phase in the Zn coating on the steel substrate surface promoted the metallurgical bonding of Mg alloy and steel, (iii) the Al_5Fe_2 phase on the steel surface resulted from the reaction between the steel substrate and the Al in the Zn coating during hot dipping, and was not related to the Al-containing Mg alloy substrate, (iv) the tensile-shear load of the FSSW Mg–steel joint reached 4.3 kN, (v) the fracture of the joint occurred along the interface on the steel substrate side and (vi) the interface between the Al_5Fe_2 layer and Mg alloy substrate was the weakest region of the Mg–steel joint.

Zhang et al. [102] investigated friction stir keyholeless spot welding (FSKSW) using a retractable pin for 1.0 mm thick galvanized mild steel and 3 mm thick AZ31B magnesium alloy in a lap configuration. The process variables were optimized in terms of the joint strength. The effects of the stacking sequence on joint formation and the joining mechanism of FSKSW AZ31B-to-mild steel joints were also analyzed. It was reported that (i) the process window and joint strength are strongly influenced by the stacking sequence of the workpieces; (ii) while the process window is narrow and unstable for FSKSW of a magnesium-to-steel stack-up, a desirable process was established for the steel-to-magnesium stacking sequence, a desirable process and higher strength joint and higher joint strength can be obtained if steel and magnesium are stacked layer by layer; and (iii) XRD phase and EPMA analyses of the FSKSW joint showed that the IMCs are formed at the steel-to-magnesium interface, and the element diffusion between the mild steel and AZ31B magnesium alloy revealed that the joining methods for FSKSW joints is the main mechanical joining along with certain metallurgical bonding. Lv et al. [103] applied the angularly exerted ultrasonic vibrations to FSW for the joining of AA 6061-T4 alloy to AZ31B at different tool rotation speeds and investigated the variations in the welding process and weld properties due to the applied acoustic field. It was reported that the process temperature was increased, the material flow path was widened and mechanical interlocking features at weld interfaces were improved in the presence of ultrasonic power. Morphology and distribution of IMCs were influenced by the added vibrations at all rotation speeds. Formation of intermetallic layers at the weld interfaces was driven by heat input; composition of the IMC was roughly unaffected but the layer thickness was reduced by the additional acoustic field; and the ultrasonic enhanced improvement in weld mechanical properties was significant at very low rotation speeds but less substantial at higher rotation speeds. Dissimilar FSW and diffusion bond welds of Al alloy 5083 and Mg alloy AZ31 were produced at similar peak and bonding temperature of 435 °C [87]. It was mentioned that (i) the weld had an irregular-shaped region in the weld center of DB weld and layered interface in friction stir weld, having a different microstructure and hardness from the two base materials; (ii) the irregular-shaped region in diffusion-bonding weld and interface of Mg and Al, in friction stir weld contained a large volume of IMC $Al_{12}Mg_{17}$ and showed significantly higher hardness in the weld center; and (iii) the present study suggests that constitutional liquation resulted in the IMC $Al_{12}Mg_{17}$ in the weld center.

Xu et al. [104] studied FSW of a 2.4 mm thick Mg–Al–Zn alloy sheets without and with the addition of 0.1 mm thick Zn interlayer and influence of interlayer addition on the microstructural features and mechanical properties of FSWed joints was investigated by optical microscope, scanning electron microscope (SEM), TEM, XRD and tensile testing. It was found that the addition of Zn interlayer resulted in complex alloying reactions between Mg substrate and Zn interlayer, forming a bonded zone composed of α-Mg, (α-Mg + MgZn) eutectoid structure and a mixture of Mg_4Zn_7 and unreacted Zn, thereby increasing the area of bonded zone and reducing the hook defects, resulting in a significant increase in tensile–shear load from 2.4 kN to about 4 kN. Using similar sample with the addition of a thin Zn interlayer, AZ31 sheet was FSWed using a pinless tool with flat, convex and concave shoulder shapes [105]. It was shown that (i) an alloying reaction took place between the Mg substrate and Zn interlayer during FSW, forming a discontinuous intermetallics layer composed of dispersive (α-Mg + MgZn) eutectic structure underneath the shoulder and a Mg–Zn intermetallics bonding zone at the outside of the joints; (ii) this alloying reaction increased the bonded area and eliminated the hook defects, thereby producing sound FSW joints with a shallow keyhole without hook defects; (iii) the increase of plunge depth was beneficial to the Mg–Zn diffusion, thereby increasing the tensile-shear load of the joints; however, excessive plunge depths resulted in a decrease of the effective sheet thickness, reducing the strength of the joints; (iv) at a small plunge depth, the convex and concave shoulders were more beneficial to the interface reaction than the flat shoulder; (v) the maximum joint load of 6.6 kN was achieved by using the concave shoulder at a plunge depth of 1.0 mm; and (vi) a postwelding heat treatment promoted the dissolution of the discontinuous reaction layer in the joints; however, it led to the occurrence of void defects, influencing the bonding strength. The evolution of temperature and thermal stresses were examined during friction stir processing of a magnesium alloy using in situ neutron diffraction [106]. It was mentioned that, at the maximum temperature of 464 °C, the compressive stress distributions (up to 52 MPa) with the tool via the thermomechanical deformation was found with the Zener-Holloman parameter of 4.51×10^{10}/s. Macroscopic nonuniform deformation is usually found in deformed joints of FSWed wrought Mg alloys, detrimental to the joint performance. Hence, Shang et al. [107] fabricated two kinds of FSW joints with different stirred zone structures for extruded AZ31 plates. It was reported that (i) the occurrence of nonuniform deformation was associated with the special texture distribution and twinning behavior in the stir zone, (ii) the shape of concave subregions in the stir zone coincided with the distribution area of extension twins, (iii) texture evolution showed that consistent lattice rotation occurred across the stir zone during tensile process, (iv) the nonuniform deformation behavior could be suppressed by modifying the texture distribution through increasing the tool rotation rate, which could improve both the tensile strength and ductility of the joints and (v) digital image correlation measurements provided detailed examination of the actual strain distribution evolved in the joints and demonstrated the dominant contribution of strain localization to the tensile properties. Welding of Mg by conventional methods is complex due to its high reactive nature which leads to oxidization or catching fire during welding. The poor corrosion resistance of Mg is also an issue that needs to be considered while designing the structures particularly intended to be used in highly corroding environments. Based on this background, Reddy et al. [108] employed FSW technique to join AZ31 Mg alloy sheets and investigated the corrosion behavior of the weld joints. The specimens were cut across the weld joint and exposed to corroding environment (3.5% NaCl solution) for 24 h, followed by the tensile testing and found that the base material has shown relatively better resistance to fracture compared with the weld joint; indicating that the corrosion-related failure must be considered as a valid input while developing structures with Mg alloys.

Liang et al. [109] joined 5A33 aluminum alloy bar with AZ31B magnesium alloy bar by continuous drive friction welding. It was obtained that the tensile strength of the joints increased with increasing friction time, and on average, the highest strength could reach up to 101 MPa when friction time was 5 s. The tensile fracture appearances showed almost flat surface, indicating brittle fracture. A new reaction layer formed on the friction interface consisted of IMCs layer and Mg solid solution layer, and the IMCs were mainly $Mg_{17}Al_{12}$ and Al_3Mg_2. Due to high microhardness of reaction layer, the microhardness value on the interface was dramatically larger than that of the Mg base material. The thickness of hardened layer in the Mg side and softened layer in the Al side increased with increasing friction time. Since the continuous IMCs at the NZ of dissimilar friction stir-welded Mg/Al joint easily become crack initiation and propagation path, deteriorating mechanical properties, it is needed to reduce or eliminate the disadvantages induced by the continuous IMCs, and Liu et al. [110] employed ultrasonic-assisted FSW based on stationary shoulder system to join 6061-T6 aluminum alloy and AZ31B magnesium alloy. It was reported that (i) defect-free joint without the shoulder marks was obtained under the synergistic effect of the stationary shoulder and the ultrasonic, (ii) vibration and acoustic streaming induced by the ultrasonic broke the continuous IMC layer near the TMAZ of advancing side into pieces or particles, (iii) fracture path from the short Al/Mg interface near the TMAZ at the advancing side of the conventional joint was changed to the long Al/Mg interface at the retreating side of the FSWed joint, improving tensile properties, (iv) the maximum values of tensile strength and EL of the joint were 152.4 MPa and 1.9%, which were 17 MPa and 0.8% higher than those of the conventional joint, respectively. FSWed Mg alloys usually exhibit an undesirable combination of strength and EL due to its strong texture develops in the weld. Thus, Xu et al. [111] applied large load FSW associated with an extremely low welding speed and rotation rate to an AZ31B Mg alloy to modify the microstructure, the texture and the mechanical properties of the joint. The twin structure in the weld provided adequate barriers for dislocation motion for strengthening and created more local sites for nucleating and accommodating dislocations, thereby elevating ductility and strain hardening of the weld, claiming that the procedure provided a simple and effective method to enhance the strength of an FSW Mg joint without ductility loss. Kumar et al. [112] studied effects of ultrasonic vibrations on different sets of rotational as well as translation speeds on FSWed AZ31B and 6061 Al alloys. It was obtained that (i) the ultrasonic vibrations assisted producing additional turbulence in the stirred zone of the weldment which causes intense plastic deformation, (ii) a considerable reduction in the magnitude of the axial force, as well as tool torque is evident in case of ultrasonic-vibrations-assisted linear FSW and (iii) tensile results depict that the ultrasonic vibrations help to reduce the defects in the weld NZ and hence improves the strength than that of conventional FSW. Shang et al. [113] reported that the yield strength of the FSWed joint of AZ31was raised from 96 to 122 MPa and the tensile strength was enhanced to be roughly equal to that of the base material with no reduction of EL.

11.5.4 AZ61 alloy

Microstructural evolution of magnesium alloy AZ61 during FSW and details of the relationship between the microstructure and mechanical properties are discussed [114, 115].

It was mentioned that the development of weld microstructure is controlled by shear deformation and thermal effects. In the weld of wrought AZ61 alloy, the crystallographic texture develops with a strong concentration of {0001} basal planes, being heterogeneously distributed in stir zone. Deformation of magnesium with hexagonal close-packed structure is controlled by a slip along {0001} basal plane; therefore, formation of this type of texture during welding affects the mechanical properties of weld. During FSW of two AZ61 plates with a thickness of 6.3 mm, both the transition and stir regions developed similar grain size, much finer than in the base alloy. Zhou et al. [116] investigated AZX612 (Mg–6% Al–1% Zn–2% Ca) noncombustive magnesium alloy joints formed by asymmetric double-sided FSW with different lower tool rotation rates. It was reported that (i) when compared with the conventional one-sided FSW, joints fabricated by the asymmetric double-sided FSW showed better tensile strength and EL values; (ii) the stir zone formed at the upper and lower tool rotation rates of 600 and 500 rpm exhibits the lowest <0001> texture intensity, thereby showing the best balance of tensile strength and ductility; and (iii) with defect-free joining parameters, the complexity of the material flow caused by the asymmetric layout of the double tools needs both a small difference between the upper and lower tool rotation rates and a proper heat input. Using self-reacting FSW technique, Li et al. [117] fabricated the welded 5-mm-thick Mg–6Al–1Zn alloy at various welding speeds. It was reported that (i) sound joints were achieved with welding speed ranging from 300 to 400 mm/min; (ii) at lower welding speed, pore defect formed in the weld NZ due to the inadequate mixing of the plastic materials; (iii) the TMAZ consisted of fine equiaxed dynamic recrystallized grains instead of the elongated and rotated grains formed in the affected zone of FSWed Mg and Al alloys; (iv) finer grains were obtained in the welded NZ, TMAZ and HAZ at higher welding speed due to the lower heat input; (v) both weld NZ and TMAZ exhibit grains with a high density of dislocations due to the straining exerted by the tool; (vi) hardness profiles show slight variation throughout the weld with the hardness values fluctuated between 50 and 68 HV; (vii) the tensile strength increased with increasing welding speed with the maximal strength efficiency reached 77%; (viii) EL at fracture was lower than that of the BM due to the inhomogeneous microstructure throughout the joint; and (ix) the impact energy of both the weld NZ and HAZ increased with increasing welding speed.

11.5.5 AZ80 and AZ91 alloys

Sevvel et al. [118] studied impact of the tool geometry on the mechanical properties of AZ80A Mg alloy by employing different axial forces during FSW. It was found that (i) joints produced using taper cylindrical pin-profiled tool under a 3 kN axial force exhibited defect-free weldments with superior mechanical properties, (ii) ideal level of heat generation and formation of grain structures with uniformly distributed and finely refined grains in the zone of FSW are found to be the dominant reasons for the formation of flawless joints with superior mechanical properties.

There are several studies done for FSWed AZ91 Mg alloys. Noncombustive Mg-9Al-Zn-Ca magnesium alloy was friction stir-welded with rotation speeds ranging from 500 to 1,250 rpm at a constant welding speed of 200 mm/min [119]. It was mentioned that (i) defect-free joints were successfully produced at rotation speeds of 750 and 1,000 rpm, (ii) the as-received hot-extruded material consisted of equiaxed α-Mg grains with β-$Mg_{17}Al_{12}$ and Al_2Ca compounds distributed along the grain boundaries; (iii) FSW produced much refined α-Mg grains accompanied by the dissolution of the eutectic β-$Mg_{17}Al_{12}$ phase, while Al_2Ca phase was dispersed homogeneously into the Mg matrix; (iv) an increase in rotation speed increased the α-Mg grain size but not significantly, while microstructure in the HAZ was almost not changed compared with the base material; (v) the hardness tests showed uniform distributed and slightly increased harness in the stir zone; and (vi) transverse tensile tests indicated that the defect-free joints fractured at the base material, while longitudinal tensile tests showed that the strength of the defect-free welds was improved due to microstructural refinement and uniform distribution of IMCs. Luo et al. [120] investigated FSW of dissimilar welds between ZG61 alloy and AZ91D alloy. It was found that (i) severe deformation and metal flow occur in the stir zone under high strain rates and high temperatures, (ii) no distinct reaction layer or IMCs are observed at the interface of two alloys, (iii) when AZ91D was arranged in the advancing side and ZG61 in the retreating side, the joints quality was very poor with all parameters and (iv) the tensile properties of the weld of joints are significantly influenced by the materials positions, grain size and crystallographic orientation. Hosseini et al. [121] studied semisolid stir welding of AZ91 with focus on the joining temperature and rotational speed with an Mg–25%Zn interlayer located between two AZ91 pieces while heating up to the semisolid state of BM and interlayer. It was found that (i) the lowest cavity content (2.1%) with the maximum ultimate shear strength (about 188 MPa) was obtained in weld with the joining temperature of 530 °C and the rotational speed of 1,600 rpm, (ii) low-quality welds and a reduction of ultimate shear strength were observed at very high or low rotational speeds and joining temperatures and (iii) the process produced close mechanical properties to those of the BM and homogenous quality throughout the joint, when the intermediate temperature and rotational speeds were employed. The influence of tool rotational speed on mechanical properties of friction stir-welded AZ91E magnesium alloy was investigated [122] with different rotational speeds of 900, 1,000, 1,100 and 1,200 rpm and at a constant axial load and transverse speed of 3 kN and 90 mm/min, respectively. It was reported that the dynamic recrystallization happened in the friction stir-welded zone; as a result, the joints fabricated at 1,000 rpm rotational speed had an increase of 110% in UTS compared to the BM. In the present work, the effect of process parameters on joining of AZ91 Mg alloy and Al6063 aluminum alloy sheets during FSW was studied [123]. It was mentioned that (i) a successful joint was achieved at 1,100 rpm tool rotational speed and 25 mm/min tool travel speed and (ii) combination of tool rotational speed and tool travel speed has observed a profound effect on the material flow mechanisms at the NZ. Li et al. [124] fabricated defect-free friction stir-welded joints between the AZ91 Mg alloy and A383 Al alloy at a welding speed of 40 mm/min and a rotational speed of 900 rpm. It was obtained that (i) the IMCs Al_3Mg_2, $Al_{12}Mg_{17}$ and Mg_2Si distributed uniformly in stir zone at a rotational speed of 900 rpm, and there is a narrow IMCs layer (~10 μm) at the interface of the two BMs; (ii) the tensile strength of the dissimilar AZ91/A383 joint is 93 MPa, which is approximately 45% of the A383 alloy; and (iii) the sufficient material intermixing and uniform distribution of second phases are helpful to the joint properties. Sameer et al. [125] fabricated FSWed AZ91 magnesium alloy and AA6082-T6 aluminum alloy. It was reported that (i) when Mg was placed on advancing side, more aluminum content was soluble in NZ than the case where Mg was placed on the retreating side, (ii) thin intermetallic layer in the joint interface of Mg/Al and thick intermetallic layer with poor adhesion of the aluminum and magnesium have been observed in the dissimilar joints varying the sides, (iii) the highest UTS of 172.3 MPa was found for Mg–Al when Mg was placed on advancing side and lower that of 156.25 MPa was obtained when Mg was placed on retreating side and (iv) hardness of 86 and 89 HV were observed in the stir zone for the dissimilar AZ91 Mg alloy and AA6082-T6 Al alloy when AZ91 Mg alloy was placed on the advancing side and on the retreating side, respectively.

11.5.6 Other Mg-based alloys

Yu et al. [126] evaluated the properties of FSWed thixomolded AE42 Mg alloy. It was reported that, according to X-ray radiography, the optimum FSW condition range of AE42 alloy exists between AZ61 and AZ31 alloys and it seems that the optimum welding condition range increases with decreasing Al content in the Mg alloys. There are mainly two kinds of compounds in the thixomolded AE42 alloy, and FSW has little influence on the grainy $Al_{10}RE_2Mn_7$ compound, but it has great influence on $Al_{11}RE_3$ phase, which is changed from lamellar eutectic to small particles after welding. The hardness in stir zone is higher than that in BM, and tensile strength and EL are both improved after welding because the stirring refines and uniforms the microstructure and IMCs.

In joining of AM20 magnesium alloy using FSW process, Sahu et al. [127] used Al and Zn alloying element at the joint interface to act as an interlayer material. It was reported that defect-free joints with sound mechanical properties are obtained with suitable alloying element at optimized parameter settings. Joints with Al and Zn interlayer results in 77% and 90% of UTS of base material, respectively; on the other hand, it is observed that without interlayer, the UTS of the joint is only 65% of the BM. Fractographically, the tensile-tested specimens reveal ductile fracture in the joints with interlayer whereas without interlayer mixed fracture is observed in the joints. The maximum flexural strength with Zn interlayer is around 87% of the BM. The microhardness increased from bottom to top surface of the weld with maximum hardness at the nugget compared to other zones and weld specimens with Al and Zn interlayer give higher hardness compared to without interlayer cases. The addition of appropriate amount of Al in Mg substrate increases the contents of Al-base solid solution namely $Al_{12}Mg_{17}$ and AlMg IMCs that eliminates stress concentration and hinders crack propagation resulting in improved tensile strength, and the addition of Zn with Mg substrate formed MgZn eutectoid structure with Mg_7Zn_3 structure and unreacted Mg resulting in improved mechanical properties.

Templeman et al. [98] studied FSW behavior of die-cast AZ50 alloy. It was found that (i) the mechanism of the recrystallization was continuous, manifested by dislocation rearrangement into subgrain boundaries and (ii) the nugget exhibited significantly higher surface potential than the BM mainly due to the higher Al concentration in the matrix of the nugget, resulting from the dissolution of Al-enrichment and β-$Mg_{17}Al_{12}$ phase.

Kim et al. [128] reported on the FSWed twin-roll cast and subsequently heat-treated Mg–6Zn–1Mn–1Al alloy sheets with a thin thickness of 1 mm that (i) the welded sheet revealed several distinct weld zones, which are closely related to plastic flow and frictional heat generation during welding and (ii) although large microstructural differences were found among the welded zones, the presence of thermally stable Al_8Mn_5 particles preexisting in the sheet appeared uninfluenced by the welding process.

Newly developed hot-extruded Mg–5Al–3Sn magnesium alloy plates were butt-welded by FSW at various welding speeds [129]. It was reported that (i) the alloy was jointed without defects; (ii) after FSW, β-$Mg_{17}Al_{12}$ phase was dissolved into α-Mg matrix while Mg_2Sn phase with high dissolution point and good thermal stability remained in the NZ; (iii) with increasing welding speed, the maximum (0002) pole intensity in the NZ first decreased and then increased, and grain size of α-Mg matrix decreased arising from lower heat input while some intermetallic particles coarsened at higher welding speed due to solid-state diffusion and less applied stress; (iv) in all cases, the tensile properties of the alloy after FSW decreased due to the softened region at the HAZ, the dissolution of β-$Mg_{17}Al_{12}$ phase, the residual stress and dislocation content in the TMAZ, the textural variation and the secondary phase changes; and (v) the elastic behavior of weld joints was different from the BM due to the dissolution of β-$Mg_{17}Al_{12}$ particles. FSW is one of those welding techniques with many parameters which have different effects on the quality of the welds. In FSW, the tool rotational speed and transverse speed influence the strength (i.e., hardness distribution) of the stirred zone. Richmire et al. [130] investigated these two factors to determine the effect they will have on the hardness in the stirred zone of the friction stir welds and how the two factors are related to one another for as-cast magnesium alloy AM60 with nominal chemical composition of Mg-(5.5–6.5) Al-(0.24–0.6)Mn-0.22Zn-0.1Si under three different tool rotational speeds and three different transverse speeds and it was mentioned that both tool rotational speed and transverse speed possess significant effects on the stir zone hardness.

Askariani et al. [131] investigated FSW of an Mg–12Li–1Al alloy containing β phase (bcc) in terms of the effects of rotating speed and welding speed on the mechanical and physical properties of the welds were studied. It was reported that (i) microstructural examinations demonstrated an increase in grain size from 19 to 73 μm when maximum temperature of the welding process changed from 333 to 426 °C, respectively, (ii) the top and root surface layers of the weld underwent transformation of Mg–Li β to Mg–Li α, whose fraction was found to decrease with increase in the heat input and (iii) the thickness of the phase-transformed layer also proved to be less than 0.2 mm.

There are still interesting works on FSW of Mg materials with different materials. This is a major problem with FSW when different alloys such as Ti and Mg alloys are used. Sundar et al. [132] investigated the effects of spindle speed, feed rate and various shapes, and it was found that (i) ignition is prone to occur at certain spindle speeds and (ii) when the feed rate and spindle speed was 90 mm/min ≤ feed rate ≤ 210 mm/min, 1,000 rpm ≤ spindle speed ≤ 2,000 rpm, respectively. Choi et al. [133] optimized dissimilar FSW of immiscible pure Ti/pure Mg using an Al filler material with a thickness of 0.05 mm through tuning welding speeds ranging from 50 to 200 mm/min at a constant tool rotation speed and a constant probe offset. It was reported that (i) with a lower welding speed, the average grain diameter in the Mg stir zone of the Ti/Mg joints became smaller even though the higher welding temperature and lower strain rate were achieved. This is because the Al concentration dissolved in the Mg matrix increased at the lower welding speed, leading to a reduction in the stacking fault energy, thereby facilitating the occurrence of dynamic recrystallization rather than dynamic recovery during the FSW. Also, (ii) the relatively high hardness value in the Mg stir zone of the Ti/Mg dissimilar joint fabricated at the lower welding speed was attributed not only by the grain refinement strengthening but also by the solid solution strengthening due to the Al dissolving in the Mg matrix, while the increase in hardness was suppressed near the weld interface in the joint fabricated at the higher welding speed due to the decreased welding temperature and stirring effect in the Mg stir zone.

11.6 Solid-state bonding

In this section, joining techniques which are mainly operated at solid state of faying materials (pure metal as well as alloys), the transient liquid phase diffusion bonding (TLPDB) involving melting interlayer(s), electromagnetic pulse welding (which is operated at solid-state condition) and cold metal transfer (CMT) welding are discussed.

11.6.1 Solid-state diffusion bonding

DB is a solid-state joining process that can join a variety of materials in the solid state below the melting point (normally less than 70 °C of melting point, T_M) under moderate pressure in inert gas atmosphere, so that the atomic migration is not accompanied by macroscopic deformation. The principle mechanism involves the interdiffusion of atoms between the mating surfaces at their interface [3, 4]. Since the process temperature does not exceed melting point, it allows to eliminate many problems associated with fusion welding such as existence of HAZ. To obtain high bonding, the surface should be clean and flat. There are three major consequent stages of the bonding progress: (1) A contact between materials occurs through the mating surfaces; during this stage, removal of surface roughness and irregularity play a significant role in ensuring good contact between the mating surfaces. (2) Diffusion within grain boundaries predominates; during this stage, microscopic plastic deformation takes place at the interface, thus eliminating pores and ensuring arrangements and migration of grain boundaries. It is followed by (3) the volume diffusion to complete the DB process. During the bonding process, mating surfaces do not undergo any metallurgical discontinuity. As a result, the mechanical and microstructural property of the joint formed normally resembles those of the base materials.

This process is frequently completed by one of the two methods: (1) the solid-state DB and (2) the TLP DB. As mentioned previously, in the solid-state DB, the BMs to be joined are heated to approximately $0.7T_M$ of the metals under the influence of static load, hence melting at the interface of the mating surfaces is prevented, however, interdiffusion of the diffusing species leads to the formation of solid-state bond. In the second TLP process, an interlayer is placed between the metals to be joined. Interdiffusion between the interlayer and the BMs facilitates the formation of a eutectic reaction which transitions from liquid to solid by isothermal solidification as the composition of the eutectic liquid changes due to diffusion [132, 134]. In either case for similar metal DB or dissimilar metal DB, the method for applying a certain level of pressure to the mating surfaces are varied. The externally applied pressure can be rolling force, extrusion force, pressing force, or plastic deformation force. Details will be discussed later in this chapter.

DB was found applicable for pure magnesium and its alloys. Somekawa et al. [135] using rolled sheet pure Mg material with an initial grain size of 85 µm, conducted the DB tests in air at the pressure range from 2 to 20 MPa and at the temperature range from 300 to 400 °C and for the times up to 72 h. It was reported that (i) the maximum of lap shear strength was 0.89 at a bonding pressure of 20 MPa and a bonding temperature of 400 °C, with a bonding time of 1 h, and (ii) in high ratio of lap shear strengths, the bond line was not identified by optical microscopy, and surface fracture after compression lap shear test was also fully ductile failure, indicating that there is a possibility to fabricate magnesium products using DB technique. During manufacturing of complex structures, DB is often combined with superplastic forming (SPF), which was first discovered and reported by Oshida et al. [136, 137]. During investigating the transformation superplasticity of cast iron under the compressive force, the faying surfaces of cast iron sample, which was intentionally broken and re-bonded since the brittle fractured surface (in terms of surface toughness and detailed disparity) of mating surfaces are ideally matches to each other, were successfully diffusion bonded. Since then, the term SPF/DB (cooccurrence of SPF and DB) was frequently used by various researchers and engineers [138, 139]. Studies on SPF/DB of Mg-based alloys were conducted by Somekawa et al. [140, 141]. The superplastic characteristic and DB behavior were investigated in a commercial AZ31 magnesium alloy sheet having equiaxed grain size with an average size of 16.8 μm at a temperature range from 350 to 450 °C [140]. It was reported the maximum of lap shear strength was 0.85 at a bonding pressure of 3 MPa and a bonding temperature of 350 °C, with a bonding time of 3 h [140]. Using the same alloy with finer grain size of 8.5 μm that was processed by hot rolling, it was reported that the material behaved in a superplastic manner at temperatures of 250 and 300 °C, and successfully diffusion bonded at these temperatures [141].

Basically, sintering process is achieved by the DB among individual powder particles in the compacted pellets (or green) at the solid-state conditions. It was also reported that the superplastic pressing can effectively assisted to produce products with higher density during the powder metallurgy technique [142]. In many circumstances, dissimilar metals have to be bonded together and the resulting joint interfaces must typically sustain mechanical and/or electrical forces without failure, which is not possible by fusion-welding processes. Although DB has been studied extensively as a method for both similar and dissimilar joining of magnesium alloys, the dissimilar joining of magnesium alloys to other metals is significantly inhibited by the differences in the properties of the materials such as melting temperature, the coefficient of thermal expansion and thermal conductivity. As mentioned here, the common combination of dissimilar couples for DB is Mg-based alloy to Al-based alloy. For bonding of unalloyed Mg and unalloyed Al, Peng et al. [143] studied characteristics of phase constitution near the interface of Mg/Al diffusion-bonded joint by means of SEM, XRD and TEM. It was mentioned that (i) the obvious diffusion zone forms near the Mg/Al interface as a result of the vacuum DB. The diffusion zone of Mg/Al diffusion-bonded joint consists of IMCs such as $Mg_{17}Al_{12}$ and Mg_2Al_3; (ii) the transition region on Mg side mainly consists of Mg crystals, and the new phase formed is Mg_3Al_2 IMCs; and (iii) this is favorable to the enhancing of the combination strength for Mg substrate/diffusion zone. The formation of these IMCs can be found in the Mg–Al equilibrium phase diagram (see Figure 11.1) [144].

Li et al. [145] investigated the microstructure and phase constitution near the DB interface of Mg/Al dissimilar materials using SEM, XRD and TEM. It was reported that (i) an obvious diffusion zone was formed near the Mg/Al interface during the vacuum DB, (ii) the diffusion-transition zone near the interface consists of various Mg_xAl_y phases and (iii) the transition region on the Mg side mainly consists of Mg crystals, and the new phase formed was the Mg_3Al_2 phase having a face-centered cubic lattice. For a bonding between Mg and Cu, the melting points of Mg and Cu have a significant difference (nearly 400 °C, as shown in Figure 11.2 [146]) and this may lead to a large difference in the microstructure and joint performance of Mg–Cu joints. However, DB can be used to join these alloys without much difficulty. Mahendan et al. [147] analyzed the effect of parameters on diffusion-layer thickness, hardness and strength of magnesium–copper dissimilar joints using three-factor, five-level, central composite rotatable design matrix to predict diffusion-layer thickness, hardness and strength using response surface methodology. It was reported that (i) bonding temperature has predominant effect on bond characteristics, and (ii) joints fabricated at a bonding temperature of 450 °C, bonding pressure of 12 MPa and bonding time of 30 min exhibited maximum shear strength and bonding strength of 66 and 81 MPa, respectively.

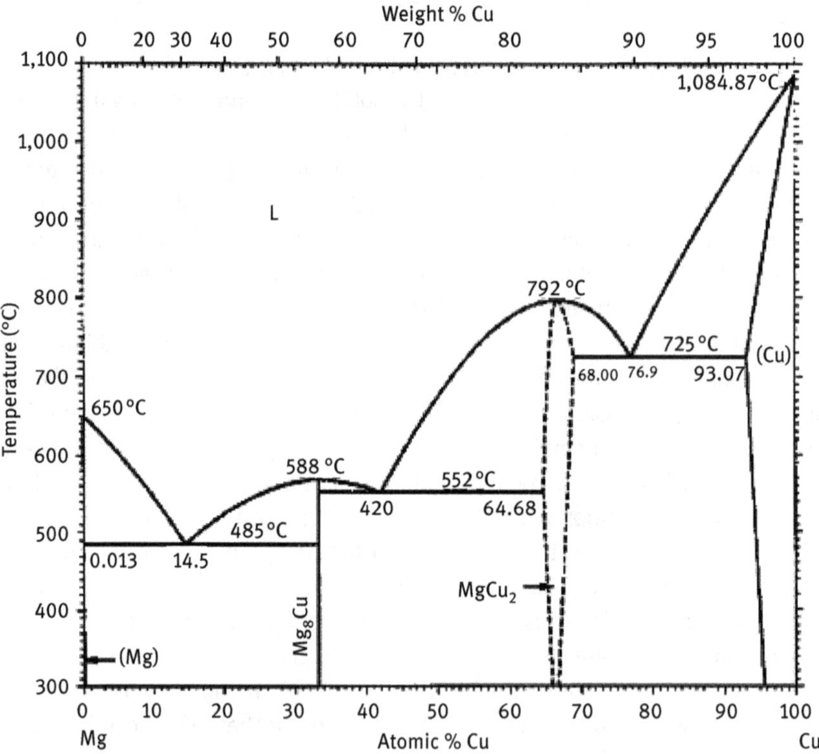

Figure 11.2: Mg–Cu phase diagram.

As we have seen for unalloyed diffusion-bonded Mg with unalloyed Al, basic research has been done on diffusion-welded joints with the overall aim of an adjusted interface design. Similarly, the phase formation of aluminum alloy/magnesium alloy bonds has been revealed by XRD, energy-dispersive spectroscopy and electron backscatter diffraction to show the presence of $Al_{12}Mg_{17}$ and Al_3Mg_2 phases in a bilayer. It was pointed out that (i) the precipitates originating from the alloys agglomerate in the bilayered welding zone, (ii) their arrangement in combination with the grain boundary evolution of the intermetallics and the change of the aluminum base solid solution in the interface region has a significant influence on the mechanical properties of the joint [148]. There are several studies on DB of AZ31 (Mg–3Al–1Zn) with different dissimilar alloys, including DB couples of AZ31 with Ti–6Al–4V [149], AZ31 with 6061 Al alloy (precipitation-hardened alloy with 96–98.5 wt% Al with small amount of Mg, SI, Fe, Cu, Cr and others) [150, 151] and AZ31 with 7075 Al alloy (5.6–6.1Zn, 2.1–2.5 Mg, 1.2–1.6Cu by wt%) [152]. The common findings are as follows: (i) diffusion zone is composed of Mg_2Al_3 layer, $Mg_{17}Al_{12}$ layer, eutectic layer of $Mg_{17}Al_{12}$ and Mg-based solid solution, and (ii) the joining temperature of about 450 °C offers the highest tensile strength of about 40 MPa, and the corresponding joint exhibits brittle fracture at the intermetallic eutectic compound layer of $Mg_{17}Al_{12}$. Very similar results can be found with AZ80 (Mg–8Al–0.5Zn by wt%) to 6061 Al alloy [153] and AZ80 to 7075 Al alloy [154].

11.6.2 Transient liquid phase diffusion bonding

Main advantage associated with TLP bonding is that resulting bonds have a higher melting point than the bonding temperature. During the TLP bonding process, on heating, the interlayer melts and the interlayer element (or a constituent of an alloy interlayer) diffuses into the substrate materials, causing isothermal solidification [155]. Therefore, the TLP bonding possesses mixed characterizations of the DB and brazing (which involves a liquid phase). As a result, it is commonly understood as a similar phenomenon as diffusion brazing and is also referred to as transient insert liquid metal bonding. Although it is not solely solid-state DB, we will discuss this technology here since it involves partially solid-state bonding.

Atieh et al. [156] performed TLP bonding of AZ31 to Ti–6Al–4V with pure thin Ni electrodeposited coat interlayer (12 µm) and investigated the effect of bonding temperature, time and pressure on microstructural developments and subsequent mechanical properties across joint interface at a temperature range from 500 to 540 °C, bonding time from 1 to 60 min and bonding pressure from 0 to 0.8 MPa. It was reported that (i) the mechanisms of bond formation varied across the joint region, with solid-state diffusion dominant at the Ti–6Al–4V interface and eutectic diffusion at the Mg–AZ31 interface, (ii) the maximum joint shear strength of 61 MPa was obtained at a temperature of 520 °C, 20 min and at a bonding pressure of 0.2 MPa, and this joint strength was three times the bond strength reported for joints made using adhesives and represents 50% of the Mg–AZ31 alloy shear strength. Xu et al. [157] reported that (i) an ultrarapid TLP bonding method was successfully used to join AZ31B Mg alloys by using pure Zn interlayers in air; (ii) the bonding time was shortened to 1 s with ultrasonic assistance; (iii) eutectic structures, MgZn and $MgZn_2$, formed at relatively low temperatures of 360 and 370 °C; (iv) $MgZn_2$ had higher hardness and modulus than those of MgZn; (v) the shear strength of joint was inversely proportional to its width; and (vi) the fractured through $MgZn_2$ at 360 and 370 °C, and through eutectoid structures at 380 °C. Mehrzad et al. [158] fabricated joints of AM60 (Mg–6Al–0.5Mn by wt%) to SS304 (Fe–18Cr–8Ni by wt%) with depositing 1 µm layer of Zn on the Mg alloy side by sputtering. It was reported that (i) through the TLP process, eutectic constituents of MgZn and Mg_7Zn_3 are solidified at the interface as the main intermetallics, (ii) based on Mg concentration in different locations of the interface, either primary Mg or MgZn crystallize before the eutectic reaction, (iii) the interlayer connection to the AM60 side is stronger than that of SS304, (iv) the bond strength has a direct relationship to the area fraction of peeled interlayer from the AM60 side, (v) at the SS304 interface, Zn reacts with steel to yield a thin ζ-FeZn phase where excess Ni was rejected into the liquid to form Mg_2Ni precipitates and (vi) the strongest joint was processed at 470 °C for 30 min.

11.6.3 Electromagnetic welding

Electromagnetic pulse welding explores a phenomenon where current-carrying conductors exert a force on each other. The force depends on the current direction and is repulsive for opposite direction flow and attractive for the same flow direction. In practice, the electric current in the coil creates an eddy current within the work piece which generates forces between the coil and the material placed within it. During the welding process, these forces cause the outer work piece to plastically deform after it accelerates toward the inner work piece, thus creating a solid-state weld [159]. Magnetic pulse welding is a solid-state joining process and has a modification called pressure seam welding. Very high currents are generated by discharging a set of charged capacitors rapidly through the coil which surrounds the component to be welded. The eddy currents oppose the magnetic field in the coil and a repulsive force is created, which drives the parts together at very high force speed and creates an explosive or impact type of weld [164]. Lee et al. [160] performed the lap joining of low-carbon steel and A6111 aluminum alloy using the magnetic pressure seam welding method. Lap joining was successfully attained in several microseconds with no temperature increase. It was reported that (i) weld interface of the lap joint showed wavy morphology and the intermediate layer was observed along the wavy interface, (ii) these microstructures are similar to that of the explosive weld lap joint, (iii) grain structure of A6111 matrix close to the weld interface was refined, (iv) the bonding strength of the joint was quite high and it failed at the parent plate and (v) the multiphase intermediate layer and grain-refined aluminum layer are considered to be the origin of high interfacial bonding strength of the lap joint. Electromagnetic compression is a suitable technology for the processing of hollow profiles made of aluminum alloys. In order to evaluate its suitability for magnesium profiles, different extruded magnesium alloys have been characterized. Important requirements on the tube material are, on the one hand, a high electrical conductivity and, on the other hand, a good formability. These modifications of magnetic welding were successfully applied for magnesium [161]. Zhu et al. [162] examined the microstructure and mechanical properties of Al/Mg welded joints after heat preservation at different temperatures. It was shown that (i) the treatment has no obvious effects on the morphology of the Al/Mg welding interface, but the morphology of the grain structure on the magnesium alloy side was improved, (ii) when the temperature was below 150 °C, there was no significant change in the microstructure and mechanical properties of Al/Mg welded joint; while, the IMC layer composed of $Al_{12}Mg_{17}$ was formed at the interface when the temperature was raised to 200 °C, (iii) the welding interface generated two IMC layers composed of $Al_{12}Mg_{17}$ and Al_3Mg_2 as the temperature reached to 250 °C, (iv) IMCs severely affected the strength of the welded joint because of greater brittleness and (v) in order to maintain reliable performance, the temperature use of the Al/Mg-welded structural parts should not exceed 150 °C.

11.6.4 Cold metal transfer welding

During welding, temperature variations in welds and parent metals have important effects on material characteristics, residual stresses as well as on dimensional and shape accuracy of welded products [163]. CMT technology has revolutionized the welding process of dissimilar metals and thicker materials, based on dip transfer welding, characterized by controlled material deposition during the short circuit of the wire electrode to the workpiece and low hear input [164, 165]. It was mentioned that, with the CMT process, (i) it is possible to do nearly spatter-free brazing of zinc-coated steel sheets and welding of thin aluminum and stainless steel materials, and (ii) in addition, it is even possible to join steel with aluminum, and reported that the droplet detachment mode of CMT process is without the aid of the electromagnetic force compared to the conventional MIG process, so the spatter can decrease [166]. Pickin et al. [164] presented the suitability of this process for welding aluminum alloy. It was found that (i) trials show that in comparison with pulsed MIG welding, CMT exhibits a higher electrode melting coefficient, (ii) by adjusting the short-circuit duration, penetration can be controlled with only a small change in electrode deposition and (iii) furthermore, by mixing pulsed MIG welding with CMT welding, the working envelope of the process is greatly extended allowing thicker material sections to be welded with improved weld bead aesthetics. Selvi et al. [165] reviewed the process, weld combinations, laser–CMT hybrid welding and applications of CMT welding. It was indicated that (i) the CMT–laser hybrid welding is more preferable to laser or laser-hybrid welding, and (ii) CMT welding has found applications in automobile industries, defense sectors and power plants as a method of additive manufacturing. Talalaev et al. [163] studied the welding of thin sheet metal products from stainless steel and aluminum by using a novel CMT process, which is an alternative to TIG, providing advantages, such as reduction of distortions and increased productivity and the optimization of the process using the existing welding equipment (robot, manipulator, etc.) and validation of the CMT process. It was reported that (i) the limiting factors for the increase of the productivity are the reduction of quality (increase of porosity, distortions and inacceptable shape of the welding bed), and (ii) practical recommendations are given for the implementation of the CMT technology for robotic welding.

There are several studies of CMT joining on magnesium materials. Mg-based alloys are used for selected aerospace structural applications due to their specific strength [167]. The manufacturing, maintenance, and repair of components made from Mg alloys require the use of welding processes that maximize strength at low structural distortion. Unfortunately, the repair of Mg alloys using conventional fusion welding processes (TIG and gas metal arc welding) is not easily performed. Mg alloys possess physical properties that make them highly susceptible to the formation of weld defects and oxides and excessive geometrical distortion, which become detrimental to the quality of welds produced. In addition, conventional welding processes do not offer sufficient repeatability, postweld strength or control of distortion to meet stringent aerospace acceptance standards with minimal postweld heat treatment. Consequently, weld behavior studies in aerospace Mg alloys continue to be a subject of rigorous research [168]. A majority of investigated Mg material is AZ31 (Mg–3Al–1Zn alloy). Cao et al. studied the CMT welding to steel [169], to Al alloy [170] and copper [171]. It was reported that (i) CMT welding of Mg to steel is possible if the steel has a zinc coating because the zinc, which has a lower melting temperature than the steel, interacts with the molten Mg alloy to provide a braze joint; (ii) the brazing interface between the Mg weld metal and galvanized mild steel primarily consists of Al, Zn and Mg intermetallics and solid solution, such as Mg solid solutions, $MgFeAlO_4$, Fe_2O_3 and Mg_2Zn_{11}; and (iii) the strength of the CMT weld-brazed, lap-shear, 1-mm-thick Mg AZ31–galvanized mild steel joint is comparable to the strength of a lap-shear 1-mm-thick Mg AZ31–Mg AZ31 welded joint [169]. Welding of 1-mm-thick AZ31B to 1 mm thick A6061-T6 using a 1.6 mm diameter aluminum filler wire 4047 was investigated [170] and it was reported that (i) although extensive efforts have been exercised to control the heat input, Mg-rich intermetallic γ-$Al_{12}Mg_{17}$ and Al-rich intermetallic β-Al_3Mg_2 were still produced in the weld, (ii) in order to improve the joint, minimizing the content of the intermetallics especially Mg-rich is essential. Cao et al. [171] studied also CMT joining of AZ31 to copper. The joint was composed of Mg–Mg welding joint formed between the Mg weld metal and the Mg BM, and Mg–Cu brazing joint formed between the Mg weld metal and the local molten Cu BM. It was reported that (i) the interfacial reaction layers of the brazing joint consisted of Mg_2Cu, $Al_6Cu_4Mg_5$,

$MgCu_2$ and $Mg_{17}Al_{12}$ intermetallic phases, and (ii) the tensile shear strength of the Mg/Cu CMT welding–brazing joint could reach 172 · 5 N/mm.

Madhavan et al. [172] reported the procedure to join A6061-T6 to AZ31B alloy using Al–5%Si filler by CMT and pulsed CMT processes and mentioned that the welding current, welding speed and the wire-feed rate had significant effect on the joint strength. Wang et al. [173] joined AZ31B and Al 6061 by CMT process with ER4043 (Al-based welding filler wire with 5% Si and small amount of Fe, Cu, Zn, Ti, Mn, Mg, Be and others) as filler metal, and the effects of the ratio of electrode positive/negative CMT cycles (EP/EN ratio: positive electrode/negative electrode ratio) on the microstructure–strength relationships of welded joints were investigated. It was reported that (i) hard brittle Mg–Al IMC layers were formed in the weld interfaces and consisted of three intermediate layers: Mg_2Al_3 layer, $Mg_{17}Al_{12}$ layer and $Mg_{17}Al_{12}$ + α-Mg solid solution eutectic layer (very thin), (ii) with decreasing EP/EN ratio from 4:1 to 1:4, the thicknesses of the Mg_2Al_3 layer and $Mg_{17}Al_{12}$ layer were reduced from 80 to 10 μm and from 105 to 80 μm, respectively, (iii) the tensile strength, which was fairly dependent on the thicknesses of these intermediate layers, increased significantly by over 100 percent and (iv) the fractures of the joints with 4:1 and 1:4 EP/EN ratio occurred primarily within the Mg_2Al_3 layer and the $Mg_{17}Al_{12}$ layer, respectively; as a result, the more EN-CMT cycles, the lower energy input, the thinner IMC layer, and the higher joint strength. Hu et al. [174] investigated the arc characteristics of CMT welding with AZ31 magnesium alloy wire were investigated. It was found that (i) for DC-CMT, stable welding process could be achieved when wire feed speed was no more than 5 m/min and for pulsed CMT, the wire feed speed should be no more than 4 m/min, (ii) the welding arc was formed between weld pool and molten droplet and exhibited as an asymmetrical bell shape, (iii) evaporation of molten droplet gave itself a recoil force, pushing it away from wire axis, (iv) at mid to upper power range, repelled droplet transfer process was observed and (v) the wire feed speed of 4 m/min under pulsed CMT mode could gain good clad appearance and a favorable contact angle, which could be capable of realizing multipass cladding of magnesium alloys.

References

[1] Liu L. Welding and Joining of Magnesium Alloys. Woodhead Pub. 2018.

[2] Czerwinski F. Welding and Joining of Magnesium Alloys. In; Czerwinski F ed., Magnesium Alloys – Design, Processing and Properties, 2011, 460–490.

[3] Cooke KO, Alhazaa A, Atieh AM. Dissimilar Welding and Joining of Magnesium Alloys: Principles and Application, IntechOpen. 2019, DOI: 10.5772/intechopen.85111; https://www.intechopen.com/online-first/dissimilar-welding-and-joining-of-magnesium-alloys-principles-and-application.

[4] https://www.tws.edu/blog/welding/what-is-tig-welding/.

[5] Peng J, Zhou C, Tao J-Q, Pan F-S. Gas tungsten arc welding of dissimilar magnesium alloys as AZ31 with AZ61. Journal of Materials Engineering. 2011, 1, 46–51.

[6] Liu X-H, Gu S-H, Wu R-Z, Leng X-S, Zhang M-L. Microstructure and mechanical properties of Mg-Li alloy after TIG welding. Transactions of Nonferrous Metals Society of China. 2011, 21, 477–81.

[7] Song G, Diao Z, Lv X, Liu L. TIG and laser-TIG hybrid filler wire welding of casting and wrought dissimilar magnesium alloy. Journal of Manufacturing Processes. 2018, 34, 204–14.

[8] Song G, Li T, Chen L. The mechanical properties and interface bonding mechanism of immiscible Mg/steel by laser–tungsten inert gas welding with filler wire. Materials Science and Engineering: A. 2018, 736, 306–15.

[9] Liu F, Wang H, Liu L. Characterization of Mg/Al butt joints welded by gas tungsten arc filling with Zn–29.5Al–0.5Ti filler metal. Materials Characterization. 2014, 90, 1–6.

[10] Dai X, Zhang H, Wang B, Ji A, Feng J. Improving weld strength of arc-assisted ultrasonic seam welded Mg/Al joint with Sn interlayer. Materials & Design. 2016, 98, 262–71.

[11] Yang F, Zhou J, Ding R. Ultrasonic vibration assisted tungsten inert gas welding of dissimilar magnesium alloys. Journal of Materials Science & Technology. 2018, 34, 2240–5.

[12] Marya M, Edwards GR. Chloride contribution in flux-assisted GTA welding of magnesium alloys. Welding Journal. 2002, 12, 291–8.

[13] Liu L, Ren D. A novel weld-bonding hybrid process for joining Mg alloy and Al alloy. Materials & Design. 2011, 32, 3730–5.

[14] Sun DX, Sun DQ, Gu XY, Xuan ZZ. Hot cracking of metal inert gas arc welded magnesium. Iron and Steel Institute of Japan, ISIJ International. 2008, 49, 270–4.

[15] Wang X-Y. Sun D-Q, Yin S-Q, Liu D-Y. Microstructures and mechanical properties of metal inert-gas arc welded Mg-steel dissimilar joints. Transactions of Nonferrous Metals Society of China. 2015, 25, 2533–42.

[16] Gaur V, Enoki M, Yomogida S. Physically short and long-crack growth behavior of MIG welded Al-5.8% Mg alloy. Engineering Fracture Mechanics. 2019, 209, 301–16.

[17] Sun DQ, Lang B Sun DX, Li JB. Microstructure and mechanical properties of resistance spot welded magnesium alloy joints, Materials Science and Engineering A. 2007, 460/461, 494–8.

[18] Shi H, Qiu R, Zhu J, Zhang K, Yu H, Ding G. Effects of welding parameters on the characteristics of magnesium alloy joint welded by resistance spot welding with cover plates, Materials & Design. 2010, 31, 4853–7.

[19] Xu W, Chen DL, Liu L, Mori H, Zhou Y. Microstructure and mechanical properties of weld-bonded and resistance spot welded magnesium-to steel dissimilar joints. Materials Science and Engineering A. 2012, 537, 11–24.

[20] Patel VK, Bhole SD, Chen DL. Fatigue life estimation of ultrasonic spot welded Mg alloy joints. Materials & Design. 2014, 62, 124–32.

[21] de Leon M, Shin H-S. Weldability assessment of Mg alloy (AZ31B) sheets by an ultrasonic spot welding method. Journal of Materials Processing Technology. 2017, 243, 1–8.

[22] Penner P, Liu L, Gerlich A, Zhou Y. Feasibility study of resistance spot welding of dissimilar Al/Mg combinations with Ni based interlayers. Science and Technology of Welding and Joining. 2013, 18, 541–50.

[23] Penner P, Liu L, Gerlich A, Zhou Y. Dissimilar resistance spot welding of aluminum to magnesium with Zn-coated steel interlayers. Welding Journal. 2014, 93, 225–31.

[24] Patel VK, Bhole SD, Chen DL. Improving weld strength of magnesium to aluminium dissimilar joints via tin interlayer during ultrasonic spot welding. Science and Technology of Welding and Joining. 2012, 17, 342–7.

[25] Patel VK, Chen DL, Bhole SD. Dissimilar ultrasonic spot welding of Mg-Al and Mg-high strength low alloy steel. Theoretical and Applied Mechanics Letters. 2014, 4; https://www.sciencedirect.com/science/article/pii/S2095034915303263.

[26] Zhang Y, Luo Z, Li Y, Liu ZM, Huang ZY. Microstructure characterization and tensile properties of Mg/Al dissimilar joints manufactured by thermo-compensated resistance spot welding with Zn interlayer. Materials & Design. 2015, 75, 166–73.
[27] Zhang K, Wu L, Tan C, Sun Y, Song X. Influence of Al-Si coating on resistance spot welding of Mg to 22MnB5 boron steel. Journal of Materials Processing Technology. 2019, 271, 23–35.
[28] Zhou J, Li L, Liu Z. CO2 and diode laser welding of AZ31 magnesium alloy. Applied Surface Science. 2005, 247, 300–6.
[29] Lei Z, Bi J, Li P, Guo T, Zhang D. Analysis on welding characteristics of ultrasonic assisted laser welding of AZ31B magnesium alloy. Optics & Laser Technology. 2018, 105, 15–22.
[30] Wahba M, Kawahito Y, Katayama S. Laser direct joining of AZ91D thixomolded Mg alloy and amorphous polyethylene terephthalate. Journal of Materials Processing Technology. 2011, 211, 1166–74.
[31] Zhao H, Debroy T. Pore formation during laser beam welding of die-cast magnesium alloy AM60B – mechanism and remedy. Welding Research Supplement. 2001, 8, 204–9.
[32] Quan Y, Chen Z, Yu Z, Gong X, Li M. Characteristics of laser welded wrought Mg-Al-Mn alloy. Materials Characterization. 2008, 59, 1799–804.
[33] Al-Kazzaz H, Medraj M, Cao X, Jahazi M. Nd: YAG laser welding of aerospace grade ZE41A magnesium alloy: Modeling and experimental investigations. Materials Chemistry and Physics. 2008, 109, 61–76.
[34] Dai J, Huang J, Li Z, Wu Y. Microstructure and mechanical properties of high power CO2 laser welded joint of Mg-Rare earth alloy NZ30K. Physics Procedia. 2010, 5, 511–516.
[35] Dai J, Huang J, Li M, Li Z, Wu Y. Effects of heat treatments on laser welded Mg-rare earth alloy NZ30K. Materials Science and Engineering: A. 2011, 529, 401–5.
[36] Yan K, Su J, Zhao Y. Microstructure and mechanical properties of the laser-welded Mg-3Nd-0.2Zn-0.4Zr (NZ30K) magnesium alloy. Optics & Laser Technology. 2107, 93, 109–17.
[37] She Q-Y, Yan H-G, Chen J-H, Su B, Yu Z-H, Chen C, Xia W-J. Microstructure characteristics and liquation behavior of fiber laser welded joints of Mg-5Zn-1Mn-0.6Sn alloy sheets. Transactions of Nonferrous Metals Society of China. 2017, 27, 812–9.
[38] Wang L, Huang J, Peng Y, Wu Y. Precipitates evolution in the heat affected zone of Mg-Gd-Y-Zr alloy in T6 condition during laser welding. Materials Characterization. 2019, 154, 386–94.
[39] Gao M, Mei S, Li X, Zeng X. Characterization and formation mechanism of laser-welded Mg and Al alloys using Ti interlayer. Scripta Materialia. 2012, 67, 193–6.
[40] Zhang C, Liu J, Tan C, Zhang K, Feng J. Laser conduction welding characteristics of dissimilar metals Mg/Ti with Al interlayer. Journal of Manufacturing Processes. 2018, 32, 595–605.
[41] Zhang K, Liu J, Tan C, Wang G, Feng J. Dissimilar joining of AZ31B Mg alloy to Ni-coated Ti-6Al-4V by laser heat-conduction welding process. Journal of Manufacturing Processes. 2018, 34A, 148–57.
[42] Liu L, Wang J, Song G. Hybrid laser-TIG welding, laser beam welding and gas tungsten arc welding of AZ31B magnesium alloy. Materials Science and Engineering A. 2004, 381, 129–33.
[43] Liu L, Liu X, Liu S. Microstructure of laser-TIG hybrid welds of dissimilar Mg alloy and Al alloy with Ce as interlayer. Scripta Materialia. 2006, 55, 383–6.
[44] Liu LM, Zhan X. Study on the weld joint of Mg alloy and steel by laser-GTA hybrid welding. Materials Characterization. 2008, 59, 1279–84.
[45] Qi X, Song G. Interfacial structure of the joints between magnesium alloy and mild steel with nickel as interlayer by hybrid laser-TIG welding. Materials & Design. 2010, 31, 605–9.
[46] Song G, Yu J, Li T, Wang J, Liu L. Effect of laser-GTAW hybrid welding heat input on the performance of Mg/Steel butt joint. Journal of Manufacturing Processes. 2018, 31, 131–8.

[47] Li L, Tan C, Chen Y, Gio W, Song F. Comparative study on microstructure and mechanical properties of laser welded–brazed Mg/mild steel and Mg/stainless steel joints. Materials & Design. 2013, 43, 59–65.
[48] Li L, Tan C, Chen Y, Guo W, Mei C. CO_2 laser welding–brazing characteristics of dissimilar metals AZ31B Mg alloy to Zn coated dual phase steel with Mg based filler. Journal of Materials Processing Technology. 2013, 213, 361–75.
[49] Chai S, Zhang D, Fan X, Yu D, Pan F. Evolution of microstructure, porosity and mechanical properties of AZ80 Mg joints during two post-weld processing routes. Materials Science and Engineering: A. 2015, 648, 392–400.
[50] Tan C, Lu Q, Chen B, Song X, Wang Y. Influence of laser power on microstructure and mechanical properties of laser welded-brazed Mg to Ni coated Ti alloys. Optics & Laser Technology. 2017, 89, 156–67.
[51] Zhang Z, Tan C, Zhao X, Chen B, Zhao H. Influence of Cu coating thickness on interfacial reactions in laser welding-brazing of Mg to Ti. Journal of Materials Processing Technology. 2108, 261, 61–73.
[52] Zhao X, Tan C, Xiao L, Hongbo X, Chen B, Song X, Li L, Feng J. Effect of the Ni coating thickness on laser welding-brazing of Mg/steel. Journal of Alloys and Compounds. 2018, 769, 1042–58.
[53] Tan C, Zang C, Zhao X, Xia H, Lu Q, Song X, Chen B, Wang G. Influence of Ni-coating thickness on laser lap welding-brazing of Mg/Ti. Optics & Laser Technology. 2018, 108, 378–91.
[54] Auwal ST, Ramesh S, Zhang Z, Liu J, Tarlochan F. Influence of electrodeposited Cu-Ni layer on interfacial reaction and mechanical properties of laser welded-brazed Mg/Ti lap joints. Journal of Manufacturing Processes. 2019, 37, 251–65.
[55] Xin Y, Hong R, Feng B, Yu H, Liu Q. Fabrication of Mg/Al multilayer plates using an accumulative extrusion bonding process. Materials Science and Engineering: A. 2015, 640, 210–6.
[56] Han T, Huang G, Ma L, Wang G, Wang L, Pan F. Evolution of microstructure and mechanical properties of AZ31 Mg alloy sheets processed by accumulated extrusion bonding with different relative orientation. Journal of Alloys and Compounds. 2019, 784, 584–91.
[57] Zhou W, Li H, Li Z, Zhu X, He L. Bonding of Zr44Ti11Cu10Ni10Be25 bulk metallic glass and AZ31B magnesium alloy by hot staking extrusion. Vacuum. 2019, 166, 240–7.
[58] Liu CY, Wang Q, Jia YZ, Jiang R, Zhang B, Ma MZ, Liu RP. Microstructures and mechanical properties of Mg/Mg and Mg/Al/Mg laminated composites prepared via warm roll bonding. Materials Science and Engineering: A. 2012, 556, 1–8.
[59] Chai S, Zhang D, Dong Y, Pan F. Effect of partial rolling on the microstructure, mechanical properties and fracture behavior of AZ31 Mg alloy joints. Materials Science and Engineering: A. 2015, 620, 1–9.
[60] Anne G, Ramesh MR, Nayaka S, Arya SB, Sahu S. Development and characteristics of accumulative roll bonded Mg-Zn/Ce/Al hybrid composite. Journal of Alloys and Compounds. 2017, 724, 146–54.
[61] Song D, Jing X, Wang J, Yang P, Zhang M. The assembly of ZSM-5 layer on Mg–Li alloy by hot-pressing using silane coupling agent as bond and its corrosion resistance. Journal of Alloys and Compounds. 2012, 510, 66–70.
[62] Arkhurst BM, Lee M, Kim JH. Effect of resin matrix on the strength of an AZ31Mg alloy-CFRP joint made by the hot metal pressing technique. Composite Structures. 2018, 201, 303–14.
[63] Chen Z, Wang D, Cao X, Yang W, Wang W. Influence of multi-pass rolling and subsequent annealing on the interface microstructure and mechanical properties of the explosive welding Mg/Al composite plates. Materials Science and Engineering: A. 2018, 723, 97–108.

[64] Zhang T, Wang W, Zhou J, Yan Z, Zhang J. Interfacial characteristics and nano-mechanical properties of dissimilar 304 austenitic stainless steel/AZ31B Mg alloy welding joint. Journal of Manufacturing Processes. 2019, 42, 257–65.
[65] Wang H, Liu L, Liu F. The characterization investigation of laser-arc-adhesive hybrid welding of Mg to Al joint using Ni interlayer. Materials & Design. 2013, 50, 463–66.
[66] Ren DX, Liu LM, Li YF. Investigation on overlap joining of AZ61 magnesium alloy: laser welding, adhesive bonding and laser weld bonding. The International Journal, Advanced Manufacturing Technology. 2012, 61, 195–204.
[67] Kay D. Brazing vs Soldering. 2013; https://vacaero.com/information-resources/vacuum-brazing-with-dan-kay/1345-brazing-vs-soldering.html.
[68] Liu L, Ren D, Liu FA. A Review of dissimilar welding techniques for magnesium alloys to aluminum alloys. Materials. 2014, 7, 3735–57.
[69] Xu ZW, Li ZW, Li JP, Ma ZP, Yan JC. Control Al/Mg intermetallic compound formation during ultrasonic-assisted soldering Mg to Al. Ultrasonics Sonochemistry. 2018, 46, 79–88.
[70] Chang S-Y, Lee J-Y, Huang Y-H, Wu A-B. Joining of AZ31 Magnesium Alloy to 6061 Aluminum Alloy with Sn-Zn Filler Metals Containing Trace Rare Earth Elements. Applied Science, 2019, 9, 2655: https://doi.org/10.3390/app9132655.
[71] Xu Z, Li Z, Zhao D, Liu X, Yan J. Effects of Zn on intermetallic compounds and strength of Al/Mg joints ultrasonically soldered in air. Journal of Materials Processing Technology. 2019, 271, 384–93.
[72] Ma L, He DY, Li XY, Jiang JM. High frequency soldering of magnesium alloy AZ31B using Zn-Al filler metal, Materials Letters. 2010, 64, 596–8.
[73] Li X, Liang W, Zhao X, Zhang Y, Fu X, Liu F. Bonding of Mg and Al with Mg-Al eutectic alloy and its application in aluminum coating on magnesium. Journal of Alloys and Compounds. 2009, 471, 408–11.
[74] Liu L, Tan J, Liu X. Reactive brazing of Al alloy to Mg alloy using zinc-based brazing alloy. Materials Letters. 2007, 61, 2373–7.
[75] Liu LM, Tan JH, Zhao LM, Liu XJ. The relationship between microstructure and properties of Mg/Al brazed joints using Zn filler metal. Materials Characterization. 2008, 59, 479–83.
[76] Elthalabawy WM, Khan TI. Microstructural development of diffusion brazed austenitic stainless steel to magnesium using nickel interlayer. Materials Characterization. 2010, 61, 703–12.
[77] Wang Z, Qu W, Zhuang H. Development of a Mg-Al filler metal for brazing magnesium alloy AZ31B. Materials Letters. 2016, 182, 75–7.
[78] Watanabe T, Komatsu S, Oohara K. Development of flux and filler metal for brazing magnesium alloy AZ31B. Welding Journal. 2005, 84, 37S-40S.
[79] Singh K, Singh G, Singh H. Review on friction stir welding of magnesium alloys. Journal of Magnesium and Alloys. 2018, 6, 399–416.
[80] Mishra RS, Ma ZY. Friction stir welding and processing. Materials Science and Engineering. 2005, 50, 1–78.
[81] Wang K, Khan HA, Li Z, Lyu S, Li J. Micro friction stir welding of multilayer aluminum alloy sheets. Journal of Materials Processing Technology. 2018, 260, 137–45.
[82] Radj BM, Senthivelan T. Analysis of mechanical properties on friction stir welded magnesium alloy by applying Taguchi Grey based approach. Materials Today: Proceedings. 2018, 5, 8025–32.
[83] Boccarusso L, Astarita A, Carlone P, Scherillo F, Squillace A. Dissimilar friction stir lap welding of AA 6082 – Mg AZ31: Force analysis and microstructure evolution. Journal of Manufacturing Processes. 2019, 44, 376–88.

[84] Ji S, Niu S, Liu J, Meng X. Friction stir lap welding of Al to Mg assisted by ultrasound and a Zn interlayer. Journal of Materials Processing Technology. 2019, 267, 141–51.
[85] Dong Z, Song Q, Zi X, Lv Z. Effect of joining time on intermetallic compound thickness and mechanical properties of refill friction stir spot welded dissimilar Al/Mg alloys. Journal of Manufacturing Processes. 2019, 42, 106–12.
[86] Meng X, Jin Y, Ji S, Yan D. Improving friction stir weldability of Al/Mg alloys via ultrasonically diminishing pin adhesion. Journal of Materials Science & Technology. 2018, 34, 1817–22.
[87] Mofid MA, Loryaei E. Investigating microstructural evolution at the interface of friction stir weld and diffusion bond of Al and Mg alloys. Journal of Materials Research and Technology. 2019, 8, 3872–7.
[88] Mofid MA, Abdollah-Zadeh A, Malek Ghaini F, Gur CH. Submerged friction-stir welding (SFSW) underwater and under liquid nitrogen: an improved method to join Al alloys to Mg alloys. Metallurgy of Materials Transactions A. 2012, 43, 5106–14.
[89] Firouzdor V, Kou S. Al-to-mg friction stir welding effect of material position, travel speed, and rotation speed. Metallurgy of Materials Transactions A. 2010, 41, 2914–35.
[90] Suhuddin UFH, Fischer V, Dos Santos JF. The thermal cycle during the dissimilar friction spot welding of aluminum and magnesium alloy. Scripta Materialia. 2013, 68, 87–90.
[91] Chang W-S, Rajesh SR, Chun C-K, Kim H-J. Microstructure and Mechanical Properties of Hybrid Laser-Friction Stir Welding between AA6061-T6 Al Alloy and AZ31 Mg Alloy. Journal of Materials Science & Technology. 2011, 27, 199–204.
[92] Liu D, Nishio H, Nakata K. Anisotropic property of material arrangement in friction stir welding of dissimilar Mg alloys. Materials & Design. 2011, 32, 4818–24.
[93] Choi D-H, Kim S-K, Jung S-B. The microstructures and mechanical properties of friction stir welded AZ31 with CaO Mg alloys. Journal of Alloys and Compounds. 2013, 554, 162–8.
[94] Xin R, Sun L, Liu D, Zhou Z, Liu Q. Effect of subsequent tension and annealing on microstructure evolution and strength enhancement of friction stir welded Mg alloys. Materials Science and Engineering: A. 2014, 602, 1–10.
[95] Xin R, Liu D, Shu X, Li B, Liu Q. Influence of welding parameter on texture distribution and plastic deformation behavior of as-rolled AZ31 Mg alloys. Journal of Alloys and Compounds. 2016, 670, 64–71.
[96] Suhuddin U, Fischer V, Kroeff F, Dos Santos JF. Microstructure and mechanical properties of friction spot welds of dissimilar AA5754 Al and AZ31 Mg alloys. Materials Science and Engineering: A. 2014, 590, 384–9.
[97] Singh I, Cheema GS, Kang AS. An Experimental Approach to Study the Effect of Welding Parameters on Similar Friction Stir Welded Joints of AZ31B-O Mg alloy. Procedia Engineering. 2014, 97, 837–46.
[98] Templeman Y, Hamu GB, Meshi L. Friction stir welded AM50 and AZ31 Mg alloys: Microstructural evolution and improved corrosion resistance. Materials Characterization. 2017, 126, 86–95.
[99] Kim MS, Jung JY, Song YM, Choi S-H. Simulation of microtexture developments in the stir zone of friction stir-welded AZ31 Mg alloys. International Journal of Plasticity. 2017, 94, 24–43.
[100] Shang Q, Ni DR, Xue P, Xiao BL, Ma ZY. Evolution of local texture and its effect on mechanical properties and fracture behavior of friction stir welded joint of extruded Mg-3Al-1Zn alloy. Materials Characterization. 2017, 128, 14–22.
[101] Xu RZ, Ni DR, Yang Q, Xiao BL, Liu CZ, Ma ZY. Influencing mechanism of Al-containing Zn coating on interfacial microstructure and mechanical properties of friction stir spot welded Mg–steel joint. Materials Characterization. 2018, 140, 197–206.

[102] Zhang Z-K, Wang X-J, Wang P-C, Zhao G. Friction stir keyholeless spot welding of AZ31Mg alloy-mild steel. Transactions of Nonferrous Metals Society of China. 2014, 24, 1709–16.

[103] Lv X, Wu CS, Yang C, Padhy GK. Weld microstructure and mechanical properties in ultrasonic enhanced friction stir welding of Al alloy to Mg alloy. Journal of Materials Processing Technology. 2018, 254, 145–57.

[104] Xu RZ, Ni DR, Yang Q, Liu CZ, Ma ZY. Influencing mechanism of Zn interlayer addition on hook defects of friction stir spot welded Mg–Al–Zn alloy joints. Materials & Design. 2015, 69, 163–9.

[105] Xu RZ, Ni DR, Yang Q, Liu CZ, Ma ZY. Pinless Friction Stir Spot Welding of Mg–3Al–1Zn Alloy with Zn Interlayer. Journal of Materials Science & Technology. 2016, 32, 76–88.

[106] Woo W, Feng Z, Clausen B, David SA. In situ neutron diffraction analyses of temperature and stresses during friction stir processing of Mg-3Al-1Zn magnesium alloy. Materials Letters. 2017, 196, 284–7.

[107] Shang Q, Ni DR, Xue P, Xiao BL, Ma ZY. Improving joint performance of friction stir welded wrought Mg alloy by controlling non-uniform deformation behavior. Materials Science and Engineering: A. 2017, 707, 426–34.

[108] Reddy GPK, Sunil BR, Balakroshna B. Joining of AZ31 Mg alloy sheets by friction stir welding and investigating corrosion initiated failure. Materials Today: Proceedings. 2017, 4, 6712–7.

[109] Liang Z, Qin G, Geng P, Yang F, Meng X. Continuous drive friction welding of 5A33 Al alloy to AZ31B Mg alloy. Journal of Manufacturing Processes. 2017, 25, 153–62.

[110] Liu Z, Meng X, Ji S, Li Z, Wang L. Improving tensile properties of Al/Mg joint by smashing intermetallic compounds via ultrasonic-assisted stationary shoulder friction stir welding. Journal of Manufacturing Processes. 2018, 31, 552–9.

[111] Xu N, Song Q, Fujii H, Bao Y, Shen J. Mechanical properties' modification of large load friction stir welded AZ31B Mg alloy joint. Materials Letters. 2018, 219, 93–6.

[112] Kumar S, Wu CS. A novel technique to join Al and Mg alloys: Ultrasonic vibration assisted linear friction stir welding. Materials Today: Proceedings. 2018, 5, 18142–51.

[113] Shang Q, Ni DR, Xue P, Xiao BL, Ma ZY. An approach to enhancement of Mg alloy joint performance by additional pass of friction stir processing. Journal of Materials Processing Technology. 2019, 264, 336–45.

[114] Park SHC, Sato YS, Kokawa H. Basal plane texture and flow pattern in friction stir weld of a magnesium alloy. Metallurgical and Materials Transactions A. 2003, 34, 987–94.

[115] Park SHC, Sato YS, Kokawa H. Effect of micro-texture on fracture location in friction stir weld of Mg alloy AZ61 during tensile test. Scripta Materialia. 2003, 49, 161–6.

[116] Zhou M, Morisada Y, Fujii H, Ishikawa T. Mechanical properties optimization of AZX612-Mg alloy joint by double-sided friction stir welding. Journal of Materials Processing Technology. 2018, 254, 91–9.

[117] Li G, Zhou L, Luo S, Huang Y, Guo N, Zhao H, Song X. Effect of self-reacting friction stir welding on microstructure and mechanical properties of Mg-Al-Zn alloy joints. Journal of Manufacturing Processes. 2019, 37, 1–10.

[118] Sevvel P, Jaiganesh V. Effects of axial force on the mechanical properties of AZ80A Mg alloy during friction stir welding. Materials Today: Proceedings. 2017, 4, 1312–20.

[119] Zhou L, Nakata K, Liao J, Tsumura T. Microstructural characteristics and mechanical properties of non-combustive Mg-9Al-Zn-Ca magnesium alloy friction stir welded joints. Materials & Design. 2012, 42, 505–12.

[120] Luo C, Li X, Song D, Zhou N, Qi W. Microstructure evolution and mechanical properties of friction stir welded dissimilar joints of Mg–Zn–Gd and Mg–Al–Zn alloys. Materials Science and Engineering: A. 2016, 664, 103–13.

[121] Hosseini VA, Aashuri H, Kokabi AH. Effect of welding parameters on semisolid stir welding of Mg-9Al-1Zn magnesium alloy. Transactions of Nonferrous Metals Society of China. 2016, 26, 2586–94.
[122] Jaiganesh V, Govind Vignesh S, Vignesh SM. Investigation on Micro structural and Mechanical Properties of Friction Stir Welded AZ91E Mg Alloy. Materials Today: Proceedings. 2017, 4, 6704–11.
[123] Prasad BL, Neelaiah G, Krishna MG, Ramana SVV, Prakash KS, Sarika G, Pradeep G, Reddy K, Dumpala R, Sunil BR. Joining of AZ91 Mg alloy and Al6063 alloy sheets by friction stir welding. Journal of Magnesium and Alloys. 2018, 6, 71–6.
[124] Li P, You G, Wen H, Guo W, Li S. Friction stir welding between the high-pressure die casting of AZ91 magnesium alloy and A383 aluminum alloy. Journal of Materials Processing Technology. 2019, 264, 55–63.
[125] Sameer MD, Anil KB. Mechanical and metallurgical properties of friction stir welded dissimilar joints of AZ91 magnesium alloy and AA 6082-T6 aluminium alloy, Journal of Magnesium and Alloys. 2019, 7, 264–71.
[126] Yu L, Nakata K, Liao J. Microstructural modification and mechanical property improvement in friction stir zone of thixo-molded AE42 Mg alloy. Journal of Alloys and Compounds. 2009, 480, 340–6.
[127] Sahu PK, Pal S. Influence of metallic foil alloying by FSW process on mechanical properties and metallurgical characterization of AM20 Mg alloy. Materials Science and Engineering: A. 2017, 684, 442–55.
[128] Kim B, Park SS, Lee JG, Bae GT, Kim NJ. Microstructure and mechanical properties of twin-roll cast Mg-6Zn-1Mn-1Al alloy joined by surface-friction welding. Materials Characterization. 2017, 124, 8–13.
[129] Pan F, Xu A, Deng D, Ye J, Ran Y. Effects of friction stir welding on microstructure and mechanical properties of magnesium alloy Mg-5Al-3Sn. Materials & Design. 2016, 110, 266–74.
[130] Richmire S, Hall K, Haghshenas. Design of experiment study on hardness variations in friction stir welding of AM60 Mag alloy. Journal of Magnesium and Alloys. 2018, 6, 215–28.
[131] Askariani SA, Pishbin H, Moshref-Javadi M. Effect of welding parameters on the microstructure and mechanical properties of the friction stir welded joints of a Ma-12Li-1Al alloy. Journal of Alloys and Compounds. 2017, 724, 859–68.
[132] Sundar Singh Sivam SP, Loganathan GB, Saravanan K, Umasekar VG. Experimental study and ignition fire risk mapping on friction stir welding parameters of dissimilar alloys for the benefits of environment. Materials Today: Proceedings. 2019, 22, 342–6.
[133] Choi J-W, Liu H, Ushioda K, Fujii H. Effect of an Al filler material on interfacial microstructure and mechanical properties of dissimilar friction stir welded Ti/Mg joint. Materials Characterization. 2019, 155; https://doi.org/10.1016/j.matchar.2019.109801.
[134] Maharana HS, Ashok A, Pal S, Basu A. Surface-mechanical properties of electrodeposited Cu-Al_2O_3 composite coating and effects of processing parameters. Metallurgical and Materials Transactions A. 2016, 47, 388–99.
[135] Somekawa H, Hosokawa H, Watanabe H, Higashi K. Experimental study of diffusion bonding in pure magnesium. Materials Transactions. 2001, 42, 2075–8.
[136] Oshida Y, Takase S. Application of Dynamic Superplasticity to Solid-State Bonding of Cast Irons to Different Ferrous Alloys. Journal of Japan Institution of Casting Ironsactions 1976, 48, 349–54.
[137] Oshida Y, Takase S. On the Micro-Structures of Superplastic Solid-State Bonded Parts in Cast Irons. Journal of Japan Institution of Casting Ironsactions 1976, 48, 763–8.

[138] Li ZQ, Li XH. The Applications of SPF/DB Combined with Welding Technologies. Materials Science Forum. 2007, 551/552, 49–54.
[139] Shao J, Li ZQ, Han XQ, Han XN, Deng Y. Application of SPF/DB New Structure to Titanium Main-Load Carrying Components. Materials Science Forum. 2012, 735, 210–4.
[140] Somekawa H, Hosokawa H, Watanabe H, Higashi K. Diffusion bonding in superplastic magnesium alloys. Materials Science and Engineering A. 2003, 339, 328–33.
[141] Somekawa H, Watanabe H, Mukai T, Higashi K. Low temperature diffusion bonding in a superplastic AZ31 magnesium alloy. Scripta Materialia. 2003, 48, 1249–54.
[142] Oshida Y. An Application of Superplasticity to Powder Metallurgy. Journal of Japan Society of Powder and Powder Metallurgy. 1975, 22, 147–53.
[143] Peng L, Yajiang L, Haoran G, Juan W. A study of phase constitution near the interface of Mg/Al vacuum diffusion bonding. Materials Letters. 2005, 59, 2001–5.
[144] Wang M, Jia P, Lv D, Geng H. Study on the microstructure and liquid–solid correlation of Al–Mg alloys. Physics and Chemistry of Liquids. 2015, 54, 1–8.
[145] Li Y, Liu P, Wang J, Ma H. XRD and SEM analysis near the diffusion bonding interface of Mg/Al dissimilar materials, Vacuum. 2007, 82, 15–19.
[146] Gupta K. The Cu-Mg-Ni (Copper-Magnesium-Nickel) System. Chemistry. 2004: DOI:10.1007/s11669-004-0143-4.
[147] Mahendran G, Balasuramanian V, Senthilvelan T. Influences of diffusion bonding process parameters on bond characteristics of Mg-Cu dissimilar joints. Transactions of Nonferrous Metals Society of China. 2010, 20, 997–1005.
[148] Dietrich D, Nickel D, Krause M, Lampke T, Coleman MP, Randle V. Formation of intermetallic phases in diffusion welded joints of aluminium and magnesium alloys. Journal of Materials Science. 2011, 46, 357–64.
[149] Duygulu O, Kaya AA, Oktay G, Sahin FC. Diffusion Bonding of Magnesium, Zirconium and Titanium as Implant Material. Materials Science Forum. 2007, 546/549, 417–20.
[150] Shang J, Wang KH, Zhou Q, Zhang DK, Huang J, Ge JQ. Effect of joining temperature on microstructure and properties of diffusion bonded Mg/Al joints. Transactions of Nonferrous Metals Society of China. 2012, 22, 1961–6.
[151] Jafarian M, Saboktakin Rizi M, Jafarian M, Honarmand M, Javadinejad HR, Ghaheri A, Bahramipour MT, Ebrahimian. Effect of thermal tempering on microstructure and mechanical properties of Mg-AZ31/Al-6061 diffusion bonding. Materials Science and Engineering: A. 2016, 666, 372–9.
[152] Azizi A, Alimardan H. Effect of welding temperature and duration on properties of 7075 Al to AZ31B Mg diffusion bonded joint. Transactions of Nonferrous Metals Society of China. 2016, 26, 85–92.
[153] Fernandus MJ, Senthilkumar T, Balasubramanian V, Rajakumar S. Optimizing diffusion bonding parameters in AA6061-T6 aluminum and AZ80 magnesium alloy dissimilar joints. Journal of Materials Engineering and Performance. 2012, 21, 2303–15.
[154] Nimal RJGR, Sivakumar M, Raj SG, Vendan SA, Esakkimuthu G. Microstructural, mechanical and metallurgical analysis of Al interlayer coating on Mg-Al alloy using diffusion bonding. Materials Today: Proceedings. 2018, 5, 5886–90.
[155] Cook GO, Sorensen CD. Overview of transient liquid phase and partial transient liquid phase bonding. Journal of Materials Science. 2011, 46, 5305–23.
[156] Atieh AM, Khan TI. TLP bonding of Ti-6Al-4V and Mg-AZ31 alloys using pure Ni electro-deposited coats. Journal of Materials Processing Technology. 2014, 214, 3158–68.
[157] Xu Z, Li Z, Peng L, Yan J. Ultra-rapid transient liquid phase bonding of Mg alloys within 1 s in air by ultrasonic assistance. Materials & Design. 2019, 161, 72–9.

[158] Mehrzad M, Sadeghi A, Farahani M. Microstructure and properties of transient liquid phase bonding of AM60 Mg alloy to 304 stainless steel with Zn interlayer. Journal of Materials Processing Technology. 2019, 266, 558–68.
[159] Sapanathan T, Raoelison RN, Buiron N, Rachik M. Magnetic Pulse Welding: An Innovative Joining Technology for Similar and Dissimilar Metal Pairs, Joining Technologies 2016, IntechOpen. https://www.intechopen.com/books/joining-technologies/magnetic-pulse-welding-an-innovative-joining-technology-for-similar-and-dissimilar-metal-pairs.
[160] Lee KJ, Kumai S, Arai T, Aizawa T. Interfacial microstructure and strength of steel/aluminum alloy lap joint fabricated by magnetic pressure seam welding. Materials Science and Engineering A. 2007, 471, 95–101.
[161] Psyk V, Beerwald C, Klaus A, Kleiner M. Characterization of extruded magnesium profiles for electromagnetic joining. Journal of Materials Processing Technology. 2006, 177, 266–9.
[162] Zhu C, Sun L, Gao W, Li G, Cui J. The effect of temperature on microstructure and mechanical properties of Al/Mg lap joints manufactured by magnetic pulse welding. Journal of Materials Research and Technology. 2019, 8, 3270–80.
[163] Talalaev R, Veinthal R, Laansoo A, Sarkans M. Cold metal transfer (CMT) welding of thin sheet metal products. Estonian Journal of Engineering. 2012, 18, 243–50.
[164] Pickin CG, Young K. Evaluation of cold metal transfer (CMT) for welding aluminium alloy. Science and Technology of Welding and Joining. 2006, 11, 583–5.
[165] Selvi S, Vishvaksenan A, Rajasekar E. Cold metal transfer (CMT) technology – An overview. Defence Technology. 2018, 14, 28–44.
[166] Schierl A. The CMT-process – a revolution in welding technology. Weld World. 2005, 49; https://www.researchgate.net/publication/279573285_The_CMT_-_Process_-_A_Revolution_in_welding_technology.
[167] Smola B, Stulikova I, Von Buch F, Mordike BL. Structural aspects of high performance Mg alloys design. Materials of Science and Engineering A. 2002, 324, 113–7.
[168] Ola OT, Valdez RL, Oluwasegun KM, Olo OA, Chan K, Birur A, Cuddy J. Process variable optimization in the cold metal transfer weld repair of aerospace ZE41A-T5 alloy using central composite design. The International Journal, Advanced Manufacturing Technology. 2019, 105, 4827–35.
[169] Cao R, Yu JY, Chen JH, Wang P-C. Feasibility of cold-metal-transfer welding magnesium AZ31 to galvanized mild steel. Welding Journal. 2013, 92, 274s-82s.
[170] Cao R, Wen BF, Chen JH, Wang P-C. Cold Metal Transfer joining of magnesium AZ31B-to-aluminum A6061-T6. Materials Science and Engineering. A, Structural Materials: Properties, Microstructure and Processing. 2013, 560, 256–66.
[171] Cao R, Feng JZ, Chen JH. Cold metal transfer welding–brazing of magnesium to pure copper. Journal of Science and Technology of Welding and Joining. 2014, 19, 451–60.
[172] Madhavan S, Kamaraj M, Vijayaraghavan L. Cold metal transfer welding of aluminium to magnesium: microstructure and mechanical properties. Journal of Science and Technology of Welding and Joining. 2016, 21, 310–6.
[173] Wang P, Hu S, Shen J, Liang Y, Pang J. Effects of electrode positive/negative ratio on microstructure and mechanical properties of Mg/Al dissimilar variable polarity cold metal transfer welded joints. Materials Science and Engineering: A. 2016, 652, 127–35.
[174] Hu S, Zhang H, Wang Z, Liang Y, Liu Y. The arc characteristics of cold metal transfer welding with AZ31 magnesium alloy wire. Journal of Manufacturing Processes. 2016, 24, 298–306.

Chapter 12 Hydrophobicity and wettability

For certain applicable areas of Mg-based alloys, unique surface behavior is required such as hydrophobicity or hydrophilicity to control surface chemical and/or electrochemical activities. It is generally believed that superhydrophobic coating, known as a material surface with a contact angle greater than 150°, has been gradually used as a protect film on the surface of metallic material in recent studies. These are particularly important when Mg materials are used in biomedical applications because they normally exhibit poor anticorrosion property and uncontrolled biodegradation and hydrogen evolution due to high hydrogen overpotential. Hydrophobic surfaces can be developed by chemical, electrochemical and physical surface treatments, which could facilitate the formation of coatings or surface roughening on Mg alloys [1]. In an area where the biocompatibilities including hemocompatibility and cytocompatibility are required, the surface is modified to exhibit a hydrophilic nature. For these surface hydrophilic modifications, to which cytocompatibility or hemocompatibility are essential, chemical, electrochemical, mechanical and/or thermal treatments are employed [2].

Figure 12.1 illustrates gradual changes in contact angle, adhesiveness and wettability from superhydrophilic surface to superhydrophobic surface [3].

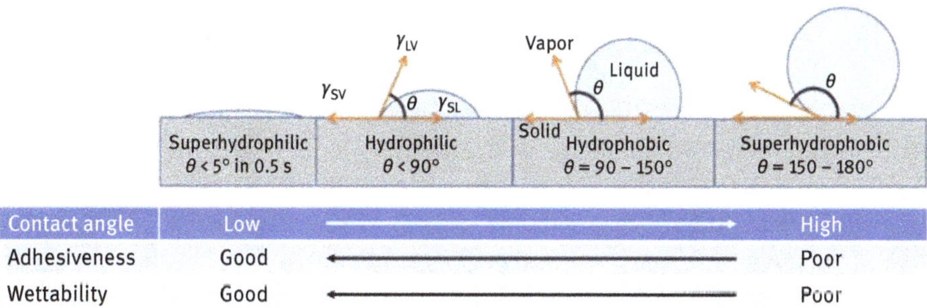

Figure 12.1: Schematic diagram representing water contact angle on different surface energy levels [3].

12.1 Coating

Kuang et al. [4] fabricated a superhydrophobic coating based on a Mg–Mn layered double hydroxide (LDHs) film on pure Mg by an in situ growth method and chemical modification by adsorption of myristic acid ($CH_3(CH_2)_{12}COOH$). It was found that (i) the static contact angle of the superhydrophobic surface was about 152.2°, (ii) the electrochemical impedance of the superhydrophobic coating sample at low

https://doi.org/10.1515/9783110676945-012

frequency is approximately 20,000 $\Omega \cdot cm^2$ which is more than twice that of the LDHs film and ten times that of the pure Mg substrate and (iii) the superhydrophobic coating can effectively protect the Mg from corrosion in the simulated body fluid for a long time. Wang et al. [5] fabricated superhydrophobic nickel coating deposited on the surface of Mg alloy with good anticorrosion property through combing methods of etching, electroplating and chemical modification. It was reported that (i) the as-prepared nickel-coated etched Mg alloy had a multiscaled structure, (ii) combined with chemical modification, the water contact angle on the surface of the nickel-coated etched Mg alloy modified with stearic acid with the lowest sliding angle (SA) of 7.2° was the highest and reached 153°, showing superhydrophobic property, compared with that of the bare Mg alloy and etched Mg alloy with and without modification and (iii) the results also showed that the nickel-coated etched Mg alloy modified with stearic acid presented the best corrosion resistance and long-term durability in 3.5 wt% NaCl solution, suggesting that it may be due to the good anticorrosion property of nickel coating and the superhydrophobic surface which help to reduce the contact area of surface with NaCl solution. Luo et al. [6] prepared a hydrophobic surface on the surface of an extruded Mg–5Sn–1Zn (TZ51) alloy by microarc oxidation (MAO) with a subsequent stearic acid modification. It was reported that (i) the maximum water contact angle of 122.5° can be obtained by the MAO at 400 V for 5 min with the stearic acid modification, which can be attributed to the rough island structures and volcano-like structures with the formation of the stearic acid coating, (ii) both the hydrophobic surface and MAO coating effectively inhibit the corrosion of the extruded TZ51 alloy and (iii) the corrosion current decreases from 8.9 to 0.07 $\mu A/cm^2$ and the polarization resistance increases from 2.11 to 434.30 11 $k\Omega \cdot cm^2$ without changing corrosion potential (−1.53 V (vs SCE)) after MAO at 400 V for 5 min MAO with subsequent steric acid treatment, indicating the effective corrosion inhibition of hydrophobic surface and the MAO coating. A composite coating consisting of polyphenylene sulfide (PPS), polytetrafluoroethylene (PTFE) and 40 nm silicon dioxide (SiO_2) nanoparticles (PPS–PTFE/SiO_2) with SiO_2 in the range of 0–4 g/L was successfully prepared on AZ31 Mg alloys by a simple spray process [7]. It was found that (i) microsized protrusions distribute on the surface of the coatings, and a fibrous-network structure of PTFE arranges on the protrusions; (ii) water contact angles of the PPS–PTFE/SiO_2 (0–4 g/L) coating are in the range of (152°–145.5°) ± 0.3° and the SAs are less than 5°; (iii) the water contact angles of the unabraded and 10 m abraded-on-sandpaper PPS–PTFE/SiO_2 (4 g/L) coating are 145.5° ± 0.3° and 142.5° ± 0.3°, respectively, implying the PPS–PTFE/SiO_2 coating is a robust superhydrophobic one with good wear resistance; (iv) due to the superhydrophobic characteristics, the PPS–PTFE-based coatings show superior corrosion resistance in 3.5 wt% NaCl solution to pristine AZ31 Mg alloys; and (v) owing to the excellent superhydrophobicity, wear resistance and corrosion resistance properties, the robust PPS–PTFE/SiO_2 coating is regarded to possess great potential to be applied in automobiles and navigation industries in future. Ji et al. [8]

deposited a high hydrophobic Ni–Cu–SiC coating with a graded nanostructure on the Mg–Li alloy via electroplating and stearic acid modification. It was reported that after stearic acid modification, the as-prepared Ni–Cu–SiC coating displays high hydrophobicity with contact angle of 156.0°. Ishizuka et al. [9] developed direct growth of anticorrosive magnesium hydroxide films containing Mg–Al LDH with anion exchangeability on magnesium alloy by a chemical-free steam coating method. It was mentioned that (i) the films had thicknesses ranging from 2 to 68 μm depending on the preparation conditions with two distinct crystal structures of crystalline $Mg(OH)_2$ and carbonate Mg–Al LDH and (ii) the corrosion tests in 5 wt% NaCl aqueous solution by electrochemical measurements indicated an inhibiting effect on the corrosion reaction.

Wang et al. [10] prepared the rough surface structure by electrodeposition of copper, followed by changing from hydrophilic to superhydrophobic via modification with lauric acid. It was reported that the superhydrophobic coatings have ultralow slide angles (2°) and contact angles of 154°. Li et al. [11] prepared the organophosphonate molecules self-assembled onto a hydrophilic plasma electrolytic oxidation (PEO) coated Mg–Li alloy surface. It was indicated that (i) the superhydrophobic composite coating exhibits excellent nonwetting and superior corrosion resistance properties, making corrosive ions nearly nonpermeable and (ii) the superhydrophobic composite coating does not deteriorate obviously after prolonged exposure to air, resulting in exceptional corrosion tolerance as well as long-term durability in air. La et al. [12] mentioned that the Mg-based switchable mirrors can reversibly change their optical properties between the transparent and the reflective state as a result of hydrogenation and dehydrogenation and these films can potentially be applied as new energy-saving windows, by controlling the transmittance of solar radiation through the regulation of their reflective state. Based on this background, La et al. [13] prepared Mg–Y alloy thin films using a DC magnetron sputtering method. For further improving the films' switching durability, luminous transmittance and the surface functionalization, PTFE was coated with thermal vacuum deposition for use as the top layer of Mg–Y/Pd switchable mirrors. It was mentioned that the PTFE layer had a porous network structure and exhibited a superhydrophobic surface with a water contact angle of approximately 152°. By characterization, PTFE thin films show an excellent protection role against the oxidization of Mg, and the switching durability of the films were improved 3 times, and also show that the antireflection role of the luminous transmission of films was enhanced by 7% through the top covered with PTFE.

Certain types of polymers show its effectiveness to obtain superhydrophobicity on Mg surface by coating [1, 14], including polyvinyl chloride, polystyrene, polypropylene, poly (methyl methacrylate), polycarbonate, and polyether-based polyurethaneurea [1, 13–15].

12.2 Deposition

Chemical or electrochemical deposition is one of the most significant methods to fabricate hydrophobic surfaces. In this category, chemical processes involve chemical salts deposition, conversion coatings, sol–gel process and (electro)chemical vapor deposition [1]. Song et al. [16] adopted a simple immersion approach in aqueous $CuSO_4$ solution for fabricating superhydrophobic Mg alloy surfaces. It was reported that (i) after modification with stearic acid, the as-prepared micro/nanometer-scale rough structures and the micrometer-scale lump-like rough structures all show superhydrophobicity, (ii) the contact angles (which is a function of surface energy) of the water droplet on the aforementioned two structures are 151.3° and 161.8°, respectively, and (iii) the rolling angles are 3° and 13°, respectively, indicating that the cooperation of suitable rough structures and stearic acid modification is responsible for the obtained superhydrophobicity on the Mg alloy surfaces.

A superhydrophobic surface was successfully fabricated on magnesium alloy by electrodeposition of Zn–Co coating from choline chloride-based ionic liquid and subsequent surface modification [17]. It was mentioned that (i) the water contact angle was measured to be as high as 152°, (ii) the corrosion resistant performance of magnesium alloy in 0.1 mol/L NaCl solution was improved and (iii) the superhydrophobic coating exhibited high stability in aqueous solution, the rough surface textures were retained and the coating still exhibited a large contact angle after mechanical destroy. Qiu [18] used magnetic Fe_3O_4 nanoparticles treated with hexadecyltrimethoxysilane as immobilization material. It was reported that (i) the hierarchical rough surfaces on the substrates form a superhydrophobic coating with a water contact angle as high as 157° and (ii) the coating significantly decreased the corrosion rate compared with the pristine magnesium alloy in 3.5 wt% NaCl solution. Liu et al. [19] fabricated the superamphiphobic surfaces by combining the nickel-plating process and modification with perfluorocaprylic acid. Superamphiphobic (both superhydrophobic and superoleophobic) surfaces have attracted great interests in the fundamental research and practical application. It was mentioned that (i) the contact angles of water/oil have reached up to 160.2 ± 1°/152.4 ± 1°, respectively, (ii) the electrochemical measurements of superamphiphobic surfaces revealed that the surface corrosion inhibition was improved significantly and (iii) superamphiphobic surfaces exhibited superior stability in the solutions with a large pH range, also could maintain excellent performance after storing for a long time in the air. Through the nickel electrodeposition approach, a superhydrophobic surface, which possess self-cleaning feature, was succeeded to be deposited on AZ31 Mg alloy [20]. It was noted that the water contact angle is 151.7°. Jia et al. [21] fabricated a superhydrophobic film on magnesium alloys using chemical silvering and self-assembly treatments. It was reported that (i) the treated magnesium alloy surface exhibits high hydrophobicity with an apparent contact angle of 153° and contact angle hysteresis of 4° and (ii) comparing with untreated magnesium alloys, the corrosion resistance of treated magnesium alloy in 0.1 mol/L NaCl aqueous solution is significantly improved by the superhydrophobic film, and the film is positive enough to prevent the pitting corrosion.

12.3 Electrochemical conversion coatings

A stable superhydrophobic surface with self-cleaning property was obtained on Mg-3Al-1Zn alloy surface through a process combining both electrodeposition and post-modification with stearic acid [22]. It was mentioned that (i) a static water contact angle was 156.2 ± 0.6° and a SA was as low as 1.0°, (ii) corrosion resistance of magnesium alloy in 3.5 wt% NaCl solution was improved, (iii) the superhydrophobic surface showed good chemical stability for the liquids with high salinity and corrosive effect and (iv) the as-prepared surface could maintain superhydrophobicity after mechanical abrasion for 900 mm, showing high mechanical stability. The superhydrophobic surface could maintain good corrosion resistance even after abrasion for 1,100 mm indicating that the presented method is of significant value for the industrial fabrication of mechanically robust, corrosion resistant and self-cleaning superhydrophobic surfaces. She et al. [23] fabricated a highly anticorrosion and self-cleaning superhydrophobic surface with hierarchical flowerlike structures on AZ91D magnesium alloy through electrodeposition of Ni–Co alloy coating, followed by modification of stearic acid. It was found that (i) a superhydrophobic surface with a water contact angle as high as 167.3 ± 1.3° and an ultralow SA of about 1° was achieved, (ii) the superhydrophobic surface can present an excellent anticorrosion effect (in neutral 3.5 at% NaCl solution) with the inhibition efficiency of 99.99% to the bare magnesium alloy and its corrosion rate being 0.06% of that of bare magnesium alloy and (iii) the as-prepared superhydrophobic surface possessed good chemical stability and self-cleaning effect. Liu [24] developed a simple, one-step method to produce a superhydrophobic surface by electrodepositing Mg–Mn–Ce magnesium plate in an ethanol solution containing cerium nitrate hexahydrate and myristic acid. It was reported that (i) the shortest electrodeposition time to obtain a superhydrophobic surface was about 1 min, and the as-prepared superhydrophobic surfaces had a maximum contact angle of 159.8° and a SA of less than 2° and (ii) potentiodynamic polarization and electrochemical impedance spectroscopy measurements demonstrated that the superhydrophobic surface greatly improved the corrosion properties of magnesium alloy in 3.5 wt% aqueous solutions of NaCl, Na_2SO_4, $NaClO_3$ and $NaNO_3$.

Khaselev et al. [25] studied constant voltage anodizing of binary Mg–Al alloys containing 2%, 5%, 8% and 12% of aluminum in the process of anodizing conducted in a bath containing 3 M KOH + 0.6 M KF + 0.21 M Na_3PO_4 with additions of 0.013, 0.064, 0.13 and 0.4 M of $Al(OH)_3$. It was mentioned that (i) a thin amorphous film was formed during the first stage of anodizing and prolonged anodizing caused local breakdown and crystallization of the initially formed anodic films, (ii) the elements in the film were mainly magnesium, aluminum and oxygen, (iii) Al element penetrated into the film both from the electrolyte and from the Mg–Al alloy substrate and (iv) the phase composition of the anodic films was found to be a mixture of MgO and $MgA1_2O_4$. Mizutani et al. [26] investigated the electrochemical behaviors of 99.95 mass% magnesium and its alloys, that is, AZ31 and AZ91, in NaOH alkaline solution. Mg and Mg alloy specimens were anodized for 10 min at 3, 10 and 80 V in 1 mol/dm^3 NaOH alkaline solution. It was mentioned that (i) the films anodized at 3 V on Mg and Mg alloys had the best effective corrosion resistance and these films consisted of comparatively thick magnesium hydroxide and (ii) corrosion resistances of the films anodized at 80 V on Mg and Mg alloys were higher than those at 10 V and lower than those at 3 V, from results of the anodic polarization measurement in 0.1 mass% NaCl solution. Liu et al. [27] studied the deterioration process of a PEO coating containing zirconium oxides on AM30 magnesium alloy in 3.5 wt% NaCl solution. It was found that (i) the coating consists of an outer porous layer and an inner dense layer, (ii) the content of MgF_2 is high in the pores and an MgO-rich layer is evident in the inner layer and (iii) the corrosion resistance of the outer layer gradually decreases in the initial immersion stage (96 h) due to the decomposition of MgO, and the deterioration of the inner layer is delayed by the blocking effect of the outer layer.

12.4 Hydrothermal process

Wang et al. [28] constructed a superhydrophobic film comprising hierarchical structures on the surface of Mg alloy substrates by a hydrothermal process, and subsequently covered with fluoroalkylsilane (FAS) molecules. It was indicated that (i) the superhydrophobic surface exhibited a static water contact angle of 151°, due to combination of the increase of the surface roughness and reduction of the surface energy and (ii) the electrochemical measurement showed that the superhydrophobic film provided an effective corrosion resistant coating for the Mg alloy substrate. Ou et al. [29] formed microstructured oxide or hydroxide layers through hydrothermally treated in H_2O (for Mg alloy and Al alloy) or H_2O_2 (for Ti alloy) on light alloy substrates. Such surfaces served as the active layers to boost the self-assembling of perfluorooctyltriethoxysilane and finally endowed the substrates with unique wettability, that is, superhydrophobicity. Gao et al. [30] fabricated a superhydrophobic film successfully on the surface of magnesium alloy AZ31 by a rapid hydrothermal process in the presence of hydrogen peroxide without using any template and surfactant, and then covered with FAS molecules. It was reported that (i) the surface was composed of a large amount of spheres, the random stack of these spheres induces unique rough structure, and the superhydrophobic surface exhibited good water repellency with a static water contact angle of 164° and (ii) the corrosion resistance of the superhydrophobic magnesium alloy revealed that superhydrophobic film considerably improved the corrosion resistance performance of magnesium alloy. Gao et al. [31] produced the hierarchical structure fibrous szaibelyite films by a simple template-free hydrothermal synthesis method on AZ31 magnesium alloy. It was mentioned that (i) the static water contact angle was 166° and a SA less than 5° and (ii) the superhydrophobic film maintained excellent corrosion resistance performance, after immersion in a corrosive medium (3.5 wt% NaCl aqueous) for 32 days. Wang et al. [32] fabricated an anticorrosion superhydrophobic film with antibacteria adhesion effect on AZ91D Mg alloy by hydrothermal method. It was reported that (i) the as-prepared superhydrophobic film has a contact angle of 155° and a low SA of ~2°, (ii) electrochemical measurements and long-term immersion test showed that the superhydrophobic film can greatly enhance the corrosion resistance of Mg alloy in the Hank's solution, (iii) cytotoxicity test showed that the superhydrophobic film could effectively lower the toxicity of Mg alloy and (iv) the superhydrophobic film can obviously resist the adhesion of the bacteria on Mg alloy, showing a good antibacteria adhesion effect and then reducing the risk of infection in/after the implanting operation. Zhang et al. [33] produced the superhydrophobic surface on the AZ31 alloy by the combination of the hydrothermal treatment method and post modification with stearic acid. It was indicated that the superhydrophobic surface showed a static water contact angle of 157.6°. Zhang et al. [34] formed coatings of the $Mg(OH)_2$/Mg–Al LDH composite by a combined coprecipitation method and hydrothermal process on the AZ31 alloy substrate in alkaline condition followed by constructing a superhydrophobic surface to modify the composite coatings on the AZ31 alloy substrate using stearic acid. It was mentioned that the superhydrophobic coatings considerably improved the corrosion resistance performance of the LDH coatings on the AZ31 alloy substrate. Li et al. [35] prepared a superhydrophobic surface with peony-like microstructures for corrosion protection of AZ61 Mg; through (1) magnesium hydroxides with appealing peony-like microstructures were constructed on AZ61 Mg by a simple water-only hydrothermal oxidation method and (2) the surface was modified by a low-surface-energy compound, dodecafluoroheptyl-propyl-trimethoxylsilane (Actyflon G502). It was reported that (i) the water contact angle was 152.1° and (ii) the corrosion resistance of the as-prepared superhydrophobic layer is 35,149 $\Omega \cdot cm^2$, much higher than that of the hydrothermally formed sample (4,435 $\Omega \cdot cm^2$), which can decrease the corrosion current density of AZ61 Mg to about one-eighth of that of the untreated sample and to about one-fourth of that of the hydrothermally treated sample relying on the obstructive and capillary effects.

12.5 Etching

Etching is a simple and effective route to form a rough and hierarchical structure on the surface of metals and alloys, including Al [36–38], Cu [36, 37], Zn [36] and Si [39–41]. There are several researches done on Mg materials. Yin et al. [42] fabricated the superhydrophobic coating on the surface of magnesium alloy AZ31 by chemical etching and surface modification. It was shown that (i) the rough and porous micro–nano structure was presented on the surface of magnesium alloy, and the contact angle could reach up to 157.3 ± 0.5° with SA smaller than 10° and (ii) the results of electrochemical measurements showed that anticorrosion property of magnesium alloy was improved. Wan et al. [43] constructed micro-nanometer-scale structure of nubby clusters overlay on the surface of an AZ31 magnesium alloy by a wet chemical method. It was reported that the superhydrophobicity was achieved with a water contact angle of 142° and a SA of about 5° and (ii) potentiodynamic polarization and electrochemical impedance spectroscopy tests showed that the superhydrophobic treatment could improve the corrosion resistance of magnesium alloys in phosphate-buffered saline solution and inhibit blood platelet adhesion on the surface, which implied excellent hemocompatibility with controlled degradation. Feng et al. [44] fabricated a superhydrophobic AZ91 by sulfuric acid etching, $AgNO_3$ treatment and dodecyl mercaptan modification. It was found that the water contact angle was 154° and a SA of 5°, indicating that the magnesium alloy with higher water contact angle has better corrosion resistance, while the magnesium alloy with the superhydrophobic property has the best corrosion resistance. Wang et al. [45] fabricated superhydrophobic surfaces on the AZ31 Mg alloy by etching in the $CuCl_2$ followed by immersion in the oleic acid ($C_{18}H_{34}O_2$). It was mentioned that (i) the surface water contact angle was 155°, (ii) the formation of the superhydrophobic film is due to a combination of a three-dimensional porous structure and a low surface energy film, (iii) the corrosion resistance of the samples with the superhydrophobic films has been significantly improved when compared with the corrosion resistance of the bare Mg alloy and (iv) the superhydrophobic film has good stability when exposed to air for 6 months.

12.6 Wettability

Even dealing the same Mg-based biomaterials, the surface requirements are sometimes quite opposite; namely from hydrophobility to hydrophilicity (with good wettability). The latter becomes more important when wettability of a biomaterial is expected to play a vital role in cell adhesion and proliferation.

Manne et al. [46] utilized the laser surface melting (LSM) to tailor initial corrosion rates of Mg–2.2Zn alloy implants. It was found that (i) the LSM resulted in much finer cellular microstructural features than as-cast alloy and the melted region depths between 65 and 115 μm, (ii) higher treatment depths helped to extend the corrosion protection time by suppressing the corrosion front movement, (iii) polished LSM samples resulted in overall corrosion rates of 0.5–0.62 mm/year which was about 40–50% reduction compared to the as-cast alloy and (iv) accelerated biomineralization of the surface via enhancements in the surface energy due to microstructural refinement as well as microstructural homogeneity and Zn enrichment in α-Mg favored improvement of the overall corrosion performance of LSM-treated alloy. Khadka et al. [47] examined the wetting behavior of the Mg alloy (WE54), which was tailored by LSM method. The effective change on wettability properties of WE54 after LSM process was studied under deionized water and simulated body fluid. It was reported that (i) cellular structure and some buds were observed on the laser melted surface of WE54, (ii) evaporation of Mg and enrichment of Y up to 12.10% and 13.43% were observed and (iii) the contact angle was reduced from 81° to 41.03° in deionized water after laser treatment, whereas in simulated body fluid it was reduced to 23.13° indicating that WE54 alloy also has a biowettability characteristic, which is very important for bioapplications. Sasikumar et al. [48] prepared the dicalcium phosphate dihydrate (DCPD) brushite coating with flake like crystal structure for the protection of AZX310 and AM50 magnesium (Mg) alloys through chemical deposition treatment. Chemical deposition treatment was employed using $Ca(NO_3)_2 \cdot 4H_2O$ and KH_2PO_4 along with subsequent heat treatment. It was reported that (i) hydrophilic nature of the DCPD coatings was confirmed by contact angle measurements and (ii) electrochemical immersion and in vitro studies were evaluated to measure the corrosion performance and biocompatibility performance, and the deposition of DCPD coating for HTI AM50 enables a tenfold increase in the corrosion resistance compared with AZX310, indicating that the ability to offer such significant improvement in corrosion resistance for HTI AM50 coupled with more bioactive nature of the DCPD coating is a viable approach for the development of Mg-based degradable implant materials. Ji et al. [8] mentioned that the surface wettability of Mg–Li alloy transition from high hydrophobicity to superhydrophilicity can be achieved by UV irradiation, and subsequently, the high hydrophobicity can recover to hydrophobicity via stearic acid remodification.

There are mechanical and/or a combined method of mechanical and chemical etching to create the surface hydrophilicity reported by Oshida et al. [49–51]. In particular, the hybrid roughening can be achieved by macroroughness generated by shot peening, followed by chemical treatment to microroughening. It was reported that (i) the roughness and surface water contact angle are linearly related; (ii) as shot-peened surfaces of pure Ti, Ti–6Al–4 V and NiTi are 54.8°, 50.5° and 59.2°, they have been changed to 28.7°, 32.1° and 40.2°, respectively, after treated in 1% NaCl 30 °C solution for 30 min.

References

[1] Yeganeh M, Mohammadi N. Superhydrophobic surface of Mg alloys: A review. Journal of Magnesium and Alloys. 2018, 6, 59–70.
[2] Oshida Y. Surface Engineering and Technology for Biomedical Implants. Momentum Press, New York NY, 2014.
[3] Nuraji N, Khan WS, Lei Y, Ceylan M, Asmatulu R. Superhydrophobic electrospun nanofibers. Journal of Materials Chemistry A. 2013, 1929–46.
[4] Kuang J, Ba Z, Li Z, Jia Y, Wang Z. Fabrication of a superhydrophobic Mg-Mn layered double hydroxides coating on pure magnesium and its corrosion resistance. Surface & Coatings Technology. 2019, 361, 75–82.
[5] Wang Y, Gu Z, Xin Y, Yuan N, Ding J. Facile formation of super-hydrophobic nickel coating on magnesium alloy with improved corrosion resistance. Colloids and Surfaces. A, Physicochemical and Engineering Aspects. 2018, 538, 500–5.
[6] Luo D, Liu Y, Yin X, Wang H, Ren L. Corrosion inhibition of hydrophobic coatings fabricated by micro-arc oxidation on an extruded Mg-5Sn-1Zn alloy substrate. Journal of Alloys and Compounds. 2018, 731, 731–8.
[7] Shi L, Hu J, Lin XD, Fang L, Meng FM. A robust superhydrophobic PPS-PTFE/SiO2 composite coating on AZ31 Mg alloy with excellent wear and corrosion resistance properties. Journal of Alloys and Compounds. 2017, 721, 157–63.
[8] Ji P, Long R, Hou L, Wu R, Zhang M. Study on hydrophobicity and wettability transition of Ni-Cu-SiC coating on Mg-Li alloy. Surface & Coatings Technology. 2018, 350, 428–35.
[9] Ishizaki T, Chiba S, Watanabe K, Suzuki H. Corrosion resistance of Mg–Al layered double hydroxide container-containing magnesium hydroxide films formed directly on magnesium alloy by chemical-free steam coating. Journal of Material Chemistry A 2013, 1, 8968–77.
[10] Wang Z, Li Q, She, Chen F, Li L. Low-cost and large-scale fabrication method for an environmentally-friendly superhydrophobic coating on magnesium alloy. Journal of Materials Chemistry. 2012, 22, 4097–105.
[11] Li Z, Yuan Y. Preparation and characterization of superhydrophobic composite coatings on a magnesium–lithium alloy. Royal Society of Chemistry Advances. 2016, 6, 90587–96.
[12] La M, Zhou H, Li N, Xin Y, Jin P. Improved performance of Mg–Y alloy thin film switchable mirrors after coating with a superhydrophobic surface. Applied Surface Science. 2017, 403, 23–8.
[13] Kang Z, Lai X, Sang J, Li Y. Fabrication of hydrophobic/super-hydrophobic nanofilms on magnesium alloys by polymer plating. Thin Solid Films. 2011, 520, 800–6.
[14] Yilgor I, Bilgin S, Isik M, Yilgor E. Facile preparation of superhydrophobic polymer surfaces. Polymer. 2012, 53, 1180–8.
[15] Yang N, Li J, Bai N, Xu L, Li Q. One step phase separation process to fabricate superhydrophobic PVC films and its corrosion prevention for AZ91D magnesium alloy. Material Science and Engineering B. 2016, 209, 1–9.
[16] Song J, Lu Y, Huang S, Liu X, Xu W. A simple immersion approach for fabricating superhydrophobic Mg alloy surfaces. Applied Surface Science. 2013, 266, 445–50.
[17] Chu Q, Liang J, Hao J. Facile fabrication of a robust super-hydrophobic surface on magnesium alloy. Collloids and Surfaces. A, Physicochemical and Engineering Aspects. 2014, 443, 118–22.
[18] Qiu Z, Sun J, Wang R, Zhang Y, Wu X. Magnet-induced fabrication of a superhydrophobic surface on ZK60 magnesium alloy. Surface Coating of Technology 2016, 286, 246–50.
[19] Liu Y, Li S, Wang Y, Wang H, Gao K, Han Z, Ren L. Superhydrophobic and superoleophobic surface by electrodeposition on magnesium alloy substrate: Wettability and corrosion inhibition. Journal of Colloid and Interface Science 2016, 478, 164–71.

[20] Han B, Yang Y, Fang L, Peng G, Yang C. Electrodeposition of Super-Hydrophobic Nickel Film on Magnesium Alloy AZ31 and Its Corrosion Resistance. International Journal of Electrochemical Science 2016, 11, 9206–15.
[21] Jia J, Fan J, Xu B, Dong H. Microstructure and properties of the super-hydrophobic films fabricated on magnesium alloys. Journal of Alloy Compounds 2013, 554, 142–6.
[22] Li W, Kang Z. Fabrication of corrosion resistant superhydrophobic surface with self-cleaning property on magnesium alloy and its mechanical stability. Surface Coating of Technology 2014, 253, 205–13.
[23] She Z, Li Q, Wang Z, Tan C, Zhou J, Li L. Highly anticorrosion, self-cleaning superhydrophobic Ni–Co surface fabricated on AZ91D magnesium alloy. Surface Coating of Technology 2014, 251, 7–14.
[24] Liu Q, Chen D, Kang Z. One-Step Electrodeposition Process To Fabricate Corrosion-Resistant Superhydrophobic Surface on Magnesium Alloy. ACS Applied Materials Interfaces. 2015, 7, 1859–67.
[25] Khaselev O, Yahalom J. Constant Voltage Anodizing of Mg-Al Alloys in KOH-Al(OH)3 Solutions. Journal of the Electrochemical Society 1998, 145, 190–3.
[26] Mizutani Y, Kim SJ, Ichino R, Okido M. Anodizing of Mg alloys in alkaline solutions. Surface Coating Technology. 2003, 169, 143–6.
[27] Liu F, Shan DY, Song YW, Han EH, Ke W. Corrosion behavior of the composite ceramic coating containing zirconium oxides on AM30 magnesium alloy by plasma electrolytic oxidation. Corrosion Science. 2011, 53, 3845–52.
[28] Wang J, Li D, Gao R, Liu Q, Jiang Z. Construction of superhydrophobic hydromagnesite films on the Mg alloy. Materials Chemistry and Physics. 2011, 129, 154–60.
[29] Ou J, Hu W, Xue M, Wang F, Li W. Superhydrophobic Surfaces on Light Alloy Substrates Fabricated by a Versatile Process and Their Corrosion Protection. ACS Applied Material Interface 2013, 5, 3101–7.
[30] Gao R, Wang J, Zhang X, Yan H, Yang W, Liu Q, Zhang M, Liu L, Takahashi K. Fabrication of superhydrophobic magnesium alloy through the oxidation of hydrogen peroxide. Lloids and Surfaces. A, Physicochemical and Engineering Aspects. 2013, 436, 906–11.
[31] Gao R, Liu Q, Wang J, Zhang X, Yang W, Liu J, Liu L. Fabrication of fibrous szaibelyite with hierarchical structure superhydrophobic coating on AZ31 magnesium alloy for corrosion protection. Chemical. Engineering Journal 2014, 241, 352–9.
[32] Wang Z, Su Y, Li Q, Liu Y, She Z, Chen F, Li L, Zhang X, Zhang P. Researching a highly anti-corrosion superhydrophobic film fabricated on AZ91D magnesium alloy and its anti-bacteria adhesion effect. Materials of Characterization 2015, 99, 200–9.
[33] Zhang F, Zhang C, Song L, Zeng R, Li S, Cui H. Fabrication of the Superhydrophobic Surface on Magnesium Alloy and Its Corrosion Resistance. Journal of Materials Science and Technol. 2015, 31, 1139–43.
[34] Zhang F, Zhang C, Zeng R, Song L, Guo L, Huang X. Corrosion Resistance of the Superhydrophobic $Mg(OH)_2$/Mg-Al Layered Double Hydroxide Coatings on Magnesium Alloys. Metals. 2016, 6, 85–97.
[35] Li L, He J, Lei J, Liu L, Pan F. Anticorrosive superhydrophobic AZ61 Mg surface with peony-like microstructures. Journal of the Taiwan Institute of Chemical Engineers. 2017, 75, 240–7.
[36] Qian BT, Shen ZQ. Fabrication of Superhydrophobic Surfaces by Dislocation-Selective Chemical Etching on Aluminum, Copper, and Zinc Substrates. Langmuir. 2005, 21, 9007–9.
[37] Lee JP, Choi S, Park S. Extremely Superhydrophobic Surfaces with Micro- and Nanostructures Fabricated by Copper Catalytic Etching. Langmuir. 2011, 27, 809–14.
[38] Saleema N, Sarkar D, Paynter R, Chen X-G. Superhydrophobic Aluminum Alloy Surfaces by a Novel One-Step Process. ACS Applied Materials Interfaces. 2010, 2, 2500–2.

[39] Song J, Xu W, Liu X, Y. Lu, Z. Wei, L. Wu. Ultrafast fabrication of rough structures required by superhydrophobic surfaces on Al substrates using an immersion method. Chemical. Engineering Journal 2012, 211/212, 143–52.

[40] Huang Z, Geyer N, Werner P, de Boor J, Gösele U. Metal-Assisted Chemical Etching of Silicon: A Review. Advanced Materials 2011, 23, 285–308.

[41] Xiu Y, Zhu L, Hess DW, Wong CP. Hierarchical Silicon Etched Structures for Controlled Hydrophobicity/Superhydrophobicity. Nano Letters. 2007, 7, 3388–93.

[42] Yin B, Fang L, Hu J. Preparation and properties of super-hydrophobic coating on magnesium alloy. Applied Surface Science 2010, 257, 1666–71.

[43] Wan P, Wu J, Tan L, Zhang B, Yang K. Research on super-hydrophobic surface of biodegradable magnesium alloys used for vascular stents. Materials of Science and Engineering 2013, 33, 2885–90.

[44] Feng L, Zhu Y, Fan W, Wang Y, Qiang X, Liu Y. Fabrication and corrosion resistance of superhydrophobic magnesium alloy. Applied Physics A. 2015, 120, 561–70.

[45] Wang H, Wei Y, Liang M, Hou L, Guo C. Fabrication of stable and corrosion-resisted superhydrophobic film on Mg alloy. Colloids and Surfaces. A, Physicochemical and Engineering Aspects. 2016, 509, 351–8.

[46] Manne B, Thiruvayapati H, Bontha S, Rangarasaiah RM, Balla VK. Surface design of Mg-Zn alloy temporary orthopaedic implants: Tailoring wettability and biodegradability using laser surface melting. Surface & Coatings Technology. 2018, 347, 337–49.

[47] Khadka I, Castagne S, Wang Z, Zheng H. Investigation of wettability properties of laser surface modified rare earth Mg alloy. Procedia Engineering. 2016, 141, 63–9.

[48] Sasikumar Y, Madhan Kumar A, Suresh Babu R, Mizanur Rahman M, Samyn LM, de Barros ALF. Biocompatible hydrophilic brushite coatings on AZX310 and AM50 alloys for orthopaedic implants. Journal of Materials Science. Materials in Medicine. 2018, 29; DOI: 10.1007/s10856-018-6131-8.

[49] Oshida Y, Sachdeva R, Miyazaki S. Changes in contact angles as a function of time on some pre-oxidized bio-materials. Journal of Materials Science: Materials in Medicine. 1992,3, 306–12.

[50] Oshida Y, Sachdeva R, Miyazaki S. Effects of Shot Peening on Surface Contact Angles of Biomaterials, Journal of Materials Science: Materials in Medicine. 1993, 4, 443–7.

[51] Lim YJ, Oshida Y, Barco T, Andres CJ. Surface characterization of variously treated titanium materials. International Journal of Oral & Maxillofacial Implants. 2001, 16, 333–42.

Chapter 13
Surface modifications

The surface of a material defines the boundary of an object and is not just a free end of a substance, but it is a contact and boundary zone with other substances (either in gaseous, liquid or solid). A physical system which comprises a homogeneous component such as solid, liquid or gas and is clearly distinguishable from each other is called a phase, and a boundary at which two or three of these individual phases are in contact is called an interface. Surface and interface reactions include reactions with organic or inorganic materials, vital or nonvital species and hostile or friendly environments. Surface activities may vary from mechanical actions (fatigue crack initiation and propagation, stress intensification, etc.), chemical action (discoloration, tarnishing, contamination, corrosion, oxidation, etc.), mechanochemical action (corrosion fatigue, stress-corrosion cracking, etc.), thermomechanical action (thermal fatigue), tribological and biotribological actions (wear and wear debris toxicity, friction, etc.) to physical and biophysical actions (surface contact and adhesion, adsorption, absorption, diffusion, cellular attachment, cell proliferation and differentiation, etc.). Consequently, the properties of the surface determine the interaction of the second material. The surface of an object determines various properties and reactivity (especially chemical); for example, in large objects with small surface area to volume ratio, the physical and chemical properties are primarily defined by the bulk; whilst in small objects with a large surface area to volume ratio, the properties are strongly influenced by the surface. Among various publications regarding the surface and interface and, in particular, surface modifications, there are several reviews for enhancing biofunctionality, facilitating surface chemical/electrochemical activities and improving biocompatibility as well as controlling biotribological actions [1–8].

Corrosion rate (particularly of Mg biomaterials) in biological environment (or biodegradation rate) becomes crucial and it is more difficult to control its rate since the chemical reaction of Mg at the initial stage is different from that during a long-term usage. The degradation rate of the initial state of the alloy is related to the amount of hydrogen evolution; while the degradation rate of implants during the healing time should be controlled since the required degradation rate depends on the application with lifetime and stability of the implant and the potential of the surrounding tissue to tolerate pH changes and high ion concentrations [5].

Surfaces can be modified through mechanical, chemical and electrochemical, physical, thermal methods or combination of these to meet predetermined specific aims. From a different point of view, it can be said that surfaces can be treated by

https://doi.org/10.1515/9783110676945-013

additive methods (for creating convex surfaces), such as the hydroxyapatite powder or titanium beads plasma spray coating, or they can also be modified by subtractive methods (for creating concave surfaces) such as acid pickling, acid etching, sand blasting and other small particle blasting to change the texture.

13.1 Mechanical modification

The effects of shot peening (including sand blasting, shot peening with various shot media and even laser peeing) possess several merits. They should include (i) enlargement of effective surface area, (ii) development of surface compressive residual stress (which is beneficial in mechanical behavior and prevent crack initiation and growth) and (iii) hardening surface zone to improve corrosion resistance as well as tribological resistance [9–11]. Tool-based material removal, that is, machining, is another mechanical surfacing process to improve corrosion resistance by generating a high finish on machined Mg-based implants [12]. Low plasticity burnishing, analogous to deep rolling, is a new mechanical treatment process used to improve the corrosion and the fatigue resistance of metallic alloys. It produces cold work hardening and introduces minimal plastic deformation generating compressive residual stress into the subsurface [13].

13.2 Chemical and thermal modifications

Chemical modifications are conducted to cover the surface of Mg alloys that are synthesized through chemical or electrochemical reactions [7]. Chemical modifications generally include acid etching, alkaline heat treatment, fluoride treatment, anodic oxidation and microarc oxidation (MAO) [14].

13.3 Physical modification

The modifications aim to offer a physical barrier to improve the corrosion resistance of magnesium substrates. The physical modifications can be performed by introducing apatite coatings, polymer coatings, laser surface processing, or cold spray coatings [7, 15]. Apatite is a main inorganic component of natural bone. It can remarkably promote the recovery of bone fracture due to its excellent bioactivity. Besides, apatite also could improve the degradation resistance of implants as a protective layer due to its relatively low solubility and high thermal stability [16]. Considering the limitations of single chemical and physical treatments, composite modifications that involve both chemical and physical treatments have been gaining increasing attention. It has been reported that double-modified layers effectively improve biodegradation resistance of substrates and control degradation rates over a larger range [14].

Except the mechanical manipulation, the rest of surface modification is related to coating technology. There are two types of coating preparation: conversion and deposition. Conversion coatings are generally developed via chemical or electrochemical reactions between the substrate and the external coating material or the environment. On the other hand, deposited coatings are mostly metallic-based coatings and are widely known, for example, varnishing in the automotive industry. In some cases, a conversion layer is developed on the substrate as a pretreatment before applying the final coating to increase the adhesion strength. While the conversion process is used in many applications such as automotive industries, the deposition process is a widely used and accepted process for biomedical coatings [6, 17]. Numerous types of coating materials have been employed, including fluoride, $Mg(OH)_2$ films, calcium phosphate (CaP), hydroxyapatite, diopside ($CaMgSi_2O_6$), titania (TiO_2) or zirconia (ZrO_2). These coating materials are coated via various techniques such as chemical conversion treatment, MAO, plasma electrolytic oxidation, electrochemical deposition, anodization, ion implantation or physical vapor deposition.

Table 13.1 lists these modification techniques in relation to their significant influences on Mg-based materials.

Table 13.1: Various surface modifications and their major influence(s).

	Fatigue Tribology	Corrosion degradation	Microstructure Refining	Mechanical property Strength	Ductility	Regeneration	Bioactivity	Cytocompatibility	Antibacterial reaction	Cell responses	Biomineralization	Biocompatibility	Hemocompatibility
Mechanical process													
Shot peening	[18–21]	[22, 23]	[21]										
Laser peening			[24, 25]	[26]	[27]								
Laser ablation		[28]		[28]									
Machining	[29]	[30–32]											
Friction stir		[33]	[34–37]	[33, 38, 39]	[34]								
Coating with polymeric materials													
Epoxy		[40–42]											
PCL, PLA		[43]											
DCPD		[44]											
Polyurethane		[45–47]				[47]							
PEEK							[48]						
Polypyrrole		[49]											
Chitosan						[50]							

Coating with hydroxyapatite and others										
HA	[51–59]		[60, 61]		[54]	[54]				
Sr-doped HA	[62, 63]					[64]	[65]			
F-doped HA			[66]				[67]		[68]	
HA composite	[69–71]		[69]	[70]		[71]				
Ca-P	[72–77]	[79]		[79]	[77]		[78]	[80]		
Ca-P comp	[81–85]			[85]		[86]			[86]	
TCP	[87, 88]		[88]	[89]						
Coating with metallic elements										
Ti	[90–92]									
Nd	[93]				[93]					
Al	[91, 94–96]		[96–98]							
Zr	[91]									
Hf	[91]									
Cr	[99]									
Ca			[100]							
Zn					[101]					
Ag				[102]		[102]				
Si										[103]

(continued)

Table 13.1 (continued)

	Fatigue Tribology	Corrosion degradation	Microstructure Refining	Mechanical property Strength	Ductility	Regeneration	Bioactivity	Cytocompatibility	Antibacterial reaction	Cell responses	Biomineralization	Biocompatibility	Hemocompatibility
Cu		[104]											
Coating with metallic oxides													
TiO2		[105–107]						[105]					
ZrO2		[108–112]							[112]				
V2O5		[113]											
ZnO		[114, 115]							[115]				
LDHs		[116–129]											
Minerals		[120–126]		[120]			[120]	[120]	[122]				
Coating with ceramics													
Glass-ceramic		[127, 130]											
Ceramics	[129]		[129]										
Coating with composites													
MMC		[130–134]											
CMC	[135]	[115, 136–142]	[78]					[139]	[115]	[78]			

PMC		[28, 143]				[144]			[143]		[143]
Modified via											
MAO	[145]	[145–159]	[152]	[145]	[160]	[161]	[148]	[159]		[155]	
PEO	[162]	[163–162]	[164]	[163, 164]	[165]						[166]

Note: PCL, polycaprolactone; PLA, polylactic acid; DCPD, dicalcium phosphate-dihydrate; PEEK, polyether ether ketone; LDS, layered double hydroxide; MMC, metal matrix composite; CMC, ceramic matrix composite; PMC, polymer matrix composite; MAO, microarc oxidation coating; PEO, plasma electrolytic oxidation.

References

[1] Hanawa T. Surface treatment and modification of metals to add biofunction. Dental Materials Journal. 2017, 36, 533–8.
[2] Oshida Y. Surface Engineering and Technology for Biomedical Implants. Momentum Press, New York NY, 2014.
[3] Oshida Y, Tuna EB. Science and Technology Integrated Titanium Dental Implant Systems. In: Basu B et al., ed., Advanced Biomaterials. Wiley, Hoboken, NJ, 2009, 143–177.
[4] Oshida Y, Guven Y. Biocompatible coating s for metallic biomaterials. In: Wen C ed., Surface Coating and Modification of Metallic Biomaterials. Woodhead Pub., Cambridge UK, 2015, 287–343.
[5] Gawlik MM, Wiese B, Desharnais V, Ebel T, Willumeit-Römer R. The effect of surface treatments on the degradation of biomedical Mg alloys – A Review Paper. Materials (Basel). 2018, 11; doi: 10.3390/ma11122561.
[6] Uddin MS, Hall C, Murphy P. Surface treatments for controlling corrosion rate of biodegradable Mg and Mg-based alloy implants. Science and Technology of Advanced Materials. 2015, 16; doi:10.1088/1468-6996/16/5/053501.
[7] Liu C, Ren Z, Xu Y, Pang S, Zhao X, Zhao Y. Biodegradable magnesium alloys developed as bone repair materials: a review. Scanning. 2018; https://doi.org/10.1155/2018/9216314.
[8] Asgari M, Hang R, Wang C, Yu Z, Li Z, Xiao Y, Biodegradable metallic wires in dental and orthopedic applications: a review. Metals. 2018, 8, 212; https://doi.org/10.3390/met8040212.
[9] Azar V, Hashemi B, Yazdi MR. The effect of shot peening on fatigue and corrosion behavior of 316L stainless steel in Ringer's solution. Surface & Coatings Technology. 2010, 204, 3546–51.
[10] Oshida Y, Sachdeva R, Miyazaki S. Effects of shot peening on surface contact angles of biomaterials, Journal of Materials Science: Materials in Medicine. 1993, 4, 443–7.
[11] Oshida Y, Daly J. Fatigue Damage Evaluation of Shot-Peened High Strength Aluminum Alloy, In: Meguid SA ed., Surface Engineering, Elsevier Applied Science, London. 1990, 404–16.
[12] von der Höh N, von Rechenberg B, Bormann D, Lucas A, Meyer-Lindenberg A. Influence of different surface machining treatments of resorbable magnesium alloy implants on degradation – EDX-analysis and histology results. Materialwissenshaft Und Werkstofftechnik. 2009, 40, 88–93.
[13] Disegi J, Sax C. Effect of low plasticity burnishing on the fatigue strength of spinal rods. In: Gilbert J ed., Materials and Processes for Medical Devices, Conf. and Expo; Minneapolis, MN. 2009, 220–4.
[14] Wang J, Tang J, Zhang P, Li Y, Lai Y, Qin L. Surface modification of magnesium alloys developed for bioabsorbable orthopedic implants: a general review. Journal of Biomedical Materials Research. Part B, Applied Biomaterials. 2012, 100, 1691–701.
[15] Tian P, Liu X. Surface modification of biodegradable magnesium and its alloys for biomedical applications. Regenerative Biomaterials. 2015, 2, 135–51.
[16] Narayanan R, Seshadri SK, Kwon TY, Kim KH. Calcium phosphate-based coatings on titanium and its alloys. Journal of Biomedical Materials Research. Part B, Applied Biomaterials. 2007, 85, 279–9.
[17] Hornberger H, Virtanen S, Boccaccini AR. Biomedical coatings on magnesium alloys – a review. Acta Biomaterialia. 2012, 8, 2442–55.
[18] Liu WC et al., Improvement of fatigue properties by shot peening for Mg-10Gd-3Y alloys under different conditions. Material Science and Engineering A. 2011, 528, 5935–44.

[19] Wagner L et al., On Methods for improving the fatigue performance of the wrought magnesium Alloys AZ31 and AZ80. Material Science Forum 2003, 419/422, 93-.102.
[20] Fouad Y et al., Effects of mechanical surface treatments on fatigue performance of extruded ZK60 alloy. Fatigue Amp Fract. Eng. Mater. Amp Struct. 2010, 34, 403–7.
[21] Liu W et al., Grain refinement and fatigue strengthening mechanisms in as-extruded Mg–6Zn–0.5Zr and Mg–10Gd–3Y–0.5Zr magnesium alloys by shot peening. International Journal of Plasticity. 2013, 49, 16–35.
[22] Mhaede M et al., Influence of shot peening on corrosion properties of biocompatible magnesium alloy AZ31 coated by dicalcium phosphate dihydrate (DCPD) Mater. Science Engineering C Materials Biology Application 2014, 39, 330–5.
[23] Liu C et al., Effect of severe shot peening on corrosion behavior of AZ31 and AZ91 magnesium alloys. Journal of Alloys and Compounds. 2019, 770, 500–6.
[24] Lu C et al., Effective femtosecond laser shock peening on a Mg–3Gd alloy at low pulse energy 430 μJ of 1 kHz. Journal of Magnesium and Alloys. 2019,7, 529–35.
[25] Ge M-Z et al., Effect of laser energy on microstructure of Mg-3Al-1Zn alloy treated by LSP. Journal of Alloys and Compounds. 2018, 734, 266–74.
[26] Luo KY et al., Tensile properties, residual stress distribution and grain arrangement as a function of sheet thickness of Mg–Al–Mn alloy subjected to two-sided and simultaneous LSP impacts. Applied Surface Science. 2016, 369, 366–76.
[27] Mao B et al., Enhanced room temperature stretch formability of AZ31B magnesium alloy sheet by laser shock peening. Materials Science and Engineering: A. 2019, 756, 219–25.
[28] Pan Y et al., Improvement in interlaminar strength and galvanic corrosion resistance of CFRP/Mg laminates by laser ablation. Materials Letters. 2017, 207, 4–7.
[29] Disegi J et al., Effect of low plasticity burnishing on the fatigue strength of spinal rods. Presented at the In Proc. of the ASM MPMD (Materials and Processes for Medical Devices) Conf. and Expo; Minneapolis, MN. 2009.
[30] von der Höh N et al., Influence of different surface machining treatments of resorbable magnesium alloy implants on degradation – EDX-analysis and histology results. Materialwissenschaft Und Werkstofftechnik 2009, 40, 88–93.
[31] Denkena B et al., Biocompatible magnesium alloys as absorbable implant materials – adjusted surface and subsurface properties by machining processes. CIRP Annual Manufacturing Technology 2007, 56, 113–6.
[32] Pu Z et al., Ultrafine-grained surface layer on Mg–Al–Zn alloy produced by cryogenic burnishing for enhanced corrosion resistance. Cripta Materialia 2011, 65, 520–3.
[33] Peng J et al., The effect of the inhomogeneous microstructure and texture on the mechanical properties of AZ31 Mg alloys processed by friction stir processing. Journal of Alloys and Compounds. 2019, 792, 16–24.
[34] Patel V et al., Homogeneous Grain Refinement and Ductility Enhancement in AZ31B Magnesium Alloy Using Friction Stir Processing. In: Joshi V. et al., ed., Magnesium Technology 2019. The Minerals, Metals & Materials Series. Springer, 2019, 83–87.
[35] Mertens A et al., Influence of fibre distribution and grain size on the mechanical behaviour of friction stir processed Mg–C composites. Materials Characterization. 2015, 107, 125–33.
[36] Zhang W et al., Effect of grain refinement and crystallographic texture produced by friction stir processing on the biodegradation behavior of a Mg-Nd-Zn alloy. Journal of Materials Science & Technology. 2019, 35, 777–83.
[37] Wang C et al., Improvement in grain refinement efficiency of Mg-Zr master alloy for magnesium alloy by friction stir processing. Journal of Magnesium and Alloy. 2014, 2, 239–44.

[38] Xu N et al., Enhanced strength and ductility of high pressure die casting AZ91D Mg alloy by using cold source assistant friction stir processing. Materials Letters. 2017, 190, 24–7.

[39] Han J et al., Microstructure, texture and mechanical properties of friction stir processed Mg-14Gd alloys. Materials & Design. 2017, 130, 90–102.

[40] Lu X et al., Improvement of protection performance of Mg-rich epoxy coating on AZ91D magnesium alloy by DC anodic oxidation. Progress in Organic Coatings. 2017, 104, 188–98.

[41] Xu P et al, Investigation of the surface modification of magnesium particles with stannate on the corrosion resistance of a Mg-rich epoxy coating on AZ91D magnesium alloy. Progress in Organic Coatings. 2019, 135, 591–600.

[42] Brusciotti F et al., Hybrid epoxy–silane coatings for improved corrosion protection of Mg alloy. Corrosion Science 2013, 67, 82–90.

[43] Chen Y et al., Interaction between a high purity magnesium surface and PCL and PLA coatings during dynamic degradation. Biomedical Materials. 2011; doi: 10.1088/1748-6041/6/2/025005.

[44] Zhao C et al., Enhanced corrosion resistance and antibacterial property of Zn doped DCPD coating on biodegradable Mg. Materials Letters. 2016, 180, 42–6.

[45] Wang C et al., Development of a novel biodegradable and anti-bacterial polyurethane coating for biomedical magnesium rods. Materials Science & Engineering. C, Materials for Biological Applications. 2019, 99, 344–56.

[46] Liu J et al., Arginine-leucine based poly (ester urea urethane) coating for Mg-Zn-Y-Nd alloy in cardiovascular stent applications. Colloids and Surfaces. B, Biointerfaces. 2017, 159, 78–88.

[47] Monfared A et al., Fabrication of tannic acid/poly(N-vinylpyrrolidone) layer-by-layer coating on Mg-based metallic glass for nerve tissue regeneration application. Colloids and Surfaces. B, Biointerfaces. 2018, 170, 617–26.

[48] Yu X et al., Biofunctional Mg coating on PEEK for improving bioactivity. Bioactive Materials 2018, 3, 139–43.

[49] Hatami M et al., Improvement in the protective performance and adhesion of polypyrrole coating on AZ31 Mg alloys. Progress in Natural Science: Materials International. 2015, 25, 478–85.

[50] Guo Y et al., Biocompatibility and osteogenic activity of guided bone regeneration membrane based on chitosan-coated magnesium alloy. Materials Science and Engineering: C. 2019, 100, 226–35.

[51] Yang H et al., In vitro corrosion and cytocompatibility properties of nano-whisker hydroxyapatite coating on magnesium alloy for bone tissue engineering applications. International Journal of Molecular Sciences. 2015, 16, 6113–23.

[52] Wang B et al., In vitro corrosion and cytocompatibility of ZK60 magnesium alloy coated with hydroxyapatite by a simple chemical conversion process for orthopedic applications. International Journal of Molecular Sciences. 2013, 14, 23614–28.

[53] Iskandar ME et al., The effects of nanostructured hydroxyapatite coating on the biodegradation and cytocompatibility of magnesium implants. Journal of Biomedical Materials Research. Part A. 2013, 101, 2340–54.

[54] Ji X-J et al., Corrosion resistance and antibacterial properties of hydroxyapatite coating induced by gentamicin-loaded polymeric multilayers on magnesium alloys. Colloids and Surfaces. B, Biointerfaces. 2019, 179, 429–36.

[55] Wen C et al., Characterization and degradation behavior of AZ31 alloy surface modified by bone-like hydroxyapatite for implant applications. Applied Surface Science 2009, 255, 6433–8.

[56] Mardali M et al., The effect of an MgO intermediate layer on a nanostructured HA coating fabricated by HVOF on an Mg alloy. Surface & Coatings Technology. 2019, 374, 1071–7.

[57] Prakash C et al., Multi-objective particle swarm optimization of EDM parameters to deposit HA-coating on biodegradable Mg-alloy. Vacuum. 2018, 158, 180–90.
[58] Li Q et al., Improving the corrosion resistance of ZEK100 magnesium alloy by combining high-pressure torsion technology with hydroxyapatite coating. Materials & Design 2019, 181, 5 November 2019, 181; https://doi.org/10.1016/j.matdes.2019.107933.
[59] Sankar M et al., Comparison of electrochemical behavior of hydroxyapatite coated onto WE43 Mg alloy by electrophoretic and pulsed laser deposition. Surface & Coatings Technology. 2017, 309, 840–8.
[60] Kannan MB et al., In vitro mechanical integrity of hydroxyapatite coated magnesium alloy. Biomedical Materials 2011, 6; doi: 10.1088/1748-6041/6/4/045003.
[61] Surmeneva MA et al., Enhancement of the mechanical properties of AZ31 magnesium alloy via nanostructured hydroxyapatite thin films fabricated via radio-frequency magnetron sputtering. Journal of Mechanical Behaviour Biomedicine Materials 2015, 46, 127–36.
[62] Wang T et al., One-pot hydrothermal synthesis, in vitro biodegradation and biocompatibility of Sr-doped nanorod/nanowire hydroxyapatite coatings on ZK60 magnesium alloy. Journal of Alloys and Compounds. 2019, 799, 71–82.
[63] Zhao D-P et al., Effects of Sr incorporation on surface structure and corrosion resistance of hydroxyapatite coated Mg-4Zn alloy for biomedical applications. Transactions of Nonferrous Metals Society of China. 2018, 28, 1563–70.
[64] Zhang Y et al., Composite coatings of Mg-MOF74 and Sr-substituted hydroxyapatite on titanium substrates for local antibacterial, anti-osteosarcoma and pro-osteogenesis applications. Materials Letters. 2019, 241, 18–22.
[65] Wei S et al., Strontium-doped Hydroxyapatite Coatings Deposited on Mg-4Zn Alloy: Physical-chemical Properties and in vitro Cell Response. Rare Metal Materials and Engineering. 2018, 47, 2371–80.
[66] Bakhsheshi-Rad HR et al., Deposition of nanostructured fluorine-doped hydroxyapatite–polycaprolactone duplex coating to enhance the mechanical properties and corrosion resistance of Mg alloy for biomedical applications. Materials Science and Engineering: C. 2016, 60, 526–37.
[67] Li J et al., The bioactivated interfacial behavior of the fluoridated hydroxyapatite-coated Mg-Zn alloy in cell culture environments. Bioinorganic Chemical Applied 2011; doi: DOI: 10.1155/2011/192671.
[68] Li J et al., In vitro responses of human bone marrow stromal cells to a fluoridated hydroxyapatite coated biodegradable Mg–Zn alloy. Biomaterials. 2010, 31, 5782–8.
[69] Diez M et al., Hydroxyapatite (HA)/poly-L-lactic acid (PLLA) dual coating on magnesium alloy under deformation for biomedical applications. Journal of Materials Science. Materials in Medicine. 2016, 27; DOI: 10.1007/s10856-015-5643-8.
[70] Abdal-hay A et al., Hydroxyapatite-doped poly(lactic acid) porous film coating for enhanced bioactivity and corrosion behavior of AZ31 Mg alloy for orthopedic applications. Ceramics International. 2013, 39, 183–95.
[71] Ji X-J et al., Corrosion resistance and antibacterial activity of hydroxyapatite coating induced by ciprofloxacin-loaded polymeric multilayers on magnesium ally. Progress in Organic Coatings. 2019, 135, 465–74.
[72] Moussa ME et al., Comparison study of Sn and Bi addition on microstructure and bio-degradation rate of as-cast Mg-4wt% Zn alloy without and with Ca-P coating. Journal of Alloys and Compounds. 2019, 792, 1239–47.
[73] Xia K et al., Effect of Ca/P ratio on the structural and corrosion properties of biomimetic CaP coatings on ZK60 magnesium alloy. Materials Science & Engineering. C, Materials for Biological Applications. 2017, 72, 676–81.

[74] Zhang Y et al., Effects of anodizing biodegradable Mg–Zn–Zr alloy on the deposition of Ca–P coating. Surface & Coatings Technology. 2013, 228, s111-5.

[75] Dorozhkin SV. Calcium orthophosphate coatings on magnesium and its biodegradable alloys. Acta Biomaterialia. 2014, 10, 2919–34.

[76] Cui F et al., Calcium phosphate coating on magnesium alloy for modification of degradation behavior. Frontier Materials Science China. 2008, 2, 143–8.

[77] Xu L-P et al., Biocorrosion property and cytocompatibility of calcium phosphate coated Mg alloy. Transactions of Nonferrous Metals Society of China. 2012, 22, 2014–20.

[78] Du H et al., Surface microstructure and cell compatibility of calcium silicate and calcium phosphate composite coatings on Mg–Zn–Mn–Ca alloy for biomedical application. Colloids and Surfaces. B, Biointerfaces. 2011, 83, 96–102.

[79] Zhang E et al., In vitro and in vivo evaluation of the surface bioactivity of a calcium phosphate coated magnesium alloy. Biomaterials. 2009, 30, 1512–23.

[80] Song Y et al., Electrodeposition of Ca–P coatings on biodegradable Mg alloy: In vitro biomineralization behavior. Acta Biomaterialia. 2010, 6, 1736–42.

[81] Zeng R-C et al., Influence of solution temperature on corrosion resistance of Zn-Ca phosphate conversion coating on biomedical Mg-Li-Ca alloys. Transactions of Nonferrous Metals Society of China. 2013, 23, 3293–9.

[82] Song Y et al., A novel biodegradable nicotinic acid/calcium phosphate composite coating on Mg–3Zn alloy. Materials Science and Engineering: C. 2013, 33, 78–84.

[83] Ke C et al., Interfacial study of the formation mechanism of corrosion resistant strontium phosphate coatings upon Mg-3Al-4.3Ca-0.1Mn. Corrosion Science. 2019, 151, 143–53.

[84] Jayaraj J et al., Investigation on the corrosion behavior of lanthanum phosphate coatings on AZ31 Mg alloy obtained through chemical conversion technique. Journal of Alloys and Compounds. 2019, 784, 1162–74.

[85] Zhang J et al., Degradable behavior and bioactivity of micro-arc oxidized AZ91D Mg alloy with calcium phosphate/chitosan composite coating in m-SBF. Colloids and Surfaces. B, Biointerfaces. 2013, 111, 179–87.

[86] Chang WH et al., In vitro biocompatibility and antibacterial behavior of anodic coatings fabricated in an organic phosphate containing solution on Mg–1.0Ca alloys. Surface & Coatings Technology. 2016, 289, 75–84.

[87] Lu X et al., The influence of aluminum tri-polyphosphate on the protective behavior of Mg-rich epoxy coating on AZ91D magnesium alloy. Electrochimica Acta. 2013, 93, 53–64.

[88] Liao Y et al., In vitro degradation and mechanical properties of polyporous CaHPO4-coated Mg–Nd–Zn–Zr alloy as potential tissue engineering scaffold. Materials Letters. 2013, 100, 306–8.

[89] Camiré CL et al., Material characterization and in vivo behavior of silicon substituted α-tricalcium phosphate cement. Journal of Biomedicine Material Research B Applied Biomaterials 2006, 76B, 424–31.

[90] Wu G et al., Improving corrosion resistance of titanium-coated magnesium alloy by modifying surface characteristics of magnesium alloy prior to titanium coating deposition. Cripta Materialia 2009, 61, 269–72.

[91] Zhang D et al., A comparative study on the corrosion behaviour of Al, Ti, Zr and Hf metallic coatings deposited on AZ91D magnesium alloys. Surface and Coatings Technology A. 2016, 303, 94–102.

[92] Zhao Y et al., Improved surface corrosion resistance of WE43 magnesium alloy by dual titanium and oxygen ion implantation. Thin Solid Films. 2013, 529, 407–11.

[93] Levy GK et al., Cytotoxic characteristics of biodegradable EW10X04 Mg alloy after Nd coating and subsequent heat treatment. Materials Science and Engineering: C. 2016, 62, 752–61.

[94] Tsai W-T et al. Electrodeposition of aluminum on magnesium (Mg) alloys in ionic liquids to improve corrosion resistance. Corrosion Prevention of Magnesium Alloys. 2013, 393–413.
[95] Zhao Y et al., Formation and electrochemical behavior of Al and O plasma-implanted biodegradable Mg-Y-RE alloy. Mater. Chem. Phys. 2012, 132, 187–91.
[96] Daroonparvar M et al., Microstructural characterization and corrosion resistance evaluation of nanostructured Al and Al/AlCr coated Mg–Zn–Ce–La alloy. Journal of Alloys and Compounds. 2014, 615, 657–71.
[97] Wang Q et al., The influence of cold and detonation thermal spraying processes on the microstructure and properties of Al-based composite coatings on Mg alloy. Surface & Coatings Technology. 2018, 352, 627–33.
[98] Chen E et al., Laser cladding of a Mg based Mg–Gd–Y–Zr alloy with Al–Si powders. Applied Surface Science. 2016, 367, 11–8.
[99] Xu R et al., Controllable degradation of biomedical magnesium by chromium and oxygen dual ion implantation. Materials Letters. 2011, 65, 2171–3.
[100] Moussa ME et al., Combined effect of high-intensity ultrasonic treatment and Ca addition on modification of primary Mg2Si and wear resistance in hypereutectic Mg–Si alloys. Journal of Alloys and Compounds. 2014, 615, 576–81.
[101] Liu J et al., Improved cytocompatibility of Mg-1Ca alloy modified by Zn ion implantation and deposition. Materials Letters 2017, 205, 87–9.
[102] Aktug SL et al., Surface and in vitro properties of Ag-deposited antibacterial and bioactive coatings on AZ31 Mg alloy. Surface & Coatings Technology. 2019, 375, 46–53.
[103] Li M et al., Plasma enhanced chemical vapor deposited silicon coatings on Mg alloy for biomedical application. Surface & Coatings Technology. 2013, 228, s262-5.
[104] Wang S-H et al., Electrodeposition of Cu coating with high corrosion resistance on Mg-3.0Nd–0.2Zn–0.4Zr magnesium alloy. Transactions of Nonferrous Metals Society of China. 2014, 24, 3810–7.
[105] Bakhsheshi-Rad HR et al., Fabrication, degradation behavior and cytotoxicity of nanostructured hardystonite and titania/hardystonite coatings on Mg alloys. Vacuum. 2016, 129, 9–12.
[106] Li M et al., Corrosion behavior in SBF for titania coatings on Mg–Ca alloy. Journal of Material Science 2011, 46, 2365–9.
[107] White L et al., TiO2 deposition on AZ31 magnesium alloy using plasma electrolytic oxidation. Journal of Nanomater. 2013; doi: 10.1155/2013/319437.
[108] Xin Y et al., Corrosion resistance of ZrO2–Zr-coated biodegradable surgical magnesium alloy. Journal of Material Research 2008, 23, 312–9.
[109] Wang M-J et al., Electrolytic MgO/ZrO2 duplex-layer coating on AZ91D magnesium alloy for corrosion resistance. Corrosion Science 2013, 76, 142–53.
[110] Phani AR et al., Enhanced corrosion resistance by sol-gel-based ZrO2-CeO2 coatings on magnesium alloys. Welkstoffe Und Korrosion (Material and Corrosion). 2005, 56, 77–82.
[111] Yang Q et al., Atomic layer deposited ZrO2 nanofilm on Mg-Sr alloy for enhanced corrosion resistance and biocompatibility. Acta Biomaterialia. 2017, 58, 515–26.
[112] Daroonparvar M et al., Antibacterial activities and corrosion behavior of novel PEO/nanostructured ZrO2 coating on Mg alloy. Transactions of Nonferrous Metals Society of China. 2018, 28, 1571–81.
[113] Hamdy AS et al., Vanadia-based coatings of self-repairing functionality for advanced magnesium Elektron ZE41 Mg–Zn–rare earth alloy. Surface & Coatings Technology. 2012, 206, 3686–92.
[114] Alves MM et al., In vitro degradation of ZnO flowered coated Zn-Mg alloys in simulated physiological conditions. Materials Science and Engineering: C. 2017, 70, 112–20.

[115] Bakhsheshi-Rad HR et al., Synthesis of a novel nanostructured zinc oxide/baghdadite coating on Mg alloy for biomedical application: In-vitro degradation behavior and antibacterial activities. Ceramics International. 2017, 43, 14842–50

[116] Wang X et al., Duplex coating combining layered double hydroxide and 8-quinolinol layers on Ma alloy for corrosion protection. Electrochimica Acta. 2018, 283, 1845–57.

[117] Zhang F et al., Corrosion resistance of Mg–Al-LDH coating on magnesium alloy AZ31. Surface & Coatings Technology. 2014, 258, 1152–8.

[118] Tang Y et al., A comparative study and optimization of corrosion resistance of ZnAl layered double hydroxides films intercalated with different anions on AZ31 Mg alloys. Surface & Coatings Technology. 2019, 358, 594–603.

[119] Kiang J et al., Fabrication of a superhydrophobic Mg-Mn layered double hydroxides coating on pure magnesium and its corrosion resistance. Surface & Coatings Technology. 2019, 361, 75–82.

[120] Razavi M et al., In vitro study of nanostructured diopside coating on Mg alloy orthopedic implants. Material Science and Engineering C. 2014, 41, 168–77.

[121] Du Y et al., Reduced Graphene Oxide Coating with Anticorrosion and Electrochemical Property-Enhancing Effects Applied in Hydrogen Storage System. ACS Applied Materials & Interfaces. 2017, 9, 28980–9.

[122] Zou YH et al., Corrosion resistance and antibacterial activity of zinc-loaded montmorillonite coatings on biodegradable magnesium alloy AZ31. Acta Biomaterialia. 2019, 98, 196–214.

[123] Niu J et al., Enhanced biocorrosion resistance and biocompatibility of degradable Mg–Nd–Zn–Zr alloy by brushite coating. Materials Science and Engineering: C. 2013, 33, 4833–41.

[124] Li D et al., Hydrotalcite conversion coating on Ma alloy and its corrosion resistance. Journal of Alloys and Compounds. 2010, 494, 271–4.

[125] Wang Y et al., Smart epoxy coating containing Ce-MCM-22 zeolites for corrosion protection of Mg-Li alloy. Applied Surface Science. 2016, 369, 384–9.

[126] Bakhsheshi-Rad HR et al., Synthesis and in-vitro performance of nanostructured monticellite coating on magnesium alloy for biomedical applications. Journal of Alloys and Compounds. 2019, 773, 180–93.

[127] Rau JV et al., Glass-ceramic coated Mg-Ca alloys for biomedical implant applications. Materials Science and Engineering: C. 2016, 64, 362–9.

[128] Ye X et al., Bioactive glass–ceramic coating for enhancing the in vitro corrosion resistance of biodegradable Mg alloy. Applied Surface Science. 2012, 259, 799–805.

[129] Daroonparvar M et al., Microstructural characterisation of air plasma sprayed nanostructure ceramic coatings on Mg–1%Ca alloys (bonded by NiCoCrAlYTa alloy). Ceramics International. 2016, 42, 357–71.

[130] Bakhsheshi-Rad HR et al., Enhancement of corrosion resistance and mechanical properties of Mg–1.2Ca–2Bi via a hybrid silicon-biopolymer coating system. Surface & Coatings Technology. 2016, 301, 133–9.

[131] Bakhsheshi-Rad HR et al., Fabrication and corrosion behavior of Si/HA nano-composite coatings on biodegradable Mg–Zn–Mn–Ca alloy. Surface & Coatings Technology. 2014, 258, 1090–9.

[132] Wang C et al., Effect of single $Si_{1-x}C_x$ coating and compound coatings on the thermal conductivity and corrosion resistance of Mg–3Sn alloy. Journal of Magnesium and Alloys. 2015, 3, 10–15.

[133] Ali W et al., Effect of fluoride coating on degradation behaviour of unidirectional Mg/PLA biodegradable composite for load-bearing bone implant application. Composites. Part A, Applied Science and Manufacturing. 2019, 124; https://doi.org/10.1016/j.compositesa.2019.05.032.

[134] Song Y-W et al., Study on electroless Ni–P–ZrO2 composite coatings on AZ91D magnesium alloys. Surface Engineering 2007, 23, 33–8.
[135] Shen J et al., Fabrication and characterization of TiB2-TiC-Co wear-resistant coatings on AZ91D magnesium alloy. Surface & Coatings Technology. 2019, 364, 358–68.
[136] Xie Z et al., Tribocorrosion behaviors of AlN/MoS2–phenolic resin duplex coatings on nitrogen implanted magnesium alloys. Surface Coating of Technology 2015, 266, 64–9.
[137] Johnson I et al., Nanostructured hydroxyapatite/poly(lactic-co-glycolic acid) composite coating for controlling magnesium degradation in simulated body fluid. Nanotechnology. 2013, 24; DOI: 10.1088/0957-4484/24/37/375103.
[138] Bakhsheshi-Rad HR et al., In vitro degradation behavior, antibacterial activity and cytotoxicity of TiO2-MAO/ZnHA composite coating on Mg alloy for orthopedic implants. Surface & Coatings Technology. 2018, 334, 450–60.
[139] Wang C et al., In vitro degradation and cytocompatibility of a silane/Mg(OH)2 composite coating on AZ31 alloy by spin coating. Journal of Alloys and Compounds. 2017, 714, 186–93.
[140] Córdoba LC et al., Bi-layered silane-TiO2/collagen coating to control biodegradation and biointegration of Mg alloys. Materials Science and Engineering: C. 2019, 94, 126–38.
[141] Li Y et al., Synthesis of stabilized dispersion covalently-jointed SiO2@polyaniline with core-shell structure and anticorrosion performance of its hydrophobic coating for Mg-Li alloy. Applied Surface Science. 2018, 462, 362–72.
[142] Lin JK et al., Formation of Mg, Al-hydrotalcite conversion coating on Mg alloy in aqueous HCO3–/CO32– and corresponding protection against corrosion by the coating. Corrosion Science. 2009, 51, 1181–8.
[143] Ma J et al., Sirolimus-eluting dextran and polyglutamic acid hybrid coatings on AZ31 for stent applications. Journal of Biomaterials Applications. 2015, 30, 579–88.
[144] Córdoba LC et al., Hybrid coatings with collagen and chitosan for improved bioactivity of Mg alloys. Surface & Coatings Technology. 2018, 341, 103–13.
[145] Liang J et al., Characterization of microarc oxidation coatings formed on AM60B magnesium alloy in silicate and phosphate electrolytes. Applied Surface Science. 2007, 253, 4490–6.
[146] Bakhsheshi-Rad HR et al., Fabrication and characterization of hydrophobic microarc oxidation/poly-lactic acid duplex coating on biodegradable Mg–Ca alloy for corrosion protection. Vacuum. 2016, 125, 185–8.
[147] Shi Y et al., MAO-DCPD composite coating on Mg alloy for degradable implant applications. Materials Letters. 2011, 65, 2201–4.
[148] Zeng RC et al., In Vitro Corrosion and Cytocompatibility of a Microarc Oxidation Coating and Poly(L-lactic acid) Composite Coating on Mg-1Li-1Ca Alloy for Orthopedic Implants. ACS Applied Material Interfaces 2016, 8, 10014–28.
[149] Yazici M et al., Biodegradability and antibacterial properties of MAO coatings formed on Mg-Sr-Ca alloys in an electrolyte containing Ag doped hydroxyapatite. Thin Solid Films. 2017, 644, 92–8.
[150] Guo M et al., Anticorrosion and cytocompatibility behavior of MAO/PLLA modified magnesium alloy WE42. Journal of Materials Science. Materials in Medicine. 2011, 22, 1735–40.
[151] Cui L-Y et al., Degradation mechanism of micro-arc oxidation coatings on biodegradable Mg-Ca alloys: The influence of porosity. Journal of Alloys and Compounds. 2017, 695, 2464–76.
[152] Cui X-J et al., Structure and properties of newly designed MAO/TiN coating on AZ31B Mg alloy. Surface & Coatings Technology. 2017, 328, 319–25.
[153] Seyfoori A et al., Biodegradation behavior of micro-arc oxidized AZ31 magnesium alloys formed in two different electrolytes. Applied Surface Science. 2012, 261, 92–100

[154] Luo D et al., Corrosion inhibition of hydrophobic coatings fabricated by micro-arc oxidation on an extruded Mg–5Sn–1Zn alloy substrate. Journal of Alloys and Compounds. 2018, 731, 731–8.
[155] Gu XN et al., Corrosion resistance and surface biocompatibility of a microarc oxidation coating on a Mg–Ca alloy. Acta Biomaterialia. 2011, 7, 1880–9.
[156] Zhang L et al., Advances in microarc oxidation coated AZ31 Mg alloys for biomedical applications. Corrosion Science. 2015, 91, 7–28.
[157] Wang Y et al., Role of β Phase during Microarc Oxidation of Mg Alloy AZ91D and Corrosion Resistance of the Oxidation Coating. Journal of Materials Science & Technology. 2013, 29, 1129–33.
[158] Joni MS et al., Effect of KOH concentration on the electrochemical behavior of coatings formed by pulsed DC micro-arc oxidation (MAO) on AZ31B Mg alloy. Journal of Alloys and Compounds. 2016, 661, 237–44.
[159] Chen J et al., In vitro degradation and antibacterial property of a copper-containing micro-arc oxidation coating on Mg-2Zn-1Gd-0.5Zr alloy. Colloids and Surfaces. B, Biointerfaces. 2019, 179, 77–86.
[160] Wu Y et al., In vivo study of microarc oxidation coated Mg alloy as a substitute for bone defect repairing: Degradation behavior, mechanical properties, and bone response. Colloids and Surfaces. B, Biointerfaces. 2019, 181, 349–59.
[161] Yang X et al., Enhanced in vitro biocompatibility/bioactivity of biodegradable Mg–Zn–Zr alloy by micro-arc oxidation coating contained Mg2SiO4. Surface & Coatings Technology. 2013, 233, 65–73.
[162] Ma C et al., Tribological behavior of plasma electrolytic oxidation coatings on the surface of Mg–8Li–1Al alloy. Tribology International. 2012, 47, 62–8.
[163] Cakmak E et al., The effect of substrate composition on the electrochemical and mechanical properties of PEO coatings on Mg alloys. Surface & Coatings Technology. 2010, 204, 1305–13.
[164] Aktuğ SL et al., Effect of Na2SiO3·5H2O concentration on microstructure and mechanical properties of plasma electrolytic oxide coatings on AZ31 Mg alloy produced by twin roll casting. Ceramics International. 2016, 42, 1246–53.
[165] Santos-Coquillat A et al., PEO coatings design for Mg-Ca alloy for cardiovascular stent and bone regeneration applications. Materials Science and Engineering: C. 2019, 105; https://doi.org/10.1016/j.msec.2019.110026.
[166] Kröger N et al., Hemocompatibility of plasma electrolytic oxidation (PEO) coated Mg-RE and Mg-Zn-Ca alloys for vascular scaffold applications. Materials Science and Engineering: C. 2018, 92, 819–26.

Chapter 14
Basic properties

In this chapter, we discuss the three basic properties of Mg materials, including mechanical, physical and chemical/electrochemical properties.

14.1 Properties in general

The most common properties of various Mg-based alloys are compared in Table 14.1 [1–10].

14.2 Mechanical properties

14.2.1 Alloying effects on mechanical properties

One of the important alloying effects should be improvement in mechanical properties associated with microstructural alterations. A combination of Mg-based (binary or ternary) alloys and additional alloying elements is listed in Table 14.2. It was found that among various alloying elements, Zn and Ca are the two most powerful alloying elements.

It is obvious that there is a limitation to exhibit the best alloying performance for each element. For example, alloying Zn with increasing content in a pure Mg alloy improved the mechanical properties such as yield strength, ultimate tensile strength (UTS) and elongation. As the Zn content was increased up to 4.0 wt% (which is maximum solubility limit to form a single α-Mg phase), the mechanical properties were at their highest, exhibiting a yield strength of 58.1 MPa, UTS of 216.85 MPa and elongation of 15.8%; however, after the peak, the mechanical properties declined. A reduction of the stacking fault energy in the alloy was reported to be responsible for the degradation of the properties [142, 143]. On the other hand, when up to 0.5 wt% Ca was added into Mg–4.0Zn alloy, the mechanical properties of the ternary alloy increased or remained constant, showing UTS of 215 MPa and elongation of 17.5%. A further increase of Ca content caused a decline in the mechanical properties. For example, at Ca of 2 wt% into Mg–4.0Zn, UTS and elongation were found to be 142 MPa and 1.7%, respectively. It was reported that a higher concentration of Ca led to the generation of pearl-shaped brittle fractures on the surface, hence degrading strength and elongation [142, 144, 145]. Therefore, it is important that the addition of Ca and Zn into Mg-based alloys must be kept within a certain limit so that the material has a level of ductility exhibiting an increase in flow stress under deformation. Moreover, Homayun et al. [146] investigated the

https://doi.org/10.1515/9783110676945-014

Table 14.1: Various properties of Mg-based alloys.

	Density (g/cm^3)	Elastic modulus (GPa)	Yield strength (MPa)	Ultimate tensile strength (MPa)	Elongation (%)	Poisson's ratio	Fracture toughness (MPa.m$^{1/2}$)	Melting point (°C)	Thermal conductivity (W/m.K)	Thermal expansion coeff (μm/m.K)	Electrical conductivity (MS/m)	Electrical resistivity (nΩm)
Pure Mg	1.74	45.2	165	228	7.83	0.34	18.7	650	156	25		43.9
Mg–1Al									112–117			62–84
Mg–10Al									44–55			170–189
Mg–1Zn									136–142			47–75
Mg–3Zn									123–125			55–81
Mg–6Zn									106–112			64–88
AZ31	1.77		83–200	207–269	4–12			1,116–1,169				185
AZ61			96–138	200–275	4–12			977–1,145				116
AZ63	1.82			210–276				850–1,130				123–150

AZ81	1.81		97	276	12			914–1,132				120
AZ91	1.81	45	83–138	165–457	3–11		11.6	875–1,105				99–115
AZ92	1.83		97–117	165–275	2–10			830–1,100				105–123
AM50			157									
AM60			130	220–282	6–30							
AM100A	1.81		85–150	150–275	2–10			867–1,101				
Mg–6Al–2Ca			152	269	13							
Mg–9Al–5Ca			469	540	2							
AE70	1.82	43	216	322	18	0.32		500–610	69	27	0.8	125
AE81	1.82	44	232	352	20	0.32		500–610	69	27	0.8	125
Mg–6Zn	1.84	42.3		277–281								
ZK21	1.80											
ZK51	1.81		165–172	276	8			549–640				
ZK60	1.83	45	179–250	269–350	11	0.35		520–670	78.3	27	0.64	156
ZK61	1.80		180–255	275–345	7			618				
ZE10	1.76											

(continued)

Table 14.1 (continued)

	Density (g/cm^3)	Elastic modulus (GPa)	Yield strength (MPa)	Ultimate tensile strength (MPa)	Elongation (%)	Poisson's ratio	Fracture toughness (MPa.m$^{1/2}$)	Melting point (°C)	Thermal conductivity (W/m.K)	Thermal expansion coeff (µm/m.K)	Electrical conductivity (MS/m)	Electrical resistivity (nΩm)
ZE41			131–140	193–205	3–5		15.5					
ZE62	1.84	45	190–302	295–350	4	0.32	21.0	530–635	78	27	0.64	156
ZH42	1.86		149	224	4.5			638				
ZH62	1.86		152	241	4.0			638				
WE43	1.84	45		250–277								
WE54	1.84	48	200–275	200–302	4	0.32	11.6	530–635	78	27	0.8	156
EZ33	1.83		85–105	140–160	3			543–643				
EK30	1.79							593–640				

EK40	1.81							645				
EK41	1.81							645				
EK43	1.83	44	225	340	12	0.3		540–640	57.6	26	0.68	148
Mg–10Gd	1.88			70–85								
Mg–1Ca	1.73			75–240								

Table 14.2: Effects of alloying elements on mechanical properties of Mg-based alloys.

	Al	Cu	Ni	Er	Zn	Zr	La	Sn	Ca	Y	Ti	Cr	Si	Ce	Sm	Li	Gd	Pd	B	RE	Mn	Sr	M	Sc
Mg	[11]		[12]						[13]							[14, 15]	[16]							[17]
Mg–Al		[18]	[18]	[19]	[20]		[21, 22]	[23]	[24, 25]	[26, 27]	[28]	[28]	[29]									[30]		
Mg–Al–Zn							[31]	[32]	[33–35]	[36]					[37]	[38]	[36]	[39]	[40]					
Mg–Al–Sn					[41, 42]				[43, 44]							[45]				[46]	[47]			
Mg–Al–Mn					[48]								[49]		[50]							[51]		
Mg–Al–Si								[52]	[53]								[53]		[52]					
Mg–Al–RE									[54, 55]		[56]											[54]		
Mg–Li	[57, 58]								[59]	[60]			[58]							[61]			[62]	[63]
Mg–Li–Al					[64]			[65, 66]	[67, 68]	[69–74]	[75]									[76, 77]		[78]		
Mg–Li–Zn										[79]				[79]										
Mg–Sn	[80]	[81]			[80, 82]				[83, 84]				[85]			[86]						[87]		
Mg–Sn–Ca										[88]				[89]			[90, 91]							
Mg–Sn–Zn	[92]																							[93]
Mg–Sn–Al					[94]									[95]										
Mg–Sn–Sr											[96]													

Mg–Y–Zn				[97]						
Mg–Y–RE			[98]			[99]		[99]		
Mg–Y–Zr									[100]	
Mg–Y–Nd									[101]	
Mg–Y–Mn					[102]					
Mg–Y–Sm			[103]							
Mg–Ce	[104]									
Mg–Ce–Mn			[105]		[106]					[105]
Mg–Si					[107]					
Mg–Ca		[108]								
Mg–Mn							[109, 110]			[111]
Mg–Sb									[112]	
Mg–Zr						[113]				
Mg–RE					[114]					
Mg–RE–Sn		[115]								
Mg–RE–Gd			[116]							
Mg–MM				[117]						
Mg–Nd		[118, 119]								
Mg–Sm	[120]									

(continued)

Table 14.2 (continued)

	Al	Cu	Ni	Er	Zn	Zr	La	Sn	Ca	Y	Ti	Cr	Si	Ce	Sm	Li	Gd	Pd	B	RE	Mn	Sr	M	Sc
Mg–Sm–Nd					[121]												[121]							
Mg–Sm–Gd					[122]																			
Mg–Gd				[123]	[124]																			
Mg–Gd–Y					[125–128]		[129]			[130, 131]			[132]				[131, 133]			[134, 135]				
Mg–Gd–Zn			[136]			[137]								[138]							[139]			
Mg–Gd–Mn									[140]															
Mg–Er					[141]																			

Note: RE, rare earth element; M, misch-metal (55Ce–25La–18Nd).

effect of Al addition on the mechanical properties of as-cast Mg–4Zn–0.2Ca alloy. It was reported that (i) though Al and Zn increase YS and UTS by solid solution and grain refinement strengthening, more than 3 wt% Al addition caused secondary phase ($Al_{12}Mg_{17}$) formation at grain boundaries and reduced elongation and UTS; (ii) however, compressive strength was not affected as same as UTS by increasing the amount of Al; (iii) tensile and compression stresses have different crack mechanism and the compressive strength increased due to the formation of secondary phase. Similarly, Yang et al. [147] mentioned that the Mg–2Al binary alloy foam could withstand higher stress in compression test than the binary alloy with higher Al addition, being attributed to the abundant secondary phase formation between Mg and Al that reduced mechanical integrity.

14.2.2 Ductility

Ductility is one of the most important mechanical properties and can be enhanced by appropriate alloying. Figure 14.1 compares alloying effectiveness toward improvements in different mechanical properties with variants of casting and wrought origins [148].

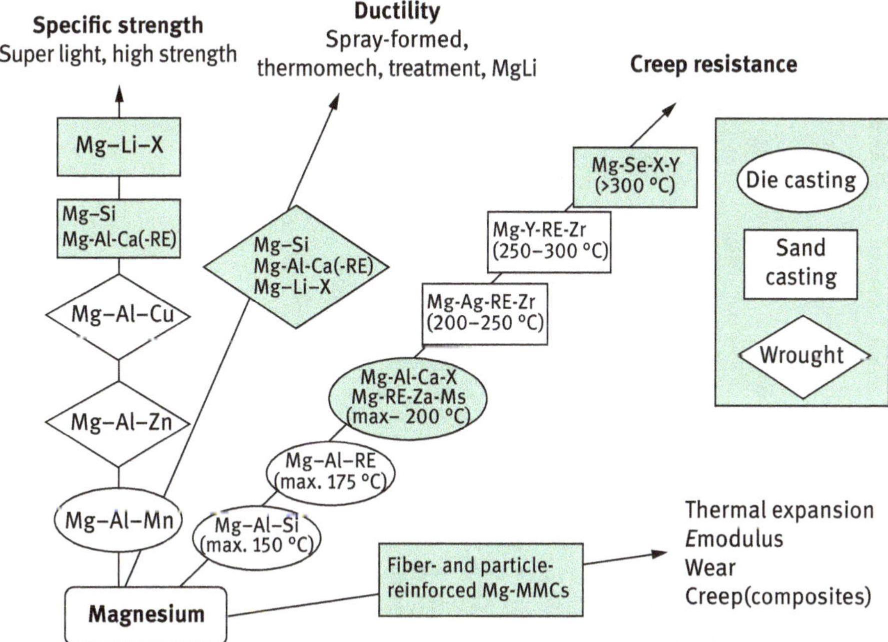

Figure 14.1: Different improvements of mechanical properties of Mg-based alloys [148].

Although Mg materials exhibit good strength with lightweight (or high specific strength), it is generally believed that Mg is relatively less ductile, making it difficult to process at room temperature (RT) and preventing its use in many applications. The poor ductility of Mg is attributed to its hexagonal close-packed crystal structure. Plastic slip in the crystallographic *c* direction is necessary for generalized plasticity, but the required easy-glide pyramidal <*c* + *a*> dislocations undergo a rapid transition to an immobile structure that limits *c*-axis plastic strain [149]. As demonstrated in Figure 14.2, such poor ductility can be improved remarkably by alloying with RE (rare earth) elements (including Y, La, Ce, Nd, Sm, Gd, Tb, Dy, Ho or Er) at very diluted concentration (i.e., ~0.03 to 1.0 at%) [149].

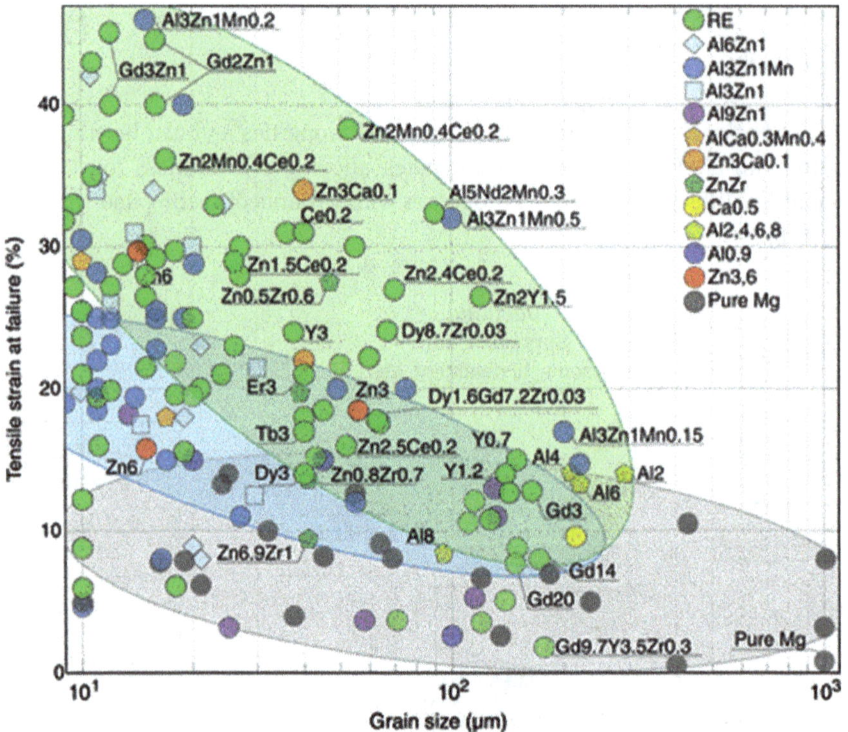

Figure 14.2: Room temperature ductility (or tensile failure strain) as a function of grain size [149].

Asgari et al. [150] and Bian et al. [151] took an interesting sight on Mg ductility. A certain type of Mg-based alloys has been recognized as biodegradable biomaterials. Because of this uniqueness, they are extensively applied in medical field, especially in tissue engineering for scaffold structure, stents and other surgical devices and orthopedic implants. Figure 14.3 shows the relationship between strength and elongation of such biodegradable Mg-based biomaterials [151]. Alloying elements shown in the figure can control the biodegradation rate and are limited as essential elements, which are possibly essential elements for human health. It is also indicated, from Figure 14.3, that extrusion can produce higher ductility and strength in comparison with rolled and casted parts.

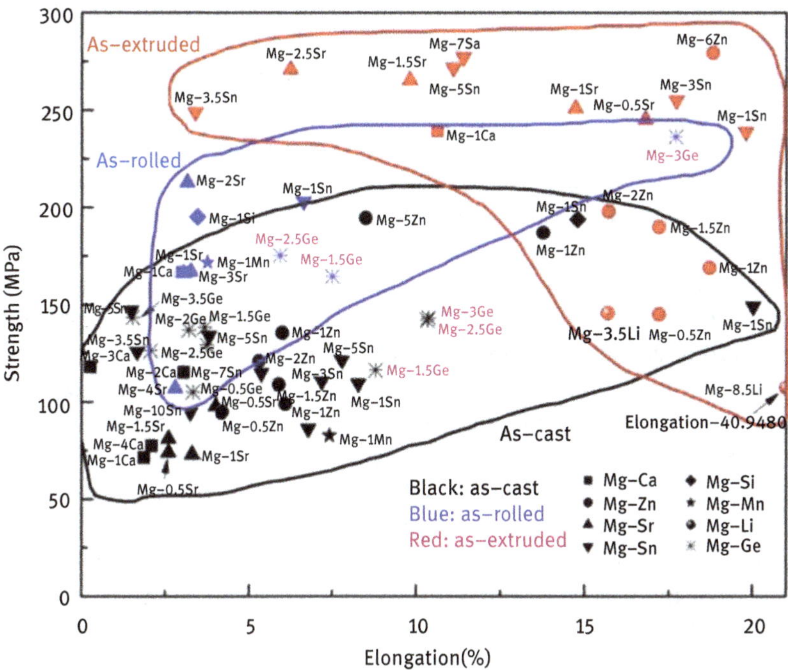

Figure 14.3: Strength and elongation relationship of various biodegradable Mg-based biomaterials [151].

Buey et al. [152] studied the ability of Y as an alloying agent to improve the ductility of magnesium using a solid solution strengthening interaction model with an edge dislocation $<c+a>$ to determine the relative strengthening effect on the available deformation modes. It was observed that (i) substituting solute atoms directly into the positions closest to the dislocation significantly changes the structure of the dislocation, making the direct calculation and representation of these interaction energies difficult, and necessitating a modification to the calculation of interaction energies and (ii) the ratio of the critical resolved shear stress of second order pyramidal $<c+a>$ slip to that of the basal slip decreases with increasing Y concentration; indicating that more isotropic plastic response is beneficial for improving the RT ductility of Mg alloys. Similar results were obtained that provide clear evidence for the occurrence of long-range motion of $<c+a>$ dislocations with relatively compact cores during plastic deformation, instead of immediate dissociation on basal planes was found [153, 154]. Sandlöbes et al. [155] investigated the mechanisms for the improved RT ductility in Mg–Y alloys compared to pure Mg by transmission electron microscopy and density functional theory. It was reported that (i) both methods show a significant decrease in the intrinsic stacking fault with the addition of Y and (ii) the mechanism is characterized by enhanced nucleation of $\langle c + a \rangle$ dislocations where the intrinsic stacking fault acts as heterogeneous source for $\langle c + a \rangle$ dislocations. With Mg–Gd–Y alloy systems, it was reported that a formation of intragranular long-period stacking ordered (LPSO) phases is important to improve the ductility [156–158]. Gao et al. [159] developed a high-ductility ZME200 (Mg–2.3Zn–0.4Mn–0.2Ce) alloy for vehicle closure and structure applications, based on an earlier ZE20 (Mg–2.0Zn–0.2Ce) alloy for extrusion applications. It was demonstrated that (i) the ZME200 alloy sheet exhibits extraordinarily higher ductility (36% in tensile elongation), much superior stretch formability (an Erichsen value of 9.5), lower anisotropy, comparable strength and corrosion resistance to AZ31 alloy and (ii) the unique rolling direction (RD)–transverse direction (TD) double split texture with remarkably reduced intensity and grain refinement gives rise to the significantly improved ductility and formability at RT. Yan et al. [160] developed new rolled Mg–1% Zn–1%Gd and Mg–2%Zn–1%Gd alloy sheets. It was reported that (i) the microstructures were characterized as fully recrystallized grains with a large amount of homogeneously distributed fine particles in the matrix, (ii) the sheets exhibit an excellent ultimate elongation of nearly 36% and an uniform elongation greater than 15%, (iii) the Mg–1%Zn–1%Gd sheet has a random basal texture and the basal pole is tilted by about 30° from the normal direction toward the transverse direction, (iv) the flow curves of the two Mg–Zn–Gd alloys display an abrupt yielding with a remarkable linear hardening at high strain rate after a plastic strain of roughly 3%, (v) the majority of grains in the tilted texture have an orientation favorable for both basal slip and tensile twining because of a high Schmid factor and (vi) the low planar anisotropy, the large uniform elongations and the high strain-hardening rate observed in the Mg–Zn–Gd sheets imply excellent RT formability.

14.2.3 Fatigue and corrosion fatigue

In this section, we will discuss both high-cycle fatigue (HCF, or low stress-level fatigue) and low-cycle fatigue (LCF, or high stress-level fatigue). Later, we will also cover environment-assisted fatigue behavior. As seen in Figure 14.4 [161], the S–N curve (stress vs numbers of cycles to fatigue failure) is conveniently divided into two regimes: HCF and LCF, although there should not be clear-cut dividing line in between. If a material has high stacking fault energy (like Al, Ni or Cu), cross slip can easily take place, so that there is no clear endurance limit, as dotted line indicates. In the figure, ultimate and yield strengths are also marked since these mechanical properties are generally obtained during the tensile stressing (which is a quarter of one full fatigue cycle).

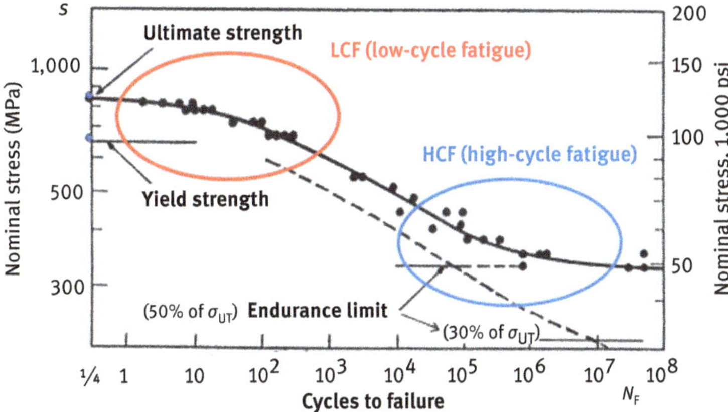

Figure 14.4: Typical S–N curves showing both HCF and LCF zones [161].

14.2.3.1 Fatigue, in general

It is stated that (1) Mg-based alloys have unique RT mechanical properties such as yielding asymmetry, anisotropy and unusual hardening response under strain path change and (2) Mg-based alloy sheets often represent inferior formability at RT due to their limited active slip systems induced by specific microstructure and texture [162]. Toscano et al. [163] investigated the multiaxial fatigue behavior of extruded AZ31B Mg alloy, which was forged at 250 °C, under axial–shear loading at phase angles of 0°, 45° and 90°. It was indicated that (i) quasistatic testing showed that the forged material retained the high yield strength of the extrusion condition with a substantial increase in failure strain, (ii) under multiaxial loading, cyclic axial strain significantly affected the shear hysteresis behavior while the effect of cyclic shear strain on the axial hysteresis was less pronounced and (iii) despite a notable change in shear hysteresis shape, fatigue life was only slightly affected by the changes in phase angle. Chen et al. [164] investigated fatigue properties and cyclic deformation behavior of an extruded AZ31 alloy by the strain-controlled LCF tests at RT. It was reported that (i) the total strain amplitude is closely related to fatigue properties and cyclic damage process, (ii) when the total strain amplitude increased from 0.3% to 0.4%, there was a noticeable change in compressive peak stress amplitude, which might correspond to the competition between twinning–detwinning process and dislocation slips and (iii) at the total strain of great amplitude, fracture surfaces were characterized by the striation-like features and dimple-like structures. Ishihara et al. [165] conducted fatigue tests under constant stress amplitudes on both die-cast and extruded Mg alloys to study their distributions of fatigue lives. It was reported that (i) during the fatigue process of the die-cast Mg alloy, cracks initiated from the casting defects inside of the specimen, and then propagated prior to final failure of the specimen, (ii) while in the extruded Mg alloy, cracks initiated from the inclusions located on the specimen surface, (iii) assuming the above defects as the initial cracks, there are common relations between the initial maximum stress intensity factors and fatigue lives, regardless of the stress amplitudes for the both Mg alloys at the constant *R* ratio (minimum stress/maximum stress) of −1, (iv) the lower the stress intensity factor, the longer the fatigue life becomes and (v) distributions of fatigue lives at the constant stress amplitudes can be represented by the Weibull distributions and dispersion as fatigue lives become larger at the lower stress amplitude than those at the higher stress amplitudes.

Cyclic deformation and fatigue of extruded RE Mg-8.0Gd-3.0Y-0.5%Zr (GW83) alloy were studied under fully reversed strain-controlled tension–compression tests along the extrusion direction with the strain amplitudes varying from 0.275% to 5.0% [166]. It was mentioned that (i) monotonic tension and compression stress–strain curves display a smooth transition from elastic to elastic–plastic deformation and exhibit a fairly yielding symmetry; (ii) with increasing number of loading cycles, a transition of stress–strain response from concave-down shape to sigmoidal shape occurs in both tension and compression reversals when the strain amplitudes are larger than 2.0%; and (iii) the strain-life fatigue curve displays a similar feature to that of conventional Mg alloys and a detectable transition from low-cycle region to high-cycle region occurs at a kink point in the vicinity of a strain amplitude of 0.75%. Using same extruded GW83 alloy, Dong et al. [167] investigated the aging effects on the deformation and fatigue behavior. It was found that (i) the aging process significantly enhances the monotonic strengths under both tension and compression; (ii) the ductility under tension is unchanged but the elongation under compression is reduced due to the aging treatment; (iii) the cyclic stress–strain curve of the aged GW83 is much higher than that of the corresponding extruded state; (iv) the strain-life fatigue curve of the aged GW83 is similar to that of the extruded GW83, but the stress-life fatigue curve of the aged GW83 is much higher, indicating an improved fatigue strength due to the aging process; and (v) similar to the other Mg alloys, a kink point in the strain-life fatigue curve was identified for the aged GW83Mg alloy, and the kink point of a strain amplitude of 0.80% for the material demarcates the activation of bulk and persistent twinning/detwinning during cyclic deformation. Tensile and strain-controlled fatigue tests were performed to investigate the influence of forging on the performance of cast AZ80 magnesium alloy [168]. It was reported that (i) the as-cast AZ80 magnesium alloy has dendritic α-Mg phase with eutectic $Mg_{17}Al_{12}$ morphology and a random texture; in contrast, the forged samples showed refined grains and a strong basal texture; (ii) the forged samples achieved comparatively longer fatigue life under strain-controlled cyclic loading; and (iii) forging caused grain refinement and texture modification, both of which enhance alloy performance by improving strength and ductility, leading to longer fatigue life.

Mg weldments are also investigated. Patel et al. [169] identified failure mode and estimated fatigue life of ultrasonic spot-welded lap joints of an AZ31B–H24 magnesium alloy. It was found that (i) the solid-state weldments exhibited a superior fatigue life compared with other welding processes; (ii) fatigue failure mode changed from interfacial failure to transverse-through-thickness crack growth with decreasing cyclic load level, depending on the welding energy; and (iii) fatigue crack initiation and propagation occurred from both the notch tip inside the faying surface. Liu et al. [170] evaluated the microstructural change and fatigue resistance of Mg/steel resistance spot welds, in comparison with Mg/Mg welds. It was mentioned that (i) the horizontal and vertical Mg hardness profiles of Mg/steel and Mg/Mg welds were similar; (ii) both Mg/steel and Mg/Mg welds were observed to have an equivalent fatigue resistance due to similar crack propagation characteristics and failure mode; (iii) both Mg/steel and Mg/Mg welds failed through thickness in the magnesium sheet under stress-controlled cyclic loading, but fatigue crack initiation of the two types of welds was different; and (iv) the crack initiation of Mg/Mg welds occurred due to a combined effect of stress concentration, grain growth in the heat-affected zone and the presence of Al-rich phases at the heat-affected zone grain boundaries, while the penetration of small amounts of Zn coating into the Mg base metal stemming from the liquid metal-induced embrittlement led to crack initiation in the Mg/steel welds.

14.2.3.2 Low-cycle fatigue

The entire fatigue life, N_T, is normally divided into two parts: fatigue crack initiation period, N_I, and crack propagation period, N_P, as illustrated in Figure 14.5 [161].

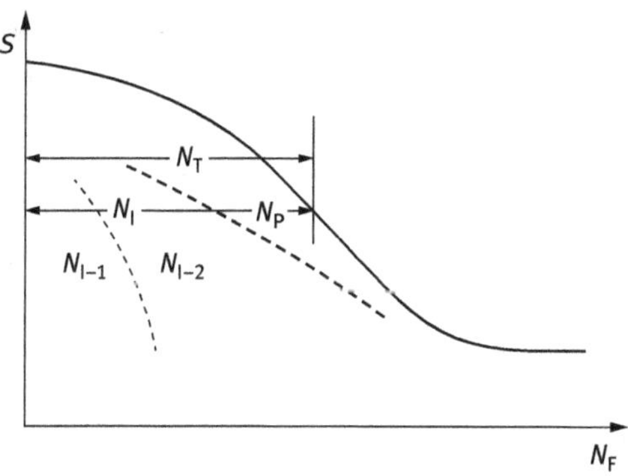

Figure 14.5: Total fatigue life consisted of crack initiation period and its propagation period [161].

Furthermore, N_I (crack initiation period) can be subdivided into N_{I-1} and N_{I-2}. During the N_{I-1} (which is called hardening and/or softening stage, depending on the original state of the materials and stress/strain amplitude) is characterized by the changes in substructure (dislocation) within the while volume of the loaded material. The N_{I-2} is called as crack nucleation stage. Microcrack nucleation at fatigue slip bands, grain boundaries or surface inclusions will take place in a small portion of the total volume, namely the surface layer. A common denominator of all types of nucleation is the stress concentration in the surface layer. The crack propagation stage, N_P, ends in the final failure. The controlling factor of crack propagation is the highly concentrated cyclic plastic deformation within the plastic zone at/ahead of the crack tip.

The proportion of these crack initiation and propagation stages for LCF and HCF is clearly different from each other. It is generally accepted that (1) in LCF regime, $N_T = N_{I+} N_P$ and $N_I \approx N_P$, and (2) for HCF regime, $N_I > N_P$. Hence, in the HCF (in other words, fatigue behavior under low stress level), the majority of fatigue life is consumed until the crack is initiated.

AZ (Mg–Al–Zn) alloy series have been subjected to LCF studies. Park et al. [171] studied LCF characteristics of rolled Mg–3Al–1Zn (AZ31) alloy by performing the LCF test along the rolling direction. It was reported that (i) the alloy has such a strong basal texture that the fatigue deformation was predominated by the alternation of twinning and detwinning during each cycle, and this made the cyclic stress response unstable and introduced a nonzero mean stress and/or strain depending on the loading condition and (ii) an energy-based concept was successfully used to predict the LCF life because a plastic strain energy density was found to have good characteristics as a fatigue parameter; it was stabilized at the early stage of fatigue life and nearly invariant through entire life. In the life prediction model, the effect of mean stress was appropriately considered. Wen et al. [172], on extruded AZ31B, studied the fatigue crack initiation and early crack growth by conducting fully reversed strain-controlled tension–compression fatigue experiments at two strain amplitudes of 1% and 0.3%. It was found that (i) at a strain amplitude of 1%, two types of twin-induced microcracks were observed; (ii) less fatigue damage can be caused by the twin-induced cracks than from slip-induced cracks; (iii) at a strain amplitude of 0.3%, slip-induced microcracks initiated from 30% to 80% of the fatigue life, and then propagated until the final failure; and (iv) no twin-induced cracks were detected at 0.3% strain amplitude. Jain et al. [173] performed the nanoindentation LCF test on AZ61Mg alloy to study the effect of cyclic loading. It was reported that (i) the cyclic load–depth curves are observed in aged and solution-treated (ST) conditions; (ii) an indentation fatigue depth propagation law is used to analyze the cyclic behavior of the alloy; and (iii) the increase in steady-state depth propagation rate with increasing stress intensity has been reported, which is qualitatively similar to the steady-state growth rate of a fatigue crack. Zhu et al. [174] studied the LCF properties of Mg–8Al–0.5Zn (AZ80) alloy as a function of precipitation state. It was found that (i) the presence of precipitates significantly reduces tension–compression yield asymmetry, compared with ST material and this decreased asymmetry significantly reduces tensile mean stress during LCF process; (ii) as the cyclic deformation progressed, an abrupt increase in the plastic strain amplitude prior to failure is observed, representing the onset of fatigue crack initiation and this increase disappears in the aged sample, which leads to the significantly decreased area of crack propagation zone, and shorter lifetime; and (iii) due to the enlarged reverse plastic zone size, the aged sample showed microscopically rough faceted fracture surfaces in the fatigue crack propagation zone. Gryguc et al. [175] conducted the stress-controlled uniaxial push–pull fatigue testing on as-received (cast and extruded) and closed-die cast-forged and extruded-forged AZ80 Mg alloy. It was reported that (i) under fatigue testing, all the materials developed some form of mean strain, with the nature and magnitude of this mean strain being dependent on primarily its texture intensity and propensity to twin in either tension or compression reversals; (ii) the type of mean strain (tensile or compressive) depends upon both the orientation and intensity of the starting texture of material; (iii) the texture-induced ratcheting and resulting mean strain evolution was most pronounced in the as-cast material and had a significant impact on the fatigue life; (iv) following forging, the material exhibited an increase in fatigue life of anywhere from 2 to 15 times for the cast then forged material and more modest yet still significant 8 times longer at stress amplitudes around 140 MPa for the extruded then forged material; (v) the extruded forged material exhibited similar fatigue lives to that of the base material at stress amplitudes that approached the yield strength; and (vi) the nature of the mean stress development and degree of fatigue life improvement depended on the processing conditions and the type of base material (cast or extruded) utilized to create the forging.

The LCF properties of extruded Mg-10Gd-2Y-0.5Zr (GW102k) was studied and compared with those of conventional extruded AZ31 magnesium alloy [176]. It was mentioned that (i) GW102k alloy contains a large amount of precipitated particles and possesses a relatively weak basal texture, which gives rise to near-symmetric yield asymmetry; (ii) different from AZ31 alloy, the GW102k alloy shows near-symmetric stress–strain hysteresis loops and marginal cyclic hardening; (iii) the symmetry significantly reduces tensile mean stress during LCF process; and (iii) due to the small reversible plastic zone size, the GW102k alloy shows rough faceted fracture surfaces in the fatigue crack propagation zone, concluding that the LCF life of GW102k alloy is found to be longer than that of AZ31 alloy.

Mohammed et al. [177] evaluated the strain-controlled LCF behavior of a high zinc-containing cast Mg–10Zn–5Al in relation to the microstructure. It was reported that (i) the addition of Zn with a Zn/Al ratio of ~2 suppressed the presence of β-$Mg_{17}Al_{12}$ phase, and the as-cast alloy consisted mainly of primary α-Mg and eutectic-like τ-$Mg_{32}(Al,Zn)_{49}$ phase in a characteristic network form, (ii) although slight cyclic softening occurred at higher strain amplitudes, cyclic stabilization basically remained; being reflected by the nearly overlapped cyclic and monotonic stress–strain curves, (iii) the fatigue crack initiated from the near-surface imperfections, and crack propagation was characterized by fatigue striation-like features along with tear ridges.

Li et al. [178] compared the LCF characteristics between the ST (T4) and peak-aged (PA, T6) Mg-3Nd-0.2Zn-0.5Zr alloys produced by semicontinuous casting. It was found that (i) the cyclic stress amplitudes of the T6-treated counterpart are higher than those of the T4-treated alloy, which is due to precipitate strengthening; (ii) at the same stress amplitude, the T4-treated alloy with higher hysteresis energies undergoes more fatigue damage, resulting in shorter fatigue lives; (iii) for the T4-treated alloy, the cyclic stress amplitude is found to increase with an increase in the cycle number, which is attributed to its soft matrix and the increased volume fraction and number density of twins under continuous loading; (iv) cyclic hardening followed by the decrease of the stress is observed in the T6-treated alloy; and (v) the cyclic deformation behavior and failure mechanism of the T4-treated alloy are dependent on the dislocations-slip plus twinning, while those of the T6-treated counterpart are dependent on the dislocations slip. Mirza et al. [179] evaluated strain-controlled cyclic deformation behavior of an extruded Mg-3Nd-0.2Zn-0.5Zr (NZ30K) alloy. It was reported that unlike the higher RE-containing Mg-10Gd-3Y-0.5Zr (GW103K) magnesium alloy, the NZ30K alloy exhibited asymmetrical hysteresis loops in tension and compression in the fully reversed strain-control tests at a strain ratio of −1, being attributed to the presence of relatively stronger crystallographic texture, precipitation-free zone and the resultant twinning–detwinning activities during cyclic deformation. While this alloy exhibited cyclic softening at lower strain amplitudes and cyclic hardening at higher strain amplitudes, it had an equivalent fatigue life to that of other extruded Mg alloys. Fatigue crack was observed to initiate from the specimen surface with some isolated facets of the cleavage-like planes near the initiation site.

14.2.3.3 High-cycle fatigue

AZs are also studied in the HCF regime. Tan et al. [180] investigated the HCF behavior of a hot-rolled AZ31 alloy at high frequencies (97.3 Hz) and different stress amplitudes (50, 60, 70, 90, 110 MPa) by using a tension–compression fatigue test at RT. It was mentioned that (i) the stress amplitude significantly influences the activation of fatigue mechanisms; (ii) when the stress amplitudes were 50 and 60 MPa, which is close to the fatigue strength, only basal dislocations were observed, no obvious twins and $<c+a>$ dislocations can be observed; and (iii) grains were refined under high cyclic numbers led by continuous dynamic recrystallization; (iv) pyramidal slip is one of the deformation mechanisms in magnesium alloy during HCF deformation when the stress amplitude is higher than the fatigue strength. Okayasu et al. [181] investigated fatigue properties and failure characteristics of a cast AZ91 alloy, which was prepared by heated-mold continuous casting (HMC) and conventional gravity casting (GC). It was reported that (i) excellent fatigue properties are obtained for the HMC alloy compared with the GC alloy; (ii) the high fatigue strength of the HMC alloy is a reflection of its improved microstructural characteristics, namely, tiny α-Mg grains and fine spherical eutectic structures (β-$Mg_{17}Al_{12}$); (iii) fatigue cracks propagate mainly in the α-Mg grains and along high-hardness β-phases in both alloys; (iv) the direction of fatigue crack growth is altered as the crack reaches the eutectic phases; (v) because the tiny eutectic phases are distributed randomly in the HMC alloy, a meandering crack path is formed, which results in high crack growth resistance, leading to the high fatigue strength; and (vi) for the HMC alloy, a striation-like failure mode can be seen in the crack growth stage, and dimple fracture is the dominant feature in the final failure stage; on the other hand, cleavage-like brittle failure with many microcracks can occur in the GC alloy.

Mg–Gd–Y alloys are also subjected to HCF evaluations. Stress-controlled HCF behaviors of cast Mg-8Gd-3Y-Zr (wt%) alloy in as-cast, ST (T4) and aged (T6) conditions were studied at RT [182]. It was mentioned that (i) during HCF, only basal slips were observed on the surface of fatigue samples under different stress amplitudes, which suggests that basal slip is the dominant fatigue damage mechanism, (ii) in the T4 alloy, a great number of basal slip planes in a single grain and most of the grains participate in the fatigue deformation, resulting higher fatigue strength (80 MPa, for 10^7 cycles) and (iii) T6 alloy showed lower fatigue strength of 70 MPa. He et al. [183] conducted HCF testing on an as-extruded (AR) Mg-10Gd-3Y-0.5Zr alloy to investigate its fatigue crack initiation and early propagation behaviors. It was found that (i) only basal slip was activated at a low cyclic stress amplitude; (ii) fatigue crack initiated from the slip bands along the basal plane, leading to the formation of cleavage-like facets on the fracture surface; and (iii) the formation of facets around the crack initiation sites consumed a vast majority of the cyclic loadings in HCF regime, and small fatigue crack propagation was significantly retarded by local microstructure heterogeneity of neighboring grains. Similarly, Dong et al. [184] investigated the influence of heat treatment (T4, T5 and T6) on HCF behavior of the AR Mg–10Gd–3Y (GW103) alloy. The five heat treatment conditions applied to the AR GW103 alloy were under-aging (T5, 225 °C × 4 h), peak-aging (T5, 225 °C × 10 h), over-aging (T5, 225 °C × 250 h), solution treatment (T4, 500 °C × 4 h), solution treatment plus artificial aging (T6, 500 °C × 4 h + 225 °C × 10 h), respectively. It was reported that (i) the T5 heat treatment can improve the fatigue behavior of the GW103 alloy, while T4 and T6 heat treatments are detrimental to the fatigue behavior of the GW103 alloy; (ii) the 10^7 cycles fatigue strength of the GW103 alloy made by peak-aging was improved by approximately 10%, compared with the AR; (iii) while the fatigue strength of the underaged (UA) and overaged (OA) GW103 alloys have no obvious difference, although fatigue life of the UA GW103 alloy is slightly higher than that of the OA GW103 alloy at high stress amplitude; and (iv) the extruded-T4 and extruded-T6 GW103 alloys exhibit similar fatigue strengths of 110 MPa. Liu et al. [185] investigated the tensile properties, HCF behavior and plane-strain fracture toughness of the sand-cast Mg–10Gd–3Y–0.5Zr alloy with comparison to that of sand-cast plus T6 heat-treated magnesium alloy, which was named after sand-cast-T6. It was shown that (i) the tensile properties of the sand-cast alloy are greatly improved after T6 heat treatment, and the fatigue strength (at 10^7 cycles) of this alloy increases from 95 to 120 MPa after T6 heat treatment, that is, the improvement of 26% in fatigue strength has been achieved and (ii) the plane-strain fracture toughness values of the sand-cast and sand-cast-T6 alloys are about 12.1 and 16.3 MPa · $m^{1/2}$, respectively. Yang et al. [186] studied very HCF behaviors of extruded Mg-12Gd-3Y-0.5Zr (GW123k) alloy and compared with that of conventional extruded AZ31 magnesium alloy. Typical postfatigue microstructure and surface morphology features are presented for both the GW123k and the AZ31 alloys in order to stand out the uniqueness of GW123k alloy. It was mentioned that (i) GW123k alloy contains a large amount of precipitated particles and possesses a relatively weak texture, which give rise to its much relieved tension–compression yield asymmetry and enhanced fatigue failure resistance and (ii) the much homogenized deformation mechanism in GW123k alloy is considered to be the underline reason for the improvement of material's fatigue performance.

Yu's research group extensively studied the HCF behavior of Mg–6Zn–1Mn (ZM61) alloy [187–189]. It was reported that all of the extruded T5-treated and double-aged ZM61 alloys exhibited more outstanding HCF strength under zero-tension load ($R = 0$) than under tension–compression load ($R = -1$) [187]. For the ZM61 alloy by servohydraulic fatigue tests with pull–push sinusoidal loading, in high stress cycles (cyclic stress ≥ 129 MPa) HCF tests promote deformation; however, in low stress cycles (cyclic stress ≤ 125 MPa) HCF tests make a contribution to RT recrystallization in this alloy [188] and for extruded and double-aged ZM61 alloy, (iii) double-aged alloy shows a deteriorative fatigue performance despite having excellent tensile strength, (iv) twinning and detwinning mechanisms play a dominant role in fatigue deformation process in double-aged alloy; however, for extruded alloy, due to the duplex grain structure, the fatigue deformation mechanism presents various deformation modes: in high stress regime (≥129 MPa) twinning takes part in fatigue process and appears in coarse grains, in low stress regime (≤125 MPa) fatigue deformation was dominated by slip [189].

Liu et al. [190] studied the HCF of as-forged T5 Mg-Zn-Y-Zr alloy at stress ratios $R = -1$ and $R = 0.1$ at ambient temperature and mentioned (i) the fatigue strength of the alloy at 10^7 cycles is strongly affected by both the heat treatment and the mean applied stress. Xu et al. [191] studied fatigue crack propagation behavior of the same alloy and found that (i) the threshold stress intensity factor ΔK_{th} values of the alloy were different and (ii) among them, the ΔK_{th} value of the T5 sample was obviously higher than that of the T6 sample.

Li et al. [192] studied the influences of casting defects on the fatigue behaviors of Mg-3Nd-0.2Zn-Zr (NZ30K) alloy using porosity-free low-pressure sand mold casting bars (LPS) and gravity permanent mold casting ingots containing a few porosities. It was shown that (i) porosities have detrimental effect on the fatigue strength and life; (ii) the samples failed from the porosities show much lower fatigue strength and life in comparison with those failed from slip bands and twin bands; (iii) the fatigue strength increases with the increase in yield strength; (iv) fatigue strength of the porosity-free T6-treated specimens made by LPS is determined by the threshold stress for basal slip, which is related to the interactions among slip bands, precipitates and grain boundaries; and (v) both grain boundary constraints and cyclic deformation irreversibly caused by twinning are the crucial factors influencing the fatigue strengths of the porosity-free T4-treated specimens made by LPS. Peng et al. [193] investigated the HCF behavior of NZ30K using porosity-free low-pressure sand mold casting bars (LSM) and reported that the LSM–NZ30K alloys show a significant response to heat treatment, achieving 51%, 39% and 17% increases in yield strength, UTS and fatigue strength, respectively, in the PA condition, compared with those of the as-cast alloy. The fatigue failure of the porosity-free LSM–NZ30K alloy is mainly originated from the localized shearing near the specimen surfaces during cyclic loading. In the T6 condition, the increased fatigue strength is attributed to the strong precipitation hardening in addition to the grain boundary constraints.

14.2.3.4 Corrosion fatigue

Fatigue crack can be initiated at localized surface sites that are crystallographic heterogeneous such as dislocation kinks or microstructural heterogeneous such as grain boundaries, inclusions or precipitates. All these heterogeneous sites are most likely subjected to localized high stress intensity. At the same time, if such surface is exposed to corrosive environment or oxidation atmosphere, these sites will act as anodic sites; hence, corrosion potential can be concentrated on these sites. As a result, crack initiation site(s) are more rapidly and aggressively attached by corrosion or oxidation reaction, causing the acceleration of the crack propagation rate. Referring to Figure 14.6(a), in a case of oxidation fatigue (or thermal fatigue), grain boundary is rapidly oxidized because oxygen bulk diffusion rate is larger than that of surface diffusion. Later, since the formed oxide is ceramic and brittle in nature, such oxide under cyclic stressing can easily be fractured to make new surface of internal material by exposure to oxidation environment. This sequence (of oxide formation and oxide fracture) can be repeated until the propagated crack becomes crucial length, as shown in Figure 14.6(b).

In biomedical applications, although biodegradable magnesium alloys have attracted research interest as matrix materials for next-generation absorbable metallic coronary stents, when they are subjected to cyclic stresses, magnesium alloy stents are prone to premature failures caused by corrosion fatigue damage [195]. For testing corrosion-assisted fatigue of Mg-based alloys, chlorine-ion containing corrosive media is commonly used, including NaCl solution, phosphate-buffered saline (PBS) or simulated body fluid (SBF). Wang et al. [196] studied the corrosion fatigue (CF) behaviors of an as-forged Mg-6.7%Zn-1.3%Y-0.6%Zr alloy before and after solid-solution treatment (T4) in 3.5 wt% NaCl solution. It was found that (i) S–N curves showed that the fatigue strength of as-forged samples corresponding to 5×10^6 cycles was 30 MPa, whereas the fatigue strength of T4 samples was 50 MPa and (ii) fracture observations showed that for the as-forged samples, fatigue cracks mainly initiated at localized corrosion sites on sample surfaces; however, for the T4 samples, the crack

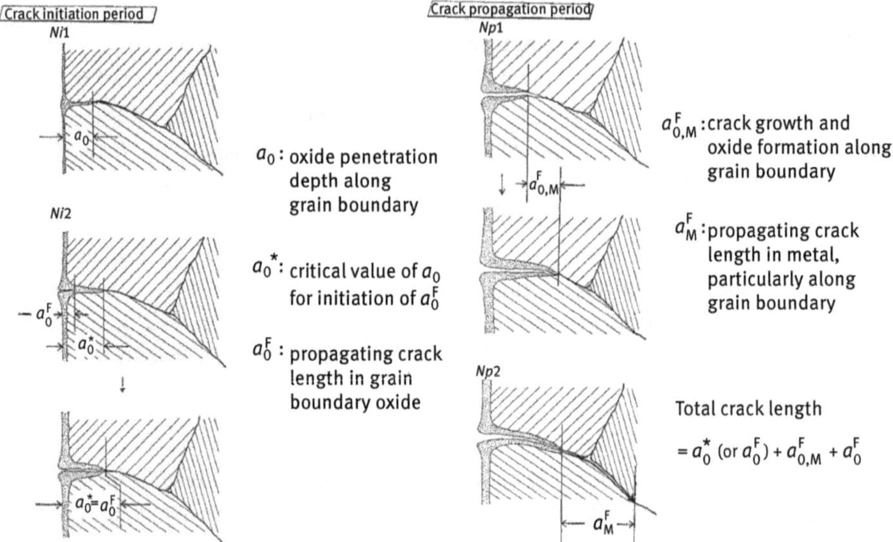

Figure 14.6: Oxidation-assisted crack initiation (a) and crack propagation (b) [194].

initiation was respectively related to the localized corrosion. The fatigue behavior of an as-cast Mg-7%Gd-5%Y-1%Nd-0.5%Zr alloy in both laboratory air and 3.5 wt% NaCl solution and the effect of corrosion attack on fatigue crack initiation were investigated [197]. It was reported that (i) the S–N curves showed that the fatigue strength in air was 120 MPa and not sensitive to the loading frequency, whereas the fatigue strength in NaCl solution decreased from 80 to 60 MPa with the loading frequency decreasing from 20 to 5 Hz; (ii) surface fractography demonstrated that in air, fatigue cracks preferentially initiated at the oxide inclusions; however, the fatigue crack initiation in NaCl solution was associated with corrosion pits; (iii) multiple fatigue cracks initiated at pits on fracture surfaces of CF failed samples when the loading frequency decreased to 5 Hz; and (iv) based on the measured defect area of oxide inclusions, the predicted fatigue strength in air could be well fitted with the experimental data; however, due to the occurrence of hydrogen embrittlement (HE) and crack initiation at multiple sites, the fatigue strength of samples tested in NaCl solution cannot be predicted.

Chen et al. [198] investigated the ratcheting and LCF behaviors of extruded AZ31B in air and in PBS. It was mentioned that (i) ratcheting fatigue interaction and fatigue corrosion were influenced by twinning and detwinning and the effect of ratcheting and corrosion environment on damage evolution of extruded AZ31B agreed well with a modified Ellyn's model. Bian et al. [199] evaluated the dynamic mechanical performances of a high-purity magnesium (99.99 wt%) and two typical promising biodegradable magnesium alloys (binary Mg–1Ca and ternary Mg–2Zn–0.2Ca) by carrying out fatigue tests in air and in SBF. It was reported that the fatigue strengths of Mg, Mg–1Ca and Mg–2Zn–0.2Ca were all around 90 MPa in air; however, they decreased to 52, 70 and 68 MPa in SBF at 4 × 10^6 cycles, respectively. The fatigue cracks initiated from the microstructural defects when tested in air, but nucleated from surface corrosion pits when tested in SBF. Cyclic loading significantly increased the corrosion rates of all the experimental materials compared to that in static SBF.

Wu et al. [200] investigated the mechanical response and failure mechanism of Mg-2.1Gd-1.1Y-0.82Zn-0.11Zr alloy (T6 peak-aging heat treatment) under a total strain-controlled low-cyclic loading at 300 °C. It was mentioned that (i) the alloy exhibits cyclic softening response at diverse total strain amplitudes and 300 °C; (ii) fractographic observations revealed that the micro-cracks initiate preferentially at the interface between long-period stacking order structures and α-Mg matrix and extend along the basal plane of α-Mg; and (iii) the massive long-period stacking order structures distributed at grain boundaries impede the transgranular propagation of cracks.

14.2.3.5 Enhancement of fatigue strength

It is well documented that when surface layer is subjected to localized forging by small particles (like sand blasting, shot peening or laser peening), the peened surface develops a beneficial compressive residual. Particularly when applying shot peening on metallic materials, their fatigue strength is enhanced [201]. Liu et al. [202] studied the influence of shot peening on the HCF performance of the Mg–10Gd–3Y alloys in four different conditions referred to as-cast, cast-T6, AR and extruded-T5, respectively. It was shown that (i) shot peening can cause different degree of enhancement of fatigue performance for Mg–10Gd–3Y alloys depending on the Almen peening intensity applied; and that the Almen intensity could always be found that conferred the optimum improvement, (ii) the effect of shot peening was quantified, and for the AR and extruded-T5 alloys it was found to be superior to that for the as-cast and cast-T6 alloys; (iii) the peened extruded-T5 Mg–10Gd–3Y alloy showed the highest fatigue strength at 10^7 cycles of 240 MPa; and (iv) microstructure affected the magnitude of the surface roughness induced by shot peening and also the maximum compressive residual stress and its relaxation during fatigue, and then determine the beneficial effect of shot peening. Similarly, Liu et al. [203] investigated the fatigue properties and fracture behavior of AR Mg–6Zn–0.5Zr and Mg-10Gd-3Y-0.5Zr alloys before and after shot peening. It was reported that (i) the stress-controlled rotating bending fatigue property improvement for Mg-10Gd-3Y-0.5Zr alloy by shot peening is significantly superior to that of Mg–6Zn–0.5Zr alloy; (ii) with the increase in peening (Almen) intensity, the fatigue crack nucleation site of Mg–6Zn–0.5Zr alloy under stress control shifted from the surface to subsurface, and then back to the surface again; (iii) meanwhile, a significantly higher number of fatigue crack initiation sites can be seen as a consequence of over-peening; however, the fatigue cracks of the peened Mg-10Gd-3Y-0.5Zr alloy initiated subsurface at all Almen intensities, showing unchanged crack initiation location with the increase in Almen intensity; (iv) the observed phenomenon is related to differences between the two alloys both in the deformation mechanisms during shot peening and the residual stress relaxation mechanisms during subsequent fatigue process; namely, in the Mg–6Zn–0.5Zr alloy twinning dominates deformation during shot peening and detwinning during fatigue and comparatively, dislocation slip dominates deformation in both shot peening and fatigue process in the Mg-10Gd-3Y-0.5Zr alloy.

14.2.4 Creep

In the plasticity, it is assumed that the plastic strain that is produced by stressing a metal with a given load has a unique value, if parameters such as temperature are held constant. This assumption is not right. There is no unique value of strain associated with a given stress. This is a consequence of the fact that plastic strain does not remain constant under a constant load. Actually, the strain increases with time and the time-dependent plastic strain that is observed in stressed materials is called the creep strain. At high temperature the amount of time-dependent plastic strain that can occur is much larger than the plastic strain produced instantaneously during the time interval, while at low temperature the amount of time-dependent strain is relatively small, even after long time intervals. Because it is small, it usually can be neglected when the stress–strain curve or the work-hardening properties of metals are being considered. It is an important consideration in the selection of materials for high temperature applications. The term high temperature is relative term and refers to a temperature ≈ $T_{MP}/2$ where T_{MP} represents the solidus temperature of the material in K scale. For most metals and alloys, creep occurs for stresses below the yield point only when the temperature is elevated. However, some nonferrous alloys and metals such as lead (T_{MP} ≈ 330 °C) exhibit creep at low stresses and RT. Creep is sensitive to both the applied load and the testing temperature (movement of thermally activated dislocation controls the creep process); increasing stress raises the level of the creep curve, and increasing temperature, which accelerates recovery processes and increases the creep rate. Creep behavior is normally presented in strain versus time as a function of constant predetermined temperature as shown in Figure 14.7 [161].

The creep rupture curve is phenomenologically divided into three distinct stages. Following the initial strain ε_o (composed of elastic strain ε_{oE} and plastic strain ε_{oP}), in the transient primary stage, the rate of work hardening is larger than creep recovery. In the secondary steady-state creep stage, it is normally that rate of work hardening is same as that of the recovery. Dislocation must be multiplied during the deformation process, resulting on increasing the dislocation density to cause the work-hardening. However, during this stage, the dislocation density was observed to be constant, suggesting that dislocations are diminished by recovery process. In the tertiary creep stage, cracks begin to form at grain boundaries and thus diminish its effective loading-carrying, cross-sectional area. Many voids are formed. Necking may begin at some points in the sample and decrease its actual

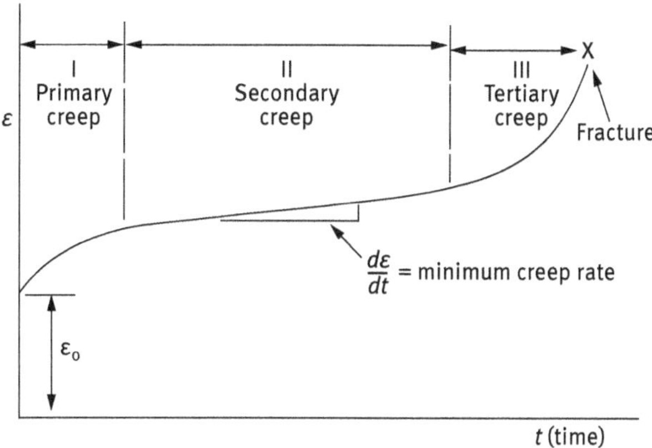

Figure 14.7: Typical creep curve [161].

load-carrying area; softening process may begin to proceed at a higher rate than work hardening. All those factors will be produced at ever-increasing rate of elongation until the sample fractures, which is called as the creep rupture.

The low creep resistance has been one of the major issues of Mg alloys, which limited their wider industrial applications in the past decades. It has been reported that the inherent creep resistance of Mg should be higher than that Al. Hence, it is highly likely that the low creep resistance of Mg alloys was attributed to the effects of alloying elements rather than Mg itself [204]. The usual commercial Mg-based alloys (such as AZ series) are relatively stable up to about 150 °C) and may be used for some applications below that temperature. Solution heat-treated castings and hard-rolled sheet in the usual alloys are unstable above 150 °C and are not suitable for use at elevated temperatures. As indicated, the ordinary Mg-based alloys used for castings or for wrought products have comparatively poor strength and poor resistance to creep at elevated temperatures. Investigations have shown that the addition of RE metals, in the form of mischmetal (MM: typical composition includes approximately 55Ce–25La–18Ne), to magnesium will yield alloys that retain much of their strength at elevated temperatures and exhibit relatively high resistance to creep over a wide range of temperature. The structural or metallographic condition having the maximum resistance to creep at elevated temperatures is produced by means of suitable heat treatment. This varies with the alloy composition and the form of the material (whether cast or wrought). The most suitable conditions for resisting creep are T2, T6 and T7. These are affected, respectively, by stabilization of as-fabricated products, solution heat treatment and aging, and solution heat treatment followed by stabilization [205]. Table 14.3 lists combination of alloying element(s) to Mg-based alloys to affect creep behaviors.

Table 14.3: Alloying effect on creep behavior of various Mg-based alloys.

	Al	Ca	Sn	Sr	Mn	RE	Mn	Si	Sr	Zn	Gd	Zr	Er	Cu	Y	Nd	Sb	La
Mg	[206]	[207]	[208–213]			[214]		[215]		[216, 217]	[218]				[219, 220]	[221, 222]		
Mg–Al		[223–228]	[229]				[230]	[233]	[228, 234]	[235–240]								
Mg–Al–Ca		[241]	[242–244]	[242–244]	[242–244]	[241, 245–247]												
Mg–Al–Ba		[248, 249]																
Mg–Al–Zn		[250]						[251]										
Mg–Zn	[252–254]	[255, 256]	[257]								[258]	[259, 260]	[261, 262]	[263]				
Mg–Li	[264]									[265]								
Mg–Ca										[266]								
Mg–Y						[267]						[268]				[269–271]		
Mg–Gd		[272]								[273, 274]		[275, 276]			[277–280]			
Mg–Gd–Y										[281, 282]						[283]		
Mg–Sn	[284–286]	[84, 287, 288]															[289]	[290, 291]
Mg–Sr					[292, 293]													
Mg–Si											[215]							
Mg–Ce							[294]											
Mg–Nd											[295, 296]							
Mg–La						[297]												

Note: RE, rare earth element.

14.2.5 Tribology

Tribology is the science and technology dealing with the wear, friction and lubrication. Hence, tribology includes the nature of surfaces from both chemical and physical points of view, including topography, the interaction of surfaces under load and changes in the interaction when tangential motion is introduced. In materials science, wear is the erosion of material from a solid surface by the action of another solid. There are four principal wear processes: adhesive wear, abrasive wear, corrosive wear and surface fatigue. Depending on the manner of applying tangential force, there are sliding wear or fretting wear involved. If the tribology action takes place in a biological environment, it is called the biotribology and an adversely synergistic effect of corrosion and tribological action is named as tribocorrosion.

14.2.5.1 Mg–Al alloy systems

A creep-resistant Mg alloy ACM720 (Mg-7Al-2Cu-Mn) was subjected to laser surface treatment using Nd:YAG laser equipped with a fiber optics beam delivery system in argon atmosphere [298] and it was reported that (i) the improved corrosion resistance was attributed to the absence of the second phase Al_2Ca at the grain boundary, microstructural refinement and extended solid solubility, particularly of Al, in α-Mg matrix owing to rapid solidification and (ii) the laser treatment also increased surface hardness 2 times and reduced the wear rate considerably due to grain refinement and solid solution strengthening. Arora et al. [299] investigated wear behavior of a Mg–4Al–2RE (AE42) alloy under as-cast as well as friction stir processed conditions and wear tests were carried out in a pin-on-disk configuration using Universal Tribometer, with the load ranging from 5 to 20 N, whereas sliding velocity from 0.33 to 3 m/s. It was reported that (i) the friction stir-processed (FSPed) AE42 alloy demonstrated significant decrease in the wear rate, which may be attributed to the microstructural refinement resulting in enhanced hardness and ductility of the FSPed alloy along with higher work hardening capability; (ii) at low loads, wear mechanism transformed from oxidation and abrasive wear at low sliding velocity to delaminationdelamination at high velocity; (iii) at intermediate loads, oxidation and abrasion characterized the worn surface at low velocity, whereas delamination and plastic deformation were found to be major wear mechanisms at high velocities; and (iv) at high loads, the corresponding mechanisms were abrasion, delamination and plastic deformation at low velocity, whereas severe plastic deformation (SPD) and delamination at high velocities [299].

14.2.5.2 Mg–Al–Zn alloy systems

There are numerous studies on wear behaviors of AZ (Mg–Al–Zn) alloys. Sun et al. [300] prepared AZ31 (Mg–3Al–1Zn) alloys containing small amounts of yttrium (<4 wt%) using an induction furnace and studied the corrosion resistance of as-cast alloys in a 3.5% NaCl solution was investigated by electrochemical polarization testing and their corrosive wear resistances in the same solution using a pin-on-disk tester. It was reported that (i) adding yttrium in Mg–3Al–1Zn alloy introduced Al_2Y precipitates and minimized the precipitation of $Mg_{17}Al_{12}$ phase with refined micro structure; (ii) the wear resistance of AZ31 was improved when yttrium was added due to the formation of uniformly distributed finer and harder Al_2Y precipitates; (iii) the yttrium addition to AZ31 alloy also enhanced the corrosion resistance, since the galvanic effect of finer and dispersed Al_2Y precipitates was weaker than that of the coarse $Mg_{17}Al_{12}$ particles and their network; and (iv) the combination of improved strength and corrosion resistance resulting from the Y addition increased the corrosive wear resistance of the material. Ge et al. [301] investigated dry RT sliding wear behavior of AZ31 alloy, which was subjected to laser shock peening (LSP) with three laser pulse energies of 6.5 J, 8.5 J and 10.5 J. It was found that (i) the grain size in the topmost surface of AZ31 alloy decreases as laser energy increases; (ii) when laser energy is 10.5 J, a nanostructured surface layer could be fabricated on sample; (iii) microhardness and surface roughness of the laser processed samples decrease with decreasing laser energy; (iv) compared with the untreated sample, the average wear rate of the laser shocked samples is decreased by 32.1%, 45.3% and 69.8% corresponding to laser energy of 6.5 J, 8.5 J and 10.5 J, respectively; and (v) the improvement of the wear resistance for laser-treated samples is mainly ascribed to the grain refinement and strain hardening generated by the LSP. Li et al. [302] mentioned that (i) although surface SPD is an approach used to nanocrystallize metallic surfaces for enhanced resistance to wear, SPD alone does not generate well-defined nanocrystalline structure but one consisting of nanosized dislocation cells with diffuse boundaries and (ii) for materials with limited slip systems such as Mg, SPD may harden the materials but deteriorate their fracture toughness; as a result, the benefit of SPD to the wear resistance of materials may not be appreciable. Based on these backgrounds, Li et al. [302] nanocrystallized the surface layer of AZ31Mg alloy by repeated hammering (HM), followed by recovery treatment to investigate the microstructure, wear behavior, grain structure and wear debris of differently treated samples, including HM, HM plus recovery treatment (HM-R) and as-received. It was reported that (i) the SPD-HR sample had a superior nanocrystalline surface exhibiting the highest wear resistance; (ii) the hammered sample was harder than the HM-HR one but its wear resistance is lower than that of the latter, though it still performed better than the as-received one; (iii) the wear debris analysis showed that the surface of the HM-R sample was tougher than that of the HM one, indicating that the wear resistance of AZ31Mg alloys depends on both hardness and toughness to which the ductility is of importance; and (iv) the recovery treatment after HM certainly helped achieving well-defined nanocrystallization for improved wear resistance of the Mg alloy. Guo et al. [303] surface-treated AZ31D alloy by plasma electrolytic oxidation in an alkaline silicate electrolyte with and without the addition of graphite and concluded that the ceramic coating with the addition of graphene exhibits better corrosion resistance and tribological performance.

Ram et al. [304] investigated the grain refinement effects of carbon on AZ81 alloys through the addition of synthetic graphite and activated charcoal inoculants on the mechanical and dry sliding wear properties. The test was conducted at a speed of 5.37 m/s and two loading (20 and 30 N) conditions in a pin-on-disk wear apparatus. It was reported that the mean grain size of the alloy is significantly reduced from about 185 to 32 μm when the carbon content is increased to 0.98% C; (ii) the wear rate decreases with the increase of carbon content in the alloy; (iii) the activated charcoal with 0.98 wt% C is found to be a better grain refiner in improving the properties of tensile behavior and wear resistance; and (iii) fractography of the fracture surfaceshowed the brittle intergranular fracture, indicating that abrasive and delamination wear mechanisms are responsible for the wear loss in the AZ81 alloy. Demirci et al. [305] processed the surface of AZ91 alloy with the microarc oxidation (MAO) in two different electrolyte solutions, namely phosphate–silicate and potassium stannate to evaluate the wear, corrosion or tribocorrosion properties. It was mentioned that the type of solution has an important role on the wear, corrosion and tribocorrosion resistance of the MAO coating.

14.2.5.3 Mg–Zn alloy systems

Liu et al. [306] investigated the wear behavior of Mg–1.5Zn–0.15Gd alloy before and after cryogenic treatment by dry sliding wear test and found that (i) the wear resistance of the alloys has been significantly improved after cryogenic treatment; (ii) abrasive wear is the main wear mechanism; (iii) the friction coefficient and wear rate decrease with the increase of cryogenic treatment duration, which is attributed to the increase in volume fraction of the secondary phase particles and its refinement due to the cryogenic treatment; and (iv) the alloy after cryogenic treatment exhibits a much smoother worn surface. Chen et al. [307] conducted a comparative study on the effects of MAO coating, Sr-P coating and Ca-P coating on the biodegradable and studied the wear properties of Mg–2Zn–1Gd–0.5Zr alloy. It was obtained that (i) the degradation deposition contained Gd on the surfaces of both MAO coating and Sr-P coating, which stabilized the coating, thereby increasing the degradation resistance of the alloy; (ii) the wear test showed that MAO coating and Ca-P coating exhibited good wear resistance; and (iii) for a 5 N loading, the sliding distances of MAO coating, Sr-P coating and Ca-P coating were 2.24, 0.29 and 9.00 m, respectively, before the coatings were completely destroyed, indicating that the MAO coating exhibits the best degradation resistance and the Ca-P coating exhibits the best wear resistance. Ramesh et al. [308] investigated the effect of multidirectional forging (MDF) on wear properties of Mg–xZn alloys ($x = 2$, 4, and 6 wt%) under a dry sliding wear test using pin on disk machine. It was mentioned that after 5 passes of MDF, the average grain size was found to be 30 ± 4, 22 ± 3 and

18 ± 3 μm, in Mg–2%Zn, Mg–4%Zn and Mg–6%Zn alloys, respectively, with significant improvement in hardness in all cases. Wear resistance was improved after MDF processing, as well as with increment in Zn content in Mg alloy; however, it decreased when the load and the sliding distance increased. Worn surface exhibited ploughing, delamination, plastic deformation and wear debris along the sliding direction, and abrasive wear was found to be the main mechanism.

14.2.5.4 Mg–Li alloy system

Ma et al. [309] applied plasma electrolytic oxidation coatings on the surface of Mg–8Li–1Al and studied the tribological behavior of the coated and uncoated Mg–Li alloy under dry friction conditions against a Si_3N_4 ball as counter-face material and reported that (i) the tribological behavior is greatly affected by the microstructure and phase compositions of the coatings and (ii) the plasma electrolytic oxidation coatings significantly improved the properties of friction and wear of Mg–Li alloy. Sikdar et al. [310] studied the fretting wear behavior of newly developed Mg–Li–Al-based alloys (Mg-Li-Al-Sn: LAT971 and Mg-Li-Al-Sn-Zn: LATZ9531) using reciprocating fretting wear testing under dry condition with varying number of cycles (10–10^4), normal load (1–10 N), oscillation frequency (1–9 Hz) and displacement amplitude (80–200 μm). It was shown that LATZ9531 elicits consistent performance, lower coeffi cient of frictioncoefficient of friction (~0.50) than conventional AZ31 (~0.69) and LAT971 (0.60); however, under the condition of high normal load (of 10 N), LAT971 shows least wear volume loss (~0.05 mm^3) as well as lower coefficient of friction (~0.26) compared to that of LATZ9531 or conventional AZ31. In addition to central cracking in LATZ9531, mainly adhesive and delamination wear mechanism are noticed. Under frequency variation LAT971 shows enhanced performance especially at high frequency (~9 Hz); however, with increase in slip amplitude (~200 μm), the major wear mechanism is observed to be abrasive and oxidative wear, wherein LATZ9531 shows least wear volume. Friction hysteresis of increasing slip amplitude shows an increase in energy consumption during fretting wear, and its shape confirms that in spite of change in stroke lengths, fretting is occurring in the gross slip regime.

14.2.5.5 Mg–Y alloy system

Goretta et al. [311] conducted solid-particle erosionsolid-particle erosion studies on a hardened Mg alloy (WE43A-T6) and the same alloy that had been anodized to produce a ≈ 12 μm oxide layer. Angular alumina particles of nominal diameter 63 or 143 μm traveling at 60 or 120 m/s impacted the targets at 20° or 90° and steady-state erosion rates were determined as weight loss of a sample per weight of impacting particles. It was reported that (i) the oxide coating on the WE43A–T6 alloy was removed quickly, (ii) weight-loss data indicated that the alloy underlying the anodized layer eroded measurably faster than the as-heat-treated alloy, but that below depths greater than ≈ 80 μm, the two alloys eroded at nearly equal rates and (iii) the near-surface more rapid erosion rates for the anodized alloy were attributed to loss of ductility due to internal oxidation from the anodizing process. The friction and wear properties of pure magnesium and the Mg–Y alloy were investigated using the pin-on-disk configuration [312] and mentioned that the friction and wear resistance of the Mg–Y alloy was superior to those of pure magnesium. The wear mechanism was abrasion under all the conditions. The formation of low-angle grain boundaries was also confirmed with an increase in the applied load in the Mg–Y alloy; on the other hand, grain refinement due to dynamic recrystallization was observed in pure magnesium as the wear test progressed. The different microstructures resulted from difference in the surface temperature during the wear test, which was estimated to be around 120 and 90 °C for pure magnesium and the Mg–Y alloy, respectively. The high increment temperature in the fine-grained alloys brought about the occurrence of grain boundary sliding, that is, material softening, which led to a decrease in the friction and wear properties, indicating that one of the methods for enhancing the friction and wear properties is to increase the dynamic recrystallization temperature. Hui et al. [313] conducted dry sliding wear tests on as-cast and cast and T6 Mg-11Y-5Gd-2Zn magnesium alloys using a ball-on-plate configuration. The wear rates were measured within a load range of 3–15 N, sliding speed range of 0.03–0.24 m/s, test temperature range of 25–200 °C and at a constant sliding distance of 400 m. It was found that (i) the wear rate of the alloys increases almost linearly with increasing applied load and decreases with increasing sliding speed; (ii) the wear rate of the as-cast alloy is higher than that of the cast + T6 alloy; (iii) the amount of $Mg_{12}Y_1Zn_1$ phase, surface oxidation and retained wear debris affect the wear rate; and (iv) the dominant wear mechanisms under the test condition are abrasion and plastic deformation.

14.2.5.6 Mg–Sn alloy system

Huang et al. [314] evaluated the fretting performance of Mg–Sn–Y alloy under fluids lubrication, and the fretting mechanism was explored in detail via analysis of wear track/debris using SEM and X-ray photoelectron spectroscopy (XPS) depth profile. It was shown that (i) the friction reduction is superior to wear resistance for lubricated Mg–Sn–Y/Steel contact under fretting conditions, mainly depending on the oil-film-induced transformation of fretting running regime and transition of fretting wear (from adhesive/oxidation wear and delamination under dry friction to abrasive wear and delamination under fluids lubrication) and (ii) fretting performance of Mg–Sn–Y alloy under fluids lubrication depends on fretting running regime and synergy of oil-film/protective film. Yadav et al. [315] studied fabricated Mg–2Sn, Mg–2Sn–1Ca and Mg–2Sn–2Ca (by wt%) alloys by the powder metallurgy and performed a dry sliding wear test on the pin-on-disk machine. It was found that (i) the cumulative weight loss of the Mg–2Sn–1Ca was lowest among all and (ii) it was attributed to high hardness of materials which follows the Archard's law and average coefficient of friction was decreasing in nature with normal load.

14.2.5.7 Mg–Gd alloy system

Zhang et al. [316] conducted dry sliding wear tests on as-cast and T6-treated Mg-3Gd-1Zn-0.4Zr (wt%, GZ31K) and Mg-6Gd-1Zn-0.4Zr (wt%, GZ61K) alloys using a ball-on-disk configuration at RT. Friction coefficient and wear rate of the alloys were measured under three different applied loads (50, 100 and 200 N, respectively). It was reported that (i) the friction coefficient of the alloys decreases with increasing load, except the as-cast GZ61K. The wear rates of the as-cast Mg-Gd-Zn-Zr alloys increase with the increase of the load; however, the wear rates of the T6-treated Mg-Gd-Zn-Zr alloys first increase because of the participation of a large amount of needle-like precipitates, but then decline due to obvious work hardening; (ii) the wear mechanisms of abrasion, plastic deformation, oxidation, adhesion and delamination are detected; and (iii) abrasion dominates the wear mechanism under the low load; whereas adhesion is the main wear mechanism under intermediate load, and plastic deformation has great effect on the wear rate under high applied load. The wear behavior of a Mg-10Gd-3Y-0.4Zr alloy during dry sliding was studied using ball-on-flat-type wear apparatus against an AISI 52100-type bearing steel ball counterface in a load range of 3–15 N, sliding speed range of 0.03–0.24 m/s, temperature range of 25–200 °C and at a constant sliding distance of 400 m [317]. It was mentioned that (i) the Mg-10Gd-3Y-0.4Zr alloy exhibited low wear rate compared with cast and T6 AC8A Al alloy under the same condition; (ii) the wear rate of as-cast Mg-10Gd-3Y-0.4Zr alloy was lower than that of cast T6 Mg-10Gd-3Y-0.4Zr alloy; (iii) the $Mg_{24}(Gd,Y)_5$ eutectic compound of as-cast Mg-10Gd-3Y-0.4Zr alloy could resist the material flow during friction and wear, and affected its wear rate; (iv) at high sliding speed, the retained wear debris was the major constituent of producing the severely deformed layers along the sliding direction; and (v) the trapped wear debris acted as a protective layer and reduced the wear rate. Hu et al. [318] performed dry sliding wear tests on a Mg-10Y-4Gd-1.5Zn-0.4Zr alloy using a ball-on-flat-type wear apparatus against an AISI 52100 type bearing steel ball counterface under the similar conditions as reported [317]. It was found that (i) the wear rates of Mg-10Y-4Gd-1.5Zn-0.4Zr alloy are lower than that of cast T6 AC9B Al alloy; (ii) the dominant mechanism of cast T6 Mg-10Y-4Gd-1.5Zn-0.4Zr alloy is abrasion wear mixed with other wear mechanisms, which tends to be an abrasion and plastic deformation wear at high normal load such as 10–25 N, abrasion and plastic deformation wears with small participation of delamination and oxidative wears at high sliding speed such as 0.12–0.3 m/s, and an oxidative and abrasion wear at high test temperature such as 100–200 °C; and (iii) the $Mg_{12}Y_1Zn_1$ phase in Mg-10Y-4Gd-1.5Zn-0.4Zr alloy plays an important role in the wear rate. Cao et al. [319] prepared a Mg-14.28Gd-2.44Zn-0.54Zr (mass fraction, %) alloy by conventional ingot metallurgy and investigated the wear behavior under oil lubricant condition by pin-on-disk configuration at a load of 40 N and sliding speeds of 30–300 mm/s with a sliding distance of 5,000 m at RT. It was reported that (i) the as-cast alloy is mainly composed of α-Mg solid solution, the lamellar 14 H-type long-period LPSO structure within matrix, and β-[$(Mg,Zn)_3Gd$] phase; however, most of the β-phase transforms to X-phase with 14 H-type LPSO structure after solution heat treatment at 500 °C for 35 h (T4) and (ii) the ST alloy presents low wear-resistance, because the hard β-phase is converted into thermally stable, ductile and soft X–$Mg_{12}GdZn$ phase with LPSO structure in the alloy.

14.2.5.8 Mg–Cu alloy system

Itoi et al. [320] studied the wear properties of $Mg_{90.5}Cu_{3.25}Y_{6.25}$ (at%) cast alloy consisting of Mg and long-period-ordered (LPO) phases by pin-on-disk-type wear tests under dry sliding, along with pure Mg, extruded AZ31 and cast AZ91 alloys. It was reported that (i) the wear loss of the $Mg_{90.5}Cu_{3.25}Y_{6.25}$ cast alloy at high-applied loads over 147 N was less than those of AZ Mg alloys, and about two-thirds of the AZ31 extruded alloy, which indicated that the $Mg_{90.5}Cu_{3.25}Y_{6.25}$ cast alloy has superior wear resistance; (ii) the basal planes (0 0 0 2) and (101¯1) were apparent in the X-ray diffraction (XRD) patterns of worn surfaces of pure Mg and Mg alloys, indicating that basal planes in both the Mg and LPO phases were aligned to worn surfaces for the pure Mg and Mg alloys; (iii) because slip deformation tends to easily occur on the Mg basal plane at a low critical resolved shear stress, formation of the basal-plane alignment on the wear surface negatively affects the wear resistance properties; and (iv) after the wear test of the $Mg_{90.5}Cu_{3.25}Y_{6.25}$ cast alloy, a kink deformation in the LPO phase was frequently observed in the worn edge section and the kink deformation in the LPO phase contributes to improve wear resistance properties by suppression of the basal-plane alignment.

14.2.5.9 Mg–Dy alloy system

Bi et al. [321] investigated the dry sliding wear behavior of extruded Mg–2Dy–0.5Zn alloy (at%) using a pin-on-disk configuration. The friction coefficient and wear rate were measured within a load range 20–760 N at a sliding velocity of 0.785 m/s. It was mentioned that (i) five wear mechanisms, namely abrasion, oxidation, delami nation, thermal softening and melting dominated the whole wear behavior with increasing applied load; (ii) the extruded Mg–2Dy 0.5Zn alloy exhibited the better wear resistance as compared with as-cast $Mg_{97}Zn_1Y_2$ alloy under the given conditions through contact surface temperature analysis; and (iii) the improved wear resistance was mainly related to fine grain size, good thermal stability of LPSO phase and excellent higher temperature mechanical properties.

14.2.5.10 Mg-based composites

Instead of alloying of Mg, Mg was incorporated with ceramics to enhance the wear resistance. Kaviti et al. [322] investigated the effect of boron nitride nanoparticles (NPs) reinforcement on dry sliding wear behavior of pure Mg and Mg nanocomposites. The fabricated nanocomposites contains varied percentages of boron nitride such as 0% (pure Mg), 0.5%, 1.5% and 2.5% were synthesized by using powder met allurgy technique and followed by a hot working process called hot extrusion. The pin on disk equipment was used for conducting the wear tests for traditional loads of 5, 7 and 10 N at different sliding speeds of 0.6, 0.9 and 1.2 m/s against the steel disk at RT. It was mentioned that (i) for all nanocomposites the wear level raises with respect to the sliding speeds and loads and (ii) Mg reinforced with 0.5% boron nitride shows lower wear rates and low friction coefficient values compare with magnesium reinforced with 1.5% boron nitride and 2.5% boron nitride nanocomposites. Zhang et al. [323] studied dry sliding wear behaviors of Mg-based nanocomposites with 15 vol% SiC NPs using the ball-on-disk wear tester. It was found that (i) the wear resistance is about 23 times higher than that of pure Mg and (ii) the delamination mechanism of Mg has been overcome by the addition of high volume fraction NPs, and the dominant wear mechanism of the Mg–SiC nanocomposites is oxidation. Banerjee et al. [324] examined the effect of process parameters on wear behavior of magnesium nanocomposites reinforced with WC NPs. It was reported that among three process parameters (wt% of WC, applied load and sliding speed), sliding speed and wt% of WC are found to be the most significant parameters.

Similarly, AZ alloy is composited with NPs. Arab et al. [325] investigated the effect of graphene nanoplatelet (GNP) content on mechanical and tribological properties of AZ31 Mg matrix composite. It was obtained that (i) hardness was increased up to 14% by applying the friction stir processing and 41% via adding GNPs due to grain refinement, dynamic recrystallization and pinning effect of GNPs; (ii) mechanical properties were improved by increasing the GNP content which act as an obstacle against dislocation glide; (iii) coefficient of friction was decreased from 25% to 45% when compared with the base metal, by adding GNPs; and (iv) the intensity of adhesive, abrasive and delamination wear mechanisms was decreased by increasing the GNPs through forming a lubricant layer which not only restricts frictional heat but also improves the load carrying capacity of nanocomposite. Kondaiah et al. [326] produced AZ31–matrix composites with fly ash as a dispersing phase by friction stir processing. It was mentioned that (i) microstructural observations have clearly showed fine grain structure in the processed zone, (ii) compared with annealed AZ31, a 30% increase in hardness was observed for the composites; however, a significant variation in the hardness was observed across the processed region (advancing, nugget and retreating regions), (iii) grain refinement and the presence of fly ash are the prime reasons that played an important role behind the increased hardness; and (iv) the AZ31–fly ash composites can be successfully produced in solid state by friction stir processing, and the effect of fly ash as a dispersing phase on enhancing the hardness and wear properties is promising.

14.2.6 Fracture and environment-assisted fracture

Fracture behavior of Mg materials, like other materials, depends on various factors including production routes (as-cast, wrought, powder metallurgy, etc.), history of heat treatment (directly related to microstructures including precipitates, segregation and grain size), testing modes (temperature and strain rate) and testing environment (such as SCC: stress corrosion cracking or HE).

14.2.6.1 Fractography

Khan et al. [327] investigated the microstructure, mechanical properties and frac ture behavior of an as-received QE22 (Mg–2Ag–2RE) alloy under different thermal conditions, including ST, UA, PA and OA conditions. Fractographically, different natures of crack initiation and propagation were observed under different thermal conditions during tensile testing at RT. It was also mentioned that (i) the mode of failure of ST sample is transgranular (TG), cleavage and twin boundary fractures and (ii) a mixed mode of transgranular, intergranular (IG), cleavage and twin boundary failure is observed in both PA and OA samples. Figure 14.8 illustrates the typical path of transgranular crack propagation (a) and intergranular propagation [328].

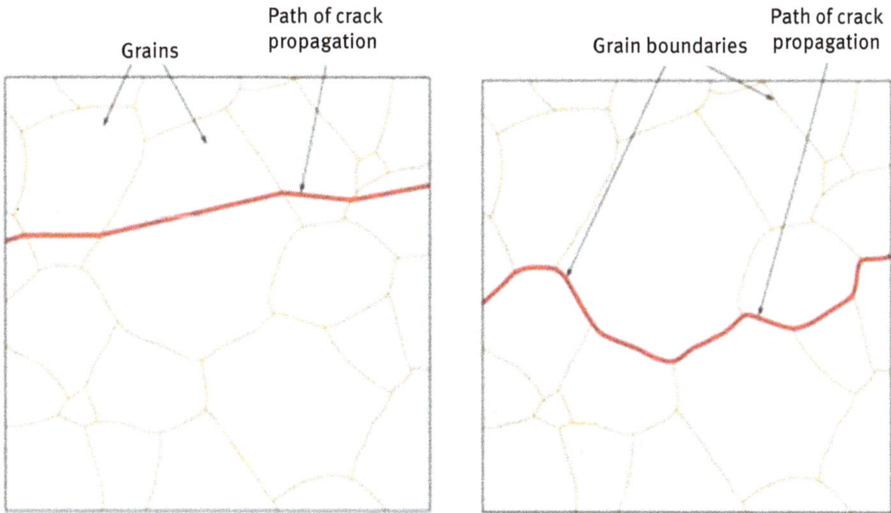

Figure 14.8: Transgranular crack propagation (a) and intergranular crack propagation [328].

Gao et al. [329] studied the fracture behavior of a permanent mold casting Mg–8.57Gd–3.72Y–0.54Zr (mas %) (GW94) alloy under different thermal conditions, including as-cast, ST, PA and OA states. It was reported that (i) during tensile test at RT, the fracture model of the as-cast GW94 alloy is quasicleavage, while that of the ST alloy is transgranular cleavage; (ii) it is a mixed pattern of transgranular and intergranular fracture for both the aged conditions; (iii) large cavities formed at grain boundaries are observed in the PA sample tested at 300 °C, corresponding to the intergranular fracture; and (iv) localized plastic deformation at grain boundaries is also observed and corresponds to the high elongation at 300 °C. Li et al. [330] processed as-cast $Mg_{97}Y_2Zn_1$ billets with a two-phase microstructure with four passes of equal channel angular extrusion (ECAE) using different routes at 350 °C to refine the microstructure. The duplex microstructure of this material consists of a Mg-rich alloy matrix with an LPSO reinforcement phase. It was mentioned that (i) localized deformation is responsible for the final failure of the ECAEed $Mg_{97}Y_2Zn_1$ alloy under both quasistatic and high strain rate loading, (ii) the grain morphology and distribution after deformation indicated that the shear localization resulted from the rotation and rearrangement of grains and (iii) cracks were found to propagate along the grain boundaries leading to final failure. Lin et al. [331] studied the effects of plastic deformation on precipitation behavior and tensile fracture behavior of Mg–10Gd–3Y–0.6Zr alloy. It was shown that (i) with increasing the plastic deformation, the microcracks occur at the interface between grain boundary precipitations and matrix, and then propagate intergranularly and (ii) when intergranular fracture combines with the formation of smoothing facets on the fracture surface, the tensile properties decrease. Ortega et al. [332] studied the tensile properties and fracture characteristics of the PA Mg–1.0 wt% Ca and Mg–1.0 wt% Ca–1.0 wt% Zn alloys in the temperature range 22–177 °C. It was found that (i) microstructure observations using scanning electron microscopy revealed that the failure mode for both alloys is transgranular combined with intergranular rupture, irrespective of the treatment and test temperature and (ii) the fractography analyses showed that the transgranular fracture changed from quasicleavage to dimple rupture with increasing temperature. Liu et al. [333] conducted tensile test of the as-cast Mg–6Zn–2Er alloy, which has coarse secondary W-phase ($Mg_3Zn_3Er_2$). It was reported that (i) the existence of the W-phase activates the stress concentrations due to the incapacity of W-phase for the load transfer, which results in the void at the inner of the W-phase and (ii) in comparison, the interface between the matrix and the secondary phase is stable; concluding that (iii) the characters of the secondary phases with respect to size, distribution, morphology and type, play an important role in the plastic deformation behavior of the alloy. Gui et al. [334] investigated the microstructures, tensile properties, fracture pathways and fracture characteristics of the as-cast, heat-treated and hot-extruded Mg-1.59Nd-2.91Zn-0.05Zr-0.35Mn (NZKM) alloys and indicated that (i) the fracture patterns changed with the evolution of the microstructures and (ii) intergranular and transgranular cleavage fractures were changed to ductile fractures by hot extrusion.

Magnesium alloy EZ10 (Mg–RE–Zn) was deformed in tension at temperatures from 20 up to 520 °C [335]. It was reported that (i) a rapid decrease of the yield and tensile strength with temperature was observed at temperatures higher than 300 °C and (ii) diffusional processes occurring at temperatures higher than 300 °C significantly influenced the deformation mechanism as well as the fracture character. Jia et al. [336] studied the deformation and fracture behaviors of as-cast AZ31B Mg alloy by uniaxial compression experiments with wide ranges of temperature and strain rate and mentioned that the observed sharp in stress caused by micro-cracks initiation and propagation can be readily produced at relatively low temperatures and high strain rates. Yu et al. [337] investigated the dynamic deformational behavior and failure mechanisms of extruded Mg–Gd–Y alloy, under high strain rates, at ambient temperature 27, 200 and 300 °C. It was found that (i) extruded Mg–Gd–Y alloy has the largest dynamic compressive strength which is 535 MPa at ambient temperature and strain rate of 2,826/s, (ii) when temperature increases, dynamic compressive strength decreases, while ductility increases, (iii) the dynamic compression fracture mechanism of extruded Mg–Gd–Y alloy is multi-crack propagation and intergranular quasicleavage fracture at both ambient temperature and high temperature and (iv) the dynamic compressive deformation mechanism of extruded Mg–Gd–Y alloy is a combination of twinning, slipping and dynamic recrystallization at both ambient temperature and high temperature. Mine et al. [338] studied the fracture behavior of extruded Mg–1Zn–2Y alloys (consisted of α-Mg and LPSO structure phases) at RT and at 200 °C using microfracture testing. It was mentioned that (i) the fracture behavior changed from brittle to ductile as the testing temperature increased, (ii) the LPSO-phase specimen remained brittle even at the elevated temperature and the intrinsic fracture toughness values obtained at both testing temperatures were nearly identical and (iii) mechanical twinning in the α-Mg phase did not occur at the elevated temperature, although it was activated at RT, suggesting that the plastic deformation mode in the α-Mg phase plays a crucial part in the enhanced crack growth resistance of the two-phase alloy at the elevated temperature.

14.2.6.2 Crack initiation and propagation

For Mg–2Gd alloy, Liu et al. [339] studied intergranular deformation anisotropy and grain boundary microcrack nucleation by tensile tests. It was mentioned that (i) a predictive fracture initiation parameter, which correlates with dislocation activity, twinning deformation and the geometrical orientation of grain boundary, has been modified to evaluate the probability of the microcrack nucleation at grain boundary and the statistical results revealed that the fracture initiation parameter which has been used to evaluate microcrack initiation in TiAl alloys can also well predict the nucleation of microcracks with this following law, that is, grain boundaries with larger fracture initiation parameter are more likely to cause microcrack nucleation. Yue et al. [340]. studied the tensile crack initiation behaviors in cast NZ30K (Mg-Ni-Zn-Zr) alloys under as-cast, T4- and T6-treated conditions. It was indicated that (i) for the as-cast alloy, the microcracks form mainly by cracking of the eutectic phases (~83%), (ii) twin grain boundaries are also found to be preferential sites for crack nucleation (~17%), (iii) the tensile failure in the T4- and T6-treated alloys is mainly caused by twin nucleation (T4–60% and T6–44%) and grain boundaries cracking (T4–28% and T6–52%) and (iv) interactions among dislocation slip, twinning and grain boundaries as well as eutectic phases determine the crack initiation behavior of cast magnesium alloys. Cui et al. [341] investigated the influence of secondary phases on the initiation and propagation of tensile crack during the fracture process in as-cast Mg–Al–Zn–Nd alloy. It was reported that (i) micro-cracks initiated in divorced eutectic $Mg_{17}Al_{12}$ phase, eutectic $Mg_{17}Al_{12}$ phase, twin boundaries and interface between $\alpha + \beta$ eutectic structure and α-Mg matrix, (ii) the breaking of the divorced eutectic $Mg_{17}Al_{12}$ phase at the grain collapsing zone edge and the decreased effective force bearing area due to grain collapsing contributed to the propagation of transgranular cracks, (iii) breaking of $Mg_{17}Al_{12}$ phase is accompanied by the formation of voids at the main crack tip, which provided a path for crack propagation and growth and (iv) formation of voids can also blunt the main crack tip and divert the crack propagation direction. Basha et al. [342] studied crack nucleation and propagation in thin foils of pure Mg and Mg–0.3 at %Y alloy under tension and mentioned that (i) during propagation along grain boundaries, twin nucleation occurred from the crack tip, (ii) in case of pure Mg, the crack did not propagate along the twin boundaries but continued along the grain boundaries and (iii) in case of Mg–0.3 at %Y alloy, in which the grain boundaries were segregated with yttrium, the crack propagated along newly formed twin boundaries nucleated at the crack tip.

14.2.6.3 Fracture toughness

A micromechanical approach for determining the fracture toughness was developed for AZ31 alloy by employing a phase-field model for grain growth to generate microstructures with varying attributes and the cohesive finite element method to quantify the interaction between a propagating crack and microstructures [343]. It was mentioned that (i) simulations show that fracture toughness increases as the average grain size decreases and that the local crack tip environment significantly affects the fracture behavior and (ii) dramatically different dependences of fracture toughness on overall strain rate are seen when two different types of cohesive laws are employed. Prasad et al. [344] investigated the effect of notch acuity on fracture behavior of rolled AZ31Mg alloy by conducting mode-I fracture experiments using four-point bend specimens with different notch root radii. It was reported that (i) that the fracture toughness Jc increases linearly with notch root radius beyond a threshold value and is almost constant below this limit and this trend is rationalized from fractographic observations near the crack initiation region which show predominantly quasibrittle features for fatigue precracked specimen and dimples of increasing size in notched specimens with enhancement in notch root radius, (ii) significant tensile twinning is noticed in the ligament for all specimens, especially near their far edge and (iii) the strong increase in Jc with notch root radius beyond a threshold is interpreted using two ductile fracture initiation models. Zindal et al. [345] studied the fracture and fracture toughness properties of the Mg–0.8Al–0.5Zn alloy. It was reported that (i) the precipitation state at the grain boundary plays an important role in deciding the exact mode of failure (i.e., intergranular or transgranular type), (ii) the role of precipitate characteristics in determining the fracture mode has been ascertained and (iii) the correlation between the various microstructural features and fracture toughness value is established following the Hornbogen and Graf model and the measured values of fracture toughness are found to be in good agreement with the values predicted by the model. Hase et al. [346] measured impact toughness of three alloys (Mg, Mg–0.3Ca–0.6Zn, and Mg–0.3Ca–0.6–Al by at%) by the impact three-point bending test. It was mentioned that the plastic deformability and impact toughness were higher in the ternary alloys than in pure Mg. The generalized stacking fault energystacking fault energy and grain boundary cohesive energy were estimated by first-principles calculations for Mg, binary Mg–Ca, ternary Mg–Ca–Zn and ternary Mg–Ca–Al alloys and the calculated results agreed with the trend in the experimental results, suggesting that addition of Ca along with Zn- or Al-reduced plastic anisotropy plastic anisotropy and strengthened the grain boundaries, leading to higher in impact toughness of Mg alloys. Wang et al. [347] studied impact toughness and plane-strain fracture toughness of sand-cast Mg-6Gd-3Y-0.5Zr (GW63) alloy in different thermal conditions, including as-cast, as-quenched and isothermal aging states. It was shown that (i) optimum heat treatment is solutionized at 490 ℃ for 12 h, and then aged at 212 ℃ for 100 h, (ii) impact values of GW63 alloy are 34.6, 50.9 and 20.3 J/cm^2 in the as-cast, as-quenched and aged states, respectively, (iii) RT impact toughness is more closely related to material ductility than strength and (iv) the plane-strain fracture toughness values of the as-cast, as-quenched and aged alloy are 16.2, 17.7 and 19.5 MPa m½, respectively, that is, the improvement of 20.4% has been achieved by aging precipitation strengthening in contrast with slight improvement of 9.3% by solid solution strengthening.

14.2.6.4 Stress corrosion cracking

SCC and HE are two typical phenomena in which fracture takes place under an adverse influence of environmental factors (which is, in most cases, corrosion actions).

Referring to Figure 14.9 [348], basic mechanism for both SCC and HE can be explained. Prior to crack initiation, surface should be locally attacked by corrosive environment; hence, the sequential cracking should proceed as follows: (1) passive film breakdown by Cl^{-1} ion attack and/or movement of slip steps, (2) formation of pit, (3) crack initiated at pit due to highly concentrated stress intensity and (4) crack propagation. During the corrosive action by Cl^{-1} ion, there are two basic

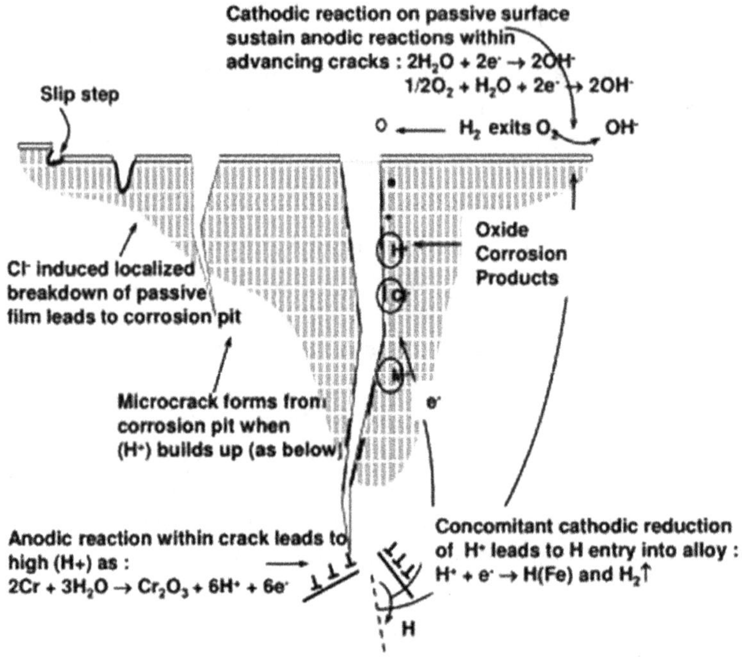

Figure 14.9: Illustration of basic reactions for both SCC and HE [348].

co-occurring reactions; namely, anodic active dissolution of element (which is the most least noble element out of elements of an alloy) and slip dissolution, and cathodic reaction with hydrogen, which is generated at the cathodic site during the corrosion reaction. Once a crack is initiated, the stress–strain condition at the crack tip turns to be favorable to advance the crack with repeated concomitant reactions of anodic dissolution and hydrogen absorption [349, 350].

There are two types of SCC, depending on the crack propagation passage, that is, IGSCC (intergranular SCC) and TGSCC (transgranular SCC). Grain boundaries possess several characteristics, including segregation and precipitation of inclusions (which cause the localized galvanic corrosion), dislocation pileups or crystallographic mismatching. All these irregularities associated with grain boundary increases chemical potential, resulting in providing itself as favorable sites for corrosion. Hence, IGSCC is typically caused by a continuous second phase along grain boundaries. The second phase accelerates corrosion of the adjacent matrix by microgalvanic corrosion; the applied stress opens the crack and allows propagation through the alloy. IGSCC can be avoided by appropriate Mg alloy design. TGSCC is the intrinsic form of SCC, caused by an interaction of hydrogen with the microstruc ture. Many Mg alloys have a threshold stress for SCC of the order of half the yield stress in common environments, including high-purity water [351–353].

Jones et al. [354] pointed out that (i) precipitation of the γ-phase ($Mg_{17}Al_{12}$) at grain boundaries of the Mg–Al alloys is a critical factor in their stress corrosion performance, (ii) γ-phase is cathodic (noble) to the matrix and (iii) this intermetallic phase produces localized galvanic-induced corrosion that leads to IGSCC and crack growth rates of 1,800 times faster than the ST condition. Wearmouth et al. [355] mentioned that (i) the correlation of the threshold stress for SCC of plain specimens and of K_{ISCC} (threshold stress intensity factor for SCC) for precracked specimens in a Mg 7% Al alloy immersed in K_2CrO_4/NaCl solutions is explicable in terms of the formation of cracks that do not propagate to total failure in plain specimens stressed below the threshold stress; (ii) whether or not a crack continues to propagate relates to the competition between the lateral film growth rate, tending to inhibit corrosion, and the strain rate, tending to create reactive bare metal; (iii) study of the effects of various strain rates has shown that SCC only occurs within a restricted range of strain rates, with ductile failures at higher or lower rates, lending support to the suggestion that if the effective strain rate is too low film growth occurs as fast as bare metal is created and stress corrosion failure does not occur; and (iv) in SCC in Mg–Al alloy and possibly some other systems, stress or stress intensity, per se, may be less important than the strain rates they produce. Makar et al. [356] investigated SCC of rapidly solidified Mg–1Al and Mg–9Al alloys in aqueous solutions of potassium chromate and sodium chloride. It was reported that (i) potential pulse and scratched electrode experiments showed that repassivation kinetics are improved both by rapid solidification and increased aluminum content; (ii) the melt-spun alloys experienced relatively uniform attack, and repassivated more rapidly and more completely than their as-cast counterparts; (iii) both failed by TGSCC in aqueous 0.21 M K_2CrO_4 containing 0.6 M NaCl at displacement rates between 5×10^{-5} and 9×10^{-3} mm/s; (iv) in 0.6 M NaCl, TGSCC occurred only near 3.6×10^{-3} mm/s, while no stress corrosion was observed in chromate solution without chloride; (v) constant displacement rate tests in air after pre-exposure to the electrolyte indicated that TGSCC probably results from a HE process; and (vi) using reasonable estimates of the diffusivity of hydrogen in magnesium, analysis of the constant displacement rate and potential pulse tests for Mg–9Al supports a model involving the formation of magnesium hydride ahead of the crack tip.

Winzer et al. [357, 358] investigated mechanisms for the SCC of the two-phase alloy AZ91 and the single-phase alloys AZ31 and AM30 in distilled water. It was found that (i) the mechanism for crack initiation in AZ31 and AM30 involves localized dissolution; (ii) the mechanisms for crack propagation in AZ31 and AM30 involve microvoid coalescence and cleavage, respectively; (iii) the mechanism for crack initiation in AZ91 is unclear, but may involve the fracture of β-particles near the surface; (iv) the mechanism for crack propagation at moderate strain rates in AZ91 is similar to that in AZ31, with β-particles acting as sources of H for mobile dislocations; (v) the fracture surface for AZ91 tested at the strain rate 3×10^{-8}/s was similar to that for specimens precharged in gaseous H_2; and (vi) the fracture surface is the result of (a) the nucleation and growth of MgH_2 particles; (b) sudden fracture through the MgH_2 particles at some critical stress; and (c) decomposition of the MgH_2 particles after fracture. Tsao [359] evaluated the SCC behavior of a commercial AZ31 magnesium alloy after T5 and T6 heat treatments under a vacuum of 10^{-3} torr via slow strain rate tensile tests in an aqueous 3.5 wt% NaCl solution. It was shown that (i) AZ31 displays a high sensitivity to SCC; (ii) the fractured surface was consistent with a significant transgranular component; (iii) double-line cracking that resulted from twinning could be readily spotted on the cleavage plane; (iv) the presence of such deformation twins accompanied by the formation of voids is the main reason for the SCC susceptibility of this alloy; and (v) the disappearance of twins after artificial aging at 260 °C for 4 h significantly improves the corrosion resistance, increases the breakdown potential difference (thus lowering the pitting tendency), and decreases the corrosion current density in a 3.5 wt% NaCl solution. Kappes et al. [360] investigated SCC of the Mg–Al–Zn (AZ31B) alloy in sodium chloride (NaCl) solutions at different potentials and NaCl concentrations using the slow strain rate technique. It was indicated that (i) stress–strain curves were similar despite changes in potential and chloride concentration; (ii) pre-exposure tests were performed in NaCl solutions at the open-circuit potential followed by immediate straining or straining after a dry air exposure delay; (iii) the dependence of ductility with pre-exposure time, the reversibility of embrittlement, and the fracture surface of preexposed samples suggested that the AZ31B alloy was susceptible to internal HE; and (iv) SCC and the pre-exposure embrittlement of AZ31B in NaCl environments are explained assuming that crack growth rate was controlled by hydrogen diffusion. Kannan et al. [361] evaluated the SCC susceptibility of sand-cast Mg–Al–Zn alloy in modified SBF using the slow strain rate test method and mentioned that the SCC susceptibility of the sand-cast magnesium alloy is not substantial and this aspect should not be a concern for its implant applications. Winzer et al. [362, 363] studied TGSCC of the AZ91 in distilled water and 5 g/L NaCl solution. It was reported that (i) the TGSCC threshold stress was 55–75 MPa in distilled water and in 5 g/L NaCl and (ii) the TGSCC velocity was 7×10^{-10} to 5×10^{-9} m/s.

Prabhu et al. [364] investigated the SCC susceptibility of Mg–4Zn alloy in SBF at different strain rates and mentioned that (i) elongation to failure and UTS decreased by 80% and 58%, respectively, when extension rate in SBF decreased from 3.6×10^{-4}/s to 3.6×10^{-6}/s; (ii) when the Mg–4Zn alloy is strained in SBF, multiple surface cracks appear on the gauge, initiated at the corrosion pits that induce mechanical overload and failure at higher strain rates; (iii) as the strain rate decreases, the increased contact time between the surface and SBF results in HE, microcrack formation and progressive transgranular failure that is evident in the fractography and (iv) the in UTS and elongation even at the highest strain rate tested indicate that the critical strain rate for SCC of Mg–4Zn alloy in SBF could be as high as 3.6×10^{-4}/s.

Li et al. [365] studied that the SCC of EV31A (Mg–3Nd–1Gd–0.5Zr) in 0.1 M Na_2SO_4 saturated with $Mg(OH)_2$ using linearly increasing stress tests, compared with pure Mg and WE43B (Mg–4Y–3RE). It was obtained that (i) all three materials were susceptible to SCC; (ii) SCC susceptibility increased with decreasing applied stress rate; (iii) the threshold stress was 0.3× (yield stress) for pure Mg, 0.6× (yield stress) for EV31A, and 0.8× (yield stress) for WE43B; and (iv) the SCC velocities at an applied stress rate of 7.3×10^{-4} MPa/s were 7.2×10^{-8} m/s for pure Mg, 5.6×10^{-9} m/s for WE43B and 1.5×10^{-9} m/s for EV31A.

Wang et al. [366] studied SCC behavior and the effect of strain rate on the SCC susceptibility of an extruded Mg-7%Gd-5%Y-1%Nd-0.5%Zr (EW75) alloy in 3.5 wt% NaCl solution with different strain rates. It was found that (i) the alloy is susceptible to SCC when the strain rate is lower than 5×10^{-6}/s, (ii) at the strain rate of 1×10^{-6}/s, the SCC susceptibility index is 0.96 and the elongation to failure is only 0.11%; (iii) fractography indicates that the brittle quasicleavage feature is very obvious and become more pronounced with decreasing the strain rate; and (iv) further analysis confirms that the cracking mode is predominantly transgranular, but the partial intergranular cracking at some localized area can also occur.

Raja et al. [367] studied the role of chlorides on SCC behavior of Mg–Mn hot rolled alloy in $Mg(OH)_2$ saturated, 0.01 and 0.1 M NaCl solutions. It was found that (i) the alloy was found to fail by HE mechanism both in the presence and absence of chlorides; however, the role of chloride has been found to be to damage the passive film, cause pitting and increasing HE tendency of the alloy and (ii) crack initiation occurred through pitting and grew in a transgranular manner involving hydrogen. Similarly, Pannindre et al. [368] investigated the role of arsenate ions and cathodic charging on the environmentally assisted cracking (EAC) behavior of a Mg–Mn alloy in 0.6 M NaCl saturated with $Mg(OH)_2$. It was reported that (i) the stability of the surface film and the repassivation kinetics have been found to play a critical role in the EAC tendency of the alloy than hydrogen-assisted mechanisms and (ii) cathodic charging was found to be beneficial in lowering the EAC tendency of the alloy.

14.2.6.5 Hydrogen embrittlement

Kappes et al. [369] pointed out that the HE is caused by various factors and concerns, including hydrogen diffusion in magnesium substrate, kinetics of hydrogen transport, hydrogen adsorption and absorption, thermodynamic stability of Mg hydrides such as $Mg(OH)_2$ or MgH_2 (Mg is a well-known hydride-forming element with applications to solid-state hydrogen storage, as discussed in Chapter 16), delayed hydride cracking, hydrogen-enhanced decohesion and hydrogen-enhanced localized plasticity.

Silverstein et al. [370] studied the effect of local hydrogen concentration and distribution in AZ31 and AZ91 alloys in regard to HE to examine the effect of microstructure on the MgH_2 reaction (or hydriding), and its decomposition (or dehydriding). The MgH_2 compound was investigated in terms of two aspects: first, as the main source for controlling the hydrogen dehydriding process; second, as a hydrogen trapping site for preventing HE process. It was mentioned that (i) the TDS (total dissolved solids) analysis revealed a certain hydrogen concentration evolving near β-$Mg_{17}Al_{12}$ phase, accompanied by H_2 desorption at a temperature range between ~200 and 300 °C and (ii) hence, β-phase plays a fundamental role in the dehydriding process, and this response is a crucial step in effecting the embrittlement behavior. Kannan et al. [371] studied the pitting corrosion susceptibility and its role on the HE behavior of AZ80 magnesium alloy using slow strain rate testing, electrochemical technique and immersion test method. It was reported that (i) the electrochemical and immersion tests in chloride-containing solution revealed severe pitting corrosion in the alloy; (ii) the slow strain rate testing results of the alloy under continuously exposed conditions in chloride-containing solution and in distilled water showed that the mechanical properties of the alloy deteriorated considerably in both the solutions; (iii) pre-exposure of the alloy in distilled water did not show any considerable change in the mechanical properties of the alloy, however, in chloride-containing solution a significant loss in the mechanical properties was noticed; (iv) cleavage facets were observed in the vicinity of the localized attacked region of the alloy preexposed in chloride-containing solution; and (v) desiccating the preexposed (in chloride-containing solution) samples reduced the loss in the mechanical properties, which could be attributed to reversible hydrogen, suggesting that pitting corrosion facilitates hydrogen entry into the alloy and causes HE. Maker et al. [372] showed that (i) rapidly solidified AZ61 exhibited better resistance to pitting than cast AZ61 in a buffered carbonate solution containing various levels of Cl^- and (ii) pit initiation of rapidly solidified AZ61 is found to take place at a higher potential and the pit growth rate was apparently lower than cast AZ61.

14.3 Physical properties

Table 14.4 lists and compares several important physical properties among pure metals (Mg, Al, Fe and Ti) and their typical alloys [373–377]. Accordingly, there are numerous studies on thermal conductivity, damping capability as well as electromagnetic wave shielding of Mg-based alloys. Improvements on formability of Mg materials are discussed in Chapter 9 and huge studies on corrosion behaviors in various environment will be discussed in the subsequent Section 14.4 of this chapter.

Table 14.4: Typical properties of common pure metals and alloys.

	Density (g/cm3)	Melting point (°C)	Thermal conductivity (W/m.K)	Specific heat (J/kg.K)	Specific strength	Damping capacity	Magnetic field shielding	Corrosion resistance	Formability
Mg	1.74	649	156	1,038	⊙	⊙	⊙	△	△
AM60	1.79	615	62						
AM31	1.80	632	77						
AM91	1.82	596	72						
Al	2.70	660	238	917	○	△	⊙	○	○
7075	2.80	635	130						
Fe	7.87	1,536	78	456	△	△	⊙	⊙	⊙
304SS	7.91	1,425	16						
Ti	4.50	1,667	22	528					
Ti-64	4.43	1,600	8						
TB340	4.50	1,668	17						

Note: ⊙: excellent, O: good, △: needs improvement.

14.3.1 Diffusion

Diffusion phenomenon can be simply defined as the movement of atoms or molecules in a material in either solid, liquid or gaseous state and point defects as well as lattice imperfections are responsible to diffusion-controlled process at solid state, including oxidation at metals ceramic interface, fluoride uptake/release, water sorption in polymers and Hg in Ag_2Hg_3 phase or tarnishing or corrosion. Surface free energy of solid surface (due to the fact that the atomic bonding is not continuous) is reduced by atomic diffusion and absorption of gaseous species. In general, the kinetic barrier to the movement of an atom through a solid lattice is greater than that to movement through a liquid or gas. This is reflected in the higher activation energy Q that is necessary for volume diffusion through a solid than through a liquid or gas. There are basically three paths for diffusion: volume diffusion, grain boundary diffusion and surface diffusion. The amount of energy necessary for each of these types of relative to one another can be summarized by $Q_{vol} > Q_{gb} > Q_{surf}$ and in general, it can be determined as the following ratios: Q_{vol}: Q_{gb}:$Q_{surf} \approx 4{:}2{:}1$ or 4:3:2. Simultaneously, typical values of D_O are $D_{Ovol} > D_{Ogb} > D_{O\,surf}$ and it is reported that the range is between 0.1 and 1.0 cm^2/s. As a result, the three coefficients of diffusion may be arranged: $D_{surf} > D_{gb} > D_{vol}$ for temperature of interest in solid-state reactions [378]. Figure 14.10 shows equal-concentration profile of surface, grain boundary and volume (bulk) diffusion in the same solid [378].

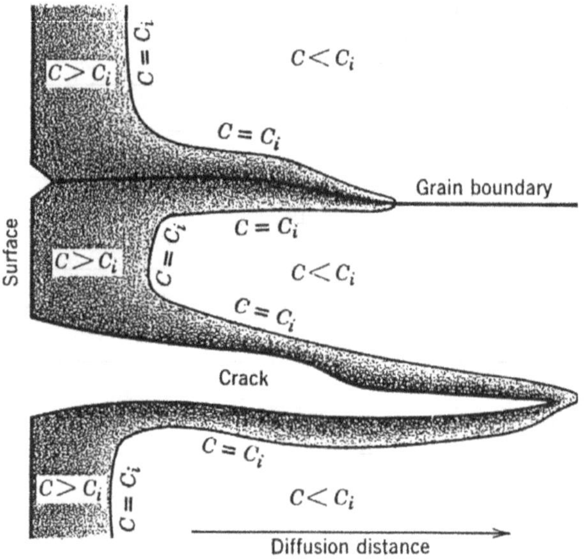

Figure 14.10: Illustration of equal-concentration profiles for surface, grain boundary and volume diffusion [378].

Grain boundary diffusion of Al in polycrystalline Mg was measured from diffusion couple experiments between 330 and 420 °C by high-resolution scanning electron microscopy microanalysis [379]. It was reported that (i) grain boundary diffusion of Al is found to increase with increasing misorientation between adjacent Mg grains, and the grain boundary diffusion coefficients of Al can be two orders of magnitude faster than the volume diffusion of Al in Mg and (ii) the difference between grain boundary and volume diffusion of Al becomes larger at lower temperatures. Wang et al. [380] studied the interdiffusion of Al in Mg at 400 and 450 °C. It was mentioned that (i) the interdiffusion coefficients generally increased with the Al content and the rotation angle with respect to the *c*-axis with a valley point around $\theta \approx 30°$ at 450 °C and (ii) diffusion along the basal plane was always faster than along the

c-axis. Wang et al. [381] computed the surface energies of $Mg_{17}Al_{12}$ β-phase with different surface configurations by using molecular dynamic simulations. Surface terminations were carefully selected to calculate the energy of β-phase. It was shown that (i) surfaces occupied by higher fraction of magnesium atoms generate lower surface energies, (ii) the interfacial energy for $Mg_{17}Al_{12}$ β-phase and Mg matrix was calculated as well based on the Burger's orientation relationship and the lowest energy surface of $Mg_{17}Al_{12}$ does not generate the lowest interfacial energy and (iii) the interfacial energy increases by ~250 mJ/m^2 due to the change in orientation relationship between $Mg_{17}Al_{12}$ and the matrix after twinning. Ouyang et al. [382] investigated the growth kinetics, diffusion kinetics and mechanical properties of intermetallics in Mg–Zn binary systems. Four intermetallic compounds including Mg_2Zn_{11}, $MgZn_2$, $Mg_{21}Zn_{25}$ and Mg_4Zn_7 are observed in the Mg–Zn diffusion zone at the temperature range of 250–320 °C. It was reported that the square of thickness for intermetallic compounds diffusion layer increases linearly with time, which is consistent with the parabolic growth law, and the growth of intermetallic compounds is controlled by diffusion.

There are numerous studies on single element diffusion into Mg substrate (Al, Ca, Ce, Gd, Mn, Sn, Zn and Y) in Mg [383], (Nd, Gd and Y) in Mg [384], (Gd) in Mg [385], (Ag, Al, As, Au, Be, Bi, Ca, Cd, Co, Cr, Cu, Fe, Ga, Ge, Hf, Hg, In, Ir, Li, Mn, Mo, Na, Nb, Ni, Os, Pb, Pd, Pt, Re, Rh, Ru, Sb, Sc, Se, Si, Sn, Sr, Ta, Tc, Te, Ti, Tl, V, W, Y, Zn and Zr) in Mg [386], (Ag, Cd, In, Sn and Sb) in Mg [387], (Ga) in Mg [388], Mn in Mg [389] and (Gd and Y) in Mg [390].

14.3.2 Thermal conductivity

The rate at which heat is transferred through a solid is determined by the thermal of the solid and the temperature gradient between heat source and heat sink. The thermal conductivity of a crystalline solid is anisotropic and differs in different crystallographic directions. Cold-rolled or drawn metals can have a texture, an alignment of the crystal axes of a majority of grains along the specific directions, resulting in some anisotropy in thermal as well as electrical conductivity [391]. In general, for metals at RT, good thermal conductivity is always accompanied by good electrical conductivity because heat transfer in metals is due mainly to free electrons [392].

Thermal conductivity is sensitive to microstructures that are influenced directly or indirectly by alloying elements, grain size, precipitates, intermetallic compounds, forming, heat treatment or fabrication. Peng et al. [393] studied the effects of extrusion on thermal conductivity of Mg-2.0Zn-1.0Mn-0.2Ce and mentioned that (i) the thermal conductivity increases when the extrusion temperature increased from 340 to 400 °C, and then decreased further increased to 430 °C; (ii) the extrusion temperature changes the microstructure and solid solution of elements, which comprehensively affect the thermal conductivity of AR alloys; and (iii) after extrusion, thermal conductivity of the AR alloy decreased and the anisotropy of thermal conductivity was observed because of the texture formed during extrusion. Similarly, Ying et al. [394] measured thermal conductivity of Mg–Zn (0.5–5.0 wt%) and compared data between as-cast and AR conditions and reported that (i) with the increase concentration of Zn, thermal conductivity decreased gradually in both as-cast and AR Mg–Zn alloys and (ii) the thermal conductivity of AR Mg–Zn alloys in the direction perpendicular to extrusion direction was similar to that in the corresponding as-cast samples, which was due to the combined effects of defects and texture.

Effect of La element was investigated in Mg–Al–La alloy system [395] and in Mg–La–Zr alloy system [396]. For Mg–Al–La alloy, it was reported that (i) the concentration of Al dissolved in α-Mg matrix decreases with the increase of La content, and the volume fraction of $Al_{11}La_3$ in the Mg–4Al–*x*La alloys increases because La tends to consume Al to form $Al_{11}La_3$ and (ii) as a consequence, thermal conductivity of the Mg–4Al–*x*La alloys in as-cast condition increase with the increasing La content; (iii) after extrusion, thermal conductivity further increase due to dynamic precipitation of $Al_{11}La_3$ which consumes the Al solutes dissolved in the α-Mg and (iv) the extruded Mg–4Al–6La alloy exhibits high thermal conductivity of 130 W/mK [395]. For Mg–La–Zr alloy, it was mentioned that (i) $Mg_{99.7}La_{0.2}Zr_{0.1}$ (136.6 W/mK) exhibits higher thermal conductivity than $Mg_{99.1}La_{0.8}Zr_{0.1}$ (113.9 W/mK) [396]. Chen et al. [397], studying thermal property of Mg–11Y–5Gd–2Zn–0.5Zr (wt%) alloy, reported that (i) the values of the thermal conductivity at RT was 23.0 W/mK and (ii) the transitional element Y has an effective influence on the thermal conductivity. Wang et al. [398] studied the thermal conductivity of Mg–3Zn–*x*Sn ($x = 0.5$, 1.5, 2.5, 3.5 in wt%) alloys and found that, with the increase in Sn content, the thermal conductivity decreases.

Thermal conductivity is influenced by distribution, volume fractions and shape of intermetallic compounds [399] and precipitation [400]. Zhong et al. [401] studied the microstructure and thermal conductivity of four groups of Mg–RE binary alloys (Mg–Ce, Mg–Nd, Mg–Y and Mg–Gd) in as-cast and as-solutionized states. It was reported that (i) the thermal conductivity of as-cast and as-solutionized Mg–RE alloys decreased with the increase of concentrations; (ii) the thermal conductivity of as-solutionized Mg–Nd, Mg–Y and Mg–Gd alloys was lower than that of as-cast alloys; (iii) the thermal conductivity of as-solutionized Mg–Ce alloys was higher than that of as-cast alloys, because of the elimination of lattice defects and fine dispersed particles during solutionizing treatment; (iv) different RE elements have different influences on the thermal conductivity of Mg alloys in the following order: $Ce < Nd < Y < Gd$; and (v) Ce element has the minimum effect on thermal conductivity of Mg alloys, because of the very low solubility of Ce in the α-Mg matrix, which might be attributed to the maximum solid solubility of elements in the α-Mg matrix. Li et al. [402] studied thermal conductivity of annealed/aged Mg–2Zn–Zr alloy. It was mentioned that (i) the average grain size is reduced to 7.8 μm after mill-annealing with a reduction of 75%; (ii) the phases of MgZn and ZnZr exist in the as-cast alloy; (iii) after aging, the main precipitated phases are ZnZr, Zn_2Zr and Zn_2Zr_3 and the precipitation of MgZn is inhibited and (iii) the thermal conductivity of the alloy is 132.1 W/mK, suggesting that the Mg–2Zn–Zr alloy after mill-annealing and subsequent aging process is a potential preferable thermal conductivity material. Zhong et al. [403] investigated the effect of Ce addition on the microstructure, thermal con ductivity and mechanical properties of Mg–0.5Mn addition. It was reported that (i) the thermal conductivity of as-cast Mg–0.5Mn–*x*Ce alloys decreased gradually with the increase of Ce content; (ii) meanwhile, the thermal conductivity of AR Mg–0.5Mn–0.3Ce alloy (139.7 W/mK) was higher than that of other AR alloys; (iii) the AR Mg–0.5Mn–*x*Ce alloys exhibited higher thermal conductivity than that of as-cast counterparts, except for Mg–0.5Mn–0.6Ce alloy, the improvement being attributed to the weakening of basal texture in wrought products.

14.3.3 Electrical and optical properties

14.3.3.1 Electrical property

The temperature dependence of electrical resistivity (ER) in pure Mg polycrystals and single crystals, and the commercial Mg–Al–Zn alloys (AZ31 and AZ80) have been studied during continuous heating from RT to 420 °C [404]. It was reported that (i) the temperature dependence of ER of the studied materials is sensitive to the amount of alloying Al atoms in the solid solution. The pure Mg polycrystal has the largest overall slope and the highest concentrated SST alloy (AZ80) has the lowest one (see Figure 14.11); (ii) dissolution of eutectic-phase $Mg_{17}Al_{12}$ in the cast AZ80 alloy reduces the overall slope of temperature dependence of ER in solid ST alloy; and (iii) grain size has no effects on the ER.

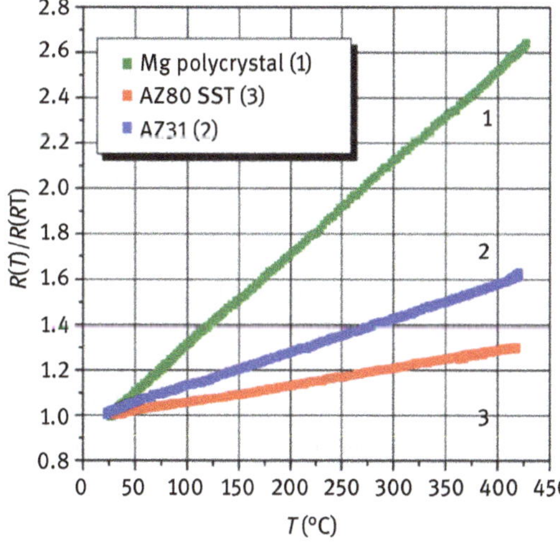

Figure 14.11: Electrical resistivity at the heating rate 25 °C/min, where SST refers to solid-solution treatment [404].

Pan et al. [405] developed Mg–Zn alloy sheets with high conductivity, refined grain structure and acceptable strength by cold rolling and the following aging treatment. It was found that (i) rolling process decreased the electrical conductivity of the extruded sheet, while the following aging would improve the corresponding conductivity remarkably and (ii) the obtained highest electrical conductivity of the Mg–Zn sheet was 20.01 (10^6 S/m), noting electrical conductivity of the pure Mg is 22.8 (10^6 S/m). Fu et al. [406] investigated electrical resistivity in amorphous $Mg_{65}Zn_{30}Ca_5$ thin films with thicknesses ranging from 49 to 1,786 nm by four-probe method at -269 °C. It was mentioned that (i) for thickness from 94 nm to 1,786 nm the Ziman–Faber diffraction model can describe temperature-dependent electrical resistivity, while for the 49 nm thick film the two-level system scattering mechanism is validated below 40 K and Ziman–Faber diffraction model above 40 K and (ii) more interface fraction between the columnar structures with enhanced heterogeneity could be the possible origin of two-level system scattering in thinnest film instead of denser atomic packing. Liu et al. [407] studied microstructure, electrical conduc tivity, and electromagnetic interference shielding effectiveness of cast Mg–*x*Zn–*y*Y ($x = 2–5$, $y = 1–10$) alloys to understand the effects of Zn and Y additions on electrical conductivity and electromagnetic shielding effectiveness of the alloys. It was obtained that (i) the electrical conductivity and shielding effectiveness of the Mg–*x*Zn–*y*Y alloys decrease with Y/Zn ratio, (ii) electrical conductivity is the main factor that affects the electromagnetic shielding properties and the variation tendency of electromagnetic shielding properties of the Mg–*x*Zn–*y*Y alloys is consistent with conductivity, (iii) valence of Y and Zn atoms, configuration of extranuclear electron and volumetric difference are main reasons for the variations in the electrical conductivity and (iv) a high density of second phase and the formation of semicontinuous network structure can also improve the shielding effectiveness value at high frequencies. Geng et al. [408] measured the resistivity of $Mg_{63.5}Zn_{34}Y_{2.5}$ alloy including icosahedral quasicrystalline phase (I-phase) and reported that (i) the quasicrystal alloy has a negative temperature coefficient of resistivity (TCR) before melting of I-phase and (ii) the temperature coefficient of resistivity shows a reversible transition at ~800 °C during heating and cooling processes, involving evolution of icosahedral short-range orders inheriting from I-phase.

Wang et al. [409] measured the electrical resistivity of NZ30K–Mg (Mg-3Nd-0.1Zn-0.4Zr) alloy at different heating rates during continuous heating to study the precipitation kinetics. It was mentioned that (i) two kinds of metastable phases, β′ and β″, formed during the heating and (ii) the precipitation kinetic parameters of NZ30K–Mg alloy can be obtained accurately using isoconversional method. Rokhlin et al. [410], using electrical resistivity and hardness measurements, investigated the recovery after aging in two Mg-based alloys (Mg–12 wt% Y and Mg–24 wt% Gd). The alloys were ST and aged up to the hardness maximum. It was found that (i) similar and different features of the recovery behavior in the two alloys were revealed with different RE metals, (ii) in both alloys a similar dependence of the recovery on the annealing temperature and time was established, (iii) the dissolution of the precipitate into the Mg matrix increased with increasing annealing temperature and passed through a maximum as the annealing time became longer and (iv) the increase of the annealing temperature and time promoted only softening of the alloys; meanwhile, in Mg–24 wt% Gd the recovery effect was significantly smaller than in Mg–12 wt% Y; indicating the higher decomposition rate of the Mg–Gd solid solution at the annealing temperatures. Jalaih et al. [411] prepared Zr and Mg cosubstituted $Ni_{0.5}Zn_{0.5}Fe_2O_4$ ferrites by the sol–gel autocombustion method. It was mentioned that (i) the same variation is found for the drift mobility and DC resistivity, (ii) the Arrhenius graphs of DC resistivity exhibit the semiconductor nature, for which the activation energy decreased with increasing the dopant concentration and (iii) as the dopant contents increased, the saturation magnetization, net magnetic moment and permeability are reduced, while the coercivity is reinforced.

Hu et al. [412, 413] studied the structural, electronic and optical properties of wurtzite Mg–Zn–O with Mg concentration ranging from 0 to 0.5. It was mentioned that (i) the lattice constants c and specific volume V of the Mg–Zn–O alloys decrease and their band gap widens as Mg concentration increases; (ii) a particular Mg concentration is found to exist at around 0.375, equals to which the corresponding Mg–Zn–O alloy has the minimum width of the top valence band; indicating that Mg concentration may be used to tune the electronic properties of Mg–Zn–O alloy, (iii) the energy response range of the optical spectrums decreases with the increase of Mg concentration and (iv) there are different energy shifts toward high energy (blue shift) of the peaks in the optical spectrums with the increase of Mg concentration, which are explained by the variations of the density of states in details; concluding that (v) the electronic and optical properties of Mg–Zn–O may be tuned through Mg concentration to develop and design of photoelectric devices.

14.3.3.2 Optical property

Yamada et al. [414, 415] improved the transmittance of Mg–Y-based switchable mirrors in the transparent state the surface which was coated with a TiO_2 thin film using e-beam evaporation. It was reported that (i) the TiO_2 films had a refractive index of ~2.1, (ii) as a result of the TiO_2 coating with a thickness of ~65 nm, the transmittance in the visible range was considerably improved and consequently the visible transmittance in the transparent state reached 68% and this result was consistent with simulation results calculated using complex refractive indices for hy drides of Pd, Mg–Y alloy, and Ta and (iii) TiO_2 is one of the best candidates for an antireflection layer to improve the optical properties of switchable mirrors. Liu et al. [416] fabricated the novel gasochromic switchable mirrors based on

Pd/Mg–TiO_2 films by magnetron sputtering and investigated their optical properties, microstructures and structure–function relationship. It was reported that (i) the mirror based on Pd/0.9 Mg–0.1TiO_2 film exhibits larger optical dynamic range at visible wavelengths and excellent structural recovery even after 100 cycles of hydrogenation and dehydrogenation compared with Pd/Mg film, (ii) the brookite TiO_2, crystalline Mg and some amorphous phases coexist in the Mg–TiO_2 layer of Pd/0.9 Mg–0.1TiO_2 film with no trace of Pd and (iii) the TiO_2 nanocrystal clusters are distributed in stripe among Mg matrix; in contrast, the Pd/0.63 Mg–0.37TiO_2 film consists of crystalline Mg and $MgTi_2O_5$ phase, where $MgTi_2O_5$ phase is derived from the reaction of superfluous TiO_2 with a part of Mg and deteriorates the optical properties of the mirror dramatically. Based on these findings, it was concluded that a novel strategy for improving optical performance of Mg-based switchable mirrors was offered by introducing metal oxides into switchable layer and uncovers a broad field to be explored.

Qi et al. [417] adjusted light scattering properties of Mg-doped ZnO nanorods by hydrothermal process through nonstoichiometric ratio ($Zn_1Mg_xO_1$, $x = 0.2–1$). It was reported that (i) Mg ions substituted the Zn sites without changing the hexagonal wurtzite structure, which was accompanied by gradually decrease in tensile stress due to increased Zn/Mg ratio from 1:0.2 to 1:0.8, (ii) the average diameter of nanorods rose from ~75 to 90 nm and turned into a plane with water ripple as Zn/Mg ratio enhanced to 1:1, (iii) the light scattering ability and optical constants of Mg–ZnO nanorods exhibited significant wavelength dependency, which exponentially declined as wavelength increased, (iv) the higher relative intensities of the visible peak recorded for Mg–ZnO nanorods testified of the elevated oxygen vacan cies density when Zn/Mg ratio enhanced from 1:0.6 to 1:1 and (v) the proposed method looked promising as facile and novel way for adjusting light-trapping abilities of Mg–ZnO NRs thin films suitable for polymer solar cells and other ZnO-based optoelectronic and photonic devices. Shi et al. [418] prepared ZnO, K-doped ZnO (KZO) and (Mg, K) codoped ZnO (MKZO) thin films using sol–gel method and studied the morphological, structural and optical properties. It was reported that (i) all the films have a preferential *c*-axis orientation and an average transmittance of over 93% in the visible range, (ii) the optical band gap decreases by K doping, but gradually increases by Mg doping at a given K doping concentration and (iii) photolumi nescence spectra show that the visible emission was enhanced, which indicates that the number of defects should be changed at Mg doping concentration of 8 mol%.

14.3.3.3 Optoelectrical property

Optoelectronics (or optronics) is the study and application of electronic devices and systems that source, detect and control light, usually considered a subfield of photon ics. In this context, light often includes invisible forms of radiation such as gamma rays, X-rays, ultraviolet and infrared, in addition to visible light. Optoelectronic devices are electrical-to-optical or optical-to-electrical transducers, or instruments that use such devices in their operation [419]. Si et al. [420] investigated the band structure, density of states and optical properties of Mg-doped and Mg–Al codoped ZnO by adopting the first-principles calculation of plane wave ultra-soft pseudo-potential technology based on the density function theory. It was mentioned that (i) by introducing the impurity atoms of Mg, the band gap increases with increasing the content of Mg but decreases in the Mg–Al codoped ZnO structure, while the electrical conductivity increases apparently, (ii) both the absorptivity and the reflectivity of the optical properties decline significantly after codoping and (iii) specifically, the blue shift arises in the absorption edge and the absorptivity decreases with the increase of Mg content in the range of 350–600 nm, indicating that the Mg–Al doping can enhance the transmittance with a certain thickness. Xu et al. [421] prepared Mg-doped $Al_xGa_{1-x}N$ (x = 0.23 and 0.35) alloys grown on GaN templates with high-temperature AlN interlayer by metalorganic chemical vapor deposition. It was found that (i) analytical data indicate the formation of more inversion domains in the high Al mole fraction Mg-doped AlGaN alloys at Mg concentration ~$10^{20}/cm^3$, (ii) for Mg-doped $Al_{0.23}Ga_{0.77}N$ epilayer, the analysis of cathodoluminescence spectra supports the existence of self-compensation effects due to the presence of intrinsic defects and Mg-related centers, (iii) the energy level of Mg is estimated to be around 193 meV from the temperature dependence of the resistivity measured by Hall effect experiments, (iv) hole concentration and mobility are measured to be $1.2 \times 10^{18}/cm^3$ and 0.56 cm^2/V at RT, (v) the reduction of acceptor activation energy and low hole mobility are attributed to inversion domains and self-compensation and (vi) impurity band conduction is dominant in carrier transport up to a relatively higher temperature in high Al content Mg-doped AlGaN alloys.

14.3.3.4 Thermoelectric property

The thermoelectric effect is the direct conversion of temperature differences to electric voltage and vice versa via a thermocouple. Thermoelectric devices create a voltage when there is a different temperature on each side. Conversely, when a voltage is applied to it, heat is transferred from one side to the other, creating a temperature difference. At the atomic scale, an applied temperature gradient causes charge carriers in the material to diffuse from the hot side to the cold side [422]. Cao et al. [423] studied thermoelectric properties of $YbCdSb_2$ doped by Mg to form p-type $YbCd_{2-x}Mg_xSb_2$ (x = 0.1, 0.2, 0.4, 0.6, 0.8) Zintl phases via melting reaction followed by suitable cooling, annealing, grinding, and spark plasma sinteringdensification processes. Electrical conductivity, Seebeck's coefficient and thermal conductivity conductivity, thermal measurements have been performed as a function of temperature from 27 to 377 °C. It was found that the XRD patterns show that the solubility limit x of Mg in the $YbCd_{2-x}Mg_xSb_2$ is less than 0.8. With increasing Mg content x, the cell parameters a and c of the $YbCd_{2-x}Mg_xSb_2$ compounds decrease. The isoelectronic substitution of Mg for Cd leads to a remarkable decrease in total thermal conductivity and an increase in Seebeck's coefficient, through a slight decease in electrical conductivity. As a result, the maximum dimensionless figure of merit ZT of 1.08 is obtained at 377 °C for $YbCd_{1.9}Mg_{0.1}Sb_2$, and when compared with the ZT of 0.78 at 377 °C in the unsubstituted $YbCd_2Sb_2$, it is improved greatly by 38%. Chen et al. [424] developed β-In_2S_3 was developed as a potential thermoelectric material and Mg-doped In_2S_3 samples were prepared by conventional solid-state reaction method followed by pulsed current sintering. It was reported that (i) for $In_{2-x}Mg_xS_3$ ($0 \le x \le 0.20$), the prepared samples maintain tetragonal β-In_2S_3 phase while α-In_2S_3 with cubic structure were obtained at $x \ge 0.30$, (ii) the both Mg and S concentrations were less than the nominal values, and the lack of S naturally lead to an effective increase of electron concentration in the bands crossing the Fermi level and (iii) the lattice thermal conductivity was reduced by the Mg-substitution, and the value of ZT reached 0.53 at 427 °C for $x = 0.05$, which is 1.4 times larger than that of non-doped sample. Nieroda et al. [425] studied the structural, microstructural and ther moelectric properties of Mg2Si synthesized by spark plasma sintering method under excessive Mg content(with 0–10 wt%). The influence of Mg content on the impedance spectrum and transport properties, that is, electrical conductivity, the Seebeck coefficient and the thermal conductivity was studied in temperature range from 27 to 447 °C and the temperature dependences of the thermoelectric figure of merit ZT were calculated. It was reported that (i) Mg excess which is in liquid phase during the sintering process gathers mostly at the grain boundaries, enhancing sintering process and decreasing total porosity of the samples, (ii) higher Mg content increases electrical and thermal conductivity of Mg_2Si, what causes simultaneous decrease of Seebeck coefficient and (iii) step change in the electrical conductivity between the samples without and with the excess of magnesium (e.g., $\sigma = 30$ S/m for 0 wt% and $\sigma = 1.26 \cdot 10^5$ S/m^1 for 10 wt%) indicates the presence of a percolating mechanism.

14.3.4 Damping characteristics

Among various characteristics required for applicable materials in transportation, other industries and even biomedical fields, damping characteristic has become one of important directions in the research and development of Mg-based alloys [426–430]. Energy dissipation of pure Mg through dislocation movements occurs primarily via an internal friction mechanism [431–433]. Vibrations of the dislocation loops around their equilibrium positions in Mg alloys are responsible for damping levels of about 10 times higher than those in pure aluminum [209]. A damping coefficient is a material property that indicates whether a material will bounce back or return energy to a system. If the bounce is caused by an unwanted vibration or shock, a high damping coefficient in the material will diminish the response. It will swallow the energy and reduce the undesired reaction. Such measures are required when evaluating material and system responses to dynamic loading conditions. Materials with high damping coefficients are used in applications of shock absorption, vibration control, noise reduction and dissipating increased heat. Engineers use damping coefficients to compare materials to see which will be the best one for the application. This number describes the behavior of the material in a damped system [434–436].

Table 14.5 lists and compares several essential properties which are directly or indirectly related to damping characteristics of major pure metals [437, 438].

A number of alloying elements that are evaluated to be effective to enhance the damping characteristics were found, as listed in Table 14.6. Since Mg–Zn was developed as an excellent damping property, Y-containing and Zn, Zr-containing Mg-based alloys have been developed.

Table 14.5: Static properties of materials under standard conditions (at 20 °C).

	Density (g/cm³)	Elastic modulus (GPa)	Shear modulus (GPa)	Poisson's ratio	Propagation velocity of longitudinal wave in a rod (m/s)	Propagation velocity of torsional wave (m/s)
Al	2.70	72	27	0.30	5,200	3,100
Fe	7.80	200	77	0.40	5,050	3,100
Cu	8.90	125	46	0.35	3,700	2,300
Mg	1.74	43	17	0.29	5,000	3,100
Ni	8.90	205	77	0.30	4,800	2,900
Zn	7.13	13.1	5.0	0.33	1,350	850
Sn	7.28	4.4	1.6	0.39	780	470

Table 14.6: Alloying effects on various damping Mg-based alloys.

	Al	Ca	Cu	Ni	Zr	Si	Ce	Y	RE	La	Mn	Nd	Zn	Sn
Mg	[439, 440]	[441–443]	[444]	[445–447]	[447–449]	[450, 451]	[452]	[453, 454]	[455]					
Mg–Al						[456]	[457, 458]			[21]				
Mg–Zn	[459]							[460, 461]						
Mg–Mn			[462, 463]											
Mg–Cu											[463, 464]			
Mg–Ni			[465]					[466]			[467]			
Mg–Zr								[113, 468]						
Mg–Li	[469]													
Mg–Zn–Y					[470–474]							[475]		
Mg–Cu–Mn								[476]					[476]	
Mg–Er–Gd													[477]	
Mg–Li–Al														[478]
Mg-Li-Al-Sn													[478]	
Mg-Zn-Y-Nd					[479, 480]									

Mg-Zn-Y-Zr	[481]	[481]	
Mg-Cu-Mn-Zn	[482–484]		
Mg-Gd-Y-Nd-Zr			[128]

Note: RE, rare earth element.

14.3.5 Magnetic field shielding

Unlike electricity, magnetic fields cannot be blocked or insulated so that magnetic field shielding is necessitated. Magnetic shielding is a process that limits the coupling of a magnetic field between two locations. This can be done with a number of materials, including sheet metal, metal mesh, ionized gas or plasma. The purpose is most often to prevent magnetic fields from interfering with electrical devices. Magnetic permeability describes the ability of a material to be magnetized. If the material used has a greater permeability than the object inside, the magnetic field will tend to flow along this material, avoiding the objects inside. Thus, the magnetic field lines are allowed to terminate on opposite poles but are merely redirected. While the materials used in magnetic shielding must have a high permeability and should not develop permanent magnetization. The most effective shielding material available is mu-metal. Mu-metal is a Ni–Fe soft ferromagnetic alloy with very high permeability (e.g., approximately 77Ni-16Fe-5Cu-2%Cr or Mo). The name came from the Greek letter mu (μ) which represents permeability in physics and engineering formulae. Mu-metal objects require heat treatment of annealing in a magnetic field in hydrogen atmosphere, which increases the magnetic permeability about 40 times. The annealing alters the material's crystal structure, aligning the grains and removing some impurities, especially carbon, which obstruct the free motion of the magnetic domain boundaries. Although mu-metal is recognized as an excellent electromagnetic field shielding material, it is expensive, resulting in developing new types of less-expensive materials including Mg-containing alloys and composites. Magnetic shielding is often employed in hospitals, where devices such as mag netic resonance imaging equipment generate powerful magnetic flux. Shielded rooms are constructed to prevent this equipment from interfering with surrounding instruments or meters [485–488].

Chiba et al. [489] studied behaviors of the microstructural and the magnetic properties of magnesium and 3d-transition metal alloys with because of which there is a difficulty of alloying thus by the conventional method a positive value of mixing enthalpy. It was mentioned that (i) the fabricated Mg–Fe alloys with a composition less than 25 at% Mg were in single phase BCC with expanded lattice parameter, (ii) the variation tendency in lattice parameter and the coercive force with Mg composition were opposite and (iii) the microstructure of Mg–Co powders implies that the alloy could be partially amorphized or they could form a nanosized morphology as expected. Li et al. [490] prepared Mg-Mn-Fe-Co-Ni-Gd alloy films by electrodeposition. It was reported that (i) the surface morphology can be controlled by deposition potential and solution composition, (ii) hollow microspheres and core-shell microspheres can be obtained and (iii) the as-deposited alloy is amorphous and the ferromagnetism to diamagnetism transition can be observed when the contents of Mg is lower than 20%.

Morozov et al. [491] prepared cubic, terraced and spherical Mg–MgO NPs, ranging in average particle size from 30 up to 80 nm through vaporization and condensation of Mg metal in mix gas flow (argon + air) at conditions of the levitation-jet aerosol synthe sis. These NPs were collected in three zones, located at different distances from an evaporator. It was indicated that (i) RT ferromagnetism with the maximum magnetization of up to 0.65 emu/g was found in the NPs, (ii) the maximum specific magnetization of the NPs depends on the value of specific surface area multiplied by oxide content in the form of two-peaks function, (iii) a clear increase in the maximum magnetization of NPs, collected in the different zones, was observed with an increase in the distance of these zones from the evaporator, (iv) the observed ferromagnetic ordering may be related to the Mg-deficient defects on the surface of NPs and (v) various values of the maximum magnetization origin from the different fabrication conditions promoting defects propagation on the surface of NPs. Pourzaki et al. [492] synthesized Co–Mg ferrites, $Co_xMg_{1-y}Fe_{2-z}O_4$ ($x = 0.0$, 0.2, 0.4, 0.6, 0.8 and 1.0, $0 < y < 0.34$ and $0 < z < 0.67$) via a standard ceramic route. It was reported that (i) the XRD patterns proved the formation of single-phase Mg ferrite in the samples with "x" contents varying from 0.0 to 0.8, (ii) the sample with $x = 1.0$ showed two phases: a spinel Mg-ferrite and a secondary (Co,Mg) O phase, (iii) a maximum bulk density of 4.94 g/cm^3 was obtained for $x = 0.8$ and (iv) magnetic properties of the sintered samples showed an increase in coercive force up to 113 Oe by increasing Co substitution up to $x = 1.0$. Kagdi et al. [493] synthesized Mg which was substituted in the X-type hexagonal ferrites with the chemical composition $Ba_2Zn_{2-x}Mg_xFe_{28}O_{46}$ ($x =$ 0.0, 0.4, 0.8, 1.2, 1.6 and 2.0) by a sol–gel autocombustion technique and investigated the effect of Mg substitution on structural, magnetic and dielec tric properties. It was reported that (i) the variations (decreasing trend) in lattice parame ters with Mg substitution indicate the incorporation of Mg substitution into the crystal structure, (ii) the average crystallite size of heated powders was found to be in the range of 16–22 nm, (iii) the saturation magnetization showed an initial decrease with $x =$ 0.4 – 1.2, and then an increase with $x > 1.2$, to the largest final values of 63.29 A m^2/kg for the fully Mg–substituted $x =$ 2.0, (iv) the value of coercivity lies in the range of 89.9–209.3 kA/m (1,130–2,630 Oe), and the magnetic results suggest that the compositions $x =$ 0.0, 0.4 and 1.2 possess multidomain microstructures, while $x =$ 0.8, 1.6 and 2.0 possess single domain microstructures and (v) a steady real permeability of around 1.2–1.5 over the whole 1–13 GHz range, and ferromagnetic resonance between 1 and 5 GHz, and ~12.5 GHz was noticed.

Li et al. [494] studied the magnetic properties of sintered Nd–Fe–B magnets, the $(PrNd)_{29.9}Dy_{0.1}B_1Co_1Cu_{0.15}Fe_{bal}$ (wt%) powders were mixed with Mg nanopow ders, as grain boundary modifiers. It was mentioned that for Nd–Fe–B magnets with 0.1–0.4 wt% Mg addition, addition amount of 0.1 wt% Mg, H_{cj} reaches the maximum value of 999.1 kA/m, Br reaches 1.436 T, $(BH)_{max}$ reaches 396.9 kJ/m^3 and magnet density is 7.42 g/cm^3, which are related to the microstructural modification of grain boundaries and the magnet density. Saritaş [495] used Mg doped zinc ferrite ($Mg{:}Zn_xFe_{3-x}O_4$) crystal to avoid the damage of Fe_3O_4 (magnetite) crystal instead of Zn^{2+}. It was mentioned that (i) because the radius of the Mg^{2+} ion in the A-site (tetrahedral) is almost equal to that of the replaced Fe^{3+} ion, (ii) inverse-spinel structure in which oxygen ions (O^{2-}) are arranged to form a face-centered cubic (FCC) lattice where there are two kinds of sublattices, namely, A-site and B-site (octahedral) interstitial sites and in which the super exchange interactions occur. Furthermore, triple and quaternary; iron oxide and zinc ferrite thin films with Mg metal dopants were grown by using spray pyrolysis technique to study the structural, electrical and magnetic properties of Mg-doped iron oxide (Fe_2O_3) and zinc ferrite ($Zn_xFe_{3-x}O_4$) thin films. It was reported that Mg-doped iron oxide thin film has huge diamagnetic and of Mg-doped zinc ferrite thin film has paramagnetic property at bigger magnetic field.

14.4 Oxidation and corrosion

14.4.1 Basic reaction

When viewed from the standpoint of partial processes of oxidation and reduction, all oxidation and corrosion (including electrochemical) can be classified into electron-generation or electron-consumption process. An oxidation process is responsible to electron generation as

$M \rightarrow M^{2+} + ne^-$, where M represents metallic element, e for electron and n for valency.

This reaction is sometimes called as an anodic reaction in particularly, electrochemical reaction. There are a few examples:

$Ag \rightarrow Ag^+ + e^-$
$Mg \rightarrow Mg^{2+} + 2e^-$
$Zn \rightarrow Zn^{2+} + 2e^-$
$Al \rightarrow Al^{3+} + 3e^-$

In each case, the number of produced electrons equals the valence of the (metallic) ion. Generated electrons should be consumed at cathodic reaction(s) and one of the following cathodic reactions can take place, depending on the pH (which is a function of hydrogen concentration:

$pH = -\log[H^+]$):
Hydrogen evolution: $2\,H^+ + 2e^- \rightarrow H_2$
Oxygen reduction: $O_2 + 4\,H^+ + 4e^- \rightarrow 2H_2O$ (in acid solutions)
$O_2 + 2H_2O + 4e^- \rightarrow 4OH^-$ (neutral or basic solutions)
Metal ion reduction: $M^{3+} + e^- \rightarrow M^{2+}$
Metal deposition: $M^+ + e^- \rightarrow M$

These anodic reaction rates (in other words, electron generation rate) should be balanced by cathodic reaction rate (or electron consumption rate) in order to continue oxidation (or corrosion) process proceed. If intentionally either one of oxidation or reduction process is interrupted to make off-balance of electrons, this entire process stops. If this action is effectively managed, such technique is called anodic or cathodic protection, depending on which action is under control.

To describe the corrosion form, there are two forms divided into general (uniform) corrosion and localized (including crevice corrosion, pitting corrosion, galvanic corrosion, filiform corrosion and intergranular corrosion). Uniform attack is the most common form of corrosion. It is normally characterized by a chemical or electrochemical reaction which proceeds uniformly over the entire exposed surface or over a large area. As a result, it would be easy to predict corrosion margin based on the empirical forum: mpy = 534 W/DAT, where mpy is mills per year, W = weight loss (mg), D = density of material (g/cm^3), A = area of material (in^2), T = exposure time (h) and number of 534 comes from the interconversion between different unit systems [496]. Unfortunately, the effectiveness of this empirical forum is so limited because most of the corrosion cases appear in the localized manner. Even when looking at one polycrystalline metal (or alloy), there are numerous sites that can act as selective anodic sites which possess normally higher chemical potential, so that they will preferentially attacked and the resultant corrosion current density should get higher. Such preferential anodic sites include grain boundaries, dislocation kinks, precipitates or other inclusions within grains. All of these metallographic irregularity sites should be exposed to corrosive environment.

Magnesium alloys corrode/degrade in aqueous materials by several different oxidation-reduction reactions, depending on alloying elements. Generally, the corrosion of magnesium in water will yield magnesium hydroxide and hydrogen gas evolution [497]. Accordingly, all necessary reactions as well as corrosion product can be expressed as follows:

An anodic reaction: $Mg\ (s) \rightarrow Mg^{2+} + 2e^-$

Reduction reaction: $2H_2O + 2e^- \rightarrow H_2 + 2OH^-$.

Net reaction from these half-cell reactions: $Mg + 2H_2O \rightarrow Mg(OH)_2 + H_2$

Corrosion byproduct formation: $Mg^{2+} + 2OH^- \rightarrow Mg(OH)_2$

14.4.2 Atmospheric corrosion

Various hazardous particulate matter suspended in air and the extent of their ill effects on sensitive devices such as electronics as well as on human beings are compared (see Table 14.7), indicating that electronics are more sensitive to environmental hazards than human beings [498–500].

In atmospheric corrosion, besides the aforementioned particles, there are two most important parameters influencing corrosion, that is, humidity and temperature.

Table 14.7: Critical allowable limit of air pollution (ppm).

Type of gas	Electronics	Human
SO_2	<30	<2,000
H_2S	<10	<10,000
NO_x	<30	<2,000
$Cl_2 + HCl$	<10	<5,500
HF	<10	
NH_3	<500	<25,000
O_2	<5	<100

Atmospheric conditions contain certain levels of water content in the form of humidity, and the corrosion of magnesium alloys increases with relative humidity (RH) [501–503]. It was reported that after 18 months of study, neither pure magnesium nor any of its alloys exhibit evidence of surface corrosion at 9.5% RH, whereas minimal corrosion occurs at 30% RH and at 80% RH, substantial surface corrosion occurs [502]. Liu et al. [504] indicated that (i) temperature increases the corrosion rate unless a protective film causes a decrease [505–507] and (ii) gaseous species such as O_2, SO_2 and NO_2 accelerate the atmospheric corrosion rate, whereas the corrosion rate is decreased by CO_2. It is obvious that many corrosion-related parameters (temperature, relative humidity, time of wetness, atmospheric composition, the presence of industrial pollutants, and the presence of inorganic salts) [504] should be involved in atmospheric corrosion, since Mg-based alloys are practically used for automobile, aerospace or telecommunication applications. These complicated corrosive environment causes more complicated influence on the corrosion behavior, and their influence is difficult to predict based on the corrosion behavior in aqueous solution, as indicated [505, 508].

Among various common Mg-based alloys, it is interestingly to find that AZ91 (Mg–9Al–1Zn) alloy has been subjected to researches. LeBozec et al. [509] conducted laboratory corrosion tests with climate parameters of relative humidity (76%, 85% and 95%), temperature (25 and 35 °C), and the amount of sodium chloride (ranging from 14 to 240 μg/cm^2 NaCl) to study the influence on the corrosion rate of magnesium alloys AZ91D and AM50 alloys. It was found that the corrosion rate of both materials increased as a function of temperature, RH, and amount of NaCl and (ii) a strong influence of the surface state, that is, as-cast or polished, was observed mainly due to the combined effect of an active surface layer and the roughness of as-cast surfaces. Jönsson et al. studied the atmospheric corrosion behavior of AZ91D in humid air at 95% RH with a deposition of 70 μg/cm^2 NaCl [510] and in the marine environment was 4.2 μm/year, and in the rural and urban environments 2.2 and 1.8 μm/year, respectively [511]. It was reported that (i) the corrosion products identified were the magnesium carbonates hydromagnesite ($Mg_5(CO_3)_4(OH)_2 \cdot 4H_2O$) and nesquehonite ($MgCO_3 \cdot 3H_2O$); (ii) the corrosion attack starts with the formation of magnesite at locations with higher NaCl contents; (iii) at 95% RH, a sequence of reactions was observed with the initial formation of magnesite, which transformed into nesquehonite after 2–3 days; and (iv) long exposures result in the formation of pits containing brucite $Mg(OH_2)$ covered with hydromagnesite crusts [510]. It was further mentioned that the main corrosion product found was magnesium carbonate hydromagnesite $Mg_5(CO_3)_4(OH)_2 \cdot 4H_2O$, which was formed at all three exposure sites. The corrosion attack started in the α-phase in larger grains at the boundary between the α-phase and the eutectic α-/β-phase and microgalvanic elements were formed with the eutectic α-/β-Mg phase as a cathodic site and the α-Mg grains as anodes [511]. Zhao et al. [512] exposed AZ91 with other Ng-based alloys to the interrupted salt spray test and found that the corrosion product was $Mg(OH)_2$. Zhou et al. [513] investigated the corrosion behavior of AZ91 alloy under NaCl particle deposition condition by gravimetric method. It was mentioned that (i) the mass gain increased rapidly at the beginning of exposure and then slowly with time, (ii) the corrosion morphologies were observed and the results showed that NaCl deposition resulted in the occurrence of localized corrosion and (iii) the corrosion product was a mixture of oxide and hydroxide of magnesium and aluminum.

14.4.3 Oxidation

14.4.3.1 Mechanisms and kinetics

In general, metallic oxides are considered as semiconductors and oxides can be classified into three groups: metal-excess semiconductor (n-type donor), metal-deficit semiconductor (p-type acceptor) and amphoteric conductors [514]. A typical magnesium oxide is formed as MgO, which is believed to be recognized as an n-type semiconductor (metal excess), so that new oxide can grow at the MgO/O interface. This can be verified by comparing the diffusion coefficient (D_o) of both ions: D_o of O into MgO was reported to be 2.5–2.9 × 10^{-6} (cm^2/s) [515] in single-crystal MgO or 4.5 × 10^{-5} (cm^2/s) [516] in polycrystalline MgO, while D_o of Mg into MgO was 2.2 × 10^{-5} (cm^2/s) [517], so that outward diffusing of Mg is faster than inward diffusing of O ions to grow new formed oxide outwardly.

The growth of thicker oxide layers is described by the Wagner theory of oxidation [518, 519]. According to this model (see Figure 14.12), oxide layers (containing both ionic and electronic resistances) grow both from the metal substrate outward and from the outer oxide layer inward. Metal atoms are oxidized to metal cations at the metal substrate, and the cations that are produced diffuse outward through the oxide film, along with a concomitant outward migration of electrons produced by

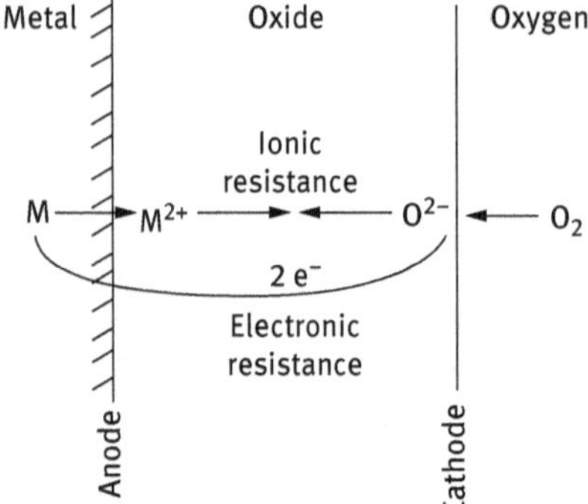

Figure 14.12: The Wagner mechanism of high-temperature oxidation [518].

the oxidation reaction. At the outermost surface of the oxide film, O_2 gas is reduced to O^{2-} ions, which then diffuse inward through the oxide film. For the growth of an oxide of MO, there are three basic reactions taking place:

At the metal/oxide interface: $M \rightarrow M^{2+} + 2e^-$
At the oxide/oxygen interface: $\frac{1}{2}O_2 + 2e^- \rightarrow O^{2-}$
Overall reaction: $M + \frac{1}{2}O_2 \rightarrow MO$

Governing oxide growth kinetics can be expressed by growing oxide thickness (y) as a function of oxidation duration (t), as shown in Figure 14.13. For a liner growth, $y = f(t)$, while for parabolic growth, $y^2 = f(t)$ and for logarithmic growth, $y = f(\log t)$. According to Kubaschewski et al. [514], MgO growth kinetic obeys logarithmic law up to about 200 °C, then parabolic growth controls the growth till approximately 500 °C and the linear-rate growth follows.

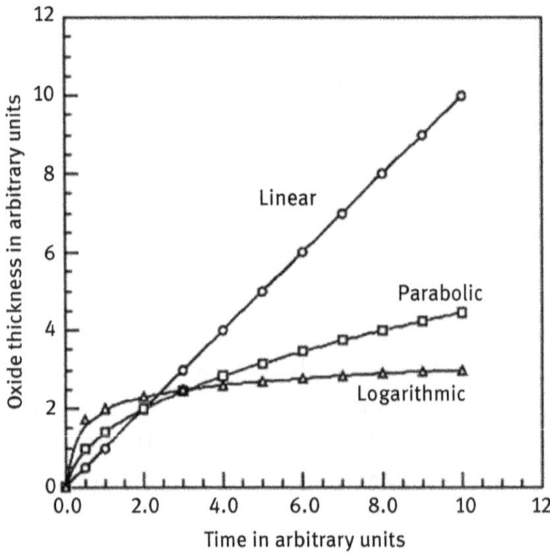

Figure 14.13: Schematic illustration of three typical oxide growth kinetics [514, 519].

At an interface between growing oxide and metal substrate, there should be lower partial oxygen pressure. Prorok et al. [520] studied internal oxidation of Mg in Ag/1.12 Mg (at%) at 450–825 °C in various oxygen partial pressures. It was mentioned that (i) measurements of O weight gain and oxidation-front velocity showed that at 450 °C the rate of O penetration into the alloy was ≈400 times slower than O diffusion in pure Ag, (ii) at 825 °C, this factor decreased to ≈60 times slower, (iii) a comparison of these results with a calculation based on a model of internal oxidation indicated that O diffusivity in pure Ag was nearly identical to O diffusivity in the alloy, (iv) the decreased O penetration rate in the alloy was attributed to O uptake by the Mg species, which are able to capture hypostoichiometric amounts of O and (v) O fixation proceeded according to predictions of the model; oxidation rate increased with partial pressure due to an increased O activity gradient; however, below ≈600 °C and at 0.08 atm partial pressure, O fixation progressed at a rate notably faster than that predicted by the model; which might be attributed to a change in Mg–O fixation stoichiometry, such that smaller amounts of O were absorbed, allowing the oxidation front to proceed more rapidly. Xu et al. [521] performed computer simulations to explain the variety of crystal orientations observed at interfaces between MgO and Mg when Mg single crystals are oxidized. It was found that a combination of interfacial chemical bonding energy and epitaxial strain stored in the oxide layers can change the relative stability of competing MgO/Mg interfaces. Jeurgens et al. [522] investigated the initial, thermal oxidation of unalloyed Mg, Mg–7.31Al alloys (at%) at 31 °C in the partial oxygen pressure range of $10^{-6} \leqslant pO_2 \leqslant 10^{-4}$ Pa. It was reported that (i) the chemical constitution of the initially grown oxide film resembles that of a MgO type of oxide with, adjacent to the alloy/oxide interface, (ii) Al enrichments were observed in both the oxide film and the subsurface region of the alloy substrate, (iii) the Al-to-Mg content of the oxide films is governed by the alloy composition in the subsurface region, which deviates from the bulk alloy composition due to sputter cleaning prior to oxidation, (iv) continued oxide film growth proceeds by the transformation of a defective surface oxide structure into the bulk oxide upon reacting with outwardly diffusing Mg cations under the influence of a surface charge field and (v) the effective rate of depletion of Mg from the alloy subsurface region is governed by the competing processes of preferential oxidation of Mg and interfacial segregation of Mg.

14.4.3.2 Characterization of formed oxides

Wang et al. [523] studied the early oxidation behaviors of Mg–Y alloys (Y = 0.82, 1.09, 4.31 and 25.00 wt%) oxidized in pure O_2. It was found that (i) the oxidation behaviors of the Mg–Y alloys (Y = 4.31 and 25.00 wt%) obeyed a parabolic law, while that of the Mg–Y (Y = 0.82 and 1.09 wt%) exhibited both parabolic and linear kinetics depending on the oxidation temperature and (ii) an oxide film with a single structure composed of MgO and Y_2O_3 had formed. Wang et al. [524] investigated the isothermal early oxidation behaviors of Mg–10Gd–3Y alloys over the temperature range of 450–600 °C in pure O_2 up to 90 min. It was reported that (i) in general, the oxidation kinetics of the Mg–10Gd–3Y alloys obeyed a parabolic rate law, and the higher the oxidation temperature was, the greater the oxidation rate was, (ii) an oxide film with a duplex structure had formed, which was composed of Gd_2O_3, Y_2O_3 and little MgO and (iii) in contrast to pure Mg, the improved oxidation resistance of the Mg–10Gd–3Y alloys can be due to the formed dense oxide film. Miral et al. [525] studied the nonisothermal early stages of surface oxidation of liquid Mg–1%Y alloy during casting under ultra-high-purity argon, dry air, and air mixed with protective fluorine-bearing gases. It was reported that a layer of smooth and tightly coherent oxidation film composed of MgO and Y_2O_3 formed on the molten Mg–Y alloy surface with 40–60 nm thickness under dry air. About the nonflammable Mg–10Al–5Ca (at%) alloy that can be melted in air without a cover gas or flux is developed, Inoue et al. [526] mentioned that (i) the alloy immediately forms a protective oxide film consisting of three layers, a fine CaO outer layer, a fine MgO intermediate layer, and a coarse MgO innermost layer, (ii) the anionic volume ratio of the CaO/MgO interface is 1.48, which is sufficiently large to suggest the generation of a strong compressive force in the CaO layer and (iii) the dense, uniform fine CaO layer may act as a protective layer preventing the diffusion of oxygen.

Hwang et al. [527] identified the oxide layer formed on AZ91 (Mg–Al–Zn) alloy by applying different voltage with $KMnO_4$ contained solution and reported the oxide layer formed on AZ91 Mg alloy in electrolyte with potassium permanganate consists of MgO and Mn_2O_3. Le et al. [528] found the outer oxide layer was mainly comprised of ZrO_2 compound while both ZrO_2 and $Mg_2Zr_5O_{12}$ compounds existed together as the main compounds in the intermediate oxide layer when AZ91 was subjected to two-step plasma electrolytic oxidation where an acid electrolyte with K_2ZrF_6. Wu et al. [529, 530] oxidizing Mg–2.1Gd–1.1Y–0.82Zn alloy at high temperatures and mentioned a formation of protective $(Gd_x,Y_{2-x})O_3$ film. Zhou et al. [531] studied the selective oxidation of Mg–Y–Ca–Ce alloy and found dense and compact oxide films composed of MgO, Y_2O_3 and CaO formed. Yu et al. [532, 533] oxidized Mg–Y–Sn, Mg–Y and Mg–Sn alloys at 500 °C and reported that the films are mainly composed of Y_2O_3 and MgO according to XRD and XPS analysis. The compact surface oxide film can effectively protect the matrix from oxidizing. Simultaneously, the electrochemical corrosion and immersion tests showed that corrosion resistance of the oxidized Mg–Y–Sn and Mg–Y alloys has been enhanced compared with the initial unoxidized alloys. Y plays a decisive role in improving the protective property of the oxide film. Aydin et al. [534, 535] studied oxidation behavior of Mg–Nd (0.3 and 0.5 wt%) alloy and identified a mixed MgO–Nd_2O_3 scale formation on the surfaces with a Nd_2O_3-rich subscale. Gunduz et al. [536] studied oxidation of Mg–Al and Mg–Zn containing atomically 2%, 4% and 8% and found a mixture of MgO–Al_2O_3. A mixture of MgO and ZnO was identified on oxidized Mg–2Zn and Mg–5ZN alloys [537]. Oxidizing $Mg_{97}Zn_1Y_2$ (at%) alloys with Ca and Ba addition, Inoue et al. [538] mentioned that (i) the formation of a thin and continuous CaO and MgO outermost layer above Y_2O_3 inner layer, what helps to prevent the internal oxidation of Y and an increased ignition temperature can be achieved and (ii) the addition of a small amount of Be also helps to suppress the internal oxidation of Y. Saini et al. [539] studied oxidation behavior of Mg-9Li-7Al-1Sn (wt%) at 50, 150 and 300 °C and identified Li_2CO_3, $MgCO_3$ and Mg-oxide, respectively.

14.4.3.3 Alloying effect

Alloying elements exhibit various effects on oxidation behavior of Mg materials, including enhancing oxidation resistance, control internal oxidation and others. Yu et al. [540] investigated the effect of Zn addition on oxidation behavior of Mg–3Y alloys at 500 and 530 °C in the dry air. It was mentioned that (i) the alloy with 2.5 wt% Zn addition showed the best oxidation resistance of all; (ii) a dense and compact Y_2O_3/MgO composite oxide film was formed on the surface of Mg–3Y–2.5Zn alloy after oxidation; (iii) in addition, the concentration of Y element in the oxide film of Mg–3Y–2.5Zn alloy was found to have a relatively high level among the test Mg–Y–Zn alloys; (iv) the appropriate addition of Zn (1–2.5 wt%) was beneficial to the enrichment of Y element in the oxide film; however, excessive addition of Zn (3.5 wt%) caused the decrease of Y content and the formation of ZnO in the oxide film, which would deteriorate the oxidation resistance of Mg–Y alloy; and (v) the concentration of Y_2O_3 increased from the outmost to the inner layer in the oxide film of Mg-3Y-2.5Zn and Mg-3Y-3.5Zn alloys, and the content of MgO ($MgCO_3$/$Mg(OH)_2$) slightly reduced from the substrate surface to inner layer. ZnO mainly existed in the outside layer in the oxide film of Mg–3Y–3.5Zn alloy. Lin et al. [541] investigated the effects of alloying element Ce on the oxidation behavior and the surface tension of Mg–1.2Ca alloy. It was shown that (i) with the increase of Ce content from 0 wt% to 1.5 wt%, the ignition point of Mg–1.2Ca alloy increases rapidly while the surface tension declines, (ii) the ignition point of Mg–1.2Ca–1.2Ce alloy can reach 780 °C, (iii) the oxidation film of Mg–1.2Ca melt becomes smooth and dense with the increase of Ce addition, which can prevent magnesium alloys from further oxidation and burning and (iv) the oxide film of Mg–1.2Ca–1.2Ce alloy consists of three layers, that is, loose MgO in the outer layer, MgO–CaO composite oxide film in the middle layer and MgO–Ce_2O_3 composite oxide film in the inner layer. Tan et al. [542] studied the Be influences on Mg alloy oxidation and mentioned that Be microalloying significantly decreased the oxidation rate at 500 °C and increased the ignition temperatures of as-cast Mg–2Zn, Mg–2Sn, AS21, and ZC63; however, Be addition had little effect on the oxidation resistance of as-cast ZK20, AM60 and Mg–2Y. Tan et al. [543] also studied oxidation behavior of AZ91 alloy under influences of Be (60 wt ppm) and Ca (0.5 wt%) elements and mentioned that the improved oxidation resistance was attributed to the formation of a Be-reinforced compact CaO–MgO composite layer on the alloy surface. Lee et al. [544] studied oxidation and burning behaviors for CaO added AM50 Mg composites which were manufactured by conventional melting and casting processes without SF_6 protective gas. CaO-added AM50 Mg composites show the stable oxidation resistance, while AM50 Mg alloys show the poor oxidation resistance. It was found that (i) with increasing CaO addition, the burning temperature

Table 14.8: Alloying effect on corrosion and electrochemical corrosion resistance.

	Al	Mn	Ca	Zn	R	Y	Sn	Nd	Ha	Sr	Ag	Ti	Gd	Cu	Pd	Er	La	Ce	M	Li	Ga	Sb	Si	Bi	Zr
Mg	[546–548]	[546]	[546, 549, 550]	[546, 550–553]	[546, 554]	[555, 556]	[557]							[558]							[559]	[560]			
Mg–Al		[561–563]	[561, 564]	[562, 565]		[561]	[562, 566]	[561, 567]		[568]						[569, 570]	[571]	[571, 572]	[573]	[574]					
Mg–Al–Zn						[575]						[576]													
Mg–Al–Mn			[577]																						
Mg–Al–Sn			[44]							[44]															
Mg–Al–Sn–Mn						[578]																			
Mg–Zn									[579]	[580]	[581]														[582]
Mg–Zn–Sr									[583]																
Mg–Zn–Ca		[584]													[585]										
Mg–Zn–Si										[586]															
Mg–Zn–Y													[587]												
Mg–Zn–Y–Nd											[588]														
Mg–Zn–Mn			[589, 590]				[589]																		
Mg–Li–Al						[591]		[592]																	
Mg–Zr–Ca							[593]			[593]															
Mg–Nd–Zn–Zr											[594, 595]														

Mg–Ca				[596]			[596]			[597]	
Mg–Ca–Zn								[598]			
Mg–Sn–Zn	[599]										
Mg–Sn–Al–Zn		[600]									
Mg–Sb									[560]		
Mg–Mn–Zn						[601]					
Mg–Mn–Ca	[602]		[602]		[602]						
Mg–Gd–Zr							[603]				
Mg–Dy			[604]					[605]			[605]

Note: R, rare earth element; Ha, hydroxyapatite; M, mischmetal (55Ce–25La–(15-18)Nd–RE).

increases under ambient, nitrogen and dry air atmospheres and (ii) the burning temperatures of small test specimen under all conditions greatly increase even by 0.3% CaO (mass fraction) addition into AM50 Mg alloys. The high reactivity of magnesium limits its extensive applications in the transportation industry for the development of lightweight vehicles and aircrafts. In addition to modification of the corrosion potential of bulk magnesium through alloying elements, tailoring its surface oxide film is an alternative approach for enhanced resistance corrosion. Based on this background, Nouri et al. [545] investigated effects of small amounts of a RE element, yttrium, on the strength of surface oxide film formed on Mg–3Al (wt%) alloy and its adherence to the substrate. It was reported that (i) the yttrium addition decreased the component ratio of hydroxides to oxides, mainly $Mg(OH)_2$ to MgO, in the surface oxide film, leading to markedly enhanced mechanical strength and resistance to scratch with stronger adherence to the substrate and (ii) meanwhile, as the nominal yttrium concentration exceeded a certain level, the beneficial effect of Y on the film was weakened.

14.4.4 Chemical corrosion

In general, there are two major areas in research on corrosion behaviors of Mg-based alloys: alloying effects (particularly, improving corrosion resistance) and testing corrosive media (simulating close to actual applicable environment). Biocorrosion (corrosion phenomenon in biological environment) and biodegradation (synergistic phenomenon of biocorrosion and degradation of structural integrity, which is particularly important in orthopedic implants and scaffold and surgical devises in medicine) will be discussed in Chapter 18.

14.4.4.1 Alloying effect

Table 14.8 lists alloying elements to Mg-based alloys mostly for enhancing corrosion resistance. Reflecting to the previously discussed on oxide formation, it appears that Ca and Zn are most effective alloying elements.

14.4.4.2 Testing media

Table 14.9 lists various media for corrosion tests, indicating that chlorine ion containing media appear to be most frequently used testing solutions.

14.4.4.3 Microstructural influencing factors on corrosion behavior

As pointed out by Atrens et al. [657], microstructural features of materials play an crucial role in corrosion behaviors of alloys and these influencing parameters should include impurity (its concentration), secondary phase(s) and intermetallics (volume fraction, size and distribution), heat treatment (its resultant microstructural

Table 14.9: Media for corrosion tests.

	NaCl solution	SBF	Hank's solution	PEMFC	SDS (0.05 M H_3BO_3 + 0.075 M $Na_2B_4O_7$ solution)	Salt spray test (ASTM-B117)	Artificial plasma	Na_2SO_4	Bile	Cell culture medium (CCM)	Aodium sulfate	Nitrates with buffers (phosphate and borate)
Mg–Al	[562, 564, 606]											
Mg–Al–Zn	[565, 607–611]	[612, 613]	[614]									[615]
Mg–Al–Zn–Ca	[616]					[617]						
Mg–Al–Zn–Mn											[618]	
Mg–Al–Si												[615]
Mg–Al–Mn	[619]											
Mg–Al–Mn–Ca	[616, 620]											
Mg–Al–Er					[569]							
Mg–Al–MM	[57[illegible]]											
Mg–Al–Pb	[621]											

(continued)

Table 14.9 (continued)

	NaCl solution	SBF	Hank's solution	PEMFC	SDS (0.05 M H_3BO_3 + 0.075 M $Na_2B_4O_7$ solution)	Salt spray test (ASTM-B117)	Artificial plasma	Na_2SO_4	Bile	Cell culture medium (CCM)	Aodium sulfate	Nitrates with buffers (phosphate and borate)
Mg-Al-Pb-Zn-Mn	[621]											
Mg–Zn	[551, 606]		[622]						[622]			
Mg-Zn-Mn-Ca		[590]										
Mg-Zn-Mn-Nd		[623]										
Mg–Zn–RE	[624, 625]		[625]					[626]				
Mg–Zn–Ca		[627, 628]	[585, 629]									
Mg–Zn–Zr		[582]										
Mg–Zn–Sr	[580]											
Mg-Zn-Gd-Y	[563]											
Mg–Li	[630]											
Mg–Li–Al	[592]											
Mg–Li–Ca			[631]									

Mg-Li-Zn-Al	[632]						
Mg–Ca	[606]	[633]	[634]				
Mg–Sn	[606, 635]						
Mg-Sn-Zn-Al	[599]						
Mg-Sn-Zn-Mn		[636]					
Mg–Y	[555, 637–639]					[555]	
Mg–Y–RE	[640]	[641, 642]				[626]	
Mg-Y-RE-Zr	[643]						
Mg-Y-Gd-Nd-Zr	[644]						
Mg–Gd–Zn	[645]						
Mg-Gd-Zn-Zr-Mn			[646]				
Mg-Gd-Y-Nd-Zr	[647]						
Mg-Gd-Ca-Zr							[648]
Mg-Nd-Zn-Zr		[594, 649]		[650]	[651]		
Mg–Ni	[652]						
Mg–Cu	[652]						
Mg–Ti	[653, 654]						
Mg–RE–Zn	[625]		[625]				
Mg–RE–Gd						[626]	

(continued)

Table 14.9 (continued)

	NaCl solution	SBF	Hank's solution	PEMFC	SDS (0.05 M H_3BO_3 + 0.075 M $Na_2B_4O_7$ solution)	Salt spray test (ASTM-B117)	Artificial plasma	Na_2SO_4	Bile	Cell culture medium (CCM)	Aodium sulfate	Nitrates with buffers (phosphate and borate)
Mg–Dy										[655]		
Mg–Mn	[606]											
Mg–Zr	[606]											[656]
Mg–Si	[606]											
Mg–Sr	[606]											

Note: RE, rare earth element; MM, mischmetal (55Ce-25La-(15–18)Nd-RE); SBF, simulated body fluid; Hank's solution, a salt solution usually used in combination with naturally occurring body substances (e.g., blood serum, tissue extracts) and/or more complex chemically defined nutritive solutions for culturing animal cells; two variation concentrations of $CaCl_2$, $MgSO_4 \cdot 7H_2O$, KCl, KH_2PO_4, $NaHCO_3$, NaCl, $Na_2HPO_4 \cdot 2H_2O$, and D-glucose; PEMFC, polymer electrolyte membrane fuel cell (0.01 M HCl + 0.01 M Na_2SO_4 solutions bubbled with O_2 or H_2); SDS, specially designed solution (0.05 M H_3BO_3 + 0.075 M $Na_2B_4O_7$ solution).

alterations), forming (extent of severity of plastic deformation) [657–659]. Microscopically, crystal orientation should exhibit remarkable influences on corrosion behavior. Jia et al. [660] characterized microstructure and crystallographic orientation of directionally solidified Mg–4 wt% Zn alloy. It was reported that {0002} oriented planes have better corrosion resistance than $\{11\bar{2}0\}$ and $\{10\bar{1}0\}$ ones, which is attributed to a synergistic effect of surface energy, atomic packing density and the stability of oxidation film. Hagihara et al. [661] examined corrosion behavior of single Mg crystal and mentioned that (i) Mg possessed a orientation-dependency in its corrosion behavior and (ii) the corrosion rates increased in the order $(0001) < (11\bar{2}0) < (10\bar{1}0) < (11\bar{2}3) < (10\bar{1}2)$. Jiang et al. [662] investigated the influences of crystallographic texture and grain size on corrosion behavior of AZ31 sheets produced in the following ways: AR, cross-rolling (CR) and unidirectional rolling (UR). It was reported that (i) the corrosion rate AZ31 sheets decreased in the following order: AR, CR, UR and (ii) the decrease in corrosion rate was attributed to an increase in basal plane intensity in the crystallographic texture and the reduced grain size.

It was mentioned that the existence of secondary phase affected adversely corrosion behavior [663–665]. Liu et al. [664] studied the influence of the quantity of the Mg_2Sn phase on the corrosion behavior of different solution temperature-treated Mg–7Sn magnesium alloy and reported that (i) the corrosion mode and corrosion rate were associated with the quantity of Mg_2Sn phases and tin concentration of the matrix; (ii) if most of the tin was present as Mg_2Sn, the corrosion mode was pitting corrosion and it accelerated the corrosion rate; and (iii) if most of tin was dissolved in matrix, the corrosion mode was filiform corrosion and it decreased the corrosion rate. Feng et al. [665] prepared Mg–xAl–(15 – x) Zn (x = 12.5, 5.6, 3.3, 1.0 wt%) two-phase alloys containing a certain amount of the different second phases, two binary compounds γ, MgZn, and two ternary second phases Φ, q to examine the effects of these secondary phases on corrosion behavior in the 3.5 wt% NaCl solution. It was found that (i) the second phases precipitated both in the Mg matrix and along the grain boundaries and acted as a microcathode, accelerating corrosion dissolution of the Mg substrate and (ii) the acceleration effect of the second phases is in the order of γ-$Mg_{17}Al_{12}$ > q-$Mg_{44}Zn_{41}Al_1$ > Φ-$Mg_{21}(Zn,Al)_{17}$ > MgZn. The volume fraction of LPSO phases were also studied on their effects on corrosion behavior of Mg materials. Li et al. [666] investigated the microstructural evolution and corrosion behavior of cast Mg–Zn–Y alloys as a function of volume fraction of LPSO phases. It was reported that (i) LPSO phases in these alloys acted as a microcathode to accelerate corrosion progress due to their nobler nature than that of α-Mg matrix and (ii) the galvanic couple effect between LPSO phases and α-Mg matrix dominated the corrosion rate of the cast Mg–Zn–Y alloys in the long-term corrosion process; as a result, ZW12 alloy displayed the best corrosion resistance due to the least volume fraction of microcathodes (i.e., LPSO phases). Cheng et al. [667] prepared three different morphologies of LPSO phase, that is, lamellar, block-like, and rod-like to examine the effect of the morphology of LPSO phase on corrosion behavior of cast

Mg-Zn-Y-Ti alloy. It was reported that (i) the alloys with the rod-like LPSO phases exhibited more uniform corrosion mode and better corrosion resistance than the alloys with the block-like LPSO phases, so the former had excellent comprehensive properties and (ii) the precipitation of the lamellar LPSO phases not only reduced the mechanical properties, but also accelerated the corrosion rate and produced severe localized corrosion.

14.4.4.4 Effects of heat treatments

The microstructural evolution, corrosion resistance and mechanical properties of an as-forged Mg-6.7%Zn-1.3%Y-0.6%Zr alloy before and after solid-solution treatment (T4) were investigated [668]. It was mentioned that the T4 treatment can improve corrosion resistance of the alloy; due to eliminated inhomogeneous distribution associated with the $MgZn_2$ precipitates formed during hot forging process. Shahri et al. [669] treated a Mg–6Zn biodegradable alloy at 350 °C for 6–48 h to evaluate the effects of resulting microstructure changes on the alloy's degradation rate and mechanisms in vitro. It was shown that (i) over 24 h solution treatment dissolves intermetallic phases in matrix and produces an almost single phase microstructure, resulting in lower cathode/anode region ratios and lowers corrosion rates and (ii) the solution treatment was suggested as a corrosion improving process for the application of Mg–Zn alloys as biodegradable implant materials. Zhang et al. [670] investigated the effect of solid-solution treatment on corrosion and electrochemical mechanisms of Mg–15Y alloy in 3.5 wt% NaCl solution. It was indicated that (i) the corrosion resistance of Mg–15Y sample gradually deteriorated with immersion time increasing, which was consistent with the observation of corrosion morphologies and (ii) the corrosion potential and corrosion rate of as-cast samples were both lower than those of solid ST samples, and both increased with increment of solid ST time.

14.4.4.5 Effects of forming

Ha et al. [671] studied the corrosion behavior of extruded Mg–(2–8 wt%) Sn alloys in aqueous chloride solutions to examine the influences of the volume fraction of Mg_2Sn intermetallics, solutionized Sn, and area fraction of grain boundaries on the corrosion behavior. It was mentioned that (i) the Sn addition up to 8 wt% increased the overall dissolution rate of the alloys, although it promoted the passivity, which resulted from the increased H_2 evolution rate and increased numbers of initiation sites for pitting corrosion and (ii) the overall corrosion behavior primarily depended on the amount of Mg_2Sn intermetallics, which promoted passivity and notably increased the H_2 evolution rate, and functioned as pitting corrosion initiation sites. Xu et al. [672] studied the influences of the hot extrusion process on the microstructure, corrosion behavior and corrosion mechanism for Mg–Y alloy. It was reported that (i) the open-circuit potential had a certain degree of improvement after extrusion, the open-circuit potential increased with increment of extrusion ratio, and the corrosion potential of the vertical section was higher than that of the same alloy in the same compression ratio, (ii) the shift rate of the corrosion potential relatively became larger with increasing of the extrusion ratio, and the cathode corrosion current corresponding to the branch migration shifted to the positive direction and (iii) the corrosion morphologies of Mg–0.25Y alloy were uniform corrosion, and the corrosion morphologies of Mg–(2.5, 5, 8 and 15) were the pitting corrosion and the small range, deep depth localized corrosion. Wu et al. [673] studied the effect of extrusion on the microstructures and corrosion properties of Mg–2Ca–xAl ($x = 0$, 2, 3, 5 wt%) alloys and mentioned that the as-cast alloys showed uniform corrosion mechanism while the AR Mg–Al–Ca alloys presented local corrosion characteristic. Zhang et al. [674] conducted double extrusion process to refine microstructure and improve mechanical properties and corrosion properties of Mg-2.25Nd-0.11Zn-0.43Zr (A1) and Mg-2.70Nd-0.20Zn-0.41Zr (A2) alloys. It was mentioned that the results of immersion experiment and electrochemical measurements in SBF show that the corrosion resistance of A1 and A2 under double extrusion was increased by 7% and 8%, respectively, compared with those under just once extrusion.

The influence of hot rolling on the corrosion of Mg–X alloys (X = Gd, Ca, Al, Mn, Sn, Sr, Nd, La, Ce, Zr or Si) was investigated by immersion tests in 3.5% NaCl solution saturated with $Mg(OH)_2$ [675]. It was found that (i) the corrosion rates for all Mg–X alloys (except Mg–0.1Zr and Mg–0.3Si) decreased after hot rolling, attributed to fine-grained alloys having a more homogeneous microstructure, and fewer, smaller second-phase particles and (ii) for Mg–0.1Zr and Mg–0.3Si, the corrosion rate increased after hot rolling. Xiang et al. [676] investigated the effect of rolling-induced microstructural changes of Mg–5Li–1Al (LA51) alloy sheet on its corrosion behavior. It was obtained that (i) the corrosion performance of LA51 alloy sheet improved as a function of rolling reduction and (ii) the notable increase in corrosion resistance of the rolled LA51 alloy sheet was attributed to its characteristic texture, texture-intensity and the formation of twins and protective oxide surface films. Seong et al. [677] studied the effective refinement and dispersion of the Mg_2Ca phase in the Mg–Ca (2–3 wt%Ca) alloys using extrusion followed by high-ratio differential speed rolling (HRDSR) and postrolling annealing, which led to the formation of homogeneous microstructures in which submicron-sized and nanosized Mg_2Ca particles were distributed over the fine-grained recrystallized matrices with grain sizes of ~6 μm. It was found that (i) rolled Mg–Ca alloy exhibited significant improvement in the corrosion resistance in Hank's solution and (ii) the annealed HRDSR-processed Mg–Ca alloys showed higher corrosion resistance and higher mechanical strength compared with pure magnesium.

The effect of MDF on corrosion behavior of Mg-4Zn-2Gd-0.5Ca alloy was studied [678]. It was reported that (i) the corrosion resistance of Mg-4Zn-2Gd-0.5Ca alloy became worse after 1 pass of MDF as compared with the as-homogenized condition because of the precipitation of I phase, (ii) the corrosion resistance of the as-MDFed

Mg-4Zn-2Gd-0.5Ca alloy deteriorated with the increasing pass of MDF and (iii) as compared with grain refinement, the precipitated I phase is thought to play a main role on the corrosion behavior of Mg–4Zn–0.5Ca alloy. Wan et al. [679] realized simultaneous improvements in strength and corrosion resistance of Mg-Gd-Y-Zr alloy were realized through forging at RT with formation of ultrafine-grained structure and mentioned that the improvement in corrosion resistance is attributed to the formation of subgrain boundaries.

Jiang et al. [680] processed ZK60 Mg alloy by multipass equal-channel angular pressing (ECAP) followed by aging to investigate the effect of grain refinement and second-phase redistribution on its corrosion behavior. It was reported that (i) the fine-grained samples after more ECAP passes have higher corrosion current densities in the polarization curves, lower charge-transfer resistance values, (ii) the SPD decreases the alloy corrosion resistance besides the well-known strengthening and toughening and (iii) the post-ECAP aging can slightly improve the corrosion resistance of the fine-grained ZK60 Mg alloy and enhance the comprehensive performances, due to the stress relief and uniform distribution of second-phase particles.

14.4.4.6 Others

Liu et al. [681] preformed severe shot peening (SP) on AZ31 and AZ91 Mg alloys to obtain a nanostructured surface layer. It was mentioned that (i) the corrosion resis tance of AZ31 alloy was improved by SP treatment, because a relatively compact passive film formed rapidly on the nanostructured surface and (ii) SP treatment played a minor role in enhancing the corrosion resistance of AZ91 alloy, because it had little effect on size and distribution of β-phases. It should be added to the above comments that there would be a possibility of surface contamination due to short media residues, which might act as potential anodic sites.

Johnston et al. [682] studied the influence of two common sterilization techniques, ethylene oxide (EO) and gamma irradiation (GI), on the corrosion rate of four Mg-based materials (high-purity (HP)-Mg, ZE41, ultra-high-purity (XHP)-Mg, and XHP-ZX00) in CO_2-bicarbonate buffered Hanks' solution. It was mentioned that (i) neither sterilization technique (EO and GI) significantly influenced the corrosion rate as measured by P_m nor P_H, being consistent across the four materials tested, as there was no interaction between the test variables of material and sterilization condition for P_m or P_H and (ii) as neither EO nor GI influenced the corrosion rates, either of these techniques warrants consideration for use on Mg-based medical implants and devices.

14.4.5 Electrochemical corrosion

In electrochemistry, the Pourbaix diagram, also known as a potential/pH diagram [EH–pH] shows possible stable (equilibrium) phases of an aqueous electrochemical system. Predominant ion boundaries are represented by lines. Referring to Figure 14.14 [683, 684], the intersecting point on potential E-axis at pH = 0 for H_2O should be 1.229 (against SHE: standard hydrogen electrode) and zone defined by two dotted lines indicates a stable zone for water. It can be also easily noticed that Mg is highly prone to aqueous corrosion in neutral and acidic pH ranges [685]. The corrosion occurs rapidly when exposed to salt water, moisture or acidic liquids with a strong inclination for the localized attack along with the production of hydrogen gas. In basic solutions, protective surface passivation film is possible by the formed hydroxide layer. Thermodynamic equilibrium cannot exist for Mg in aqueous solution: however, this is possible if the hydrogen overpotential is about 1 V and the pH is greater than 5. Corrosion potential is slightly more negative than −1.5 V/SHE in dilute chloride solutions [686]. Under a presence of OH^- ion, corrosion product might be $Mg(OH)_2$ ($\leftarrow Mg^{2+} + 2OH^-$), while if chlorine ion Cl^- exists in aqueous environment, corrosion product will be Mg $(Cl)_2$ (through $Mg(OH)_2 + 2Cl^- \rightarrow Mg(Cl)_2 + 2OH^-$).

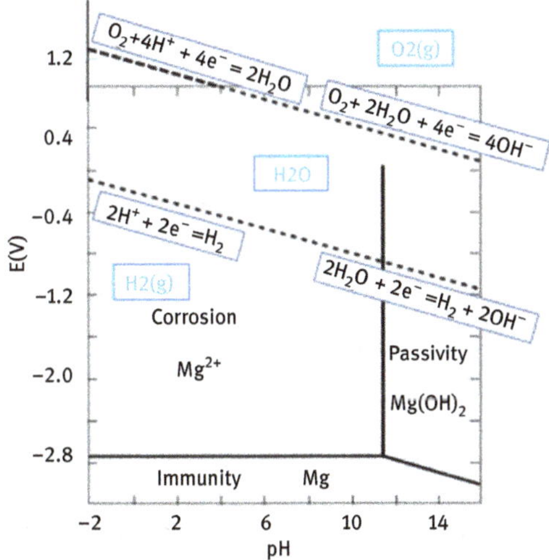

Figure 14.14: Combined Pourbaix diagrams for Mg-pH and H_2O-pH systems.

For studying electrochemical corrosion behavior of an electrode (as a metallic sample) in electrolyte (mostly corrosive environment), there are two useful methods available: that is, polarization curve and electrochemical impedance spectroscopy (EIS). The polarization curve is the basic kinetic law for any electrochemical reaction and is a plot of current density versus electrode potential for a specific electrode–electrolyte combination. Polarization curves are valuable in quantifying the behaviors of metals under various conditions. Polarization curves for passive systems may show active/passive and/or passive/transpassive transitions (if any). For example, as shown in Figure 14.15, polarization curves for individual alloys possess unique and distinct natures from each other. For this example, Zhang et al. [687] conducted systematic tests to find the best Mg–Zn alloy systems suitable and applicable as degradable biomaterial. As figure indicates, alloying effect of Zn element is clearly shown when tested in SBF. In further discussion, it was mentioned that the reason for the increased corrosion potential of Mg–*x*Zn alloys was that the Zn element had high electronegativity, but, when the Zn concentration increased, the corrosion resistance was decreased. Due to the fact that the second phase precipitated during the solid solidification processes, which accelerated the corrosion rate due to the different electrochemical behaviors of α-Mg and precipitates and the degradation rates of Mg–1.0Zn degraded were slower than Mg–5.0Zn, Mg–6.0Zn adhered to the electrochemical results.

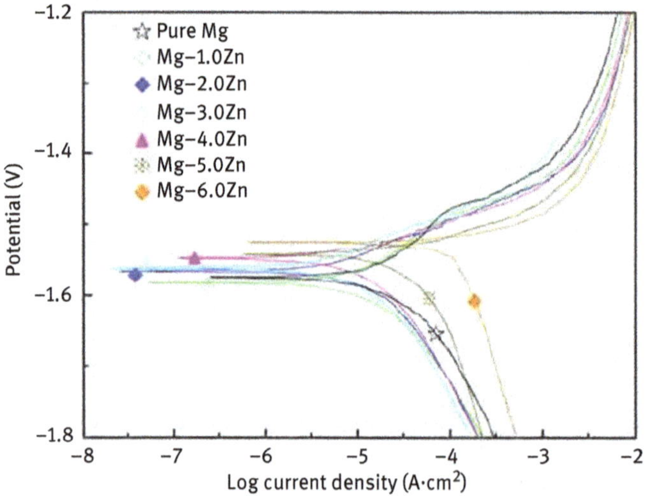

Figure 14.15: Polarizations curves of Mg alloyed with various % of Zn in SBF [687].

Figure 14.16 is another good example of comparison of various polarization curves, in which Kim et al. [688] investigated effects of surface treatment on corrosion behavior of Mg materials in SBF. Mg–2.72Al–0.87Zn (AZ31) was treated with MAO coating in alkaline electrolytes such as 1.0 M NaOH with 0.1 M glycerol and 0.1 M Na_3PO_4, followed by hydrothermal treatment in 0.1 M Ca-EDTA ($C_{10}H_{12}CaN_2Na_2O_8$) and 0.5 M NaOH solution at 90 °C for different times (6, 12, 24 and 48 h), so that by prolonging the treatment time, contents of Na and Ca incorporated in surface layer increases, while that of Mg decreases although amounts of Al and Zn did not change remarkably.

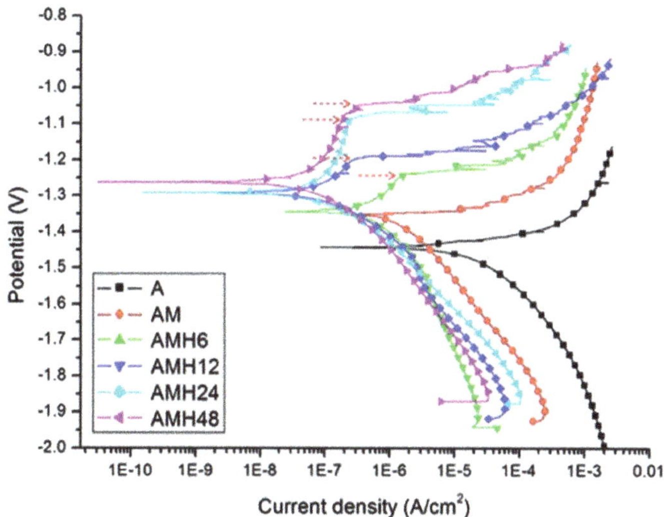

Figure 14.16: Polarization curves of treated AZ31 with different times [688].

It was further mentioned that (i) after MAO coating, the corrosion current density (I_{corr}) decreased to $1.66 \times 10 - 6A/cm^2$ and the corrosion potential (E_{corr}) increased to −1,357.39 mV; (ii) after hydrothermal treatment, it was found that the values of pitting corrosion potential (as marked with arrows) were not correlated with the treatment time; (iii) as hydrothermal treatment time increased, the current density decreased and the corrosion potential increased; (iv) a passivation area was formed after hydrothermal treatment; (v) after hydrothermal treatment for 6 h, the current density decreased to $1.37 \times 10 - 6A/cm^2$; (vi) after 12 h treatment, the current density rapidly decreased and the corrosion potential increased; (vii) in the 24 h group, the lowest current density was shown, and the pitting corrosion potential became higher rapidly; and (viii) the corrosion property of surface after the hydrothermal treatment for 48 h was similar with that for 24 h, only the corrosion potential slightly moved to the novel direction.

A portion where a transition from the cathodic polarization to anodic polarization takes place is called the Tafel slope (or Stearn Gary plot), as shown in Figure 14.17 [689]. The intersecting point of extrapolated cathodic current slope and anodic current slope defines I_{CORR} (corrosion current density) and E_{CORR} (corrosion potential). Corrosion current is related to Tafel slopes as follows:

$I_{CORR} = [\beta_A \beta_C]/[2.3(R_P)(\beta_A + \beta_C)]$, where
β_A is the anodic Tafel slope,
β_C the cathodic Tafel slope and
R_P represents polarization resistance.

If R_P increases, I_{CORR} decreases, so as corrosion rate.

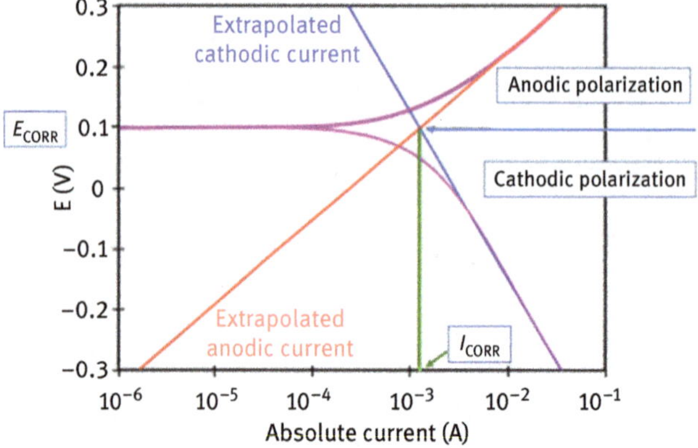

Figure 14.17: Tafel slope for estimation for corrosion rate [689].

By knowing $I_{CORR,}$ the corrosion rate in MPY (mils per year) can be empirically estimated by corrosion rate in MPY = [0.13 × I_{CORR} × EW]/[A × d], where MPY is mils (1/1,000 inch) per year, EW is equivalent weight [g/eq.] (for Mg in MgO: 24.31/2 = 12.31; $Mg^{2+} + O^{2-}$), A is exposed area (cm^2), d is density (g/cm^3) and "0.13" indicates metric and time conversion factor.

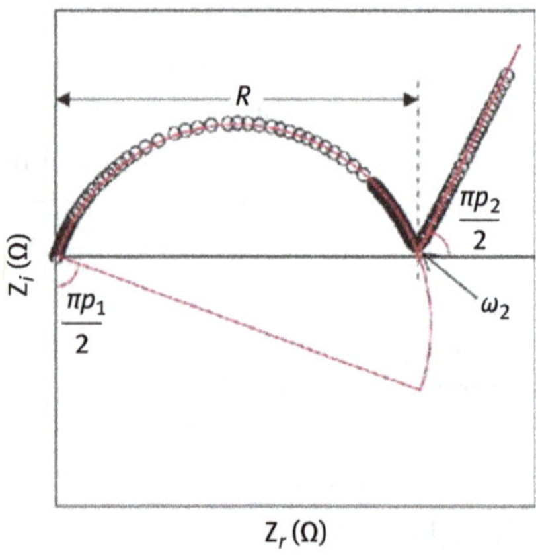

Figure 14.18: Typical Nyquist plot, obtained by EIS test [690].

From Ohm's law, there are two formulae; one is with DC condition which can be expressed as $E(V) = I \times R$, where R is resistance and the other is with AC condition which can be expressed by $E(V) = I \times Z$, where ($Z^2 = Z'^2_{real} + Z''^2_{imaginary}$) and Z is impedance. Figure 14.18 [690] shows a typical Nyquist plotting of real component Z' versus imaginary component Z''. The radius of the curve R represents R_P (polarization resistance). There are several advantages associated with EIS AC impedance method over conventional DC method, including (1) the R_P measurement takes a

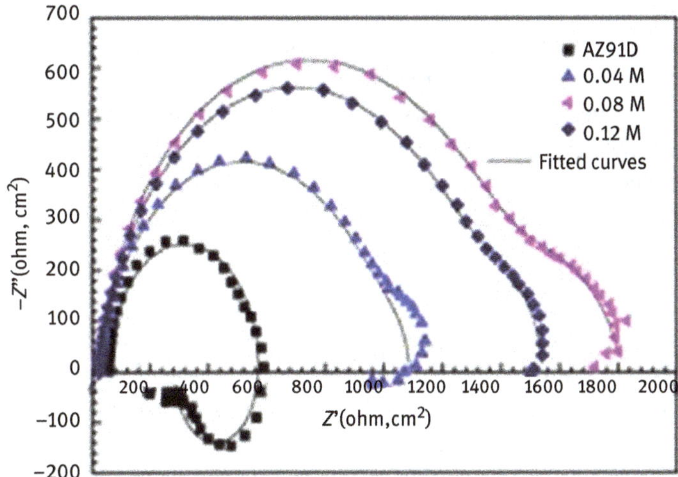

Figure 14.19: Nyquist plot of AZ91 alloys treated with different concentration of $NaVO_3$, tested in 3.5 wt% NaCl solution [691].

much shorter time to make than DC method and (2) the R_P measurement takes specimen to smaller voltages (e.g., up to maximum 10 mV), and thus does not significantly alter the surface condition.

Sun et al. [691] investigated the effects of Ca–P–V composite coating (with different concentration of $NaVO_3$) on AZ91 alloy on corrosion behavior in 3.5 wt% NaCl solution. It was reported that (i) the Ca–P–V-coated samples not only exhibit good corrosion resistance property, but also show self-healing ability, (ii) by increasing the concentration of $NaVO_3$, the capacitive loop diameter at high frequency also increases, which is related to high corrosion resistance (see Figure 14.18) and (iii) the sample coated with 0.08 M $NaVO_3$ shows the largest loop compared with other coated samples.

14.4.5.1 Mg

The influences of solute atoms (Li, Al, Mn, Zn, Fe, Ni, Cu, Y, Zr) and Cl adsorption on the anodic corrosion performance on Mg (0001) surface have been investigated [692]. It was reported that (i) at 25% surface doping rate, Y decreased the work function of Mg, while the impact of remaining doping elements on the work function of Mg was trivial due to the small surface dipole moment change, (ii) the adsorption of Cl destabilized the Mg atoms at surface by weakening the bonding between surface Mg atoms and (iii) a stronger hybridization of *d* orbits of alloying elements (e.g., Zr) with the orbits of Mg can greatly increase the local electrode potential, which even overbalances the negative effect introduced by Cl adsorbates and hence improves the corrosion resistance of Mg alloys. Gomes et al. [693] analyzed the electrochemical impedance spectra obtained for the Mg electrode during immersion in a sodium sulfate solution. It was mentioned that there are various parameters detected such as the thin oxide film thickness, the resistivity at the metal/oxide film interface and at the oxide film/electrolyte interface, the active surface area as a function of the exposure time to the electrolyte, the thickness of the thick $Mg(OH)_2$ layer and the kinetic constants of the electrochemical reaction.

14.4.5.2 Mg–Al

Corrosion of high-purity Mg–Al alloys containing 3, 6 and 9 wt% Al was investigated using electrochemical noise analysis [694]. It was reported that (i) steady-state corrosion in all alloys was highly localized, (ii) for the Mg–3%Al alloy, localized corrosion was preceded by a period of general corrosion, (iii) the corrosion rate of the as-cast Mg–9%Al alloy was less than those of the other materials but increased with solution annealing time and (iv) the results are consistent with strong galvanic coupling between Al-depleted and Al-enriched zones of the α-phase. Rosalbino et al. [695] studied the electrochemical behavior of new Mg–Al–RE (RE = Ce, Er) alloys AE91 in 0.01 M NaCl electrolyte (pH = 12) and compared with that of the most commonly used Mg alloy in the automotive field, the AZ91D. It was found that (i) AE91 alloys showed very similar microstructures characterized by a three-phase appearance: a Mg-based solid solution containing only Al and two intermetallic phases $\gamma(Mg_{17}Al_{12})$ and $(Al_{1-X}Mg_X)_3Ce$ or $(Al_{1-X}Mg_X)_2Er$, (ii) free corrosion potential measurements, potentiodynamic polarization curves and EIS revealed improved passivity behavior compared to AZ91D alloy and (iii) the apparent presence of trace amounts of RE oxides in the passive film is presumed to be the reason for the enhanced corrosion resistance of AE91 alloys in the aggressive environment considered. Mg–Al–Pb alloy is a good candidate for the anode material of magnesium seawater battery. Feng et al. [696], for improving the low current utilization efficiency of Mg–Al–Pb alloy, investigated the influence of Ce on the microstructures and electrochemical corrosion properties in a 3.5% NaCl solution. It was indicated that (i) Ce refines the grain structure of Mg–Al–Pb alloy, (ii) the formation of strip $Al_{11}Ce_3$ second phase promotes the uniform distribution of $Mg_{17}Al_{12}$ phase in Mg-Al-Pb-Ce alloy, (iii) the addition of Ce accelerates the discharge activity of Mg–Al–Pb alloy and (iv) due to a large number of cathodic $Al_{11}Ce_3$ and $Mg_{17}Al_{12}$ phases, Ce promotes the microgalvanic corrosion and leads to larger corrosion current density and hydrogen evolution rate in Mg-Al-Pb-Ce alloy than those in Mg–Al–Pb alloy; however, Mg–Al–Pb alloy expresses smaller utilization efficiency than Mg-Al-Pb-Ce alloy because of grain detachment. Medhashree et al. [697] studied the corrosion behavior of Mg-Al-Zn-Mn alloy in 30% (v/v) aqueous ethylene glycol containing chloride anions at neutral pH value. It was found that the rate of corrosion increases with the increase in chloride ion concentration and also with the increase in medium temperature. Effects of coverage layer on the electro chemical corrosion behavior of Mg–Al–Mn alloy subjected to massive LSPLSP treat ment was investigated and it was reported that (i) LSP induced an obvious improvement in electrochemical corrosion resistance with increasing coverage layer, (ii) even in a higher corrosive solution concentration, LSP could still prevent corrosion to some extent and (iii) the improvement in electrochemical corrosion resistance was due to the grain refinement and compressive residual stress induced by massive LSP treatment [698].

14.4.5.3 Mg–Al–Zn

The passivation and corrosion behaviors of Mg alloy AZ31B were investigated in chloride-free NaOH solutions with pH range from 10 to 14 [699]. It was reported that (i) various phases behave differently at different pH levels, (ii) Al–Mn intermetallics serve as strong cathode at pH ≤ 11, but dissolve at pH ≥ 13, (iii) ambient oxygen is responsible for the potential rise at pH ≥ 13 and subsequent significant potential oscillation (>1 V) is attributed to the passive film breakdown at the intergranular boundaries in the oxide film and (iv) optimal passivation is achieved at pH 12 with thin uniform passive film formed across the surface. Rolled AZ31 Mg alloy, which has great potential applications in the automobile industry, is detected to be highly crystallographic textured. It was reported that (i) its rolling surface (RS), mainly consisting of (0001) crystallographic planes, was more electrochemically stable and corrosion resistant than its cross-section surface (CS) mainly composed of crystallographic planes (1010) and (1120) in 5 wt% NaCl, (ii) the different corrosion performances of these crystallographic planes can be ascribed to their different anodic and cathodic reaction activities and (iii) the different electrochemical activities of RS and CS surfaces originate from the different surface energy levels of the (0001), (10$\bar{1}$0) and (11$\bar{2}$0) crystallographic planes [700]. Srinivasan et al. [701] carried out electrochemical polymerization of pyrrole (Py) from aqueous salicylate solution over AZ31 Mg alloy. It was found that (i) open-circuit potential measurement and potentiodynamic polarization studies revealed that the coating prepared using 0.25 M of Py had positive shift of about 120 mV in corrosion potential and lower corrosion current density (0.03 mA/cm^2) compared to other concentrations and uncoated AZ31 Mg alloy (0.25 mA/cm^2) and (ii) EIS studies of uncoated and Py-coated Mg alloy in SBF revealed three-time constants behavior with about one order of increment in impedance value for 0.25 M of Py.

Electrochemical behavior of AZ91D in aerated 3.5 wt% NaCl solution was studied to examine the possibility of anodization [702]. It was obtained that (i) the corrosion behavior of Mg alloy makes significant, characteristic changes due to anodization and (ii) impedance spectra show a regular evolution with exposure time revealing the development of corrosion damage. Zhang et al. [703] investigated the evolution of morphology, structure and composition of anodic film on Mg alloy

AZ91D with anodizing time. It was reported that (i) the development of anodic film on the Mg alloy was similar to that on high-purity Mg except that, attributed to alloying effect, hunch-like resultants replaced volcano-like ones to become predominant initial products at transitional stage of anodization, (ii) the main elements in anodizing products were Mg, O, Al and Si, indicating that both alloy substrate and electrolyte solution were involved in anodization and (iii) anodic film developed early was mainly comprised of periclase MgO and forsterite Mg_2SiO_4; however, amorphous compounds became dominant with treatment time increasing. Chelliah et al. [704] studied the electrochemical impedance and biocorrosion characteristics of AZ91 Mg alloy in Ringer's solution. As-cast AZ91 Mg-alloy was subjected to T4 heat treatment in a way to homogenize its microstructure by dissolving most of the β-$Mg_{17}Al_{12}$ phase at the vicinity of grain boundaries. It was mentioned that (i) EIS spectra showed that both microstructures exhibit similar dynamic response as a function of the immersion time; however, the value of impedance and maximum phase angle are about 50% higher in as-cast AZ91 Mg-alloy as compared to that of homogenized AZ91 Mg alloy, (ii) weight loss measurement indicated that corrosion resistance of as-cast AZ91 was significantly better than that of homogenized AZ91 and (iii) microstructural and XRD analysis revealed that as-cast AZ91 contains a passive film of $MgCO_3$ and $CaCO_3$ precipitates with near spherical morphologies, whereas homogenized AZ91 comprised mainly unstable $Mg(OH)_2$ film featured by irregular plate-like morphologies. Barbosa et al. [705] treated AZ91 in NaOH solution to form anodic oxide film and reported that (i) the anodic film consists of an inner barrier layer and an outer porous layer, (ii) the thin barrier layer is hydrated or contains $Mg(OH)_2$ and the porous layer was identified as crystalline MgO (periclase) and contains tunnels formed by breakdown/repair events, which involve plasma-electrolytic reactions and (iii) applied current density, potential limit, electrolyte concentration and alloy phase were identified as parameters which have an influence on density and diameter of the tunnels. Corrosion and passivation behavior of AZ91D was investigated in aqueous sodium borate solutions (pH 9.2) [706]. It was mentioned that (i) increasing borate concentration (0.01–0.10 M) or temperature up to 25 °C leads to increase the corrosion rate of the alloy; however, at temperatures higher than 25 °C borate anions have stronger propensity to passivate the alloy, thereby decreases its corrosion rate, (ii) for a fixed borate concentration increasing Cl^- addition is correlated with a more negative corrosion potential and a higher corrosion rate, as well as increase the vulnerability of the anodic passive film for breakdown and (iii) the influence of oxidizing potentials over the range – 1.5 V to 2.75 V (SCE: saturated calomel electrode) on the performance of the alloy in the most aggressive borate solution (0.10 M) reveals that higher potentials, induces better passivation due to formation of a rather thick and more protective n-type semiconducting film.

Tekin et al. [707] prepared ceramic-like oxide coatings on RE element containing Elektron21 (E21) and WE43 Mg alloys using plasma electrolytic oxidation (PEO) process. It was found that electrochemical corrosion test in 3.5% NaCl solution results showed that the corrosion rates of PEO-coated substrates greatly decreased when compared to that of bare Mg alloys; however, bare RE-containing alloys showed increased corrosion resistance compared to bare AZ31B alloy. Li et al. [708] investigated the microstructures and discharge products of Mg–6%Al–3%Zn and Mg–6%Al–3%Zn–0.5%In alloys. It was obtained that (i) Indium addition into Mg promotes Mg dissolution through synergistic effects, which involve increasing the second-phase amount, generating less-protective products, promoting products self-peeling, and dissolution–reprecipitation of indium and (ii) the homogenized Mg-Al-Zn-In alloy performs desirable corrosion resistance and discharge capability and thus is a promising candidate for applications as anode materials.

Badawy et al. [709] studied the electrochemical behavior of Mg, Mg–Al–Zn and Mg-Al-Zn-Mn alloys in aqueous acidic, neutral and basic solutions. It was found that (i) the rate of corrosion in acidic solution is relatively high compared to that in neutral or basic solutions, (ii) the presence of Al, Zn and Mn as alloying elements decreases the rate of corrosion of the alloy, (iii) the activation energy of the corrosion process occurring at the surface of Mg or Mg alloys in aqueous solutions is less than 40 kJ/mol and (iv) the impedance data were fitted to equivalent circuit models that explain the different electrochemical processes occurring at the electrode/electrolyte interface. The effects of sulfate ion concentration, temperature and medium pH on the corrosion of Mg-Al-Zn-Mn alloy in 30% aqueous ethylene glycol solution were investigated [710]. It was reported that (i) the nature of the polarization curves remain the same at higher concentration of sulfate ion, which indicates the insignificant role of sulfate ion on the mechanism of corrosion; however, the polarization curves shifted to higher current density region with the increase in the concentration of the sulfate ion, indicating an increase in the corrosion rate with the increase in the concentration of sulfate ion (see Figure 14.20 (a)), (ii) the polarization curves shifted to the higher current density region with the rise in temperature (Figure 14.20 (b)) and (iii) the polarization curves shift to the higher current density region with decreasing the medium pH from alkaline to acidic condition.

14.4.5.4 Mg–Zn

Abulsain et al. [711] conducted anodization on metastable, solid-solution Mg–0.8 at% Cu and Mg–1.4 at% Zn alloys up to 250 V at 10 mA/cm^2 in an alkaline phosphate electrolyte at 20 °C and studied the enriching of alloying elements beneath the anodic films. It was found that (i) Rutherford backscattering spectroscopy revealed enrichments to about 4.1×10^{15} Cu atoms cm^{-2} and 5.2×10^{15} Zn atoms/cm^2, which correlate with the higher standard Gibbs free energies per equivalent for formation of copper and zinc oxides relative to that for formation of MgO, (ii) the anodic films, composed mainly of magnesium hydroxide, contained copper and zinc species throughout their thicknesses; the Cu:Mg and Zn:Mg atomic ratios were about 18%

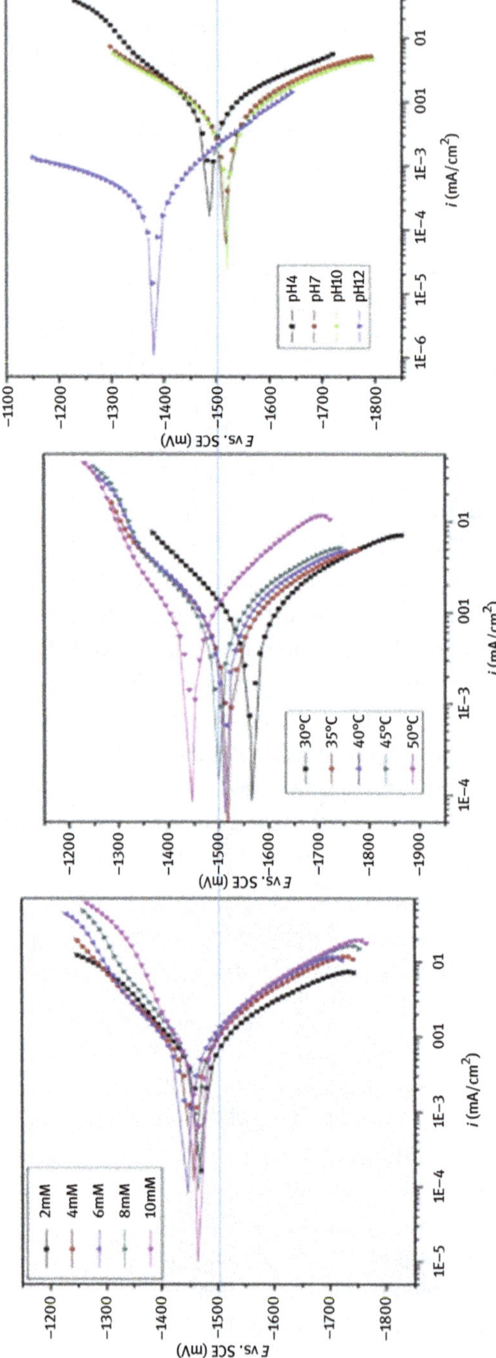

Figure 14.20: Polarization curves for the corrosion of Mg-Al-Zn-Mn alloy [710]. (a) Different concentrations of sulfate ions at 50 °C, (b) different temperatures and (c) different pH at 30 °C.

and 25% of those of the alloys, respectively, (iii) phosphorus species were present in most of the film regions, with a P:Mg atomic ratio of about 0.16 and (iv) Mg ions in the film account for about 30% of the charge passed during anodizing. Wang et al. [712] prepared dicalcium phosphate dihydrate (DCPD) and polycaprolactone (PCL) on a Mg–Zn alloy substrate to obtain a composite coating. It was reported that (i) the corrosion potential of the DCPD–PCL-coated alloy increased by 0.14 V compared to that of the DCPD-coated alloy, (ii) the corrosion current was about one third of the DCPD-coated alloy, (iii) the real impedance component of the DCPD–PCL-coated alloy was approximately 4 times as large as that of the DCPD-coated one, (iv) the immersion test implied that the integrity of the DCPD–PCL composite coating kept better in the SBF after 260 h immersion than the DCPD coating, (v) the less released hydrogen indicated that the degradation rate was reduced compared to the DCPD-coated alloy and (vi) the degradation rate rapidly increased after 150 h for the DCPD-coated alloy while 225 h for the DCPD–PCL-coated case which meant the composite coating could retard the corrosion for a longer time; all indicating that the composite coating can protect the Mg alloy more efficiently. Lamesh et al. [713] evaluated the corrosion behavior of commercially pure magnesium (CP-Mg) and ZM21 Mg alloy immersed in Ringer's solution for 92 h. It was reported that (i) the formation of a compact layer of well-developed rod-like aragonitic $CaCO_3$ crystals was observed and its subsequent thickening with increase in immersion time offers a higher corrosion protective ability for ZM21 Mg alloy was found and (ii) the formation of a mud-crack pattern and a large number of clusters of needle-like crystals offers a relatively lower corrosion resistance for CP-Mg, suggesting that ZM21 Mg alloy is a promising candidate material for the development of degradable implants.

Yamasali et al. [714] prepared corrosion-resistant nanocrystalline Mg-0.75Zn-2Y-0.5Al multiphase and Mg-0.75Zn-2*x*Y-*x*Al (at%) alloys by consolidation of rapidly solidified ribbons. It was mentioned that (i) rapid solidification brings about the grain refinement and an increase in the solid solubility of Zn, Y and Al into the magnesium matrix, enhancing microstructural and electrochemical homogeneity, which in turn enhanced corrosion resistance and (ii) the addition of Al to Mg can modify the structure and chemical composition of surface films and improves the resistance to local breakdown of the films. Ren et al. [715] investigated microstructure and biocorrosion behavior of as-cast Mg-2Zn-0.5Ca-Y series alloys for biomedical application, tested in Hank's solution and NaCl solution (3.5 wt%). It was reported that (i) the morphologies of the Mg-2Zn-0.5Ca-Y alloys indicate that the corrosion is not uniform and a lot of cracks are formed on the surface of the corrosion layer after immersion tests, (ii) the corrosion resistance of as-cast Mg-2Zn-0.5Ca-Y series alloys increases owing to the addition of the RE element Y and that of Mg-2Zn-0.5Ca-1.0Y alloy is the best, (iii) the potentiodynamic polarization curves obtained in the tests in Hank's solution and NaCl solution show current plateaus which are due to the presence of a protective corrosion product film and (iv) the EIS curves of the alloys in the test solutions have only one capacitive loop, indicating that the appearance of a capacitive loop at high frequency is caused by the stable double-layer capacitance and the capacitive loop at low frequency is attributed to diffusion control at film-free areas. Cai et al. [716] studied the microstructure evolution and corrosion behavior in SBF of Mg-2Zn-0.6Zr-*x*Nd alloys ($x = 0$, 0.2, 0.6 and 1 wt%). It was mentioned that (i) the MgZn phase in Mg–2Zn–0.6Zr alloy changed to $Mg_{60}Zn_{32}Nd_8$ (T_2) and $Mg_{35}Zn_{40}Nd_{25}$ (T_3) phases after adding 0.2–1 wt% Nd, (ii) T_2 and T_3 phases with a relative Volta potential of about −400 mV acted as microanodes, so that they were corroded preferentially during the corrosion process and (iii) because of the appropriate amount of anodic T phases and their discontinuous distribution, the alloy with 0.2 wt% Nd addition showed a uniform surface corrosion characteristic and exhibit the best corrosion resistance.

14.4.5.5 Mg–Li

There are various studies on electrochemical corrosion behaviors of Mg–Li-based alloys. Zhang et al. [717] studied the corrosion characteristic of a Mg–Li alloy with RE in alkaline NaCl solution and mentioned that (i) Cl^- concentration and pH value affected the corrosion of Mg–Li alloy, and in high Cl^- concentration was the major factor, (ii) corrosion of the alloy was slighter in the stronger alkaline solution, because corrosion current reduced, corrosion potential turned to positive direction and the capacitive loops enlarged and (iii) with increased Cl^- concentration, corrosion current increased and capacitive loops got smaller; indicating that corrosion of the alloy was more serious with the increase in Cl^- concentration. The electrochemical formation of Mg–Li alloys was examined in a molten LiCl–KCl (58–42 mol%) eutectic melt at 450 °C [718]. It was shown that (i) the cyclic voltammogram for a Mo electrode showed that the electroreduction of Li^+ proceeds in a single step and the deposition potential of Li metal was −2.40 V (vs. Ag/AgCl), (ii) for Mg electrode, the electroreduction of Li^+ takes place at less cathodic potential than that at the Mo electrode which was caused by the formation of Mg–Li alloys and (iii) phase of the deposited Mg–Li alloys could be controlled by the electrolysis potential; indicating that α-Mg and β-Li phases were obtained at −2.35 and −2.55 V, respectively. Lv et al. [719] studied the electrochemical performances of Mg, Mg-Li-Al-Ce and Mg-Li-Al-Ce-Y as the anode of Mg–hydrogen peroxide semifuel cells. It was mentioned that (i) Mg-Li-Al-Ce and Mg-Li-Al-Ce-Y electrodes are less corrosion resistant than that of Mg electrode in 0.7 mol/L NaCl solution and the corrosion current density decreases with the following order: Mg < Mg-Li-Al-Ce-Y < Mg-Li-Al-Ce, (ii) the Mg-Li-Ce-Y anode is more active than Mg-Li-Al-Ce and Mg and (iii) the Mg–hydrogen peroxide semifuel cell with Mg-Li-Al-Ce-Y anode shows better performance than that with Mg-Li-Al-Ce and Mg. Jiang et al. [720] prepared Mg–14Li–1Al (LA141), LA141–0.3Y, LA141–0.3Sr and LA141–0.3Y–0.3Sr alloys were prepared and studied their electrochemical behavior in 0.7 mol/L NaCl solutions. The effects of gallium oxide as an electrolyte additive on the potentiostatic discharge performances of these magnesium alloys were also studied. It was reported that (i) the discharge activities and utilization efficiencies of these alloys increase in the order: LA141 < LA141–0.3Sr < LA141–0.3Y < LA141–0.3Y–0.3Sr, both in the absence and the presence of Ga_2O_3, (ii) the addition of Ga_2O_3 into NaCl electrolyte solution improves the discharging current of the alloys by more than 4% and enhanced the utilization efficiencies of the alloys by more than 13%, (iii) EIS measurements show that the polarization resistances of the alloys decrease in the following order: LA141 > LA141–0.3Sr > LA141–0.3Y > LA141–0.3Y–0.3Sr and (iv) in the respect of improving the electrochemical performance Y is more obvious than Sr and it is the most significant when Y and Sr are alloyed in magnesium at the same time. Based on these findings, it was concluded that LA141–0.3Y–0.3Sr exhibits the best performance in terms of activity and utilization efficiency and the least dense oxide products on alloy surface. Chen et al. [721] studied electrochemical codeposition of Mg–Li–Yb alloys in LiCl–KCl–KF–$MgCl_2$–Yb_2O_3 melts on molybdenum. The factors of the current efficiency were investigated. It was reported that (i) electrolysis temperature had great influence on current efficiency; the highest current efficiency was obtained when electrolysis temperature was about 660 °C; (ii) the content of Li in Mg–Li–Yb alloys increased with the high current densities; (iii) the optimal electrolytic temperature and cathodic current density were around 660 °C and 9.3 A/cm^2, respectively; (iv) the intermetallic of Mg–Yb was mainly distributed in the grain boundary of the alloys, presented as reticulated structures, and refined the grains; and (v) Li and Y contents in Mg–Li–Yb alloys could be controlled by changing the concentration of $MgCl_2$ and Yb_2O_3 and the electrolysis conditions.

A Mg-10.02Li-3.86Zn-2.54Al-1.76Cu alloy was prepared and its corrosion-resistant coating was obtained in 25 g/L $K_2Cr_2O_7$ + 25 g/L H_2SO_4 solution was performed by galvanic anodizing method [722] and reported that the coating thickness increases with pH value decrease and operating temperature increase, while its corro sion resistance decreases; indicating that coatings obtained at RT with pH 4.5 and/ or pH 5.5 possess better corrosion resistance. Lv et al. [723] investigated the electro chemical oxidation behaviors of Mg-8Li-3Al-0.5Zn and Mg-8Li-3Al-1.0Zn electrodes in 0.7 mol/L NaCl solution. It was reported that (i) the Mg-8Li-3Al-0.5Zn electrode has higher discharge activity and less corrosion resistance than that of Mg-8Li-3Al-1.0Zn electrode in 0.7 mol/L NaCl solution, (ii) the Mg–H_2O_2 semifuel cell with Mg 8Li-3Al-0.5Zn anode presents a maximum power density of 100 mW/cm^2 at RT, which is higher than that of Mg-8Li-3Al-1.0Zn anode (80 mW/cm^2) and the performance of semi fuel cell with the Mg-8Li-3Al-0.5Zn electrode is better than that with Mg-8Li-3Al-1.0Zn electrode, especially at higher current density (>30 mA/cm^2). Similarly, Lv et al. [724] investigated the electrochemical performances of Mg–8Li–0.5Y and Mg–8Li–1Y electrodes in 0.7 mol/L NaCl solution. It was mentioned that (i) the Mg–8Li–1Y electrode has higher corrosion-resistant ability and electrooxida tion activity than that of Mg–8Li–0.5Y electrode; (ii) the corrosion potential of Mg–8Li–1Y electrode is 60 mV more positive than that of Mg–8Li–0.5Y electrode; (iii) the current density of Mg–8Li–1Y electrode is around 2 mA/cm^2 higher than that of Mg–8Li–0.5Y electrode at the discharge potentials of −0.8, −1.0 and −1.2 V, and it is similar to that of Mg–8Li–0.5Y electrode at –1.4 V; (iv) the Mg–H_2O_2 semifuel cell with Mg–8Li–1Y anode presents a maximum power density of 59 mW/cm^2 at RT, which is higher than that of Mg–8Li–0.5Y anode (53 mW/cm^2); and (v) the Y content obviously affects the performance of the alloys and the Y content of 1 wt% is better than 0.5 wt%. Cao et al. [725] prepared Mg–Li, Mg–Li–Al and Mg–Li–Al–Ce alloys and studied their electrochemical behavior in 0.7 M NaCl solutions. It was reported that (i) the discharge activities and utilization efficiencies of these alloys increase in the order: Mg–Li < Mg–Li–Al < Mg-Li-Al-Ce, both in the absence and presence of Ga_2O_3; (ii) these alloys are more active than commercial magnesium alloy AZ31; (iii) the addition of Ga_2O_3 into NaCl electrolyte solution improved the discharging currents of the alloys by more than 4%, and enhanced the utilization efficiencies of the alloys by more than 6%; (iv) EIS measurements showed that the polarization resis tance of the alloys decreases in the following order: Mg–Li > Mg–Li–Al > Mg-Li-Al-Ce; and (v) Mg-Li-Al-Ce exhibited the best performance in terms of activity, utilization efficiency and activation time.

14.4.5.6 Mg–Y

The effect of solid-solution treatment on corrosion and electrochemical mechanisms of Mg–15Y alloy in 3.5 wt% NaCl solution was investigated [670]. It was reported that (i) the corrosion resistance of Mg–15Y sample gradually deteriorated with immersion time increasing, which was consistent with the observation of corrosion morphologies, (ii) the solid-solution treatment decreased the amounts of second phase $Mg_{24}Y_5$ (which confirmed the result reported by Sudholz et al. [726]) and (iii) the corrosion potential and corrosion rate of as-cast samples were both lower than those of solid ST samples, and both increased with increment of solid ST time. The corrosion mechanism of Mg–Y alloys in 3.5% NaCl solution was also investigated [727] with findings (i) the corrosion potential of Mg–Y alloys in 3.5% NaCl solution increased with the increase of Y addition, (ii) the corrosion rate increased with the increase of Y addition because of the increase of $Mg_{24}Y_5$ intermetallic amounts, (iii) the corrosion gradually deteriorated with the increase of immersion time and the main solid corrosion products were $Mg(OH)_2$ and $Mg_2(OH)_3C1 \cdot 4H_2O$.

Mg–Y–RE alloy is potentially useful in biodegradable implants but the fast degradation rate in the physiological environment restrains actual applications, so that Zhao et al. [728] enhanced the corrosion resistance by aluminum and oxygen ion implantation to modify the surface of the Mg-Y–RE alloy. It was mentioned that (i) Al and O ion implantation produces an Al_2O_3-containing protection layer which improves the corrosion resistance of Mg–Y–RE alloy and (ii) after the surface treatment, localized corrosion becomes the dominant corrosion mechanism instead of general corrosion. Jamesh et al. [729] investigated the corrosion behavior of WE43 and ZK60 Mg alloys in Ringer's solution and SBF. It was reported that (i) the major protective corrosion-products formed on both Mg alloys are crystalline aragonite form of $CaCO_3$

and $Mg(OH)_2$ in Ringer's solution, whereas $Ca_{10}(PO_4)_6(OH)_2$, $Ca_3(PO_4)_2 \cdot 3H_2O$ and Mg $(OH)_2$ in SBF and (ii) EIS reveals that in the initial stage, the increase in the corrosion resistance on both Mg alloys in Ringer's solution is more than 6 times than in SBF.

Zhang et al. [730] studied the corrosion mechanism of the as-cast Mg-5Y-7Gd-1Nd-0.5Zr alloy immersed in 5% NaCl aqueous solution. It was found that (i) the corrosion resistance of Mg–5Y-7Gd-1Nd-0.5Zr alloy in 5% NaCl aqueous solution gradually deteriorates with immersion time increasing from 2, 24, 60 h to 108 h, (ii) the Cl^- anion leads to the initiation and development of the corrosion pits, and Mg-5Y-7Gd-1Nd-0.5Zr alloy exhibits filiform type of attack under significant anodic control of magnesium solution reaction and (iii) the corrosion potential becomes noble with increasing immersion time. Ninlachert et al. [731] studied electrochemical passivation of Mg–Y–Nd alloy (WE43C or Elektron 43) in 0.1 M NaOH solution with the addition of chloride from 0 to 1,000 ppm. It was reported that (i) the passive potential range typically extended to more than 1.5 V [against Ag/AgCl electrode], (ii) the transpassive potential was not dependent on the heat treatment condition of the alloy when the chloride concentration increased up to 500 ppm; however, pitting protection potential varied with the heat treatment condition when the chloride addition was 500 ppm or more and (iii) the passivated surface of the WE43C specimens indicated that the surface layer consisted of MgO, $Mg(OH)_2$, and RE oxide phases, and the heat treatment conditions did not significantly affect the composition of the surface film. Similar study on passivation kinetics of two Mg–RE alloys (Mg-Nd-Gd-Zn-Zr (EV31A) and Mg-Y-Nd-Gd-Zr (WE43C)) were conducted in two different heat-treated conditions (ST and OA) in 0.01–1.0 M NaOH solutions [732]. It was mentioned that (i) the negative reaction order was observed in dilute NaOH which transitioned to positive values as the passivation time increased and in the 1 M NaOH as well, (ii) the electrochemical impedance increased with increase in the NaOH concentration in the ST condition of both Mg–RE alloys, whereas the OA EV31A alloy showed a reverse trend, (iii) the passive layer of EV31A showed almost 100% higher charge carrier density than the film formed on the WE43C in the OA condition, (iv) a better passivation behavior was observed in the ST condition than that in the OA condition which could be attributed to the uniform distribution of the RE elements in the ST specimens and (v) the WE43C alloy revealed better corrosion resistance in the alkaline solution than the EV31A alloy.

14.4.5.7 Mg–Ca

The electrochemical behaviors and discharge performance of an AR Mg–1.5 wt%Ca alloy anode were investigated [733]. It was reported that (i) the as-extruded Mg–1.5 wt %Ca anode exhibits a superior discharge performance than the as-extruded CP-Mg anode, (ii) the fine dynamic recrystallized grains (15 ± 2 μm) and the active Mg2Ca particles around grain boundaries are responsible for the promoted discharge performance, (iii) the fine and dispersive Mg2Ca particles are favor of the uniform consumption of Mg anode during discharge and (iv) the detachment of discharge products of Mg–1.5 wt%Ca anode is more difficult than that of pure Mg, resulting an early failure of discharge at 80 mA/cm^2. Pan et al. [734] coated calcium phosphate (CaP) ce ramicon pure Mg and Mg–0.6Ca, Mg–0.55Ca–1.74Zn alloys by MAO and mentioned that (i) Mg–0.55Ca–1.74Zn alloy exhibits the highest mechanical strength and electrochemical corrosion resistance in SBF among the three alloys and (ii) the MAO-coated Mg–0.55Ca–1.74Zn alloy has the potential to be served as a biodegradable implant.

14.4.5.8 Mg–Sn

Anodic oxidation behavior of Mg–Sn alloys was studied to elucidate the effect of Sn content in Mg alloy on the formation of anodic films in alkaline solutions [735]. It was reported that (i) the anodic films become less resistive by the presence of Sn in Mg in 0.1 M NaOH, while the anodic films formed in 0.1 M NaOH + 0.1 M KF becomes more resistive with increasing Sn content in Mg, (ii) generation of microarcs during the anodizing was observed only in a fluoride-containing solution for Mg–6Sn and Mg–8Sn and (iii) corrosion resistance of the anodized Mg–Sn alloys in the fluoride-containing solution increased with increasing Sn content in Mg. Ha et al. [736] investigated corrosion behavior of extruded Mg and Mg–5Sn (in wt%) alloy in a 0.6 M NaCl solution. It was mentioned that (i) corrosion of the Mg was significantly faster than the Mg–5Sn alloy, and vigorous H_2 evolution was accompanied with the severe corrosion of Mg and (ii) polarization tests confirmed that cathodic reaction was inhibited in the Mg–5Sn alloy.

14.4.6 Corrosion protection

Main corrosion product formed on Mg materials during (electro)chemical corrosion process is $Mg(OH)_2$ and the formed hydroxide is not dense enough to protect the substrate from further corrosion. In addition, if the corrosive environment contains chlorine ion, $MgCl_2$ will be formed through the $Mg(OH)_2 + 2Cl^- \rightarrow MgCl_2 + 2OH^-$. To protect Mg materials from undesired corrosion reaction, there are various ways proposed and practiced [737–740]. Before going this topic in details, it should be noted two important issues associated with Mg. Mg is well-known metal serving as a sacrificial anode to protect structures made of other metals. Mg is also employed in particular area of medicine (e.g., scaffold structure in tissue engineering) because Mg is prone to exhibit biodegradation if its degradation rate is well-controlled. These two phenomena are typical examples in which Mg are utilized positively through corrosion behavior.

Corrosion behavior of Mg materials can be improved through (i) alloying effect with more noble element(s), (ii) heat treatment for altering microstructures, (iii) thermal or mechanical surface modification through SPD, (iv) physiochemical surface manipulation to alter surface energy and (v) coating technique with various oxides, composites, polymeric materials or hybrids.

14.4.6.1 Alloying effect

As pointed out [741–743], appropriate selection of alloying effect should improve corrosion behavior of Mg materials. For details, Table 14.8 suggests possible combination for alloying elements to various Mg-based alloys.

14.4.6.2 Heat treatment

As pointed out [679, 735–749], heat treatment and its resultant alteration of microstructures as well as secondary phase evolution assist to improve corrosion behavior of Mg-based alloys and also we have discussed in both Sections 14.4.4.3 and 14.4.4.4 previously. Differing from as-cast and solid-solution alloys with coarse eutectic phases ($Mg_{17}Al_{12}$), Feng et al. [750] employed ultra-high-pressure solid-solution treatment (at 800 °C and under 4 GPa) to Mg–25Al (wt%) to produce the nanoscaled $Mg_{17}Al_{12}$ particles. It was reported that, due to the formation of Al-rich oxide layer, wherein residual stress and pitting corrosion are eliminated, such treated Mg–Al exhibited good corrosion resistance, which overwhelms the majority of Mg-based alloys reported so far, near to high-purity Mg. Zhang et al. [751] prepared ZM61 (Mg–Zn–Mn) alloy by conventional casting and rapidly solidification and studied the corrosion resistance in 3.5% NaCl solution. It was reported that the rapidly solidified ZM61 alloy performs better in corrosion resistance than the extruded ZK60 and pure Mg alloys, suggesting that the rapid solidification technique is a promising way to improve the strength and corrosion resistance of magnesium alloy for the structural and corrosive media utilization.

14.4.6.3 Surface modification

Microstructural modification is not necessary conducted on entire body of materials when the corrosion resistance improvement is considered since corrosion phenomenon is limited to the surface reaction. Heat treatment is not exceptions for this category. Ma et al. [752] laser-modified Mg–Gd–Ca alloy which was subjected to immersion corrosion test. It was mentioned that (i) the enhanced corrosion resistance was found to be caused by the combined effect of the dissolution of secondary phase and the decrease of galvanic corrosion in the laser-modified zone and (ii) results of direct cell culturing suggested that the laser-modified surface exhibited good cell adhesion property, spreading performance and proliferation capacity. Liu et al. [747] investigated the microstructure modifications and corrosion behaviors of a Mg–4Sm alloy treated by high current pulsed electron beam with different number of pulses. It was reported that (i) the dissolution of large $Mg_{41}Sm_5$ segregates, the formation of $Mg_{41}Sm_5$ nanoprecipitates and twins in the surface layers after treatments, (ii) EIS and polarization tests in the 3.5 wt% NaCl solution showed that the 15 pulses treated Mg–4Sm alloy sample exhibited the lowest corrosion current density, highest corrosion po tential; due to the homogeneous microstructure and composition with fewer defects in the surface layer after sufficient number of high current pulsed electron beam pulses.

Yin et al. [753] studied the effects of the second phases on corrosion resistance of AZ91–*x*Gd alloys treated with ultrasonic vibration. It was found that (i) the addition of Gd led to the formation of many fine Al_2Gd/Al–Mn–Gd particles that consumed Al and reduced the volume fraction of β-$Mg_{17}Al_{12}$ phase; meanwhile, the β-$Mg_{17}Al_{12}$ phase morphology in ultrasound-treated AZ91–Gd alloys changed from semicontinuous reticular structure to rod-shaped and granular structure, (ii) the ultrasound-treated AZ91–1.0 wt% Gd alloy with fine granular β-$Mg_{17}Al_{12}$ phase and Al_2Gd/Al–Mn–Gd particles showed better corrosion resistance than other ultrasound-treated alloys, (iii) microgalvanic corrosion was formed and rapidly extended to the matrix alloy interior along local coarser reticular β-$Mg_{17}Al_{12}$ phase, then causing localized serious corrosion and (iv) the finer and dispersed rod-shaped β-$Mg_{17}Al_{12}$ phase and Al_2Gd/Al–Mn–Gd particles led to microgalvanic corrosion uniformly distribute on the surface of alloys, and formed a uniform corrosion layer with 18 μm thickness.

There are several studies on effects of SPD on corrosion behaviors of Mg-based alloys. Mineta et al. [754] studied corrosion resistance of Mg–Li–Al (LA143) alloy, which was subjected to SPD and found that SPD was an effective way to simultaneously improve the hardness and corrosion resistance of LA143 alloy specimens in 3.5 mass% NaCl aqueous solution. Huo et al. [755] applied the sliding friction treatment (SFT) to Mg–3Al–1Zn (AZ31) and studied corrosion resistance of 3.5% NaCl. It was mentioned that (i) the hydrogen evolution rate during 80 h immersion in 3.5% NaCl is reduced from 0.44 to 0.17 mL/cm^2/h after SFT treatment and (ii) the improvement in corrosion resistance might be correlated with SFT-induced grain refinement, good surface quality, second-phase particles fragmentation and strong basal texture. Zhang et al. [756] processed Mg-Gd-Nd-Zn-Zr alloy ECAP at 375 °C to obtain the grain size of ~2.5 μm with the spherical precipitates (β_1-phase) distributing in the matrix. It was mentioned that the corrosion rate of the ECAPed magne sium alloy in SBF dramatically decreased from 0.236 to 0.126 mm/a due to the strong basal texture and refined microstructure, indicating that this wrought magnesium alloy shows potentials in biomedical application. The double extrusion process was adopted to refine microstructure and improve mechanical properties of Mg-2.25Nd-0.11Zn-0.43Zr (alloy 1) and Mg-2.70Nd-0.20Zn-0.41Zr (alloy 2) alloys to test the corrosion resistance [674]. It was mentioned that the results of immersion experiment and electrochemical measurements in SBF show that the corrosion resistance of alloy 1 and alloy 2 under double extrusion was increased by 7% and 8%, respectively, compared with those under just once extrusion.

14.4.6.4 Physicochemical surface manipulation

Recently, nanocomposite coatings, hydrophobic coatings and organic–inorganic hybrids have been shown to increase the life of materials prone to oxidation/corrosion; potentially possessing a wide range of applications such as marine, pipeline, aerospace, automobiles and construction industries [757]. Li et al. [758] fabricated a hydrotalcite/hydromagnesite conversion coating with hierarchical structure on a Mg alloy substrate by in situ hydrothermal crystallization method. It was mentioned that (i) polarization measurements have shown that the hydrophobic conversion coating exhibited a low corrosion current density value of 0.432 $\mu A/cm^2$, which means that the hydrophobic conversion coating can effectively protect Mg alloy from corrosion and (ii) EIS showed that the impedance of the hydrophobic conversion coating was 9 kΩ, indicating that the coating served as a passive layer with high charge transfer resistance. Cui et al. [759] fabricated a hydrophobic surface through the MAO and subsequent stearic acid surface modification of AZ31 Mg alloy, achieving a maximum water contact angle of 151.5° after 10 h of modification. It was reported that (i) the obtained hydrophobicity is ascribed to a combination of the MAO coating's rough micropore structure and the formation of a stearic acid monolayer through bidentate bonding, (ii) the hydrophobic MAO coating effectively inhibits corrosion of the Mg alloy, especially pitting corrosion. A superhydrophobic coating film of Mg–Mn LDHs (layered double hydrox ides) was fabricated on pure Mg by an in situ growth method and chemical modification by adsorption of myristic acid (MA, $CH_3(CH_2)_{12}COOH$) [760]. It was reported that (i) the static contact angle of the superhydrophobic surface was about 152.2°, (ii) the impedance of the superhydrophobic coating sample at low frequency is approximately $20{,}000\ \Omega \cdot cm^2$ which is more than twice of that of the LDHs film and 10 times of that of pure Mg substrate and (iii) the superhydrophobic coating can effectively protect the Mg from corrosion in SBF for a long time. Qian et al. [761] prepared silica-based superhydrophobic coatings on AZ31B Mg alloy surfaces by a spraying method. It was reported that in contrast with the bare magnesium alloy AZ31B, after coating, the corrosion current density shows more than three orders of magnitude smaller value, and the water contact angle increases from ~32° to over 155°. Solution pH and coexisted NaCl, $MgCl_2$, NaI and CH_3COONa salts have little effect on the wetting properties of the prepared superhydrophobic surfaces. On the contrary, coexisted C_2H_5OH, $C_{17}H_{33}COONa$ or sodium dodecylbenzene sulfonate have an obvious effect on the wetting properties, and the differences in the wetting properties were explained by considering the interactions between the superhydrophobic surfaces and the surfaces of the solution droplets.

14.4.6.5 Coating

Various types of materials (such as oxides, hydroxides, nitrides, carbide, fluoride, phosphates, ceramics, polymers, composites or hybrids) are coated on Mg substrates for improving corrosion resistance. Table 14.10 lists coating materials of oxides and others.

Table 14.10: Coating of oxides, hydroxides, nitrides, phosphates on Mg substrates.

	ZnO composites	Ti-O or TiO_2	V_2O_5 of vanadate	$Mg(OH)_2$	LDHs	Hydroxyapatite	Phosphates with Ca and P	$Pr(NO_3)_3$	Fluoride	NbN	TaN	SIN	Mg–Al intermetallics	Glass-ceramic	SIC
AZ31	[762]	[763]			[764]	[765]						[766]	[767]	[768]	
AZ91				[769]	[770]								[771]		
Mg–Al–Ca–Mn							[772]								
Mg–Al–Zn–Nd								[773]							
Mg–Ca	[774]					[775, 776]									
Mg–Zn						[777]									
Mg–Zn–Ca														[778]	
Mg–Zn–Y–Nd		[779, 780]													
Mg–Zn–Er									[781]						
Mg–Zn–Zr									[782]						

ZE41	[624]												
ZEK100				[783]									
Mg–Li–Al–Ce	[784]												
Mg–Li–Ca					[785, 786]								
Mg–Sn													[787]
Mg–Sr					[788]								
Mg–Y–RE								[789]	[790] ·				

Note: LDHs, layered double hydroxides.

Metallic elements are also coated to protect surfaces of Mg materials. Apart from the alloying effect of metallic elements, plating of metals on Mg surface possesses several technical problems, including (1) high susceptibility to the degradation reactions such as galvanic corrosioncorrosion, galvanic in the plating processes [791] and (2) adhesive strength (or coating strength) and (3) surface hydrophobicity. Table 14.11 lists a combination of coating metals and Mg-based alloy substrate.

Table 14.11: Metallic element coating on Mg alloys.

	Cu	Ni	Ni/Cu/Ni	Al	Ti	Zr	Hf	Ta	Mg	Zn	Ag	Se
Mg										[792]		
Mg-Nd-Zn-Zr	[793]											
AZ31		[794]							[795]		[796]	[797]
AZ91		[798]		[799]	[800]	[800]	[800]					
Mg–Li			[801]									
ZK60								[802]				

There are a variety of studies conducted and reported on coating with polymers, composites and hybrids on Mg substrates.

For AZ31 (Mg–3Al–1Zn) alloy, coating materials include superhydrophobic PPS–PTFE/SiO_2 composite [803], hydroxyapatite (HA)-doped poly(lactic acid) porous film [804], metal-organic framework (bio-MOF-1) composite [805], composite of β-tricalcium phosphate and $Mg(OH)_2$ composite [806], silane/graphene oxide/silane composite [807], hybrid epoxy-silane coating [808] or polymeric coating obtained from a phytocompound [809].

For AZ91 (Mg–9Al–1Zn) alloy, there are Mg-rice epoxy resin [810], amino acids and montmorillonite NP composites [811], 8-hydroxyquinoline [812] or HA/Fe_3O_4/CS composite [813].

For Mg–Zn alloy systems, they include biodegradable polymer for Mg–6Zn–Ca [814], fluorine-doped HA–PCL duplex coating for Mg–2Zn–3Ce [815] or Si/HA nanocomposite for Mg–Zn–Mn–Ca alloy system [816].

For Mg–Ca alloy systems, coating materials are NiCrAlY/nano-YSZ duplex composite for Mg–1.2Ca–3Zn [817], octacalcium phosphate and HA as an underlayer and PCL as an overlayer for Mg–1.2Ca–2Zn [818], hybrid silicon biopolymer for Mg–1.2Ca–2Bi [819] or nano-AL/PCL composite for Mg–Ca–Bi alloy systems [820].

For Mg–Li alloy systems, coating materials include polyaniline/graphene for Mg-9Li-7Al-1Sn and Mg-9Li-5Al-3SN-1Zn alloys [821] and polyaniline containing epoxy resin for Mg–5Li [822].

14.4.6.6 MAO/ PEO

MAO or PEO is an electrochemical process of oxidation that is performed by creating microdischarges on the surface of components immersed in an electrolyte, hence, is a combined nature of a plasma chemical and electrochemical process. The process results in the formation of a physically protective oxide film on the metal surface to enhance mechanical, tribological, thermal, dielectric and corrosion properties. It is especially suitable for the surface oxidation and pigmentation of aluminum, titanium, niobium, zirconium, magnesium and their alloys. The treated components are used in buildings, mechanics, transportations, energy sectors and biological environments.

A variety of electrolyte has been employed for MAO or PEO coating process.

For AZ31 alloy, alkaline silicate electrolyte [823] or alkaline electrolyte containing ethylenediaminetetraacetic acid disodium (EDTA-2Na) [824] was utilized as effective electrolyte for MAO/PEO coating process.

For AZ91 alloy, the following electrolytes were used; silicate electrolyte [825], $Na_5P_3O_{10}$ and K_2ZrF_6 solution [826], silicate-containing alkaline electrolyte [663] or K_2ZrF_6-based electrolyte solution [827].

For Mg–Al–Mn alloy systems, phosphate-silicate mixture electrolyte was used for AMX 602 (Mg-Al-Mn-Ca) [828] and potassium fluoride (KF) solution [829] or alkaline electrolyte containing inert SiO_2 and La_2O_3 particles [830] was employed for AM50 alloy.

For Mg–Zn–Ca alloy system, phosphate-based electrolyte [831] or electrolyte containing 15 g/L $Na_3PO_4 \bullet 12H_2O$ and 10 g/L KF [832] was used.

For Mg–Li–Ca alloy, a stearic acid was used [833].

For Mg–Ca alloy, KF-silicate (Si coating), KF-phosphate (P coating) and KF-silicate phosphate (SiP coating) electrolytes were investigated for MAO coating [834].

For Mg–5SN–1ZN (TZ51) alloy, modified stearic acid was employed [835].

14.4.7 Sacrificial anode cathodic protection

Cathodic protection is the most important of all approaches to corrosion control. Be externally applied electric current, corrosion is reduced virtually to zero, and a metal surface can be maintained in a corrosive environment without deterioration for a prolong service time. Cathodic protection requires a source of direct current and an auxiliary electrode (anode having more less noble potential than that of metal-to-be-protected), as shown in Figure 14.21 [836]. The d-c source is connected with positive terminal to the auxiliary electrode (scrap iron or graphite) and negative terminal to the pipeline, so that current flows from electrode through the electrolyte to the pipeline structure. The externally impressed current is provided by the rectifier.

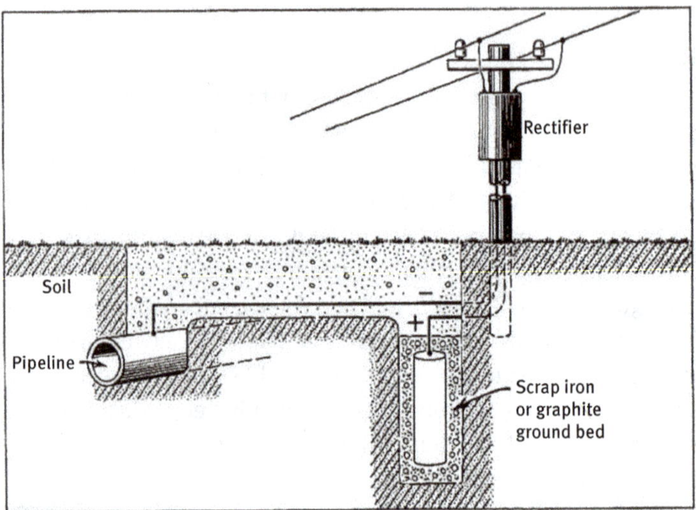

Figure 14.21: Sketch of cathodically protected underground pipeline [836].

If the impressed current flow using the rectifier is omitted and the electrode in this situation is called a sacrificial anode, as seen in Figure 14.22 [837].

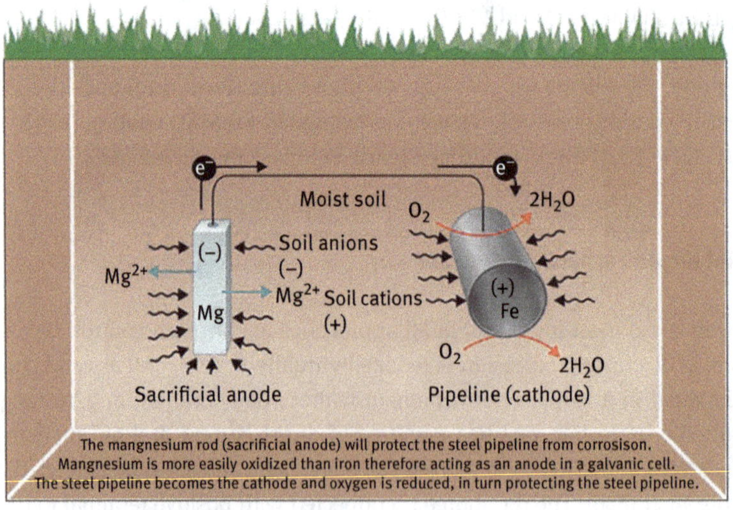

Figure 14.22: Illustration of protecting pipeline by sacrificial anode cathodic protection [837].

Magnesium is electrochemically the most active metal employed in common structural alloys of iron and aluminum. Mg is widely used as a sacrificial anode to provide cathodic protection of underground and undersea metallic structures, ships, submarines, bridges, decks, aircraft and ground transportation systems. Sacrificial anodes serve essentially as sources of portable electrical energy. Figure 14.23 shows how to install sacrificial Mg anode plates to protect screw propeller on ocean-going tankers and cruise ships [838, 839].

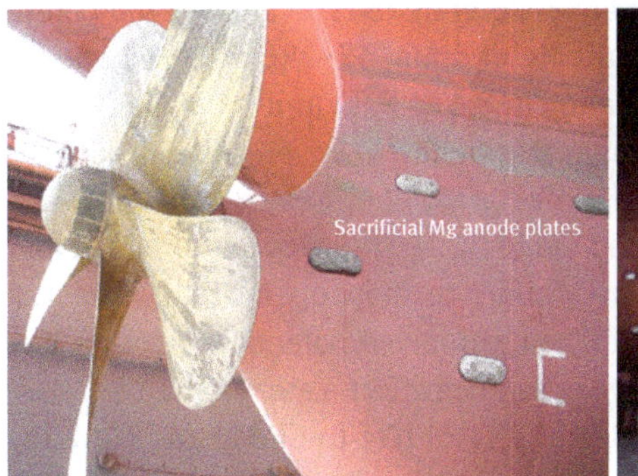

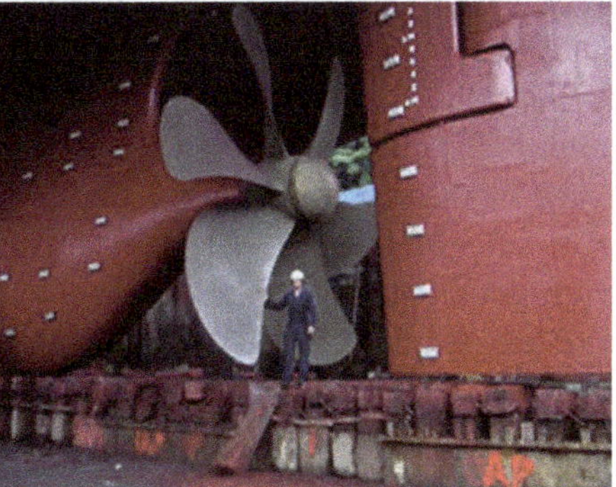

Figure 14.23: Typical examples of Mg sacrificial anodes installed on stern area to protect screw propeller [838, 839].

Mg and Zn are two most frequently used as sacrificial anode metals. The selection between two is dependent on difference in open-circuit potential with that of the metal to be protected. Fe (of main element of protected structure) has an open-circuit potential of −0.55 V (against the reference electrode of Ag/AgCl), while Mg has −1.5 V and Zn has −1.05 V. Hence, the potential difference ΔE (Mg/Fe) of 0.95 V is larger and more effective than that of ΔE (Zn/Fe) with 0.9 V as a sacrificial anode metal [840, 841].

Yan et al. [842] mentioned that (i) corrosivity of simulated concrete pore solution (SCPS) contaminated by chloride was automatically detected and corrosion of steel in SCPS was intelligently prevented by AZ91 alloy, (ii) Mg of AZ91 alloy could act as effective sacrificial anode to cathodically protect steel from corrosion attack once the SCPS was polluted by chlorides and (iii) Al alloying could enhance the sensitivity of Mg anode to chloride contamination and further improve its cathodic protection effect, and thus enhanced its intelligence level as corrosivity detector and corrosion protector. Tokuda et al. [843] determined the effects of Mg on the anodic dissolution behavior of the 55Al–Zn coating layer by in situ observation during galvanostatic polarization. It was reported that (i) the Zn-rich phases were observed to corrode at lower potentials than the dissolution potential region of the Al-rich matrix phases, and the dissolution duration of the Zn-rich phases was prolonged by

Mg addition and (ii) the corrosion products of the 55Al–Zn–Mg coating layer were suggested to inhibit the oxygen reduction reaction on the steel substrate.

Glover et al. [844] evaluated three solid solution Mg–*x*Sn ($x = 1$, 5, 10 wt%) alloys as candidates for the sacrificial cathodic protection of AZ31B–H24 in 0.6 M aqueous NaCl solution. It was found that (i) Mg–1Sn was shown to galvanically protect AZ31B–H24 for 24 h with 95% efficiency, (ii) polarity reversal was observed for Mg–5Sn during the initial 10 h, after which protection was offered; and Mg–10Sn provided no protection and (iii) self-corrosion rates of 60% and 52% were observed for Mg–1Sn and Mg–5Sn alloys, respectively. Cain et al. [845] evaluated the potential range for sacrificial Mg (including pure Mg and Mg–4Y–3RE: WE43B) anodes for the cathodic protection of AZ31B–H24 alloy in 0.6 M NaCl and 0.1 M $MgCl_2$ electrolytes. It was reported that (i) a wide range of potentials for practical or kinetic-based sacrificial cathodic protection is possible for Mg alloys but a practical range of potentials for substantial cathodic protection in 0.1 M TRIS was not observed and (ii) residual corrosion rates at potentials cathodic to their open-circuit potential were greater than expectations from electrochemical mixed potential corrosion theory interpreted to be a result of the negative difference effect. Zero resistance ammeter (ZRA) testing was performed on couples of AZ31B–H24 to CP-Mg and Mg alloy WE43B–T5 to validate the range of protection for AZ31B–H24 and to evaluate their suitability for the protection of AZ31B–H24. It was furthermore mentioned that (iii) gravimetric mass loss of AZ31B–H24 from ZRA-coupled samples revealed only a 2 × to 12 × decrease in anodic charge density compared to that at open-circuit potential, (iv) coupled WE43B possessed a lower self-corrosion fraction than coupled pure Mg because it possesses a larger potential difference between its open-circuit potential and galvanic couple potential and (v) anode–cathode polarity reversal was not observed for couples of AZ31B–H24 to CP Mg and WE43B.

Due to active electrochemical reaction of Mg material, as will be described in Chapter 16, Mg alloys are also recognized as an effective anode electrode in Mg–air batteries [846].

References

[1] Overview of materials for Magnesium Alloy; http://www.matweb.com/search/datasheet_print.aspx?matguid=4e6a4852b14c4b12998acf2f8316c07c.

[2] Wang WLE, Gupta M. Using Microwave Energy to Synthesize Light Weight/Energy Saving Magnesium Based Materials: A Review. Technologies. 2015, 3, 1–18.

[3] Haghshenas M. Mechanical characteristics of biodegradable magnesium matrix composites: A review. Journal of Magnesium and Alloys. 2017,5, 189–201.

[4] Biodegradation Properties of Magnesium Alloys; Total Materia; https://www.totalmateria.com/page.aspx?ID=CheckArticle&site=ktn&NM=370

[5] Ren L, Fan L, Zhou M, Guo Y, Zhang Y, Boehlert CJ, Quan G. Magnesium application in railway rolling stocks: A new challenge and opportunity for lightweighting. International Journal of Lightweight Materials and Manufacture. 2018, 1, 81–88.

[6] Luthringer BJC, Feyerabend F, Willumeit-Römer R. Magnesium-based implants: a mini-review. Magnesium Research. 2014, 27, 142–54.

[7] Mechanical properties Magnesium alloy and plate at room temperature; http://aviationandaccessories.tpub.com/TM-43-0106/css/TM-43-0106_216.htm.

[8] Watanabe H, Yamaguchi M, Takigawa Y, Higashi K. Mechanical properties of Mg-Al-Ca alloy processed by hot extrusion; http://www.1m-foundation.or.jp/englsih/abstratct-vol40/abstract/58.html.

[9] Kojima Y. Mechanical Properties of Magnesium. Surface Treatment. 1993,44, 866–73; jstage.ist.go.jp/article/sfj1989/44/11/44_11_866/_pdf.

[10] Pan H, Pan F, Wang X, Peng J, Gou J, She J, Tang A. Correlation on the electrical and thermal conductivity for binary Mg–Al and Mg–Zn alloys. International Journal of Thermophysics. 2013, 34, 1336–46.

[11] Zhang L et al. Effect of Al content on the microstructures and mechanical properties of Mg–Al alloys. Materials Science and Engineering: A. 2009, 508, 129–33.

[12] Yang X et al. Effects of Ni levels on microstructure and mechanical properties of Mg-Ni-Y alloy reinforced with LPSO structure. Journal of Alloys and Compounds. 2017, 726, 276–83.

[13] Seong JW et al. Mg-Ca binary alloy sheets with Ca contents of ≤1wt.% with high corrosion resistance and high toughness. Corrosion Science. 2015, 98, 372–81.

[14] Pavlic O et al. Design of Mg alloys: The effects of Li concentration on the structure and elastic properties in the Mg-Li binary system by first principles calculations. Journal of Alloys and Compounds. 2017, 691, 15–25.

[15] Zeng Y et al. Effect of Li content on microstructure, texture and mechanical behaviors of the as-extruded Mg-Li sheets. Materials Science and Engineering: A. 2017, 700, 59–65.

[16] Xu Y et al. Effects of Gd solutes on hardness and yield strength of Mg alloys. Progress in Natural Science: Materials International. 2018, 28, 724–30.

[17] Silva CJ et al. The effect of Sc on plastic deformation of Mg–Sc binary alloys under tension. Journal of Alloys and Compounds. 2018, 761, 58–70.

[18] Al-Samman T. Effect of heavy metal impurities in secondary Mg alloys on the microstructure and mechanical properties during deformation. Materials & Design (1980–2015). 2015, 65, 983–88.

[19] Seetharaman S et al. Effect of erbium modification on the microstructure, mechanical and corrosion characteristics of binary Mg–Al alloys. Journal of Alloys and Compounds. 2015, 48, 759–70.

[20] Razzaghi M et al. Unraveling the effects of Zn addition and hot extrusion process on the microstructure and mechanical properties of as-cast Mg–2Al magnesium alloy. Vacuum. 2019, 167, 214–22.

[21] Kumar A et al. Lanthanum effect on improving CTE, damping, hardness and tensile response of Mg-3Al alloy. Journal of Alloys and Compounds. 2017, 695, 3612–20.
[22] Liu YF et al. Effect of La content on microstructure, thermal conductivity and mechanical properties of Mg–4Al magnesium alloys. Journal of Alloys and Compounds. 2019, 806, 71–78.
[23] Suh B-C et al. Effect of Sn addition on the microstructure and deformation behavior of Mg-3Al alloy. Acta Materialia. 2017, 124, 268–79.
[24] Jiang H et al. The influence of Ca and Gd microalloying on microstructure and mechanical property of hot-rolled Mg-3Al alloy. Procedia Engineering. 2017, 207, 932–37.
[25] Li ZT et al. Effect of Ca/Al ratio on microstructure and mechanical properties of Mg-Al-Ca-Mn alloys. Materials Science and Engineering: A. 2017, 682, 423–32.
[26] Nouri M et al. Beneficial effects of yttrium on the performance of Mg–3%Al alloy during wear, corrosion and corrosive wear. Tribology International. 2013, 67, 154–63.
[27] Wang J et al. The effect of Y content on microstructure and tensile properties of the extruded Mg–1Al-xY alloy. Materials Science and Engineering: A. 2019, 765; https://doi.org/10.1016/j.msea.2019.138288.
[28] Can Kurnaz et al. Influence of titanium and chromium addition on the microstructure and mechanical properties of squeeze cast Mg–6Al alloy. Journal of Alloys and Compounds. 2011, 509, 3190–96.
[29] Wang H et al. Effect of Si addition on the microstructure and mechanical properties of ECAPed Mg–15Al alloy. Materials Science and Engineering: A. 2014, 589, 119–24.
[30] Fan J et al. Effect of Sr/Al ratio on microstructure and properties of Mg-Al-Sr alloy. Rare Metal Materials and Engineering. 2012, 41, 1721–24.
[31] Singh K et al. The effect of lanthanum on Microstructure & Mechanical properties of stir casted Mg alloy. Materials Today: Proceedings. 2018, 5, 6360–69.
[32] Park SH et al. Influence of Sn addition on the microstructure and mechanical properties of extruded Mg–8Al–2Zn alloy. Materials Science and Engineering: A. 2015, 626, 128–35.
[33] Wang F et al. Effects of alloying composition on the microstructures and mechanical properties of Mg-Al-Zn-Ca-RE magnesium alloy. Vacuum. 2019, 159, 400–09.
[34] Wang F et al. Effects of Al and Zn contents on the microstructure and mechanical properties of Mg-Al-Zn-Ca magnesium alloys. Materials Science and Engineering: A. 2017, 704, 57–65.
[35] Song L et al. The effect of Ca addition on microstructure and mechanical properties of extruded AZ31 alloys. Vacuum. 2019, 168; https://doi.org/10.1016/j.vacuum.2019.108822.
[36] Bu F et al. Study on the assemblage of Y and Gd on microstructure and mechanical properties of hot extruded Mg–Al–Zn alloy. Materials Science and Engineering: A. 2015, 639, 198–207.
[37] Li KJ et al. Effects of Sm addition on microstructure and mechanical properties of Mg-6Al-0.6Zn alloy. Scripta Materialia. 2009, 60, 1101–04.
[38] Qian XY et al. Study on mechanical behaviors and theoretical critical shear strength of cold-rolled AZ31 alloy with different Li additions. Materials Science and Engineering: A. 2019, 742, 241–54.
[39] Kim B et al. Effect of Pd on microstructures and tensile properties of as-cast Mg–6Al–1Zn alloys. Materials Letters. 2011, 65, 122–25.
[40] Suresh M et al. Influence of boron addition on the grain refinement and mechanical properties of AZ91 Mg alloy. Materials Science and Engineering: A. 2009, 525, 207–10.
[41] Wang H-Y et al. Effects of Zn on the microstructure and tensile properties of as-extruded Mg-8Al-2Sn alloy. Materials Science and Engineering: A. 2017, 698, 249–55.
[42] Jiang L et al. Effects of Zn addition on the aging behavior and mechanical properties of Mg8Al2Sn wrought alloy. Materials Science and Engineering: A. 2019, 752, 145–51.

[43] Kim BH et al. Investigations of the properties of Mg–4Al–2Sn–1Ca–xCe alloys. Materials Science and Engineering: A. 2010, 527, 6372–77.
[44] Kim BH et al. Effect of Ca and Sr additions on high temperature and corrosion properties of Mg–4Al–2Sn based alloys. Materials Science and Engineering: A. 2011, 528, 808–14.
[45] Kim Y-H et al. Effects of Li addition on microstructure and mechanical properties of Mg–6Al–2Sn–0.4Mn alloys. Transactions of Nonferrous Metals Society of China. 2016, 26, 697–703.
[46] Majd AM et al. Effect of RE elements on the microstructural and mechanical properties of as-cast and age hardening processed Mg–4Al–2Sn alloy. Journal of Magnesium and Alloys. 2018, 6, 309–17.
[47] Zhu T et al. Effects of Mn addition on the microstructure and mechanical properties of cast Mg–9Al–2Sn (wt.%) alloy. Journal of Magnesium and Alloys. 2014, 2, 27–35.
[48] Wang J et al. Effect of zinc and mischmetal on microstructure and mechanical properties of Mg-Al-Mn alloy. Journal of Rare Earths. 2010, 28, 794–97.
[49] Evangelista E et al. Analysis of the effect of Si content on the creep response of an Mg–5Al–Mn alloy. Materials Science and Engineering: A. 2005, 410/411, 62–66.
[50] Wang J et al. Effects of samarium on microstructures and tensile properties of Mg–5Al–0.3Mn alloy. Materials Science and Engineering: A. 2011, 528, 4115–19.
[51] Şevik H et al. The effect of strontium on the microstructure and mechanical properties of Mg–6Al–0.3Mn–0.3Ti–1Sn. Journal of Magnesium and Alloys. 2014, 2, 214–19.
[52] Hu T et al. Effects of B and Sn additions on the microstructure and mechanical property of Mg-3Al-1Si alloy. Journal of Alloys and Compounds. 2019, 796, 1–8.
[53] Liu J et al. Effect of Gd–Ca combined additions on the microstructure and creep properties of Mg–7Al–1Si alloys. Journal of Alloys and Compounds. 2015, 620, 74–79.
[54] Zhang Y et al. Effect of Ca and Sr on microstructure and compressive creep property of Mg–4Al–RE alloys. Materials Science and Engineering: A. 2014, 610, 309–14.
[55] Wu X et al. Effect of Ca addition on the microstructure and tensile property of AE42 alloy. Materials Letters. 2019, 252, 150–54.
[56] Braszczyńska-Malik KN et al. The influence of Ti particles on microstructure and mechanical properties of Mg-5Al-5RE matrix alloy composite. Journal of Alloys and Compounds. 2017, 728, 600–06.
[57] Pugazhendhi BS et al. Effect of aluminium on microstructure, mechanical property and texture evolution of dual phase Mg-8Li alloy in different processing conditions. Archives of Civil and Mechanical Engineering. 2018, 18, 1332–44.
[58] Zhao Z et al. Influence of Al and Si additions on the microstructure and mechanical properties of Mg-4Li alloys. Materials Science and Engineering: A. 2017, 702, 206–17.
[59] Li HB et al. Microstructure and mechanical properties of Mg-Li alloy with Ca addition. Acta Metallurgica Sinica (English Letters). 2006, 19, 355–61.
[60] Dong H et al. Effect of Y on microstructure and mechanical properties of duplex Mg–7Li alloys. Journal of Alloys and Compounds. 2010, 506, 468–74.
[61] Wang T et al. Influence of Rare Earth Elements on Microstructure and Mechanical Properties of Mg-Li Alloys. Journal of Rare Earths. 2006, 24, 797–800.
[62] Li Y et al. Effect of mischmetal on microstructure and mechanical properties of superlight Mg-Li Alloys. Rare Metal Materials and Engineering. 2017, 46, 1775–81.
[63] Sha G et al. Effects of Sc addition and annealing treatment on the microstructure and mechanical properties of the as-rolled Mg-3Li alloy. Journal of Materials Science & Technology. 2011, 27, 753–58.
[64] Li J et al. Effects of Cu addition on the microstructure and hardness of Mg–5Li–3Al–2Zn alloy. Materials Science and Engineering: A. 2010, 527, 2780–83.

[65] Xiang Q et al. Influence of Sn on microstructure and mechanical properties of Mg–5Li–3Al–2Zn alloys. Journal of Alloys and Compounds. 2009, 477, 832–35.
[66] Kim Y-H et al. Microstructure and mechanical properties of Mg–xLi–3Al–1Sn–0.4Mn alloys (x=5, 8 and 11wt%). Journal of Alloys and Compounds. 2014, 583, 15–20.
[67] Wang T et al. Effects of calcium on the microstructures and tensile properties of Mg–5Li–3Al alloys. Materials Science and Engineering: A. 2011, 528, 5678–84.
[68] Kim JT et al. Effect of Ca addition on the plastic deformation behavior of extruded Mg-11Li-3Al-1Sn-0.4Mn alloy. Journal of Alloys and Compounds. 2016, 687, 821–26.
[69] Cui C et al. Influence of yttrium on microstructure and mechanical properties of as-cast Mg–5Li–3Al–2Zn alloy. Journal of Alloys and Compounds. 2011, 509, 9045–49.
[70] Wu R et al. Effects of the addition of Y in Mg–8Li–(1,3)Al alloy. Materials Science and Engineering: A. 2009, 516, 96–99.
[71] Sun Y et al. Effects of Sn and Y on the microstructure, texture, and mechanical properties of as-extruded Mg-5Li-3Al-2Zn alloy. Materials Science and Engineering: A. 2018, 733, 429–39.
[72] Peng X et al. Effect of Y on microstructure and mechanical properties as well as corrosion resistance of Mg-9Li-3Al alloy. Rare Metal Materials and Engineering. 2013, 42, 1993–98.
[73] Zhao J et al. Effect of Y content on microstructure and mechanical properties of as-cast Mg–8Li–3Al–2Zn alloy with duplex structure. Materials Science and Engineering: A. 2016, 650, 240–47.
[74] Zhu T et al. Influence of Y and Nd on microstructure, texture and anisotropy of Mg–5Li–1Al alloy. Materials Science and Engineering: A. 2014, 600, 1–7.
[75] Kim JT et al. Microstructure and mechanical properties of the as-cast and warm rolled Mg-9Li-x(Al-Si)-yTi alloys with x = 1, 3, 5 and y = 0.05 wt.%. Journal of Alloys and Compounds. 2017, 711, 243–49.
[76] Peng X et al. Effects of Ce-rich RE on microstructure and mechanical properties of as-cast Mg-8Li-3Al-2Zn-0.5Nd alloy with duplex structure. Progress in Natural Science: Materials International. 2019, 29, 103–09.
[77] Wu L et al. Effects of Ce-rich RE additions and heat treatment on the microstructure and tensile properties of Mg–Li–Al–Zn-based alloy. Materials Science and Engineering: A. 2011, 528, 2174–79.
[78] Xu T-C et al. Effect of Sr content on microstructure and mechanical properties of Mg-Li-Al-Mn alloy. Transactions of Nonferrous Metals Society of China. 2014, 24, 2752–60.
[79] Ji Q et al. Effect of Y and Ce addition on microstructures and mechanical properties of LZ91 alloys. Journal of Alloys and Compounds. 2019, 800, 72–80.
[80] Son H-T et al. Effects of Al and Zn additions on mechanical properties and precipitation behaviors of Mg–Sn alloy system. Materials Letters. 2011, 65, 1966–69.
[81] Jayalakshmi S et al. Effect of Ag and Cu trace additions on the microstructural evolution and mechanical properties of Mg–5Sn alloy. Journal of Alloys and Compounds. 2013, 565, 56–65.
[82] El Mahallawy N et al. Effect of Zn addition on the microstructure and mechanical properties of cast, rolled and extruded Mg-6Sn-xZn alloys. Materials Science and Engineering: A. 2017, 80, 47–53.
[83] Keyvani M et al. Effect of Bi, Sb, and Ca additions on the hot hardness and microstructure of cast Mg–5Sn alloy. Materials Science and Engineering: A. 2010, 527, 7714–18.
[84] Nayyeri G et al. The microstructure, creep resistance, and high-temperature mechanical properties of Mg-5Sn alloy with Ca and Sb additions, and aging treatment. Materials Science and Engineering: A. 2010, 527, 5353–59.
[85] Karakulak E et al. Effect of Si addition on microstructure and wear properties of Mg-Sn as-cast alloys. Journal of Magnesium and Alloys. 2018, 6, 384–89.

[86] Jiang Y et al. Effect of Li on microstructure, mechanical properties and fracture mechanism of as-cast Mg–5Sn alloy. Materials Science and Engineering: A. 2015, 641, 256–62.
[87] Liu mH et al. Effects of strontium on microstructure and mechanical properties of as-cast Mg–5wt.%Sn alloy. Journal of Alloys and Compounds. 2010, 504, 345–50.
[88] Yang M et al. Effects of Y addition on as-cast microstructure and mechanical properties of Mg–3Sn–2Ca (wt.%) magnesium alloy. Materials Science and Engineering: A. 2009, 525, 112–20.
[89] Yang M-B et al. Effects of little Ce addition on as-cast microstructure and creep properties of Mg-3Sn-2Ca magnesium alloy. Transactions of Nonferrous Metals Society of China. 2009, 19, 1087–92.
[90] Yang M et al. Effects of Gd addition on as-cast microstructure and mechanical properties of Mg–3Sn–2Ca magnesium alloy. Materials Science and Engineering: A. 2011, 528, 1721–26.
[91] Shi B-Q et al. Effect of element Gd on phase constituent and mechanical property of Mg-5Sn-1Ca alloy. Transactions of Nonferrous Metals Society of China. 2010, 20, s341–s345.
[92] Kim S-H et al. Controlling the microstructure and improving the tensile properties of extruded Mg-Sn-Zn alloy through Al addition. Journal of Alloys and Compounds. 2018, 751, 1–11.
[93] Wang P et al. The influence of Sc addition on microstructure and tensile mechanical properties of Mg–4.5Sn–5Zn alloys. Journal of Magnesium and Alloys. 2019, 7, 456–65.
[94] Chen Y et al. Effect of Zn on microstructure and mechanical property of Mg–3Sn–1Al alloys. Materials Science and Engineering: A. 2014, 612, 96–101.
[95] Kim S-H et al. Effect of Ce addition on the microstructure and mechanical properties of extruded Mg-Sn-Al-Zn alloy. Materials Science and Engineering: A. 2016, 657, 406–12.
[96] Yang M et al. Effects of minor Ti addition on as-cast microstructure and mechanical properties of Mg–3Sn–2Sr (wt.%) magnesium alloy. Journal of Alloys and Compounds. 2013, 579, 92–99.
[97] Gao J et al. Effect of Sn element on the formation of LPSO phase and mechanical properties of Mg-6Y-2Zn alloy. Materials Science and Engineering: A. 2018, 711, 334–42.
[98] Li J et al. Effect of Zr modification on solidification behavior and mechanical properties of Mg–Y–RE (WE54) alloy. Journal of Magnesium and Alloys. 2013, 1, 346–51.
[99] Luo K et al. Effect of Y and Gd content on the microstructure and mechanical properties of Mg–Y–RE alloys. Journal of Magnesium and Alloys. 2019, 7, 345–54.
[100] Xu X et al. Effect of Nd on microstructure and mechanical properties of as-extruded Mg-Y-Zr-Nd alloy. Journal of Materials Science & Technology. 2017, 33, 926–34.
[101] Liu H-H et al. Effect of Dy addition on microstructure and mechanical properties of Mg-4Y-3Nd-0.4Zr alloy. Transactions of Nonferrous Metals Society of China, 2017, 27, 797–803.
[102] Yang M et al. Effects of minor Ca addition on as-cast microstructure and mechanical properties of Mg–4Y–1.2Mn–1Zn (wt.%) magnesium alloy. Journal of Alloys and Compounds. 2013, 574, 165–73.
[103] Zhao Y et al. Effect of zinc addition on microstructure and mechanical properties of Mg–7Y–3Sm–0.5Zr alloy. Transactions of Nonferrous Metals Society of China. 2012, 22, 1924–29.
[104] Jiang Z et al. Role of Al modification on the microstructure and mechanical properties of as-cast Mg–6Ce alloys. Materials Science and Engineering: A. 2015, 645, 57–64.
[105] Pan F et al. Effects of minor Zr and Sr on as-cast microstructure and mechanical properties of Mg–3Ce–1.2Mn–0.9Sc (wt.%) magnesium alloy. Materials Science and Engineering: A. 2011, 528, 4292–99.
[106] Yang M et al. Effects of Ca addition on as-cast microstructure and mechanical properties of Mg–3Ce–1.2Mn–1Zn (wt.%) magnesium alloy. Materials & Design (1980–2015). 2013, 52, 274–83.

[107] Moussa ME et al. Effect of Ca addition on modification of primary Mg2Si, hardness and wear behavior in Mg–Si hypereutectic alloys. Journal of Magnesium and Alloys. 2014, 2, 230–38.
[108] Du H et al. Effects of Zn on the microstructure, mechanical property and bio-corrosion property of Mg–3Ca alloys for biomedical application. Materials Chemistry and Physics. 2011, 125, 568–75.
[109] Ma N et al. Effects of cerium on microstructures, recovery behavior and mechanical properties of backward extruded Mg–0.5Mn alloys. Materials Science and Engineering: A. 2013, 564, 310–16.
[110] Zhong L et al. Effect of Ce addition on the microstructure, thermal conductivity and mechanical properties of Mg–0.5Mn alloys. Journal of Alloys and Compounds. 2016, 661, 402–10.
[111] Borkar H et al. Effect of strontium on the texture and mechanical properties of extruded Mg–1%Mn alloys. Materials Science and Engineering: A. 2012, 549, 168–75.
[112] Yang Y et al. Effect of neodymium on microstructure and mechanical properties of Mg-Sb alloy. Journal of Rare Earths. 2006, 24, 376–78.
[113] Niu R-L et al. Effect of yttrium addition on microstructures, damping properties and mechanical properties of as-cast Mg–based ternary alloys. Journal of Alloys and Compounds. 2019, 785, 1270–78.
[114] Zhang J-S et al. The effect of Ca addition on microstructures and mechanical properties of Mg-RE based alloys. Journal of Alloys and Compounds. 2013, 554, 110–14.
[115] Huang S et al. Effect of Sn on the formation of the long period stacking ordered phase and mechanical properties of Mg–RE–Zn alloy. Materials Letters. 2014, 137, 143–46.
[116] Zhang K et al. Effect of Gd content on microstructure and mechanical properties of Mg-Y-RE-Zr alloys. Transactions of Nonferrous Metals Society of China. 2008, 18, s12–s16.
[117] Lim HK et al. Effects of alloying elements on microstructures and mechanical properties of wrought Mg–MM–Sn alloy. Journal of Alloys and Compounds. 2009, 468, 308–14.
[118] Li J-H et al. Effect of gadolinium on aged hardening behavior, microstructure and mechanical properties of Mg-Nd-Zn-Zr alloy. Transactions of Nonferrous Metals Society of China. 2008, 18, s27–s32.
[119] Wang WH et al. Effect of solute atom concentration and precipitates on serrated flow in Mg-3Nd-Zn alloy. Journal of Materials Science & Technology. 2018, 34, 1236–42.
[120] Wang C et al. Effect of Al additions on grain refinement and mechanical properties of Mg–Sm alloys. Journal of Alloys and Compounds. 2015, 620, 172–79.
[121] Che C et al. The effect of Gd and Zn additions on microstructures and mechanical properties of Mg-4Sm-3Nd-Zr alloy. Journal of Alloys and Compounds. 2017, 706, 526–37.
[122] Yuan M et al. Effects of Zn on the microstructures and mechanical properties of Mg–3Sm–0.5Gd–xZn–0.5Zr (x=0, 0.3 and 0.6) alloy. Journal of Alloys and Compounds. 2014, 590, 355–61.
[123] Liu XQ et al. Effect of Er contents on the microstructure of long period stacking ordered phase and the corresponding mechanical properties in Mg-Dy-Er-Zn alloys. Materials Science and Engineering: A. 2018, 718, 461–67.
[124] Hoseini MM et al. Effect of Zn addition on dynamic recrystallization behavior of Mg-2Gd alloy during high-temperature deformation. Journal of Alloys and Compounds. 2019, 806, 1200–06.
[125] Zhao D et al. Simultaneously improving elastic modulus and damping capacity of extruded Mg-Gd-Y-Zn-Mn alloy via alloying with Si. Journal of Alloys and Compounds. 2019, 810; https://doi.org/10.1016/j.jallcom.2019.151857.
[126] Wang Y et al. Effect of Zn content on the microstructure and mechanical properties of Mg-Gd-Y-Zr alloys. Materials Science and Engineering: A. 2019, 745, 149–58.

[127] Chi YQ et al. Effect of trace zinc on the microstructure and mechanical properties of extruded Mg-Gd-Y-Zr alloy. Journal of Alloys and Compounds. 2019, 789, 416–27.
[128] Yuan J et al. Effect of Zn content on the microstructures, mechanical properties, and damping capacities of Mg–7Gd–3Y–1Nd–0.5Zr based alloys. Journal of Alloys and Compounds. 2019, 773, 919–26.
[129] Peng Q et al. The effect of La or Ce on ageing response and mechanical properties of cast Mg–Gd–Zr alloys. Materials Characterization. 2008, 59, 435–39.
[130] Wang J et al. Effect of Y for enhanced age hardening response and mechanical properties of Mg–Gd–Y–Zr alloys. Materials Science and Engineering: A. 2007, 456, 78–84.
[131] Huang S et al. Effect of Gd and Y contents on the microstructural evolution of long period stacking ordered phase and the corresponding mechanical properties in Mg–Gd–Y–Zn–Mn alloys. Materials Science and Engineering: A. 2014, 612, 363–70.
[132] Zhang X et al. Effects of Si addition on microstructure and mechanical properties of Mg–8Gd–4Y–Nd–Zr alloy. Materials & Design. 2013, 43, 74–79.
[133] Jafari HR et al. Effect of Gd content on high temperature mechanical properties of Mg–Gd–Y–Zr alloy. Materials Science and Engineering: A. 2016, 651, 840–47.
[134] Zhang X et al. Effect of Nd on the microstructure and mechanical properties of Mg–8Gd–5Y–2Zn–0.5Zr alloy. Materials Science and Engineering: A. 2013, 586, 19–24.
[135] Yu Z et al. Fabrication of a high strength Mg–11Gd–4.5Y–1Nd–1.5Zn–0.5Zr (wt%) alloy by thermomechanical treatments. Materials Science and Engineering: A. 2015, 622, 121–30.
[136] Zhang R et al. Substitution of Ni for Zn on microstructure and mechanical properties of Mg–Gd–Y–Zn–Mn alloy. Journal of Magnesium and Alloys. 2017, 5, 355–61.
[137] Fu W et al. Effects of Zr addition on the multi-scale second-phase particles and fracture behavior for Mg-3Gd-1Zn alloy. Journal of Alloys and Compounds. 2018, 747, 197–210.
[138] Li B et al. Effects of 0.5 wt% Ce addition on microstructures and mechanical properties of a wrought Mg–8Gd–1.2Zn–0.5Zr alloy. Journal of Alloys and Compounds. 2018, 763, 120–33.
[139] Wang Y et al. Effects of Mn addition on the microstructures and mechanical properties of the Mg-15Gd-1Zn alloy. Journal of Alloys and Compounds. 2017, 698, 1066–76.
[140] Yang M et al. Comparison about effects of minor Zr, Sr and Ca additions on microstructure and tensile properties of Mg–5Gd–1.2Mn–0.4Sc (wt%) magnesium alloy. Materials Science and Engineering: A. 2012, 545, 201–08.
[141] Wang Q-F et al. Effect of Zn addition on microstructure and mechanical properties of as-cast Mg–2Er alloy. Transactions of Nonferrous Metals Society of China. 2014, 24, 3792–96.
[142] Zhang S, Zhang X, Zhao C, Li J, Song Y, Xie C, Tao H, Zhang Y, He Y, Jiang Y, Bian Y. Research on an Mg–Zn alloy as a degradable biomaterial. Acta Biomaterialia. 2010, 6, 626–40.
[143] Uddin MS, Hall C, Murphy P. Surface treatments for controlling corrosion rate of biodegradable Mg and Mg-based alloy implants. Science and Technology of Advanced Materials. 2015, 16: DOI: 10.1088/1468-6996/16/5/053501.
[144] Hassel T, Bach FW, Krause C. Influence of alloy composition on the mechanical and electrochemical properties of binary Mg-Ca alloys and its corrosion behavior in solutions at different chloride concentrations. In: Kainer KU ed., Magnesium Alloys and Their Applications, Hoboken, NJ: Wiley; 2007, 789–95.
[145] Drynda A, Hassel T, Hoehn R, Perz A, Bach F-W, Peuster M. Development and biocompatibility of a novel corrodible fluoride-coated magnesium-calcium alloy with improved degradation kinetics and adequate mechanical properties for cardiovascular applications. Journal of Biomedical Materials Research Part A. 2010, 93, 763–75.
[146] Homayun B, Afshar A. Microstructure, mechanical properties, corrosion behavior and cytotoxicity of Mg–Zn–Al–Ca alloys as biodegradable materials. Journal of Alloys and Compounds. 2014, 607, 1–10.

[147] Yang D, Hu Z, Chen W, Lu J, Chen J, Wang H, Wang L, Jiang J, Ma A. Fabrication of Mg-Al alloy foam with close-cell structure by powder metallurgy approach and its mechanical properties. Journal of Advanced Manufacturing and Processing. 2016, 22, 290–96.
[148] Magnesium Alloys. http://www.dierk-raabe.com/magnesium-alloys/.
[149] Wu Z, Ahmad R, Yin B, Sandlöbes S, Curtin WA. Mechanistic origin and prediction of enhanced ductility in magnesium alloys. Science. 2018, 359, 447–52.
[150] Asgari M, Hang R, Wang C, Yu Z, Li Z, Xiao Y, Biodegradable metallic wires in dental and orthopedic applications: a review. Metals. 2018, 8, 212; https://doi.org/10.3390/met8040212.
[151] Bian D, Zhou W, Deng J, Liu Y, Li W, Chu X, Xiu P, Cai H, Kou Y, Jiang B, Zheng Y. Development of magnesium-based biodegradable metals with dietary trace element germanium as orthopaedic implant applications. Acta Biomater. 2017, 64, 421–36.
[152] Buey D, Hector Jr LG, Ghazisaeidi M. Core structure and solute strengthening of second-order pyramidal <c+a> dislocations in Mg-Y alloys. Acta Materialia. 2018. 147, 1–9.
[153] Hu WW, Yang ZQ, Ye HQ. <c+a> dislocations and their interactions with other crystal defects in a Mg alloy. Acta Materialia. 2017, 124, 372–82.
[154] Ahmad R, Yin B, Wu Z, Curtin WA. Designing high ductility in magnesium alloys. Acta Materialia. 2019, 172, 161–84.
[155] Sandlöbes S, Friák M, Zaefferer S, Dick A, Raabe D. The relation between ductility and stacking fault energies in Mg and Mg–Y alloys. Acta Materialia. 2012, 60, 3011–21.
[156] Yang HJ, An ZH, Shao XH, Zhang ZF. Enhancing strength and ductility of Mg–12Gd–3Y–0.5Zr alloy by forming a bi-ultrafine microstructure. Materials Science and Engineering: A. 2011, 528, 4300–11.
[157] Zhou X, Liu C, Gao Y, Jiang S, Chen Z. Improved workability and ductility of the Mg-Gd-Y-Zn-Zr alloy via enhanced kinking and dynamic recrystallization. Journal of Alloys and Compounds. 2018, 749, 878–86.
[158] Sun J, Jin L, Dong J, Wang F, Luo AA. Towards high ductility in magnesium alloys – The role of intergranular deformation. International Journal of Plasticity. 2019, 123, 121–32.
[159] Gao L, Yan H, Luo J, Luo AA, Chen R. Microstructure and mechanical properties of a high ductility Mg–Zn–Mn–Ce magnesium alloy. Journal of Magnesium and Alloys. 2013, 1, 283–91.
[160] Yan H, Chen RS, Han EH. Room-temperature ductility and anisotropy of two rolled Mg–Zn–Gd alloys. Materials Science and Engineering: A. 2010, 527, 3317–22.
[161] Oshida Y. Lecture note, Manufacturing Engineering, Syracuse University, 2007.
[162] Lee CA, Lee M-G, Seo OS, Nguyen N-T, Kim HY. Cyclic behavior of AZ31B Mg: Experiments and non-isothermal forming simulations. International Journal of Plasticity. 2015, 75, 39–62.
[163] Toscano D, Shaha SK, Behravesh B, Jahed H, Williams B. Multiaxial Cyclic Response of Low Temperature Closed-Die Forged AZ31B Mg Alloy. In: Joshi V. et al. ed., Magnesium Technology. The Minerals, Metals & Materials Series. Springer, 2019, 289–96.
[164] Chen C, Liu T, Lv C, Lu L, Luo D. Study on cyclic deformation behavior of extruded Mg–3Al–1Zn alloy. Materials Science and Engineering: A. 2012, 539, 223–29.
[165] Ishihara S, Namito T, Yoshifuji S, Goshima T. On fatigue lives of diecast and extruded Mg alloys. International Journal of Fatigue. 2012, 35, 56–62.
[166] Wang F, Dong J, Jiang Y, Ding W. Cyclic deformation and fatigue of extruded Mg–Gd–Y magnesium alloy. Materials Science and Engineering: A. 2013, 561, 403–10.
[167] Dong S, Wang F, Wan Q, Dong J, Jiang Y. Aging effects on cyclic deformation and fatigue of extruded Mg–Gd–Y–Zr alloy. Materials Science and Engineering: A. 2015, 641, 1–9.
[168] Gryguc A, Shaha SK, Behravesh SB, Jahed H, Su X. Monotonic and cyclic behaviour of cast and cast-forged AZ80 Mg. International Journal of Fatigue. 2017, 104, 136–49.

[169] Patel VK, Bhole SD, Chen DL. Fatigue life estimation of ultrasonic spot welded Mg alloy joints. Materials & Design. 2014, 62, 124–32.

[170] Liu L, Xiao L. Chen DL, Feng JC, Zhou Y. Microstructure and fatigue properties of Mg-to-steel dissimilar resistance spot welds. Materials & Design. 2013, 45, 336–42.

[171] Park SH, Hong S-G, Lee BH, Bang W, Lee CH. Low-cycle fatigue characteristics of rolled Mg–3Al–1Zn alloy. International Journal of Fatigue. 2010, 32, 1835–42.

[172] Wen B, Wang F, Jin L, Dong J. Fatigue damage development in extruded Mg-3Al-Zn magnesium alloy. Materials Science and Engineering: A. 2016, 667, 171–78.

[173] Jain S, Gokhale A, Jain J, Singh SS, Hariharan K. Fatigue behavior of aged and solution treated AZ61 Mg alloy at small length scale using nanoindentation. Materials Science and Engineering: A. 2017, 684, 652–59.

[174] Zhu R, Li W, Wu Y, Cai X, Yu Y. Effect of aging treatment on low-cycle fatigue behavior of extruded Mg–8Al–0.5Zn alloys. Materials & Design. 2012, 41, 203–07.

[175] Gryguc A, Behravesh SB, Shaha SK, Jahed H, Su X. Low-cycle fatigue characterization and texture induced ratcheting behaviour of forged AZ80 Mg alloys. International Journal of Fatigue. 2018, 116, 429–38.

[176] Zhu R, Cai X, Wu Y, Liu L, Hua B. Low-cycle fatigue behavior of extruded Mg–10Gd–2Y–0.5Zr alloys. Materials & Design. 2014, 53, 992–97.

[177] Mohammed SMAK, Li DJ, Zeng XQ, Chen DL. Cyclic deformation behavior of a high zinc-containing cast magnesium alloy. International Journal of Fatigue. 2019, 125, 1–10.

[178] Li Z, Zou H, Dai J, Feng X, Peng L. A comparison of low-cycle fatigue behavior between the solutionized and aged Mg-3Nd-0.2Zn-0.5Zr alloys. Materials Science and Engineering: A. 2017, 695, 342–49.

[179] Mirza FA, Chen DL, Li DJ, Zeng XQ. Low cycle fatigue of an extruded Mg–3Nd–0.2Zn–0.5Zr magnesium alloy. Materials & Design. 2014, 64, 63–73.

[180] Tan L, Zhang X, Sun Q, Yu J, Liu Q. Pyramidal slips in high cycle fatigue deformation of a rolled Mg-3Al-1Zn magnesium alloy. Materials Science and Engineering: A. 2017, 699, 247–53.

[181] Okayasu M, Takeuchi S. Mechanical strength and failure characteristics of cast Mg–9%Al–1%Zn alloys produced by a heated-mold continuous casting process: Fatigue properties. Materials Science and Engineering: A. 2014, 600, 211–20.

[182] Pan J, Fu P, Peng L, Hu B, Luo AA. Basal slip dominant fatigue damage behavior in a cast Mg-8Gd-3Y-Zr alloy. International Journal of Fatigue. 2019, 118, 104–16.

[183] He C, Shao X, Yuan S, Peng L, Chen Q. Small crack initiation and early propagation in an as-extruded Mg-10Gd-3Y-0.5Zr alloy in high cycle fatigue regime. Materials Science and Engineering: A. 2019, 744, 716–23.

[184] Dong J, Liu WC, Song X, Zhang P, Korsunsky AM. Influence of heat treatment on fatigue behaviour of high-strength Mg–10Gd–3Y alloy. Materials Science and Engineering: A. 2010, 527, 6053–63.

[185] Liu W, Jiang L, Cao L, Mei J, Ding W. Fatigue behavior and plane-strain fracture toughness of sand-cast Mg–10Gd–3Y–0.5Zr magnesium alloy. Materials & Design. 2014, 59, 466–74.

[186] Yang F, Lv F, Yang XM, Li SX, Wang QD. Enhanced very high cycle fatigue performance of extruded Mg–12Gd–3Y–0.5Zr magnesium alloy. Materials Science and Engineering: A. 2011, 528, 2231–38.

[187] Yu D, Zhang D, Dai Q, Lan W, Pan F. Effect of stress ratio on high cycle fatigue properties in Mg-6Zn-1Mn alloy. Materials Science and Engineering: A. 2018, 711, 624–32.

[188] Yu D, Zhang D, Luo Y, Sun J, Pan F. Microstructure evolution during high cycle fatigue in Mg–6Zn–1Mn alloy. Materials Science and Engineering: A. 2016, 658, 99–108.

[189] Yu D, Zhang D, Sun J, Luo Y, Pan F. High cycle fatigue behavior of extruded and double-aged Mg-6Zn-1Mn alloy. Materials Science and Engineering: A. 2016, 662, 1–8.
[190] Liu Z-H, Han E-H, Liu L. High-cycle fatigue behavior of Mg–Zn–Y–Zr alloy. Materials Science and Engineering: A. 2008, 483/484, 373–75.
[191] Xu DK, Liu L. Xu YB, Han EH. The fatigue crack propagation behavior of the forged Mg–Zn–Y–Zr alloy. Journal of Alloys and Compounds. 2007, 431, 107–11.
[192] Li ZM, Fu PH, Peng LM, Wang YX, Wu GH. Comparison of high cycle fatigue behaviors of Mg–3Nd–0.2Zn–Zr alloy prepared by different casting processes. Materials Science and Engineering: A. 2013, 579, 170–79.
[193] Peng LM, Fu PH, Li ZM, Yue HY, Wang YX. High cycle fatigue behaviors of low pressure cast Mg-3Nd-0.2Zn-2Zr alloys. Materials Science and Engineering: A. 2014, 611, 170–76.
[194] Oshida Y, Tominaga T. NiTi Materials: Biomedical Applications. De Gruyter Pub., Berlin, 2020, pp.726–28.
[195] Shen Z, Zhao M, Zhou X, Yang H, Yang JA. A numerical corrosion-fatigue model for biodegradable Mg alloy stents. Acta Biomaterialia. 2019, 97, 671–80.
[196] Wang BJ, Xu DK, Wang SD, Sheng LY, Han E-H. Influence of solution treatment on the corrosion fatigue behavior of an as-forged Mg-Zn-Y-Zr alloy. International Journal of Fatigue. 2019, 120, 46–55.
[197] Wang SD, Xu DK, Wang BJ, Han EH, Dong C. Effect of corrosion attack on the fatigue behavior of an as-cast Mg–7%Gd–5%Y–1%Nd–0.5%Zr alloy. Materials & Design. 2015, 84, 185–93.
[198] Chen G, Lu L-T, Cui Y, Xing R-S, Chen X. Ratcheting and low-cycle fatigue characterizations of extruded AZ31B Mg alloy with and without corrosive environment. International Journal of Fatigue. 2015, 80, 364–71.
[199] Bian D, Zhou W, Liu Y, Li N, Sun Z. Fatigue behaviors of HP-Mg, Mg–Ca and Mg–Zn–Ca biodegradable metals in air and simulated body fluid. Acta Biomaterialia. 2016, 41, 351–60.
[200] Wu L-Y, Li H-T, Yang Z. Microstructure evolution during heat treatment of Mg–Gd–Y–Zn–Zr alloy and its low-cycle fatigue behavior at 573 K. Transactions of Nonferrous Metals Society of China. 2017, 27, 1026–35.
[201] Oshida Y, Daly J. Fatigue damage evaluation of shot peened high strength aluminum ally. In: Meguid SA ed., Surface Engineering. Elsevier, New NY, 1990, 404–16.
[202] Liu WC, Zhang DP, Korsunsky AM, Ding WJ. Improvement of fatigue properties by shot peening for Mg–10Gd–3Y alloys under different conditions. Materials Science and Engineering: A. 2011, 528, 5935–44.
[203] Liu W, Wu G, Zhai C, Ding W, Korsunsky AM. Grain refinement and fatigue strengthening mechanisms in as-extruded Mg–6Zn–0.5Zr and Mg–10Gd–3Y–0.5Zr magnesium alloys by shot peening. International Journal of Plasticity. 2013, 49, 16–35.
[204] Mo N, Tan Q, Bermingham M, Huang Y, Zhang M-X. Current development of creep-resistant magnesium cast alloys: A review. Materials & Design. 2018, 155, 422–42.
[205] Magnesium Alloys Properties on Elevated Temperatures, Total Materia; https://www.totalmateria.com/page.aspx?ID=CheckArticle&site=ktn&NM=45.
[206] Spigarelli S. Constitutive equations in creep of Mg–Al alloys. Materials Science and Engineering: A. 2008, 492, 153–60.
[207] Terada Y et al. Creep characteristics of a hypoeutectic Mg–Ca binary alloy with a near-fully lamellar microstructure. Scripta Materialia. 2011, 64, 1039–42.
[208] Liu H et al. The microstructure, tensile properties, and creep behavior of as-cast Mg–(1–10)% Sn alloys. Journal of Alloys and Compounds. 2007, 440, 122–26.
[209] Kang DH et al. Effect of nano-particles on the creep resistance of Mg–Sn based alloys. Materials Science and Engineering: A. 2007, 449/451, 318–21.

[210] Nayyeri G et al. Enhanced creep properties of a cast Mg–5Sn alloy subjected to aging-treatment. Materials Science and Engineering: A. 2010, 18/19, 4613–18.
[211] Liu H et al. Tensile and indentation creep behavior of Mg–5% Sn and Mg–5% Sn–2% Di alloys. Materials Science and Engineering: A. 2007, 464, 124–28.
[212] Gibson MA et al. The effect of precipitate state on the creep resistance of Mg–Sn alloys. Scripta Materialia. 2010, 63, 899–902.
[213] Wei S et al. Compressive creep behavior of as-cast and aging-treated Mg–5wt% Sn alloys. Materials Science and Engineering: A. 2008, 492, 20–23.
[214] Choudhuri D et al. Role of Zn in enhancing the creep resistance of Mg–RE alloys. Scripta Materialia. 2014, 86, 32–35.
[215] Tanhaee Z et al. The microstructure and creep characteristics of cast Mg–3Si and Mg–3Si–1Gd alloys. Materials Science and Engineering: A. 2016, 673, 148–57.
[216] Alizadeh R et al. Creep mechanisms in an Mg–4Zn alloy in the as-cast and aged conditions. Materials Science and Engineering: A. 2013, 564, 423–30.
[217] Spigarelli S et al. Constitutive equations in creep of wrought Mg–Zn alloys. Materials Science and Engineering: A. 2009, 527, 126–31.
[218] Wang J et al. Creep behaviors of a highly concentrated Mg-18 wt%Gd binary alloy with and without artificial aging. Journal of Alloys and Compounds. 2019, 774, 1036–45.
[219] Bhatia MA et al. Atomic-scale investigation of creep behavior in anocrystalline Mg and Mg–Y alloys. Acta Materialia. 2015, 99, 382–91.
[220] Xiao Z et al. Influence of pre-straining on creep behaviors of Mg–2Y alloy sheets. Journal of Alloys and Compounds. 2019, 806, 19–32.
[221] Choudhuri D et al. Role of applied uniaxial stress during creep testing on precipitation in Mg–Nd alloys. Materials Science and Engineering: A. 2014, 612, 140–52.
[222] Yan J et al. Creep behavior of Mg–2wt.%Nd binary alloy. Materials Science and Engineering: A. 2009, 524, 102–07.
[223] Terada Y et al. Assessment of creep rupture life of heat resistant Mg–Al–Ca alloys. Journal of Alloys and Compounds. 2010, 504, 261–64.
[224] Saddock ND et al. Grain-scale creep processes in Mg–Al–Ca base alloys: Implications for alloy design. Scripta Materialia. 2010, 63, 692–97.
[225] Homma T et al. Unexpected influence of Mn addition on the creep properties of a cast Mg–2Al–2Ca (mass%) alloy. Acta Materialia. 2011, 59, 7662–72.
[226] Xiao D et al. Microstructure, mechanical and creep properties of high Ca/Al ratio Mg-Al-Ca alloy. Materials Science and Engineering: A. 2016, 660, 166–71.
[227] Samimi G et al. Improvement in impression creep property of as-cast AC515 Mg alloy by Mn addition. Materials Science and Engineering: A. 2013, 587, 213–20.
[228] Bai J et al. Effect of extrusion on microstructures, and mechanical and creep properties of Mg–Al–Sr and Mg–Al–Sr–Ca alloys. Scripta Materialia. 2006, 55, 1163–66.
[229] Kim BH et al. Microstructure, tensile properties and creep behavior of Mg–4Al–2Sn containing Ca alloy produced by different casting technologies. Materials Science and Engineering: A. 2012, 535, 40–47.
[230] Terada Y et al. Creep life assessment of a die-cast Mg–5Al–0.3Mn alloy. Materials Science and Engineering: A. 2013, 584, 63–66.
[231] Bai J et al. Microstructures and creep properties of Mg–4Al–(1–4) La alloys produced by different casting techniques. Materials Science and Engineering: A. 2012, 552, 472–80.
[232] Yang Q et al. Creep behavior of high-pressure die-cast Mg-4Al-4La-0.4Mn alloy under medium stresses and at intermediate temperatures. Materials Science and Engineering: A. 2016, 650, 190–96.

[233] Zhu Sm et al. Analysis of the creep behaviour of die-cast Mg–3Al–1Si alloy. Materials Science and Engineering: A. 2013, 578, 377–82.

[234] Bai J et al. Microstructures and creep behavior of as-cast and annealed heat-resistant Mg–4Al–2Sr–1Ca alloy. Materials Science and Engineering: A. 2012, 531, 130–40.

[235] Somokawa H et al. Dislocation creep behavior in Mg–Al–Zn alloys. Materials Science and Engineering: A. 2005, 407, 53–61.

[236] Ansary Sh et al. Creep of AZ31 Mg alloy: A comparison of impression and tensile behavior. Materials Science and Engineering: A. 2012, 556, 9–14.

[237] Mahmudi R et al. Shear punch creep characteristics of Mg–3Al–1Zn thin sheets. Materials Science and Engineering: A. 2013, 561, 441–44.

[238] Lee TJ et al. Importance of diffusional creep in fine grained Mg–3Al–1Zn alloys. Materials Science and Engineering: A. 2013, 580, 133–41.

[239] Sambhava K et al. Model based phenomenological and experimental investigation of nanoindentation creep in pure Mg and AZ61 alloy. Materials & Design. 2016, 105, 142–51.

[240] Unigovski YB et al. Corrosion creep and fatigue behavior of magnesium (Mg) alloys. corrosion of magnesium alloys. Woodhead Publishing Series in Metals and Surface Engineering. 2011, 365–402.

[241] Yang Q et al. Deteriorated tensile creep resistance of a high-pressure die-cast Mg–4Al–4RE–0.3Mn alloy induced by substituting part RE with Ca. Materials Science and Engineering: A. 2018, 716, 120–28.

[242] Mondal K et al. Correlation of microstructure and creep behaviour of MRI230D Mg alloy developed by two different casting technologies. Materials Science and Engineering: A. 2015, 631, 45–51.

[243] Amberger D et al. On the importance of a connected hard-phase skeleton for the creep resistance of Mg alloys. Acta Materialia. 2012, 60, 2277–89.

[244] Lamm S et al. Impact of Mn on the precipitate structure and creep resistance of Ca containing magnesium alloys. Materials Science and Engineering: A. 2019, 761; https://doi.org/10.1016/j.msea.2019.05.094.

[245] Zhu SM et al. The influence of minor Mn additions on creep resistance of die-cast Mg–Al–RE alloys. Materials Science and Engineering: A. 2017, 682, 535–41.

[246] Zhu SM et al. Microstructural analysis of the creep resistance of die-cast Mg–4Al–2RE alloy. Scripta Materialia. 2008, 58, 477–80.

[247] Zhang Y et al. Effect of Ca and Sr on the compressive creep behavior of Mg–4Al–RE based magnesium alloys. Materials & Design. 2014, 63, 439–45.

[248] Wittke P et al. Corrosion fatigue assessment of creep-resistant magnesium alloy Mg–4Al–2Ba–2Ca in aqueous sodium chloride solution. International Journal of Fatigue. 2016, 83, 59–65.

[249] Wittke P et al. Mechanism-oriented characterization of the load direction-dependent cyclic creep behavior of the magnesium alloys Mg-4Al-2Ba-2Ca and AE42 at room temperature. Engineering Failure Analysis. 2019, 103, 124–31.

[250] Majhi J et al. Microstructure and impression creep characteristics of squeeze-cast AZ91 magnesium alloy containing Ca and/or Bi. Materials Science and Engineering: A. 2019, 744, 691–703.

[251] Geranmayeh AR et al. Compressive and impression creep behavior of a cast Mg–Al–Zn–Si alloy. Materials Chemistry and Physics. 2013, 139, 79–86.

[252] Zou H-H. Effects of microstructure on creep behavior of Mg-5%Zn-2%Al(-2%Y) alloy. Transactions of Nonferrous Metals Society of China. 2008, 18, 580–87.

[253] Peng L et al. Impression creep of a Mg-8Zn-4Al-0.5Ca alloy. Materials Science and Engineering: A. 2005, 410/411, 42–47.

[254] Wan X-F et al. Microstructure, mechanical properties and creep resistance of Mg–(8%–12%) Zn–(2%–6%)Al alloys. Transactions of Nonferrous Metals Society of China. 2013, 23, 896–903.
[255] Yang M et al. Effects of Gd addition on as-cast microstructure, tensile and creep properties of Mg–3.8 Zn–2.2Ca (wt%) magnesium alloy. Materials Science and Engineering: A. 2013, 587, 132–42.
[256] Naghdi F et al. Threshold creep behaviour of an aged Mg–Zn–Ca alloy. Materials Science and Engineering: A. 2017, 696, 536–43.
[257] Wei J et al. Microstructure, tensile properties and creep resistance of sub-rapidly solidified Mg-Zn-Sn-Al-Ca alloys. Rare Metal Materials and Engineering. 2014, 43, 2602–08.
[258] Jono Y et al. Quantitative evaluation of creep strain distribution in an extruded Mg–Zn–Gd alloy of multimodal microstructure. Acta Materialia. 2015, 82, 198–211.
[259] Spigarelli S et al. Enhanced plasticity and creep in an extruded Mg–Zn–Zr alloy. Scripta Materialia. 2010, 63, 617–20.
[260] Zheng J et al. Effect of Sm on the microstructure, mechanical properties and creep behavior of Mg–0.5Zn–0.4Zr based alloys. Materials Science and Engineering: A. 2010, 527, 1677–85.
[261] Li J et al. Tensile and creep behaviors of Mg–5Zn–2.5Er alloy improved by icosahedral quasicrystal. Materials Science and Engineering: A. 2010, 527, 1255–59.
[262] Li H et al. Creep properties and controlled creep mechanism of as-cast Mg-5Zn-2.5Er alloy. Transactions of Nonferrous Metals Society of China. 2010, 20, 1212–16. Mg-Zn-Cu-Re.
[263] Golmakaniyoon S et al. Microstructure and creep behavior of the rare-earth doped Mg–6Zn–3Cu cast alloy. Materials Science and Engineering: A. 2011, 528, 1668–77.
[264] Jiang B et al. Creep behaviors of Mg–5Li–3Al–(0,1)Ca alloys. Materials & Design. 2012, 34, 863–66.
[265] Mahmudi R et al. Effect of Li content on the indentation creep characteristics of cast Mg-Li-Zn alloys. Materials & Design. 2015, 75, 184–90.
[266] Gao X et al. Precipitation-hardened Mg–Ca–Zn alloys with superior creep resistance. Scripta Materialia. 2005, 53, 1321–26.
[267] Kielbus A et al. Mechanical and creep properties of Mg-4Y-3RE and Mg-3Nd-1Gd magnesium alloy. Procedia Engineering. 2011, 10, 1835–40.
[268] Wang S et al. On the evolution of β' precipitate during creep in a Mg–3.3Y–0.1Zr(at.%) alloy. Materials Characterization. 2019, 147, 414–20.
[269] Fang Z et al. Creep behaviors of hot compressed Mg-4Y-2Nd-0.2Zn-0.5Zr alloy with and without aging. Materials Science and Engineering: A. 2017, 708, 460–68.
[270] Bhattacharyya JJ et al. Deformation and fracture behavior of Mg alloys, WE43, after various aging heat treatments. Materials Science and Engineering: A. 2017, 705, 79–88.
[271] Kang YH et al. Creep behavior and microstructure evolution of sand–cast Mg–4Y–2.3Nd–1Gd–0.6Zr alloy crept at 523–573 K. Journal of Materials Science & Technology. 2017, 33, 79–89.
[272] Li R et al. Different precipitation hardening behaviors of extruded Mg–6Gd–1Ca alloy during artificial aging and creep processes. Materials Science and Engineering: A. 2018, 715, 186–93.
[273] Srinivasan A et al. Creep behavior of Mg–10Gd–xZn (x=2 and 6wt%) alloys. Materials Science and Engineering: A. 2016, 649, 158–67.
[274] Xu C et al. Improving creep property of Mg–Gd–Zn alloy via trace Ca addition. Scripta Materialia. 2017, 139, 34–38.
[275] Xu WF et al. Formation of denuded zones in crept Mg–2.5Gd–0.1Zr alloy. Acta Materialia. 2015, 84, 317–29.

[276] Liu H et al. A simulation study of the distribution of β′ precipitates in a crept Mg-Gd-Zr alloy. Computational Materials Science. 2017, 130, 152–64.
[277] Liu X-B et al. Creep behavior of ageing hardened Mg-10Gd-3Y alloy. Transactions of Nonferrous Metals Society of China. 2010, 20, s545–s549. Mg-Gd-Y-Zr.
[278] Chen X et al. Tensile creep behavior and microstructure evolution of Mg-11Gd-2Y-0.5Zr alloy. Vacuum. 2019, 167, 421–27.
[279] Wang H et al. The impression creep behavior and microstructure evolution of cast and cast-then-extruded Mg–10Gd–3Y–0.5Zr (wt%). Materials Science and Engineering: A. 2016, 649, 313–24.
[280] Yuan J et al. Creep behavior of Mg–9Gd–1Y–0.5Zr (wt.%) alloy piston by squeeze casting. Materials Characterization. 2013, 78, 37–46.
[281] Xu C et al. Enhancing strength and creep resistance of Mg–Gd–Y–Zn–Zr alloy by substituting Mn for Zr. Journal of Magnesium and Alloys. 2019, 7, 388–99.
[282] Zhu X et al. Microstructure and creep behaviour of Mg-12Gd-3Y-1Zn-0.4Zr alloy. Journal of Rare Earths. 2013, 31, 186–91.
[283] Yuan L et al. Effect of heat treatment on elevated temperature tensile and creep properties of the extruded Mg–6Gd–4Y–Nd–0.7Zr alloy. Materials Science and Engineering: A. 2016, 658, 339–47.
[284] Poddar P et al. Creep behaviour of Mg–8% Sn and Mg–8% Sn–3% Al–1% Si alloys. Materials Science and Engineering: A. 2012, 545, 103–10.
[285] Lee SG et al. Investigation on microstructure and creep properties of as-cast and aging-treated Mg–6Sn–5Al–2Si alloy. Materials Science and Engineering: A. 2011, 528, 5394–99.
[286] Kang DH et al. Development of creep resistant die cast Mg–Sn–Al–Si alloy. Materials Science and Engineering: A. 2005, 413/414, 555–60.
[287] Khalipour H et al. The microstructure and impression creep behavior of cast Mg–4Sn–4Ca alloy. Materials Science and Engineering: A. 2016, 652, 365–69.
[288] Nayyeri G et al. The microstructure and impression creep behavior of cast, Mg–5Sn–xCa alloys. Materials Science and Engineering: A. 2010, 527, 2087–98.
[289] Nayyeri G et al. Effects of Sb additions on the microstructure and impression creep behavior of a cast Mg–5Sn alloy. Materials Science and Engineering: A. 2010, 527, 669–78.
[290] Zhang X-P et al. Microstructure, tensile properties and compressive creep resistance of Mg-(5–8.5)%Sn-2%La alloys. Transactions of Nonferrous Metals Society of China. 2008, 18, s299–s305.
[291] Wei S et al. Compressive creep behavior of Mg–Sn–La alloys. Materials Science and Engineering: A. 2009, 508, 59–63.
[292] Celikin M et al. Microstructural investigation and the creep behavior of Mg–Sr–Mn alloys. Materials Science and Engineering: A. 2012, 550, 39–50.
[293] Celikin M et al. Dynamic co-precipitation of α-Mn /Mg12Ce in creep resistant Mg-Sr-Mn-Ce alloys. Materials Science and Engineering: A. 2018, 719, 199–205.
[294] Celikin M et al. Effects of manganese on the microstructure and dynamic precipitation in creep-resistant cast Mg–Ce–Mn alloy. Scripta Materialia. 2012, 66, 737–40.
[295] Yang H et al. Influences of Al and high shearing dispersion technique on the microstructure and creep resistance of Mg-2.85Nd-0.92Gd-0.41Zr-0.29Zn alloy. Materials Science and Engineering: A. 2019, 764; https://doi.org/10.1016/j.msea.2019.138215.
[296] Han W et al. Creep properties and creep microstructure evolution of Mg-2.49Nd-1.82Gd-0.19Zn-0.4Zr alloy. Materials Science and Engineering: A. 2017, 684, 90–100.
[297] Garvas S et al. On the microstructural factors affecting creep resistance of die-cast Mg–La-rare earth (Nd, Y or Gd) alloys. Materials Science and Engineering: A. 2016, 675, 65–75.

[298] Mondal AK, Kumar S, Blawert C, Dahorte NB. Effect of laser surface treatment on corrosion and wear resistance of ACM720 Mg alloy. Surface and Coatings Technology. 2008, 202, 3187–98.
[299] Arora HS, Singh H, Dhindaw BK. Wear behaviour of a Mg alloy subjected to friction stir processing. Wear. 2013, 303, 65–77.
[300] Sun X, Nouri M, Wang Y, Li DY. Corrosive wear resistance of Mg–Al–Zn alloys with alloyed yttrium. Wear. 2013, 302, 1624–32.
[301] Ge M-Z, Xiang J-Y, Tang Ym, Ye Xm Zhang XH. Wear behavior of Mg-3Al-1Zn alloy subjected to laser shock peening. Surface and Coatings Technology. 2018, 337, 501–09.
[302] Li Q, Lu H, Li DY. Effect of recovery treatment on the wear resistance of surface hammered AZ31 Mg alloy. Wear 2019, 426/427, 981–88.
[303] Guo P, Tang M, Zhang C. Tribological and corrosion resistance properties of graphite composite coating on AZ31 Mg alloy surface produced by plasma electrolytic oxidation. Surface and Coatings Technology. 2019, 359, 197–205.
[304] Ram PT. Effect of synthetic graphite and activated charcoal addition on the mechanical, microstructure and wear properties of AZ 81 Mg alloys. Journal of Materials Research and Technology. 2016, 5, 259–67.
[305] Demirci EE, Arslan E, Ezirmik KV, Baran Ö, Efeoglu İ. Investigation of wear, corrosion and tribocorrosion properties of AZ91 Mg alloy coated by micro arc oxidation process in the different electrolyte solutions. Thin Solid Films. 2013, 528, 116–22.
[306] Liu Y, Shao S, Xu C, Yang X, Lu D. Enhancing wear resistance of Mg–Zn–Gd alloy by cryogenic treatment. Materials Letters. 2012, 76, 201–04.
[307] Chen J, Lu S, Tan L, Etim IP, Yang K. Comparative study on effects of different coatings on biodegradable and wear properties of Mg-2Zn-1Gd-0.5Zr alloy. Surface and Coatings Technology. 2018, 352, 273–84.
[308] Ramesh S, Anne G, Nayaka HS, Sahu S, Ramesh MR. Investigation of dry sliding wear properties of multi-directional forged Mg–Zn alloys. Journal of Magnesium and Alloys. 2019; 7, 444–55.
[309] Ma C, Zhang M, Yuan Y, Jing X, Bai X. Tribological behavior of plasma electrolytic oxidation coatings on the surface of Mg–8Li–1Al alloy. Tribology International. 2012, 47, 62–68.
[310] Sikdar K, Shekhar S, Balani K. Fretting wear of Mg–Li–Al based alloys. Wear. 2014, 318, 177–87.
[311] Goretta KC, Cunningham AJ, Chen N, Singh D, Rateick Jr RG. Solid-particle erosion of an anodized Mg alloy. Wear. 2007, 262, 1056–60.
[312] Somekawa H, Maeda S, Hirayama T, Matsuoka T, Mukai T. Microstructural evolution during dry wear test in magnesium and Mg–Y alloy. Materials Science and Engineering: A. 2013, 561, 371–77.
[313] Hu M-L, Wang Q-D, Li C, Ding W-J. Dry sliding wear behavior of cast Mg–11Y–5Gd–2Zn magnesium alloy. Transactions of Nonferrous Metals Society of China. 2012, 22, 1918–23.
[314] Huang Z, Li W, Fan X, Zeng Y, Zhu M. Probing fretting behavior of Mg–Sn–Y alloy under high-performance fluids lubrication. Tribology International. 2019, 138, 125–39.
[315] Yadav L, Dondapati S. Effect of calcium on mechanical and tribological properties of Mg-Sn alloy system fabricated by powder metallurgy (PM) process. Materials Today: Proceedings. 2018, 5, 3735–44.
[316] Zhang J, Zhang X, Liu Q, Yang S, Wang Z. Effects of Load on Dry Sliding Wear Behavior of Mg-Gd-Zn-Zr Alloys. Journal of Materials Science & Technology. 2017, 33, 645–51.
[317] Hu M, Wang Q, Chen C, Yin D, Li Z. Dry sliding wear behaviour of Mg–10Gd–3Y–0.4Zr alloy. Materials & Design. 2012, 42, 223–29.

[318] Hu M-L, Wang Q-D, Ji Z-S, Xu H-Y, Ma G-R. Wear behavior of Mg–10Y–4Gd–1.5Zn–0.4Zr alloy. Transactions of Nonferrous Metals Society of China. 2016, 26, 406–13.
[319] Cao L-J. Wu Y-J, Peng L-M, Wang Q-D, Ding W-J. Microstructure and tribological behavior of Mg–Gd–Zn–Zr alloy with LPSO structure. Transactions of Nonferrous Metals Society of China. 2014, 24, 3785–91.
[320] Itoi T, Gonda K, Hirohashi M. Relationship of wear properties to basal-plane texture of worn surface of Mg alloys. Wear. 2011, 270, 606–12.
[321] Bi G, Li Y, Huang X, Chen T, Hao Y. Dry sliding wear behavior of an extruded Mg–Dy–Zn alloy with long period stacking ordered phase. Journal of Magnesium and Alloys. 2015, 3, 63–69.
[322] Kaviti RVP, Jeyasimman D, Parande G, Gupta M, Narayanasamy R. Investigation on dry sliding wear behavior of Mg/BN nanocomposites. Journal of Magnesium and Alloy. 2018, 6, 263–76.
[323] Zhang L, Luo X, Liu J, Leng Y, An L. Dry sliding wear behavior of Mg-SiC nano-composites with high volume fractions of reinforcement. Materials Letters. 2018, 228, 112–15.
[324] Banerjee S, Poria S, Sutradhar G, Sahoo P. Wear performance of Mg-WC metal matrix nanocomposites using Taguchi methodology. Materials Today: Proceedings. 2019, 19, 177–81.
[325] Arab M, Marashi SPH. Effect of graphene nanoplatelets (GNPs) content on improvement of mechanical and tribological properties of AZ31 Mg matrix nanocomposite. Tribology International. 2019, 132, 1–10.
[326] Kondaiah VV, Pavanteja P, Afzal Khan P, Kumar A, Sunil BR. Microstructure, hardness and wear behavior of AZ31 Mg alloy – fly ash composites produced by friction stir processing. Materials Today: Proceedings. 2017, 4, 6671–77.
[327] Khan MD F, Panigrahi SK. Age hardening, fracture behavior and mechanical properties of QE22 Mg alloy. Journal of Magnesium and Alloys. 2015, 3, 210–17.
[328] https://www.slideserve.com/arella/fracture-toughness-fatigue-and-creep.
[329] Gao L, Chen R-S, Han E-H. Fracture behavior of high strength Mg-Gd-Y-Zr magnesium alloy. Transactions of Nonferrous Metals Society of China. 2010, 20, 1217–21.
[330] Li J, Suo T, Li Y, Kecskes LJ, Wei Q. Mechanical properties and failure of ECAE processed Mg97Y2Zn1 at different strain rates. Materials Science and Engineering: A. 2019, 762; https://doi.org/10.1016/j.msea.2019.138094.
[331] Lin D, Wang L, Liu Y, Cui J-Z, Le Q-C. Effects of plastic deformation on precipitation behavior and tensile fracture behavior of Mg-Gd-Y-Zr alloy. Transactions of Nonferrous Metals Society of China. 2011, 21, 2160–67.
[332] Ortega Y, Luguey T, Pareja R. Tensile fracture behavior of aging hardened Mg–1Ca and Mg–1Ca–1Zn alloys. Materials Letters. 2008, 62, 3893–95.
[333] Liu K, Wang Q-F, Du W-B, Li S-B, Wang Z-H. Failure mechanism of as-cast Mg-6Zn-2Er alloy during tensile test at room temperature. Transactions of Nonferrous Metals Society of China. 2013, 23, 3193–99.
[334] Gui Z, Kang Z, Li Y. Evolution of the microstructure and fracture characteristics of a Mg-Nd-Zn-Zr-Mn alloy through heat treatment and extrusion. Journal of Alloys and Compounds. 2018, 765, 470–79.
[335] Trojanpvá Z, Donič T, Lukáč P, Palček P, Bašťovanský R. Tensile and fracture properties of an Mg-RE-Zn alloy at elevated temperatures. Journal of Rare Earths. 2014, 32, 564–72.
[336] Jia W, Ma L, Le Q, Zhi C, Liu P. Deformation and fracture behaviors of AZ31B Mg alloy at elevated temperature under uniaxial compression. Journal of Alloys and Compounds. 2019, 783, 863–76.
[337] Yu J-C, Liu Z, Dong Y, Wang Z. Dynamic compressive property and failure behavior of extruded Mg-Gd-Y alloy under high temperatures and high strain rates. Journal of Magnesium and Alloys. 2015, 3, 134–41.

[338] Mine Y, Yoshimura H, Matsuda M, Takashima K, Kawamura Y. Microfracture behaviour of extruded Mg–Zn–Y alloys containing long-period stacking ordered structure at room and elevated temperatures. Materials Science and Engineering: A. 2013, 570, 63–69.
[339] Liu C, Jin L, Dong J, Wang F. The use of the fracture initiation parameter F1 to predict microcrack nucleation at grain boundaries in Mg-2%Gd alloy. Materials & Design. 2016, 111, 369–74.
[340] Yue H, Fu P, Li Z, Peng L. Tensile crack initiation behavior of cast Mg–3Nd–0.2Zn–0.5Zr magnesium alloy. Materials Science and Engineering: A. 2016, 673, 458–66.
[341] Cui X, Yu Z, Liu F, Du Z, Bai P. Influence of secondary phases on crack initiation and propagation during fracture process of as-cast Mg-Al-Zn-Nd alloy. Materials Science and Engineering: A. 2019, 759, 708–14.
[342] Basha DA, Somekawa H, Singh A. Crack propagation along grain boundaries and twins in Mg and Mg–0.3 at.%Y alloy during in-situ straining in transmission electron microscope. Scripta Materialia. 2018, 142, 50–54.
[343] Guo X, Chang K, Chen LQ, Zhou M. Determination of fracture toughness of AZ31 Mg alloy using the cohesive finite element method. Engineering Fracture Mechanics. 2012, 96, 401–15.
[344] Prasad NS, Narasimhan R, Suwas S. Effect of notch acuity on the fracture behavior of AZ31 Mg alloy. Engineering Fracture Mechanics. 2018, 187, 241–61.
[345] Zindal A, Jain J, Prasad R, Singh SS, Cizek P. Correlation of grain boundary precipitate characteristics with fracture and fracture toughness in an Mg-8Al-0.5 Zn alloy. Materials Science and Engineering: A. 2017, 706, 192–200.
[346] Hase T, Ohtagaki T, Yamaguchi M, Ikeo N, Mukai T. Effect of aluminum or zinc solute addition on enhancing impact fracture toughness in Mg–Ca alloys. Acta Materialia. 2016, 104, 283–94.
[347] Wang Q, Xiao L, Liu W, Zhang H, Wu G. Effect of heat treatment on tensile properties, impact toughness and plane-strain fracture toughness of sand-cast Mg-6Gd-3Y-0.5Zr magnesium alloy. Materials Science and Engineering: A. 2017, 705, 402–10.
[348] https://www.slideserve.com/tayte/14-stress-corrosion-cracking-scc.
[349] Scully JC. The interaction of strain-rate and repassivation rate in stress corrosion crack propagation. Corrosion Science. 1980, 20, 997–1016.
[350] Takano M, Nagata T. Hydrogen Indused Stress Corrosion Cracking of Al-4.5 Zn-1.5 Mg Alloy. Corrosion Engineering. 1983, 32, 456–62.
[351] Atrens A, Winzer N, Dietzel W, Srinivasan PB, Song G-L. Stress corrosion cracking (SCC) of magnesium (Mg) alloys. Corrosion of Magnesium Alloys. Woodhead Publishing Series in Metals and Surface Engineering. 2011, pp.299–364.
[352] Jafari S, Harandi SE, Raman RKS. A review of stress-corrosion cracking and corrosion fatigue of magnesium alloys for biodegradable implant applications. Journal of Metals. 2015, 67, 1143–53.
[353] Winzer N, Atrens A, Dietzel W, Song G, Kainer KU. Evaluation of the delayed hydride cracking mechanism for transgranular stress corrosion cracking of magnesium alloys. Materials Science and Engineering: A. 2007, 466, 18–31.
[354] Jones RH, Vetrano JS, Windisch Jr. CF. Stress corrosion cracking of Al-Mg and Mg-Al alloys. Corrosion. 2004, 60, 1144–54.
[355] Wearmouth WR, Dean GP, Parkins RN. Role of stress in the stress corrosion cracking of a Mg-Al alloy. Corrosion. 1973, 29, 251–60.
[356] Makar GL, Kruger J, Sieradzki K. Stress corrosion cracking of rapidly solidified magnesium-aluminum alloys. Corrosion Science. 1993, 34, 1311–42.

[357] Winzer N, Atrens A, Dietzel W, Song G, Kainer KU. Fractography of stress corrosion cracking of Mg-Al alloys. Metallurgical and Materials Transactions A. 2008, 39, 1157–73.
[358] Winzer N, Atrens A, Dietzel W, Song G, Kainer KU. Stress corrosion cracking (SCC) in Mg-Al alloys studied using compact specimens. Advanced Engineering Materials. 2008, 10, 453–58.
[359] Tsao LC. Stress-corrosion cracking susceptibility of AZ31 alloy after varied heat-treatment in 3.5 wt.% NaCl solution. International Journal of Materials Research. 2010, 101, 1166–71.
[360] Kappes M, Iannuzzi M, Carranza RM. Pre-exposure embrittlement and stress corrosion cracking of magnesium alloy AZ31B in chloride solutions. Corrosion. 2014, 70, 667–77.
[361] Kannan MB, Raman RKS. Evaluating the stress corrosion cracking susceptibility of Mg–Al–Zn alloy in modified-simulated body fluid for orthopaedic implant application. Scripta Materialia. 2008, 59, 175–78.
[362] Winzer N, Atrens A, Dietzel W, Song G, Kainer KU. (2008) Comparison of the linearly increasing stress test and the constant extension rate test in the evaluation of transgranular stress corrosion cracking of magnesium. Materials Science and Engineering: A. 2008, 472, 97–106.
[363] Winzer N, Atrens A, Dietzel W, Song G, Kainer KU. Stress corrosion cracking in magnesium alloys: characterization and prevention. Journal of Metals. 2007, 59, 49–53.
[364] Prabhu DB, Dhamotharan S, Sathishkumar G, Gopalakrishnan P, Ravi KR. Stress corrosion cracking of biodegradable Mg-4Zn alloy in simulated body fluid at different strain rates – A fractographic investigation. Materials Science and Engineering: A. 2018, 730, 223–31.
[365] Li Y, Zhou Y, Shi Z, Venezuela J, Atrens A. Stress corrosion cracking of EV31A in 0.1 M Na2SO4 saturated with Mg(OH)2. Journal of Magnesium and Alloys. 2018, 6, 337–45.
[366] Wang SD, Xu DK, Han EH, Dong C. Stress corrosion cracking susceptibility of a high strength Mg-7%Gd-5%Y-1%Nd-0.5%Zr alloy. Journal of Magnesium and Alloys. 2014, 2, 335–41.
[367] Raja VS, Padekar BS. Role of chlorides on pitting and hydrogen embrittlement of Mg–Mn wrought alloy. Corrosion Science. 2013, 75, 176–83.
[368] Pannindre AM, Raja VS, Krishnan A. Explanation for anomalous environmentally assisted cracking behaviour of a wrought Mg–Mn alloy in chloride medium. Corrosion Science. 2017, 115, 8–17.
[369] Kappes M, Iannuzzi M, Carranza RM. Hydrogen Embrittlement of Magnesium and Magnesium Alloys: A Review. Journal of Electrochemical Society. 2013, 160, C168–78.
[370] Silverstein R, Eliezer D, Kamilyan M. Hydrogen trapping and hydrogen embrittlement of Mg alloys. Journal of Materials Science. 2017, 52, 11091–100.
[371] Kannan MB, Dietzel W. Pitting-induced hydrogen embrittlement of magnesium–aluminium alloy. Materials & Design. 2012, 42, 321–26.
[372] Makar GL, Kruger J. Corrosion studies of rapidly solidified magnesium alloys. Journal of the Electrochemical Society. 1990, 137; https://iopscience.iop.org/article/10.1149/1.2086455/meta.
[373] https://www.nipponkinzoku.co.jp/corporate/business/magnesium-alloy.
[374] http://www.tokai.or.jp/tokai/kog/MG/M01.html.
[375] https://cafediecast.com/magnesium-diecast-chemical-composition-and-mechanical-physical-property/.
[376] https://www.ofic.co.jp/mg/magne.htm.
[377] https://material.st-grp.co.jp/technology/magnesium/alloytype/index.html.
[378] Brophy JH, Rose RM, Wulff J. The Structure and Properties of Materials. Vol. II Thermodynamics of Structure. John Wiley & Sons, New York, NY, 29164, pp.75–95.
[379] Das SK, Brodusch N, Gauvin R, Jung I-H. Grain boundary diffusion of Al in Mg. Scripta Materialia. 2014, 80, 41–44.

[380] Wang J, Zheng W, Xu G, Llorca J, Cui Y. High-throughput extraction of the anisotropic interdiffusion coefficients in hcp Mg–Al alloys. Journal of Alloys and Compounds. 2019, 805, 237–46.
[381] Wang F, Li B. Surface and Interfacial Energies of $Mg_{17}Al_{12}$–Mg System. In: Orlov D. et al., ed., Magnesium Technology 2018. TMS 2018. The Minerals, Metals & Materials Series. Springer, 2018, 55–62.
[382] Ouyang Y, Liu K, Peng C, Chen H, Du Y. Investigation of diffusion behavior and mechanical properties of Mg-Zn system. Calphad. 2019, 65, 204–11.
[383] Zhong W, Zhao J-C. Measurements of diffusion coefficients of Ce, Gd and Mn in Mg. Materialia 2019, 7; https://doi.org/10.1016/j.mtla.2019.100353.
[384] Paliwal M, Das SK, Kim J, Jung I-H. Diffusion of Nd in hcp Mg and interdiffusion coefficients in Mg–Nd system. Scripta Materialia. 2015, 108, 11–14.
[385] Zheng W-W, Li X-G, Li Y-J, Shi G-L. Reactive diffusion in Mg–Gd binary system at 773 K. Transactions of Nonferrous Metals Society of China. 2015, 25, 3904–08.
[386] Zhou B-C, Shang S-L, Wang Y, Liu Z-K. Data set for diffusion coefficients of alloying elements in dilute Mg alloys from first-principles. Data in Brief. 2015, 5, 900–12.
[387] Combronde J, Brebec G. Diffusion of Ag, Cd, In, Sn and Sb in magnesium. Acta Metallurgica.. 1972, 20, 37–44.
[388] Stloukal I, Čermák J. Grain boundary diffusion of ^{67}Ga in polycrystalline magnesium. Scripta Materialia. 2003, 49, 557–62.
[389] Fujikawa SI. Impurity diffusion of manganese in magnesium. Journal of Japan Institute of Light Metals. 1992, 42, 826–27.
[390] Das SK, Kang YB, Ha T, Jung IH. Thermodynamic modeling and diffusion kinetic experiments of binary Mg–Gd and Mg–Y systems. Acta Mater. 2014, 71, 164–75.
[391] Yuan J, Zhang K, Li T, Li X, Hao Y. Anisotropy of thermal conductivity and mechanical properties in Mg–5Zn–1Mn alloy. Materials & Design. 2012, 40, 257–61.
[392] Wang C, Cui Z, Liu H, Chen Y, Xiao S. Electrical and thermal conductivity in Mg–5Sn Alloy at different aging status. Materials & Design. 2015, 84, 48–52.
[393] Peng J, Zhong L, Wang Y, Lu Y, Pan F. Effect of extrusion temperature on the microstructure and thermal conductivity of Mg–2.0Zn–1.0Mn–0.2Ce alloys. Materials & Design. 2015, 87, 914–19.
[394] Ying T, Zheng MY, Li ZT, Qiao XQ, Xu SW. Thermal conductivity of as-cast and as-extruded binary Mg–Zn alloys. Journal of Alloys and Compounds. 2015, 621, 250–55.
[395] Liu YF, Jia XJ, Qiao XG, Xu SW, Zheng MY. Effect of La content on microstructure, thermal conductivity and mechanical properties of Mg–4Al magnesium alloys. Journal of Alloys and Compounds. 2019, 806, 71–78.
[396] Zhu W-F, Luo Q, Zhang J-Y, Li Q. Phase equilibria of Mg-La-Zr system and thermal conductivity of selected alloys. Journal of Alloys and Compounds. 2018, 731, 784–95.
[397] Chen CJ, Wang QD, Yin DD. Thermal properties of Mg–11Y–5Gd–2Zn–0.5Zr (wt.%) alloy. Journal of Alloys and Compounds. 2009, 487, 560–63.
[398] Wang C, Chen Y, Xiao S, Ding W, Liu X. Thermal Conductivity and Mechanical Properties of as-Cast Mg-3Zn-(0.5–3.5)Sn Alloys. Rare Metal Materials and Engineering. 2013, 42, 2019–22.
[399] Su C, Li D, Luo AA, Ying T, Zeng X. Effect of solute atoms and second phases on the thermal conductivity of Mg-RE alloys: A quantitative study. Journal of Alloys and Compounds. 2018, 747, 431–37.
[400] Peng J, Zhong L, Wang Y, Yang J, Pan F. Effect of Ce addition on thermal conductivity of Mg–2Zn–1Mn alloy. Journal of Alloys and Compounds. 2015, 639, 556–62.

[401] Zhong L, Peng J, Sun S, Wang Y, Pan F. Microstructure and thermal conductivity of As-Cast and As-solutionized Mg–rare earth binary alloys. Journal of Materials Science & Technology. 2017, 33, 1240–48.
[402] Li B, Hou L, Wu R, Zhang J, Sun B. Microstructure and thermal conductivity of Mg-2Zn-Zr alloy. Journal of Alloys and Compounds. 2017, 722, 772–77.
[403] Zhong L, Peng J, Li M, Wang Y, Pan F. Effect of Ce addition on the microstructure, thermal conductivity and mechanical properties of Mg–0.5Mn alloys. Journal of Alloys and Compounds. 2016, 661, 402–10.
[404] Yakubtsov IA. Effects of composition and microstructure on behaviors of electrical resistivity during continuous heating above room temperature in Mg-based alloys. Journal of Alloys and Compounds. 2010, 492, 153–59.
[405] Pan H, Pan F, Peng J, Gou J, Dong H. High-conductivity binary Mg–Zn sheet processed by cold rolling and subsequent aging. Journal of Alloys and Compounds. 2013, 578, 493–500.
[406] Fu Y, Cao QP, Wang XD, Zhang DX, Jiang JZ. Thickness dependent electrical resistivity in amorphous Mg-Zn-Ca thin films. Thin Solid Films. 2019, 672, 182–85.
[407] Liu L. Chen X, Wang J, Qiao L, Pan F. Effects of Y and Zn additions on electrical conductivity and electromagnetic shielding effectiveness of Mg-Y-Zn alloys. Journal of Materials Science & Technology. 2019, 35, 1074–80.
[408] Geng J, Teng X, Zhou G, Zhao D. Temperature dependence of the electrical resistivity of Mg–Zn–Y quasicrystal alloy. Materials Letters. 2014, 132, 334–37.
[409] Wang X-N, Han L-Z, Gu J-F. Precipitation kinetics of NZ30K-Mg alloys based on electrical resistivity measurement. Transactions of Nonferrous Metals Society of China. 2014, 24, 1690–97.
[410] Rokhlin LL, Nikitina NI. Recovery after ageing of Mg–Y and Mg–Gd alloys. Journal of Alloys and Compounds. 1998, 279, 166–70.
[411] Jalaih K, Mouli C, Babu V, Krishnaiah RV. Structural, electrical and magnetic properties of Mg-Zr co-substituted Ni0.5Zn0.5Fe2O4. Journal of Science: Advanced Materials and Devices. 2019, 4, 310–18.
[412] Hu Y, Cai B, Hu Z, Liu Y, Zeng H. The impact of Mg content on the structural, electrical and optical properties of MgZnO alloy: A first principles study. Current Applied Physics. 2015, 15, 423–28.
[413] Hu Y, Zeng H, Du J, Hu Z, Zhang S. The structural, electrical and optical properties of Mg-doped ZnO with different interstitial Mg concentration. Materials Chemistry and Physics. 2016, 182, 15–21.
[414] Yamada Y, Miura M, Tajima K, Okada M, Yoshimura K. Optical indices of switchable mirrors based on Mg-Y alloy thin films in the transparent state. Thin Solid Films. 2014, 571, 712–14.
[415] Yamada Y, Kitamura S, Miura M, Yoshimura K. Improving the optical properties of switchable mirrors based on Mg–Y alloy using antireflection coatings. Solar Energy Materials and Solar Cells. 2015, 141, 337–40.
[416] Liu Y, Chen J, Peng L, Han J, Chen W. Improved optical properties of switchable mirrors based on Pd/Mg-TiO2 films fabricated by magnetron sputtering. Materials & Design. 2018, 144, 256–62.
[417] Qi S, Yu X, Yu X, Zhang J, Wei J. Effects of non-stoichiometric ratio on optical characteristics of Mg-doped ZnO nanorods. Optical Materials. 2019, 90, 180–86.
[418] Shi S, Xu J, Li L. Effect of Mg concentration on morphological, structural and optical properties of Mg-K co-doped ZnO thin films prepared by sol-gel method. Materials Letters. 2018, 229, 178–81.
[419] Koch N. Supramolecular Materials for Opto-Electronics. Royal Society of Chemistry, Cambridge 2015; https://pubs.rsc.org/en/content/ebook/978-1-78262-694-7.

[420] Si X, Liu Y, Lei W, Xu J, Zheng L. First-principles investigation on the optoelectronic performance of Mg doped and Mg–Al co-doped ZnO. Materials & Design. 2016, 93, 128–32.
[421] Xu Q, Zhang S, Liu B, Tao T, Zhang R. Influence of high Mg doping on the microstructural and opto-electrical properties of AlGaN alloys. Superlattices and Microstructures. 2018, 119, 150–56.
[422] https://www.britannica.com/science/thermoelectricity
[423] Cao Q, Zheng J, Zhang K, Ma G. Thermoelectric properties of YbCd2Sb2 doped by Mg. Journal of Alloys and Compounds. 2016, 680, 278–82.
[424] Chen YX, Yamamoto A, Takeuchi T. Doping effects of Mg for In on the thermoelectric properties of β-In2S3 bulk samples. Journal of Alloys and Compounds. 2017, 695, 1631–36.
[425] Nieroda P, Kolezynski A, Leszczynski J, Nieroda J, Pasierb P. The structural, microstructural and thermoelectric properties of Mg2Si synthesized by SPS method under excess Mg content conditions. Journal of Alloys and Compounds. 2019, 775, 138–49.
[426] Wen LH, Ji ZS, Hu ML, Ning HY. Microstructure and mechanical properties of Mg-3.0Nd-0.4Zn-0.4Zr magnesium alloy. Journal of Magnesium and Alloys. 2014, 2, 85–91.
[427] Wang J, Wu Z, Gao S, Lu R, Qin D, Yang W, Pan F. Optimization of mechanical and damping properties of Mg–0.6Zr alloy by different extrusion processing. Journal of Magnesium and Alloys. 2015, 3, 79–85.
[428] Jun JH. Damping behaviors of as-cast and solution-treated AZ91–Ca magnesium alloys. Journal of Alloys and Compounds. 2014, 610, 169–72.
[429] Li T, He Y, Zhang H, Wang X. Microstructure, mechanical property and in vitro biocorrosion behavior of single-phase biodegradable Mg-1.5Zn-0.6Zr alloy. Journal of Magnesium and Alloys. 2014, 2, 181–89.
[430] Yuan J, Li T, Zhang K, Li M, Shi G. Effect of Zn content on the microstructures, mechanical properties, and damping capacities of Mg–7Gd–3Y–1Nd–0.5Zr based alloys. Journal of Alloys and Compounds. 2019, 773, 919–26.
[431] Niu R-L, Yan F-J, Wang Y-S, Duan D-P, Yang X-M. Effect of Zr content on damping property of Mg–Zr binary alloys. Materials Science and Engineering: A. 2018, 718, 418–26.
[432] Chowdhury ASMF, Mari D, Schaller R. The effect of the orientation of the basal plane on the mechanical loss in magnesium matrix composites studied by mechanical spectroscopy. Acta Mater. 2010, 58, 2555–63.
[433] Wan D, Wang J. Internal Friction Peaks in Mg-0.6% Zr and Mg-Ni High Damping Magnesium Alloys. Rare Metal Materials and Engineering. 2017, 46, 2790–93.
[434] Alciatore DG. Introduction to Mechatronics and Measurement (3rd ed.). McGraw Hill. 2007.
[435] Rao M, Qiu H. Process control engineering: a textbook for chemical, mechanical and electrical engineers. CRC Press. 1993, p.96.
[436] Golnaraghi F, Kuo BC. Automatic Control Systems (9th ed.). NY: Wiley. 2003, pp.236–37.
[437] Cremer L, Heckl M. Structure-Borne Sound: Structural Vibrations and Sound Radiation at Audio Frequencies, Springer-Verlag, New York, 1988.
[438] Irvine T. Damping Properties of Materials. 2010; http://vibrationdata.com/tutorials_alt/damping.pdf.
[439] Du G et al. Damping properties of a novel porous Mg–Al alloy coating prepared by arc ion plating. Surface and Coatings Technology. 2014, 238, 139–42.
[440] Hu Z-S et al. Effect of small tensile deformation on damping capacities of Mg-1%Al alloy. Transactions of Nonferrous Metals Society of China. 2010, 20, s444–s447.
[441] Wan D. Near spherical α-Mg dendrite morphology and high damping of low-temperature casting Mg–1wt.%Ca alloy. Materials Characterization. 2011, 62, 8–11.
[442] Motoyama T et al. Mechanical and damping properties of equal channel angular extrusion-processed Mg–Ca alloys. Materials Letters. 2017, 201, 144–47.

[443] Wan D et al. Damping properties of Mg–Ca binary alloys. Physica B: Condensed Matter. 2008, 403, 2438–42.
[444] Wan D-Q et al. High damping capacities of Mg-Cu based alloys. Transactions of Nonferrous Metals Society of China. 2010, 20, s448–s452.
[445] Hu XS et al. A study of damping capacities in pure Mg and Mg-Ni alloys. Scripta Materialia. 2005, 52, 1141–45.
[446] Wan D-Q et al. Effect of eutectic phase on damping and mechanical properties of as-cast Mg-Ni hypoeutectic alloys. Transactions of Nonferrous Metals Society of China. 2009, 19, 45–49.
[447] Wan D et al. Internal Friction Peaks in Mg-0.6% Zr and Mg-Ni High Damping Magnesium Alloys. Rare Metal Materials and Engineering. 2017, 46, 2790–93.
[448] Wang J et al. Optimization of mechanical and damping properties of Mg–0.6Zr alloy by different extrusion processing. Journal of Magnesium and Alloy. 2015, 3, 79–85.
[449] Niu R-L et al. Effect of Zr content on damping property of Mg–Zr binary alloys. Materials Science and Engineering: A. 2018, 718, 418–26.
[450] Hu XS et al. Low frequency damping capacities and mechanical properties of Mg–Si alloys. Materials Science and Engineering: A. 2007, 452/453, 374–79.
[451] Wan D et al. High damping properties of Mg–Si binary hypoeutectic alloys. Materials Letters. 2009, 63, 391–93.
[452] Wu Z et al. Enhanced damping capacities of Mg–Ce alloy by the special microstructure with parallel second phase. Journal of Materials Science & Technology. 2017, 33, 941–46.
[453] Tang YT et al. Effects of Y content and temperature on the damping capacity of extruded Mg-Y sheets. Journal of Magnesium and Alloy. 2019, 7, 522–28.
[454] Ren LB et al. Effect of heat treatment and pre-deformation on damping capacity of cast Mg-Y binary alloys. Journal of Alloys and Compounds. 2017, 699, 976–82.
[455] Ma N et al. Effect of microalloying with rare-earth on recrystallization behaviour and damping properties of Mg sheets. Journal of Alloys and Compounds. 2014, 592, 24–34.
[456] Liao L et al. Precipitation behavior and damping characteristic of Mg–Al–Si alloy. Materials Letters. 2005, 59, 2702–05.
[457] Wu J et al. Microstructure evolution, damping capacities and mechanical properties of novel Mg-xAl-0.5Ce (wt%) damping alloys. Journal of Alloys and Compounds. 2017, 729, 545–55.
[458] Wang J et al. Microstructure evolution, damping capacities and mechanical properties of novel Mg-xAl-0.5Ce (wt%) damping alloys. Journal of Alloys and Compounds. 2017, 729, 545–55.
[459] Jun J-H. Damping behavior of Mg–Zn–Al casting alloys. Materials Science and Engineering: A. 2016, 665, 86–89.
[460] Wan D et al. Microstructure and high damping properties of Mg-Zn-Y alloys containing LPSO phase and I phase. Rare Metal Materials and Engineering. 2015, 44, 2651–55.
[461] Lu R et al. Effects of heat treatment on the morphology of long-period stacking ordered phase, the corresponding damping capacities and mechanical properties of Mg–Zn–Y alloys. Journal of Alloys and Compounds. 2015, 639, 541–46.
[462] Chen S et al. Effects of Cu on microstructure, mechanical properties and damping capacity of high damping Mg–1%Mn based alloy. Materials Science and Engineering: A. 2012, 551, 87–94.
[463] Zhang Z-Y et al. Effects of Cu and Mn on mechanical properties and damping capacity of Mg-Cu-Mn alloy. Transactions of Nonferrous Metals Society of China. 2008, 18, s55–s58.
[464] Zhou H et al. Influence of rolling on internal friction peak of Mg-3Cu-1Mn alloy. Transactions of Nonferrous Metals Society of China. 2013, 23, 1610–16.
[465] Chen SQ et al. Effects of Cu on microstructure, mechanical properties and damping capacity of as-cast Mg–3%Ni alloy. Advanced Materials Research. 2012, 463/464, 52–57.

[466] Qin D et al. Effect of long period stacking ordered structure on the damping capacities of Mg–Ni–Y alloys. Materials Science and Engineering: A. 2015, 624, 9–13.
[467] Wan D et al. Effect of Mn on damping capacities, mechanical properties, and corrosion behaviour of high damping Mg–3wt.%Ni based alloy. Materials Science and Engineering: A. 2008, 494, 139–42.
[468] Wan D et al. A study of the effect of Y on the mechanical properties, damping properties of high damping Mg–0.6%Zr based alloys. Materials Science and Engineering: A. 2009, 517, 114–17.
[469] Wang J-F et al. Damping properties of as-cast Mg–xLi–1Al alloys with different phase composition. Transactions of Nonferrous Metals Society of China. 2014, 24, 334–38.
[470] Ma R et al. Effect of quasicrystal phase on mechanical properties and damping capacities of Mg–Zn–Y–Zr alloys. Materials Science and Engineering: A. 2013, 587, 328–35.
[471] Ma Q et al. Mechanical and damping properties of thermal treated Mg–Zn–Y–Zr alloys reinforced with quasicrystal phase. Materials Science and Engineering: A. 2014, 602, 11–18.
[472] Yan B et al. Effects of heat treatment on microstructure, mechanical properties and damping capacity of Mg–Zn–Y–Zr alloy. Materials Science and Engineering: A. 2014, 594, 168–77.
[473] Tang Y et al. Effect of long period stacking ordered structure on mechanical and damping properties of as-cast Mg–Zn–Y–Zr alloy. Materials Science and Engineering: A. 2015, 640, 287–94.
[474] Wang J et al. Effects of phase composition on the mechanical properties and damping capacities of as-extruded Mg–Zn–Y–Zr alloys. Journal of Alloys and Compounds. 2011, 509, 8567–72.
[475] Feng H et al. Effect of precipitates on mechanical and damping properties of Mg–Zn–Y–Nd alloys. Materials Science and Engineering: A. 2015, 639, 1–7.
[476] Wang J-F et al. Effects of Y and Zn on mechanical properties and damping capacity of Mg-Cu-Mn alloy. Transactions of Nonferrous Metals Society of China. 2010, 20, 1846–50.
[477] Xu C et al. Microstructure, mechanical and damping properties of Mg–Er–Gd–Zn alloy reinforced with stacking faults. Materials & Design. 2015, 79, 53–59.
[478] Gupta A et al. Abridgment of nano and micro length scale mechanical properties of novel Mg–9Li–7Al–1Sn and Mg–9Li–5Al–3Sn–1Zn alloys using object oriented finite element modeling. Journal of Alloys and Compounds. 2015, 634, 24–31.
[479] Feng H et al. Influence of W-phase on mechanical properties and damping capacity of Mg–Zn–Y–Nd–Zr alloys. Materials Science and Engineering: A. 2014, 609, 7–15.
[480] Feng S et al. Microstructure, mechanical properties and damping capacity of heat-treated Mg–Zn–Y–Nd–Zr alloy. Materials Science and Engineering: A. 2014, 609, 283–92.
[481] Lan A et al. Effect of substitution of minor Nd for Y on mechanical and damping properties of heat-treated Mg–Zn–Y–Zr alloy. Materials Science and Engineering: A. 2016, 651, 646–56.
[482] Wang J et al. Preparation and properties of Mg–Cu–Mn–Zn–Y damping magnesium alloy. Materials Science and Engineering: A. 2011, 528, 6484–88.
[483] Wang J et al. Effect of long period stacking ordered (LPSO) structure on the damping capacities of Mg–Cu–Mn–Zn–Y alloys. Journal of Alloys and Compounds. 2012, 537, 1–5.
[484] Huang X et al. A transmission electron microscopy investigation of defects in an Mg-Cu-Mn-Zn-Y damping alloy. Journal of Alloys and Compounds. 2012, 516, 186–91.
[485] https://www.wisegeek.com/what-is-magnetic-shielding.htm.
[486] https://www.kjmagnetics.com/blog.asp?p=shielding-materials.
[487] https://en.wikipedia.org/wiki/Mu-metal.
[488] Zhang Z-H, Pan F-S, Chen X-H, Liu J. Electromagnetic shielding properties of magnesium alloys. Journal of Materials Engineering. 2013, 3, 52–57.

[489] Chiba M, Hotta H, Nobuki T, Sotoma A, Kuji T. Microstructure dependence of the magnetic properties in fine Mg–Tm (Tm: Co, Fe) particles by using a mechanical alloying technique. Journal of Magnetism and Magnetic Materials. 2007, 316, e454–e457.
[490] Li H, Sun H, Wang C, Wei B, Ma H. Controllable electrochemical synthesis and magnetic behaviors of Mg–Mn–Fe–Co–Ni–Gd alloy films. Journal of Alloys and Compounds. 2014, 598, 161–65.
[491] Morozov IG, Sathasivam S, Belousova OV, Parkin IP, Kuznetcov MV. Effect of synthesis conditions on room-temperature ferromagnetic properties of Mg-O nanoparticles. Journal of Alloys and Compounds. 2018, 765, 343–54.
[492] Pourzaki M, Kavkhani R, Kianvash A, Hajalilou A. Structure, magnetic and transmission characteristics of the Co substituted Mg ferrites synthesized via a standard ceramic route. Ceramics International. 2019, 45, 5710–16.
[493] Kagdi AR, Solanki NP, Carvalho FE, Meena SS, Jotania RB. Influence of Mg substitution on structural, magnetic and dielectric properties of X-type bariumzinc hexaferrites Ba2Zn2-xMgxFe28O46. Journal of Alloys and Compounds. 2018, 741, 377–91.
[494] Li Z-J, Wang X-E, Li J-Y, Wang H-Z. Effects of Mg nanopowders intergranular addition on the magnetic properties and corrosion resistance of sintered Nd-Fe-B. Journal of Magnetism and Magnetic Materials. 2017, 442, 62–66.
[495] Saritaş S, Sakar BC, Kundakci M, Yildirim M. The effect of Mg dopants on magnetic and structural properties of iron oxide and zinc ferrite thin films. Results in Physics. 2018, 9, 416–23.
[496] Fontana MG, Greene ND. Corrosion Engineering. McGraw-Hill, New York NY, 1967.
[497] Persaud-Sharma D, McGoron A. Biodegradable magnesium alloys: a review of material development and applications. Journal of Biomimetics, Biomaterials, and Tissue Engineering. 2012, 12, 25–39.
[498] https://www.epa.gov/sites/production/files/2015-10/documents/ace3_criteria_air_pollutants.pdf.
[499] http://www.creativemethods.com/airquality/ambient/index.htm.
[500] https://www.epa.gov/criteria-air-pollutants/naaqs-table.
[501] Saw BA. Corrosion Resistance of Magnesium Alloys. ASM Handbook. 2003,13, 692–96.
[502] Craig B, Anderson D. Handbook of Corrosion Data. 2nd Edition. ASM International; 1995. p. 998.
[503] Song G-L. Corrosion of Magnesium Alloys. Woodhead Pub, 2011.
[504] Liu H, Cao F, Song G-L, Zheng D, Atens A. Review of the atmospheric corrosion of magnesium alloys. Journal of Materials Science & Technology. 2019, 35, 2003–16.
[505] Song G, Hapugoda S, John DS. Degradation of the surface appearance of magnesium and its alloys in simulated atmospheric environments. Corrosion Science. 2007, 49, 1245–65.
[506] Esmaily E, Svensson JE, Fajardo S, Birbilis N, Frankel GS, Virtanen S, Arrabal R, Thomas S, Johansson LG. Fundamentals and advances in magnesium alloy corrosion. Progress in Materials Science. 2017, 89, 92–193.
[507] Esmaily E, Shahabi-Navid M, Svensson JE, Halvarsson M, Nyborg L, Cao Y, Johansson LG. Influence of temperature on the atmospheric corrosion of the Mg–Al alloy AM50. Corrosion Science. 2015, 90, 420–33.
[508] Song G-L, Liu M. The effect of surface pretreatment on the corrosion performance of Electroless E-coating coated AZ31. Corrosion Science. 2012, 62, 61–72.
[509] LeBozec N, Jonsson M, Thierry D. Atmospheric corrosion of magnesium alloys: influence of temperature, relative humidity, and chloride deposition. Corrosion. 2004, 60, 356–61.
[510] Jönsson M, Persson D, Thierry D. Corrosion product formation during NaCl induced atmospheric corrosion of magnesium alloy AZ91D. Corrosion Science. 2007, 49, 1540–58.

[511] Jönsson M, Persson D, Leygraf C. Atmospheric corrosion of field-exposed magnesium alloy AZ91D. Corrosion Science. 2008, 50, 1406–13.

[512] Zhao M-C, Schmutz P, Brunner S, Liu M, Song G-L, Atrens A. An exploratory study of the corrosion of Mg alloys during interrupted salt spray testing. Corrosion Science. 2009, 51, 1277–92.

[513] Zhou W-Q, Shan D-Y, Han E-H, Ke W. Influence of NaCl deposition on atmospheric corrosion behavior of AZ91 magnesium alloy. Transactions of Nonferrous Metals Society of China. 2010, 20, s670–s673.

[514] Kubaschewski O, Hopkins BE. Oxidation of Metals and Alloys. Butterworths, London, 1962.

[515] Yoo H-L, Wuensch BJ, Petuskey WT. Oxygen self-diffusion in single-crystal MgO: secondary-ion mass spectrometric analysis with comparison of results from gas–solid and solid–solid exchange. Solid State Ionics. 2002, 150, 207–21.

[516] Reddy KPR, Cooper AR. Oxygen Diffusion in MgO and alpha-Fe2O3. Journal of the American Ceramic Society. 2006, 66, 664–66.

[517] Vočadlo L, Wall A, Parker SC, Price GD. Absolute ionic diffusion in MgO computer calculations via lattice dynamics. Physics of the Earth and Planetary Interiors. 1995, 88, 193–210.

[518] Kofstad P. High Temperature Corrosion. 1988. Elsevier Applied Science, London.

[519] McCafferty E. High-Temperature Gaseous Oxidation. In: Introduction to Corrosion Science. 2010. Springer, New York, NY.

[520] Prorok BC, Goretta KC, Park J-H, Balachandran U, McNallan MJ. Oxygen diffusion and internal oxidation of Mg in Ag/1.12at.%Mg. Physica C: Superconductivity. 2002, 370, 31–38.

[521] Xu W, Horsfield AP, Wearing D, Lee PD. Diversification of MgO//Mg interfacial crystal orientations during oxidation: A density functional theory study. Journal of Alloys and Compounds. 2016, 688, 1233–40.

[522] Jeurgens LPH, Vinodh MS, Mittenmeijer EJ. Initial oxide-film growth on Mg-based MgAl alloys at room temperature. Acta Materialia. 2008, 56, 4621–34.

[523] Wang XM, Zeng XQ, Zhou Y, Wu GS, Lai YJ. Early oxidation behaviors of Mg–Y alloys at high temperatures. Journal of Alloys and Compounds. 2008, 460, 368–74.

[524] Wang X, Wu W, Tang Y, Zeng X, Yao S. Early high temperature oxidation behaviors of Mg–10Gd–3Y alloys. Journal of Alloys and Compounds. 2009, 474, 499–504.

[525] Miral AR, Davidson CJ, Taylor JA. Study on the early surface films formed on Mg-Y molten alloy in different atmospheres. Journal of Magnesium and Alloys. 2015, 3, 173–79.

[526] Inoue S-I, Yamasaki M, Kamasaki M, Kawamura Y. Formation of an incombustible oxide film on a molten Mg-Al-Ca alloy. Corrosion Science. 2017, 122, 118–22.

[527] Hwang D-Y, Shin K-R, Yoo B, Park D-Y, Lee D-H. Characterization of plasma electrolytic oxide formed on AZ91 Mg alloy in KMnO4 electrolyte. Transactions of Nonferrous Metals Society of China. 2009, 19, 829–34.

[528] Lee KM, Ko YG, Shin DH. Microstructural characteristics of oxide layers formed on Mg–9wt% Al–1wt%Zn alloy via two-step plasma electrolytic oxidation. Journal of Alloys and Compounds. 2014, 615, s418–s422.

[529] Wu L, Yang Z. Oxidation behaviour of Mg–2.1Gd–1.1Y–0.82Zn–0.11Zr alloy at high temperatures. Journal of Alloys and Compounds. 2015, 626, 194–202.

[530] Wu L, Li H. Effect of selective oxidation on corrosion behavior of Mg–Gd–Y–Zn–Zr alloy. Corrosion Science. 2018, 142, 238–48.

[531] Zhou N, Zhang Z, Dong J, Jin L, Ding W. Selective oxidation behavior of an ignition-proof Mg-Y-Ca-Ce alloy. Journal of Rare Earths. 2013, 31, 1003–08.

[532] Yu X, Jiang B, Yang H, Yang Q, Pan F. High temperature oxidation behavior of Mg-Y-Sn, Mg-Y, Mg-Sn alloys and its effect on corrosion property. Applied Surface Science. 2015, 353, 1013–22.

[533] Yu X, Jiang B, He J, Liu B, Pan F. Oxidation resistance of Mg-Y alloys at elevated temperatures and the protection performance of the oxide films. Journal of Alloys and Compounds. 2018, 749, 1054–62.
[534] Aydin DS, Bayindir Z, Hoseini M, Pekguleryuz MO. The high temperature oxidation and ignition behavior of Mg–Nd alloys part I: The oxidation of dilute alloys. Journal of Alloys and Compounds. 2013, 569, 35–44.
[535] Aydin DS, Bayindir Z, Pekguleryuz MO. The high temperature oxidation behavior of Mg–Nd alloys. Part II: The effect of the two-phase microstructure on the on-set of oxidation and on oxide morphology. Journal of Alloys and Compounds. 2014, 584, 558–65.
[536] Gunduz KO, Oter ZC, Tarakci M, Gencer Y. Plasma electrolytic oxidation of binary Mg-Al and Mg-Zn alloys. Surface and Coatings Technology. 2017, 323, 72–81.
[537] Song Y, Han E-H, Dong K, Shan D, You BS. Microstructure and protection characteristics of the naturally formed oxide films on Mg–xZn alloys. Corrosion Science. 2013, 72, 133–43.
[538] Inoue S-I, Yamasaki M, Kawamura Y. Oxidation behavior and incombustibility of molten Mg-Zn-Y alloys with Ca and Be addition. Corrosion Science. 2019, 149, 133–43.
[539] Saini SP, Kumar S, Barman R, Dixit A, Kumar V. Oxidation Study of Mg-Li-Al based Alloy. Materials Today: Proceedings. 2016, 3, 3035–44.
[540] Yu X, Jiang B, He J, Liu B, Pan F. Effect of Zn addition on the oxidation property of Mg-Y alloy at high temperatures. Journal of Alloys and Compounds. 2016, 687, 252–62.
[541] Lin Q, Jian D, Weimin Z, Zheng F. Oxidation Behavior and Surface Tension of Mg-1.2Ca Alloy with Ce Addition. Rare Metal Materials and Engineering. 2016, 45, 23–27.
[542] Tan Q, Moc N, Lin C-L, Zhao Y, Zhang M-X. Generalisation of the oxide reinforcement model for the high oxidation resistance of some Mg alloys micro-alloyed with Be. Corrosion Science. 2019, 147, 357–71.
[543] Tan Q, Mo N, Jiang B, Pan F, Zhang M-X. Combined influence of Be and Ca on improving the high-temperature oxidation resistance of the magnesium alloy Mg-9Al-1Zn. Corrosion Science. 2017, 122, 1–11.
[544] Lee J-K, Kim SK. Effect of CaO composition on oxidation and burning behaviors of AM50 Mg alloy. Transactions of Nonferrous Metals Society of China. 2011, 21, s23–s27.
[545] Nouri M, Liu Z, Li D, Yan X, Chen D. The role of minor yttrium in tailoring the failure resistance of surface oxide film formed on Mg alloys. Thin Solid Films. 2016, 615, 29–37.
[546] Agrawal S et al. Biodegradable magnesium alloys for orthopaedic applications: A review on corrosion, biocompatibility and surface modifications. Materials Science and Engineering: C. 2016, 68, 948–63.
[547] Abady GM et al. Effect of Al content on the corrosion behavior of Mg–Al alloys in aqueous solutions of different pH. Electrochimica Acta. 2010, 55, 6651–58.
[548] Hagihara K et al. Crystal-orientation-dependent corrosion behaviour of single crystals of a pure Mg and Mg-Al and Mg-Cu solid solutions. Corrosion Science. 2016, 109, 68–85.
[549] Zeng R-C et al. In vitro corrosion of as-extruded Mg–Ca alloys – The influence of Ca concentration. Corrosion Science. 2015, 96, 23–31.
[550] Zander D et al. Influence of Ca and Zn on the microstructure and corrosion of biodegradable Mg–Ca–Zn alloys. Corrosion Science. 2015, 93, 222–33.
[551] Němec M et al. Influence of alloying element Zn on the microstructural, mechanical and corrosion properties of binary Mg-Zn alloys after severe plastic deformation. Materials Characterization. 2017, 134, 69–75.
[552] Song Y et al. The effect of Zn concentration on the corrosion behavior of Mg–xZn alloys. Corrosion Science. 2012, 65, 322–30.
[553] Cai S et al. Effects of Zn on microstructure, mechanical properties and corrosion behavior of Mg–Zn alloys. Materials Science and Engineering: C. 2012, 32, 2570–77.

[554] Liu D et al. Mechanical properties, corrosion resistance and biocompatibilities of degradable Mg-RE alloys: A review. Journal of Materials Research and Technology. 2019, 8, 1538–49.
[555] Liu M et al. The influence of yttrium (Y) on the corrosion of Mg–Y binary alloys. Corrosion Science. 2010, 52, 3687–701.
[556] Liu X et al. Influence of yttrium element on the corrosion behaviors of Mg–Y binary magnesium alloy. Journal of Magnesium and Alloys. 2017, 5, 26–34.
[557] Zhao C et al. Microstructure, corrosion behavior and cytotoxicity of biodegradable Mg–Sn implant alloys prepared by sub-rapid solidification. Materials Science and Engineering: C. 2015, 54, 245–51.
[558] Yan X et al. Corrosion and biological performance of biodegradable magnesium alloys mediated by low copper addition and processing. Materials Science and Engineering: C. 2018, 93, 565–81.
[559] Mohedano M et al. Characterization and corrosion behavior of binary Mg-Ga alloys. Materials Characterization. 2017, 128, 85–99.
[560] Rajeshkumar R et al. Investigation on the microstructure, mechanical properties and corrosion behavior of Mg-Sb and Mg-Sb-Si alloys. Journal of Alloys and Compounds. 2017, 691, 81–88.
[561] Ningo B et al. Corrosion of Mg-9Al alloy with minor alloying elements (Mn, Nd, Ca, Y and Sn). Materials & Design. 2017, 130, 48–58.
[562] Nam ND. Corrosion behavior of Mg–5Al based magnesium alloy with 1 wt.% Sn, Mn and Zn additions in 3.5 wt.% NaCl solution. Journal of Magnesium and Alloys. 2014. 2, 190–95.
[563] Zhang J et al. Effect of Gd addition on microstructure and corrosion behaviors of Mg–Zn–Y alloy. Journal of Magnesium and Alloys. 2016, 4, 319–25.
[564] Kim KH et al. Effect of calcium addition on the corrosion behavior of Mg–5Al alloy. Intermetallics. 2011, 19, 1831–38.
[565] Nam ND et al. Corrosion behavior of Mg–5Al–xZn alloys in 3.5wt.% NaCl solution. Journal of Alloys and Compounds. 2014, 616, 662–68.
[566] Metalnikov P et al. Role of Sn in microstructure and corrosion behavior of new wrought Mg-5Al alloy. Journal of Alloys and Compounds. 2019, 777, 835–49.
[567] Zhang J et al. Effect of Nd on the microstructure, mechanical properties and corrosion behavior of die-cast Mg–4Al-based alloy. Journal of Alloys and Compounds. 2008, 464, 556–64.
[568] Sadeghi A et al. Corrosion behaviour of AZ31 magnesium alloy containing various levels of strontium. Corrosion Science. 2018, 141, 117–26.
[569] Rosalbino F. Effect of erbium addition on the corrosion behaviour of Mg–Al alloys. Intermetallics. 2005, 13, 55–60.
[570] Seetharaman S et al. Effect of erbium modification on the microstructure, mechanical and corrosion characteristics of binary Mg–Al alloys. Journal of Alloys and Compounds. 2015, 648, 759–70.
[571] Zhang J et al. Microstructures, tensile properties and corrosion behavior of die-cast Mg–4Al-based alloys containing La and/or Ce. Materials Science and Engineering: A. 2008, 489, 113–19.
[572] Zhang J et al. Effect of Ce on microstructure, mechanical properties and corrosion behavior of high-pressure die-cast Mg–4Al-based alloy. Journal of Alloys and Compounds. 2011, 509, 1069–78.
[573] Nam ND et al. Effect of mischmetal on the corrosion properties of Mg–5Al alloy. Corrosion Science. 2009, 51, 2942–49.

[574] Li Y et al. Effects of Li on Microstructures and Corrosion Behaviors of Mg–Li–Al Alloys. In: Joshi V. et al., ed., Magnesium Technology 2019. The Minerals, Metals & Materials Series. Springer, 2019, 127–34.
[575] Jia R et al. Correlative change of corrosion behavior with the microstructure of AZ91 Mg alloy modified with Y additions. Journal of Alloys and Compounds. 2015, 634, 263–71.
[576] Choi JY et al. Significant effects of adding trace amounts of Ti on the microstructure and corrosion properties of Mg-6Al-1Zn magnesium alloy. Journal of Alloys and Compounds. 2014, 614, 49–55.
[577] Yang J et al. Effect of Ca addition on the corrosion behavior of Mg–Al–Mn alloy. Applied Surface Science. 2016, 369, 92–100.
[578] Hu Y et al. Microstructure, mechanical and corrosion properties of Mg-4Al-2Sn-xY-0.4Mn alloys. Journal of Alloys and Compounds. 2017, 727, 491–500.
[579] Jaiswal S et al. Mechanical, corrosion and biocompatibility behaviour of Mg-3Zn-HA biodegradable composites for orthopaedic fixture accessories. Journal of the Mechanical Behavior of Biomedical Materials. 2018, 78, 442–54.
[580] Cheng M et al. Effects of minor Sr addition on microstructure, mechanical and bio-corrosion properties of the Mg-5Zn based alloy system. Journal of Alloys and Compounds. 2017, 691, 95–102.
[581] Ben-Hamu G et al. Microstructure and corrosion behavior of Mg–Zn–Ag alloys. Materials Science and Engineering: A. 2006, 435/436, 579–87.
[582] Jamesh MI et al. Effects of zirconium and oxygen plasma ion implantation on the corrosion behavior of ZK60 Mg alloy in simulated body fluids. Corrosion Science. 2014, 82, 7–26.
[583] Li J-X et al. Effect of trace HA on microstructure, mechanical properties and corrosion behavior of Mg-2Zn-0.5Sr alloy. Journal of Materials Science & Technology. 2018, 34, 299–310.
[584] Cho DH et al. Effect of Mn addition on corrosion properties of biodegradable Mg-4Zn-0.5Ca-xMn alloys. Journal of Alloys and Compounds. 2017, 695, 1166–74.
[585] González SE et al. Improved mechanical performance and delayed corrosion phenomena in biodegradable Mg–Zn–Ca alloys through Pd-alloying. Journal of the Mechanical Behavior of Biomedical Materials. 2012, 6, 53–62.
[586] Mengqi C et al. Corrosion behavior of as-cast Mg-6Zn-4Si alloy with Sr addition. Rare Metal Materials and Engineering. 2017, 46, 2405–10.
[587] Metalnikov P et al. The relation between Mn additions, microstructure and corrosion behavior of new wrought Mg-5Al alloys. Materials Characterization. 2018, 145, 101–15.
[588] Feng Y et al. Fabrication and characterization of biodegradable Mg-Zn-Y-Nd-Ag alloy: Microstructure, mechanical properties, corrosion behavior and antibacterial activities. Bioactive Materials. 2018, 3, 225–35.
[589] Du W et al. Effects of trace Ca/Sn addition on corrosion behaviors of biodegradable Mg–4Zn–0.2Mn alloy. Journal of Magnesium and Alloys. 2018, 6, 1–14.
[590] Zhang Y et al. Effects of calcium addition on phase characteristics and corrosion behaviors of Mg-2Zn-0.2Mn-xCa in simulated body fluid. Journal of Alloys and Compounds. 2017, 728, 37–46.
[591] Pemg X et al. Effect of Y on microstructure and mechanical properties as well as corrosion resistance of Mg-9Li-3Al alloy. Rare Metal Materials and Engineering. 2013, 42, 1993–98.
[592] Dinesh P et al. Effect of Nd on the microstructure and corrosion behaviour of Mg-9Li-3Al magnesium alloy in 3.5 wt.% NaCl solution. Materials Today: Proceedings. 2019, 15, 126–31.
[593] Zhang W et al. Effects of Sr and Sn on microstructure and corrosion resistance of Mg–Zr–Ca magnesium alloy for biomedical applications. Materials & Design. 2012, 39, 379–83.

[594] Zhang X et al. Influence of silver addition on microstructure and corrosion behavior of Mg-Nd-Zn-Zr alloys for biomedical application. Materials Letters. 2013, 100, 188–91.
[595] Mao L et al. Enhanced bioactivity of Mg–Nd–Zn–Zr alloy achieved with nanoscale MgF_2 surface for vascular stent application. ACS Applied Materials & Interfaces. 2015, 7, 5320–30.
[596] Liu Y et al. Influence of biocompatible metal ions (Ag, Fe, Y) on the surface chemistry, corrosion behavior and cytocompatibility of Mg–1Ca alloy treated with MEVVA. Colloids and Surfaces B: Biointerfaces. 2015, 133, 99–107.
[597] Tok HY et al. The role of bismuth on the microstructure and corrosion behavior of ternary Mg–1.2Ca–xBi alloys for biomedical applications. Journal of Alloys and Compounds. 2015, 640, 335–46.
[598] Kania A et al. Mechanical and Corrosion Properties of Mg-Based Alloys with Gd Addition. Materials (Basel). 2019, 12; https://www.ncbi.nlm.nih.gov/pmc/articles/PMC6600794/pdf/materials-12-01775.pdf.
[599] Kim HJ et al. Influence of alloyed Al on the microstructure and corrosion properties of extruded Mg–8Sn–1Zn alloys. Corrosion Science. 2015, 95, 133–42.
[600] Liu Q et al. The role of Ca on the microstructure and corrosion behavior of Mg–8Sn–1Al–1Zn–Ca alloys. Journal of Alloys and Compounds. 2014, 590, 162–67.
[601] Zhou Y-L et al. Microstructures, mechanical and corrosion properties and biocompatibility of as extruded Mg–Mn–Zn–Nd alloys for biomedical applications. Materials Science and Engineering: C. 2015, 49, 93–100.
[602] Bahmani A et al. Corrosion behavior of Mg–Mn–Ca alloy: Influences of Al, Sn and Zn. Journal of Magnesium and Alloys. 2019, 7, 38–46.
[603] Zhang Y et al. Quasi-in-situ STEM-EDS insight into the role of Ag in the corrosion behaviour of Mg-Gd-Zr alloys. Corrosion Science. 2018, 136, 106–18.
[604] Bi G et al. Microstructure, mechanical and corrosion properties of Mg–2Dy–xZn (x=0, 0.1, 0.5 and 1 at.%) alloys. Journal of Magnesium and Alloys. 2014, 2, 64–71.
[605] Yang L et al. Microstructure, mechanical and corrosion properties of Mg–Dy–Gd–Zr alloys for medical applications. Acta Biomaterialia. 2013, 9, 8499–508.
[606] Cao F et al. Corrosion behaviour in salt spray and in 3.5% NaCl solution saturated with Mg (OH)2 of as-cast and solution heat-treated binary Mg–X alloys: X=Mn, Sn, Ca, Zn, Al, Zr, Si, Sr. Corrosion Science. 2013, 76, 60–97.
[607] Huo WT et al. Simultaneously enhanced strength and corrosion resistance of Mg–3Al–1Zn alloy sheets with nano-grained surface layer produced by sliding friction treatment. Journal of Alloys and Compounds. 2017, 720, 324–31.
[608] Jiang B et al. Influence of crystallographic texture and grain size on the corrosion behaviour of as-extruded Mg alloy AZ31 sheets. Corrosion Science. 2017, 126, 374–80.
[609] Xin R et al. Influence of texture on corrosion rate of AZ31 Mg alloy in 3.5wt.% NaCl. Materials & Design. 2011, 32, 4548–52.
[610] Singh IB et al. A comparative corrosion behavior of Mg, AZ31 and AZ91 alloys in 3.5% NaCl solution. Journal of Magnesium and Alloys. 2015, 3, 142–48.
[611] Shahar IA et al. Mechanical and corrosion properties of AZ31 Mg alloy processed by equal-channel angular pressing and aging. Procedia Engineering. 2017, 184, 423–31.
[612] Wilke BM et al. Corrosion performance of MAO coatings on AZ31 Mg alloy in simulated body fluid vs Earle's Balance Salt Solution. Applied Surface Science. 2016, 363, 328–37.
[613] Xin R et al. Texture effect on corrosion behavior of AZ31 Mg alloy in simulated physiological environment. Materials Letters. 2012, 72, 1–4.
[614] Wang BJ et al. Effect of corrosion product films on the in vitro degradation behavior of Mg-3% Al-1%Zn (in wt%) alloy in Hank's solution. Journal of Materials Science & Technology. 2018, 34, 1756–64.

[615] El Sawy EN et al. Corrosion of Mg, AS31 and AZ91 alloys in nitrate solutions. Journal of Alloys and Compounds. 2010, 492, 69–76.
[616] Choi YI et al. Temperature-dependent corrosion behaviour of flame-resistant, Ca-containing AZX911 and AMX602 Mg alloys. Corrosion Science. 2016, 103, 181–88.
[617] Manivannan S et al. Investigation and corrosion performance of cast Mg–6Al–1Zn + XCa alloy under salt spray test (ASTM-B117). Journal of Magnesium and Alloys. 2015, 3, 86–94.
[618] Shetty S et al. Influence of sulfate ion concentration and pH on the corrosion of Mg-Al-Zn-Mn (GA9) magnesium alloy. Journal of Magnesium and Alloys. 2015, 3, 258–70.
[619] Eamaily M et al. Influence of temperature on the atmospheric corrosion of the Mg–Al alloy AM50. Corrosion Science. 2015, 90, 420–33.
[620] Liao J et al. Improved corrosion resistance of a high-strength Mg–Al–Mn–Ca magnesium alloy made by rapid solidification powder metallurgy. Materials Science and Engineering: A. 2012, 544, 10–20.
[621] Wang N-G et al. Corrosion behavior of Mg-Al-Pb and Mg-Al-Pb-Zn-Mn alloys in 3.5% NaCl solution. Transactions of Nonferrous Metals Society of China. 2010, 20, 1936–43.
[622] Chen Y et al. In vitro and in vivo corrosion measurements of Mg–6Zn alloys in the bile. Materials Science and Engineering: C. 2014, 42, 116–23.
[623] Zhang Y et al. Microstructure, mechanical properties, corrosion behavior and film formation mechanism of Mg-Zn-Mn-xNd in Kokubo's solution. Journal of Alloys and Compounds. 2018, 730, 458–70.
[624] Hamdy AS et al. Vanadia-based coatings of self-repairing functionality for advanced magnesium Elektron ZE41 Mg–Zn–rare earth alloy. Surface and Coatings Technology. 2012, 206, 3686–92.
[625] AbdelGawad M et al. The Influence of Temperature and Medium on Corrosion Response of ZE41 and EZ33. In: Joshi V. et al., ed., Magnesium Technology 2019, 159–67.
[626] Leleu S et al. Corrosion rate determination of rare-earth Mg alloys in a Na2SO4 solution by electrochemical measurements and inductive coupled plasma-optical emission spectroscopy. Journal of Magnesium and Alloys. 2019, 7, 47–57.
[627] Lu Y et al. Effects of secondary phase and grain size on the corrosion of biodegradable Mg–Zn–Ca alloys. Materials Science and Engineering: C. 2015, 48, 480–86.
[628] González S et al. Improved mechanical performance and delayed corrosion phenomena in biodegradable Mg–Zn–Ca alloys through Pd-alloying. Journal of the Mechanical Behavior of Biomedical Materials. 2012, 6, 53–62.
[629] Ly XN et al. Influence of current mode on microstructure and corrosion behavior of micro-arc oxidation (MAO) biodegradable Mg-Zn-Ca alloy in Hank's solution. Surface and Coatings Technology. 2019, 358, 331–39.
[630] Song Y et al. Corrosion characterization of Mg–8Li alloy in NaCl solution. Corrosion Science. 2009, 51, 1087–94.
[631] Zeng R-C et al. Corrosion and characterisation of dual phase Mg–Li–Ca alloy in Hank's solution: The influence of microstructural features. Corrosion Science. 2014, 79, 69–82.
[632] Yang L et al. Corrosion behavior of Mg–8Li–3Zn–Al alloy in neutral 3.5% NaCl solution. Journal of Magnesium and Alloys. 2016, 4, 22–26.
[633] Bakhsheshi Rad HR et al. Microstructure analysis and corrosion behavior of biodegradable Mg–Ca implant alloys. Materials & Design. 2012, 33, 88–97.
[634] Seong JW et al. Development of biodegradable Mg–Ca alloy sheets with enhanced strength and corrosion properties through the refinement and uniform dispersion of the Mg2Ca phase by high-ratio differential speed rolling. Acta Biomaterialia. 2015, 11, 531–42.
[635] Cain TW et al. The corrosion of solid solution Mg-Sn binary alloys in NaCl solutions. Electrochimica Acta. 2019, 297, 564–75.

[636] Hou L et al. Microstructure, mechanical properties, corrosion behavior and biocompatibility of as-extruded biodegradable Mg–3Sn–1Zn–0.5Mn alloy. Journal of Materials Science & Technology. 2016, 32, 874–82.
[637] Zhang X et al. Effect of solid-solution treatment on corrosion and electrochemical behaviors of Mg-15Y alloy in 3.5 wt.% NaCl solution. Journal of Rare Earths. 2012, 30, 1158–67.
[638] Zhang X et al. Corrosion behavior of Mg–Y alloy in NaCl aqueous solution. Progress in Natural Science: Materials International. 2012, 22, 169–74.
[639] Zhang K et al. Relationship between extrusion, Y and corrosion behavior of Mg–Y alloy in NaCl aqueous solution. Journal of Magnesium and Alloys. 2013, 1, 134–38.
[640] Chu P-W et al. Linking the microstructure of a heat-treated WE43 Mg alloy with its corrosion behavior. Corrosion Science. 2014, 101, 94–104.
[641] Ascencio M et al. An investigation of the corrosion mechanisms of WE43 Mg alloy in a modified simulated body fluid solution: The influence of immersion time. Corrosion Science. 2014, 87, 489–503.
[642] Ascencio M et al. Corrosion behaviour of polypyrrole-coated WE43 Mg alloy in a modified simulated body fluid solution. Corrosion Science. 2018, 133, 261–75.
[643] Ben-Hamu G et al. The relation between microstructure and corrosion behavior of Mg–Y–RE–Zr alloys. Journal of Alloys and Compounds. 2007, 431, 269–76.
[644] Zhang X et al. Comparative study on corrosion behavior of as-cast and extruded Mg–5Y–7Gd–1Nd–0.5Zr alloy in 5% NaCl aqueous solution. Transactions of Nonferrous Metals Society of China. 2012, 22, 1018–27.
[645] Srinivasan A et al. Corrosion behavior of Mg–Gd–Zn based alloys in aqueous NaCl solution. Journal of Magnesium and Alloys. 2014, 2, 245–56.
[646] Gui Z et al. Mechanical and corrosion properties of Mg-Gd-Zn-Zr-Mn biodegradable alloy by hot extrusion. Journal of Alloys and Compounds. 2016, 685, 222–30.
[647] Zhang Jin NNZR. Mg-7Gd-5Y-Nd-Zr Alloy Plate Corrosion-resistance Property to Chloride Ion. Physics Procedia. 2013, 50, 397–404.
[648] Shi L-L et al. Mechanical properties and corrosion behavior of Mg–Gd–Ca–Zr alloys for medical applications. Journal of the Mechanical Behavior of Biomedical Materials. 2015, 47, 38–8.
[649] Zhang X et al. Improvement of mechanical properties and corrosion resistance of biodegradable Mg–Nd–Zn–Zr alloys by double extrusion. Materials Science and Engineering: B. 2012, 177, 1113–19.
[650] Feng K et al. Evaluation of Mg-Nd-Zn-Zr magnesium alloy as bipolar plate in simulated polymer electrolyte membrane fuel cell environments. International Journal of Hydrogen Energy. 2016, 41, 14191–206.
[651] Mao L et al. A novel biodegradable Mg-Nd-Zn-Zr alloy with uniform corrosion behavior in artificial plasma. Materials Letters. 2012, 88, 1–4.
[652] Ong MS et al. The influence of heat treatment on the corrosion behaviour of amorphous melt-spun binary Mg–18 at.% Ni and Mg–21 at.% Cu alloy. Materials Science and Engineering: A. 2001, 304/306, 510–14.
[653] Mitchell T et al. Characterisation of corrosion products formed on PVD in situ mechanically worked Mg–Ti alloys. Journal of Alloys and Compounds. 2005, 392, 127–41.
[654] Song G-L et al. The corrosion and passivity of sputtered Mg–Ti alloys. Corrosion Science. 2016, 104, 36–46.
[655] Yang L et al. Element distribution in the corrosion layer and cytotoxicity of alloy Mg–10Dy during in vitro biodegradation. Acta Biomaterialia. 2013, 9, 8475–87.
[656] El-Moneim AA et al. Corrosion behaviour of sputter-deposited Mg–Zr alloys in a borate buffer solution. Corrosion Science. 2011, 53, 2988–93.

[657] Atrens A, Liu M, Zainal Abidin NI, Song G-L. 3: Corrosion of magnesium (Mg) alloys and metallurgical influence. Corrosion of Magnesium Alloys. 2011, 117–65.

[658] Abdel-Gawad SA, Shoeib MA. Corrosion studies and microstructure of Mg–Zn–Ca alloys for biomedical applications. Surfaces and Interfaces. 2019, 14, 108–16.

[659] Rajeshkumar R, Jayaraj J, Srinivasan A, Pillai UTS. Investigation on the microstructure, mechanical properties and corrosion behavior of Mg-Sb and Mg-Sb-Si alloys. Journal of Alloys and Compounds. 2017, 691, 81–88.

[660] Jia H, Feng X, Yang Y. Effect of crystal orientation on corrosion behavior of directionally solidified Mg-4 wt% Zn alloy. Journal of Materials Science & Technology. 2018, 34, 1229–35.

[661] Hagihara K, Okubo M, Yamasaki M, Nakano T. Crystal-orientation-dependent corrosion behaviour of single crystals of a pure Mg and Mg-Al and Mg-Cu solid solutions. Corrosion Science. 2016, 109, 68–85.

[662] Jiang B, Xiang Q, Atrens A, Song J, Pan F. Influence of crystallographic texture and grain size on the corrosion behaviour of as-extruded Mg alloy AZ31 sheets. Corrosion Science. 2017, 126, 374–80.

[663] Chen Y, Yang Y, Zhang W, Zhang T, Wang F. Influence of second phase on corrosion performance and formation mechanism of PEO coating on AZ91 Ag alloy. Journal of Alloys and Compounds. 2017, 718, 92–103.

[664] Liu X, Shan D, Song Y, Chen R, Han E. Influences of the quantity of Mg2Sn phase on the corrosion behavior of Mg–7Sn magnesium alloy. Electrochimica Acta. 2011, 56, 2582–90.

[665] Feng H, Liu S, Du Y, Lei T, Yuan T. Effect of the second phases on corrosion behavior of the Mg-Al-Zn alloys. Journal of Alloys and Compounds. 2017, 695, 2330–38.

[666] Li CQ, Xu DK, Zeng ZR, Wang BJ, Han EH. Effect of volume fraction of LPSO phases on corrosion and mechanical properties of Mg-Zn-Y alloys. Materials & Design. 2017, 121, 430–41.

[667] Cheng P, Zhao Y, Lu R, Hou H. Effect of the morphology of long-period stacking ordered phase on mechanical properties and corrosion behavior of cast Mg-Zn-Y-Ti alloy. Journal of Alloys and Compounds. 2018, 764, 226–38.

[668] Wang SD, Xu DK, Chen XB, Han EH, Dong C. Effect of heat treatment on the corrosion resistance and mechanical properties of an as-forged Mg–Zn–Y–Zr alloy. Corrosion Science. 2015, 92, 228–36.

[669] Shahri SMG, Idris MH, Jafari H, Gholampour B, Assadian M. Effect of solution treatment on corrosion characteristics of biodegradable Mg–6Zn alloy. Transactions of Nonferrous Metals Society of China. 2015, 25, 1490–99.

[670] Zhang X, Zhang K, Li X, Deng X, Shi Y. Effect of solid-solution treatment on corrosion and electrochemical behaviors of Mg-15Y alloy in 3.5 wt.% NaCl solution. Journal of Rare Earths. 2012, 30, 1158–67.

[671] Ha H-Y, Kang J-Y, Kim SG, Kim B, You BS. Influences of metallurgical factors on the corrosion behaviour of extruded binary Mg–Sn alloys. Corrosion Science. 2014, 82, 369–79.

[672] Xu H, Zhang X, Zhang K, Shi Y, Ren J. Effect of extrusion on corrosion behavior and corrosion mechanism of Mg-Y alloy. Journal of Rare Earths. 2016, 34, 315–27.

[673] Wu P-P, Xu F-J, Deng K-K, Han F-Y, Gao R. Effect of extrusion on corrosion properties of Mg-2Ca-χAl (χ=0, 2, 3, 5) alloys. Corrosion Science. 2017, 127, 280–90.

[674] Zhang X, Wang Z, Yuan G, Xue Y. Improvement of mechanical properties and corrosion resistance of biodegradable Mg–Nd–Zn–Zr alloys by double extrusion. Materials Science and Engineering: B. 2012, 177, 1113–19.

[675] Cao F, Shi Z, Song GL, Liu M, Atrens A. Influence of hot rolling on the corrosion behavior of several Mg–X alloys. Corrosion Science. 2015, 90, 176–91.

[676] Xiang Q, Jiang B, Zhang Y, Chen X, Pan F. Effect of rolling-induced microstructure on corrosion behaviour of an as-extruded Mg-5Li-1Al alloy sheet. Corrosion Science. 2017, 119, 14–22.
[677] Seong JW, Kim WJ. Development of biodegradable Mg–Ca alloy sheets with enhanced strength and corrosion properties through the refinement and uniform dispersion of the Mg2Ca phase by high-ratio differential speed rolling. Acta Biomaterialia. 2015, 11, 531–42.
[678] Cao F-F, Deng K-K, Nie K-B, Kang J-W, Niu H-Y. Microstructure and corrosion properties of Mg-4Zn-2Gd-0.5Ca alloy influenced by multidirectional forging. Journal of Alloys and Compounds. 2019, 770, 1208–20.
[679] Wan Y, Xu S, Liu C, Gao Y, Chen Z. Enhanced strength and corrosion resistance of Mg-Gd-Y-Zr alloy with ultrafine grains. Materials Letters. 2018, 213, 274–77.
[680] Jiang J-H, Zhao Y-H, Ma A-B, Zhu Y-T. Effect of equal-channel angular pressing and aging on corrosion behavior of ZK60 Mg alloy. Transactions of Nonferrous Metals Society of China. 2015, 25, 3909–20.
[681] Liu C, Zheng H, Gu X, Jiang B, Liang J. Effect of severe shot peening on corrosion behavior of AZ31 and AZ91 magnesium alloys. Journal of Alloys and Compounds. 2019, 770, 500–06.
[682] Johnston S, Shi Z, Hoe C, Uggowitzer PJ, Cihova M, Löffler JF, Dargusch MS, Atrens A. The influence of two common sterilization techniques on the corrosion of Mg and its alloys for biomedical applications. Journal of Biomedical Materials Research Part B: Applied Biomaterials. 2018, 106, 1907–17.
[683] Pourbaix M. Atlas of electrochemical equilibria in aqueous solutions. 2d English ed. 1974, Houston, TX.: National Association of Corrosion Engineers.
[684] https://en.wikipedia.org/wiki/Pourbaix_diagram.
[685] Saji VS. Review of rare-earth-based conversion coatings for magnesium and its alloys. Journal of Materials Research and Technology. 2019, 8, 5012–35.
[686] Ghali E. Activity and passivity of magnesium (Mg) and its alloys. Corrosion of Magnesium Alloys. 2011, 66–114; https://doi.org/10.1533/9780857091413.1.66.
[687] Zhang S, Zhang X, Zhao C, Li J, Song Y, Xie C, Tao H, Zhang Y, He Y, Jiang Y, Bian Y. Research on an Mg-Zn alloy as a degradable biomaterial. Acta Biomaterialia. 2009, 6, 626–40.
[688] Kim S-Y, Kim Y-K, Ryu M-H, Bae T-S, Lee M-H. Corrosion resistance and bioactivity enhancement of MAO coated Mg alloy depending on the time of hydrothermal treatment in Ca-EDTA solution. Scientific Reports 2017, 7, 1–10.
[689] https://www.gamry.com/Framework%20Help/HTML5%20-%20Tripane%20-%20Audience%20A/Content/DC/Introduction_to_DC_Corrosion/Quantitative%20Corrosion%20Theory.htm
[690] Arof AK, Amirudin S, Yusof SZ, Noor IM. A method based on impedance spectroscopy to determine transport properties of polymer electrolytes. Physical Chemistry Chemical Physics. 2014, 16, 1856–67.
[691] Sun R, Yang S, Lv T. Corrosion behavior of AZ91D magnesium alloy with a calcium–phosphate–vanadium composite conversion coating. Coatings. 2019, 9, 379; https://doi.org/10.3390/coatings9060379.
[692] Luo Z, Zhu H, Ying T, Li D, Zeng X. First principles calculations on the influence of solute elements and chlorine adsorption on the anodic corrosion behavior of Mg (0001) surface. Surface Science. 2018, 672/673, 68–74.
[693] Gomes MP, Costa I, Pébère N, Rossi JL, Vivier V. On the corrosion mechanism of Mg investigated by electrochemical impedance spectroscopy. Electrochimica Acta. 2019, 306, 61–70.
[694] Casajús P, Winzer N. Electrochemical noise analysis of the corrosion of high-purity Mg–Al alloys. Corrosion Science. 2015, 94, 316–26.
[695] Rosalbino F, Angelini E, De Negri S, Saccone A, Delfino S. Electrochemical behaviour assessment of novel Mg-rich Mg–Al–RE alloys (RE=Ce, Er). Intermetallics. 2006, 14, 1487–92.

[696] Feng Y, Liu L, Wang R-C, Peng C-Q, Wang N-ZG. Microstructures and electrochemical corrosion properties of Mg–Al–Pb and Mg–Al–Pb–Ce anode materials. Transactions of Nonferrous Metals Society of China. 2016, 26, 1379–87.
[697] Medhashree H, Shetty AN. Electrochemical corrosion study of Mg–Al–Zn–Mn alloy in aqueous ethylene glycol containing chloride ions. Journal of Materials Research and Technology. 2017, 6, 40–49.
[698] Luo KY, Wang CY, Cui CY, Lu JZ, Lu YF. Effects of coverage layer on the electrochemical corrosion behaviour of Mg-Al-Mn alloy subjected to massive laser shock peening treatment. Journal of Alloys and Compounds. 2019, 782, 1058–75.
[699] Li S, Bacco AC, Birbilis N, Cong H, Li J. Passivation and potential fluctuation of Mg alloy AZ31B in alkaline environments. Corrosion Science. 2016, 112, 596–610.
[700] Song G-L. Mishra R, Xu ZQ. Crystallographic orientation and electrochemical activity of AZ31 Mg alloy. Electrochemistry Communications. 2010, 12, 1009–12.
[701] Srinivasan A, Ranjani P, Rajendran N. Electrochemical polymerization of pyrrole over AZ31 Mg alloy for biomedical applications. Electrochimica Acta. 2013, 88, 310–21.
[702] Zhang Y, Yan C, ang F, Li W. Electrochemical behavior of anodized Mg alloy AZ91D in chloride containing aqueous solution. Corrosion Science. 2005, 47, 2816–31.
[703] Zhang Y, Yan C. Development of anodic film on Mg alloy AZ91D. Surface and Coatings Technology. 2006, 201, 2381–86.
[704] Chelliah NM, Padaikathan P, Kumar R. Evaluation of electrochemical impedance and biocorrosion characteristics of as-cast and T4 heat treated AZ91 Mg-alloy in Ringer's solution. Journal of Magnesium and Alloys. 2019, 7, 134–43.
[705] Barbosa DP, Knörnschild G. Anodization of Mg-alloy AZ91 in NaOH solutions. Surface and Coatings Technology. 2009, 203, 1629–36.
[706] El-Taib Heakal F, Fekry AM, Abd El-Barr Jibril M. Electrochemical behaviour of the Mg alloy AZ91D in borate solutions. Corrosion Science. 2011, 53, 1174–85.
[707] Tekin KC, Malayoğlu U, Shrestha S. Electrochemical behavior of plasma electrolytic oxide coatings on rare earth element containing Mg alloys. Surface and Coatings Technology. 2013, 236, 540–49.
[708] Li J, Zhang B, Wei Q, Wang N, Hou B. Electrochemical behavior of Mg-Al-Zn-In alloy as anode materials in 3.5wt.% NaCl solution. Electrochimica Acta. 2017, 238, 156–67.
[709] Badawy WA, Hilal NH, El-Rabiee M, Nady H. Electrochemical behavior of Mg and some Mg alloys in aqueous solutions of different pH. Electrochimica Acta. 2010, 55, 1880–87.
[710] Medhashree H, Shetty AN. Electrochemical investigation on the effects of sulfate ion concentration, temperature and medium pH on the corrosion behavior of Mg–Al–Zn–Mn alloy in aqueous ethylene glycol. Journal of Magnesium and Alloys. 2017, 5, 64–73.
[711] Abulsain M, Berkani A, Bonilla FA, Liu Y, Habazaki H. Anodic oxidation of Mg–Cu and Mg–Zn alloys. Electrochimica Acta. 2004, 49, 899–904.
[712] Wang H, Zhao C, Chen Y, Li J, Zhang X. Electrochemical property and in vitro degradation of DCPD–PCL composite coating on the biodegradable Mg–Zn alloy. Materials Letters. 2012, 68, 435–38.
[713] Lamesh M, Kumar S, Sankara Narayanan TSN. Corrosion behavior of commercially pure Mg and ZM21 Mg alloy in Ringer's solution – Long term evaluation by EIS. Corrosion Science. 2011, 53, 645–54.
[714] Yamasaki M, Izumi S, Kawamura Y, Habazaki H. Corrosion and passivation behavior of Mg–Zn–Y–Al alloys prepared by cooling rate-controlled solidification. Applied Surface Science. 2011, 257, 8258–67.

[715] Ren X, Li X, Yang Y, Yang Y, Wu H. Corrosion behavior and electrochemical properties of as-cast Mg-2Zn-0.5Ca-Y series magnesium alloys in hank's solution and NaCl solution. Rare Metal Materials and Engineering. 2017, 46, 45–50.
[716] Cai C, Song R, Wang L, Li J. Effect of anodic T phase on surface micro-galvanic corrosion of biodegradable Mg-Zn-Zr-Nd alloys. Applied Surface Science. 2018, 462, 243–54.
[717] Zhang C, Huang X, Zhang M, Gao L, Wu R. Electrochemical characterization of the corrosion of a Mg–Li Alloy. Materials Letters. 2008, 62, 2177–80.
[718] Zhang ML, Chen Z, Han W, Lv YZ, Wang J. Electrochemical formation and phase control of Mg–Li alloys. Chinese Chemical Letters. 2007, 18, 1124–28.
[719] Lv Y, Xu Y, Cao D. The electrochemical behaviors of Mg, Mg–Li–Al–Ce and Mg–Li–Al–Ce–Y in sodium chloride solution. Journal of Power Sources. 2011, 196, 8809–14.
[720] Jiang B, Liu Y, Li R, Xianf Q, Pan F. Effects of Yttrium and Strontium addition on electrochemical behavior of Mg-14Li-1Al alloys. Rare Metal Materials and Engineering. 2013, 42, 1999–2003.
[721] Chen L, Zhang M, Han W, Yan Y, Cao P. Electrochemical study on preparation of Mg-Li-Yb alloys in LiCl-KCl-KF-MgCl2-Yb2O3 melts. Journal of Rare Earths. 2012, 30, 159–63.
[722] Li JF, Zheng ZQ, Li SC, Ren Wd, Zhang Z. Preparation and galvanic anodizing of a Mg–Li alloy. Materials Science and Engineering: A. 2006, 433, 233–40.
[723] Lv Y, Liu M, Xu Y, Cao D, Feng J. The electrochemical behaviors of Mg–8Li–3Al–0.5Zn and Mg–8Li–3Al–1.0Zn in sodium chloride solution. Journal of Power Sources. 2013, 225, 124–28.
[724] Lv Y, Liu M, Xu Y, Cao D, Zhang M. The electrochemical behaviors of Mg–8Li–0.5Y and Mg–8Li–1Y alloys in sodium chloride solution. Journal of Power Sources. 2013, 239, 265–68.
[725] Cao D, Wu L, Sun Y, Wang G, Lv Y. Electrochemical behavior of Mg–Li, Mg–Li–Al and Mg–Li–Al–Ce in sodium chloride solution. Journal of Power Sources. 2008, 177, 624–30.
[726] Sudholz AD, Gusieva K, Chen XB, Muddle BC, Birbilis N. Electrochemical behaviour and corrosion of Mg–Y alloys. Corrosion Science. 2011, 53, 2277–82.
[727] Zhang X, Li Y-J, Zhang K, Wang C-S, Zhang B-D. Corrosion and electrochemical behavior of Mg–Y alloys in 3.5% NaCl solution. Transactions of Nonferrous Metals Society of China. 2013, 23, 1226–36.
[728] Zhao Y, Wu G, Pan H, Yeung KWK, Chu PK. Formation and electrochemical behavior of Al and O plasma-implanted biodegradable Mg-Y-RE alloy. Materials Chemistry and Physics. 2012, 132, 187–91.
[729] Jamesh MI, Wu G, Zhao Y, McKenzie DR, Chu PK. Electrochemical corrosion behavior of biodegradable Mg–Y–RE and Mg–Zn–Zr alloys in Ringer's solution and simulated body fluid. Corrosion Science. 2015, 91, 160–84.
[730] Zhang X, Zhang K, Li X-G, Wang C, Deng X. Corrosion and electrochemical behavior of as-cast Mg-5Y-7Gd-1Nd-0.5Zr magnesium alloys in 5% NaCl aqueous solution. Progress in Natural Science: Materials International. 2011, 21, 314–21.
[731] Ninlachart J, Karmiol Z, Chidambaram D, Raja KS. Effect of heat treatment conditions on the passivation behavior of WE43C Mg–Y–Nd alloy in chloride containing alkaline environments. Journal of Magnesium and Alloys. 2017, 5, 147–65.
[732] Ninlachart J, Raja KS. Passivation kinetics of Mg-Nd-Gd-Zn-Zr (EV31A) and Mg-Y-Nd-Gd-Zr (WE43C) in NaOH solutions. Journal of Magnesium and Alloys. 2017, 5, 254–70.
[733] Liu X, Xue J, Zhang D. Electrochemical behaviors and discharge performance of the as-extruded Mg-1.5 wt%Ca alloys as anode for Mg-air battery. Journal of Alloys and Compounds. 2019, 790, 822–28.
[734] Pan Y, He S, Wang D, Huang D, Chen C. In vitro degradation and electrochemical corrosion evaluations of microarc oxidized pure Mg, Mg–Ca and Mg–Ca–Zn alloys for biomedical applications. Materials Science and Engineering: C. 2015, 47, 85–96.

[735] Moon S, Nam Y. Anodic oxidation of Mg–Sn alloys in alkaline solutions. Corrosion Science. 2012, 65, 494–501.
[736] Ha H-Y, Kang J-Y, Yang J, Yim CD, You BS. Role of Sn in corrosion and passive behavior of extruded Mg-5 wt%Sn alloy. Corrosion Science. 2016, 102, 355–62.
[737] Zheludkevich ML, Lamaka SV, Chen Y, Hoeche D, Blawert C, Kainer KU. Towards Active Corrosion Protection of Mg Alloys Using Corrosion Inhibition Approaches. In: Orlov D. et al., ed., Magnesium Technology 2018. TMS 2018. The Minerals, Metals & Materials Series. Springer, 2018, 19–20.
[738] Chen T, Yuan Y, Wu J, Liu T, Chen X, Tang A, Pan F. Alloy Design Strategies of the Native Anti-corrosion Magnesium Alloy. In: Joshi V. et al., ed., Magnesium Technology 2019. The Minerals, Metals & Materials Series. Springer, 2019, 169–73.
[739] Li L, Zhang M, Li Y, Zhao J, Qin L, Lai Y. Corrosion and biocompatibility improvement of magnesium-based alloys as bone implant materials: a review. Regenerative Biomaterials. 2017, 4, 129–37.
[740] Chen X-B, Easton A, Birbilis N, Yang H-Y, Abbott TB. Corrosion-resistant coatings for magnesium (Mg) alloys. Corrosion Prevention of Magnesium Alloys. 2013, Pages 282–312
[741] Arrabal R, Pardo A, Merino MC, Mohedano M, Casajús P, Paucar K, Garcés G. Effect of Nd on the corrosion behaviour of AM50 and AZ91D magnesium alloys in 3.5 wt.% NaCl solution. Corrosion Science. 2012, 55, 301–12.
[742] Liu M, Schmutz P, Uggowitzer PJ, Song G, Atrens A. The influence of yttrium (Y) on the corrosion of Mg–Y binary alloys. Corrosion Science. 2010, 52, 3687–701.
[743] Song Y, Shan D, Han E-H. Pitting corrosion of a Rare Earth Mg alloy GW93. Journal of Materials Science & Technology. 2017, 33, 954–60.
[744] Liu J, Yang L, Zhang C, Zhang B, Wang F. Role of the LPSO structure in the improvement of corrosion resistance of Mg-Gd-Zn-Zr alloys. Journal of Alloys and Compounds. 2019, 782, 648–58.
[745] Lu F, Ma A, Jiang J, Guo Y, Chen J. Significantly improved corrosion resistance of heat-treated Mg–Al–Gd alloy containing profuse needle-like precipitates within grains. Corrosion Science. 2015, 94, 171–78.
[746] Fan Y, Wu G, Zhai C. Influence of cerium on the microstructure, mechanical properties and corrosion resistance of magnesium alloy. Materials Science and Engineering A. 2006, 433, 208–15.
[747] Liu YR, Zhang KM, Zou JX, Liu DK, Zhang TC. Effect of the high current pulsed electron beam treatment on the surface microstructure and corrosion resistance of a Mg-4Sm alloy. Journal of Alloys and Compounds. 2018, 741, 65–75.
[748] Zhang J, Xu J, Cheng W, Chen C, Kang J. Corrosion behavior of Mg–Zn–Y alloy with long-period stacking ordered structures. Journal Materials Science & Technology. 2012, 28, 1157–62.
[749] Liu J, Yang L, Zhang C, Zhang B, Wang F. Significantly improved corrosion resistance of Mg-15Gd-2Zn-0.39Zr alloys: Effect of heat-treatment. Journal of Materials Science & Technology. 2019, 35, 1644–54.
[750] Feng J, Li H, Deng K, Fernandez C, Peng Q. Unique corrosion resistance of ultrahigh pressure Mg-25Al binary alloys. Corrosion Science. 2018, 143, 229–39.
[751] Zhang HJ, Zhang DF, Ma CH, Guo SF. Improving mechanical properties and corrosion resistance of Mg-6Zn-Mn magnesium alloy by rapid solidification. Materials Letters. 2013, 92, 45–48.
[752] Ma C, Peng G, Niw L, Liu H, Guan Y. Laser surface modification of Mg-Gd-Ca alloy for corrosion resistance and biocompatibility enhancement. Applied Surface Science. 2018, 445, 211–16.

[753] Yin Z, Chen Y, Yan H, Zhou G-H, Hu Z. Effects of the second phases on corrosion resistance of AZ91-xGd alloys treated with ultrasonic vibration. Journal of Alloys and Compounds. 2019, 783, 877–85.
[754] Mineta T, Sato H. Simultaneously improved mechanical properties and corrosion resistance of Mg-Li-Al alloy produced by severe plastic deformation. Materials Science and Engineering: A. 2018, 735, 418–22.
[755] Huo WT, Zhang W, Lu JW, Zhang YS. Simultaneously enhanced strength and corrosion resistance of Mg–3Al–1Zn alloy sheets with nano-grained surface layer produced by sliding friction treatment. Journal of Alloys and Compounds. 2017, 720, 324–31.
[756] Zhang J, Kang Z, Wang F. Mechanical properties and biocorrosion resistance of the Mg-Gd-Nd-Zn-Zr alloy processed by equal channel angular pressing. Materials Science and Engineering: C. 2016, 68, 194–97.
[757] Singh BP, KumarJena B, Bhattacharjee S, Besra L. Development of oxidation and corrosion resistance hydrophobic graphene oxide-polymer composite coating on copper. Surface and Coatings Technology. 2013, 232, 475–81.
[758] Li D, Liu Q, Yin X, Zhang M. Fabrication of hydrophobic surface with hierarchical structure on Mg alloy and its corrosion resistance. Electrochimica Acta. 2010, 55, 6897–906.
[759] Cui X-J, Lin X-Z, Liu C-H, Yang R-S, Gong M. Fabrication and corrosion resistance of a hydrophobic micro-arc oxidation coating on AZ31 Mg alloy. Corrosion Science. 2015, 90, 402–12.
[760] Kuang J, Ba Z, Li Z, Jia Y, Wang Z. Fabrication of a superhydrophobic Mg-Mn layered double hydroxides coating on pure magnesium and its corrosion resistance. Surface and Coatings Technology. 2019, 361, 75–82.
[761] Qian Z, Wang S, Ye X, Liu Z, Wu Z. Corrosion resistance and wetting properties of silica-based superhydrophobic coatings on AZ31B Mg alloy surfaces. Applied Surface Science. 2018, 453, 1–10.
[762] Kim et al. Enhanced corrosion resistance and biocompatibility of AZ31 Mg alloy using PCL/ZnO NPs via electrospinning. Applied Surface Science. 2017, 396, 249–58.
[763] Cui L-Y et al. Electrodeposition of TiO2 layer-by-layer assembled composite coating and silane treatment on Mg alloy for corrosion resistance. Surface and Coatings Technology. 2017, 324, 560–68.
[764] Tang Y et al. A comparative study and optimization of corrosion resistance of ZnAl layered double hydroxides films intercalated with different anions on AZ31 Mg alloys. Surface and Coatings Technology. 2019, 358, 594–603.
[765] Ji X-J et al. Corrosion resistance and antibacterial properties of hydroxyapatite coating induced by gentamicin-loaded polymeric multilayers on magnesium alloys. Colloids and Surfaces B: Biointerfaces. 2019, 179, 429–36.
[766] Zhu H et al. Corrosion resistance improvement of Mg alloy AZ31 by combining bilayer amorphous DLC:H/SiNx film with N+ ions implantation. Journal of Alloys and Compounds. 2018, 762, 171–83.
[767] Zwng R-C et al. Corrosion resistance of in-situ Mg–Al hydrotalcite conversion film on AZ31 magnesium alloy by one-step formation. Transactions of Nonferrous Metals Society of China. 2015, 25, 1917–25.
[768] Ye X et al. Bioactive glass–ceramic coating for enhancing the in vitro corrosion resistance of biodegradable Mg alloy. Applied Surface Science. 2012, 259, 799–805.
[769] Feng J et al. In-situ hydrothermal crystallization Mg(OH)2 films on magnesium alloy AZ91 and their corrosion resistance properties. Materials Chemistry and Physics. 2013, 143, 322–29.
[770] Hou L et al. Enhancement corrosion resistance of MgAl layered double hydroxides films by anion-exchange mechanism on magnesium alloys. Applied Surface Science. 2019, 487, 101–08.

[771] He MF et al. Novel multilayer Mg–Al intermetallic coating for corrosion protection of magnesium alloy by molten salts treatment. Transactions of Nonferrous Metals Society of China. 2012, 22, s74–s78.
[772] Ke C et al. Interfacial study of the formation mechanism of corrosion resistant strontium phosphate coatings upon Mg-3Al-4.3Ca-0.1Mn. Corrosion Science. 2019, 151, 143–53.
[773] Jamali SS et al. Corrosion protection afforded by praseodymium conversion film on Mg alloy AZNd in simulated biological fluid studied by scanning electrochemical microscopy. Journal of Electroanalytical Chemistry. 2015, 739, 211–17.
[774] Yajid MAM et al. Corrosion resistance investigation of nanostructured Si- and Si/TiO2-coated Mg alloy in 3.5% NaCl solution. Vacuum. 2014, 108, 61–65.
[775] Rau JV et al. Hydroxyapatite coatings on Mg-Ca alloy prepared by pulsed laser deposition: properties and corrosion resistance in simulated body fluid. Ceramics International. 2018, 44, 16678–87.
[776] Bakhsheshi-Rad HR et al. In-vitro corrosion inhibition mechanism of fluorine-doped hydroxyapatite and brushite coated Mg–Ca alloys for biomedical applications. Ceramics International. 2014, 40, 7971–82.
[777] Zhao D-P et al. Effects of Sr incorporation on surface structure and corrosion resistance of hydroxyapatite coated Mg-4Zn alloy for biomedical applications. Transactions of Nonferrous Metals Society of China. 2018, 28, 1563–70.
[778] Pan Y et al. Dissolution and precipitation behaviors of silicon-containing ceramic coating on Mg–Zn–Ca alloy in simulated body fluid. Colloids and Surfaces B: Biointerfaces. 2014, 122, 746–51.
[779] Guan SK et al. In vitro corrosion behavior of Ti-O film deposited on fluoride-treated Mg–Zn–Y–Nd alloy. Applied Surface Science. 2012, 258, 3571–77.
[780] Hou SS et al. In vitro corrosion behavior of Ti-O film deposited on fluoride-treated Mg–Zn–Y–Nd alloy. Applied Surface Science. 2012, 258, 3571–77.
[781] Panemangalore DB et al. Effect of fluoride coatings on the corrosion behavior of Mg-Zn-Er alloys. Surfaces and Interfaces. 2019, 14, 72–81.
[782] Li Z et al. In vitro and in vivo corrosion, mechanical properties and biocompatibility evaluation of MgF2-coated Mg-Zn-Zr alloy as cancellous screws. Materials Science and Engineering: C. 2017, 75, 1268–80.
[783] Li Q et al. Improving the corrosion resistance of ZEK100 magnesium alloy by combining high-pressure torsion technology with hydroxyapatite coating. Materials & Design. 2019, 181; https://doi.org/10.1016/j.matdes.2019.107933.
[784] Ma Y et al. Characteristics and corrosion studies of vanadate conversion coating formed on Mg–14wt%Li–1wt%Al–0.1wt%Ce alloy. Applied Surface Science. 2012, 261, 59–67.
[785] Zeng R-C et al. Influence of solution temperature on corrosion resistance of Zn-Ca phosphate conversion coating on biomedical Mg-Li-Ca alloys. Transactions of Nonferrous Metals Society of China. 2013, 23, 3293–99.
[786] Cui L-Y et al. In vitro corrosion resistance and antibacterial performance of novel tin dioxide-doped calcium phosphate coating on degradable Mg-1Li-1Ca alloy. Journal of Materials Science & Technology. 2019, 35, 254–65.
[787] Wang C et al. Effect of single Si1-xCx coating and compound coatings on the thermal conductivity and corrosion resistance of Mg-3Sn alloy. Journal of Magnesium and Alloys. 2015, 3, 10–15.
[788] Shangguan Y et al. Investigation of the inner corrosion layer formed in pulse electrodeposition coating on Mg-Sr alloy and corresponding degradation behavior. Journal of Colloid and Interface Science. 2016, 481, 1–12.

[789] Jin W et al. Improved corrosion resistance of Mg-Y-RE alloy coated with niobium nitride. Thin Solid Films. 2014, 572, 85–90.
[790] Jin W et al. Tantalum nitride films for corrosion protection of biomedical Mg-Y-RE alloy. Journal of Alloys and Compounds. 2018, 764, 947–58.
[791] Azumi K, Elsentriecy HH, Tang J. Plating techniques to protect magnesium (Mg) alloys from corrosion. Corrosion Prevention of Magnesium Alloys. 2013, 347–69.
[792] Zhao C et al. Enhanced corrosion resistance and antibacterial property of Zn doped DCPD coating on biodegradable Mg. Materials Letters. 2016, 180, 42–46.
[793] Wang S-H et al. Electrodeposition of Cu coating with high corrosion resistance on Mg-3.0Nd-0.2Zn-0.4Zr magnesium alloy. Transactions of Nonferrous Metals Society of China. 2014, 24, 3810–17.
[794] Wang Y et al. Facile formation of super-hydrophobic nickel coating on magnesium alloy with improved corrosion resistance. Colloids and Surfaces A: Physicochemical and Engineering Aspects. 2018, 538, 500–05.
[795] Lee WJ et al. Improved corrosion resistance of Mg alloy AZ31B induced by selective evaporation of Mg using large pulsed electron beam irradiation. Journal of Materials Science & Technology. 2019, 35, 891–901.
[796] Phuong NV et al. Corrosion protection utilizing Ag layer on Cu coated AZ31 Mg alloy. Corrosion Science. 2018, 136, 201–09.
[797] Saranya K et al. Selenium conversion coating on AZ31 Mg alloy: A solution for improved corrosion rate and enhanced bio-adaptability. Surface and Coatings Technology. 2019, 378; https://doi.org/10.1016/j.surfcoat.2019.124902.
[798] Zarebidaki A et al. Microstructure and corrosion behavior of electrodeposited nano-crystalline nickel coating on AZ91 Mg alloy. Journal of Alloys and Compounds. 2014, 615, 825–30.
[799] Tsai WT et al. Electrodeposition of aluminum on magnesium (Mg) alloys in ionic liquids to improve corrosion resistance. Corrosion Prevention of Magnesium Alloys. 2013, 393–413.
[800] Zhang D et al. A comparative study on the corrosion behaviour of Al, Ti, Zr and Hf metallic coatings deposited on AZ91D magnesium alloys. Surface and Coatings Technology. 2016, 303, 94–102.
[801] Chen D et al. Corrosion resistance of Ni/Cu/Ni–P triple-layered coating on Mg–Li alloy. Surface and Coatings Technology. 2014, 254, 440–46.
[802] Jin W et al. Corrosion resistance and cytocompatibility of tantalum-surface-functionalized biomedical ZK60 Mg alloy. Corrosion Science. 2017, 114, 45–56.
[803] Shi L, Hu J, Lin X-D, Fang L, Meng F-M. A robust superhydrophobic PPS-PTFE/SiO2 composite coating on AZ31 Mg alloy with excellent wear and corrosion resistance properties. Journal of Alloys and Compounds. 2017, 721, 157–63.
[804] Abdal-hay A, Barakat NAM, Lim JK. Hydroxyapatite-doped poly(lactic acid) porous film coating for enhanced bioactivity and corrosion behavior of AZ31 Mg alloy for orthopedic applications. Ceramics International. 2013, 39, 183–95.
[805] Liu W, Yan Z, Zhang Z, Zhang Y, Li Z. Bioactive and anti-corrosive bio-MOF-1 coating on magnesium alloy for bone repair application. Journal of Alloys and Compounds. 2019, 788, 705–11.
[806] Lin Y, Cai S, Jiang S, Xie D, Xu G. Enhanced corrosion resistance and bonding strength of Mg substituted β-tricalcium phosphate/Mg(OH)2 composite coating on magnesium alloys via one-step hydrothermal method. Journal of the Mechanical Behavior of Biomedical Materials. 2019, 90, 547–55.

[807] Wang Y, Gu Z, Liu J, Jiang J, Ding J. An organic/inorganic composite multi-layer coating to improve the corrosion resistance of AZ31B Mg alloy. Surface and Coatings Technology. 2019, 360, 276–84.
[808] Brusciotti F, Snihirova DV, Xue H, Montemor MF. Hybrid epoxy–silane coatings for improved corrosion protection of Mg alloy. Corrosion Science. 2013, 67, 82–90.
[809] Bertuola M, Miñán A, Grillo CA, Cortizo MC, Lorenzo de Mele MAF. Corrosion protection of AZ31 alloy and constrained bacterial adhesion mediated by a polymeric coating obtained from a phytocompound. Colloids and Surfaces B: Biointerfaces. 2018, 172, 187–96.
[810] Xu P, Lu X, Cheng H, Feng X, Shi X. Investigation of the surface modification of magnesium particles with stannate on the corrosion resistance of a Mg-rich epoxy coating on AZ91D magnesium alloy. Progress in Organic Coatings. 2019, 135, 591–600.
[811] Ashassi-Sorkhabi H, Moradi-Alavian S, Jafari R, Kazempour A, Asghari E. Effect of amino acids and montmorillonite nanoparticles on improving the corrosion protection characteristics of hybrid sol-gel coating applied on AZ91 Mg alloy. Materials Chemistry and Physics. 2019, 225, 298–308.
[812] Shen S, Zuo Y, Zhao X. The effects of 8-hydroxyquinoline on corrosion performance of a Mg-rich coating on AZ91D magnesium alloy. Corrosion Science. 2013, 76, 275–83.
[813] Singh S, Singh G, BAla N. Corrosion behavior and characterization of HA/Fe3O4/CS composite coatings on AZ91 Mg alloy by electrophoretic deposition. Materials Chemistry and Physics. 2019, 237; https://doi.org/10.1016/j.matchemphys.2019.121884.
[814] Gaur S, Singh Raman RK, Khanna AS. In vitro investigation of biodegradable polymeric coating for corrosion resistance of Mg-6Zn-Ca alloy in simulated body fluid. Materials Science and Engineering: C. 2014, 42, 91–101.
[815] Bakhsheshi-Rad HR, Hamzah E, Kasiri-Asgarani M, Jabbarzare S, Abdul Kadir MR. Deposition of nanostructured fluorine-doped hydroxyapatite–polycaprolactone duplex coating to enhance the mechanical properties and corrosion resistance of Mg alloy for biomedical applications. Materials Science and Engineering: C. 2016, 60, 526–37.
[816] Bakhsheshi-Rad HR, Hamzah E, Daroonparvar M, Yajid MAM, Medraj M. Fabrication and corrosion behavior of Si/HA nano-composite coatings on biodegradable Mg–Zn–Mn–Ca alloy. Surface and Coatings Technology. 2014, 258, 1090–99.
[817] Bakhsheshi-Rad HR, Hamzah E, Ismail AF, Daroonparvar M, Medraj M. Microstructural, mechanical properties and corrosion behavior of plasma sprayed NiCrAlY/nano-YSZ duplex coating on Mg–1.2Ca–3Zn alloy. Ceramics International. 2015, 41, 15272–77.
[818] Bakhsheshi-Rad HR, Hamzah E, Ismail AF, Sharer Z, Medraj M. Synthesis and corrosion behavior of a hybrid bioceramic-biopolymer coating on biodegradable Mg alloy for orthopaedic implants. Journal of Alloys and Compounds. 2015, 648, 1067–71.
[819] Bakhsheshi-Rad HR, Hamzah E, Daroonparvar M, Abdul Kadir MR, Staiger MP. Enhancement of corrosion resistance and mechanical properties of Mg–1.2Ca–2Bi via a hybrid silicon-biopolymer coating system. Surface and Coatings Technology. 2016, 301, 133–39.
[820] Bakhsheshi-Rad HR, Hamzah E, Abdul-Kadir MR, Daroonparvar M, Medraj M. Corrosion and mechanical performance of double-layered nano-Al/PCL coating on Mg–Ca–Bi alloy. Vacuum. 2015, 119, 95–98.
[821] Maurya R, Siddiqui AR, Katiyar PK, Balani PK. Mechanical, tribological and anti-corrosive properties of polyaniline/graphene coated Mg-9Li-7Al-1Sn and Mg-9Li-5Al-3Sn-1Zn alloys. Journal of Materials Science & Technology. 2019, 35, 1767–78.
[822] Shao Y, Huang H, Zhang T, Meng G, Wang F. Corrosion protection of Mg–5Li alloy with epoxy coatings containing polyaniline. Corrosion Science. 2009, 51, 2906–15.

[823] Guo P, Ang M, Zhang C. Tribological and corrosion resistance properties of graphite composite coating on AZ31 Mg alloy surface produced by plasma electrolytic oxidation. Surface and Coatings Technology. 2019, 359, 197–205.
[824] Li C-Y, Fan X-L, Zeng R-C, Cui L-Y, Guan S-K. Corrosion resistance of in-situ growth of nano-sized Mg(OH)2 on micro-arc oxidized magnesium alloy AZ31 – Influence of EDTA. Journal of Materials Science & Technology. 2019, 35, 1088–98.
[825] Jiang J, Zhou Q, Yu J, Ma A, Chen J. Comparative analysis for corrosion resistance of micro-arc oxidation coatings on coarse-grained and ultra-fine grained AZ91D Mg alloy. Surface and Coatings Technology. 2013, 216, 259–66.
[826] Yao Z, Xu Y, liu Y, Wang D, Wang F. Structure and corrosion resistance of ZrO2 ceramic coatings on AZ91D Mg alloys by plasma electrolytic oxidation. Journal of Alloys and Compounds. 2011, 509, 8469–74.
[827] Ur Rehman Z, Shin SH, Hussain I, Koo BH. Structure and corrosion properties of the two-step PEO coatings formed on AZ91D Mg alloy in K2ZrF6-based electrolyte solution. Surface and Coatings Technology. 2016, 307, 484–90.
[828] Mori Y, Koshi A, Liao J. Corrosion resistance of plasma electrolytic oxidation layer of a non-ignitable Mg–Al–Mn–Ca magnesium alloy. Corrosion Science. 2016, 104, 207–16.
[829] Liu F, Yu J, Song Y, Shan D, Han E-H. Effect of potassium fluoride on the in-situ sealing pores of plasma electrolytic oxidation film on AM50 Mg alloy. Materials Chemistry and Physics. 2015, 162, 452–60.
[830] Lu X, Blawert C, Kainer KU, Zheludkevich ML. Investigation of the formation mechanisms of plasma electrolytic oxidation coatings on Mg alloy AM50 using particles. Electrochimica Acta. 2016, 196, 680–91.
[831] Shahri Z, Allahkaram SR, Soltani R, Jafari H. Study on corrosion behavior of nano-structured coatings developed on biodegradable as cast Mg–Zn–Ca alloy by plasma electrolyte oxidation. Surface and Coatings Technology. 2018, 347, 225–34.
[832] Shahri Z, Allahkaram SR, Soltani R, Jafari H. Optimization of plasma electrolyte oxidation process parameters for corrosion resistance of Mg alloy. Journal of Magnesium and Alloys. 2020, 8, 431–40.
[833] Zhang CL, Zhang F, Song L, Zeng RC, Han EH. Corrosion resistance of a superhydrophobic surface on micro-arc oxidation coated Mg-Li-Ca alloy. Journal of Alloys and Compounds. 2017, 728, 815–26
[834] Jia ZJ, Li M. Liu Q, Xu XC, Wei SC. Micro-arc oxidization of a novel Mg–1Ca alloy in three alkaline KF electrolytes: Corrosion resistance and cytotoxicity. Applied Surface Science. 2014, 292, 1030–39.
[835] Luo D, Liu Y, Yin X, Wang H, Ren L. Corrosion inhibition of hydrophobic coatings fabricated by micro-arc oxidation on an extruded Mg–5Sn–1Zn alloy substrate. Journal of Alloys and Compounds. 2018, 731, 731–38.
[836] Uhlig HH. Corrosion and Corrosion Control: An introduction to corrosion science and engineering. John Wiley & Sons, New York NY, 1963.
[837] http://www.otds.co.uk/products/40/sacrificial-anode-cathodic-protection-sacp.
[838] https://www.marineinsight.com/tech/understanding-sacrificial-anodes-on-ships/.
[839] https://en.wikipedia.org/wiki/Propeller#/media/File:Ship-propeller.jpg.
[840] Sundjono, Priyotomo G, Nuraini L. The selection of magnesium alloys as sacrificial anode for the cathodic protection of underground steel structure. International Journal of Engineering Trends and Technology (IJETT). 2017, 51, 78–82.
[841] Umoru LE, Ige OO. Effects of Tin on Aluminum-Zinc-Magnesium Alloy as Sacrificial Anode in Seawater. Journal of Minerals & Materials Characterization & Engineering. 2007, 7, 105–13.

[842] Yan L, Song G-L, Zheng D. Magnesium alloy anode as a smart corrosivity detector and intelligent sacrificial anode protector for reinforced concrete. Corrosion Science. 2019, 155, 13–28.
[843] Tokuda S, Muto I, Sugawara Y, Takahashi M, Hara N. Micro-electrochemical investigation on the role of Mg in sacrificial corrosion protection of 55mass%Al-Zn-Mg coated steel. Corrosion Science. 2017, 129, 126–35.
[844] Glover CF, Cain TW, Scully JR. Performance of Mg-Sn surface alloys for the sacrificial cathodic protection of Mg alloy AZ31B-H24. Corrosion Science 2019, 149, 195–206.
[845] Cain TW, Melia MA, FitzGerald JM, Scully JR. Evaluation of the Potential Range for Sacrificial Mg Anodes for the Cathodic Protection of Mg Alloy AZ31B-H24. Corrosion. 2017, 73, 544–62.
[846] Richey FW, McCloskey BD, Luntz AC. Mg Anode Corrosion in Aqueous Electrolytes and Implications for Mg-Air Batteries, Journal of The Electrochemical Society. 2016, 163, A958–A963.

Chapter 15
Superelasticity and superplasticity

15.1 Superelasticity

The term SMAs stands for shape-memory materials that exhibit a shape memory effect. However, strictly speaking, it does not describe the manner that such SMA shows an interesting phenomenon, rather it refers to the recovery of shape (or strain) after apparent "permanent" deformation which is previously induced at relatively cold temperatures by heating above a characteristic transformation temperature. Accordingly, it should be called as shape recovery effect. SMAs are hence said to exhibit a crystallographically reversible martensitic transformation. Considering NiTi material as an example, at high temperatures, the SMA possesses an austenite phase (the parent or memory phase) with long-range order. On cooling below the transformation temperature, the austenite transforms to a thermoelastic martensite whose structure has many variants, typically sheared platelets. Because the martensitic structure is self-accommodating, the deformation on transformation to martensite is zero. The martensite deforms by a twinning mechanism that transforms the different variants to the variant that can accommodate the maximum elongation in the direction of the applied force. The interfaces between platelets in the martensite phase slip very readily and the material is deformed at low applied stresses. The austenite phase has only one possible orientation; thus when heated, all the possible deformed structures of the martensite phase must revert to this orientation of the austenite memory phase and the material recovers its original shape.

The term superelasticity (SE) implies that the extent of elasticity is great (super), from a viewpoint of phenomenology. However, it does not describe the fact that material's elasticity is super, rather it should refer to the isothermal recovery of relatively large (apparent elastic) strains during a mechanical load–unload cycle that occurs at temperatures above a characteristic transformation temperature, so that it should be called as pseudoelasticity. SMAs also display SE, which is a mechanical type of shape memory. This effect is observed when alloys are strained just above their transformation temperature. The mechanical properties of SMAs vary over the temperature range spanning their transformation. At low temperatures, the material exists as martensite and is deformed by a relatively small applied force; it also exhibits shape memory on heating. At high temperatures, the material exists as austenite, which is not easily deformed, and, on heating, no shape memory occurs because there is no phase change. However, if the material is tested just above its transformation temperature to austenite, the applied stress transforms the austenite to martensite and the material exhibits increasing strain at constant applied stress, that is, considerable deformation occurs for a relatively small applied stress. When the stress is removed, the martensite reverts to austenite and the material recovers its original shape. This effect, which makes the

https://doi.org/10.1515/9783110676945-015

alloy appear extremely elastic, is known as SE or pseudoelasticity [1]. Gathering information on superelastic materials, nonferrous materials can include Ag–Cd, Au–Cd, Cu-based alloys with Zn, Al–Ni, Sn and Au–Zn, Ni–Al, Ti–Ni, In–Tl and In–Cd, Mn–Cu, while Fe-based materials alloyed with Pt, Pd, Ni–C, Ni–Co–Ti, Mn–Si are reported as ferrous superelastic alloys. Of these alloys, only Cu–Zn–Al, Cu–Al–Ni and Ni–Ti alloys are presently of commercial importance as superelastic materials [2–6].

Recently, Koike et al. [3, 7–10] developed a new Mg alloy, claiming that it is a superelastic Mg–Sc lightweight alloy at room temperature. Investigating the stress–strain behavior of Mg–18.7 at % Sc alloy sheets at room temperature with martensitic transformation starting temperature of approximately −90 °C, and it was found that the SE of the alloy strongly depends on the grain size, and a distinct room-temperature SE (~3% superelastic strain) in the alloy with a large grain size and the obtained maximum superelastic strain was smaller than that expected from the orientation dependence of the transformation strain, suggesting that the stress-induced martensite phase was stabilized because of the introduction of slip defects. Ogawa et al. [9] examined the stress-induced (or athermal) martensitic transformation and thermally induced martensitic transformation of the β-type Mg–Sc alloy. They also investigated the crystal structure of the thermally induced martensite phase based on in situ X-ray diffraction measurements. Based on the lattice correspondence between body-centered cubic and orthorhombic structures such as that in the case of β-Ti shape-memory alloys (SMAs), it was estimated that the transformation strain of the β-Mg–Sc alloy and the transformation strains along the <001>, <011> and <111> directions in the β-phase were calculated to be +5.7%, +8.8% and +3.3%, respectively. Figure 15.1 compares the extent of SE (in %) of various alloys. It is expected to develop a wide range of superelastic Mg-based alloys in future.

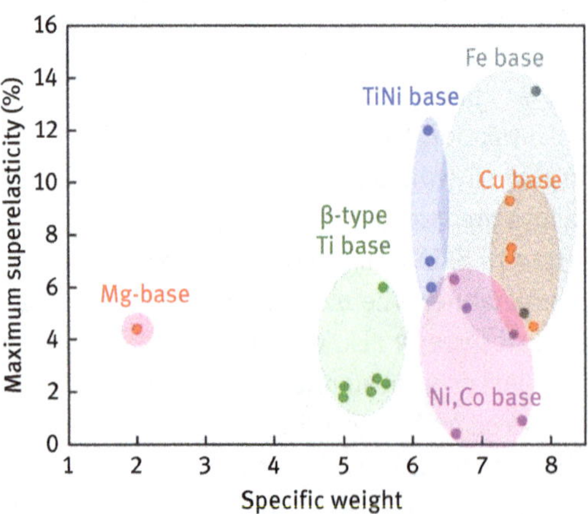

Figure 15.1: Comparison of the extent of superelasticity of various alloys versus specific weight is defined as the ratio of the density of the material (g/cm^3) to the density of water (1 g/cm^3) [3].

SMAs, which display shape recovery upon heating, as well as SE, offer many technological advantages in various applications. Those distinctive behaviors have been observed in many polycrystalline alloy systems such as nickel titanium (TiNi)-, copper-, iron-, nickel-, cobalt- and Ti-based alloys but not in lightweight alloys such as magnesium (Mg) and aluminum alloys. It was shown that an Mg SMA exhibits SE of 4.4% at −150 °C and shape recovery upon heating. The shape-memory properties are caused by reversible martensitic transformation. This Mg alloy includes lightweight scandium, and its density is about 2 g/cm^3, which is one-third less than that of practical TiNi SMAs. This finding raises the potential for development and application of lightweight SMAs across a number of industries [3]. In addition, it was also reported that an Mg–Sc alloy with 18.3 at% scandium showed shape recovery upon heating from −30 °C to room temperature. The researchers believe that this could have a significant impact on the aerospace industry. The lighter the components, the more fuel efficient the rockets and spacecraft. Hence, the lightweight magnesium-based SMA has great potential in aerospace applications such as self-deployable space habitat frames and damping devices on spacecraft systems [11].

15.2 Superplasticity

15.2.1 Phenomenon

Superplasticity is a deformation phenomenon characterized by both large neck-free elongation and vanishing flow stress, observed in a critical processing temperature range. There appear to be two types of superplastic flow, though it has not been shown that their mechanisms differ. First, there is "micrograin" plasticity, in which very fine-grained materials (1–3 μm) exhibit superplastic flow within a narrow temperature range at low strain rates ($\dot{e} \approx 10^{-5}$–10^{-3} s^{-1}); second, there is "transformation" plasticity, which occurs in allotropic materials during a phase change. Superplasticity occurs only at high homologous temperatures ($T/T_M > 0.5$; T, deformation temperature; T_M, melting point), where the dominant deformation mechanism changes from the dislocations activity to thermally activated mechanisms such as diffusional processes (e.g., volume and grain boundary diffusion) and grain boundary sliding and grain rotation. Transformation plasticity is generally rationalized in terms of deformation during structural rearrangements associated with a phase transformation [12], where the transformation front behaves like a Newtonian viscous flow through the Nabarro-Herring creep theory [13–15]. Figure 15.2 shows the basic metallographic views explaining (a) grain boundary sliding of Mg alloy (AZ31) [16] and (b) grain rotation mechanism of Al–Mg–Mn alloy [17] for the micrograin superplasticity. With ordinary materials, depending on the elongation, grains are stretched along the stressing axis, while grains remain as equiaxed structure even under a large superplastic elongation. Grain boundary sliding with diffusional

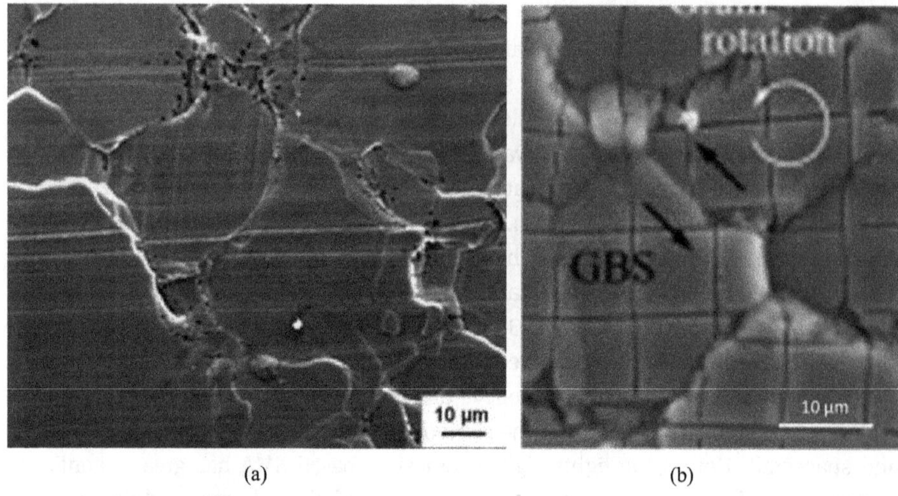

Figure 15.2: Two main mechanisms for superplastic straining: (a) grain boundary sliding of Mg alloy and (b) grain rotation of Al alloy.

accommodation model was introduced to explain a large amount of superplastic elongation. Moreover, if the "*m*" value is larger, intragrain deformation varnishes.

When work-hardening exponent (*n*) and strain rate sensitivity index (*m*) are included in the complete stress–strain relationship, the constitutive equation can be expressed as $\sigma = Ke^n\dot{e}^m$, where σ is stress, *e* is strain and $\dot{e}$ is strain rate. The "*m*" value is a macroscopic material constant. Each superplastic material has its own "*m*" value under a specific strain rate range and temperature. Since stress–strain curve during the superplastic deformation is characterized by a normal stress–strain curve under low applied stress, there does not occur any work hardening; thus, the "*n*" exponent is zero. Hence, the earlier equation, in the case of superplastic deformations, can be reduced to $\sigma = K\dot{e}^m$. It is generally believed that the smaller the grain size, the higher the "*m*" value. For superplastic deformation the range of 0.1–0.2. For superplastic deformation, "*m*" value is $0.3 < m < 1.0$, and $m = 1$ indicates the viscous flow. Under a slight change of "*m*" value, σ changes largely according to changes in strain rate ($\dot{e}$); when the local necking starts to take place, the strain rate of the portion increases, so that σ is also increased, thereby preventing the necking phenomenon. As given in Table 15.1, "*m*" has twofold characters: temperature dependency and grain size dependency. Hence, severe plastic forming methods (such as FSP, ECAP, HPR, HRDSR, MDF, MDIF, CGF) listed as footnote of Table 15.1 are conducted to produce ultra-fine grain size microstructures.

15.2.2 Superplastic metallic materials

Although superplastic materials are not limited to metallic materials, they can include ceramics such as fine-grained ZrO_2 [18] or fine-grained ZrO_2–Al_2O_3 composite [19], and plastics including PVC, PTFE, PMMA, PA66, ABS, PC, POM resins [20], the majority of superplastic materials are polycrystalline fine-grained metallic materials. During a history of research activities on both micrograin superplasticity and transformation superplasticity, most materials should include Al alloy, Bi alloy, Cd alloy, Co alloy, Cr alloy, Cu alloy, Ni alloy, Pb alloy, Sn alloy, Ti alloy, W alloy, Zn alloy, Zr alloy and Fe alloy. Mg-based alloys are listed in the following section. Several parameters common to all superplastic materials are (1) "*m*" value is in the range from nearly 0.5 to close to 1.0, and (2) most metallographic structure at a starting condition is the eutectic (lamellar) structure with a few cases of the eutectoid structure. Hence, these structures are needed to subject to a combination of appropriate heat treatment and working (such as extrusion or rolling) to achieve ultra-fine-grained structure to accommodate the best conditions for superplasticity. The required grain structure (with grain size of ~2 μm) could be obtained by several procedures, hot extrusion with a high extrusion ratio, severe plastic deformation via equal channel angular extrusion, consolidation of machined chip and/or powder metallurgy (PM) processing of rapidly solidified powders [21].

15.2.3 Superplastic Mg materials

The table lists the most updated information on superplastic Mg-based alloys, which are normally subjected to various working processes to refine the grain structure.

Table 15.1: List and principles parameters of superplastic Mg materials.

Mg-based alloy types	*m*-Index	$\dot{\varepsilon}$ (strain rate) (s^{-1})	Elongation (%)	Temperature (°C)	Grain size (μm)	Process	Ref.
Mg–Al–Zn alloy systems							
Mg–Al–Zn (AZ31)		5×10^{-4}	1,050	450	11.4	FSPed	[22]
Mg–Al–Zn (AZ31)		5×10^{-2}	268	450		FSPed	[22]
Mg–Al–Zn (ZK60)	0.5	3×10^{-4}	2,040	220		ECAPed	[23]
Mg–Al–Zn (ZK60)		3×10^{-3}	1,400	220		ECAPed	[23]
Mg–Al–Zn (AZ61)		1×10^{-3}	400	400	5	Cast	[24]

Table 15.1 (continued)

Mg-based alloy types	*m*-Index	$\dot{e}$ (strain rate) (s^{-1})	Elongation (%)	Temperature (°C)	Grain size (μm)	Process	Ref.
Mg–Al–Zn (AZ61)		2×10^{-4}	560	400	5	Cast	[24]
Mg–Al–Zn (AZ75)		1×10^{-3}	615	300	6	HPRed	[25]
Mg–Al–Zn (AZ91)	0.4	1×10^{-2}–1×10^{-4}		225–300		FSPed	[26]
Mg–Al–Zn (AZ91)			1,000	275–300		Cast	[27]
Mg–Al–Zn (AZ91)		3×10^{-3}	570			ECAPed	[28]
Mg–Al–Zn (AZ91)		1×10^{-2}–1×10^{-4}		225–300		FSPed	[27]
Mg–Zn alloy systems							
Mg–Zn–Zr (ZK30)			360		1–5	Extruded	[29]
Mg–Zn–Zr (ZK60)	0.5	3×10^{-3}	810			ECAPed	[30]
Mg–Zn–Zr (ZK61)		1×10^{-2}	800	250	1.6	Extruded	[31]
Mg-7Zn-5Gd-0.6Zr	0.45	1.67×10^{-3}	863	250	3.01	Extruded	[32]
Mg–13Zn–1.55Y (ZW132)		1×10^{-3}	455	200		HRDSRed	[33]
Mg–13Zn–1.55Y (ZW132)		1×10^{-3}	1,021	250		HRDSRed	[33]
Mg–Li alloy systems							
Mg–8Li	0.37		440	0.35Tm		Extruded	[34]
Mg–8Li		5×10^{-5}	164.5	290	10	Extruded	[35]
Mg–Li–Zn	0.5	1×10^{-3}	1,400	200		Extruded/ rolled	[36]
Mg–Li–Zn	0.5	1×10^{-2}	600	200		Extruded/ rolled	[36]
Mg–Li–Zn	0.5	1×10^{-3}	720	150		Extruded/ rolled	[36]
Mg–Li–Zn (LZ81)	0.51	3×10^{-3}–1×10^{-1}		275	4	MDFed	[37]
Mg–Li–Zn (LZ81)	0.55	1.5×10^{-4}	758	290		Extruded	[38]
Mg–Li–Zn (LZ82)	0.55	1×10^{-3}	430	225		Extruded/ rolled	[39]
Mg–Li–Al (LA91)	0.68		621.1	275–300		Cast	[40]

Table 15.1 (continued)

Mg-based alloy types	*m*-Index	$\dot{\varepsilon}$ (strain rate) (s^{-1})	Elongation (%)	Temperature (°C)	Grain size (μm)	Process	Ref.
Mg–Li–Al (LA91)			564	300		Extruded	[41]
Mg-10.2Li-2.1Al-2.23Zn-0.2Sr	0.88	1.7×10^{-3}	712	350		MDFed	[42]
Mg–Gd alloy systems							
Mg–2Gd	0.49			400	4.3	CGPed	[43]
Mg–3Gd–1Zn (GZ31)	0.51			400	1.7	ECAPed	[44]
Mg-Gd-Y-Zr alloy		2×10^{-4}	410	450	10	Extruded	[45]
Mg-Gd-Y-Zr alloy	0.32	5×10^{-4}	300	450		MDIFed	[46]
Mg-5Gd-4Y-0.4Zr (GW54)	0.5			450	2–5	ECAPed	[47]
Mg-10Gd-3Y-0.5Zr (GW103)		1.0×10^{-3}	1,110	415		FSPed	[48]
Mg–Y alloy systems							
Mg–Y–Nd		3×10^{-3}	967	460	1.3	FSPed	[49]
Mg-1.2Y-7.12Zn-0.84Zr		1×10^{-2}	1,110	450		FSPed	[50]
Mg-1.7Y-7.6Zn-1.8Zr		5×10^{-4}	780	450		Extruded/ rolled	[51]
Mg–7Y–4Gd–1Zn		1.7×10^{-4}	700	470		Extruded	[52]
Others							
Mg-8Sn-3Al-1Zn		5×10^{-4}–5×10^{-3}	450–1,050	250		Extruded	[53]

FSP, friction stir processing; ECAP, equal-channel angular pressing; HPR, hard plate rolling; HRDSR, high-ratio differential speed rolling; MDF, multidirectional forging; MDIF, multidirectional impact forging; CGP, constrained groove pressing.

15.2.4 Superplastic forming and superplastic forming–diffusion bonding

An inherent limitation of conventional metals is that they are unstable when plastically deformed by stretching forces, being responsible for the catastrophic necking observed in the tension mode. Considerable engineering attention has recently been focused on the exploitation of superplastic metals, which are relatively stable when deformed in tension. This behavior derives from the fact that flow stress of superplastic materials, under appropriate conditions, is very sensitive to the rate of deformation. In the equation $\sigma = K\dot{\varepsilon}^m$, the exaggerated strain rate sensitivity "m" of superplastic materials is usually confined to relatively low rates of strain. Under such conditions, the flow stress of the material is low compared with conventional materials. Accordingly, the forming rate is slow. The typical SPF (superplastic forming) products are shown in Figure 15.3. It is clearly indicated that SPF technique is suitable for near-net shape forming.

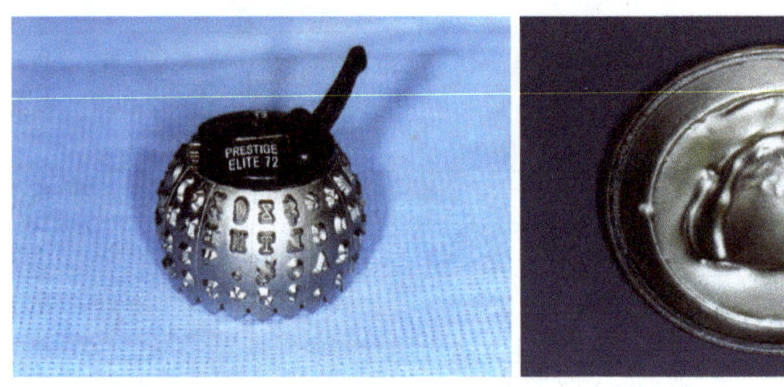

(a) IBM typewriter ball head (b) Full denture base

Figure 15.3: Typical examples of SPFed products: (a) IBM typewrite ball head made of Zn alloy and (b) SPFed full denture made of commercial pure titanium grade III.

During studying the transformation superplasticity behaviors of cast iron, Oshida et al. [54–56] discovered the possibility of diffusion bonding (DB) phenomena with higher interdiffusion coefficient, indicating pioneer studies of SPF/DB technique. Welding processes can be classified into two main categories: (1) liquid-phase welding, for example, all fusion welding processes such as conventional arc welding, laser welding and electron beam welding, and (2) solid-state welding, for example, forge welding, friction stir welding, explosive welding and solid-state DB. Diffusion welding is the only welding technique by means of which full cross-sectional welds, also of internal structures, can be obtained. Normally, there is no liquid phase and the monolithic compound is formed completely under solid-state conditions. For the conditions to be appropriate, mechanical properties across the joined part are comparable to the bulk material. Due to heating of the whole parts, no distinct heat-affected zone (HAZ) is formed. Since then, many researches on R&D of SPF and DB has been reported and SPF/DB becomes to be a well-established process for the manufacture of components almost exclusively from Ti-6Al-4V (Ti64) sheet material. The SPF/DB with gas pressure control for honeycomb structure is fabricated from Ti64 alloy as shown in Figure 15.4 [57].

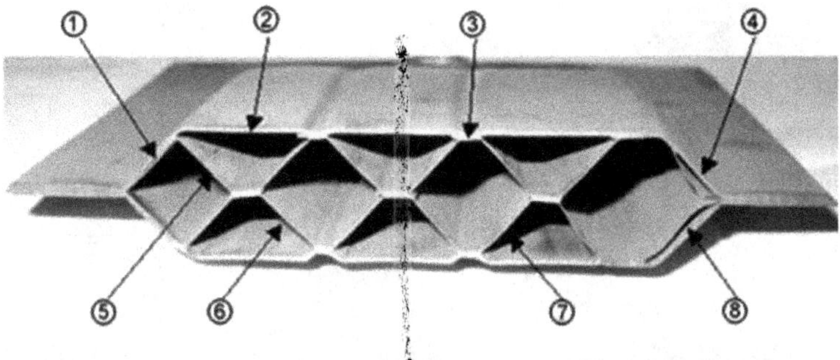

Figure 15.4: SPF/DBed honeycomb structure with a high stiffness-to-weight ratio.

Du et al. [58] fabricated the multilayer structure of Ti_2AlNb-based alloy by the SPF/dB and investigated properties of SPF/DB of Ti–22Al–27Nb alloy. It was reported that (i) the uniaxial tensile experiment showed that the tensile elongation reached up to 236% at the temperature of 970 °C with the strain rate of 3×10^{-4}/s; (ii) combining the microstructure of bonding interface with shear strength of different joints, the DB parameter for the best bonded combination was 970 °C/10 MPa/2 h, as shown in Figure 15.5, indicating an excellent solid-state bonding without any voids and remarkable distortion of grains along the mating interfaces.

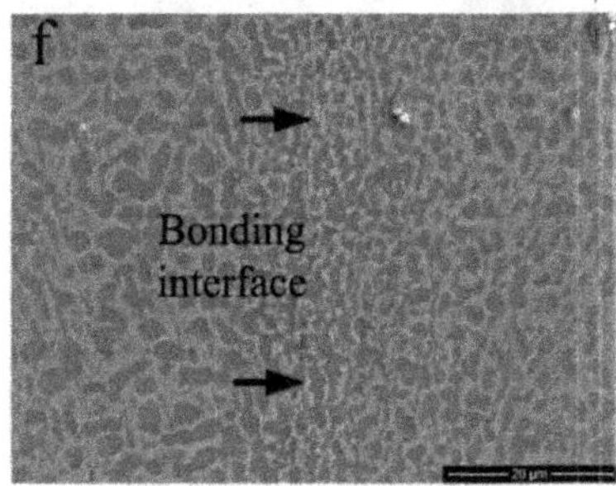

Figure 15.5: SPF/DBed Ti–22Al–27Nb alloy at 970 °C under 10 MPa pressure for 2 h [58].

Saotome et al. [59] successfully fabricated double gears made of $Pd_{40}Cd_{30}Ni_{10}P_{20}$ for millimachines by a combination of PM (DB) and superplastic forging (SPF), as shown in Figure 15.6.

15.2.5 SPF and SPF–DB of Mg materials

Magnesium alloys are of emerging interest in the automotive, aerospace and electronics industries due to their lightweight, high specific strength, damping capacity and others [60]. Cold working is known to be a difficult process for conducting the plastic working of Mg alloys since the deformability of the alloys is extremely small at room

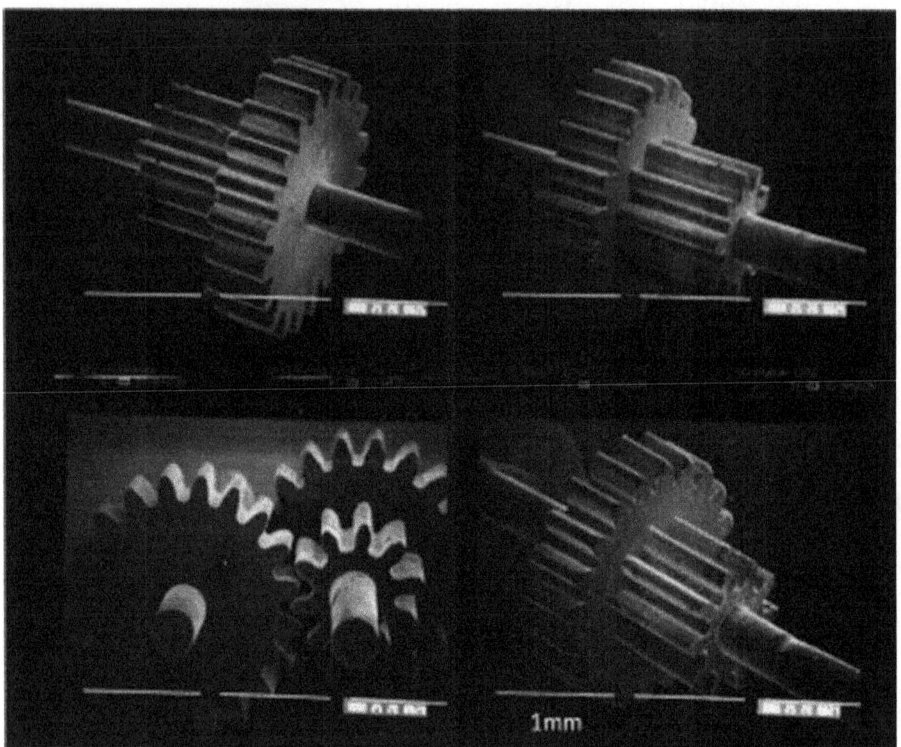

Figure 15.6: SPF–DBed minigear for millimachines [59].

temperature. Such poor formability at room temperature is affected by the lack of slip systems and the formation of basal texture, both of whose characteristics are attributed to the hexagonal close-packed structure of Mg alloys [61, 62]. However, Mg alloys with a slip system other than the basal slip system can become more active; this results in a lower deformation resistance and a considerable increase in expansion when the deformation temperature increases. Therefore, considering the product precision and formability, plastic working of Mg alloy members is conducted mostly at high temperatures [63]. There are many reports on the strength, elongation and superplasticity of Mg alloys [64–66], and data are presented in Table 15.1.

SPF has been commercially used to fabricate the complex parts from different Ni-based, Fe-based, Ti-based and Al-based alloys with high-dimensional accuracy in a single-cycle process and without any machining. SPF of Mg-based alloys is gradually receiving significant attention because of high strength-to-weight ratio of the alloys and their potential applications in automobile and aerospace industries, but low plasticity of Mg-based alloys at room temperature is still their main drawbacks for structural applications [67]. Kubota et al. [68] prepared ultrafine-grained Mg-based alloys through equal-channel angular extrusion processing (ECAP) to obtain grain size of less than 1 μm. It was reported that fine-grained Mg-based materials exhibit superplastic behavior at high stain rates (≥10^{-1} s^{-1}) or low temperatures (≤200 °C). Muraki et al. [69] mentioned that the required grain size for high strain rate SPF was estimated to be ~2 μm, which can be achieved by several procedures, hot extrusion with a high extrusion ratio, severe plastic deformation via equal channel angular extrusion, consolidation of machined chip and/or PM processing of rapidly solidified powders, on a laboratory scale. Edalati et al. [70], who studied the room-temperature superplasticity of ultrafine-grained Mg–8Li (wt%) alloy, reported that the severe plastic deformation demonstrated 440% elongation at room temperature (0.35 T_m) with a strain rate sensitivity (*m* value) of 0.37. These unique properties were associated with enhanced grain boundary sliding, which was approximately 60% of the total elongation, by the fast grain boundary diffusion caused by the Li segregation along the grain boundaries and the formation of Li-rich interphases, providing a new approach for controlling the room-temperature superplasticity by engineering grain boundary composition and diffusion, which is of importance in metal forming technology without heating. Shim et al. [60] investigated superplastic phenomena and possible application of SPF technique on commercialized AZ (Mg–Al–Zn) or ZK (Mg–Zn–Zr) series alloys and mentioned that (i) these alloys exhibit superplastic behavior and show very large tensile ductility, which means that these materials have potential application to SPF of magnesium alloy sheets; (ii) the SPF technique offers many advantages such as near-net shaping, design flexibility, simple process and low die cost; (iii) superplasticity occurs in materials having very small grain sizes of less than 10 μm and these small grains in magnesium alloys can be achieved by thermomechanical treatment in conventional rolling or extrusion processes; and (iv) some coarse-grained magnesium alloys are reported to have superplasticity when grain refinement occurs through recrystallization during deformation in the initial stage.

Moving to SPF/DB of Mg materials, Watanabe et al. [71] characterized parametric dependencies for superplastic flow in PM magnesium alloys and composites to elucidate the deformation mechanism. It was reported that the mechanism was proposed to be slip-accommodated grain boundary sliding; however, the PMed alloys and composites were strengthened at low temperatures below ~280 °C and were different from the case in ingot magnesium alloys, which behaved identically over a wide range of temperatures. The critical strain rate, below which the effect of intragranular particle was lost, was developed by considering the dislocation–particle interaction during slip accommodation process, suggesting that the diffusional relaxation around the intragranular oxide particles was not completed during the slip accommodation process at low temperatures, and this caused the dislocation pile-up at the intragranular particles. It was also expected that the dislocation pile-up at the intragranular particles would contribute to the strengthening at low temperatures in PM alloys and PM composites [71]. Somekawa et al. [72] investigated the superplastic characteristic and DB behavior in a commercial AZ31 (Mg–Al–Zn) sheet having equiaxed grain size with an average size of 16.8 μm. It was mentioned that the alloy behaved in a superplastic manner from 350 to 450 °C, and the maximum of lap shear strength was 0.85 at a bonding pressure of 3 MPa and a bonding temperature of 400 °C, with a bonding time of 3 h. Yu et al. [73] proposed a new SPF/DB technology using gasification agent as a pressurization mediator. ZK60 (Mg–Zn–Zr) alloy with a thickness of 1 mm and grain size of 7.9 µm was selected to conduct the experiment of SPF/DB and it was reported that corrugated ZK60 magnesium alloy parts were well formed under the temperature between 380 and 400 °C and forming time of 50 min. Yu et al. [74] applied the penalty function method to analyze the contact problem associated with the SPF/DB process of magnesium alloy corrugated part by FEM software (MARC) with a three-dimensional finite element model. The distribution of the wall thickness and the deformation characteristic during the forming process were analyzed, and also the location of the risky point was predicted by tracing the wall thickness and analyzing the friction between the die and the part. It was reported that ZK60 Mg alloy corrugated part was produced successfully by SPF/DB, and the results of FEM simulation were in good agreement with that of the experiment. It was observed that the cavities are growing with the increase in the deformation amount, and the cavity size and percentage get maximum values (9 µm and 7.7%, respectively) at the corner region of the part, in which the wall thickness decreases sharply and thereby leading to the fracture of the part.

References

[1] Oshida Y, Tominaga T. Nickel-Titanium Materials: Biomedical Applications. De Gruyter Pub, 2020.

[2] Bidaus J-E, Gotthardt R. Elastic Behavior: Superelasticity. In: J.-E. Bidaux, R. Gotthardt, in Reference Module in Materials Science and Materials Engineering, 2016Encyclopedia of Materials: Science and Technology. 2001, 2423–2425; https://doi.org/10.1016/B978-0-12-803581-8.02942-8.

[3] Ogawa Y, Ando D, Sutou Y, Koike J. A lightweight shape-memory magnesium alloy. Science. 2016, 353, 368–70.

[4] Tanaka Y, Himuro Y, Kainuma R, Sutou Y, Omori T, Ishida K. Ferrous polycrystalline shape-memory alloy showing huge superelasticity. Science. 2010, 327, 1488–90.

[5] Lee D, Omori T, Kainuma R. Ductility enhancement and superelasticity in Fe-Ni-Co-Al-Ti-B polycrystalline alloy. Journal of Alloys Compd. 2014, 617, 120–3.

[6] Tanaka Y, Oikawa K, Sutou Y, Omori T, Kainuma R, Ishida K. Martensitic transition and superelasticity of Co-Ni-Al ferromagnetic shape memory alloys with β + γ two-phase structure. Materials Science Engineering A. 2006, 438/440, 1054–60.

[7] Ogawa Y, Ando D, Sutou Y, Koike J. Aging effect of Mg-Sc alloy with α + β two-phase microstructure. Materials Transactions 2016, 57, 1119–23.

[8] Ogawa Y, Ando D, Sutou Y, Yoshimi K, Koike J. Determination of α/β phase boundaries and mechanical characterization of Mg-Sc binary alloys. Material Science Engineering A 2016, 670, 335–41.

[9] Ogawa Y, Ando D, Sutou Y, Somekawa H, Koike J. Martensitic transformation in a β-type Mg–Sc alloy. Shape Memory and Superelasticity. 2018, 4, 167–73.

[10] Yamagishi K, Ogawa Y, Ando D, Sutou Y, Koike J. Room temperature superelasticity in a lightweight shape memory Mg alloy. Scripta materialia 2019, 168, 114–8.

[11] Magnesium-scandium alloys show superelastic and shape memory properties, ASM International. 2017; http://www.tohoku.ac.jp/en/press/new_lightweight_shape_shifting_alloy.html.

[12] Oshida Y. Transformation Plasticity of Steels and Titanium Alloys in Compression. MS Thesis, L. C. Smith College of Engineering, Syracuse University, Syracuse NY, 1967.

[13] Langdon, T. G. A unified approach to grain boundary sliding in creep and superplasticity. Metallurgica et Materialia 1994, 42, 2437–43.

[14] Greenwodd GW. An analysis of the effect of multiaxial stresses and grain shape on Nabarro-Herring creep. Journal of Philosophical Magazine A. 1985, 51, 537–42.

[15] Oelschlägel D, Weiss V. Superplasticity of steel during the ferrite → austenite transformation. Transactions ASM.1966, 59, 143–54.

[16] Korla R, Chokshi AH. A constitutive equation for grain boundary sliding: an experimental approach. Metallurgical and Materials Transactions A. 2014, 45, 698–708.

[17] Masuda H, Kanazawa T, Tobe H, Sato E. Dynamic anisotropic grain growth during superplasticity in Al–Mg–Mn alloy. Scripta materialia 2018, 149, 84–7.

[18] Wakai F. Superplasticity of ceramics. Ceramics International. 1991, 17, 153–63.

[19] Chokshi AH. Superplasticity in fine grained ceramics and ceramic composites: current understanding and future prospects. Materials Science and Engineering: A. 1993, 166, 119–33.

[20] Oshida Y, Nakamura J. On the abnormal plastic phenomena of thermoplastic resins. Plasticity and Forming. 1975, 16, 928–34.

[21] Mukai T, Watanabe H, Higashi K. Application of superplasticity in commercial magnesium alloy for fabrication of structural components. Journal Materials Science and Technology. 2000, 16, 1314–9.

[22] Zhang D-T et al., Superplasticity of AZ31 magnesium alloy prepared by friction stir processing. Transactions of Nonferrous Metals Society of China. 2011, 21, 1911–6.

[23] Cottam R, et al., Extraordinary superplastic ductility of magnesium alloy ZK60. Journal of Materials Science. 2005, 20, 1375–8.

[24] Kim WJ, et al., Superplasticity in fine-grained AZ61 magnesium alloy. Et al., Metals and Materials. 2000, 6, 255; https://doi.org/10.1007/BF03028220June 2000, 6:255.

[25] Rong J, et al., Development of a novel strength ductile Mg-7Al-5Zn alloy with high superplasticity processed by hard-plate rolling (HPR). Journal of alloys and compounds. 2018, 738, 246–54.

[26] Cavaliere P, et al., Superplastic behaviour of friction stir processed AZ91 magnesium alloy produced by high pressure die cast. Journal of Materials Processing Technology. 2007, 184, 77–83.

[27] Solberg JK, et al., Superplasticity in magnesium alloy AZ91. Materials Science and Engineering: A. 1991, 134, 1201–3.

[28] Chuvil'deev VN, et al., Superplasticity and internal friction in microcrystalline AZ91 and ZK60 magnesium alloys processed by equal-channel angular pressing. Journal of alloys and compounds. 2004, 378, 253–7.

[29] Álvarez-Leal M, et al., Superplasticity in a commercially extruded ZK30 magnesium alloy. Materials Science and Engineering: A. 2018, 710, 240–4.

[30] Lee S, et al., Inter-granular liquid phase aiding grain boundary sliding in superplastic deformation of fine-grained ZK60 Mg Alloy. Transactions of Nonferrous Metals Society of China. 2010, 20, s576–s579.

[31] Kim B, et al., High-strain-rate superplasticity of fine-grained Mg–6Zn–0.5Zr alloy subjected to low-temperature indirect extrusion. Scripta materialia. 2017, 141, 138–42.

[32] Yin S, et al., Achieving excellent superplasticity of Mg-7Zn-5Gd-0.6Zr alloy at low temperature regime. Scientific reports. 2019, 9, 4365; https://doi.org/10.1038/s41598-018-38420-7.
[33] Kwak TY, et al., Superplastic behavior of an ultrafine-grained Mg-13Zn-1.55Y alloy with a high volume fraction of icosahedral phases prepared by high-ratio differential speed rolling. Journal of Materials Science & Technology. 2017, 33, 919–25.
[34] Edalati K, et al., Room-temperature superplasticity in an ultrafine-grained magnesium alloy. Scientific Report. 2017, 7, 2662; https://doi.org/10.1038/s41598-017-02846-2.
[35] Qu Z, et al., The superplastic property of the as-extruded Mg–8Li alloy. Materials Science and Engineering: A. 2010, 527, 3284–7.
[36] Zhang T, et al., Low temperature superplasticity of a dual-phase Mg-Li-Zn alloy processed by a multi-mode deformation process. Materials Science and Engineering: A. 2018, 737, 61–8.
[37] Mehrabi A, et al., Superplasticity in a multi-directionally forged Mg–Li–Zn alloy. Materials Science and Engineering: A. 2019, 765; https://doi.org/10.1016/j.msea.2019.138274.
[38] Liu X, et al., Superplasticity in a two-phase Mg–8Li–2Zn alloy processed by two-pass extrusion. Materials Science and Engineering: A. 2011, 528, 6157–62.
[39] Liu X, et al., Superplasticity at elevated temperature of an Mg–8%Li–2%Zn alloy. Journal of alloys and compounds 2012, 541, 372–5.
[40] Yang HP, et al., Investigation on the enhanced maximum strain rate sensitivity (m) superplasticity of Mg-9Li-1Al alloy by a two-step deformation method. Materials Science and Engineering: A. 2019, 764; https://doi.org/10.1016/j.msea.2019.138219.
[41] Yang HP, et al., Investigation on the maximum strain rate sensitivity (m) superplastic deformation of Mg-Li based alloy. Materials & design. 2016, 112, 151–9.
[42] Cao F, et al., Superplasticity of a dual-phase-dominated Mg-Li-Al-Zn-Sr alloy processed by multidirectional forging and rolling. Materials Science and Engineering: A. 2017, 704, 360–74.
[43] Hoseini-Athar MM, et al., Microstructural evolution and superplastic behavior of a fine-grained Mg–Gd alloy processed by constrained groove pressing. Materials Science and Engineering: A. 2019, 754, 390–9.
[44] Sarebanzadeh M, et al., Enhancement of superplasticity in a fine-grained Mg–3Gd–1Zn alloy processed by equal-channel angular pressing. Materials Science and Engineering: A. 2015, 646, 249–53.
[45] Zhang X, et al., Superplasticity and microstructure in Mg–Gd–Y–Zr alloy prepared by extrusion. Journal of alloys and compounds. 2009, 481, 296–300.
[46] Li JL, et al., Superplasticity of multi-directional impact forged Mg–Gd–Y-Zr alloy. Journal of alloys and compounds. 2016, 672, 27–35.
[47] Alizadeh R, et al., Microstructural evolution and superplasticity in an Mg–Gd–Y–Zr alloy after processing by different SPD techniques. Materials Science and Engineering: A. 2107, 682, 577–85.
[48] Yang Q, et al., Enhanced superplasticity in friction stir processed Mg–Gd–Y–Zr alloy. Journal of alloys and compounds. 2013, 551, 61–6.
[49] Cao G, et al., Superplastic behavior and microstructure evolution of a fine-grained Mg–Y–Nd alloy processed by submerged friction stir processing. Materials Science and Engineering: A. 2015, 642, 157–66.
[50] Yang, Q, et al., Achieving high strain rate superplasticity in Mg-Zn-Y-Zr alloy produced by friction stir processing. Scripta materialia 2011, 65, 335–8.
[51] Bae, DH, et al., Thermally stable quasicrystalline phase in a superplastic Mg-Zn-Y-Zr alloy. Materials letters. 60, 2190–2193 (2006).
[52] Zhang L, et al., Investigation of high-strength and superplastic Mg–Y–Gd–Zn alloy. Materials & design. 2014, 61, 168–76.

[53] Kim B, et al., Superplasticity and load relaxation behavior of extruded Mg–8Sn–3Al–1Zn alloy at 250°C. Materials Science and Engineering: A. 2016, 656, 234–40.
[54] Oshida Y. An Application of Superplasticity to Powder Metallurgy. Journal of Japan Soceity of Powder and Powder Metallurgy. 1975, 22, 147–53.
[55] Oshida Y, Takase S. Application of dynamic superplasticity to solid-state bonding of cast irons to different ferrous alloys. Journal Japan Institutions of Casting Irons. 1976, 48, 349–54.
[56] Oshida Y, Takase S. On the micro-structures of superplastic solid-state bonded parts in cast irons. Journal Japan Institutions of Casting Irons. 1976, 48, 763–8.
[57] Han W, Zhang K, Wang G. Superplastic forming and diffusion bonding for honeycomb structure of Ti–6Al–4V alloy. Journal of Materials Processing Technology 2007, 183, 450–5.
[58] Du Z, Jiang S, Zhang K, Lu Z, Li B, Zhang D. The structural design and superplastic forming/ diffusion bonding of Ti_2AlNb based alloy for four-layer structure. Materials & design2016, 104, 242–50.
[59] Saotome Y, Itoh A, Amada S (1993) Superplastic micro forming of double gear for milli-machines. Proceedings of the 4th ICTP, Beijing. 2000–5.
[60] Shim J-D, Byun J-Y. Superplasticity of Magnesium Alloys and SPF Applications. Korean Journal of Materials Research. 2017, 27, 53–61.
[61] Noda M, Mori H, Funami K. Transition in deformation mechanism of AZ31 magnesium alloy during high-temperature tensile deformation. Journal of Metallurgy. 2011; https://doi.org/10.1155/2011/165307.
[62] Yoshinaga H, Horiuchi R. On the flow stress of α solid solution Mg-Li alloy single crystals. Transactions of the Japan Institute of Metals. 1963, 4, 134–41.
[63] Takara A, Nishikawa Y, Watanabe H, Somekawa H, Mukai T, Higashi K. New forming process of three-dimensionally shaped magnesium parts utilizing high-strain-rate superplasticity. Materials Transactions. 2004, 45, 2531–6.
[64] Boileau JM, Friedman PA, Houston DQ, Luckey SG. Superplastic response of continuously cast AZ31B magnesium sheet alloys. Journal of materials engineering and performance 2010, 19, 467–80.
[65] Liu M, Yuan G, Wang Q, Wei Y, Ding W, Zhu Y. Superplastic behavior and microstructural evolution in a commercial Mg-3Al-1Zn magnesium alloy. Materials Transactions. 2002, 43, 2433–6.
[66] Panicker R, Chokshi AH, Mishra RK, Verma R, Krajewski PE. Microstructural evolution and grain boundary sliding in a superplastic magnesium AZ31 alloy. Acta materialia 2009, 57, 3683–93.
[67] Paton NE, Hamilton CH. Superplastic Forming of Structural Alloys. The Metallurgical Society of AIME, AIME, Warrendale PA, USA, 1982.
[68] Kubota K, Mabuchi M, Higashi K. Review Processing and mechanical properties of fine-grained magnesium alloys. Journal of Materials Science. 1999, 34, 2255–62.
[69] Muraki T, Watanabe H, Higashi K. Application of superplasticity in commercial magnesium alloy for fabrication of structural components. Materials Science and Technology. 2000, 16, 1314–9.
[70] Edalati K, Masuda T, Arita M, Furui M, Sauvage X, Horita Z, Valiev RZ. Room-temperature superplasticity in an ultrafine-grained magnesium alloy. Scientific reports 2017, 7, 2662; https://doi.org/10.1038/s41598-017-02846-2.
[71] Watanabe H, Mukai T, Mabuchi M, Higashi K. Superplastic deformation mechanism in powder metallurgy magnesium alloys and composites. Acta materialia 2001, 49, 2027–37.
[72] Somekawa H, Hosokawa H, Watanabe H, Higashi K. Diffusion bonding in superplastic magnesium alloys. Materials Science and Engineering: A. 2003, 339, 328–33.

[73] Yu YD, Wang CW, Yin DL. SPF/DB Research in ZK60 Alloy with Gasification Agent as Pressurization Mediator. In: Zhang KF ed., Superplasticity in Advanced Materials – ICSAM; Materials Science Forum. 2006, 551/552, 241–4.

[74] Yu Y, Li C, Feng J. Finite element simulation of SPF/DB process for ZK60 magnesium alloy corrugated part. Proceedings of 2011 International Conference on Electronic & Mechanical Engineering and Information Technology, Harbin. 2011, 1654–7.

Chapter 16
Nonmedical applications

16.1 In general

The practical materials can be, in general, divided into two groups: structural materials and functional materials. Structural (or engineering) materials are those that bear load with required key properties of materials in relation to load bearing including elastic modulus, yield strength, ultimate tensile strength, hardness, ductility, fracture toughness, fatigue and creep resistance. In addition, if materials corrode or wear, their ability to carry load will be degraded. Furthermore, any stress-assisted corrosive activities such as stress-corrosion cracking, corrosion fatigue or hydrogen embrittlement also cause Mg materials to deteriorate much faster than the predicted time. In general, magnesium applications are motivated by the lightweight, high strength, high damping capacity, close dimensional tolerance and ease of fabrication of its alloys. Applications include hand tools, sporting goods, luggage frames, cameras, household appliances, business machines and automobile parts. The aerospace industry employs magnesium alloys in the manufacture of aircraft, rockets and space satellites. Magnesium is also used in tooling plates and, because of its rapid and controlled etching characteristics, in photoengraving [1]. Functional materials display a physical property, which is of use. There is a huge range of functional materials. The following will be covered in this chapter: optical (including lasers, Raman scattering, fluorescence and phosphorescence), electrical (including semiconducting devices and superconductors), dielectrics (piezoelectrics, ferroelectrics, optical fibers, the photocopying process and liquid crystals), magnetics and thermal materials. To these lists, biofunctionality as well as biodegradation should be added as we will be discussing later. Moreover, Mg alloys are flammable as a result of the activated metal in the alloy. When Mg is alloyed with Ca, it was reported that the addition of Ca results in an oxide film and raises the ignition temperature from 27 to 127 °C [2].

Magnesium materials have been utilized equally as structural materials and functional materials. In this chapter, we discuss structural magnesium materials in transportation area and functional magnesium materials employed in variety of areas including energy-related engineering, air-battery applications or home appliances. Our discussion is limited for nonmedical applications.

16.2 Transportation

The unique value of the high specific strength makes magnesium alloys ideal materials for the transportation industry. As far as fuel efficiency and environmental disruption are concerned, not only Mg materials but also any materials possessing high specific

https://doi.org/10.1515/9783110676945-016

strength (such as Al-based alloys and Ti-based alloys) should be material's first choice. Due to the inherent difficulty of eased deformation because of the few active slip systems available, which is characteristic of their hexagonal close-packed (HCP) lattice, wrought magnesium alloys are difficult to deform. As a result, the most of the commercially available magnesium alloys are Mg–Al-based binary system used in casting processes. The mechanical properties of magnesium improve when it is alloyed with small amounts of other metals. In most cases, the alloying elements form intermetallic compounds that permit heat treatment for enhanced mechanical properties.

16.2.1 Automobiles

As the social demands on new materials' developments exhibiting accommodating to environment necessities for pollution and reduction of fuel consumption [3], new Mg materials have been developed with a classical question on the question of whether established forming processes for aluminum and steel can be changed to magnesium and its alloys. Table 16.1 lists required mechanical parameters for transportation applications [4, 5]. Based on these requirements, it was pointed out that Mg-based wrought alloys including Mg–Al–Zn, Mg–Zn–Zr–Re and Mg–Y–Re are recommended [4, 5].

Table 16.1: Mechanical requirements for Mg-based materials for transportation applications.

Properties	*T* (°C)	Materials	
		Structural applications	**System applications**
Tensile ultimate strength	RT	450 MPa	275–350 MPa
Tensile yield strength	RT	350 MPa	200–300 MPa
Elongation to fracture	RT	16–18%	12–16%
Yield strength	150	0.9 YTS	0.9 YTS
Compressive yield strength	RT	1.1 YTS to 0.9 YTS	1.1 YTS to 0.9 YTS
Failure under compression	RT	Alike: Al 2024 T3	Alike: Al 5083
Specific weight	RT	1.75	1.75
Residual strength	RT	Alike to 2024 T3	n. a.
Fatigue crack growth	RT	Alike to 2024 T3	n. a.
Fatigue limit ($K_t = 1.0$, $R = 0.1$)	RT	140 MPa	160 MPa

RT, room temperature.

Lightweight materials are important in technology that can improve passenger vehicle fuel efficiency by 6–8% for each 10% reduction in weight [6]. Reducing vehicle weight improves the fuel efficiency, driving dynamics and performance of vehicles ranging from traditional internal combustion engine powered to battery electric vehicles, fuel cell vehicles and the full range of hybrids [7]. Although cast and wrought magnesium have long been identified as a key pathway to automotive lightweighting and improved energy efficiency [8], cast magnesium components have been extensively used in the automotive industry but only niche applications are known to exist for magnesium sheets to this date. This limitation is due to inherent HCP-structured material's deformation property. By utilizing the twin-roll casting technique [9, 10], novel Mg-Zn-Ca-Zr (ZXK) alloy sheets were developed with improved formability as a result of a texture weakening effect [9]. For developing heat-resistant magnesium alloys for automotive powertrain application, Mg-4Al-2Sn-1Ca alloy with Ce addition have been developed with microstructures of $Mg_{17}Al_{12}$, Mg_2Sn, CaMgSn (causing grain refining) and $Al_{11}Ce_3$ phases and the deformation mechanism was observed in the twin deformation [11].

Figure 16.1 depicts Mg material forging and casting for automobile applications. Although some of these applications are duplicated in two figures, several components are still individually illustrated.

16.2.2 Aircrafts

There is a continuous history of magnesium casting alloy developments for aircraft applications as shown in Figure 16.2 [14]. Same as the automobile applications, materials for air-born structures require lightweight and strength [15, 16].

Ribs and brackets are important components in structuring aircrafts and made of forged AZ31 Mg–Al–Zn alloy, as shown in Figure 16.3 [17]. Besides these, another aircrafts' interior parts including seat back frame, cross-tube, spreader bar baggage bar or set leg assembly are fabricated by Mg-based alloys [18]. Figure 16.4 shows magnesium materials applied as the aircraft components [12].

16.2.3 Bike

The basic properties of magnesium alloys propose that they would keenly find use in bicycles. Magnesium alloys have low density and a high strength-to-weight ratio and are readily extrudable, and some alloys are highly weldable. Most bicycle industry believes that magnesium is not weldable and is very much brittle. But some alloys are weldable, and it has been recognized that the ductility of common magnesium alloys [19] is equivalent to that of aluminum alloys (such as 6061 and 7075 aluminum alloys) [3]. Magnesium frames may be manufactured by die casting or by

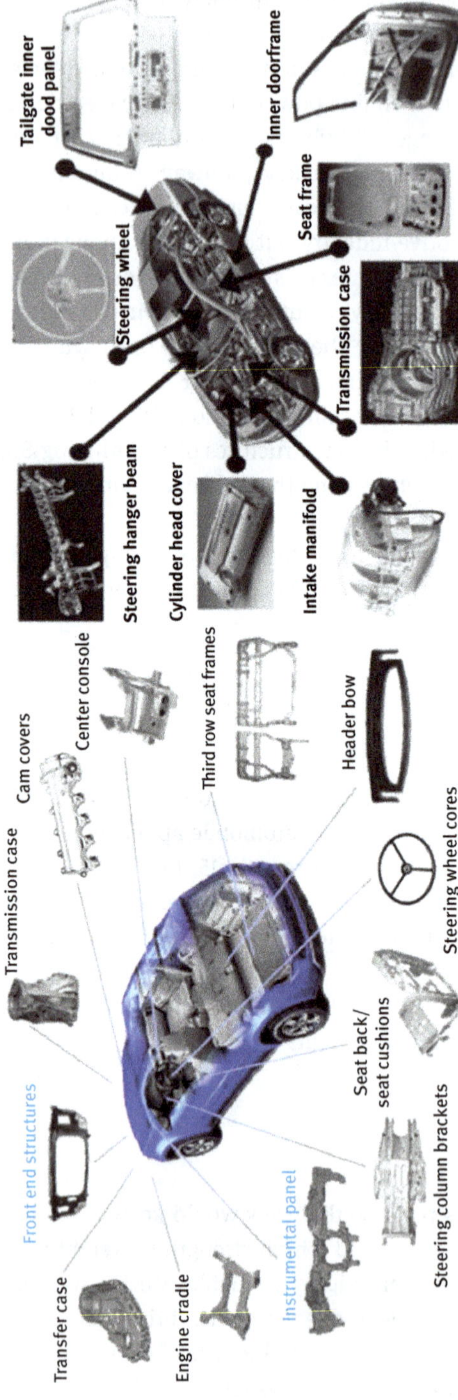

Figure 16.1: Mg applications for automobiles [12, 13].

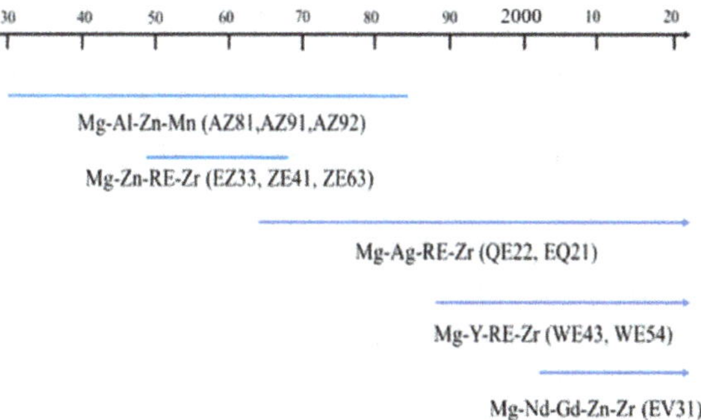

Figure 16.2: History of Mg alloys for aircraft applications [14].

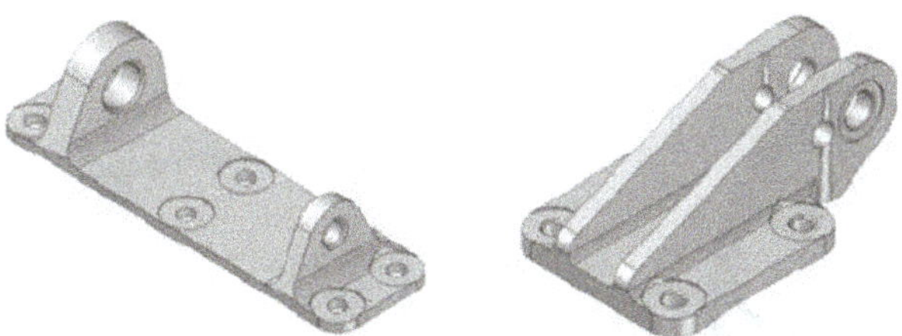

Figure 16.3: Forged Mg-based alloy for robs and brackets.

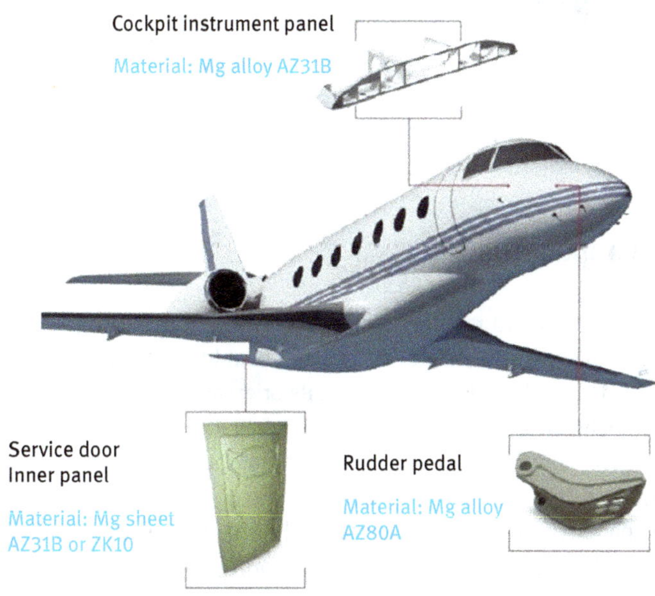

Figure 16.4: Mg-based alloys for aircraft components [12].

welding extruded and welded tubes. The wrought magnesium alloys generally offer improved elongation and superior forms. Among the high damping properties and low density of magnesium, it can easily exceed any of the current metals in ride quality leading to an improved fatigue life [3, 16, 20, 21]; mostly, AE81 and AE70 (good weldability and excellent strength and elongation), ZE2 (forged products with excellent elongation and strength) and WE54 (excellent castability and machinability with excellent elevated temperature strength).

The most popular application of Mg materials in bike section, it should be the mountain bike for which a wheel [22, 23] and a main structural frame [24]. Figure 16.5 shows a typical wheel [23] and a main frame [24], both are important components in mountain bikes, as shown in Figures 16.5 and 16.6.

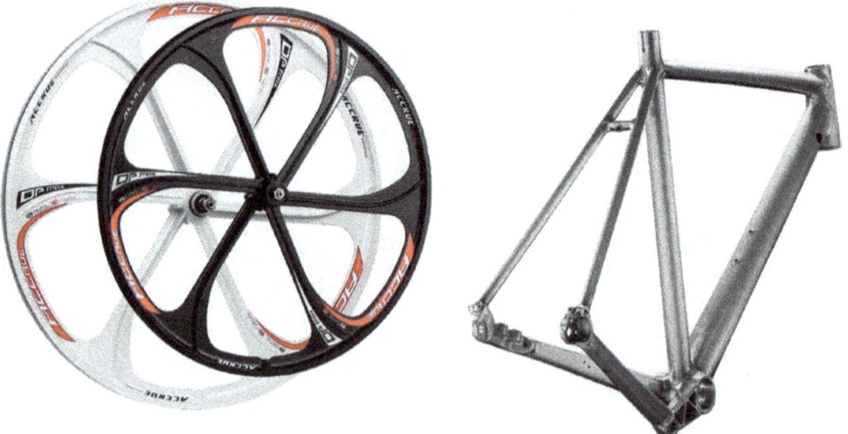

Figure 16.5: Magnesium bike wheel.

Figure 16.6: Magnesium bike frame.

16.3 Energy-related applications

Magnesium material plays an important role for complete recycling from serving as hydrogen energy storage through converting useful energy and heat to reducing the reactant product of Mg oxide and/or hydroxide to free Mg at its original starting point. The utilization includes thermochemical (combustion), photochemical, electrochemical (fuel cells) and nuclear conversion of hydrogen, hydrogen isotopes and/or hydrogen carriers to thermal, mechanical and electrical energies, and their applications in transportation (including aerospace), industrial, commercial and residential sectors. During these sequences, hydriding/dehydriding as well as absorption/desorption are crucial for determining its efficiency and efficacy since these are considered as a function of time, temperature and pressure explicitly [25, 26].

Mg-based materials are thought to be promising candidates for future hydrogen storage applications due to the low cost, abundant resources and large hydrogen storage capacity. However, they (particularly MgH_2) suffer from the challenges of sluggish kinetics and large volume change after hydriding/dehydriding process [27–29].

16.3.1 Hydrogen storage

Hydrogen can be stored physically as either a gas or a liquid. Storage of hydrogen as a gas typically requires high-pressure tanks. Storage of hydrogen as a liquid requires cryogenic temperatures because the boiling point of hydrogen at one atmosphere pressure is −252.8 °C. Hydrogen can also be stored on the surfaces of solids (by adsorption) or within solids (by absorption) [30, 31], as shown in Figure 16.7.

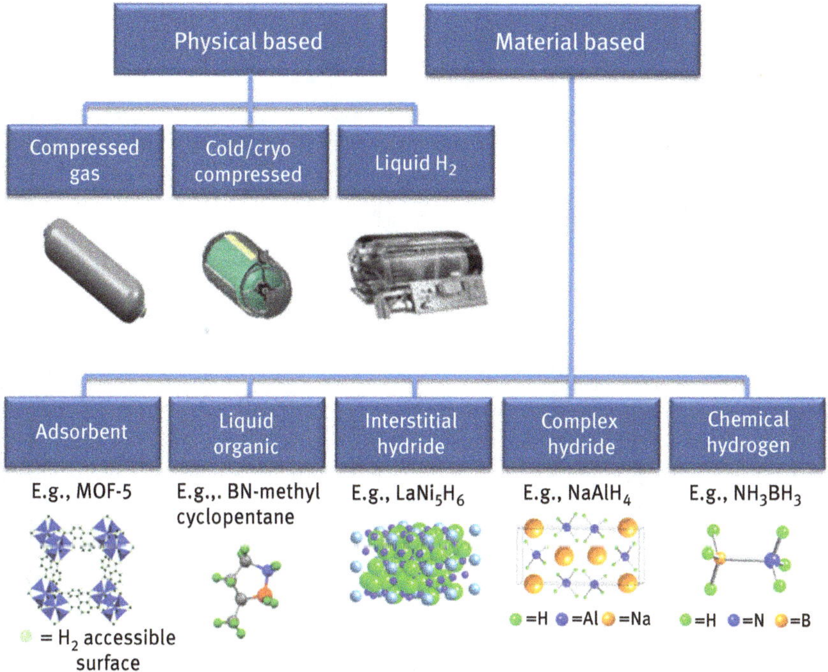

Figure 16.7: Hydrogen physical storage and chemical storage [30].

Table 16.2 lists Mg-based alloy system employed for hydrogen storage. To basic binary Mg alloys on left columns, various additional alloying elements listed on top row are added.

Table 16.2: Combination of hydrogen storage basic materials and additional element(s).

	Al	C	Li	Zn	Ni	Ti	Pr	V	Zr	H	Cr	Y	M	Ox	La	Ce	Cu	Nb	Sn
Mg–X binary alloy bases																			
–Li	[32] [33]	[34]																	
–Al	[35–43]	[44, 45]	[46–48]	[49, 50]	[51]	[52]	[53]							[54, 55]					
–Ca								[56]											
–Ti	[43, 57]				[58]				[59]	[60–62]	[63]								
–Mn	[64]				[65]														
–Fe	[43]					[66]													
–Co	[67–70]																		
–Ni	[71–85]	[86]				[87–89]		[90, 91]				[92–98]	[99–103]	[104]	[105–110]	[111–115]	[116–123]	[124]	
–Cu	[42, 125]				[92]							[126]							
–Zn	[50, 127]				[128]														[129]
–Y	[130–133]				[97, 117, 134]	[135]								[136]					
–Zr					[137]														
–Pd	[138]																		
–Sn																			
–La					[108, 141]														
–Ce					[112, 142–145]														
–Nd	[146]				[147]														
–Gd	[148]																		

Notes: C represents carbon, graphite and graphene; M, mischmetal (45Ce-38La-12Nd-4Pr); Ox, oxides.

Besides these metallic-based hydrogen storage systems (listed in Table 16.2), there are several different types of R&D materials for hydrogen storage systems.

16.3.1.1 Intermetallic compounds and composites

These should include Mg_2Ni and Mg_2Cu [149], Mg–Mg_2Ni [150, 151], Mg–Mg_2Sn [152], Mg–Mg_2Si [153, 154] or hybrids such Mg–$LaNi_3$–Cu [155], $Mg_{14}TMAlH_{32}$ and $Mg_{14}TMLiH_{32}$ (TM = Ti, Sc, Zn) [156] or $(Mg_{1-x}M_x)2Ni/M'$ ($x = 0, 0.5$; M = Al, Mn; M′ = C, Pd) [157].

16.3.1.2 Hydrides and composites

These are MgH_2 [158], M–MgH_2 [159, 160], Mg–$(BH_4)_2$ [161, 162], Mg_2CoH_5 and Mg_3CoH_5 [163], $MgH_2CeH_{2.73}$ [164] and MgH_2–Mg_2NiH_4–YH_2 or MgH_2–$MgCu_2$–YH_2 [165].

16.3.1.3 Oxides and composites

These include MgO–$Mg(OH)_2$ [166], Mg–Nb_2O_5–CNT (carbon nanotubes) [167] Mg–7.5Fe_2O_3–7.5Ni [168] and Mg–(Fe_2O_3, CaO, MoO_3, Fe_3O_4, Nb_2O_5 and TiO_2) [169].

16.3.1.4 Fluorides and composites

These are Mg–5NbF_5 [170] and Mg–5TaF_5 [171].

16.3.2 Battery

Magnesium–air battery is a kind of air battery, having metallic magnesium as a negative electrode, oxygen in air as a positive electrode with a saline solution as an electrolyte, which would exhibit higher than 90% of efficiency and be operative in temperatures ranging from −20 to 55 °C [172, 173] (see Figure 16.8) [172].

In order to prevent the self-discharge phenomenon, if the electrolyte is changed to be alkaline, magnesium will react to form a passive film of magnesium hydroxide accompanied with unnecessary heat generated. However, if Mg is alloyed with Ca element, occurrence of reaction of either Mg or Ca element with OH^- ion is shared with each other, resulting in dissolving Mg is controlled. Magnesium is the eighth most abundant element and constitutes about 2% of the Earth's crust as several ores, including dolomite, magnesite, brucite, carnallite and olivine. It is the third most plentiful element dissolved in seawater, with a concentration averaging 0.13% (which can be converted to approximately 18,200 trillion tons). A new concept has been developed as to the magnesium recycling society, in which energy stored using magnetism is utilized as a battery of fuel and reactant product (mostly magnesium oxide and/or hydroxide) that can be reduced to metallic magnesium under natural energy such as solar energy and reduced magnesium can be reused for

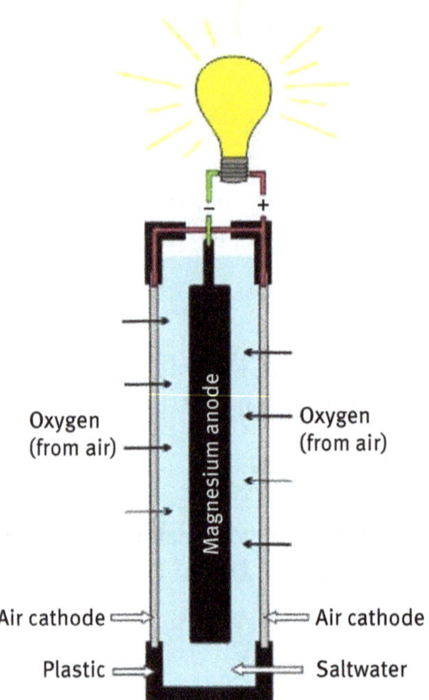

Figure 16.8: Schematic illustration of the typical magnesium air battery.

energy storage. Table 16.3 lists a combination of Mg-based binary alloys with additional alloying elements for Mg–air battery.

Table 16.3: Anode electrode Mg-based alloys for Mg–air battery.

		Hg	Zn	Al	Pb	Mn	Sn	Ca
Mg–Ga		[174, 175]						
Mg–Al			[176–179]		[180–183]	[184]	[185, 186]	
Mg–Li				[179]				
Mg–Ca	[187–189]							
Mg–Bi								[190]

16.3.3 Others

16.3.3.1 Thermal energy storage

Risueño et al. [191, 192] investigated materials for the latent heat energy storage in concentrated solar power applications [191, 192]. Such thermal energy should include latent heat, melting/solidification temperatures, thermal conductivity and specific heat. Accordingly, the materials should exhibit high thermal conductivity.

It was mentioned that Mg–Zn–Al ternary alloys (including $Mg_{71}Zn_{28.9}Al_{0.1}$, $Mg_{70}Zn_{24.9}Al_{5.1}$ and $Mg_{70}Zn_{24.4}Al_{5.6}$) are promising.

16.3.3.2 Superconductor

Rahul et al. [193] fabricated Mg–Si alloy which has uniformly distributed Mg_2Si particles casting technique. It was reported that (i) peaks of Mg_2Si in all Si-containing samples were identified and a microstructure with distinctly smaller grains and reduced crystallinity in doped samples were observed; and (ii) doping has not severely affected the transition temperature of the samples and at the same time enhanced the in-field critical current density. Güner et al. [194] prepared a series of bulk samples of $MgB_2 + x$ wt% of Mg ($x = 0, 5, 10, 15, 20$ and 30) by solid-state reaction method. It was mentioned that the maximum repulsive and attractive force values of 15 wt% of excess magnesium MgB_2 sample compared to the other samples imply that the intergranular connection between grains enhanced while pore and microcrack density decreased, which brings an increase in the values of the radius of a shielding current loop and the critical current density. It was determined to set the optimum excess content of Mg was 15 wt% in order to obtain the enhancement of the micro- and macro-structural properties, since the optimum content might cause the higher critical current density and the maximum levitation and lateral force values.

16.4 Home appliances

Magnesium materials are so versatile in many types of home appliances.

Case structural frame for a smartphone is magnesium-made (see Figure 16.9 [195]).

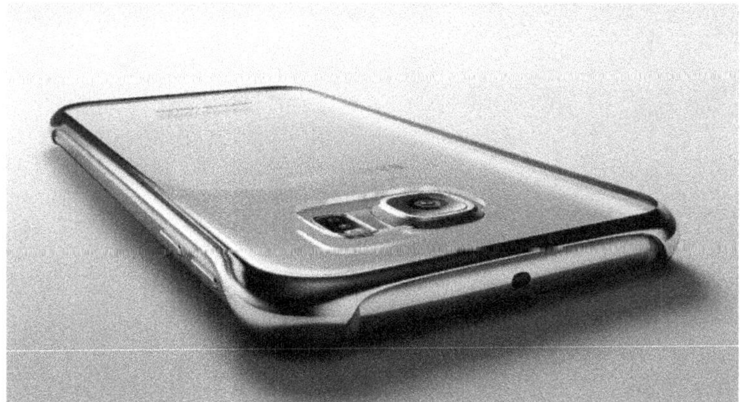

Figure 16.9: Mg case frame for smartphone.

Optical eyeglass frame (Figure 16.10 [196]) and suitcase (Figure 16.11 [197]) are made of magnesium alloy. Figure 16.12 shows light case with heatsink device [200] and Figure 16.13 shows a case for camera made of magnesium [200].

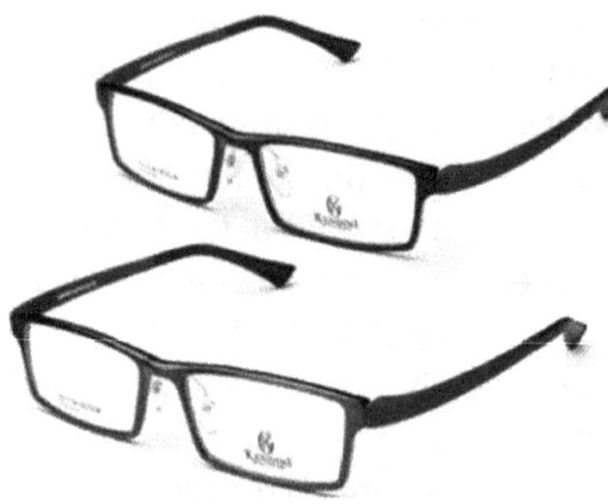

Figure 16.10: Magnesium eyeglass frame.

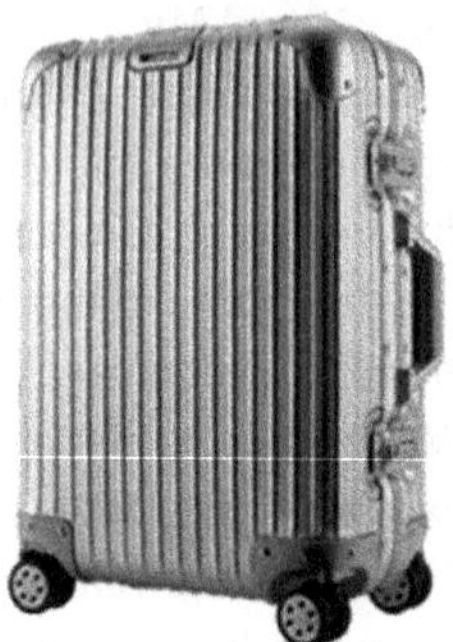

Figure 16.11: Magnesium suitcase: a combination of light case with heatsink function is made from magnesium material, as shown in Figure 16.12 [198, 199].

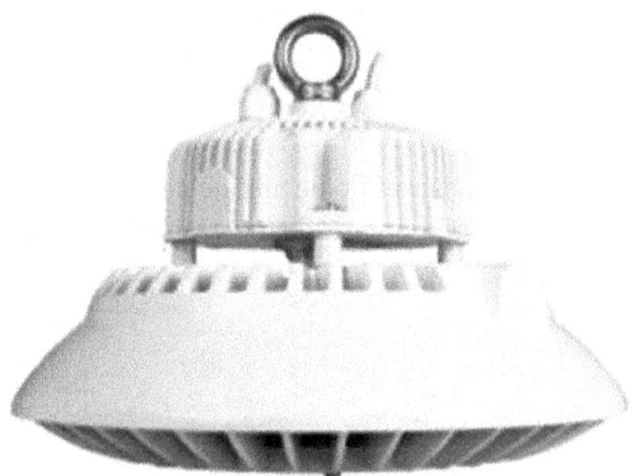

Figure 16.12: Light case with heatsink devices. Case for camera is made of magnesium, too (Figure 16.14 [200]).

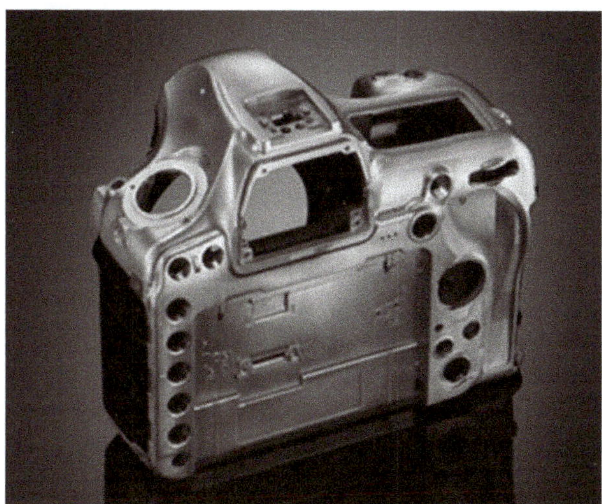

Figure 16.13: Magnesium camera case.

To support injured anterior or posterior cruciate ligament and medial meniscus, magnesium supporter can be effective, as shown in Figure 16.14 [201].

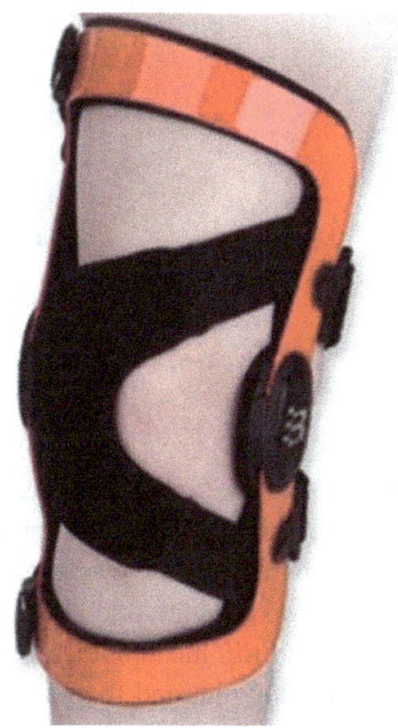

Figure 16.14: Magnesium knee supporter [202].

16.5 Miscellaneous

16.5.1 Switchable mirror

Switchable mirrors are a new generation of electrochromic windows that can alternate between a reflecting state and a transparent or absorbing state when a small voltage is applied, as demonstrated in Figure 16.15 [202]. A typical device consists of a thin reflective film of an active material such as antimony applied to a glass substrate. The electrolyte may be solid, liquid or polymer. A counter electrode supplies positive lithium ions and may be transparent, opaque, reflecting or electrochromic, depending on the application. When a potential is applied, electrons flow into the active metallic layer. At the same time, lithium ions are taken up by the metal to form a new transparent compound. The transition may be stopped or reversed at any point to achieve a desired level of transparency or reflectivity [203, 204].

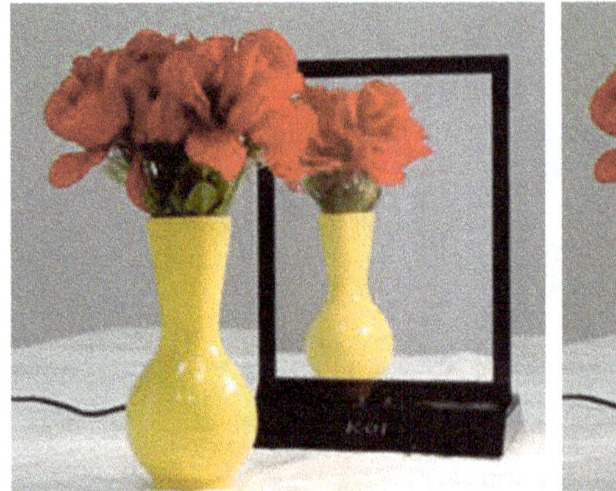

In reflection state

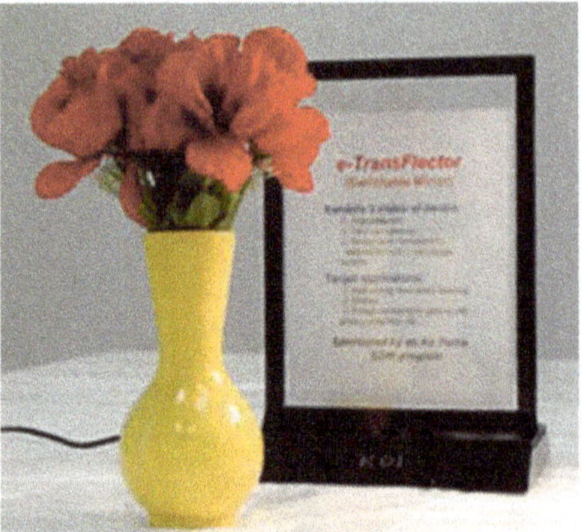

In transparent state

Figure 16.15: Demonstration of switchable mirror.

Slack et al. [205] fabricated Pd-coated Mg–Mn–Ni films exhibiting as gasochromic switchable mirrors and reported that (i) the cycling stability of the optical switching depends upon preservation of the integrity of the Pd catalyst overlayer; (ii) alloying between Mg and Pd causes interdiffusion of the two elements and leads to degradation in switching speed and eventual deactivation; and (iii) incorporation of a thin Nb-oxide barrier layer between the active magnesium alloy film and the Pd layer substantially improves the cycling stability of the mirror. Tajima et al. [206] developed gasochromic and electrochromic switchable mirrors that contain a ternary Mg–Zr–Ni alloy instead of binary Mg-based alloy including Mg–Ni, Mg–Ti or Mg–Ca. It was mentioned that the additional elements in the Mg alloys improve the optical switching properties, and hydrogen-permeable Zr–Ni alloy membranes do not become embrittled by hydrogen and have a high hydrogen permeation rate. Both types of switchable mirror with the Mg–Zr–Ni thin film exhibited optical switching properties, which depend strongly on the composition of the thin film. In both the gasochromic and electrochromic mirrors, the switching speed increased as the Zr and Ni contents of the film increased, although the maximum transmittance decreased and the environmental durability of the electrochromic mirror increased with the Zr and Ni contents of the alloy thin film, and films with a high Mg content degraded more rapidly. La et al. [207] prepared Mg–Y alloy thin films using a DC magnetron sputtering method. In order to improve the films switching durability, luminous transmittance and the surface functionalization, polytetrafluoroethylene (PTFE) was coated with thermal vacuum deposition for use as the top layer of Mg–Y/Pd switchable mirrors. It was found that (i) the PTFE layer had a porous network structure and exhibited a superhydrophobic surface with a water contact angle of approximately 152° and (ii) by characterization, PTFE thin films show the excellent protection role against the oxidization of Mg, the switching durability of the films were improved 3 times and also show the antireflection role the luminous transmission of films was enhanced by 7% through the top covered with PTFE. For the past two decades, the reported magnesium-based gasochromic switchable mirrors have been limited to magnesium alloys. Because of the excellent catalytic property of TiO_2 for the magnesium–hydrogen reaction, Liu et al. [208] fabricated the novel gasochromic switchable mirrors based on Pd/Mg–TiO_2 films by magnetron sputtering. It was reported that (i) the mirror based on Pd/0.9 Mg–0.1TiO_2 film exhibits larger optical dynamic range at visible wavelengths and excellent structural recovery even after 100 cycles of hydrogenation and dehydrogenation compared with Pd/Mg film; (ii) the brookite TiO_2, crystalline Mg and some amorphous phases coexist in the Mg–TiO_2 layer of Pd/0.9 Mg–0.1TiO_2 film with no trace of Pd; and (iii) the TiO_2 nanocrystal clusters are distributed in stripe among Mg matrix; however, the Pd/0.63 Mg–0.37TiO_2 film consists of crystalline Mg and $MgTi_2O_5$ phase, where $MgTi_2O_5$ phase is derived from the reaction of superfluous TiO_2 with a part of Mg and deteriorates the optical properties of the mirror dramatically.

16.5.2 Sensors

Mukherjee et al. [209] prepared a photodetector based on Mg/$ZnSnP_2$/Sn structure on p-type silicon (100) to operate in the wavelength range of 450–850 nm. It was indicated that (i) the device showed strong photoresponse in both the forward and reverse bias configurations, and the current–voltage curve shifted to the fourth quadrant under illumination; (ii) the maximum values of responsivity, photosensitivity and detectivity were found to be 22.76 mA/W, 57.00 cm^2/W and 6.34×10^{10} cm $Hz^{1/2}$/W in the forward bias and 3.48 mA/W, 48.22 cm^2/W and 2.25×10^{10} cm $Hz^{1/2}$/W in the reverse bias, respectively, at illumination of 850 nm wavelength and (iii) the photodetector showed a fast response time of 47 µs and multiple recovery times of 725 µs, 1.2 ms and 1.3 ms, respectively.

Bolokang et al. [210] studied the gas-sensing properties of novel ball-milled and nitrided Mg–TiO_2 prepared powder, which was ball-milled for 60 h to reduce crystallite sizes, followed by annealing in nitrogen at 650 °C. It was reported that (i) the nitrided powder sample exhibited various morphologies including nanorods as well as nanoparticles showing porous behavior; (ii) the atomic force microscopy and Brunauer–Emmett–Teller analyses showed high roughness and surface area for 60 h milled Mg–TiO_2 nanostructures; and (iii) the Mg–TiO_2 60 h sensing material showed high sensing response to NH_3, disclosing fast response-recovery time and high selectivity to NH_3.

16.5.3 Drone

The same requirements for aircrafts, structural as well as component materials for drone are chosen from materials' group having a high specific strength. As shown in Figures 16.16 and 16.17, magnesium has been extensively utilized.

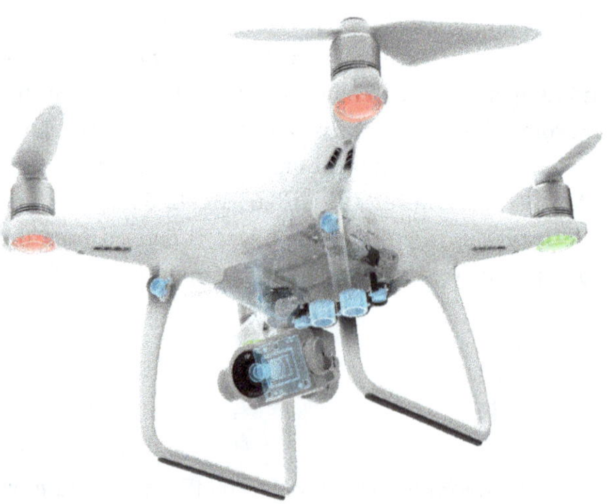

Figure 16.16: Typical drone made of Mg and Al materials [211].

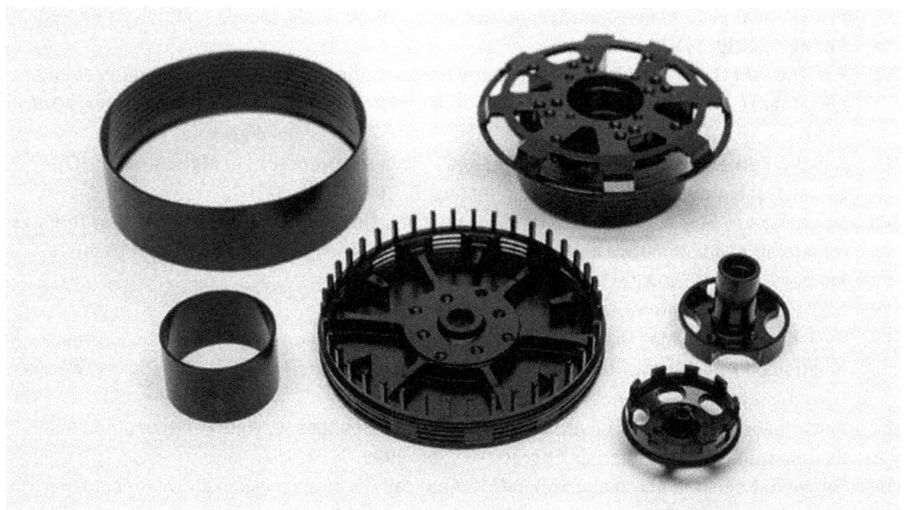

Figure 16.17: Drone parts manufactured from magnesium alloy [24].

References

[1] Encyclopædia Britannica. Magnesium Processing; https://www.britannica.com/technology/magnesium-processing/The-metal-and-its-alloys.

[2] Ito T, Saito G, Uehigashi N, Mori H. Mechanical properties of a flame-resistant Ma alloy as a next-generation transportation structural material. Energy Procedia. 2016, 89, 6–14.

[3] Monteiro WA, Buso SJ, da Silva LV. Application of magnesium alloys in transport, new features on magnesium alloys, Waldemar Alfredo Monteiro, IntechOpen. 2012, DOI: 10.5772/48273. Available from: https://www.intechopen.com/books/new-features-on-magnesium-alloys/application-of-magnesium-alloys-in-transport.

[4] Hombergsmeier E. AEROMAG- Magnesium suitable for aeronautic applications? Proceedings of the Sixth European Aeronautics Days- Aerodays. World Magnesium Conference. 2009, 66, 143–52.

[5] Knüwer M, Guillan A, Besuchet P, Busch H-P, Entelmann W, Hombergsmeier E. Development of Magnesium Alloy Parts for Airbus Air- crafts. Proceedings of IMA Annual World Magnesium Conference. 2009, 66, 153–60.

[6] Joost W. Reducing vehicle weight and improving U.S. Energy efficiency using integrated computational materials engineering. Journal of Metals. 2012, 64, 1032–8.

[7] Joost WJ. Targeting High Impact R&D for Automotive Magnesium Alloys. In: Solanki K. et al. ed. Magnesium Technology 2017. The Minerals, Metals & Materials Series. Springer, 2017, 5–6.

[8] Kleinbaum S. Magnesium for Automotive Lightweighting: Status and Challenges. In: Joshi V. et al., ed., Magnesium Technology 2019. The Minerals, Metals & Materials Series. Springer, 2019, 13–14.

[9] Klaumünzer D, Victoria Hernandez J, Yi S, Letzig D, Kim S-H, Kim JJ, Seo MH, Ahn K. Magnesium Process and Alloy Development for Applications in the Automotive Industry. In:

Joshi V. et al., ed., Magnesium Technology 2019. The Minerals, Metals & Materials Series. Springer, 2019, 15–20.
[10] Romanowski C. Magnesium Alloy Sheet for Transportation Applications. In: Joshi V. et al., ed., Magnesium Technology 2019. The Minerals, Metals & Materials Series. Springer, 2019, 3–12.
[11] Kim BH, Park KC, Park YH, Park IM. Investigations of the properties of Mg–4Al–2Sn–1Ca–xCe alloys. Materials Science and Engineering: A. 2010, 527, 6372–7.
[12] Dziubińska A, Surdacki P, Dziubiński M, Barszcz M. The forming of magnesium alloy forgings for aircraft and automotive applications. Advances in Science and Technology, Research Journal 2016; DOI: 10.12913/22998624/64003.
[13] http://apac.totalmateria.com
[14] Gwynne B, Lyon P. Magnesium Alloys in Aerospace Applications, Past Concerns, Current Solutions. https://www.fire.tc.faa.gov/2007conference/files/Materials_Fire_Safety/WedAM/GwynneMagnesium/GwynneMagnesiumPres.pdf.
[15] Immarigeon JP, Holt RT, Koul AK, Zhao L, Wallace W, Beddoes JC. Lightweight materials for aircraft applications. Materials Characterization. 1995, 35, 41–67.
[16] Furuya H, Kogiso N, Matunaga S, Senda K. Applications of magnesium alloys for aerospace structure systems. Materials Science Forum. 1999, 350, 341–8.
[17] Dziubińska A, Surdacki P. A new method for producing magnesium alloy twin-rib aircraft brackets. Aircraft Engineering and Aerospace Technology. 2015, 87, 180–8.
[18] Davis B. The Applications of Magnesium Alloys in Aircraft Interiors. In: Manuel MV et al., ed. Magnesium Technology 2015, TMS (The Minerals, Metals & Materials Society), 2015.
[19] Avadesian M, Baker H. Magnesium and Magnesium Alloys, ASM Specialty Handbook (Materials Park, OH: ASM International) 1999.
[20] Deetz J. The use of wrought magnesium in bicycles. Journal of Metals 2005, 57, 50–3.
[21] Easton M, Beer A, Barnett M, Davies C, Dunlop G, Durandet Y, Blacket S, Hilditch T, Beggs P. Magnesium alloy applications in automotive structures. Journal of Metals. 2008, 60, 57–62.
[22] Barber J. Your Next Mountain Bike Could Be Made from Super Magnesium. September 20, 2018; https://www.singletracks.com/mtb-gear/your-next-mountain-bike-could-be-made-from-super-magnesium/.
[23] https://mediativereading.blogspot.com/2019/04/1-pair-mtb-wheelset-rims-26-275-29er.html.
[24] McCoy S. Declassified: 'Super Magnesium' Lighter Than Titanium, Stronger Than Steel. 2018; https://gearjunkie.com/allite-super-magnesium.
[25] Shao H, Xin G, Zheng J, Li X, Akiba E. Nano Energy. 2012, 1, 590–601.
[26] Liu W, Setijadi E, Crema L, Bartali R, Speranza G. Carbon nanostructures/Mg hybrid materials for hydrogen storage. Diamond and Related Materials. 2018, 82, 19–24.
[27] Li J, Li B, Yu X, Zhao H, Shao H. Geometrical effect in Mg-based metastable nano alloys with BCC structure for hydrogen storage. International Journal of Hydrogen Energy 2019, 44, 29291–6.
[28] Zhang J, Zhu Y, Yao L, Xu C, Li L. State of the art multi-strategy improvement of Mg-based hydrides for hydrogen storage. Journal of Alloys and Compounds. 2019, 782, 796–823.
[29] Luo Q, Li J, Li B. Liu B, Li Q. Kinetics in Mg-based hydrogen storage materials: Enhancement and mechanism. Journal of Magnesium and Alloys. 2019, 7, 58–71.
[30] Hydrogen Storage. https://www.energy.gov/eere/fuelcells/hydrogen-storage
[31] Züttel A. Materials for hydrogen storage. Materials Today. 2003, 6, 24–33.
[32] Liang G. Synthesis and hydrogen storage properties of Mg-based alloys. Journal of Alloys and Compounds. 2004, 370, 123–8.

[33] Leeflang MA et al. Long-term biodegradation and associated hydrogen evolution of duplex-structured Mg–Li–Al–(RE) alloys and their mechanical properties. Materials Science and Engineering: B. 2011, 176, 1741–5.
[34] Huajian W et al. Catalytic effect of graphene on the hydrogen storage properties of Mg-Li alloy. Materials Chemistry and Physics. 2018, 207, 221–5.
[35] El-Amoush AS. An X-ray investigation of hydrogenated Mg–30Al magnesium alloy. Journal of Alloys and Compounds. 2007, 441, 278–83.
[36] Andreasen A et al. Interaction of hydrogen with an Mg–Al alloy. Journal of Alloys and Compounds. 2005, 404/406, 323–6.
[37] Andreasen A. Hydrogenation properties of Mg–Al alloys. International Journal of Hydrogen Energy. 2008, 33, 7489–97.
[38] Zhong HC et al. Improving the hydrogen storage properties of MgH2 by reversibly forming Mg–Al solid solution alloys. International Journal of Hydrogen Energy. 2014, 39, 3320–6.
[39] Zou M-S et al. Preparation and characterization of hydro-reactive Mg–Al mechanical alloy materials for hydrogen production in seawater. Journal of Power Sources. 2012, 219, 60–4.
[40] Chiu C et al. Improving hydrogen storage performance of AZ31 Mg alloy by equal channel angular pressing and additives. Journal of Alloys and Compounds. 2018, 743, 437–47.
[41] Tanniru M et al. A study of stability of MgH2 in Mg–8at%Al alloy powder. International Journal of Hydrogen Energy. 2010, 35, 3555–64.
[42] Cho YH et al. Correlation between hydrogen migration and microstructure in cast Mg alloys. Journal of Alloys and Compounds. 2011, 509, s621-4.
[43] Kalisvaart WP et al. Hydrogen storage in binary and ternary Mg-based alloys: A comprehensive experimental study. International Journal of Hydrogen Energy. 2010, 35, 2091–103.
[44] Niyomsoan S et al. Effects of graphite addition and air exposure on ball-milled Mg–Al alloys for hydrogen storage. International Journal of Hydrogen Energy. 2019, 44, 23257–66.
[45] Shang H et al. Influence of adding nano-graphite powders on the microstructure and gas hydrogen storage properties of ball-milled Mg90Al10 alloys. Carbon. 2019, 149, 93–104.
[46] Ning H et al. Enhanced hydrogen sorption on Mg17Al12 alloy induced adding Li: A first principle study. Applied Surface Science 2019, 471, 239–45.
[47] Lan Z et al. Preparation and hydrogen storage properties of Mg-Al-Li solid solution. International Journal of Hydrogen Energy. 2016, 41, 6134–8.
[48] Abdessameud S et al. Thermodynamic analysis of dehydrogenation path of Mg–Al–Li–Na alloys. Calphad. 2016, 54, 54–66.
[49] Hu L et al. Microstructure nanocrystallization of a Mg–3 wt%Al–1 wt%Zn alloy by mechanically assisted hydriding–dehydriding. Materials Letters 2008, 62, 2984–7.
[50] Brady MP et al. Tracer study of oxygen and hydrogen uptake by Mg alloys in air with water vapor. Scripta Materialia. 2015, 106, 38–41.
[51] Bououdina M et al. Comparative study of mechanical alloying of (Mg+Al) and (Mg+Al+Ni) mixtures for hydrogen storage. Journal of Alloys and Compounds. 2002, 336, 222–31.
[52] Kral L et al. Improvement of hydrogen storage properties of Mg by catalytic effect of Al-containing phases in Mg-Al-Ti-Zr-C powders. International Journal of Hydrogen Energy. 2019, 44, 13561–8.
[53] Zhou J et al. Improved cycle durability of hydrogen absorption and desorption in melt-spun Mg86Pr3Al11 alloy. Materials Letters 2019, 255: https://doi.org/10.1016/j.matlet.2019.126548.
[54] Crivello J-C et al. Improvement of Mg–Al alloys for hydrogen storage applications. International Journal of Hydrogen Energy. 2009, 34, 1937–43.

[55] Li Y et al. Effects of adding nano-CeO2 powder on microstructure and hydrogen storage performances of mechanical alloyed Mg90Al10 alloy. International Journal of Hydrogen Energy. 2019, 44, 1735–49.

[56] Kondo T et al. Hydrogen absorption–desorption properties of Mg–Ca–V BCC alloy prepared by mechanical alloying. Journal of Alloys and Compounds. 2006, 417, 164–8.

[57] Calizzi M et al. Mg–Ti nanoparticles with superior kinetics for hydrogen storage. International Journal of Hydrogen Energy. 2016, 41, 14447–54.

[58] Denys RV et al. Phase equilibria in the Mg–Ti–Ni system at 500 °C and hydrogenation properties of selected alloys. Intermetallics. 2013, 32, 167–75.

[59] Anik M et al. Electrochemical hydrogen storage performance of Mg–Ti–Zr–Ni alloys. International Journal of Hydrogen Energy. 2009, 34, 9765–72.

[60] Vermeulen P et al. Ternary MgTiX-alloys: a promising route towards low-temperature, high-capacity, hydrogen-storage materials. Chemistry. 2007, 13, 9892–8.

[61] Iliescu I et al. Dehydrogenation process and thermal stability of Mg-Ti-H films in-situ hydrogenated by microwave reactive plasma-assisted co-sputtering technique. Journal of Alloys and Compounds. 2018, 768, 157–65.

[62] Rousselot S et al. Synthesis of fcc Mg–Ti–H alloys by high energy ball milling: Structure and electrochemical hydrogen storage properties. Journal of Power Sources. 2010, 195, 4370–4.

[63] Zhang J et al. Synthesis, hydrogen storage properties and thermodynamic destabilization of Mg-TixCr0.8-xV0.2 (x=0.25, 0.35, 0.45, 0.55) nanocomposites. Journal of Alloys and Compounds. 2019, 798, 597–605.

[64] Raja VS et al. Role of chlorides on pitting and hydrogen embrittlement of Mg–Mn wrought alloy. Corrosion Science. 2013, 75, 176–83.

[65] Denys RV et al. New Mg–Mn–Ni alloys as efficient hydrogen storage materials. Intermetallics. 2010, 18, 1579–85.

[66] Meyer M et al. Mechanically alloyed Mg–Ni–Ti and Mg–Fe–Ti powders as hydrogen storage materials. International Journal of Hydrogen Energy. 2012, 37, 14864–9.

[67] Zhang Y et al. The study on binary Mg–Co hydrogen storage alloys with BCC phase. Journal of Alloys and Compounds. 2005, 393, 147–53.

[68] Shao H et al. Hydrogen storage and thermal conductivity properties of Mg-based materials with different structures. International Journal of Hydrogen Energy. 2014, 39, 9893–8.

[69] Kravchenko OV et al. Formation of hydrogen from oxidation of Mg, Mg alloys and mixture with Ni, Co, Cu and Fe in aqueous salt solutions. International Journal of Hydrogen Energy. 2014, 39, 5522–7.

[70] Shao H et al. Phase and morphology evolution study of ball milled Mg–Co hydrogen storage alloys. International Journal of Hydrogen Energy. 2013, 38, 7070–6.

[71] Hou X et al. Synergetic catalytic effect of MWCNTs and TiF3 on hydrogenation properties of nanocrystalline Mg-10wt%Ni alloys. International Journal of Hydrogen Energy. 2013, 38, 12904–11.

[72] Bendersky LA et al. Effect of rapid solidification on hydrogen solubility in Mg-rich Mg–Ni alloys. International Journal of Hydrogen Energy. 2011, 36, 5388–99.

[73] Oh SK et al. Design of Mg–Ni alloys for fast hydrogen generation from seawater and their application in polymer electrolyte membrane fuel cells. International Journal of Hydrogen Energy. 2016, 41, 5296–303.

[74] Ha W et al. Hydrogenation and degradation of Mg–10wt% Ni alloy after cyclic hydriding–dehydriding. International Journal of Hydrogen Energy. 2007, 32, 1885–89.

[75] Shao H et al. Preparation and hydrogen storage properties of nanostructured Mg–Ni BCC alloys. Journal of Alloys and Compounds. 2009, 477, 301–6.

[76] Tran XQ et al. In-situ synchrotron X-ray diffraction investigation of the hydriding and dehydriding properties of a cast Mg–Ni alloy. Journal of Alloys and Compounds. 2015, 636, 249–56.
[77] Huang J et al. Hydrogenation and crystallization of amorphous phase: A new mechanism for the electrochemical capacity and its decay in milled MgNi alloys. Electrochimica Acta. 2019, 305, 145–54.
[78] Yuan JG et al. Preparation and hydrogen storage property of Mg-based hydrogen storage composite embedded by polymethyl methacrylate. International Journal of Hydrogen Energy. 2017, 42, 22366–72.
[79] Yim CD et al. Hydriding properties of Mg–xNi alloys with different microstructures. Catalysis Today. 2007, 120, 276–80.
[80] Révész Á et al. Hydrogen storage of nanocrystalline Mg–Ni alloy processed by equal-channel angular pressing and cold rolling. International Journal of Hydrogen Energy. 2014, 39, 9911–7.
[81] Gajdics M et al. Characterization of a nanocrystalline Mg–Ni alloy processed by high-pressure torsion during hydrogenation and dehydrogenation. International Journal of Hydrogen Energy. 2016, 41, 9803–9.
[82] de Rango P et al. Fast Forging: A new SPD method to synthesize Mg-based alloys for hydrogen storage. International Journal of Hydrogen Energy. 2020, 45, 7912–6.
[83] Ağaoğlu GH et al. Elaboration and electrochemical characterization of Mg–Ni hydrogen storage alloy electrodes for Ni/MH batteries. International Journal of Hydrogen Energy. 2017, 42, 8098–108.
[84] Zhu M et al. Composite structure and hydrogen storage properties in Mg-base alloys. International Journal of Hydrogen Energy. 2006, 31, 251–7.
[85] Cho YH et al. The effect of transition metals on hydrogen migration and catalysis in cast Mg–Ni alloys. International Journal of Hydrogen Energy. 2011, 36, 4984–92.
[86] Palumbo O et al. Study of the hydrogenation/dehydrogenation process in the Mg–Ni–C–Al system. Journal of Alloys and Compounds. 2015, 645, s239–41.
[87] Li Y et al. Hydrogen storage of casting MgTiNi alloys. Catalysis Today. 2018, 318, 103–6.
[88] Zhang Y et al. Microstructure characterization and hydrogen storage properties study of Mg2Ni0.92M0.08 (M = Ti, V, Fe or Si) alloys. Progress in Natural Science: Materials International. 2018, 28, 464–9.
[89] Zhang Y et al. The study on the electrochemical performance of mechanically alloyed Mg–Ti–Ni-based ternary and quaternary hydrogen storage electrode alloys. International Journal of Hydrogen Energy. 2001, 26, 801–6.
[90] Skamoto T et al. Hydrogen absorption/desorption characteristics of Mg-V-Ni hydrogen storage alloys. Fusion Engineering and Design. 2019, 138, 6–9.
[91] Xie X et al. Synergistic catalytic effects of the Ni and V nanoparticles on the hydrogen storage properties of Mg-Ni-V nanocomposite. Chemical Engineering Journal. 2018, 347, 145–55.
[92] Kalinichenka S et al. Hydrogen desorption properties of melt-spun and hydrogenated Mg-based alloys using in situ synchrotron X-ray diffraction and TGA. Journal of Alloys and Compounds. 2011, 509, s629–32.
[93] Kalinichenka S et al. Structural and hydrogen storage properties of melt-spun Mg–Ni–Y alloys. International Journal of Hydrogen Energy. 2009, 34, 7749–55.
[94] Zhang T et al. Surface valence transformation during thermal activation and hydrogenation thermodynamics of Mg–Ni–Y melt-spun ribbons. Applied Surface Science 2016, 371, 35–43.
[95] Zhang Y et al. An investigation on electrochemical hydrogen storage performances of Mg-Y-Ni alloys prepared by mechanical milling. Journal of Rare Earths. 2015, 33, 874–83.
[96] Zhang Y et al. Structure and hydrogen storage characteristics of as-spun Mg-Y-Ni-Cu alloys. Journal of Materials Science & Technology. 2019, 35, 1727–34.

[97] Zhang Y et al. Improved hydrogen storage performances of Mg-Y-Ni-Cu alloys by melt spinning. Renewable Energy. 2019, 138, 263–71.
[98] Sun Y et al. Hydrogen storage properties of ultrahigh pressure Mg12NiY alloys with a superfine LPSO structure. International Journal of Hydrogen Energy. 2019, 44, 23179–87.
[99] Spassov T et al. Hydrogenation of amorphous and nanocrystalline Mg-based alloys. Journal of Alloys and Compounds. 1999, 287, 243–50.
[100] Vojtěch D et al. Study of the diffusion kinetics and mechanism of electrochemical hydriding of Mg–Ni–Mm alloys. International Journal of Hydrogen Energy. 2011, 36, 6689–97.
[101] Knotek V et al. Electrochemical hydriding of Mg–Ni–Mm (Mm = mischmetal) alloys as an effective method for hydrogen storage. International Journal of Hydrogen Energy. 2013, 38, 3030–40.
[102] Vojtěch D et al. Hydrogen storage by direct electrochemical hydriding of Mg-based alloys. Journal of Alloys and Compounds. 2010, 494, 456–62.
[103] Yuan JG et al. The effect of Mm content on microstructure and hydrogen storage properties of the as-cast Mg-10Ni-xMm (x = 1, 2, 3 At.%) Alloys. International Journal of Hydrogen Energy. 2017, 42, 6118–26.
[104] Hong S-H et al. Hydrogen-storage properties of gravity cast and melt spun Mg–Ni–Nb2O5 alloys. International Journal of Hydrogen Energy. 2009, 34, 1944–50.
[105] Fan Y et al. Modifying microstructures and hydrogen storage properties of 85mass% Mg–10mass% Ni–5mass% La alloy by ultra-high pressure. Journal of Alloys and Compounds. 2014, 596, 113–7.
[106] Jurczyk M et al. Hydrogen storage by Mg-based nanocomposites. International Journal of Hydrogen Energy 2012, 37, 3652–8.
[107] Wu D et al. Microstructural investigation of electrochemical hydrogen storage in amorphous Mg–Ni–La alloy. Materials Science and Engineering: B. 2010, 175, 248–52.
[108] Guo F et al. Composition dependent microstructure evolution, activation and de-/hydrogenation properties of Mg–Ni–La alloys. International Journal of Hydrogen Energy. 2019, 44, 16745–56.
[109] Ren H-P et al. Influence of the substitution of La for Mg on the microstructure and hydrogen storage characteristics of Mg20–xLaxNi10 (x=0–6) alloys. International Journal of Hydrogen Energy. 2009, 34, 1429–36.
[110] Lass EA. Hydrogen storage measurements in novel Mg-based nanostructured alloys produced via rapid solidification and devitrification. International Journal of Hydrogen Energy. 2011, 36, 10787–96.
[111] Hou X et al. Enhanced hydrogen generation behaviors and hydrolysis thermodynamics of as-cast Mg–Ni–Ce magnesium-rich alloys in simulate seawater. International Journal of Hydrogen Energy. 2019, 44, 24086–97.
[112] Zhang Y et al. Electrochemical hydrogen storage behaviors of as-milled Mg-Ce-Ni-Al-based alloys applied to Ni-MH battery. Applied Surface Science 2019, 494, 170–8.
[113] Zhang Y et al. Effects of milling duration on electrochemical hydrogen storage behavior of as-milled Mg–Ce–Ni–Al-based alloys for use in Ni-metal hydride batteries. Journal of Physics and Chemistry of Solids. 2019, 133, 178–86.
[114] Li J et al. Microstructure and absorption/desorption kinetics evolutions of MgNiCe alloys during hydrogenation and dehydrogenation cycles. International Journal of Hydrogen Energy. 2018, 43, 8404–14.
[115] Xie L et al. Microstructure and hydrogen storage properties of Mg-Ni-Ce alloys with a long-period stacking ordered phase. Journal of Power Sources. 2017, 338, 91–102.

[116] Song MY et al. Preparation of Mg–23.5Ni–10 (Cuor La) hydrogen-storage alloys by melt spinning and crystallization heat treatment. International Journal of Hydrogen Energy. 2008, 33, 87–92.
[117] Sun H et al. Gas hydrogen absorption and electrochemical properties of Mg24Ni10Cu2 alloys improved by Y substitution, ball milling and Ni addition. International Journal of Hydrogen Energy. 2019, 44, 5382–8.
[118] Hong S-H et al. Hydrogen storage characteristics of melt spun Mg–23.5Ni–5Cu alloys mixed with LaNi5 and/or Nb2O5. Journal of Industrial and Engineering Chemistry. 2012, 18, 61–4.
[119] Hong SH et al. Hydrogen-storage characteristics of Cu, Nb2O5, and NbF5-added Mg–Ni alloys. Materials Research Bulletin. 2012, 47, 172–8.
[120] Luo Q et al. The hydriding kinetics of Mg–Ni based hydrogen storage alloys: A comparative study on Chou model and Jander model. International Journal of Hydrogen Energy. 2010, 35, 7842–9.
[121] Dou B et al. Hydrogen sorption and desorption behaviors of Mg-Ni-Cu doped carbon nanotubes at high temperature. Energy. 2019, 167, 1097–106.
[122] Ding X et al. Dependence and mechanism of hydrogenation behavior on absorption conditions in hypo-eutectic Mg–Ni–Cu alloy. International Journal of Hydrogen Energy. 2018, 43, 16617–22.
[123] Bu W et al. Hydrogen storage properties of amorphous and nanocrystalline (Mg24Ni10Cu2) 100-xNdx (x = 0–20) alloys. International Journal of Hydrogen Energy. 2019, 44, 5365–73.
[124] Aminorroaya S et al. Hydrogen storage properties of Mg-10 wt% Ni alloy co-catalysed with niobium and multi-walled carbon nanotubes. International Journal of Hydrogen Energy. 2011, 36, 571–9.
[125] Oh SK et al. Design of Mg-Cu alloys for fast hydrogen production, and its application to PEM fuel cell. Journal of Alloys and Compounds. 2018, 741, 590–6.
[126] Chen R et al. In-situ hydrogen-induced evolution and de-/hydrogenation behaviors of the Mg93Cu7-xYx alloys with equalized LPSO and eutectic structure. International Journal of Hydrogen Energy. 2019, 44, 21999–2010.
[127] Webb TA et al. In-situ neutron powder diffraction study of Mg-Zn alloys during hydrogen cycling. International Journal of Hydrogen Energy. 2015, 40, 8106–9.
[128] Yin Y et al. Microstructure and improved hydrogen storage properties of Mg85Zn5Ni10 alloy catalyzed by Cr2O3 nanoparticles. Journal of Physics and Chemistry of Solids. 2019, 134, 295–306.
[129] Jiang W et al. Low hydrogen release behavior and antibacterial property of Mg-4Zn-xSn alloys. Materials Letters 2019, 241, 88–91.
[130] Wang Y et al. Superior electrochemical hydrogen storage properties of binary Mg–Y thin films. International Journal of Hydrogen Energy. 2014, 39, 4373–9.
[131] Yang T et al. Improved hydrogen absorption and desorption kinetics of magnesium-based alloy via addition of yttrium. Journal of Power Sources. 2018, 378, 636–45.
[132] Peng Q et al. Microstructures, aging behaviour and mechanical properties in hydrogen and chloride media of backward extruded Mg–Y based biomaterials. Journal of the Mechanical Behavior of Biomedical Materials. 2013, 17, 176–85.
[133] Shi X et al. Study on hydrogenation behaviors of a Mg-13Y alloy. International Journal of Hydrogen Energy. 2014, 39, 8303–10.
[134] Yang T et al. Characterization of microstructure, hydrogen storage kinetics and thermodynamics of a melt-spun Mg86Y10Ni4 alloy. International Journal of Hydrogen Energy. 2019, 44, 6728–37.
[135] Zlotea C et al. Hydrogen sorption properties of a Mg–Y–Ti alloy. Journal of Alloys and Compounds. 2010, 489, 375–8.

[136] Long S et al. A comparison study of Mg–Y2O3 and Mg–Y hydrogen storage composite powders prepared through arc plasma method. Journal of Alloys and Compounds. 2014, 615, s684–8.
[137] Bambhaniya KG et al. Fast hydriding Mg–Zr–Mn–Ni alloy compositions for high capacity hydrogen storage application. International Journal of Hydrogen Energy. 2012, 37, 3671–6.
[138] Ogawa S et al. Hydrogen storage of binary nanoparticles composed of Mg and Pd. International Journal of Hydrogen Energy. 2015, 40, 11895–901.
[139] Ha H-Y et al. Role of hydrogen evolution rate in determining the corrosion rate of extruded Mg–5Sn–(1–4wt%)Zn alloys. Corrosion Science. 2014, 89, 275–85.
[140] Zhong HC et al. Tuning the de/hydriding thermodynamics and kinetics of Mg by mechanical alloying with Sn and Zn. International Journal of Hydrogen Energy. 2019, 44, 2926–33.
[141] Li Q et al. Structures and properties of Mg–La–Ni ternary hydrogen storage alloys by microwave-assisted activation synthesis. International Journal of Hydrogen Energy. 2014, 39, 14247–54.
[142] Lin H-J et al. Controlling nanocrystallization and hydrogen storage property of Mg-based amorphous alloy via a gas-solid reaction. Journal of Alloys and Compounds. 2016, 685, 272–7.
[143] Lin H-J et al. Hydrogenation properties of five-component Mg60Ce10Ni20Cu5X5 (X= Co, Zn) metallic glasses. Intermetallics. 2019, 108, 94–9.
[144] Lin HJ et al. Room temperature gaseous hydrogen storage properties of Mg-based metallic glasses with ultrahigh Mg contents. Journal of Non-Crystalline Solids. 2012, 358, 1387–90.
[145] Zhang C et al. Effect of Cu on dehydrogenation and thermal stability of amorphous Mg-Ce-Ni-Cu alloys. Progress in Natural Science: Materials International. 2017, 27, 622–6.
[146] Lu ZW et al. Electrochemical hydrogen storage of ball-milled Mg-rich Mg–Nd alloy with Ni powders. Journal of Alloys and Compounds. 2007, 433, 269–73.
[147] Zhang Y et al. Hydrogen storage characteristics of the nanocrystalline and amorphous Mg–Nd–Ni–Cu-based alloys prepared by melt spinning. International Journal of Hydrogen Energy. 2014, 39, 3790–8.
[148] Vlček M et al. Hydrogen absorption in Mg-Gd alloy. International Journal of Hydrogen Energy. 2017, 42, 22598–604.
[149] Aydınlı A, Aktekin B, Öztürk T. Size reduction in Mg rich intermetallics via hydrogen decrepitation. Journal of Alloys and Compounds. 2015, 645, s27–s31.
[150] Gupta A, Shervani S, Faisal M, Balani K, Subramaniam A. Hydrogen storage in Mg–Mg2Ni–carbon hybrids. Journal of Alloys and Compounds. 2015, 645, s397–9.
[151] Nogita K, McDonald SD, Duguid A, Tsubota M, Gu QF. Hydrogen desorption of Mg-Mg2Ni hypo-eutectic alloys in air, Ar, CO2, N2 and H2. Journal of Alloys and Compounds. 2013, 580, s140–3.
[152] Zhong HC, Wang H, Ouyang LZ, Zhu M. Microstructure and hydrogen storage properties of Mg–Sn nanocomposite by mechanical milling. Journal of Alloys and Compounds. 2011, 509, 4268–72.
[153] Tan Z, Ouyang L, Liu J, Wan H, Zhu M. Hydrogen generation by hydrolysis of Mg-Mg2Si composite and enhanced kinetics performance from introducing of MgCl2 and Si. International Journal of Hydrogen Energy 2018, 43, 2903–12.
[154] Cermak J, Kral L. Hydrogen storage behavior of Mg@Mg2Si and Mg@Mg17Al12 alloys with additions of carbon allotropes and talc. Journal of Alloys and Compounds. 2018, 744, 252–9.
[155] Li F, Zhuo H, Lijun J, Jun D, Feng Z. Hydrogenation properties of Mg-based composites prepared by reactive mechanical alloying. International Journal of Hydrogen Energy 2007, 32, 1855–9.

[156] Bhihi M, El Khatabi M, Lakhal M, Naji S, Loulidi M. First principle study of hydrogen storage in doubly substituted Mg based hydrides. International Journal of Hydrogen Energy 2015, 40, 8356–61.

[157] Jurczyk M, Smardz L, Okonska I, Jankowska E, Smardz K. Nanoscale Mg-based materials for hydrogen storage. International Journal of Hydrogen Energy 2008, 33, 374–80.

[158] Liu T, Wang C. Wu Y. Mg-based nanocomposites with improved hydrogen storage performances. International Journal of Hydrogen Energy. 2014, 39, 14262–74.

[159] Galey B, Auroux A, Sabo-Etienne S, Grellier M, Postole G. Enhancing hydrogen storage properties of the Mg/MgH2 system by the addition of bis(tricyclohexylphosphine)nickel(II) dichloride. International Journal of Hydrogen Energy 2019, 44, 11939–52.

[160] Shen C, Aguey-Zinsou K-F. Electrochemical deposited Mg-PPy multilayered film to store hydrogen. International Journal of Hydrogen Energy 2018, 43, 22385–90.

[161] Zheng J, Xiao X, Zhang L, He Y, Chen L. Study on the dehydrogenation properties and reversibility of Mg(BH4)2AlH3 composite under moderate conditions. International Journal of Hydrogen Energy 2017, 42, 8050–6.

[162] Jiang Z, Yuan J, Han H, Wu Y. Effect of carbon nanotubes on the microstructural evolution and hydrogen storage properties of Mg(BH4)2. Journal of Alloys and Compounds. 2018, 743, 11–6.

[163] Lu C, Zou J, Zeng X, Ding W. Hydrogen storage properties of core-shell structured Mg@TM (TM = Co, V) composites. International Journal of Hydrogen Energy 2017, 42, 15246–55.

[164] Xie L, Li J, Zhang T, Song L. Dehydrogenation steps and factors controlling desorption kinetics of a MgCe hydrogen storage alloy. International Journal of Hydrogen Energy 2017, 42, 21121–30.

[165] Xu C, Lin H-J, Wang Y, Zhang P, Zhu Y. Catalytic effect of in situ formed nano-Mg2Ni and Mg2Cu on the hydrogen storage properties of Mg-Y hydride composites. Journal of Alloys and Compounds. 2019, 782, 242–50.

[166] Song G-L, Unocic KA. The anodic surface film and hydrogen evolution on Mg. Corrosion Science. 2015, 98, 758–65.

[167] Gajdics M, Spassov T, Kis VK, Scahfler E, Révész Á. Microstructural and morphological investigations on Mg-Nb2O5-CNT nanocomposites processed by high-pressure torsion for hydrogen storage applications. International Journal of Hydrogen Energy 2019, 45, 7917–28.

[168] Song MY, Kwon SN, Mumm DR, Hong S-Y. Development of Mg-oxide–Ni hydrogen-storage alloys by reactive mechanical grinding. International Journal of Hydrogen Energy 2007, 32, 3921–8.

[169] Huang M, Ouyang L, Chen Z, Peng C, Zhu M. Hydrogen production via hydrolysis of Mg-oxide composites. International Journal of Hydrogen Energy 2017, 42, 22305–11.

[170] Lee SH, Kwak YJ, Park HR, Song MY. Preparation and characterization of NbF5-added Mg hydrogen storage alloy. International Journal of Hydrogen Energy 2014, 39, 16486–92.

[171] Kwak YJ, Lee SH, Song MY. Development of an Mg-Based Alloy with High Hydriding and Dehydriding Rates and Large Hydrogen Storage Capacity by Adding TaF_5. Journal of Nanoscience and Nanotechnology 2018, 18, 6040–6.

[172] Messina J. Magnesium: Alternative Power Source. PhyOrg. 2010, https://phys.org/news/2010-04-magnesium-alternative-power-source.html.

[173] NHK. Science Zero. 2002; https://ja.wikipedia.org/wiki/%E3%82%B5%E3%82%A4%E3%82%A8%E3%83%B3%E3%82%B9ZERO.

[174] Zhao J et al. Discharge behavior of Mg–4wt%Ga–2wt%Hg alloy as anode for seawater activated battery. Electrochimica Acta. 2011, 56, 8224–31.

[175] Yu K et al. Microstructure effects on the electrochemical corrosion properties of Mg – 4.1% Ga – 2.2% Hg alloy as the anode for seawater-activated batteries. Corrosion Science. 2011, 53, 2035–40.
[176] Huang G et al. Performance of Mg–air battery based on AZ31 alloy sheet with twins. Materials Letters 2013, 113, 46–9.
[177] Zhao Y et al. Effect of phosphate and vanadate as electrolyte additives on the performance of Mg-air batteries. Materials Chemistry and Physics. 2018, 218, 256–61.
[178] Zhao Y et al. Effect of Texture on the Performance of Mg-air Battery Based on Rolled Mg-3Al-1Zn Alloy Sheet. Rare Metal Materials and Engineering. 2018, 47, 1064–8.
[179] Liu X et al. Discharge performance of the magnesium anodes with different phase constitutions for Mg-air batteries. Journal of Power Sources. 2018, 396, 667–74.
[180] Wang N et al. Discharge behaviour of Mg-Al-Pb and Mg-Al-Pb-In alloys as anodes for Mg-air battery. Electrochimica Acta. 2014, 149, 193–205.
[181] Wen L et al. Composition optimization and electrochemical properties of Mg-Al-Pb-(Zn) alloys as anodes for seawater activated battery. Electrochimica Acta. 2016, 194, 40–51.
[182] Shi Y et al. Enhancement of discharge properties of an extruded Mg-Al-Pb anode for seawater-activated battery by lanthanum addition. Journal of Alloys and Compounds. 2017, 721, 392–404.
[183] Wang N et al. Wrought Mg-Al-Pb-RE alloy strips as the anodes for Mg-air batteries. Journal of Power Sources. 2019, 436; https://doi.org/10.1016/j.jpowsour.2019.226855.
[184] Yuasa M et al. Discharge properties of Mg–Al–Mn–Ca and Mg–Al–Mn alloys as anode materials for primary magnesium–air batteries. Journal of Power Sources. 2015, 297, 449–56.
[185] Xiong H et al. Effects of microstructure on the electrochemical discharge behavior of Mg-6wt %Al-1wt%Sn alloy as anode for Mg-air primary battery. Journal of Alloys and Compounds. 2017, 708, 652–61.
[186] Zheng T et al. Composition optimization and electrochemical properties of Mg-Al-Sn-Mn alloy anode for Mg-air batteries. Materials & Design. 2018, 137, 245–55.
[187] Deng M et al. Mg-Ca binary alloys as anodes for primary Mg-air batteries. Journal of Power Sources. 2018, 396, 109–18.
[188] Deng M et al., Revealing the impact of second phase morphology on discharge properties of binary Mg-Ca anodes for primary Mg-air batteries. Corrosion Science. 2019, 153, 225–35.
[189] Liu X et al. Electrochemical behaviors and discharge performance of the as-extruded Mg-1.5 wt %Ca alloys as anode for Mg-air battery. Journal of Alloys and Compounds. 2019, 790, 822–8.
[190] Cheng S-M et al. Discharge properties of low-alloyed Mg–Bi–Ca alloys as anode materials for Mg–air batteries: Influence of Ca alloying. Journal of Alloys and Compounds. 2020, 823; https://doi.org/10.1016/j.jallcom.2020.153779.
[191] Risueño E, Faik A, Rodríguez-Aseguinolaza J, Blanco-Rodríguez P, D'Aguanno B. Mg-Zn-Al Eutectic Alloys as Phase Change Material for Latent Heat Thermal Energy Storage. Energy Procedia 2015, 69, 1006–13.
[192] Risueño E, Doppiu S, Rodríguez-Aseguinolaza J, Blanco P, D'Aguanno B. Experimental investigation of Mg-Zn-Al metal alloys for latent heat storage application. Journal of Alloys and Compounds. 2016, 685, 724–32.
[193] Rahul S, Syju T, Devadas KM, Neson V, Syamaprasad U. Tackling the agglomeration of Mg2Si dopant in MgB2 superconductor using cast Mg–Si alloy. Materials Research Bulletin. 2017, 93, 296–302.
[194] Güner SB, Savaşkan B, Öztürk K, Çelik Ş, Yanmaz E. Investigation on superconducting and magnetic levitation force behaviour of excess Mg doped-bulk MgB2 superconductors. Cryogenics. 2019, 101, 131–6.

[195] https://www.phonearena.com/news/Magnesium-vs-aluminum-or-why-a-Samsung-Galaxy-S7-made-of-magnesium-would-be-awesome_id76835.
[196] https://alexnld.com/.
[197] https://www.amazon.co.jp/dp/B072JTM3DG/ref=sspa_dk_detail_0?psc=1.
[198] https://www.manufacturer.lighting/products/373/.
[199] http://www.wuxifumei.com/en/PRODUCTS/Magnesium_alloy_LED_ele/.
[200] https://www.nikonusa.com/en/nikon-products/d850-technical.page.
[201] http://www.bledsoebrace.com/products/z–12/.
[202] http://kentoptronics.com/switchable.html.
[203] Richardson TJ. New Electrochromic Mirror Systems. Solid State Ionics. 2003, 165, 305–8.
[204] Farangis B, Nachimuthu P, Richardson TJ, Slack JL, Meye BK, Perera RCC, Rubin MD. Structural and electronic properties of magnesium–3D transition metal switchable mirrors. Solid State Inonics. 2003, 165, 309–14.
[205] Slack JL, Locke JCW, Song S, Ona J, Richardson TJ. Metal hydride switchable mirrors: Factors influencing dynamic range and stability. Solar Energy Materials Solar Energy Materials and Solar Cells. 2006, 90, 485–90.
[206] Tajima K, Yamada Y, Yoshimura K. Switchable mirror glass with a Mg–Zr–Ni ternary alloy thin film. Solar Energy Materials and Solar Cells. 2014, 126, 227–36.
[207] La M, Zhou H, Li N, Xin Y, Jin P. Improved performance of Mg–Y alloy thin film switchable mirrors after coating with a superhydrophobic surface. Applied Surface Science 2017, 403, 23–8.
[208] Liu Y, Chen J, Peng L, Han J, Chen W. Improved optical properties of switchable mirrors based on Pd/Mg-TiO2 films fabricated by magnetron sputtering. Materials & Design. 2018, 144, 256–62.
[209] Mukherjee S, Maitra T, Pradhan A, Mukherjee S, Nayak A. Rapid responsive Mg/ZnSnP2/Sn photodetector for visible to near-infrared application. Solar Energy Materials and Solar Cells. 2019, 189, 181–7.
[210] Bolokang AS, Dhonge BP, Swart HC, Arendse CJ, Motaoung DE. Structural and optical characterization of mechanically milled Mg-TiO2 and nitrided Mg-TiOx-Ny nanostructures: Possible candidates for gas sensing application. Applied Surface Science 2016, 360, 1047–58.
[211] https://www.dji.com/jp/phantom-4-adv.

Chapter 17
Biological behaviors

17.1 Metabolism and homeostasis

In this section, we deal with Mg element as a bioabsorbable element, instead of biodegradable one. There are several ways to consider the composition of the human body, including the elements, type of molecule or type of cells. Most of the human body is made up of water, with cells consisting of 65–90% water by weight. Therefore, it is not surprising that most of the human body's mass is oxygen [1, 2]. Carbon, the basic unit for organic molecules, comes second. A total of 99% of mass of the human body is made up of just six elements: oxygen, carbon, hydrogen, nitrogen, calcium and phosphorus, as shown in Figure 17.1 [3].

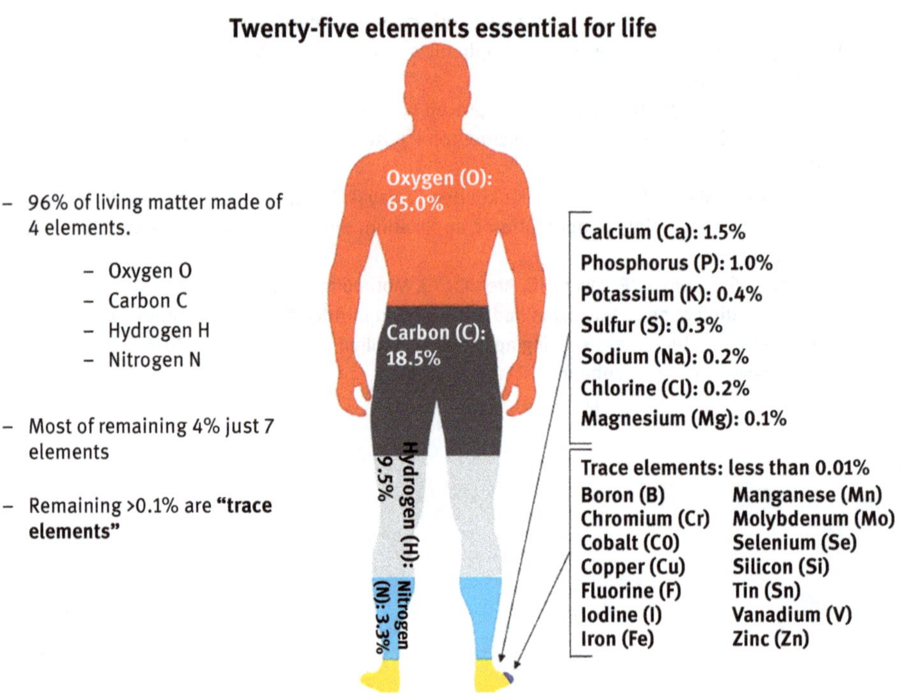

Figure 17.1: Distribution of essential elements in human body [3].

Not all of the elements found within the body are essential for life. Some are considered contaminants that appear to do no harm but serve no known function. Examples include cesium and titanium. Others are actively toxic, including mercury, cadmium and

https://doi.org/10.1515/9783110676945-017

the radioactive elements. Arsenic is considered to be toxic to humans, but serves as a function in other mammals (goats, rats and hamsters) in trace amounts. Aluminum is interesting because it is the third most common element in the Earth's crust yet serves no known function in living cells. While fluorine is used by plants to produce protective toxins, it serves no essential biological role in human beings [2]. Magnesium is an essential element to human body and is involved in over 300 metabolic reactions. Mg is used to build the structure of muscles and bones and is an important cofactor in enzymatic reactions. The recommended daily allowance for Mg depends on age and gender and the National Institutes of Health (NIH) recommended the following Mg intake [4]: 80 mg/day for ages between 1 and 3, 130 mg/day for ages from 4 to 8 and 240 mg/day for ages from 9 to 13. From 14 years, the requirements are different for men and women as follows: males aged 14–18 years: 410 mg/day, males aged 19 years and over: 400–420 mg/day, females aged 14–18 years: 360 mg/day, females aged 19 years and over: 310–320 mg/day, during pregnancy: 350 to 400 mg/day and during breast feeding: 310–360 mg/day.

As to the metabolism of magnesium, it is reported that an adult has 22–26 g of magnesium, with 60% in the skeleton, 39% intracellular (20% in skeletal muscle) and 1% extracellular. Serum levels are typically 0.7–1.0 mmol/L or 1.8–2.4 mEq/L. Serum magnesium levels may be normal even when intracellular magnesium is deficient. The mechanisms for maintaining the magnesium level in the serum show varying gastrointestinal absorption and renal excretion. Intracellular magnesium is correlated with intracellular potassium. Increased magnesium lowers calcium and can either prevent hypercalcemia or cause hypocalcemia depending on the initial level. Both low and high protein intake conditions inhibit magnesium absorption, as does the amount of phosphate, phytate and fat in the gut. Unabsorbed dietary magnesium is excreted in feces; absorbed magnesium is excreted in urine and sweat [5]. An average diet contains around 300 mg of magnesium, of which two-thirds is absorbed. As shown in Figure 17.2 [6], half of the absorbed magnesium is excreted by the kidneys, which can regulate the amount within a range of 1–150 mmol/day. This control is subject to the influences of the parathyroid hormone parathormone and the thyroid hormone calcitotonin. Magnesium is important to neuromuscular transmission. It is also an important cofactor in the enzymic processes that form the matrix of bone and in the synthesis of nucleic acid. Magnesium deficiency can result from the overuse of diuretics and from chronic renal failure, chronic alcoholism, uncontrolled diabetes mellitus and intestinal malabsorption [6, 7].

Magnesium has an inverse relationship with calcium. Thus, if food is deficient in magnesium, more of the calcium in the food is absorbed. If the blood level of magnesium is low, calcium is mobilized from bone. The treatment of hypocalcemia due to malabsorption includes administration of magnesium supplements [8]. Hence, the dietary balance of Ca/Mg ratio is very important [8–11]. Figure 17.3 shows how the dietary Ca/Mg ratio influences the death incidence due to ischemic heart disease [11].

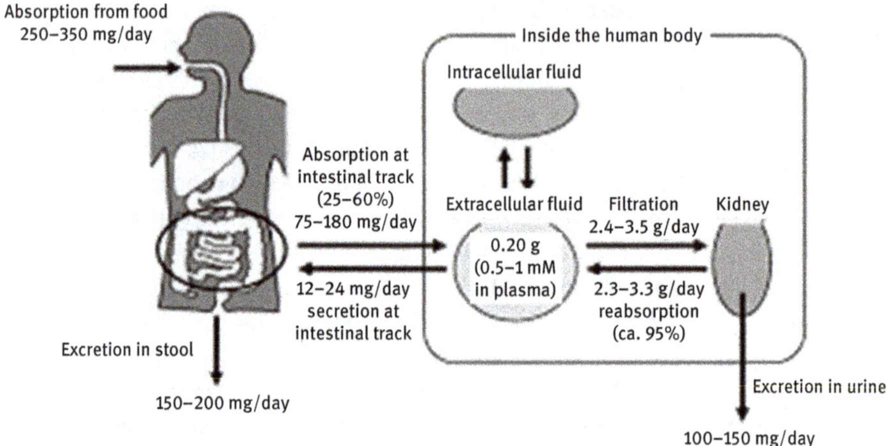

Figure 17.2: Metabolic path for taken magnesium element [6].

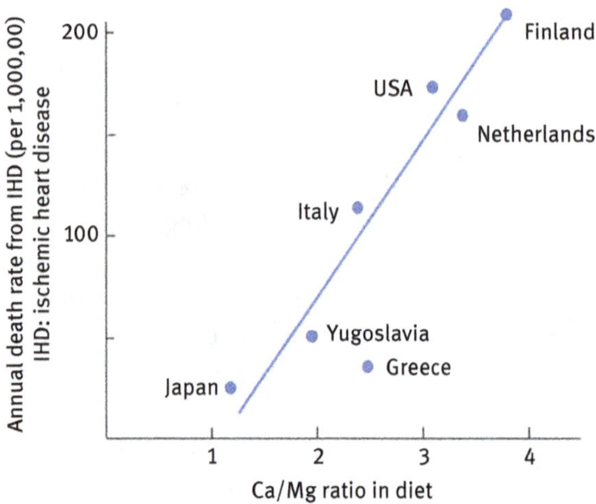

Figure 17.3: Relationship between the incidence of death from the ischemic heart disease and the dietary Ca/Mg ratio [11].

It is reported that magnesium deficiency, also known as hypomagnesemia, is often overlooked. While less than 2% of Americans have been estimated to experience magnesium deficiency, one study suggests that up to 75% are not meeting their recommended intake, as described previously [12]. There are at least seven common symptoms of magnesium deficiency, including (i) muscle twitches and cramps, (ii) mental disorders, (iii) osteoporosis [13], (iv) fatigue and muscle weakness, (v) high blood pressure, (vi) asthma and (vii) irregular heartbeat [14]. On the other hand, overdose from dietary sources alone is unlikely because excess magnesium in the blood is promptly filtered by the kidneys, as shown in Figure 17.2 and overdose is more likely in the presence of impaired renal function. The most common symptoms of overdose are nausea, vomiting and diarrhea; other symptoms include hypotension, confusion, slowed heart and respiratory rates, deficiencies of other minerals, coma, cardiac arrhythmia and death from cardiac arrest [15].

As iron is an essential element to carry oxygen inside our body, magnesium element is also essential to control healthy physical condition as well as feeling. The best sources of magnesium are nuts and seeds, dark green vegetables, whole grains and legumes. Magnesium is also added to some breakfast cereals and other fortified foods. Magnesium is lost as wheat is refined, so it is best to choose cereals and bread products made with whole grains. Most common fruits, meat and fish are low in magnesium. Here are some good sources of magnesium [4] (see Figure 17.4 [16]): sunflower seeds, dry roasted (1 cup: 512 mg); almonds, dry-roasted (1 cup: 420 mg); sesame seeds, roasted whole (1 ounce: 101 mg); spinach, boiled (1 cup: 78 mg); cashews, dry-roasted (1 ounce: 74 mg); shredded wheat cereal (two large biscuits: 61 mg); soymilk, plain (1 cup: 61 mg); black beans, cooked (1 cup: 120 mg); oatmeal, cooked (1 cup: 58 mg); broccoli, cooked (1 cup: 51 mg); edamame, shelled, cooked (1 cup: 100 mg); peanut butter, smooth (2 tablespoons: 49 mg); shrimp, raw (4 ounces: 48 mg); black-eyed peas, cooked (1 cup: 92 mg); brown rice, cooked (1 cup: 84 mg); kidney beans, canned (1 cup: 70 mg); cow's milk, whole (1 cup: 33 mg); banana (one medium: 33 mg); and bread, whole-wheat (one slice: 23 mg).

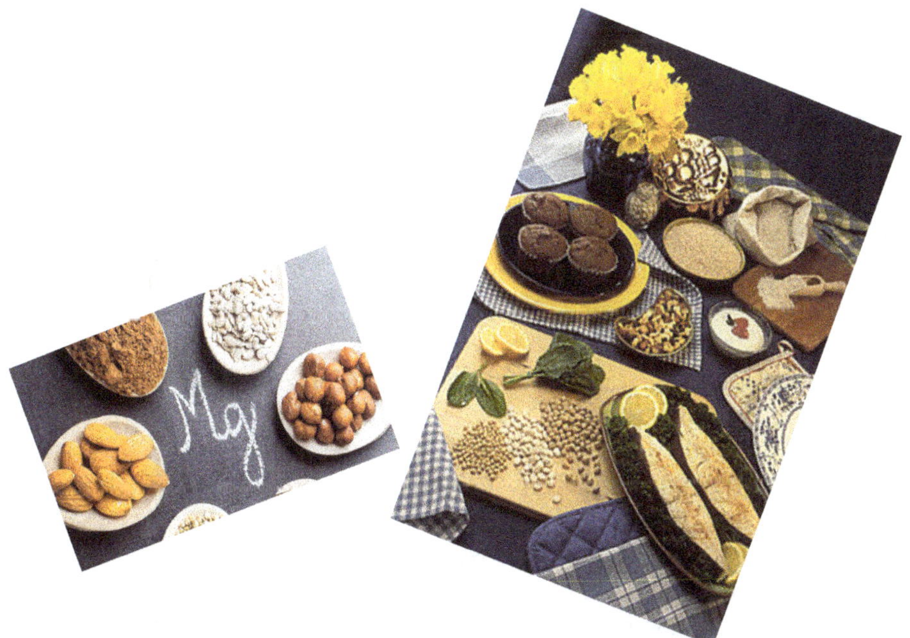

Figure 17.4: Typical Mg-rich foods [16].

Source of bioabsorbable Mg element is not limited from foods but from biodegradable Mg medical devices too. Biodegradable Mg-based metals are promising orthopedic implants for treating challenging bone diseases, attributed to their desirable mechanical and osteopromotive properties. Wang et al. [17] investigated the metabolism of taken biodegraded Mg element and mentioned that (i) as the fourth most prevalent mineral in the human body, Mg is involved in hundreds of biochemical reactions and acts as an essential element in the construction of bone and soft tissue [15]; (ii) a healthy adult restores 24–30 g of Mg for maintaining regular functions and the recommended daily allowance for Mg is 310–420 mg to maintain health [15]; (iii) excessive Mg ions are permissible as they can be transported via the circulatory system and promptly excreted by way of urine and faces, without causing any adverse effects, as shown in Figure 17.5 [17]; and (iv) Mg-based metals can be defined as a type of novel absorbable metallic material.

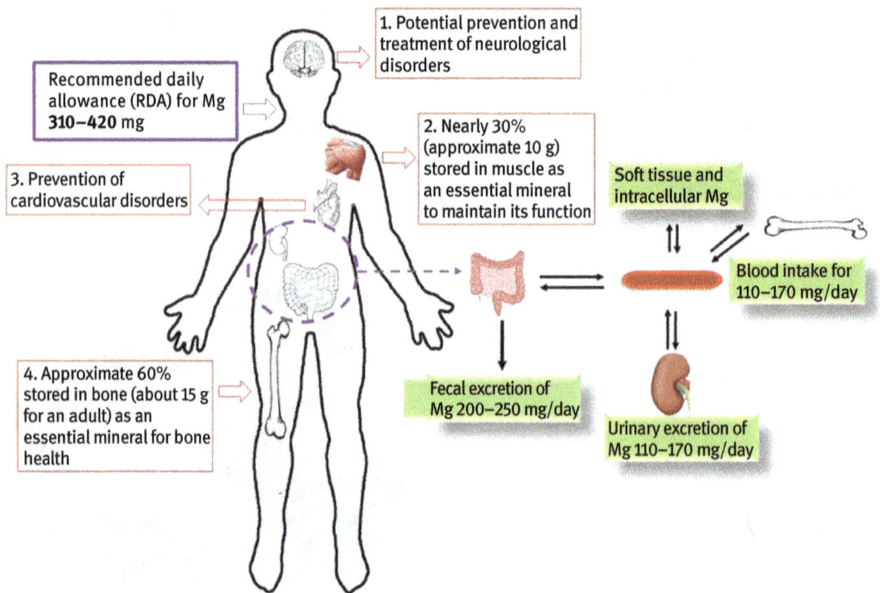

Figure 17.5: Good biocompatibility of biodegradable Mg-based orthopedic implants [17].

17.2 Biological reaction

Mg is one of the most important and essential metallic elements for human body where it is involved in various enzymatic reactions. It was reported that Mg takes place in synthesis processes of protein and nucleic acid, stabilization of plasma membrane and many other cellular activities. Amount of Mg in an average adult human body is around 21–28 g and more than 50% of which is present in bone tissue and soft tissues contain 35–40% of this content and less than 1% is sequestered in serum [18, 19]. It was further mentioned that (i) Mg element, which is sequestered in bone, acts as a reservoir for acute change in Mg levels of serum; (ii) Mg^{2+} ions play an important role in determining bone fragility; (iii) Mg^{2+} ion takes place in transformation process of immature bone into a mature bone; (iv) Mg ion content in bone mineral is around 6 mol% but this content decreases during maturation process of bone (see Figure 17.5); (v) cartilage and immature bone tissues contain high concentration of Mg^{2+} ion but this concentration changes depending on the aging; and (vi) Mg in bone composition increases the elasticity of bone [18, 19]. As internal fixing devices (like bone plates or fixing screws) for fractured bone structures, permanent metals or resorbable polymeric materials have been selected as a material choice. Although permanent metals normally exhibit enough mechanical strength and good biocompatibility, they might cause long-term complications and may require removal. Resorbable polymers reduce long-term complications but are unsuitable for many load-bearing applications. Based on these advantages and disadvantages associated with conventional materials, biologically degradable Mg alloys have been developed for craniofacial and orthopedic applications. Chaya et al. [20] reported that, by conducting fracture fixing assessment with pure Mg device using rabbit ulna fracture model, (i) device degradation was observed; (ii) the calculated corrosion rate was 0.40 ± 0.04 mm/year after 8 weeks, (iii) fracture healing by 8 weeks and maturation after 16 weeks were recognized and (iv) Mg degradation led to the release of Mg^{2+} ions to surrounding tissue which resulted in stimulation of local cells to bone formation. Hydrogen gas that is released during degradation process of Mg and its alloys can be tolerated by human body; however, high amount of hydrogen gas release can result in complication at healing period and the corrosion rate of Mg should be controlled to decrease risk of gas accumulation, suggesting that Mg devices provide stabilization to facilitate healing, while degrading and stimulating new bone formation.

Effects of biological reactions of human tissue to the Mg element can be found in diverse areas. We will discuss further these individual reactions including cytocompatibility, hemocompatibility, biocompatibility and osseointegration as well.

17.3 Antibacterial reaction

Magnesium alloys are attracting increasing attention and interest as orthopedic applications (such as bone reconstruction or bone graft substitution) on account of their superior biocompatibility and biodegradability. Although favorable osteogenic activity and antibacterial ability are highly desired for hard tissue repair and replacement materials, the aforementioned clinical applications of Mg materials have been limited by their high (sometimes uncontrollable) degradation rate, inadequate antibacterial ability and potential toxicity in physiological environment.

There are researches reported on alloying or coating to improve the antibacterial ability of Mg-based alloys. Qin et al. [21] fabricated Mg-Nd-Zn-Zr by alloying with neodymium (Nd), zinc (Zn) and zirconium (Zr). It was reported that (i) newly developed Mg-based alloy improved its corrosion resistance, (ii) the results of the in vitro and in vivo antibacterial capability of microbiological counting and histopathology in vivo consistently indicated the alloy enhanced the antibacterial activity and (iii) the significantly improved cytocompatibility was found in this alloy, suggesting Mg-Nd-Zn-Zr alloy effectively enhances the corrosion resistance, biocompatibility and antimicrobial properties. Feng et al. [22] prepared biodegradable magnesium Mg-Zn-Y-Nd-Ag, followed by extruding for further densification purpose. It was mentioned that (i) the results of a systematic investigation of the in vivo antibacterial capability of *Staphylococcus aureus* and *Escherichia coli* indicated that all Mg-Zn-Y-N-xAg ($x = 0.2, 0.4, 0.6, 0.8$) alloys exhibited certain antibacterial property, which increased with the increase of Ag content and (ii) overall the antimicrobial property of the as-extruded alloy containing 0.4 wt% Ag exhibited the relatively better antimicrobial properties and mechanical property with the relatively small loss in corrosion resistance, indicating the potential utility of as-extruded Mg-Zn-Y-N-0.4Ag in treating orthopedic infections. Gao et al. [23] employed Mg alloys containing microlevel concentrations of Ga and/or Sr (0.1 wt%) employed as model materials to evaluate their controlling ability release of antibacterial species. Biodegradation progress of metal specimens is examined through pH and mass loss measurements, and inductively coupled plasma-atomic emission spectrometry (ICP-AES) as a function of immersion time in trypticase soy broth solution under physiological conditions. In vitro biocompatibility and antibacterial performance are characterized through MTT (3-(4,5-dimethylthiazol-2-yl)-2,5-diphenyltetrazolium bromide) proliferation assay with human mesenchymal stem cells (MSCs) and the spread plate method with three representative bacterial strains, that is, *S. aureus*, *E. coli* and *Staphylococcus epidermidis*. Animal tests are performed through implanting target metal rods into femurs of Sprague-Dawley rats, accompanied with injection of *S. aureus* to build a model of osteomyelitis. It was mentioned that (i) such lean additions of Ga and/or Sr reduce the degradation kinetics of Mg matrix and the release of Ga^{3+} ions plays a crucial role in disabling the viability of all selected bacterial strains; (ii) the histological tests confirm that the growth of fibrous tissue has been accelerated in the vicinity of Mg-based implants; and (iii) the smallest number density of *S. aureus* bacteria is on the surface of the retrieved Ga-containing Mg rod implants.

Sun et al. [24] deposited self-assembled colloidal particles onto magnesium surfaces in ethanol by a simple and effective electrophoretic deposition (EPD) method. The colloidal particles were poly(isobornyl acrylate-*co*-dimethylaminoethyl methacrylate)/tannic acid (P(ISA-*co*-DMA)/TA) colloidal particles. It was reported that the electrochemical test, pH value and Mg ion concentration data show that the corrosion resistance of Mg samples is enhanced appreciably after surface treatment. The in vitro cellular response and antibacterial capability of the modified Mg substrates are performed and found that significantly increased cell adhesion and viability are observed from the coated Mg samples, and the amounts of adherent bacteria on the treated Mg surfaces diminish remarkably compared to the bare Mg. The uncoated and coated Mg samples were implanted in New Zealand white rabbits for 12 weeks to examine the in vivo long-term corrosion performance and in situ inflammation behavior and obtained that the results confirmed that compared with uncoated Mg substrate, the corrosion and foreign-body reactions of the coated Mg samples were suppressed, suggesting that the coatings, which effectively enhance the biocompatibility, antimicrobial properties and corrosion resistance of Mg substrate, provide a simple and practical strategy to expedite clinical acceptance of biodegradable Mg and its alloys. Bakhsheshi-Rad et al. [25] coated a poly-L-lactic acid (PLLA)-åkermanite (AKT)-doxycycline (DOXY) nanofiber coating, created using the electrospinning method, to enhance the corrosion resistance, antibacterial performance and cytocompatibility of Mg alloys. It was reported that the PLLA-based nanofiber coatings are smooth and uniform with fiber diameters ranging from 300 to 350 nm. An in vitro drug release profile of PLLA-AKT nanofibers containing DOXY shows that the nanofibers allow rapid release of drug in the initial stage to provide antibacterial effects as well as sustained release over the long term to prevent infection and the implants coated with PLLA-AKT nanofibers containing DOXY have excellent antibacterial performance against Gram-positive (*S. aureus*) and Gram-negative (*E. coli*) bacteria; those coated with PLLA and PLLA-AKT without DOXY have poor antibacterial performance. Cytotoxicity tests show that PLLA and PLLA-AKT nanofiber coatings considerably enhance the cytocompatibility of Mg alloys, while incorporation of a high concentration of DOXY (10 wt%) into the PLLA-AKT coating has adverse effects on cytocompatibility and PLLA-AKT nanofiber coatings containing low concentrations of DOXY can be employed to control the degradation rate and enhance the antibacterial performance and biocompatibility of Mg alloys as applied to bone infection treatments, providing essential information to direct the development of future orthopedic applications.

Cui et al. [26] employed an SnO_2-doped calcium phosphate (Ca–P–Sn)-coating material on Mg–1Li–1Ca alloy by a hydrothermal process. It was reported that (i) a triple-layered structure, which is composed of $Ca_3(PO_4)_2$, $(Ca, Mg)_3(PO_4)_2$, SnO_2 and $MgHPO_4 \cdot 3H_2O$, is evident and leads to the formation of $Ca_{10}(PO_4)_6(OH)_2$ in Hank's solution; (ii) the corrosion resistance and antibacterial activity were improved through the coating treatment; and (iii) the embedded SnO_2 nanoparticles (NPs) enhanced crystallization of the coating. Ji et al. [27] prepared the HA coating induced by ciprofloxacin-loaded polymeric multilayers on Mg alloy via the combination of layer-by-layer assembly and hydrothermal treatment. It was indicated that the as-prepared HA coating with a compact topography showed favorable corrosion resistance, antibacterial activity (against *S. aureus* and *E. coli*) and cell compatibility (via an indirect extraction test for MC3T3-E1 preosteoblasts).

In order to achieve a proper degradation rate, acceptable biocompatibility and good antibacterial ability, Chang et al. [28] modified the surface of Mg alloys by microarc oxidation (MAO) with electrolyte of sodium phytate ($Na_{12}Phy$), which is one of the natural organic substances and widely used as a food additive. It was found that magnesium phosphate is developed in the MAO coatings, suggesting that $Na_{12}Phy$ is decomposed into inorganic phosphates and lower myoinositol phosphate esters due to spark discharge. The in vitro biocompatibility evaluated by L-929 cells indicates that both the substrate and MAOed samples do not induce toxicity to the cells, meeting the need for use as biomaterials; the MAOed samples achieve the antibacterial effect of 99.99% against *S. aureus* and 99.98% against *E. coli*. After 24 h immersion in *E. coli* suspensions, the MAO samples have been corroded, indicating that they achieve the excellent antibacterial ability due to their corrosion in the tested suspensions. Yazici et al. [29] prepared Mg–Sr–Ca ternary alloys in a vacuum/atmosphere-controlled furnace and coated by MAO process for 5 min to decrease the degradation rate and enhance the biocompatibility. Moreover, Ag-doped hydroxyapatite nanopowder (Ag-HA) was also added to alkaline MAO solution by amount of 1 and 10 g/l to improve the antibacterial properties, while enhancing their bioactivity in one single process. It was reported that the addition of more Ag-HA increased the HA formation both before and after simulated body fluid (SBF) immersion test and enhanced their antibacterial properties; however, Ag-HA addition decreased the corrosion resistance of the coated alloys in SBF compared to Ag-HA-free coating, indicating that the Ag-HA nanopowder added MAO coating is a good combination to enhance the corrosion resistance, bioactivity and the antibacterial properties of Mg-based biodegradable alloys. Aktug et al. [30] fabricated Ag-based bioceramic coatings on AZ31 Mg alloy by combining the MAO and physical vapor deposition (PVD) methods. As a first step, AZ31 Mg surfaces were coated using MAO using a solution consisting of sodium silicate and potassium hydroxide. As a second step, an Ag layer was accumulated on the MAOed surfaces using the PVD method. It was obtained that (i) the X-ray diffraction (XRD) patterns identified the presence of Mg, Si, M_2SiO_4 (forsterite) and MgO (periclase) on the Ag-deposited MAOed surfaces; (ii) surfaces of both coatings were porous due to the existence of discharge channels; (iii) the Ag-deposited MAOed surfaces were found to have hydrophobic properties with respect to plain MAOed surfaces; (iv) newly formed layers consisted of $Ca_{15}(SiO_4)_6(PO_4)_2$, $Ca_3(PO_4)_2$ and $Ca_{10}(PO_4)_6(OH)_2$ as produced on plain MAOed and Ag-deposited MAOed surfaces by immersion in SBF. These layers were more homogeneous on Ag-deposited MAO coatings than ones on plain MAO. For *E. coli* and *S. aureus* bacteria, the numbers of active bacterial colonies on Ag-deposited MAOed surfaces were significantly reduced with respect to plain MAOed surfaces. Yan et al. [31] examined the MAOed Mg–0.06Cu alloy and mentioned that the solution treatment significantly decreased the corrosion rate compared with the as-cast condition due to the decrease of the amount of cathodic Mg_2Cu-phase particles. MAO produced a coating layer that separated the substrate from the solution so that the MAO-treated condition had a corrosion rate that was 1/76 of that of the as-cast condition and antibacterial test revealed that MAO coating on as-cast and solution-treated conditions possessed excellent antibacterial ability, which might be attributed to the porous structure of the coating and the presence of a trace amount of copper.

17.4 Biocompatibility

Biological compatibility (or in short, biocompatibility) of biomaterial or medical/dental device can be defined as an ability to perform its intended biofunction, with the desired degree of incorporation in the host, without eliciting any undesirable local or systemic effects (such as inflammation, toxicity, carcinogenicity or injurious effects) on that host system [32]. Hence, the biocompatibility deals with systemic safety covering tissue and cells (relating to the cytocompatibility), bloods (affecting the hemocompatibility) and bones (responding to the biomechanical compatibility and osseointegration). Mg and its alloys are considered attractive metallic materials for the development of potential medical implants; biocompatibility is the most essential aspect for consideration [33–35], so that there are numerous researches conducted for enhancement or improving biocompatibility of Mg-based alloys by alloying, coating or microstructural alterations [36–39].

17.4.1 Mg

Binary Mg-based alloys with nine alloying elements (Al, Ag, In, Mn, Si, Sn, Y, Zn and Zr) were prepared to evaluate their alloying effects on mechanical properties, corrosion properties and in vitro biocompatibilities (cytotoxicity and hemocompatibility) by scanning electron microscopy (SEM), XRD, tensile test, immersion test, electrochemical corrosion test in both SBF and Hank's solutions, cell culture and platelet adhesion test [40]. Pure magnesium was used as control. It was reported that (i) the addition of alloying elements could influence the strength and corrosion resistance of Mg and (ii) the cytotoxicity tests indicated that Mg–1Al, Mg–1Sn and Mg–1Zn alloy extracts showed no significant reduced cell viability to fibroblasts (L-929 and NIH3T3) and osteoblasts (MC3T3-E1); Mg–1Al and Mg–1Zn alloy extracts indicated no negative effect on viabilities of blood vessel-related cells, ECV304 and VSMC. In hemolysis assays, Mg–1In, Mg–1Mn, Mg–1Si and Mg–1Y alloys had low ratios of hemolysis of less than 5% and adhered platelets are approximately round in shape and have slight spreading of pseudopodia, but fewer were adhered for alloys compared to the pure Mg control, indicating that an appropriate selection of alloying element to Mg becomes a crucial factor for controlling biocompatibility.

17.4.2 Mg–Al alloy system

To improve biocompatibility of AZ31 (Mg–Al–Zn alloy), there are several coatings developed and investigated. Chai et al. [41] coated β-tricalcium phosphate (β-TCP) on AZ31 by phosphating process and implanted coated AZ31 alloy into the femurs of rats after predrilling with 1 mm hand-operated drills to evaluate implant osteogenesis and biodegradability. It was reported that in vitro, the human osteosarcoma cell line ($SaOS_2$) showed significantly good adherence and proliferation on the surface of the β-TCP-coated Mg alloy after 24 h incubation and the growth factor bone morphogenetic protein-2 (BMP-2) was highly expressed in $SaOS_2$ cultured with the β-TCP-coated Mg alloy by Western blot analysis. In vivo, the newborn bone at the implant/bone interface was formed at week 1 and matured at week 4 postimplantation and villous tissue was found at the implant/bone interface at week 12 postimplantation; the contents of phosphorus and calcium on the surface of the β-TCP-coated Mg alloy were decreased at week 4 and week 12 postimplantation, respectively. Immunohistochemical analysis of the experimental results demonstrated that the β-TCP-coated Mg alloy implants provided a high BMP-2 expression during the first 4 weeks postimplantation. Compared with the uncoated AZ31 alloy which was degraded for 33% in vivo, only 17% of the β-TCP-coated Mg alloy was degraded at week 12 postimplantation. The in vitro cell tests showed that the β-TCP coating provided the Mg alloy with a significantly better surface cytocompatibility, and in vivo results also confirmed that the β-TCP coating exhibited greatly improved osteoconductivity and osteogenesis in the early 12-week postoperation period. The in vivo experiment demonstrated that the β-TCP coating layer could slow down the degradation of the uncoated AZ31 at the early stage of implantation. Peng et al. [42] treated porous surface structure of plasma electrolytic oxidation (PEOed) AZ31 with Mg–Al-layered double hydroxide (LDH) via hydrothermal treatment. It was mentioned that (i) PEO/LDH composite coating possesses a two-layer structure, an inner layer made up of PEO coating (~5 μm) and an outer layer of Mg-Al LDH (~2 μm); (ii) electrochemical and hydrogen evolution tests suggest preferable corrosion resistance of the PEO/LDH coating; (iii) cytotoxicity, cell adhesion, live/dead staining and proliferation data of rat bone marrow stem cells demonstrate that PEO/LDH coating remarkably enhances the cytocompatibility of the substrate, indicating a potential application in orthopedic surgeries; (iv) hemolysis rate (HR) value of PEO/LDH coating is $1.10 \pm 0.47\%$, fulfilling the request of clinical application; and (v) the structure of Mg–Al LDH on the top of PEO coating shows excellent drug delivery ability. Pan et al. [43] modified surface of AZ31B by the alkali-heating treatment followed by the self-assembly of 3-phosphonopropionic acid, 3-aminopropyltrimethoxysilane (APTMS) and dopamine, respectively. It was found that an excellent hydrophilic surface was obtained after the alkali-heating treatment and the water contact angle increased to some degree after the self-assembly of dopamine, APTMS and 3-phosphonopropionic acid; however, the hydrophilicity of the modified samples was better than that of the pristine magnesium substrate. Due to the formation of the passivation layer after the alkali-heating treatment, the corrosion resistance of AZ31 was obviously improved and the corrosion rate further decreased to varying degrees after the self-assembly surface modification. The blood compatibility of the pristine magnesium was significantly improved after the surface modification; the hemolysis rate (HR) was reduced from 56% of the blank magnesium alloy to 18% of the alkali-heating treated sample and the values were further reduced to about 10% of dopamine-modified sample and 7% of APTMS-modified sample and the HR was below 5% for the 3-phosphonopropionic acid-modified sample. The modified samples showed good cytocompatibility; endothelial cells exhibited the improved proliferative profiles in terms of CCK-8 assay as compared to those on the pristine magnesium alloy; and the modified samples showed better endothelial cell adhesion and spreading than the pristine magnesium alloy. Based on these findings, it was indicated that the surface modification can be used to modify the magnesium alloy surface to improve the corrosion resistance and biocompatibility simultaneously. Kim et al. [44] coated AZ31 with polycaprolactone (PCL) and (Zn) oxide NPs (ZnO NPs) composite coatings by electrospinning technique. It was mentioned that (i) the increase in the content of ZnO NPs in the composite coatings not only improved the coating adhesion of composite coatings on Mg alloys, but also increased the corrosion resistance and (ii) the biocompatibility of MC3T3-E1 osteoblasts of the PCL/ZnO composite-coated samples was superior to the biocompatibility of the bare samples. Applying PCL/ZnO composite coating to the magnesium alloys has suggested suitable potential in biomedical applications. Hou et al. [45] applied the ultrasonic nanocrystal surface modification (UNSM) (which is developed to induce plastic strain on metal surfaces) to an AZ31B alloy. It was obtained that (i) significant improvement in hardness, yield stress and wear resistance was achieved after the UNSM treatment; (ii) the corrosion behavior of UNSM-treated AZ31B was not compromised compared with the untreated samples, as demonstrated by the weight loss and released element concentrations of Mg and Al after immersion in alpha-minimum essential medium (α-MEM) for 24 h; and (iii) the in vitro biocompatibility of the AZ31B Mg alloys toward adipose-derived stem cells (ADSCs) before and after UNSM processing was also evaluated using a cell culture study to show that UNSM could significantly improve the mechanical properties of Mg alloys without compromising their corrosion rate and biocompatibility in vitro. UNSM is a promising method to treat biodegradable Mg alloys for orthopedic applications. Lu et al. [46] treated AZ31B by laser surface treatments via the employment of a continuous-wave Nd:YAG laser using laser fluences in the range of 1.06–4.24 J/mm^2 (250–1,000 W) and it was indicated that the potential of laser surface engineering to realize AZ31B alloy as a viable biodegradable bone implant material.

17.4.3 Mg–Zn alloy system

For Mg–4Zn–0.2Ca alloy, both cytotoxicity and *in vivo* biocompatibility were studied and will be discussed in the next cytocompatibility Section (5). Ding et al. [48] fabricated Mg–Zn–Ca alloy operative clip by combining hot extrusion and blanking processing and evaluated the in vitro and in vivo biocompatibility by L-929 cells and SD rat model. It was mentioned that (i) Mg–Zn–Ca alloy exhibited noncytotoxic to L-929 cells, (ii) the in vivo implantation showed that the newly designed Mg–Zn–Ca clip can successfully ligate carotid artery and no blood leakage occurred postsurgery, (iii) during the period of the clip degradation, a small amount of H_2 gas formation and no tissue inflammation around the clips were observed, (iv) the degradation rate of the clip near the heart ligated the arteries faster than that of clip far away the heart due do the effect of arterial blood and (v) histological analysis and various blood biochemical parameters in rat serum samples collected at different times after clip implantation showed no tissue inflammation around the clips [47]. Wong et al. [48] evaluated the biocompatibility of Mg–35Zn–5Ca bulk metallic glass composite (BMGC) implanted by a rabbit tendon-bone interference fixation model. It was found that (i) the biocomposite may be classed as slightly toxic on the basis of the standard ISO (International Organization for Standardization) 10993-5 and (ii) in vivo test, a rabbit tendon–bone interference fixation model was established to determine the biocompatibility and osteogenic potential of the bio-composite in a created bony tunnel for a period of up to 24 weeks. Mg–35Zn–5Ca BMGC induced considerable new bone formation at the implant site in comparison with conventional titanium alloy after 24 weeks of implantation. Based on these results, it was concluded that Mg–35Zn–5Ca bulk metallic glass composite demonstrated adequate biocompatibility and exhibited significant osteogenic potential both in vitro and in vivo, as a promising future application of implants. Zhao et al. [49] evaluated MgZnCaY-1RE, MgZnCaY-2RE, MgYZr-1RE and MgZnYZr-1RE alloys for cardiovascular stents applications regarding their mechanical strength, corrosion resistance, hemolysis, platelet adhesion/activation and endothelial biocompatibility. It was mentioned that (i) the mechanical properties of all alloys were significantly improved, (ii) potentiodynamic polarization showed that the corrosion resistance of four alloys was at least 3–10 times higher than that of pure Mg control, (iii) hemolysis test revealed that all the materials were nonhemolytic while little to moderate platelet adhesion was found on all material surfaces, (iv) no significant cytotoxicity was observed in human aorta endothelial cells cultured with magnesium alloy extract solution for up to seven days and (v) direct endothelialization test showed that all the alloys possess significantly better capability to sustain endothelial cell attachment and growth, demonstrating the promising potential of these alloys for stent material applications in the future.

For Mg–Zn–Zr alloy systems, Dziuba et al. [50] developed a new degradable Mg alloy, ZEK100 (Mg-1Zn-0.5Zr-0.3RE) and explored its long-term degradation and biocompatibility in adult female New Zealand white rabbits. Five rabbits each with intramedullary tibia implants were examined over 9 and 12 months. Three legs were left without an implant to serve as negative controls. Numerous examinations were performed in the follow-up (clinical examinations, serum analysis and radiographic and in vivo micro-CT investigations) and after death (ex vivo micro-CT, histology and implant analysis) to assess the in vivo degradation and biocompatibility. It was mentioned that ZEK100 degrades slowly in vivo; however, favorable in vivo degradation is not necessarily associated with good biocompatibility and the absence of general pathological disorders does not definitively indicate that Mg implants have acceptable biocompatibility. Although ZEK100 provided a very high initial stability and positive biodegradation, it must be excluded from further biomedical testing as it showed pathological effects on the host tissue following complete degradation. Li et al. [51] prepared four Mg-1.5Zn-0.6Zr-*x*Sc (x = 0, 0.2, 0.5, 1.0 wt%) alloys and studied their hydrophilicity, cytotoxicity and hemocompatibility. It was found that (i) the contact angle measurements revealed that addition of Sc improved the hydrophilicity of the alloys; (ii) for biodegradable alloys, perfect hydrophilicity could promote the tissue attaching on implant surface, establishing a benign biological reaction and improving the therapeutic effectiveness; (iii) the viabilities of L-929 cells and SP2/0 cells for all the alloys were about 100% and 90% compared to negative control, respectively; (iv) no obvious differences existed in cell viabilities between different Sc contents; and (v) with increasing addition of Sc, the hemolysis percentages and the degree of platelet activation increased. Wang et al. [52] studied biocompatibility of Sr-doped nanorod/nanowire hydroxyapatite (HA) coatings on ZK60 (Mg-5Zn-0.5Zr) alloy. It was shown that with the addition of Sr element, the shape of the fabricated HA turned from nanorods into nanowires and the morphology of the coatings changed from a flower-like structure to a network structure. The electrochemical and immersion tests showed that the Sr doping can enhance the corrosion resistance of the HA coatings and BMSCs (bone marrow stromal cells) cell culture results suggested that the addition of the trace element Sr can promote the cell adhesion and proliferation of HA-coated biodegradable Mg alloys. A simple and efficient way to fabricate nanowired HA coating on biodegradable Mg alloys with improved biocompatibility and osteogenicity was provided and the Sr-doped HA coatings on biodegradable Mg alloys have shown a great potential for the orthopedic application. Gu et al. [53] investigated the feasibility of ZK60 alloy for biomedical applications through microstructure characterization, corrosion tests in different biological media, and cell proliferation, differentiation and adhesion tests. It was reported that (i) corrosion tests showed the ZK60 alloy in the as-extruded state with finer grain sizes exhibited slower corrosion rates than the same alloy in the as-cast state; (ii) the tests conducted in different biological fluids showed that the corrosion rates of the as-cast and as-extruded ZK60 alloy in DMEM (Dulbecco's modified Eagle's medium) + FBS (fetal bovine serum) were the highest, while those in Hank's solution were the lowest; The corrosion rate of the as-extruded ZK60 alloy was similar to the corrosion rates of other commercial magnesium alloys, namely, the die-cast AZ91D, die-cast AM50, extruded AZ31 and extruded WE43 alloys. The indirect cytotoxicity evaluation showed that the 100% concentrated cast and extruded ZK60 alloy extracts resulted in significantly reduced cell numbers and total protein amounts, as compared to the negative control. The cell number and total protein amount increased with the gradual dilution of the extracts, but the protein-normalized alkaline phosphatase (ALP) activity showed an opposite trend and for the direct assay, L-929 and MG63 cells exhibited good adhesion with spread pseudopod on the surface of extruded ZK60 alloy samples after 24 h culture, summarizing that the as-extruded ZK60 alloy could be a good candidate material for biodegradable implants.

Zhang et al. [54] implanted Mg–Zn–Mn alloy into rats to investigate the in vivo degradation of Mg alloy, response of the bone to the biodegradable Mg implant and effect of the degradation of Mg alloy on blood composition and organs. It was mentioned that (i) Mg–Zn–Mn alloy was found to degrade at different rates in the marrow cavity and cortical bone and (ii) new bone tissue formed around the magnesium implants after 6 weeks implantation but no fibrous capsule was found and on Mg implant side, crystalline magnesium calcium phosphate formed on the surface of the implant due to the reaction between the implant and blood or body fluid. The new bone tissue side was 10–30 μm membrane comprising two distinct layers with many fibroblasts in the layer close to the new bone tissue. The new bone was in tight contact with the implant through the membrane and phosphate layer due to the good osteoconductivity of the phosphate layer. After 10 and 26 weeks postimplantation, more new bone tissues as well as the membrane were found around the implant; however, no apparent increase in the thickness of the membrane was observed with the increasing of the implantation duration and blood examination has shown that the degradation of the magnesium implant caused little change to blood composition but no disorder to liver or kidneys.

Jaiswal et al. [55] investigated mechanical, corrosion and biocompatibility behavior of Mg–3Zn–HA biodegradable composites for orthopedic fixture accessories. It was mentioned that (i) addition of 5 wt% HA is found effective in reducing the corrosion rate by 42% and improvement in the compressive yield strength of biodegradable magnesium alloy by 23%, (ii) the in vitro evaluation, up to 56 days, reveal improved resistance to degradation with HA reinforcement to Mg and (iii) osteoblast cells show better growth and proliferation on HA-reinforced surfaces of the composite. Mg-HA composite structure shows impressive potential to be used in orthopedic fracture fixing accessories.

Scheideler et al. [56] stated that (i) the standard cell culture tests according to ISO 10993 have only limited value for the biocompatibility screening of degradable biomaterials such as Mg alloys, (ii) the correlation between in vitro and in vivo results is poor and (iii) standard cytotoxicity tests mimic the clinical situation to only a limited extent, since in vivo proteins and macromolecules in the blood and interstitial liquid will influence the corrosion behavior and, hence, biocompatibility of Mg alloys to a significant extent. Based on these controversial issues, Scheideler et al. [56] modified cytotoxicity test simulating the in vivo conditions by use of bovine serum as the extraction vehicle instead of the cell culture medium routinely used in standard cytotoxicity testing according to ISO 10993-5 and applied to Mg alloys. Cytotoxicity was assayed by inhibition of cell metabolic activity. It was reported that (i) when extraction of the alloy samples was performed in serum instead of cell culture medium, the metabolic activity was significantly less inhibited for six of the eight alloys and (ii) the reduction in apparent cytotoxicity under serum extraction conditions was most pronounced for Mg–1Zn (109% relative metabolic activity with serum extracts vs 26% in DMEM), for MgY4 (103% in serum vs 32% in DMEM) and for Mg–3Al–1Zn (84% vs 17%), resulting in a completely different cytotoxicity ranking of the tested materials when serum extraction was used. The modified test system has the potential to enhance the predictability of in vivo corrosion behavior and biocompatibility of Mg-based materials for biodegradable medical devices.

17.4.4 Mg–Ca alloy system

An in vitro corrosion assessment of Mg–Ca (0.8 wt% of Ca) in Hank's balanced salt solution (HBSS) was conducted by immersion, hydrogen evolution and electrochemical behavior was studied as well as the cytotoxicity of the degradation products [57]. It was mentioned that immersion degradation resulted in the formation of the needle-shaped carbonated HA, which was similar to the biological apatite in the human bone. Degradation kinetics showed that Mg–0.8Ca alloy had approximately threefold faster degradation rate than the pure Mg (1.08 ± 0.38 mm/year for Mg–0.8Ca and 0.35 ± 0.17 mm/year for pure Mg), as observed in two independent experiments. Both pure Mg and Mg–0.8Ca alloys were biocompatible, generating no cytotoxic degradation products against human-derived HEK 293 cells and the Mg–0.8Ca alloy was found to be a promising biodegradable implant in terms of bioactivity and compatibility with human cell lines. The desired degradation rate of an implant can be controlled by the Mg–Ca composition of such alloys, depending on the application of the implant and the estimated healing time of the bone. Li et al. [58] fabricated binary Mg–xCa ($x = 1$–3 wt%) alloys with various Ca contents, having two phases of α(Mg) and Mg_2Ca. It was found that (i) the in vitro corrosion test in SBF indicated that the microstructure and working history of Mg–xCa alloys strongly affected their corrosion behaviors, (ii) an increasing content of Mg_2Ca phase led to a higher corrosion rate whereas hot rolling and hot extrusion could reduce it and (iii) the cytotoxicity evaluation using L-929 cells revealed that Mg–1Ca alloy did not induce toxicity to cells, and the viability of cells for Mg–1Ca alloy extraction medium was better than that of control. After implanted into the left and right rabbit femoral shafts, high activity of osteoblast and osteocytes were observed around the Mg–1Ca alloy pins as shown by hematoxylin and eosin (HE)-stained tissue sections and both the in vitro and in vivo corrosions suggested that a mixture of $Mg(OH)_2$ and HA formed on the surface of Mg–1Ca alloy with the extension of immersion/implantation time. Mg–1Ca alloy concluded the acceptable biocompatibility as a new kind of biodegradable implant material. Fernandes et al. [59] investigated the mechanical strength and biocompatibility of Mg–2Ca–2Gd and Mg–1Ca–2Nd (wt%) alloys developed for biomedical application as implantable bioabsorbable devices. Samples were implanted in New Zealand rabbits tibia for 3, 6 and 8 weeks and compatibility analysis involved whole blood test, biochemistry, histopathology, histology and radiographs. It was mentioned that refinement in grains were observed in Mg_2Ca_2Gd alloy; and Mg_5Gd, $Mg_{41}Nd_5$, α-Mg and Mg_2Ca phases were identified. Polarization curves revealed easier oxidation of Mg–2C–a2Gd alloy, smaller values of corrosion rate and a higher polarization resistance of Mg–1Ca–2Nd; adequate compatibility of both alloys was identified with preosteoblast stem cells; red and white cells stayed compatible with reference ranges; enzymes from liver and kidneys stayed at regular values and samples from kidneys and liver tissues presented similar organization to control animals; histological displays from implantation sites disclosed well-structured tissues with evidences of bone cells activities compatible with the new bone tissues observed; Mg–2Ca–2Gd alloy demonstrated faster degradation; and adequate biocompatibility was observed in Mg–Ca alloys with RE addition, being potential candidates for development of metallic implantable bioabsorbable devices. Harandi et al. [60] studied effect of calcium addition on microstructure, hardness value and corrosion behavior of five different Mg–*x*Ca binary alloys ($x = 0.7$, 1, 2, 3, 4 wt%). It was reported that refinement in microstructure of the alloy occurred with increasing calcium content. In addition, more uniform distribution of Mg_2Ca phase was observed in α-Mg matrix resulted in an increase in hardness value. The in vitro corrosion examination using SBF showed that the addition of calcium shifted the fluid pH value to a higher level similar to those found in pure commercial Mg. High pH value amplified the formation and growth of bone-like apatite; higher percentage of Ca resulted in needle-shaped growth of the apatite; and electrochemical measurements in the same solution revealed that increasing Ca content led to higher corrosion rates due to the formation of more cathodic Mg_2Ca precipitate in the microstructure. Mg–0.7Ca with the minimum amount of Mg_2Ca is a good candidate for bio-implant applications.

17.4.5 Mg–Li alloy system

Although Mg–Li-based alloys are considered as future cardiovascular stent application as they possess excellent ductility, the alloys exhibit reduced mechanical strengths due to the presence of lithium. Hence, to improve the mechanical strengths of Mg–Li binary alloys, aluminum and rare earth (RE) elements were added to form Mg–Li–Al ternary and Mg-Li-Al-RE quaternary alloys [61]. It was reported that (i) microstructure characterization revealed that grain sizes were moderately refined by the addition of RE elements; (ii) electrochemical and immersion tests showed reduced corrosion resistance caused by intermetallic compounds distributed throughout the magnesium matrix in the RE-containing Mg–Li alloys; (iii) cytotoxicity assays, hemolysis tests as well as platelet adhesion tests were performed to evaluate in vitro biocompatibilities of the Mg–Li-based alloys and the results of cytotoxicity assays clearly showed that the Mg-3.5Li-2Al-2RE, Mg-3.5Li-4Al-2RE and Mg-8.5Li-2Al-2RE alloys suppressed vascular smooth muscle cell (VSMC) proliferation after 5-day incubation, while the Mg–3.5Li, Mg–8.5Li and Mg–8.5Li–1Al alloys were proven to be tolerated; (iv) in the case of human umbilical vein endothelial cells (HUVEC), the Mg–Li-based alloys showed no significantly reduced cell viabilities except for the Mg-8.5Li-2Al-2RE alloy, with no obvious differences in cell viability between different culture periods; and (v) with the exception of Mg-8.5Li-2Al-2RE, all of the other Mg-Li-(Al)-(RE) alloys exhibited acceptable hemolysis ratios, and no sign of thrombogenicity was found. The potential of Mg-Li-(Al)-(RE) alloys indicated biomaterials for future cardiovascular stent application and the worthiness of investigating their biodegradation behaviors in vivo.

17.4.6 Mg–Mn alloy system

Corrosion behavior as well as biocompatibility of extruded Mg-1Mn-2ZN-xNd ($x = 0.5$, 1.0 and 1.5 mass%) were studied [62]. The extrusion on the alloys was performed at temperature of 350 °C with an extrusion ratio of 14.7 under an average extrusion speed of 4 mm/s. The biocompatibility was evaluated using osteoblast-like $SaOS_2$ cells. It was found that all extruded Mg-1Mn-2Zn-xNd alloys are composed of both α-Mg and a compound of Mg_7Zn_3 with very fine microstructures, and show good ductility and much higher mechanical strength than that of cast pure Mg and natural bone. The extruded alloys show good biocompatibility and much higher corrosion resistance than that of cast pure Mg, indicating that the extruded Mg-1Mn-2Zn-1.0Nd alloy shows a great potential for biomedical applications due to the combination of enhanced mechanical properties, high corrosion resistance and good biocompatibility. Wang et al. [63] investigated in vitro cellular responses and degradation of the Mg alloy M1A (Mg–1.42 wt% Mn) in SBF and albumin-containing SBF (A-SBF, 40 g/L). It was reported that (i) the corrosion of M1A was strongly affected by the presence of albumin due to the synergistic effects of albumin adsorption and chelation and (ii) M1A samples had well-spread cells and good cell viability, implying that M1A Mg alloy has the potential to serve biodegradable implants.

17.4.7 Mg–Zr alloy system

Li et al. [64] developed Mg–Zr–Sr alloys use as biodegradable implant materials, which were prepared by mixing and diluting both Mg–Zr and Mg–Sr master alloys with commercially pure Mg. The in vitro biocompatibility was assessed using osteoblast-like $SaOS_2$ cells and MTS and hemolysis tests. The in vivo bone formation and biodegradability were studied in a rabbit model. It was found that (i) both Zr and Sr are excellent candidates for Mg alloying elements in manufacturing biodegradable Mg alloy implants; (ii) Zr addition refined the grain size, improved the ductility, smoothed the grain boundaries and enhanced the corrosion resistance of Mg alloys; and (iii) Sr addition led to an increase in compressive strength, better in vitro biocompatibility, and significantly higher bone formation in vivo, suggesting that Mg–xZr–ySr alloys with x and y 5 wt% would make excellent biodegradable implant materials for load-bearing applications.

17.4.8 Mg–Gd alloy system

The capability of laser surface modification for better corrosion resistance of Mg–Gd–Ca alloy was demonstrated to avoid rapid degradation, which helps to enhance the biocompatibility [65]. Microstructure of both as-received surface and laser-modified surface was analyzed carefully by scanning electron microscopy and X-ray diffraction. It was mentioned that (i) the enhanced corrosion resistance was found to be caused by the combined effect of the dissolution of secondary phase and the decrease of galvanic corrosion in the laser-modified zone and (ii) results of direct cell culturing suggested that the laser-modified surface exhibited good cell adhesion property, spreading performance and proliferation capacity. Zhang et al. [66] demonstrated a hybrid laser surface modification method including melting and surface texturing on Mg–Gd–Ca alloy to improve mechanical properties and control cell behavior. The in vitro adhesion and growth behavior were studied using MC3T3-E1 cells. It was reported that (i) the laser surface modification can improve the hardness and wear resistance without deteriorating elastic modulus of Mg–Gd–Ca alloy, (ii) on the laser-melted and laser-induced periodic surface structures (LIPSS) surface, the cells were elongated along the direction of LIPSS, due to the anisotropic and persistent mechanical stimulus effect and (iii) while on the laser-melted and microgroove surface, the cells exclusively attach to the laser-melted surfaces and completely avoid the surrounding the microgroove, due to the cell-repellent effect of the microstructures. Based on these results, it was indicated that the enhanced mechanical properties and biocompatibility accompanied with the simplicity of fabrication makes laser surface modification a promising candidate method for biomedical applications in biomedical devices.

17.4.9 Mg–Nd alloy system

Mg-Nd-Zn-Zr was fabricated by alloying with neodymium (Nd), zinc (Zn) and zirconium (Zr). Magnesium (Mg) does not compromise the antibacterial activity in order to improve the corrosion resistance. It was mentioned that the results of microbiological counting, SEM in vitro, and microbiological cultures, histopathology in vivo consistently show Mg–Nd–Zn–Zr alloy enhanced the antibacterial activity and the significantly improved cytocompatibility is observed, suggesting that the alloy effectively enhances the corrosion resistance, biocompatibility and antimicrobial properties of Mg by alloying with the proper amount of Zn, Zr and Nd. Mao et al. [68] evaluated corrosion properties by immersion test and electrochemical measurement of Mg-2.5Nd-0.21Zn-0.44Zr. It was mentioned that the alloy exhibits less susceptibility to pitting corrosion and lower corrosion rate, as compared with AZ31 alloy. The corrosion products do not cause significant adverse effect on the cell viability and growth during in vitro cytotoxicity test of the Mg extract via human vascular endothelial cells and *the* in vivo degradation assessment via implantation of Mg-Nd-Zn-Zr stent in an animal model confirmed long-term stability and structural integrity of the stent in blood vessel, indicating that Mg-2.5Nd-0.21Zn-0.44Zr alloy with excellent biocompatibility and long-term stability and durability in vivo represents a significant advance in the development of biodegradable implants. Niu et al. [69] coated a biodegradable calcium phosphate coating (Ca-P coating) with high bonding strength developed using a novel chemical deposition method onto Mg-Nd-Zn-Zr alloy. The main composition of the Ca-P coating was brushite ($CaHPO_4 \cdot 2H_2O$). It was mentioned that (i) the in vitro corrosion tests indicated that the Ca–P treatment improved the corrosion resistance of the alloy in Hank's solution, (ii) Ca-P treatment significantly reduced the HR from 48% to 0.68%, and induced nontoxicity to MC3T3-E1 cells, (iii) the in vivo implantation experiment in New Zealand's rabbit tibia showed that the degradation rate was reduced obviously by the Ca-P treatment and less gas was produced from Ca-P treated Mg-Nd-Zn-Zr alloy bone plates and screws in early stage of the implantation, and at least 10 weeks degradation time can be prolonged by the present coating techniques. Both Ca-P-treated and -untreated alloys induced bone growth, indicating that the Ca–P treatment is a promising technique for the degradable Mg-based biomaterials for orthopedic applications. Peng et al. [70] treated Mg-Nd-Zn-Zr alloy with $Mg(OH)_2$ coating by introducing magnesium–aluminum-LDH (Mg-Al LDH). It was reported that (i) the anions in the interlayer of Mg–Al LDH can be replaced by chloride ions, resulting in a relatively low chloride ion concentration near the surface of the coating, (ii) the favorable corrosion resistance of the coating was proved by polarization curves and hydrogen collection test, (iii) the Mg–Al LDH significantly promoted cell adhesion, migration and proliferation in vitro, (iv) the coating almost fulfilled the request of the clinical application in the hemolysis ratio test and (v) the in vivo results indicated that the coating offered the greatest long-lasting protection from corrosion and triggered the mildest inflammation comparing to the pure $Mg(OH)_2$ coatings and untreated magnesium alloy. Based on these findings, it was concluded that $Mg(OH)_2$ coating containing Mg–Al LDH exhibits a promising application in improving anticorrosion and biocompatibility of Mg alloys and might act as a platform for a further modification of Mg alloys ascribed to its special layer structure.

17.4.10 Mg–Sr alloy system

The corrosion rate in SBF of a series of Mg–*x*Sr (x = 0.3–2.5 wt%) was studied [71]. It was found that (i) Mg–0.5Sr alloy showed the slowest corrosion rate, (ii) the degradation rate from this alloy indicated that the daily Sr intake from a typical stent would be 0.01–0.02 mg/day, which is well below the maximum daily Sr intake levels of 4 mg/day and (iii) indirect cytotoxicity assays using human umbilical vascular endothelial cells indicated that Mg–0.5Sr extraction medium did not cause any toxicity or detrimental effect on the viability of the cells. A tubular Mg–0.5Sr stent sample, along with a WE43 control stent, was implanted into the right and left dog femoral artery. It was mentioned that no thrombosis effect was observed in the Mg–0.5Sr stent after 3 weeks of implantation while the WE43 stent thrombosed, XRD demonstrated the formation of HA and $Mg(OH)_2$ as a result of the degradation of Mg–0.5Sr alloy after 3 days in SBF and X-ray photoelectron spectroscopy (XPS) further showed the possibility of the formation of a HA Sr-substituted layer that presents as a thin layer at the interface between the Mg–0.5Sr alloy and the corrosion products. Based on these conclusions, Bornapour et al. [72] examined the biodegradation mechanism of Mg–0.3Sr–0.3Ca, to identify the exact nature of its protective layer and to evaluate the in vitro and in vivo biocompatibility of the alloy for cardiovascular applications. To better simulate the physiological environment, the alloy was immersed in SBF which was daily refreshed. It was found that (i) Raman spectroscopy and XPS confirmed the formation of a thin, Sr-substituted HA layer at the interface between the alloy and the corrosion products and (ii) the in vitro biocompatibility evaluated via indirect cytotoxicity assays using HUVECs showed no toxicity effect and ions extracted from Mg–0.3Sr–0.3Ca in fact increased the viability of HUVECs after 1 week. The in vivo tests were performed by implanting a tubular Mg–0.3Sr–0.3Ca stent along with a WE43 control stent into the right and left femoral arteries of a dog. It was further mentioned that postimplantation and histological analyses showed no thrombosis in the artery with Mg–0.3Sr–0.3Ca stent after 5 weeks of implantation while the artery implanted with WE43 stent was extensively occluded and thrombosed and microscopic observation of the Mg–0.3Sr–0.3Ca implant–tissue interface confirmed the in situ formation of Sr-substituted HA on the surface during in vivo test. The interfacial layer protects the surface of the Mg–0.3Sr–0.3Ca alloy both in vitro and in vivo and is the key factor in the biocorrosion resistance of the alloy. Yang et al. [73] fabricated a compact zirconia (ZrO_2) nanofilm on the surface of a Mg–Sr alloy by the atomic layer deposition method, which can regulate the thickness of the film precisely and thus also control the corrosion rate. It was shown that (i) corrosion tests reveal that the ZrO_2 film can effectively reduce the corrosion rate of Mg–Sr alloys that is closely related to the thickness of the film and (ii) the cell culture test shows that this kind of ZrO_2 film can also enhance the activity and adhesion of osteoblasts on the surfaces of Mg–Sr alloys.

17.5 Cytocompatibility and cytotoxicity

Cytology (or cell biology) is a branch of biology dealing with the structure, function, multiplication, pathology and life history of cells and its ability to be compatible to human body is called as cytological compatibility (in short, cytocompatibility).

Biodegradable magnesium and its alloys are advantageous over existing biodegradable materials such as polymers, ceramics and bioactive glasses in load-bearing applications where sufficient strength (high specific strength), modulus of elasticity close to that of the bone are required. Hence, Mg biomaterials have been extensively employed as orthopedic implants, surgical devices (such as cardiovascular stents) and scaffold frame structures. However, rapid corrosion rate in the early stage of the degradation process in physiological environment and resultant potential toxicity greatly influences the cytocompatibility and hinters their clinical application.

During the corrosion (oxidation) process of Mg in physiological environment (inside human body), Mg reacting with water results in forming magnesium hydroxide and hydrogen evolution. Hence, biological degradation of these Mg alloys results in ion release, which may cause severe cytotoxicity and undesirable complications after implantation, and the biocompatibility of Mg biodegradable implants compromises strong hydrogen evolution (depending on the localized hydrogen overpotential) and surface alkalization due to high initial corrosion rates of Mg materials in the physiological environment. Metal ions and generated hydrogen gas as well as pH value are recognized as cells' hazards. When designed for medical applications, these alloys must have suitable degradation properties, that is, their degradation rate should not exceed the rate at which the degradation products can be excreted from the body. Hence, the degradation rate should be controlled, for example, of orthopedic applications, uncontrolled fast degradation rate leads to premature deterioration of biofunctionality.

Same as for improvement of biocompatibility, there are studies on improving cytocompatibility of Mg biomaterials by alloying, surface treating or coating.

17.5.1 Mg

Surface topology might affect the surface physicochemistry. Gu et al. [74] prepared the lotus-type porous pure magnesium using a metal/gas eutectic unidirectional solidification method. It was mentioned that (i) the porous pure Mg indicates better corrosion resistance than that of compact pure Mg in the SBF at 37 °C and (ii) with larger exposed surface area, porous pure Mg shows higher Mg concentration in the extract than that of compact pure Mg, leading to a higher osmotic pressure to cells and might affect its indirect cytotoxicity assay result. Addition to requirements of sufficient strength of mechanical properties, ideally, Mg-based medical devices should biodegrade no faster than the degradation products can be excreted efficiently from the body. Liu et al. [75] characterized Mg surface and investigated the effects of two surface conditions (the presence vs absence of surface oxides) on Mg degradation and MSC adhesion, and the effects of two essential aqueous environments (the presence vs absence of physiological ions and proteins) on Mg degradation. It was demonstrated that (i) original surface (oxidized vs polished) conditions had a less pronounced effect on regulating initial cell adhesion but did affect surface morphology and composition of the Mg samples after 24 h of cell culture and (ii) the presence versus absence of biological ions and proteins had a significant effect on Mg degradation mode and rate, concluding that (iii) the material surface and anatomical sites of implantation dependent on the intended applications must be carefully considered while assessing Mg alloys in vitro or in vivo for medical applications.

For a purpose of improving the corrosion resistance meanwhile do not compromise other excellent performance, Sun et al. [24] deposited self-assembled colloidal particles on magnesium surfaces in ethanol by a simple and effective EPD method. The coating colloids were P(ISA-*co*-DMA)/TA colloidal particles. It was reported that (i) the electrochemical test, pH value and Mg ion concentration data show that the corrosion resistance of Mg samples is enhanced appreciably after surface treatment and (ii) test of the in vitro cellular response and antibacterial capability of the modified Mg substrates showed that increased cell adhesion and viability are observed from the coated Mg samples, and the amounts of adherent bacteria on the treated Mg surfaces diminish remarkably compared to the bare Mg. The uncoated and coated Mg samples were implanted in New Zealand white rabbits for 12 weeks to examine the in vivo long-term corrosion performance and in situ inflammation behavior. It was indicated that compared with uncoated Mg substrate, the corrosion and foreign-body reactions of the coated Mg samples were suppressed. Based on these results, it was suggested that the coatings effectively enhance the biocompatibility, antimicrobial properties and corrosion resistance of Mg substrate. Geng et al. [76] prepared biodegradable and bioactive β-tricalcium phosphate (β-TCP) coatings on Mg substrate in order to improve its biocompatibility by a chemical method. The cytocompatibility of β-TCP-coated Mg was studied by using human osteoblast-like MG63 cells. It was mentioned that the MG63 cells could grow well on the surface of β-TCP-coated Mg and the cell viability on β-TCP-coated Mg was above 80% during the cocultivation of MG63 cells and β-TCP-coated Mg for 10 days, indicating no cytotoxicity. The β-TCP-coated Mg had good cytocompatibility and a bone-like apatite continually formed on the surface of the sample with the degradation of both Mg substrate and β-TCP coating in Hank's solution (an SBF). Xu et al. [77] prepared biodegradable polymer films by spin coating in order to improve the early corrosion resistance and cytocompatibility of Mg. Coated films were uniform, nonporous, amorphous PLLA and semicrystalline PCL films. It was reported that PLLA film shows better adhesion strength to Mg substrate than that of PCL film. For both PLLA and PCL, low-molecular-weight film is thinner and exhibits better adhesion strength than high-molecular-weight one. The $SaOS_2$ cells show significantly good attachment and high growth on the polymer-coated Mg, demonstrating that all the polymer films can significantly improve the cytocompatibility in the 7-day incubation. The pH measurement of the immersion medium and the quantification of released Mg^{2+} during the cell culture clearly indicate that the corrosion resistance of Mg substrate is improved by the polymer films to different extents. Both PLLA and PCL films are promising protective coatings for improving the initial corrosion resistance and cytocompatibility. Wang et al. [78] cultured two tumor cells (MG63 and KB) directly on a pure Mg with and without MAO coating to evaluate their cytotoxic effects on the tumor cells. It was obtained that both MG63 cells and KB cells adhered better on the surface of the coated Mg samples than those on the pure Mg samples; however, the survivals of two kinds of tumor cells were obviously inhibited on both Mg samples with and without coating, compared with that on the pure titanium. The survival of MG63 cells was more susceptive to the Mg degradation compared with the KB cells, suggesting that the application of such effect should take into account of the fact that the degradation of Mg-based metal may result in different cytotoxic effect on different cells. Wagener et al. [79] coated Mg substrate with organic coatings of aminopropyltriethoxysilane + vitamin C (AV), carbonyldiimidazole (CDI) or stearic acid (SA), which reduced initial corrosion and to enhance protein adsorption and hence cell adhesion on magnesium surfaces. Endothelial cells (DH1 +/+) and osteosarcoma cells (MG63) were cultured on coated samples for up to 20 days. To quantify Mg corrosion, electrochemical impedance spectroscopy (EIS) was measured after 1, 3 and 5 days of cell culture. The speed of initial cell spreading after seeding using fluorescently labeled fibroblasts (NIH/3T3) was also studied. It was reported that hydrogen evolution after contact with cell culture medium was markedly decreased on AV- and SA-coated Mg compared to uncoated Mg. The coatings showed improved cell adhesion and spreading after 24 h of culture comparable to tissue-treated plastic surfaces, and on AV-coated cp Mg, a confluent layer of endothelial cells formed after 5 days and remained intact for up to 20 days, indicating that surface coating with AV is a viable strategy for improving long-term biocompatibility of cp Mg-based implants.

Li et al. [80] conducted corrosion tests on Mg in SBF with and without Cl^- ions to examine the cytotoxicity. It was mentioned that (i) alkali and heat-treated magnesium has relatively high corrosion resistance in SBF, compared to untreated samples, (ii) calcium-phosphate apatites were identified on the treated samples after they had been soaked in SBF for 14 days and (iii) in cytotoxicity tests, no signs of morphological changes on cells or inhibitory effect on cell growth were detected. Tavares et al. [81] produced dense granules of tricalcium phosphate (β-TCP) and Mg-substituted β-TCP (or β-TCMP with Mg/Ca ratio of 0.15 mol), in order to evaluate the impact of Mg incorporation on the physicochemical parameters and in vitro biocompatibility. It was found that (i) XRD profile presented the main peaks of β-TCP and β-TCMP, (ii) the ICP results of β-TCMP granules extract showed a precipitation of calcium and release of Mg into the culture medium and (iii) regarding the cytotoxicity assays, β-TCMP dense granules did not significantly affect the mitochondrial activity and relative cell density in relation to β-TCP dense granules, despite the release of Mg from granules into the cell culture medium. β-TCMP granules were successfully produced and were able to release Mg into media without cytotoxicity, indicating the suitability of this promising material for further biological studies on its adequacy for bone therapy.

17.5.2 Mg–Al alloy system

AZ31 (Mg–3Al–1Zn) and AZ91 (Mg–9Al-–Zn) have been extensively subjected to examine the cytocompatibility under influences of surface modifications. A Si-containing coating was fabricated on AZ31B Mg alloy to evaluate cytocompatibility [82]. Effects of a number of incubation variables on the sensitivity and reproducibility of the hemolysis test were also examined by using positively and negatively responding biomaterials. It was reported that cytocompatibility testing results indicated that cell condition, cell adherence, cell proliferation and extracellular matrix secretion of the coated alloy were improved compared with those of the uncoated alloy for different extraction and coculture time. After the hemolysis test, it was mentioned that 1 day in vitro degradation of the uncoated AZ31B alloy had no destructive effect on erythrocyte and as for the coated AZ31B alloy at any time point, the HR was much lower than 5%, the safe value for biomaterials. The Si-containing coating is effective to improve the cytocompatibility and hemolysis behaviors of AZ31B alloy during its degradation [82]. Wang et al. [83] coated a new organic–inorganic composite coating on AZ31 alloy surface with the sol–gel method to improve the anticorrosion and biocompatibility in the physiological environment. It was found that the silane/$Mg(OH)_2$ composite coating significantly enhanced the anticorrosion ability and slowed down the degradation of AZ31 alloy under in vitro condition. The composite coating was uniform and defect free and MTT (cytotoxicity testing assay) and ALP tests indicated that the composite coating greatly enhanced the cell proliferation and osteogenic differentiation of osteoblasts on the AZ31 alloy surface. Mochizuki et al. [84] investigated the in vitro cytocompatibility of AZ31 by culturing cells directly on it. Investigations were carried out in terms of the cell viability along with the use of scanning electron microscopy to observe its morphology. The cell lines used were derived from fibroblast, endothelial and smooth muscle cells. The viability of cells on the metal samples and on the margin area of a multiwell plate was investigated. It was reported that (i) Mg^{2+}, Zn^{2+} and Al^{3+} ions were less toxic at the investigated concentrations and (ii) these factors will not produce negative effects on cells. Zhu et al. [85] prepared HA/TA coating on AZ31 alloys via chemical conversion and biomimetic methods. It was mentioned that the TA as an inducer increased the number of nucleation centers of HA and rendered the morphology more uniform. Compared to uncoated AZ31 alloys, the corrosion current density of the HA/TA-coated magnesium alloys decreased two orders of magnitude, and the corrosion potential of the HA/TA-coated Mg alloys increased by about 158 mV, indicating that the HA/TA coating was effectively protecting the AZ31 against corrosion in SBF and MC3Te-E1 cell proliferation assays and cell morphology observations results showed that the HA/TA coating was not toxic to the MC3T3-E1 cells.

Lopes et al. [86] evaluated the effect of the high-pressure torsion (HPT) processing on cytotoxicity and corrosion behavior in Hank's solution by using samples of commercial purity in Mg, AZ31, AZ91 and ZK60 alloys. All samples are subjected to electrochemical testing and hydrogen evolution testing before and after processing by HPT. It was reported that the HPT processing improves the corrosion resistance of pure magnesium, has no significant effect on the AZ31 and AZ91 alloys but reduces the corrosion resistance of the ZK60 alloy. The in vitro cytotoxicity tests demonstrate that HPT processing may be used to improve the performance of magnesium and its alloys as biodegradable implants. The cytological effects of Mg alloys containing varying amounts of Al, Zn, Nd and Y were studied [87], which were incubated either directly or indirectly with the endothelial cell line EA.hy926 or primary endothelial cells from different patients, and cell viability was measured. In addition, the concentrations of released metal ions from the alloys were determined. It was reported that (i) dependent on the magnesium alloys used and the incubation period, direct or indirect contact with endothelial cells led to various reactions in cell viability; (ii) only the AZ91 alloy was found to exhibit tolerable cytotoxicity on all endothelial cells tested; and (iii) the in vitro study revealed that the cytocompatibility of biodegradable magnesium alloys is not predictable only by determining the ion release or by testing the alloys with immortalized cell lines. cytocompatibility properties of new biodegradable material should be tested using primary cells of various donors in order to guarantee safe in vivo application and avoid interindividual differences. Xin et al. [88] deposited a stable and dense hydrogenated amorphous silicon coating (a-Si:H) with desirable bioactivity on AZ91 alloy using magnetron sputtering deposition. It was found that (i) the coating is mainly composed of hydrogenated amorphous silicon, (ii) the hardness of the coated alloy is enhanced significantly and the coating is quite hydrophilic as well, (iii) potentiodynamic polarization results show that the corrosion resistance of the coated alloy is enhanced dramatically and (iv) the cytocompatibility of the coated Mg is evaluated for the first time using hFOB1.19 cells and favorable biocompatibility is observed.

17.5.3 Mg–Zn alloy system

17.5.3.1 Mg–Zn binary alloy

A binary Mg–4Zn alloy surface was coated with the highly biocompatible HA and Sr (strontium)-doped HA coatings by electrochemical deposition [89]. It was mentioned that (i) the incorporation of Sr in the HA coatings leads to lattice distortion and decreased crystallinity, (ii) the smaller amount of Mg ion release of the Sr-doped HA-coated samples suggests a better corrosion resistance, (iii) the improved protein adsorption and initial adhesion of MSCs of the Sr-doped samples should be due to their higher surface roughness and wettability and (iv) the introduction of Sr leads to comparable cell proliferation behavior, but significantly improved osteogenic differentiation, concluding that (v) the Sr-doped HA coatings are promising candidates for the protective biocompatible coating on Mg-based implants. Zhang et al. [90] investigated pure Mg and an Mg–6Zn alloy on the in vitro corrosion behavior in 37 °C SBF, and the in vivo degradation and histocompatibility through implantation into the bladders of Wistar rats. It was mentioned that the alloying element Zn elevated the passivation potential and increased the cathodic current density. Both in vitro and in vivo degradation tests showed a faster corrosion rate for the Mg–6Zn alloy and tissues stained with HE suggested that both pure Mg and Mg–6Zn alloy exhibited good histocompatibility in the bladder indwelling implantation and no differences between pure Mg and Mg–6Zn groups were found in bladder, liver and kidney tissues during the 2 weeks implantation.

17.5.3.2 Mg–Zn–Zr alloy

An Mg metal matrix composite (MMC) was fabricated using Mg-2.9Zn-0.7Zr alloy as the matrix and 1 wt% nano-HA (n-HA) particles as reinforcements [91] to study the in vitro corrosion behavior in SBF and cytocompatibility of an Mg-Zn-Zr/*n*-HA composite and an Mg–Zn–Zr alloy. It was found that the average corrosion rate of MMC is 0.75 mm/year after immersion in SBF for 20 days, and the surface of MMC is covered with white Ca-P apatite precipitates. The cocultivation of MMC with osteoblasts results in the adhesion and proliferation of cells on the surface of the composite. The maximum cell density is calculated to be $(1.85 \pm 0.15) \times 10^4$/L after 5 days of coculture with osteoblasts and (iv) the average cell numbers for two groups after culturing for 3 and 5 days are significantly different. The Mg–Zn–Zr/*n*-HA composite can be potentially used as biodegradable bone fixation material. Huan et al. [92] investigated the degradation rate, hydrogen evolution, ion release, surface layer and in vitro cytotoxicity of two Mg–Zn–Zr alloys (ZK30 and ZK60) and a WE-type alloy (Mg-Y-RE-Zr) by means of long-term static immersion testing in Hank's solution, nonstatic immersion testing in Hank's solution and cell–material interaction analysis. It was reported that (i) among these three magnesium alloys, ZK30 had the lowest degradation rate and the least hydrogen evolution (as shown in Figure 17.6),

(ii) a magnesium calcium phosphate layer was formed on the surface of ZK30 sample during nonstatic immersion and its degradation caused minute changes in the ion concentrations and pH value of Hank's solution and (iii) the ZK30 alloy showed insignificant cytotoxicity against BMSCs as compared with biocompatible HA and the WE-type alloy. After prolonged incubation for 7 days, a stimulatory effect on cell proliferation was observed. ZK30 could be a promising material for biodegradable orthopedic implants and worth further investigation to evaluate its in vitro and in vivo degradation behavior.

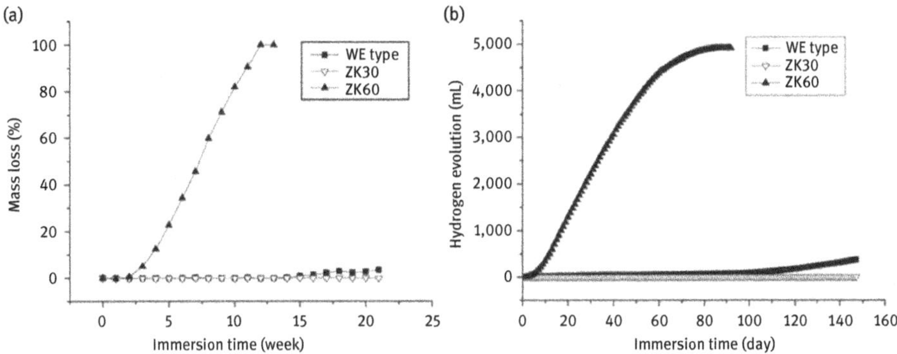

Figure 17.6: Mass loss (a) and hydrogen evolution (b) as a function of immersion time of three Mg-based alloys [92].

Tantalum (Ta) was introduced to the surface of the ZK60 Mg alloy by reactive magnetron sputtering to enhance the corrosion resistance and cytocompatibility [93]. It was found that the surface layer composed of Ta_2O_5, Ta suboxide, and Ta increases the corrosion resistance of ZK60 while simultaneously improving cell attachment, spreading and proliferation in vitro. Hong et al. [94] investigated Mg–4Zn–0.5Zr (ZK40) alloy as a candidate material for biodegradable metallic implants in terms of its biocorrosion resistance, mechanical properties and cytocompatibility. The corrosion characteristics of ZK40 alloy were assessed by potentiodynamic polarization and immersion testing in DMEM + 10% FBS solution. It was found that the corrosion rates of ZK40 alloy in as-cast and solution treatment (T4) condition were slightly higher than those of pure Mg or as-drawn AZ31. In order to examine the in vitro cytocompatibility of ZK40 alloy, live/dead cell viability assay and indirect MTT assay were performed using a murine osteoblast-like cell line (MC3T3) and it was found that after 3 days of direct culture of MC3T3 on ZK40 alloys the live/dead assay indicated favorable cell viability and attachment. The degradation product of ZK40 also showed minimal cytotoxicity when assessed in indirect MTT assay. Based on these findings, it was concluded that e ZK40 alloy exhibited favorable cytocompatibility, biocorrosion and mechanical properties rendering it a potential candidate for degradable implant applications. Yang et al. [95]

coated nanowhisker/wire-like HA (nHA) coatings on ZK60 substrates for controlling the biodegradation of Mg alloy while improving its cytocompatibility for orthopedic applications, using a simple one-step hydrothermal treatment process in aqueous solution. It was mentioned that (i) the biodegradation of ZK60 alloy was greatly restrained by the nanowhisker/wire-like HA coatings and (ii) improved cytocompatibility was observed in nanowhisker/wire-like HA-coated ZK60 samples and the cytotoxicity of ZK60 samples coated for 2 and 2.5 h are in grade 1. The coatings with nanowhisker/wire-like HA are promising for improving the in vitro biodegradation and cytocompatibility properties of Mg-based orthopedic implants and devices. Wang et al. [96] developed an HA coating on ZK60 magnesium alloy substrates to mediate the rapid degradation of Mg while improving its cytocompatibility for orthopedic applications via a simple chemical conversion process. Murine fibroblast L-929 cells were harvested and cultured with coated and noncoated ZK60 samples to determine cytocompatibility. It was mentioned that (i) the degradation results suggested that the HA coatings decreased the degradation of ZK60 alloy, (ii) no significant deterioration in compression strength was observed for all the uncoated and coated samples after 2 and 4 weeks' immersion in SBF. The cytotoxicity test indicated that the coatings, especially HA coating, improved cytocompatibility of ZK60 alloy for L-929 cells.

17.5.3.3 Mg–Zn–Mn alloy

Four kinds of biodegradable polymers (poly-L-lactide (PLLA), poly(3-hydroxybutyrate) (PHB), poly(3-hydroxybutyrate-*co*-3-hydroxyvalerate) (PHBV) or poly(lactic-*co*-glycolic) acid (PLGA)) were used for preparation of bioresorbable coatings on Mg–2.0Zn–0.98Mn (ZM21) alloy to understand the relationship between polymer characteristics, protective effects on substrate corrosion, cytocompatibility and cell functionality [97]. After 4 weeks of immersion into cell culture medium, degradation of PLGA and PLLA coatings was confirmed by ATR-FTIR observation. It was found that the coatings of PLLA, PHB and PHBV (which have lower water permeability and slower degradation than PLGA) provide better suppression of initial ZM21 degradation and faster promotion of human osteosarcoma cell growth and differentiation. He et al. [98] investigated the in vitro degradation behavior and biological performance of the extruded and aged Mg–6Zn–Mn alloys by electrochemical measurement and immersion test in SBF, cell culture cytotoxicity test and hemolytic ability evaluation. It was reported that the cytotoxicity test shows no significant deleterious effects on HUVECs for Mg–6Zn–Mn alloys, indicating a good in vitro cytocompatibility. HRs of the extruded and aged alloys are far lower than the safe value of 5% according to ISO 10993-4, suggesting that the present Mg–6Zn–Mn alloys are promising materials for biodegradable implants. Li et al. [99] prepared the extracts of Mg–Zn–Mn alloy and examined their effects on the angiogenesis of HUVECs. It was obtained that the DNA synthesis capacity, the cell viability and the tube formation capacity of HUVECs could be significantly induced by 6.25% Mg alloy extract, while the ratios of p-FGFR/FGFR, p-PI3K/PI3K and p-AKT/AKT were significantly increased by 6.25% Mg alloy extract treatment and decreased by FGFR/FGFR signaling pathway inhibitor BFJ398, indicating that 6.25% Mg alloy extract could promote the angiogenesis of HUVECs via activating FGF/FGFR signaling pathway. It was hence concluded that 6.25% Mg–Zn–Mn alloy extract induces the angiogenesis of HUVECs via FGF signaling pathway. Du et al. [100] coated a calcium silicate and calcium phosphate ($CaSiO_3/CaHPO_4 \cdot 2H_2O$) composite coating to Mg-Zn-Mn-Ca alloy to improve its biocompatibility. It was mentioned that (i) XRD identified that the reaction layer was mainly composed of $CaHPO_4 \cdot 2H_2O$ and a small amount of $CaSiO_3$, (ii) the in vitro cell experiments indicated that *osteoblasts* showed good adhesion, high growth rates and proliferation characteristics on the coated Mg-Zn-Mn-Ca alloy, indicating that the surface cytocompatibility of Mg-Zn-Mn-Ca alloy was significantly improved by the calcium phosphate coating.

17.5.3.4 Mg–Zn–Sr alloy

The Mg–1Zn–*x*Sr ($x = 0.2$, 0.5, 0.8 and 1 wt%) alloys were prepared by zone purifying solidification followed by backward extrusion (BE). It was shown that (i) the grain size was reduced and the hardness was improved with the increased concentration of strontium (Sr) after BE, (ii) extruded Mg–1Zn–0.8Sr alloy was mostly composed of fine precipitates (MgZn and $Mg_{17}Sr_2$) and Mg matrix, (iii) the degradation rate is significantly increased when Sr content is over 0.8 wt% and the homogenous degradation rate is achieved and (iv) the degradation products show good biocompatibility evaluated by MTT method using L929 cell line, indicating that the microalloying element of Sr is a potential approach to develop novel Mg–Zn based biomaterials [101]. Cipriano research group [102–104] conducted extensive studies on Mg–Zn–Sr alloys. It was reported that four distinct ZSr41 alloys with varied strontium compositions (0.15, 0.5, 1 and 1.5 wt%) were tested with culturing with hESCs and found that the Mg–Zn–Sr alloy with 0.15 wt% Sr provided slower degradation and improved cytocompatibility as compared with pure Mg control [102]. Using the same alloys, the early-stage inflammatory response in cultured HUVECs as indicated by the induction of vascular cellular adhesion molecule-1 (VCAM-1) was studied. It was shown that the 24 h in vitro degradation of the ZSr41 alloys containing a β-phase with a Zn/Sr at% ratio ~1.5 was significantly faster than the ZSr41 alloys with Zn/Sr at% ~1 and the adhesion density of HUVECs in the direct culture but not in direct contact with the ZSr41 alloys for up to 24 h was not adversely affected by the degradation of the alloys. Neither culture media supplemented with up to 27.6 mM Mg^{2+} ions nor media intentionally adjusted up to alkaline pH 9 induced any detectable adverse effects on HUVEC responses and in contrast, the significantly higher, yet noncytotoxic, Zn^{2+} ion concentration from the degradation of ZSr41D alloy was likely the cause for the initially higher VCAM-1 expression on cultured HUVECs [103]. Moreover, the behaviors of bone-marrow-derived MSCs (BMSCs) in the direct culture with four Mg–4Zn–*x*Sr alloys ($x = 0.15, 0.5, 1.0, 1.5$ wt%) and a systematic comparison on the degradation of the ZSr41 alloys and their biological impact in the direct culture with different cell types in their respective media were studied. It was found that BMSCs adhered and remained viable on the surfaces of all ZSr41 alloys, but the faster degrading ZSr41A and ZSr41B alloys showed a significantly lower amount of viable BMSCs adhered to their surfaces. The BMSCs adhered to the culture plate surrounding the samples were unaffected by the solubilized degradation products from the ZSr41 alloys. The results from the comparison study showed that the in vitro degradation rates of Mg-based biomaterials in different culture systems might be mostly affected by media buffer capacity (i.e., HCO^{3-} concentration), and to a lesser extent, d-glucose concentration. The comparison study also indicated that BMSCs were more robust than H9 human embryonic stem cells and HUVECs for screening the cytocompatibility of Mg-based biomaterials, suggesting that the adhesion and viability of BMSCs at the cell-material interface were inversely proportional to the alloy degradation rates [104]. Tian et al. [105] investigated Mg–4Zn–*x*Sr (ZSr41) alloys ($x = 0.15, 0.5, 1.0$ and 1.5 Sr wt%) as a potential ureteral stent application. The cytocompatibility and degradation behaviors of Mg–4Zn–*x*Sr alloys were studied by culturing with human urothelial cells (HUCs) for 24 and 48 h using exposure culture method. It was reported that ZSr41 with 0.5Sr showed a better cytocompatibility with HUCs among all the Mg–4Zn–*x*Sr alloys in both 24 and 48 h cultures. The cytocompatibility of insoluble degradation products of Mg (namely, MgO and $Mg(OH)_2$) was also investigated by culturing different concentrations of MgO and $Mg(OH)_2$ NPs with HUCs for 24 and 48 h. It was mentioned that the concentration of MgO and $Mg(OH)_2$ particles at 0.5 mg/mL and above showed a significant decrease of cell density and cell size after 24 and 48 h cultures and the concentration of MgO and $Mg(OH)_2$ at 1.0 mg/mL and above showed no viable cells after 24 h culture.

17.5.3.5 Mg–Zn—Ca alloy

The corrosion behavior and cytotoxicity of Mg–Zn–*x*Ca ($x = 1$, 2 and 3 wt%) were studied to understand the in vitro biocompatibility by culturing ASCs for 24 and 72 h in contact with 10%, 50% and 100% extraction of all alloys prepared in DMEM [106]. It was mentioned that (i) the cytotoxicity results showed that all alloys had no significant adverse effects on cell viability in 24 h, (ii) after 72 h, cell viability and proliferation increased in the cells exposed to pure Mg and Mg–2Zn–1Ca extracts and (iii) the release of Mg, Zn and Ca ions in culture media had no toxic impacts on ASCs viability and proliferation. The Mg–2Zn–1Ca alloy can be suggested as a good candidate to be used in biomedical applications. Sun et al. [107] studied the mechanical properties, in vitro degradation and cytotoxicity of Mg–4.0Zn–0.2Ca alloy and mentioned that the in vitro corrosion test in SBF revealed that the addition of Zn and Ca into Mg matrix could enhance the corrosion potential and reduced the degradation rate and the in vitro cytotoxicity of the alloy was disclosed that Mg–4.0Zn–0.2Ca alloy has suitable biocompatibility. Homayun et al. [108] assessed cytotoxicity, indicating the good biocompatibility of the Mg–4Zn–0.2Ca alloy, making it a suitable candidate for further considerations as a degradable metallic biomaterial. Xia et al. [109] investigated the in vitro cytotoxicity and the in vivo compatibility of Mg–4.0Zn–0.2Ca alloy are studied. The cytotoxicity was examined by MTT method on osteoblast cells and the in vivo behavior was studied on rabbits. It was reported that (i) Mg–4.0Zn–0.2Ca alloy extract has no cytotoxicity on osteoblast cells and (ii) 3 months after in vivo experiment, about 35–38% magnesium alloy implant has been degraded and a degradation layer which is composed of Ca, P, O and Mg has been formed on the magnesium alloy implants. The histological analysis showed that new bone is observed around magnesium implant without inflammation reaction and in vitro and in vivo tests indicated that the Mg–4.0Zn–0.2Ca alloy has good biocompatibility. Pellicer et al. [110] investigated the evolution of microstructure and mechanical properties of almost fully amorphous $Mg_{72}Zn_{23}Ca_5$ and crystalline Mg-23Zn-5Ca-2Pd alloys during immersion in HBSS, as well as their cytocompatibility, in order to assess the feasibility of both materials as biodegradable implants. It was found that (i) after 22 h immersion, the concentration of Mg ions in the HBSS medium containing the Mg-23Zn-5Ca-2Pd sample is 6 times larger than for Mg–23Zn–5Ca; (ii) due to the Zn enrichment and the incipient porosity, the mechanical properties of the Mg–23Zn–5Ca sample improve within the first stages of biodegradation (i.e., hardness increases while the Young's modulus decreases, thus rendering an enhanced wear resistance) and (iii) cytocompatibility studies reveal that neither Mg–23Zn–5Ca nor Mg-23Zn-5Ca-2Pd are cytotoxic, although preosteoblast cell adhesion is to some extent precluded, particularly onto the surface of Mg-23Zn-5Ca-2Pd, because of the relatively high hydrophobicity, indicating that the use of the Pd-free alloy in temporary implants such as screws, stents and sutures is envisioned.

17.5.3.6 Mg–Zn–Y alloy

The Mg-Zn-Y-Nd alloy is a new type of degradable material for biomedical application. Kang et al. [111] fabricated Mg-6Zn-1.2Y-0.8Nd alloy, followed by extrusion and heat treatment were conducted to optimize its mechanical properties and cytocompatibility. It was reported that the degradation behavior of the as-cast alloy and extruded alloys does not show much difference, but improves slightly in extruded and heat treated alloy, because the heat treatment has homogenized the microstructure and released the residual stress in the alloy. The directly and indirectly cell viability tests indicate that alloy extrude and heat-treated alloy exhibits the best cytocompatibility, which should be ascribed to its relative uniform degradation and low ion releasing rate. Based on these results, it was concluded that the combination of hot extrusion and heat treatment could optimize the mechanical property and cytocompatibility of the Mg-Zn-Y-Nd alloy together, which is beneficial for the future application of the alloy. Song et al. [112] evaluated the cytocompatibility of Mg-Zn-Y-Nd-Zr alloy through in vitro cell culture method. MTT assay was applied to evaluate the cytotoxicity of Mg-Zn-Y-Nd-Zr alloy and no toxic effect was observed on L929 and MC3T3-E1 cells followed the protocol of ISO 10993 standard. The cytotoxic effect of accumulated metallic ions during the alloy degradation by extending the extract preparation time was also investigated. It was reported that when the extract preparation time was prolonged to 1,440 h, the accumulated metallic ions leaded to severe cell apoptosis, of which the combined ion concentration was determined as 39.5–65.8 μM of Mg^{2+}, 3.5–5.9 μM of Zn^{2+}, 0.44–0.74 μM of Y^{3+}, 0.3–0.52 μM of Nd^{3+} and 0.11–0.18 μM of Zr^{4+} for L929 and 65.8–92.2 μM of Mg^{2+}, 5.9–8.3 μM of Zn^{2+}, 0.74–1.04 μM of Y^{3+}, 0.52–0.73 μM of Nd^{3+} and 0.18–0.25 μM of Zr^{4+} for MC3T3-E1 cells. It was also mentioned that besides the cell viability assessment, high expression of ALP activity and calcified nodules implied that metal elements in Mg-Zn-Y-Nd-Zr alloys can promote the osteogenic differentiation; accordingly, excellent cytocompatibility has equipped Mg-Zn-Y-Nd-Zr alloy as a promising candidate for orthopedic implant application, which can remarkably guide the magnesium-based alloy design and provide scientific evidence for clinical practice in future.

17.5.3.7 Mg–Zn–Sn alloy

Jiang et al. [113] studied the mechanical properties and biocorrosion behaviors of as-extruded Mg–4Zn–1.5Sn alloy. It was found that (i) a small amount of Sn addition to Mg–4Zn alloy slightly improved the mechanical properties for solid solution strengthening, and significantly controlled the biocorrosion rates; (ii) Sn participating in the outer layer film formation as SnO/SnO_2 resisted the biocorrosion proceeding; (iii) especially, Mg–4Zn–1.5Sn alloy, with a weight loss rate of 0.45 mm/year and hydrogen evolution rate of 0.099 $mL/cm^2/day$, showed cytotoxicity grade of 0 to MC3T3-E1 cells; and (iv) the perfect alliance of cytocompatibility, suitable mechanical properties and low bio-corrosion rate demonstrates that this Mg–4Zn–1.5Sn alloy is a promising biodegradable magnesium alloy for orthopedic implants.

17.5.4 Mg–Ca alloy system

A newly developed Mg–1Ca (wt%) alloy was treated by MAO in various electrolytes including KF-silicate, KF-phosphate and KF-silicate-phosphate to study the microstructure, composition and corrosion resistance [114]. Electrochemical analysis and immersion test in Hanks' solution and MTT assay for in vitro toxicity against MG63 cells were conducted and it was reported that all the three MAO coatings contributed to the improvement of corrosion resistance and cytocompatibility of substrate; however, P coating outperformed the two others due to its specific microstructure and composition. Zhao et al. [115] fabricated a rough, hydrophobic and ZrO_2-containing surface film on Mg–Ca and Mg–Sr alloys by dual Zr and oxygen ion implantation for purpose of improving the corrosion resistance. It was obtained that weight loss measurements and electrochemical corrosion tests show that the corrosion rate of the Mg–Ca and Mg–Sr alloys is reduced appreciably after surface treatment. A systematic investigation of the in vitro cellular response and antibacterial capability of the modified binary magnesium alloys is performed and it was mentioned that the amounts of adherent bacteria on the Zr–O-implanted and Zr-implanted samples diminish remarkably compared to the nonimplanted control; significantly enhanced cell adhesion and proliferation are observed from the Zr–O-implanted sample. Based on these findings, it was suggested that dual Zr and oxygen ion implantation (which effectively enhances the corrosion resistance, the in vitro biocompatibility and antimicrobial properties of Mg–Ca and Mg–Sr alloys) provides a simple and practical means to expedite clinical acceptance of biodegradable magnesium alloys. Liu et al. [116] implanted Mg–1Ca samples with biocompatible alloy ions Ag, Fe and Y, respectively, with a dose of 2×10^{17} ions/cm^2 by metal vapor vacuum arc technique. It was mentioned that surface changes were observed after all three kinds of elemental ion implantation; the modified layer was composed of two sublayers, including an outer oxidized layer with mixture of oxides and an inner implanted layer, after Ag and Fe ion implantation. Y ion implantation induced an Mg/Ca-deficient outer oxidized layer and the distribution of Y along with depth was more homogeneous. Both electrochemical test and immersion test revealed accelerated corrosion rate of Ag-implanted Mg–1Ca and Fe-implanted Mg–1Ca, whereas Y ion implantation showed a short period of protection since enhanced corrosion resistance was obtained by electrochemical test, but accelerated corrosion rate was found by long-period immersion test and indirect cytotoxicity assay indicated good cytocompatibility of Y-implanted Mg–1Ca. Liu et al. [117] modified Mg–1Ca alloy by Zn ion implantation and deposition using metal vapor vacuum arc plasma source. The surface characteristics, corrosion behavior and cytocompatibility were investigated. It was shown that (i) the auger electron spectroscopy results showed that an uniform ZnO layer was formed on the surface of Mg–1Ca alloy and (ii) the electrochemical measurements revealed that the corrosion potential has been increased, and a comparable corrosion current density in the SBF was obtained for the Zn-modified Mg–1Ca alloy. The indirect cell viability evaluation and direct cell culture results indicated that the cytocompatibility of MC3T3-E1 cells on the Mg-1Ca alloy was improved by the ZnO layer on the surface. Neacsu et al. [118] synthesized Mg-1Ca-0.2Mn-0.6Zr alloy and coated cellulose acetate (CA) to improve its performance as a temporary bone implant. It was mentioned that the potentiodynamic polarization test revealed that the CA coating significantly improved the corrosion resistance of the Mg alloy. The in vitro experiments demonstrated that the media containing their extracts showed good cytocompatibility on MC3T3-E1 preosteoblasts in terms of cell adhesion and spreading, viability, proliferation and osteogenic differentiation and the in vivo studies conducted in rats revealed that the intramedullary-coated implant for fixation of femur fracture was more efficient in inducing bone regeneration than the uncoated one, suggesting that the CA-coated Mg-based alloy holds promise for orthopedic applications.

Bakhsheshi research group [119–121] studied various coatings on Mg–Ca alloy systems to improve the degradation behavior and enhance the cytocompatibility. Nanostructured hardystonite (HT) and titania (TiO_2)/HT dual-layered coatings [119] were deposited on biodegradable Mg–Ca–Zn alloy via PVD combined with EPD. It was reported that although a single layer nano-HT coating can decrease the corrosion rate from 1.68 to 1.02 mm/year, due to the presence of porosities and microcracks, the nano-HT layer cannot sufficiently protect the Mg substrate. However, the corrosion resistance of nano-HT coating is further improved by using nano-TiO_2 underlayer since it was a smooth, very uniform and compact layer with higher contact angle (52.30°) and the MTT assay showed the viability of MC3T3-E1 on the nano-HT and nano-TiO_2/HT coatings, indicating that the two-step surface modification improved both corrosion resistance and the cytocompatibility of the Mg alloy, hence making it feasible for orthopedic applications. Gelatin-ciprofloxacin (Gel-Cip) nanofibers containing various amounts of Cip (0, 2, 4 and 8 wt%) [120] were fabricated on the surface of Mg-1Ca alloy via an electrospinning process. It was found that prolonged drug release was attained from Gel-Cip nanofibers coating along with initial rapid drug release of around 20–22% during 12 h, followed by a slow release stage that can effectively control the infection. The incorporation of 2–4 wt% Cip into Gel nanofibers coating significantly increased the antibacterial performance and corrosion resistance of the uncoated Mg–Ca alloy without showing an inhibitory influence on the cytocompatibility characteristic. It is potentially appropriate as the novel electrospun nanofibers coating material for bone regeneration application. Moreover, Mg–Ca–TiO_2 (MCT) composite scaffolds loaded with different concentrations of doxycycline (DOXY) with a network of interconnected pores with good compressive strength (5 ± 0.1 MPa) were fabricated via space holder method [121]. It was reported that (i) MCT-DC scaffolds possess a porosity and pore size in the range of 65–67% and 600–800 μm, respectively, (ii) the bioactivity results exhibited the apatite formation on the MCT-DC scaffold surface, indicating that DOXY did not obstruct the bioactivity of MCT, (iii) the MCT-DC scaffolds drug release profiles show the initial burst and sustained drug release (55–75%) and the release rate could be adjusted via altering the DC concentration, (iv) the MCT loaded with 1 and 5% DC did not indicate cytotoxic behavior against MG63 cells while further DC loading resulted in some toxicity and (v) antimicrobial properties of MCT-DC scaffolds against *S. aureus* and *E. coli* bacteria were examined and the results reveal oblivious inhibition zone around each MCT-DC scaffold whereas no obvious inhibition is observed around the MCT scaffold. Therefore, MCT-DC composite scaffolds with low concentration of DC could be alternative candidates for infection prevention and bone tissue engineering.

17.5.5 Mg–Li alloy system

The characteristics of a MAO, prepared in phytic acid, and PLLA composite coating, fabricated on a novel Mg–1Li–1Ca alloy, were studied [122]. The corrosion behaviors of the samples were evaluated via hydrogen evolution, potentiodynamic polarization and EIS in Hanks' solution. It was found that (i) the MAO/PLLA composite coatings significantly enhanced the corrosion resistance of the Mg–1Li–1Ca alloy and (ii) MTT and ALP assays using MC3T3 osteoblasts indicated that the MAO/PLLA coatings greatly improved the cytocompatibility, and the morphology of the cells cultured on different samples exhibited good adhesion. Hemolysis tests showed that the composite coatings endowed the Mg–1Li–1Ca alloys with a low hemolysis ratio and the increased solution pH resulting from the corrosion of magnesium could be tailored by the degradation of PLLA, suggesting that the MAO/PLLA composite coating may be appropriate for applications on degradable Mg-based orthopedic implants. Liu et al. [123] developed a novel Mg–(3.5, 6.5 wt%)Li–(0.5, 2, 4 wt%)Zn ternary alloys as biodegradable metallic materials with potential for stent application. It was reported that among the alloys studied, the Mg–3.5Li–2Zn and Mg–6.5Li–2Zn alloys exhibited comparable corrosion resistance in Hank's solution to pure magnesium and better corrosion resistance in a cell culture medium than pure magnesium. The corrosion products observed on the corroded surface were composed of $Mg(OH)_2$, $MgCO_3$ and Ca-free Mg/P inorganics and Ca/P inorganics. The in vitro cytotoxicity assay revealed different behaviors of HUVECs and human aorta VSMCs to material extracts and HUVECs showed increasing nitric oxide release and tolerable toxicity, whereas VSMCs exhibited limited decreasing viability with time. Platelet adhesion, hemolysis and coagulation tests of these Mg–Li–Zn alloys showed different degrees of activation behavior, in which the hemolysis of the Mg–3.5Li–2Zn alloy was lower than 5%, indicating the potential of the Mg–Li–Zn alloys as good candidate materials for cardiovascular stent applications.

17.5.6 Mg–Ag alloy system

Three Mg–Ag alloys (Mg–2Ag, Mg–4Ag and Mg–6Ag by wt%) were cast and processed with solution (T4) and aging (T6) heat treatment [124]. It was mentioned that all alloys contained Mg_4Ag as the dominant β-phase, and after heat treatment, the mechanical properties of all Mg–Ag alloys were significantly improved and the corrosion rate was also significantly reduced, due to the presence of silver. $Mg(OH)_2$ and MgO present the main magnesium corrosion products, while AgCl was found as the corresponding primary silver corrosion product. It was further reported that immersion tests, under cell culture conditions, demonstrated that the silver content did not significantly shift the pH and magnesium ion release and the in vitro tests, with both primary osteoblasts and cell lines (MG63, RAW 264.7), revealed that Mg–Ag alloys show negligible cytotoxicity and sound cytocompatibility. Antibacterial assays, performed in a dynamic bioreactor system, proved that the alloys reduce the viability of two common pathogenic bacteria, *S. aureus* (DSMZ 20231) and *S. epidermidis* (DSMZ 3269), and the results showed that the killing rate of the alloys against tested bacteria exceeded 90%. Based on these findings, it was summarized that biodegradable Mg–Ag alloys are cytocompatible materials with adjustable mechanical and corrosion properties and show promising antibacterial activity, which indicates their potential as antibacterial biodegradable implant materials. Mostofi et al. [125] investigated the effect of biodegradable Mg and Mg alloys (Mg–2Ag and Mg–10Gd) on selected properties of MC3T3-E1 cells elicited by direct cell/material interaction. It was mentioned that (i) cells did not survive when cultured on 3-day precorroded pure Mg and Mg–2Ag, indicating crystal formation to be particular detrimental in this regard; (ii) cell viability was not affected when cells were cultured on noncorroded Mg and Mg alloys for up to 12 days, suggesting that corrosion associated changes in surface morphology and chemical composition significantly hamper cell viability and, thus, that noncorroded surfaces are more conducive to cell survival. An analysis of the differentiation potential of MC3T3-E1 cells cultured on noncorroded samples based on measurement of collagen I and Runx2 expression, revealed a downregulation of these markers within the first 6 days following cell seeding on all samples, despite persistent survival and proliferation and cells cultured on Mg10Gd, however, exhibited a pronounced upregulation of collagen I and Runx2 between days 8 and 12, indicating an enhancement of osteointegration by this alloy that could be valuable for in vivo orthopedic applications. Liu et al. [126], with a purpose of enhancing the antibacterial property, studied the influence of the microstructure and silver content on degradation, cytocompatibility and antibacterial properties of Mg–Ag alloys in vitro. It was indicated that (i) a higher silver content can increase the degradation rate of Mg–Ag alloys; however, the degradation rate could be reduced by eliminating the precipitates in the Mg–Ag alloys via T4 treatment and (ii) by controlling the microstructure and increasing the silver content, Mg–Ag alloys obtained good antibacterial properties in harsh and dynamic conditions but had almost equivalent cytocompatibility to human primary osteoblasts as pure Mg.

17.5.7 Mg–Y alloy system

The microstructure, mechanical properties, in vitro degradation assessments and in vitro cytotoxicity evaluations of the as-cast state, as-heat-treated state and as-extruded state of Mg-1.5Y-1.2Zn-0.44Zr alloy were conducted [34]. It was mentioned that (i) the microstructure of the alloy is mainly composed of the matrix α-Mg phases and the $Mg_{12}ZnY$ secondary phases (LPS structure), (ii) the results of immersion tests and electrochemical measurements in the SBF indicate that a protective film precipitated on the alloy's surface with the extension of degradation, (iii) the protective film contains

$Mg(OH)_2$ and HA which can reinforce osteoblast activity and promote good biocompatibility and (iv) no significant cytotoxicity towards L-929 cells was detected and the immersion extracts of alloy samples could enhance the cell proliferation with time in the cytotoxicity evaluations, implying that the Mg-1.5Y-1.2Zn-0.44Zr alloys have the potential to be used for biomedical applications. Chou et al. [127] prepared Mg-Y(1–4 wt%)-Ca-Zr alloys by conventional melting and casting techniques, followed by T4 solution treatment. The in vitro cytocompatibility tests on MC3T3-E1 preosteoblast cells were conducted. It was noted that (i) the Mg-Y-Ca-Zr alloys demonstrated excellent in vitro cytocompatibility and normal in vivo host response and (ii) the mechanical, corrosion and biological evaluations performed in this study demonstrated that Mg-Y-Ca-Zr alloys, especially with the 4 wt% Y content, would perform well as orthopedic and craniofacial implant biomaterials. Li et al. [128] investigated mechanical property, degradation behavior and cytocompatibility of Mg-2Y-1Zn-0.4Zr (which was subjected to heat treatment and extrusion). The cytotoxicity was evaluated using the methylthiazolyl diphenyltetrazolium bromide method via mouse fibroblast L929 cells. It was mentioned that (i) the cytocompatibility of Mg-2Y-1Zn-0.4Zr alloy was enhanced by heat treatment and extrusion and (ii) as-extruded alloy showed favorable mechanical property, the best degradation behavior and cytocompatibility which suggests that as-extruded may be a good candidate to be used in biomedical applications. Guo et al. [129] fabricated a composite MAO/PLLA coating on the surface of the magnesium alloy WE42 to improve its corrosion resistance and the cytocompatibility of the modified materials. It was obtained that (i) the PLLA coating effectively sealed the microcracks and micropores on the surface of the MAO coating by physical interlocking to interfere the corrosion ions and (ii) the corrosion rate was decreased and the cytotoxicity test showed that the MAO/PLLA composite coating WE42 had good cytocompatibility. Smola et al. [130] studied the microstructure, corrosion resistance and cytocompatibility of Mg-5Y-4RE-0.5 Zr (WE54) alloy prepared by powder metallurgy. Open-circuit potential and polarization resistance in the isotonic saline (9 g/L $NaCl/H_2O$) were monitored for 24 h. It was found that (i) the corrosion rate of the T4- and T6-treated alloys was about 80 times lower than that of commercial Mg, (ii) both alloys prepared by powder metallurgy exhibited approximately eight times higher corrosion resistance than commercial Mg, (iii) the human MG-63 osteoblast-like cells spreading and division in the extracts (0.28 g in 28 mL of EMEM) of all four alloys were monitored by cinemicrography for 24 h. The MG-63 cells proliferate without cytotoxicity in all extracts.

17.5.8 Mg–Sn alloy system

The alloying effects of Sn and Zn elements to Mg base have attracted attention since they belong to the group of basic elements in the human body if such alloys are exposed to biodegradable environment. When these elements form a certain ratio of alloy with Mg, they have a significant effect on the microstructure, corrosion resistance and biocompatibility [131]. There is a limitation of adding amount; Sn addition up to 5% by weight increases corrosion properties; however, with addition of Sn above this value, toxic effects occur in cells, and the corrosion resistance decreases [132, 133]. Zhao et al. [134] fabricated biodegradable Mg–Sn alloys by subrapid solidification and investigated their microstructure, corrosion behavior and cytotoxicity. It was indicated that (i) the microstructure of Mg-1Sn alloy was almost equiaxed grain, while the Mg–Sn alloys with higher Sn content (Sn ≥ 3 wt%) displayed α-Mg dendrites, and the secondary dendrite arm spacing of the primary α-Mg decreased significantly with increasing Sn content, (ii) the Mg-Sn alloys consisted of primary α-Mg matrix, Sn-rich segregation and Mg_2Sn phase, and the amount of Mg_2Sn phases increased with increasing Sn content, (iii) potentiodynamic polarization and immersion tests revealed that the corrosion rates of Mg–Sn alloys increased with increasing Sn content and (iv) cytotoxicity test showed that Mg–1Sn and Mg–3Sn alloys were harmless to MG-63 cells, suggesting that Mg–1Sn and Mg–3Sn alloys were promising to be used as biodegradable implants. Ercetin et al. [131] prepared Mg–5Sn–*x*Zn ($x = 0$, 1, 2, 3, 4 and 5 wt%) alloys by a mixing technique which prevents contact of magnesium with oxygen has been applied in order to produce Mg–Sn–Zn alloys by hot pressing. It was mentioned that (i) a homogeneous microstructure could be obtained, and the formed secondary phases were uniformly distributed at the grain boundaries, (ii) addition of Zn had a grain refiner effect on microstructure, leading to increased corrosion resistance, (iii) apatite structures were formed on specimen surfaces during degradation as protective layers, (iv) the highest corrosion resistance was obtained from TZ54 (Mg–5Sn–4Zn) alloy, in which the apatite structures formed intensively and (v) the addition of Zn to the alloys had no toxic effects on human neuron cells in terms of biocompatibility, but was effective for cell growth.

17.5.9 Mg–RE alloy system

RE elements have been added to Mg base as effective alloying element(s) improve the corrosion resistance of degradable Mg alloys for medical applications. However, good biocompatibility of the elements released by Mg alloys during biodegradation is crucial when such Mg materials are used as orthopedic implants, so that the effects of ions released at the biological interface are needed to be full understood. Levy et al. [135] investigated the cell cytotoxicity effects during corrosion of a novel magnesium alloy, EW10X04 (Mg-1.2Nd-0.5Y-0.5Zr-0.4Ca), following diffusion coating (DC) and heat treatment to reduce the corrosion rate. Cells were exposed either to corrosion products or to the corroding scaffold surface, in vitro. It was reported that (i) cell viability, growth and adhesion were all improved when cultured on the EW10X04 + DC surface or under corrosion product extracts due to lower corrosion rates relative to the EW10X04 control samples and (ii) the tested alloy after Nd coating and heat treatment may introduce a good balance between its biodegradation characteristics and cytotoxic effects towards cells. Grillo et al. [136] studied the in vitro toxicological effects of two RE Mg-alloying elements, La and Gd, as individual ions and in mixtures with and without Mg ions. Different combinations (Mg + Gd, Mg + La and Mg + Gd + La) were used to evaluate their possible synergistic effects on CHO-K1 cells. Two sets of experiments were designed to assess (i) the cytogenotoxic effect of La and Gd ions by neutral red (NR) technique, Reduction of tetrazolium salt (MTT), Viability with Acridine Orange staining, Clonogenic test and Comet assay; and, (ii) the possible synergistic toxicological effect of La and Gd ions in mixtures, and the influence of osmolarity increase on cellular response. It was reported that (i) cytotoxic effects of RE were found at concentrations ≥200 μM RE while DNA damage was detected for doses ≥1,500 μM and ≥1,600 μM for La and Gd, respectively, and (ii) when mixtures of ions were evaluated, neither synergistic cytotoxic effects nor biological damage related to osmolarity increase were detected.

Using several different in vitro assays, Weizbauer et al. [137] investigated a new biodegradable Mg–2La alloy as a possible implant material for biomedical applications. It was mentioned that (i) an in vitro cytotoxicity test, according to EN ISO 10993-5/12, with L929 and human osteoblastic cells identified no toxic effects on cell viability at physiological concentrations (at 50% dilutions and higher), (ii) the metabolic activity of human osteoblasts in the 100% extract was decreased to <70% and was therefore rated as cytotoxic and (iii) the degradation rates of Mg–2La were evaluated in phosphate-buffered saline and four different cell culture media and the degradation rates were shown to be influenced by the composition of the solution, and the addition of fetal bovine serum slightly accelerated the corrosive process, suggesting that (iv) Mg–2La is a promising candidate for use as an orthopedic implant material.

Yang et al. [138] studied the corrosion behavior in a cell culture medium (CCM) under cell culture conditions close to the in vivo environment, the element distribution in the corrosion layer and the cytocompatibility of alloy Mg–10Dy evaluated by MTT, cell adhesion and live/dead staining tests. It was found that (i) the corrosion layer was enriched in Dy, while the P and Ca content gradually decreased from the surface to the bottom of the corrosion layer, (ii) large amounts of $MgCO_3 \cdot 3H_2O$ formed in the corrosion layer after 28 days immersion and (iii) both extracts and the Dy-enriched corrosion layer of alloy Mg-10Dy showed no cytotoxicity to primary human osteoblasts.

The cytological effects of various Mg alloys on cells that play an important role in bone repair were investigated [139]. Eight different magnesium alloys containing varying amounts of Al, Zn, Nd and Y were either incubated directly or indirectly with the osteosarcoma cell line $SaOS_2$ or with uninduced and osteogenically induced human MSCs isolated from bone marrow specimens obtained from the femoral shaft of patients undergoing total hip replacement. Cell viability, cell attachment and the release of ions were investigated at different time points in vitro. It was reported that (i) during direct or indirect incubation different cytotoxic effects of the Mg alloys on $SaOS_2$ cells and osteogenically induced or uninduced MSCs were observed, (ii) the concentration of degradation products released from the Mg alloys differed and (iii) Mg alloys including Mg–2Nd, Mg–4Y, Mg–9Al–1Zn and Mg–4Y–2Nd exhibit good cytocompatibility. Based on the obtained results, it was concluded that (iv) the necessity of cytocompatibility evaluation of new biodegradable magnesium alloys with cells that will get in direct contact to the implant material. Zhang et al. [140] developed a patent magnesium alloy Mg-Nd-Zn-Zr alloy for cardiovascular stent application which was treated by immersion in hydrofluoric acid. A 1.5 μm thick MgF_2 layer was prepared. It was mentioned that (i) the MgF_2 layer slowed down in vitro degradation rate, but lost the protection effect after 10 days, (ii) the treatment enhanced human albumin adsorption while no difference of human fibrinogen adsorption amount was observed, (iii) direct cell adhesion test showed many more live HUVECs retained than bare magnesium alloy and (iv) both treated and untreated Mg-Nd-Zn-Zr showed no adverse effect on HUVEC viability and spreading morphology. Using the same alloy, Qin et al. [67] conducted a systematic investigation of the in vitro and in vivo antibacterial capability. It was found that (i) the results of microbiological counting, confocal laser scanning microscopy (CLSM), SEM in vitro, and microbiological cultures, histopathology in vivo consistently show JDBM enhanced the antibacterial activity and (ii) the significantly improved cytocompatibility is observed from Mg-Nd-Zn-Zr alloy, suggesting that the alloy effectively enhances the corrosion resistance, biocompatibility and antimicrobial properties of Mg by alloying with the proper amount of Zn, Zr and Nd. Jin et al. [141] used two inflammatory cell lines, that is, THP-1 cells and THP-1 macrophages, to evaluate the effect of Mg-Nd-Zn-Zr alloy extracts on cell viability, death modes, cell cycle, phagocytosis, differentiation, migration and inflammatory response. It was reported that (i) high-concentration extract induced necrosis and complete damage of cell function, (ii) for middle-concentration extract, cell apoptosis and partially impaired cell function were observed, (iii) TNF-α expression of macrophages was upregulated by coculture with extract in 20% concentration, but was down-regulated in the same concentration in the presence of LPS stimulation, (iv) the production of TNF-α decreased when macrophages were cultured in middle and high concentration extracts independent of LPS and (v) cell viability was also negatively affected by magnesium ions in JDBM extracts, which was a potential factor affecting cell function. Levy et al. [135] investigated the cell cytotoxicity effects during corrosion of anovel magnesium alloy, Mg-1.2Nd-0.5Y-0.5Zr-0.4Ca (EW10X04), followed by diffusion coating and heat treatment to reduce the corrosion rate. Cells were exposed either to corrosion products or to the corroding scaffold surface, in vitro. It was obtained that the cell viability, growth and adhesion were all improved when cultured on the EW10X04 + diffusion coating surface or under corrosion product extracts due to lower corrosion rates relative to the EW10X04 control samples, indicating that the alloy after Nd coating and heat treatment may introduce a good balance between its biodegradation characteristics and cytotoxic effects towards cells.

To control the biodegradation rate, Shangguan et al. [142] employed three commonly used coatings on Mg–Sr alloy, including MOA coating, electrodeposition coating and chemical conversion coating, and compared these coatings for requirements of favorable degradation and biological performances, how each of these coating systems has performed and mentioned that the MOA coating on Mg–Sr alloy exhibited the best corrosion resistance and cell response among these coatings, and is proved to be more suitable for the orthopedic application. Zhao et al. [143] studied as-extruded Mg–Sr alloys for orthopedic application on their microstructure, mechanical properties, biocorrosion properties and cytotoxicity. It was reported that (i) as-extruded Mg–Sr alloys were composed of α-Mg and $Mg_{17}Sr_2$ phases, and the content of $Mg_{17}Sr_2$ phases increased with increasing Sr content, (ii) immersion and electrochemical tests showed that as-extruded Mg–0.5Sr alloy exhibited the best anticorrosion property, and the anticorrosion property of as-extruded Mg–Sr alloys deteriorated with increasing Sr content, which was greatly associated with galvanic couple effect and (ii) the cytotoxicity test revealed that as-extruded Mg–0.5Sr alloy did not induce toxicity to cells, indicating that (iii) as-extruded Mg–0.5Sr alloy with suitable mechanical properties, corrosion resistance and good cytocompatibility was potential as a biodegradable implant for orthopedic application.

Microstructure, biocorrosion behavior and cytotoxicity of an as-extruded Mg-11.3Gd-2.5Zn-0.7Zr (wt%) alloy were studied to develop new biodegradable magnesium alloy [144]. It was obtained that (i) the corrosion rate in Hanks' solution is only 0.17 mm/year and the corrosion mode of the alloy is uniform corrosion, which is much better than that of as-extruded Mg-10.2Gd-3.3Y-0.6Zr alloy and (ii) the cell toxicity grade of this alloy is grade 1 (i.e., only slightly having cytotoxicity), suggesting that (iii) the Mg-Gd-Zn-Zr alloy with LPSO structure will become one of novel promising high-strength biodegradable magnesium alloys. Sanchez et al. [145] evaluated the in vitro differentiation of ATDC5 cells under the influence of pure Mg, Mg–10Gd and Mg–2Ag degradation products (extracts) and direct cell culture on the materials. It was shown that (i) gene expression showed an inhibitory effect on ATDC5 mineralization with the three extracts and a chondrogenic potential of Mg–10Gd, (ii) cells cultured in Mg–10Gd and Mg–2Ag extracts showed the same proliferation and morphology than cells cultured in growth conditions, (iii) Mg–10Gd induced an increase in production of ECM and a bigger cell size, similar to the effects found with differentiation conditions, (iv) an increased metabolic activity was observed in cells cultured under the influence of Mg–10Gd extracts, indicated by an acidic pH during most of the culture period and (v) after 7 days of culture on the materials, ATDC5 growth, distribution and ECM synthesis were higher on Mg–10Gd samples, followed by Mg–2Ag and PMg, which was influenced by the homogeneity and composition of the degradation layer. Based on these findings, it was concluded that (vi) the tolerance of ATDC5 cells to Mg-based materials and a chondrogenic effect of Mg–10Gd was confirmed.

17.5.10 Mg composites

The cell culture tests for examining the in vitro cytocompatibility property were conducted on a new generation bioactive ceramic, based on $MgKPO_4$ (magnesium potassium phosphate) for biomedical applications [146] and it was mentioned that the results reveal good cell adhesion and spreading of L929 mouse fibroblast cells and (ii) MTT assay analysis with L929 cells confirmed noncytotoxic behavior of magnesium potassium phosphate containing ceramics and the results are comparable with sintered HAP ceramics. The indirect cytotoxicity tests were performed on Mg (0.97, 1.98, 2.5)–TiO_2, Mg (0.58, 0.97, 1.98)–TiC and Mg (0.58, 0.97, 1.98)–TiN (by vol%) to determine the cytotoxicity of low-volume nanoparticulate reinforcement on magnesium [147]. It was reported that (i) results of the indirect MTT assay on day 3 and day 5 indicate that 2.5 vol% TiO_2, TiC and TiN has little effect on the cytotoxicity when added as low volume fraction reinforcement to magnesium, (ii) while (0.97, 1.98)-TiO_2 negatively affected the cytotoxicity when added to Mg and (iii) the modulus of elasticity of the materials was found to remain close to that of cortical bone which would suggest that the stress shielding effect would be reduced as the increase in modulus of elasticity was mitigated by the low volume addition of reinforcements. The cytocompatibility of pure Mg and Mg–*x*HAP biocomposites ($x = 5$, 10 and 15 wt%) fabricated by powder metallurgy routes was investigated [148]. The materials were produced from raw HA powders with particle mean sizes of 6 µm (S-*x*HA) or 25 µm (L-*x*HA). The biocompatibility study has been performed for MC3T3 cells (osteoblasts/osteoclasts) and L929 fibroblasts. It was mentioned that (i) S–Mg, S-10HA and L-10HA composites are the materials with the best biocompatibility, (ii) the ability of *S. aureus* bacteria to assemble biofilms was also evaluated, (iii) biofilm formation assays showed that these materials are not particular prone to colonization and biofilm assembly is strain dependent, (iv) the corrosion resistance of S–Mg, S-10HA and L-10HA materials immersed in the media used for the cells culture has also been analyzed and (v) different trends in the corrosion resistance have been found: S–Mg and S-10HA show a very high resistance to corrosion whereas the corrosion of L-10HA steadily increases with time. Mg–Ca–TiO_2 (MCT) composite scaffolds loaded with different concentrations of doxycycline (DC) with a network of interconnected pores were fabricated via space holder method and characterized [121]. It was mentioned that (i) MCT-DC scaffolds possess a porosity and pore size in the range of 65–67% and 600–800 µm respectively, (ii) the bioactivity results exhibited the apatite formation on the MCT-DC scaffold surface, indicating that DC did not obstruct the bioactivity of MCT, (iii) MCT-DC scaffolds drug release profiles show the initial burst and sustained drug release (55–75%) and the release rate could be adjusted via altering the DC concentration, (iv) MCT loaded with 1 and 5% DC did not indicate cytotoxic behavior against MG63 cells while further DC loading resulted in some toxicity and (v) antimicrobial properties of MCT-DC scaffolds against *S. aureus* and *E. coli* bacteria were examined and the results reveal oblivious inhibition zone around each MCT-DC scaffold whereas no obvious inhibition is observed around the MCT scaffold, indicating that (vi) MCT-DC composite scaffolds with low concentration of DC could be alternative candidates for infection prevention and bone tissue engineering. In order to reduce the degradation rate, TiO_2-incorporated MAO (TM) coatings were prepared on Mg- Ca alloy using MAO [149]. Subsequently, Zn-doped HA (ZH) coating was deposited by EPD on the MAO coating. It was reported that (i) the electrochemical test results demonstrated that the deposition of ZH composite coatings on Mg alloy significantly reduces its corrosion rate and improves its charge transfer resistance, (ii) antibacterial activity of the coating against *E. coli* was studied using disk-diffusion and spread plate methods, (iii) the number of *E. coli* colonies reduces to 92% after ZH coating implying its good antibacterial properties and (iv) the cytotoxicity test indicated that cell viability of MG63 osteoblast cells cultured with ZH extracts was higher compared to the TM coating and bare Mg alloy, indicating that (v) Mg alloy coated by TM/ZH exhibits high corrosion resistance, antibacterial activity and favorable bioactivity and cytocompatibility, indicating their substantial potentials for biomedical applications.

17.6 Hemocompatibility

The chemical composition of human blood and urine has provided valuable insight into biochemical and physiological processes and the understanding of many human diseases. Hemocompatibility evaluates the material's compatibility with red blood cells. In particular, thrombogenic property or changes in red blood cells content in a blood stream flowing over the biomaterials are assessed and a better thrombus material should ideally show limited thrombus formation. Hemocompatibility can define the limit for clinical applicability of blood-contacting biomaterials (which should include catheters, guidewires, dialyzer, oxygenators (artificial lungs), heart-supporting systems, cardiac pacemaker, vascular grafts, stents, heart valves, micro-, NPs and others), which come in close or direct contact with blood, which is a complex organ comprising of 55% plasma, 44% erythrocytes and 1% leukocytes and platelets [150]. Thus, adverse interactions between newly developed materials and blood should be extensively analyzed to prevent activation and destruction of blood components. The initially adsorbed protein layer on the biomaterial surface mainly triggers the adverse reactions, such as the activation of coagulation via intrinsic pathway, the activation of leukocytes, which results in inflammation, and the adhesion and activation of platelets, resulting in making the number of blood cells decrease and a thrombus can be formed [151]. Prior to clinical application, the hemocompatibility of blood-contacting medical materials have to be analyzed and therefore, a guidance is developed by the ISO 10993-4. According this guideline, five different categories, thrombosis, coagulation, platelets, hematology and immunology (complement system and leukocytes), are indicated for hemocompatibility evaluation. The devices are divided into three categories concerning blood contact: (i) externally communicating devices with indirect blood contact, for example, cannulas and blood collection sets; (ii) externally communicating devices with direct blood contact, for example, catheters and hemodialysis equipment; (iii) implant devices, for example, heart valves, stents and vascular grafts [150]. Erythrocytes are the most abundant blood cells with $4–6 \times 10^6$ cells/μL and they are important for the transport of oxygen (O_2) from the lung to all tissues and cells and carbon dioxide (CO_2) from tissues back to the lung. Since erythrocytes are the most rigid cells in the blood, they are sensitive to rupture and hemolysis due to shear stress and changes in osmotic pressure. Blood platelets are the smallest (1–3 μm) and the second abundant cell type in the blood with $1.5–3.5 \times 10^5$ cells/μL, which can rapidly recognize foreign surfaces and initiate blood coagulation. Furthermore, human blood contains $4.3–10 \times 10^3$ leukocytes/μL, such as granulocytes, lymphocytes, monocytes, dendritic and natural killer cells. Monocytes account for 1–6% of all leukocytes and neutrophil granulocytes are the most abundant leukocytes in the blood, comprising 50–70% of all leukocytes. These immune cells are belonging to the innate immune system and they can be rapidly activated upon recognition of a foreign invader such as a pathogen or a foreign material. Furthermore, blood plasma contains high amounts of plasma proteins, such as albumin, coagulation factors and immunoglobulins [150, 152].

Lu et al. [153] fabricated a biocompatible MAO/PLLA composite coating on the magnesium alloy WE42 (Mg-4Y-2RE) substrate and evaluated magnesium ions release, biocorrosion and hemocompatibility. The SEM images were used to demonstrate the morphology of the samples before and after being submerged in hanks solution for 4 weeks. The degradation was evaluated through the magnesium ions release rate and EIS test. The biocompatibility of the samples was demonstrated by coagulation time and hemolysis behavior. It was reported that (i) the PLLA effectively improved the corrosion resistance by sealing the microcracks and microholes on the surface of the MAO coating and (ii) the modified samples had good compatibility. Ma et al. [154] introduced a concept "bio-adaption" between the Mg alloy stent and the local tissue microenvironment after implantation. The healing responses of stented blood vessel can be generally described in three overlapping phases: inflammation, granulation and remodeling and the ideal bio-adaption of the Mg alloy stent, once implanted into the blood vessel, needs to be a reasonable function of the time and the space/dimension. It was pointed out (i) a very slow degeneration of mechanical support is expected in the initial four months in order to provide sufficient mechanical support to the injured vessels and (ii) once the Mg alloy stent being degraded, the void space will be filled by the regenerated blood vessel tissues and the degradation of the Mg alloy stent should be 100% completed with no residues, and the degradation products (e.g., ions and hydrogen) will be helpful for the tissue reconstruction of the blood vessel. Chen et al. [155], for purpose of improving corrosion resistance and hemocompatibility of Mg alloy, fabricated a polymerized 2-methacryloyloxyethyl phosphorycholine (PMPC) coating via surface thiol-ene photopolymerization onto Mg alloy treated by cathodic plasma electrolytic deposition (CPED). It was mentioned that (i) potentiodynamic polarization test and EIS illustrated that the corrosion resistance of Mg alloy in SBF was significantly enhanced after the formation of CPED/PMPC composite coating and (ii) platelets adhesion measurement indicated that CPED/PMPC treated Mg alloy possesses promising hemocompatibility. Assuring the hemocompatibility and foremost assessing the thrombogenicity of new biomaterials prior to their use is essential in order to avoid adverse effects, it is important to assess thrombocyte adhesion on coated Mg–RE and Mg–Zn–Ca alloys [156]. Static experiments with human blood were carried out on the plasma electrolytically treated or corresponding untreated Mg alloy in order to assess quantity and quality of thrombocyte adhesion via standardized SEM imaging. It was mentioned that (i) a new parallel plate flow chamber design simulating blood circulation was successfully established, enabling the further assessment of platelet adhesion on bioabsorbable materials under dynamic flow conditions, (ii) static and dynamic experiments showed, that plasma-electrolytically treated specimens showed low thrombocyte adhesion on both alloys, proposing their potential use in vascular scaffolds and (iii) the uncoated magnesium alloys showed rapid degradation along with gas formation due to the chemically active surface and therefore give concern regarding their safety and suitability for vascular applications [156]. Rezaei et al. [157] modified surface of severely plastic deformed titanium implants with fine Mg hydride powder to form Mg-rich islands with varying sizes ranging from 100 to 1,000 nm to be integrated inside a thin surface layer (100–500 μM) of the implant. It was found that (i) selective etching of the surface forms a fine structure of surface pores which their average size varies in the range of 200–500 nm depending on the processing condition and (ii) the in vitro biocompatibility and hemocompatibility assays show that the Mg-rich islands and the induced surface pores significantly enhance cell attachment and biocompatibility without an adverse effect on the cell viability, indicating that (iii) severe plastic integration of Mg-rich islands on titanium surface accompanying with porosification is a new and promising procedure with high potential for nanoscale modification of biomedical implants. Wang et al. [158] immobilized a silk fibroin blended with heparin and GREDVY (Gly-Arg-Glu-Asp-Val-Tyr) peptide on a HF-pretreated Mg-Zn-Y-Nd alloy surface via a polydopamine layer to improve its corrosion resistance, blood compatibility and endothelialization. It was reported that (i) standard electrochemical measurements along with the long-term immersion results indicated that the functionalized Mg-Zn-Y-Nd alloy had preferable anticorrosion abilities compared with the untreated alloy, (ii) the modified surface exhibited outstanding hemocompatibility with reduced platelet adhesion, HR and prolonged blood coagulation time and (iii) HUVEC and VSMC coculture results revealed more attached HUVECs on the functionalized samples than on the Mg-Zn-Y-Nd alloy surfaces, indicating that the excellent corrosion retardation, hemocompatibility and re-endothelialization of the multifunctional coating indicate a promising method in the field of biodegradable magnesium-based implantable cardiovascular stents.

17.7 Osseointegration

Broadly speaking about the mechanism for the placed metallic implant to fuse (or integrate) with receiving vital hard tissue, two types of anchorage mechanisms have been described: biomechanical and biochemical. Biomechanical binding is when bone ingrowth occurs into micrometer sized surface irregularities. The term osseointegration is probably, realistically, this biomechanical phenomenon. Biochemical bonding may occur with certain bioactive materials where there is primarily a chemical bonding, with possible supplemental biomechanical interlocking. The distinct advantage with the biochemical bonding is that the anchorage is accomplished within a relatively short period of time, while biomechanical anchorage takes weeks to develop. This would clinically translate into the possibility of earlier restorative loading of implants. Most commercially available implants depend on biomechanical interlocking for anchorage. All implants must exhibit biomechanical as well as morphological compatibility [159, 160]. As we have seen previously, Ti implants coated with calcium phosphate, or inorganic or organic bone-like apatite possess both anchorage mechanisms, because (i) coated surfaces are normally rough which can facilitate the biomechanical anchorage (morphological compatibility), and (ii) coated materials per se accommodate biochemical bonding (biological compatibility). Bone fusing to titanium was first reported in 1940 by Bothe et al. [161]. Brånemark began extensive experimental studies in 1952 on the microscopic circulation of bone marrow healing. These studies led to dental implant application in early 1960, 10-year implant integration was established in dogs without significant adverse reactions to hard or soft tissues. Studies in humans began in 1965, were followed for 10 years, and reported in 1977 [162]. Osseointegration, as first defined by Brånemark, denotes at least some direct contact between vital bone with the surface of an implant at the light microscopic level of magnification [163]. The percentage of direct bone–implant contact is variable. To determine osseointegration, the implant must be removed and evaluated under a microscope. Rigid fixation defines the clinical aspect of this microscopic bone contact with an implant and is the absence of mobility with 1 to 500 g force applied in a vertical or horizontal direction. Rigid fixation is the clinical result of a direct bone interface but has also been reported with fibrous tissue interfaces [164]. Osseointegration was originally defined as a direct structural and functional connection between ordered living bone and the surface of a load-carrying artificial implant (which is typically made of titanium materials). It is now said that an implant is regarded as osseointegrated when there is no progressive relative movement between the implant and the bone with which it has direct contact. In practice, this means that in osseointegration there is an anchorage mechanism, whereby nonvital components can be reliably and predictably incorporated into living bone and that this anchorage can persist under all normal conditions of loading. Bioactive (or biochemical) retention can be achieved in cases where the implant is coated with bioactive materials, like HA. These bioactive materials stimulate bone formation leading, to a physicochemical bond. If it is recognized that the implant is ankylosed with the bone, it is sometimes called a biointegration instead of osseointegration [164]. In cementless fixation systems, surface character is an important factor.

Mg-based alloys, as a potential orthopedic implant, can self-degrade to avoid second operation for its remove, and enable to promote bone repair; however, the underlying molecular mechanisms remain unclear. Accordingly, Zhang et al. [165] examined the effect of Mg ions on osteogenesis, chemotaxis and antialkaline stress in hFOB1.19 human osteoblast cells to simulate bone-repairing effect of a biodegradable Mg-based alloy implant in vitro, and explored the regulatory role of the transient receptor potential melastatin 7 (TRPM7)/phosphoinositide 3-kinase (PI3K) signaling pathway in the process of Mg ion-induced bone repair by knockdown of TRPM7 and antagonizing PI3K activity. It was reported that (i) Mg ions up-regulated the expression of Runx2 and ALP through TRPM7/PI3K signaling pathway, which could significantly enhance the osteogenic activity of human osteoblasts, (ii) the expression levels of MMP2, MMP9 and vascular endothelial growth factor were increased by TRPM7/PI3K signaling pathway, which recruits osteoblasts from low- to high-Mg ion environments by inducing cell migration, (iii) although an alkaline environment has antibacterial effects, alkaline stress can cause cytotoxicity and induce cell death and (iv) Mg ions could activate PI3K phosphorylation to promote cell growth and survival, protecting cells against the alkaline-stress-induced cytotoxicity caused by the degradation of Mg-based alloy implants, indicating that (v) it was not only revealed the molecular mechanism of Mg in promoting bone repair but also explained the protective effects of Mg ions on osteoblasts in an alkaline environment, which provides a theoretical basis and new directions for the application of Mg-based alloy implant material in orthopedics fixations and osteosarcoma treatment. Castellani et al. [166] investigated whether bone–implant interface strength and osseointegration of a novel biodegradable magnesium alloy (Mg-Y-Nd-HRE, based on WE43) is comparable to that of a titanium control (Ti–6Al–7Nb) currently in clinical use. Biomechanical push-out testing, microfocus computed tomography (CT) and scanning electron microscopy were performed in 72 Sprague-Dawley rats 4, 12 and 24 weeks after implantation to address this question. Additionally, blood smears were obtained from each rat at sacrifice to detect potential systemic inflammatory reactions. It was found that (i) push-out testing revealed highly significantly greater maximum push-out force, ultimate shear strength and energy absorption to failure in magnesium alloy rods than in titanium controls after each implantation period, (ii) microfocus CT showed significantly higher bone-implant contact and bone volume per tissue volume in magnesium alloy implants as well and (iii) no systemic inflammatory reactions were observed in any of the animals, concluding that (iv) the tested biodegradable implant is superior to the titanium control with respect to both bone–implant interface strength and osseointegration and (v) the investigated biodegradable magnesium alloy not only achieves enhanced bone response but also excellent interfacial strength and thus fulfils two critical requirements for bone implant applications.

Trincă et al. [167] mentioned that Mg–Ca alloys as a typical example are biocompatible substrates with mechanical properties similar to those of bones and the biodegradable alloys of Mg–Ca provide sufficient mechanical strength in load carrying applications as opposed to biopolymers and also they avoid stress shielding and secondary surgery inherent with permanent metallic implant materials. However, as have been discussed previously, the main issue facing a biodegradable Mg alloys such as Mg–Ca alloy is the fast degradation in the aggressive physiological environment of the body. The alloy's corrosion is proportional with the dissolution of the Mg in the body: the reaction with the water generates magnesium hydroxide and hydrogen. The thus generated hydrogen might cause cytotoxic reaction. The accelerated corrosion will lead to early loss of the alloy's mechanical integrity. The degradation rate of an alloy can be improved mainly through tailoring the composition and by carrying out surface treatments, as we have seen before. Based on this background, the ability to adjust degradation rate of Mg–Ca alloys by an original method and studies the biological activity of the resulted specimens was examined [167]. A new Mg–Ca alloy, with a Si gradient concentration from the surface to the interior of the material, was prepared. The in vivo degradation behavior, biological compatibility and activity of Mg–Ca alloys with/without Si gradient concentration were studied with an implant model (subcutaneous and bony) in rats. It was reported that the results sustained that Si gradient concentration can be used to control the rate of degradation of the Mg–Ca alloys for enhancing their biologic activity in order to facilitate bone tissue repair.

Mushahary et al. [168] coated Mg–Zr–Ca alloy implants with collagen type I (Coll-I) and assessed for their rate and efficacy of bone mineralization and implant stabilization. The corrosion behavior was established by their hydrogen production rate in SBF. The coated alloys were implanted into the femur bones of male New Zealand white rabbits. It was mentioned that (i) upon surface coating with Coll-I, the alloys demonstrated high surface energy showing enhanced performance as an implant material that is suitable for rapid and efficient new bone tissue induction with optimal mineral content and cellular properties and (ii) Coll-I-coated Mg–Zr–Ca alloys have a tendency to form superior trabecular bone structure with better osteoinduction around the implants and higher implant secondary stabilization, through the phenomenon of contact osteogenesis, compared to the control and uncoated ones in shorter periods of implantation, indicating that (iii) Coll-I surface coating of Mg–Zr–Ca alloys is a promising method for expediting new bone formation in vivo and enhancing osseointegration in load bearing implant applications. Li et al. [169] studied the in vitro responses of bone-forming MC3T3-E1 preosteoblasts to Mg-Zn-Ca-Sr BMGs in order to assess their feasibility to serve as orthopedic implants. It was mentioned that (i) Mg-Zn-Ca-Sr BMGs were much more capable of supporting cell adhesion and spreading in comparison with crystalline AZ31B Mg alloy, (ii) Mg-Zn-Ca-Sr BMG extracts showed no cytotoxicity to and slightly stimulated the proliferation of preosteoblasts, (iii) the cells cultured in 100% BMG extracts exhibited lower ALP activity as compared with that in negative control, which could be mainly ascribed to the inhibition of high concentrations of Zn ions on cell differentiation, (iv) with decreasing the extract concentration, the inhibitory effect was diminished and the 5% BMG extract exhibited slight stimulation in cell differentiation and mineralization and (v) the high corrosion resistance of BMGs contributed to smaller environmental variations, compared with AZ31B alloy, thus lowering the unfavorable influences on cellular responses. Torroni et al. [170] tested the WE43 Mg alloy (as-cast and T-5 treated) to assess their biological behavior and degradation pattern when implanted as endosteal implants on a calvarial bone sheep model. Six implants in form of cylindrical disks were tested in six sheep, one per composition of each disk was placed in two monocortical cranial defect created with high speed trephine bur in the parietal bone. After euthanasia at 6 weeks histomorphological analysis of the bone/implant specimens was performed. It was reported that (i) WE43-as cast showed higher degradation rate, increased bone remodeling, gas pockets formation and osteolysis compared with the T5 alloy and (ii) WE43-T5 showed greater bone/implant interface stability and seemed to be more suitable for fabrication of endosteal bone screws.

17.8 Magnetic resonance imaging compatibility

17.8.1 In general

Magnetic resonance imaging (MRI) is probably the most innovative and revolutionary imaging technology, with the exception of compound tomography. MRI is a three-dimensional (3D) imaging technique used to image the protons of the body by employing magnetic fields, radio frequencies, electromagnetic detectors and computers [171]. For millions of patients worldwide, MRI examinations provide essential and potentially life-saving information. Some devices, such as pacemakers and neurostimulator, have limitations related to MRI safety and may be contraindicated for use with MRI. Other internal devices such as stents, vena cava filters and some types of catheters and guidewires, are safe for use with MRI but have limited MRI image compatibility. Some of these devices are simply not well imaged under MRI. Others have properties that interfere with the MRI image by causing an image artifact (distortion) in the area and around the device, limiting the effectiveness of MRI for assisting placement or diagnostic follow-up on these implants. It may be contraindicated in certain situations because the magnetic field present in the MRI environment may, under certain circumstances, result in movement or heating of a metallic orthopedic implant device. Further, metals that exhibit magnetic attraction in the MRI setting may be subject to movement (deflection) during the procedure. Both magnetic and nonmagnetic metallic devices of certain geometries may be subjected to heating caused by interactions with the magnetic field. There are currently several researchers and an American Society for Testing and Materials committee exploring methods for accurately assessing the MRI compatibility of implant devices. The primary focus of their research has been the measurement of implant movement in response to a magnetic field. Shellock et al. [172–174] conducted several studies in which the movement/deflection of various orthopedic implants was measured in the high magnetic field (0.3–1.5 T) region of MRI units. The results of these studies show no measurable movement of implants fabricated from cobalt, titanium and stainless steel alloys [175]. Ferromagnetic metals will cause a magnetic field inhomogeneity, which, in turn, causes a local signal void, often accompanied by an area of high signal intensity, as well as a distortion of the image. They create their own magnetic fields and dramatically alter precession frequencies of protons in the adjacent tissues. Tissues adjacent of ferromagnetic components become influenced by the induced magnetic field of the metal hardware rather than the parent field and, therefore, either fail to process or do so at a different frequency and hence do not generate useful signal. Two components contribute to the susceptibility artifact: induced magnetism in the ferromagnetic component itself and induced magnetism in protons adjacent to the component. Artifacts from metal may have varied appearance on MRI scans due to different types of metal or configuration of the piece of metal. In relation to MRI, titanium alloys are less ferromagnetic than both cobalt and stainless steel, induce less susceptibility to artifacts, and result in less marked image degradation [174–177].

17.8.2 Artifacts

MRI is widely used as an important diagnostic tool, especially for orthopedic and brain surgery. This method has remarkable advantages for obtaining various cross-sectional views and for diagnosis of the human body with no invasion and no exposure of the human body to X-ray radiation. However, MRI diagnosis is inhibited when metals are implanted in the body, since metallic implants, such as stainless steels, Co–Cr alloys and Ti alloys become magnetized in the intense magnetic field of the MRI instrument, and artifacts occur in the image [178–181]. Metallic objects produce artifacts on magnetic resonance (MR) images. Elison et al. [180] evaluated cranial MRI distortion caused by various orthodontic brackets. Ten subjects received five consecutive cranial MR scans. A control scan was conducted with Essix trays (GAC International, Bohemia, NY) fitted over the maxillary and mandibular teeth. Four experimental MR scans of the head were conducted with plastic, ceramic, titanium and stainless steel brackets incorporated into the Essix tray material. It was found that (i) there is a statistically significant difference between the mean distortion scores of stainless steel brackets and the mean distortion scores of the other experimental MR scans; (ii) interrater and intrarater agreement was high; (iii) the study showed that plastic, ceramic and titanium brackets cause minimal distortion of cranial MR images (similar to the control); on the other hand, stainless steel brackets cause significant distortion, rendering several cranial regions nondiagnostic; (iv) areas with the most distortion were the body of the mandible, the hard palate, the base of the tongue, the globes, the nasopharynx and the frontal lobes; (v) in general, the closer the stainless steel appliance was to a specific anatomic region, the greater the distortion of the MR image. Orthodontic appliances are often prophylactically removed prior to MRI examinations, although they are sometimes left in situ (out of ignorance). Blankenstein et al. [182] measured the size of experimental artifacts created by orthodontic devices and to develop criteria using sound material science research for making MRI more compatible, thereby supporting radiologists and orthodontists in their efforts. Sixteen orthodontic small device and wire specimens made of different steel and titanium or CoCr alloys were placed in a chambered water-filled phantom for MRI. Each was subjected to spin-echo and gradient-echo sequences at 1.5 and 3 T. It was observed that (i) artifact formation depends on the material properties (specimen size, crystalline structure, manufacture-related processing) and on the specifications of the MRI system used (main field strength, sequence type), (ii) artifact radii ranged from 14 mm (spin echo at 1.5 T) to 51 mm (gradient echo at 3 T), and (iii) no artifacts occurred at 1.5 T around the titanium and Co–Cr specimens; the same observation was made with one of the steel grades. Based on these results, it was concluded that (iv) artifact size cannot be predicted merely from the designation steel, (v) nor did the crystalline structure of the baseline material from which a steel device had been produced have major implications for artifact size, (vi) relevant, however, was the magnetic permeability (or susceptibility) of the final products, which is not disclosed by the manufacturers, and it cannot be measured on fixed intraoral appliances, and (vii) the present investigation reveals that some steel devices can remain in situ without triggering adverse consequences.

Sonnow et al. [183] evaluated the imaging properties of a magnesium Herbert compression screw and studied the optimal imaging parameters in order to achieve maximal artifact reduction and image quality with in vivo applicable imaging modalities. A CE-approved magnesium Herbert screw (MAGNEZIX®) and a titanium screw of the same dimensions (3.2 × 20 mm) were imaged using different modalities: digital radiography (DX), multidetector CT (MDCT), high-resolution flat panel CT (FPCT) and MRI. The screws were scanned in vitro and after implantation in a fresh chicken tibia in order to simulate surrounding bone and soft tissue. The images were quantitatively evaluated with respect to the overall image quality and the extent and intensity of artifacts. It was found that (i) in all modalities, the artifacts generated by the magnesium screw had a lesser extent and were less severe as compared to the titanium screw (mean difference of artifact size of solo scanned screws in DX: 0.7 mm, MDCT: 6.2 mm, FPCT: 5.9 mm and MRI: 4.73 mm), (ii) in MDCT and FPCT multiplanar reformations and 3D reconstructions were superior as compared with the titanium screw and the metal-bone interface after implanting the screws in chicken cadavers was more clearly depicted and (iii) while the artifacts of the titanium screw could be effectively reduced using metal-artifact reduction sequences in MRI (WARP, mean reduction of 2.5 mm), there was no significant difference for the magnesium screw. Based on these results, it was concluded that (iv) magnesium Herbert screws show significantly fewer artifacts in DX, MDCT, FPCT and MRI in comparison to conventional titanium, (v) since biodegradable magnesium implants are commercially available in Europe and will now be increasingly used this knowledge is very important for postoperative imaging and (vi) further in vivo studies are required in order to depict and understand the degradation and resorption process. Intervertebral spacers are made of different materials, which can affect the postfusion MRI scans. Susceptibility artifacts especially for metallic implants can decrease the image quality. Accordingly, Ernstberger et al. [184] determined whether magnesium as a lightweight and biocompatible metal is suitable as a biomaterial for spinal implants based on its MRI artifacting behavior. To compare artifacting behaviors, different test spacers made of magnesium, titanium and carbon-fiber-reinforced thermoplastics (CFRP) were implanted into one cadaveric spine, as shown in Figure 17.7. All test spacers were scanned using two T1-TSE MRI sequences. The artifact dimensions were traced on all scans and statistically analyzed. MRI was performed with a 1.5 T MRI (Magnetom Symphony, Siemens AG Medical Solutions, Erlangen, Germany). The T1w-TSE sequences were used to acquire a slice thickness of 3 mm (see Figure 17.7) which included a first sequence (TR 600, TE 14, flip angle 15, band width 150) and a second sequence (TR 2,260, TE 14, flip angle 15, band width 150). A matrix of 512 × 512 pixels combined with a field of view of 500 mm was chosen for the study. It was reported that the total artifact volume and median artifact area of the titanium spacers were statistically significantly larger than magnesium spacers, while magnesium and CFRP spacers produced almost identical artifacting behaviors, suggesting that (i) spinal implants made with magnesium alloys will behave more like CFRP devices in MRI scans, (ii) given its osseoconductive potential as a metal, implant alloys made with magnesium would combine the advantages to the two principal spacer materials currently used but without their limitations, at least in terms of MRI artifacting.

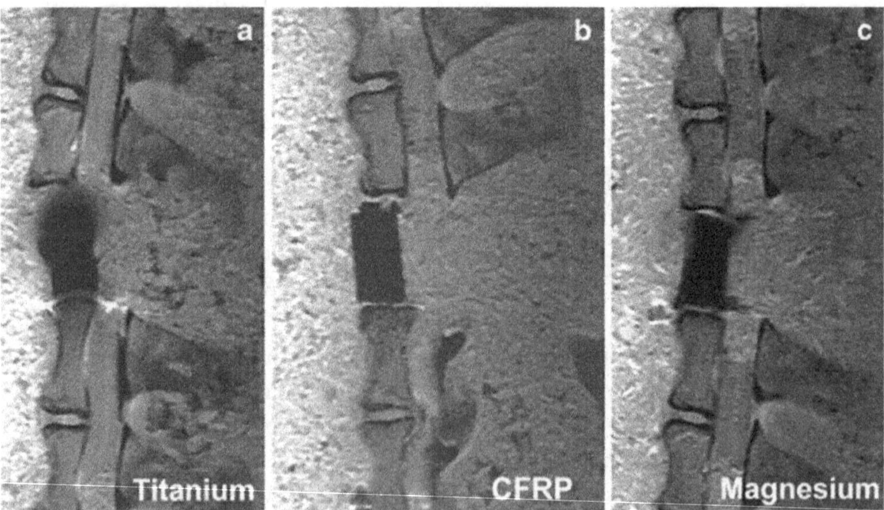

Figure 17.7: Median MRI artifact range depicted in a selection of three large test implants: (a) Ti-6Al-4V, (b) CFRP (carbon-fiber reinforced thermoplastic) and (c) AM50 (Mg-5Al-0.5Mn-0.2Zn) [184].

17.8.3 Indications and contraindications

There are different types of contraindications that would prevent a person from being examined with an MRI scanner. MRI systems use strong magnetic fields that attract any ferromagnetic objects with enormous force. Caused by the potential risk of heating, produced from the radio frequency pulses during the MRI procedure, metallic objects like wires, foreign bodies and other implants needs to be checked for compatibility. High field MRI requires particular safety precautions. In addition, any device or MRI equipment that enters the magnet room has to be MR compatible. MRI examinations are safe and harmless, if these MRI risks are observed. Safety concerns in MRI include: the magnetic field strength, possible missile effects caused by magnetic forces, the potential for heating of body tissue due to the application of radio frequency energy, the effects on implanted active devices such as cardiac pacemakers or insulin pumps, magnetic torque effects on indwelling metal (clips etc.), the audible acoustic noise, danger due to cryogenic liquids and the application of contrast medium.

MRI use is contraindicated for the following devices (except where noted) [185]:

- Cardiac pacemakers: are absolutely contraindicated; however, MRI-compatible pacemakers are being developed. A few pacemaker patients have been scanned for life-threatening situations or inadvertently. Subsequently, their pacemakers must be meticulously checked for function. Some deaths have been reported.
- Intracranial aneurysm clips: are contraindicated, unless the specific type of MRI-compatible clip can be absolutely documented.
- Neurostimulators/spinal-fusion stimulators: are generally contraindicated. There are two manufactures that are seeking FDA approval for usage of their product in MRI, but under strict guidelines.
- Drug fusion pumps: are generally contraindicated. There are two models (Synchro Med and Synchro Med EL) that are currently FDA approved with specific guidelines.
- Metallic foreign bodies: may or may not preclude MRI scanning depending on the type, size and location. These patients must be screened by X-ray. Detection should also target possible orbital metallic foreign bodies.
- Cochlear implants: contraindicated.
- Other otologic implants: generally, these are nonferromagnetic and MRI compatible. The exception is the McGee stapedectomy piston prosthesis – it is not MRI compatible.
- Dental implants: are generally compatible, except for those that contain magnetically activated components.
- Ocular implants: some are MRI compatible.
- Intravascular stents, filters and coils: most of these are compatible 6–8 weeks following placement, unless they are made of nonferrous metal, for example, titanium, in which case they can be imaged right after the placement. Drug-eluting

stents must be cleared by the implanting physician if they have been in less than 3 months.
- Vascular access ports and catheters: are compatible, excluding the Swan Ganz catheter.
- Penile implants: these are of mixed compatibility and should be checked.
- Orthopedic implants/prosthesis: are compatible, though MRI may cause local heating and MRI will cause local image artifact.
- Heart valve prosthesis: is compatible, but there is a prototype electromagnetically controlled heart valve that is being developed, which is contraindicated.
- Pacer wires (without pacemaker): to having an MRI compatibility is controversial, but they are probably fine at low MRI fields but questionable at high-field imaging. All patients must have a chest X-ray prior to having an MRI to ensure that the wires are not looped or crossed.
- Holter monitor: contraindicated.
- Ventricular-peritoneal shunts: compatible, except SOPHY-adjustable pressure valve type.
- Swan Ganz catheter: contraindicated. The thermal dilutor may melt.
- Dermal patches: can cause burns during MRI study and should be removed.
- Pessary and diaphragm: compatible, but it will produce local image artifact.
- Hearing aids: must be removed.
- Permanent eyeliner/tattoos: can cause local burns.
- Body rings/spikes: can cause local burns, dislodgment or artifacts. It is suggested to remove these devices under normal MRI or the use under low-field MR.
- Breast tissue expanders: not compatible.
- Bullets, shrapnel and pellets: depends on the foreign body's location and duration of the MRI. An X-ray is required before an MRI can be done.

References

[1] Trumbo P, Yates AA, Schlicker S, Poos M. Dietary reference intakes: vitamin A, vitamin K, arsenic, boron, chromium, copper, iodine, iron, manganese, molybdenum, nickel, silicon, vanadium, and zinc. Journal of the American Dietetic Association. 2001, 101, 294–301.
[2] Helmenstine AM. What Are the Elements in the Human Body? 2020; https://www.thoughtco.com/elements-in-the-human-body-p2-602188.
[3] https://steemkr.com/science/@techlife/how-the-essential-elements-for-life-were-created.
[4] Ware M. Why do we need magnesium? Medical News Today. 2020; https://www.medicalnewstoday.com/articles/286839.php.
[5] https://en.wikipedia.org/wiki/Magnesium#cite_note-57.
[6] Yamamoto A, Hiromoto S. Effect of inorganic salts, amino acids and proteins on the degradation of pure magnesium in vitro. Materials Science & Engineering C: Materials in Biological Applications. 2009, 29, 1559–68.

[7] Zheng Y. Magnesium Alloys as Degradable Biomaterials. CRC Press, Taylor & Francis, New York NY, 2016.
[8] Cocchioni M, Pellegrini MG, Grappasonni I, Vitali C, Marsili G. Daily intake of macro and trace elements in the diet. 4. Sodium, potassium, calcium, and magnesium. Annali Di Igiene. 1989, 1, 923–42.
[9] Seelig MS, Rosanoff A. The Magnesium Factor: How One Simple Nutrient Can Prevent, Treat, and Reverse High Blood Pressure, Heart Disease, Diabetes, and Other Chronic Conditions. Penguin Group, New York NY, 2003.
[10] Kalsner S. The effect of magnesium deficiency and excess on bovine coronary artery tone and responses to agonists. British Journal of Pharmacology. 1983, 78, 629–38.
[11] Karppanen H, Pennanen R, Passinen L. Minerals, coronary heart disease and sudden coronary death. Advanced Cariology. 1978, 25, 9–24.
[12] https://www.healthline.com/nutrition/magnesium-deficiency-symptoms.
[13] Strause L, Saltman P, Glowacki J. The effect of deficiencies of manganese and copper on osteoinduction and on resorption of bone particles in rats. Calcified Tissue International. 1987, 41, 145–50.
[14] Leone N, Courbon D, Ducimetiere P, Zureik M. Zinc, copper, and magnesium and risks for all-cause, cancer, and cardiovascular mortality. Epidemiology. 2006, 17, 308–14.
[15] Saris N-E, Mervaala E, Karppanen H, Khawaja JA, Lewenstam A. Magnesium. An update on physiological, clinical and analytical aspects. Clinica Chimica Acta. 2000, 294, 1–26.
[16] https://fcl-education.com/nutrition/nutrient/fcl-mineraru-magunesiumu/.
[17] Wang JL, Xu J-K, Hopkins C, Chow DHK, Qin L. Biodegradable Magnesium-Based Implants in Orthopedics – A General Review and Perspectives. Advanced Science. 2020; https://doi.org/10.1002/advs.201902443.
[18] Sezer N, Evis Z, Kayhan SM, Tahmasebifar A, Koç M. Review of magnesium-based biomaterials and their applications. Journal of Magnesium and Alloys. 2018, 6, 23–43.
[19] Walker J, Shadanbaz S, Woodfield TGF, Staiger MP, Dias GJ. Magnesium biomaterials for orthopedic application: A review from a biological perspective. Journal of Biomedical Materials Research B. 2014, 102, 1316–31.
[20] Chaya A, Yoshizawa S, Verdelis K, Myers N, Costello BJ, Chou D-T, Pal S, Maiti S, Kumta PN, Sfeir C. *In vivo* study of magnesium plate and screw degradation and bone fracture healing. Acta Biomaterialia. 2015, 18, 262–9.
[21] Qin H, Zhao Y, An Z, Cheng M, Yuan G. Enhanced antibacterial properties, biocompatibility, and corrosion resistance of degradable Mg-Nd-Zn-Zr alloy. Biomaterials. 2015, 53, 211–20.
[22] Feng Y, Zhu S, Wang L, Chang L, Guan S. Fabrication and characterization of biodegradable Mg-Zn-Y-Nd-Ag alloy: Microstructure, mechanical properties, corrosion behavior and antibacterial activities. Bioactive Materials. 2018, 3, 225–35.
[23] Gao Z, Song M, Liu R-L, Shen Y, Liu X. Improving in vitro and in vivo antibacterial functionality of Mg alloys through micro-alloying with Sr and Ga. Materials Science and Engineering: C. 2019, 104; https://doi.org/10.1016/j.msec.2019.109926.
[24] Sun J, Zhu Y, Meng L, Chen P, Zheng Y. Electrophoretic deposition of colloidal particles on Mg with cytocompatibility, antibacterial performance, and corrosion resistance. Acta Biomaterialia. 2016, 45, 387–98.
[25] Bakhsheshi-Rad HR, Akbari M, Ismail AF, Aziz M, Chen X. Coating biodegradable magnesium alloys with electrospun poly-L-lactic acid-åkermanite-doxycycline nanofibers for enhanced biocompatibility, antibacterial activity, and corrosion resistance. Surface & Coatings Technology. 2019, 377; https://doi.org/10.1016/j.surfcoat.2019.124898.

[26] Cui L-Y, Wei G-B, Han Z-Z, Zeng R-C, Guan S-K. In vitro corrosion resistance and antibacterial performance of novel tin dioxide-doped calcium phosphate coating on degradable Mg-1Li-1Ca alloy. Journal of Materials Science & Technology. 2019, 35, 254–65.
[27] Ji X-J, Gao L, Liu J-C, Jiang R-Z, Wang Z-L. Corrosion resistance and antibacterial activity of hydroxyapatite coating induced by ciprofloxacin-loaded polymeric multilayers on magnesium alloy. Progress in Organic Coatings. 2019, 135, 465–74.
[28] Chang WH, Qu B, Laio AD, Zhang SF, Xiang JH. In vitro biocompatibility and antibacterial behavior of anodic coatings fabricated in an organic phosphate containing solution on Mg–1.0Ca alloys. Surface & Coatings Technology. 2016, 289, 75–84.
[29] Yazici M, Gulec AE, Gurbuz M, Gencer Y, Tarakci M. Biodegradability and antibacterial properties of MAO coatings formed on Mg-Sr-Ca alloys in an electrolyte containing Ag doped hydroxyapatite. Thin Solid Films. 2017, 644, 92–8.
[30] Aktug SL, Surdu S, Aktas S, Yalcin E, Usta M. Surface and in vitro properties of Ag-deposited antibacterial and bioactive coatings on AZ31 Mg alloy. Surface & Coatings Technology. 2019, 375, 46–53.
[31] Yan X, Zhao M-C, Yang Y, Tan L, Atrens A. Improvement of biodegradable and antibacterial properties by solution treatment and micro-arc oxidation (MAO) of a magnesium alloy with a trace of copper. Corrosion Science. 2019, 156, 125–38.
[32] Oshida Y. Bioscience and Bioengineering of Titanium Materials. Elsevier, London UK, 2007.
[33] Wolff M, Schaper JG, Suckert MR, Dahms M, Ebel T, Willumeit-Römer R, Klassen T. Magnesium Powder Injection Molding (MIM) of Orthopedic Implants for Biomedical Applications. JOM. 2016, 68, 1191–7.
[34] Fan J, Qiu X, Niu X, Tian Z, Sun W, Liu X, Li Y, Li W, Meng J. Microstructure, mechanical properties, in vitro degradation and cytotoxicity evaluations of Mg–1.5Y–1.2Zn–0.44Zr alloys for biodegradable metallic implants. Materials Science and Engineering: C. 2013, 33, 2345–52.
[35] Huang Y, Liu D, Anguilano L, You D, Chen M. Fabrication and characterization of a biodegradable Mg–2Zn–0.5Ca/1β-TCP composite. Materials Science and Engineering: C. 2015, 54, 120–32.
[36] Charyeva O, Dakischew O, Sommer U, Heiss C, Schnettler R, Lips KS. Biocompatibility of magnesium implants in primary human reaming debris-derived cells stem cells in vitro. Journal of Orthopaedics and Traumatology : Official Journal of the Italian Society of Orthopaedics and Traumatology. 2016, 17, 63–73.
[37] Qiao LY, Gao JC, Wang Y, Wang SL, Wu S. Xue Y. Biocompatibility Evaluation of Magnesium-Based Materials. Materials Science Forum. 2006, 546/549, 459–62.
[38] Virtanen S, Fabry B. Corrosion, Surface Modification, and Biocompatibility of Mg and Mg Alloys. In: Sillekens et al. ed., Essential Readings in Magnesium Technology. Springer, Cham. 2016, pp 625–628.
[39] Tang M, Yan Y, Yang JO, Yu K, Liu C, Zhou X, Wang Z, Deng Y, Shuai C. Research on corrosion behavior and biocompatibility of a porous Mg–3%Zn/5%β-$Ca_3(PO_4)_2$ composite scaffold for bone tissue engineering. Journal of Applied Biomaterials & Functional Materials. 2019, 17; DOI: 10.1177/2280800019857064.
[40] Gu X, Zheng Y, Cheng Y, Zhong S, Xi T. In vitro corrosion and biocompatibility of binary magnesium alloys. Biomaterials. 2009, 30, 484–98.
[41] Chai H, Guo L, Wang X, Gao X, Liu K, Fu Y. Guan J, Tan L. In vitro and in vivo evaluations on osteogenesis and biodegradability of a β-tricalcium phosphate coated magnesium alloy. Journal of Biomedical Materials Research: A. 2012, 100, 293–304.

[42] Peng F, Wang D, Tian Y, Cao H, Qiao H, Liu X. Sealing the pores of PEO coating with Mg–Al layered double hydroxide: enhanced corrosion resistance, cytocompatibility and drug delivery ability. Scientific Reports. 2017, 7; https://doi.org/10.1038/s41598-017-08238-w.
[43] Pan CJ, Hou Y, Wang YN, Gao F, Liu T, Hou YH, Zhu YF, Ye W, Wang LR. Effects of self-assembly of 3-phosphonopropionic acid, 3-aminopropyltrimethoxysilane and dopamine on the corrosion behaviors and biocompatibility of a magnesium alloy. Materials Science & Engineering C-Materials for Biological Applications. 2016, 67, 132–43.
[44] Kim J, Mousa HM, Park CH, Kim CS. Enhanced corrosion resistance and biocompatibility of AZ31 Mg alloy using PCL/ZnO NPs via electrospinning. Applied Surface Science. 2017, 396, 249–58.
[45] Hou X, Qin H, Gao H, Mankoci S, Ye C. A systematic study of mechanical properties, corrosion behavior and biocompatibility of AZ31B Mg alloy after ultrasonic nanocrystal surface modification. Materials Science and Engineering: C. 2017, 78, 1061–71.
[46] Lu JZ, Joshi SS, Pantawane MV, Ho Y-H, Dahotre NB. Optimization of biocompatibility in a laser surface treated Mg-AZ31B alloy. Materials Science and Engineering: C, 2019, 105; https://doi.org/10.1016/j.msec.2019.110028.
[47] Ding P, Liu Y, He X, Liu D, Chen M. In vitro and in vivo biocompatibility of Mg–Zn–Ca alloy operative clip. Bioactive Materials. 2019, 4, 236–44.
[48] Wong CC, Wong PC, Tsai PH, Jang JS, Cheng CK, Chen HH, Chen CH. Biocompatibility and osteogenic capacity of Mg-Zn-Ca bulk metallic glass for rabbit tendon-bone interference fixation. International Journal of Molecular Sciences. 2019, 20; doi: 10.3390/ijms20092191.
[49] Zhao N, Watson N, Xu Z, Chen Y, Waterman J, Sankar J, Zhu D. In vitro biocompatibility and endothelialization of novel magnesium-rare Earth alloys for improved stent applications. PLoS One. 2014, 9; doi: 10.1371/journal.pone.0098674.
[50] Dziuba D, Meyer-Lindenberg A, Seitz JM, Waizy H, Angrisani N, Reifenrath J. Long-term in vivo degradation behaviour and biocompatibility of the magnesium alloy ZEK100 for use as a biodegradable bone implant. Acta Biomaterialia. 2013, 9, 8548–60.
[51] Li T, He Y, Zhou J, Tang S, Wang X. Effects of scandium addition on biocompatibility of biodegradable Mg–1.5Zn–0.6Zr Alloy. Materials Letters. 2015, 215, 200–2.
[52] Wang T, Yang G, Zhou W, Hu J, Lu W. One-pot hydrothermal synthesis, in vitro biodegradation and biocompatibility of Sr-doped nanorod/nanowire hydroxyapatite coatings on ZK60 magnesium alloy. Journal of Alloys and Compounds. 2019, 799, 71–82.
[53] Gu XN, Li N, Zheng YF, Ruan L. In vitro degradation performance and biological response of a Mg–Zn–Zr alloy. Materials Science and Engineering: B. 2011, 176, 1778–84.
[54] Zhang E, Xu L, Pan F, Yang K. In vivo evaluation of biodegradable magnesium alloy bone implant in the first 6 months implantation. Journal of Biomedical Materials Research. Part A. 2009, 90A, 882–93.
[55] Jaiswal S, Kumar RM, Gupta P, Kumaraswamy M, Lahiri D. Mechanical, corrosion and biocompatibility behaviour of Mg-3Zn-HA biodegradable composites for orthopaedic fixture accessories. Journal of the Mechanical Behavior of Biomedical Materials. 2018, 78, 442–54.
[56] Scheideler L, Füger C, Schille C, Rupp F, Geis-Gerstorfer J. Comparison of different in vitro tests for biocompatibility screening of Mg alloys. Acta Biomaterialia. 2013, 9, 8740–5.
[57] Mohamed A, El-Aziz AM, Breitinger H-G. Study of the degradation behavior and the biocompatibility of Mg–0.8Ca alloy for orthopedic implant applications. Journal of Magnesium and Alloys. 2019, 7, 249–57.
[58] Li Z, Gu X, Lou S, Zheng Y. The development of binary Mg–Ca alloys for use as biodegradable materials within bone. Biomaterials. 2008, 29, 1329–44.

[59] Fernandes D, Resende C, Cavalcanti J, Liu D, Elias C. Biocompatibility of bioabsorbable Mg-Ca alloys with rare earth elements addition. Journal of Materials Science. Materials in Medicine. 2019, 30, 134; doi: 10.1007/s10856-019-6330-y.

[60] Harandi SE, Mirshahi M, Koleini S, Idris MH, Jafari S, Kadir MRA. Effect of calcium content on the microstructure, hardness and in-vitro corrosion behavior of biodegradable Mg-Ca binary alloy. Materials Research. 2013, 16; http://dx.doi.org/10.1590/S1516-14392012005000151.

[61] Zhou WR, Zheng YF, Leeflang MA, Zhou J. Mechanical property, biocorrosion and in vitro biocompatibility evaluations of Mg–Li–(Al)–(RE) alloys for future cardiovascular stent application. Acta Biomaterialia. 2013, 9, 8488–98.

[62] Zhou Y-L, Li Y, Luo D-M, Ding Y, Hodgson P. Microstructures, mechanical and corrosion properties and biocompatibility of as extruded Mg–Mn–Zn–Nd alloys for biomedical applications. Materials Science and Engineering: C. 2015, 49, 93–100.

[63] Wang Y, Lim CS, Lim CV, Yong MS, Teo EK, Moh LN. In vitro degradation behavior of M1A magnesium alloy in protein-containing simulated body fluid. Materials Science & Engineering. C, Materials for Biological Applications. 2011, 31, 579–87.

[64] Li Y, Wen C, Mushahary D, Sravanthi R, Harishankar N, Pande G, Hodgson P. Mg–Zr–Sr alloys as biodegradable implant materials. Acta Biomaterialia. 2012, 8, 3177–88.

[65] Ma C, Peng G, Nie L, Liu H, Guan Y. Laser surface modification of Mg-Gd-Ca alloy for corrosion resistance and biocompatibility enhancement. Applied Surface Science. 2018, 445, 211–6.

[66] Zhang J, Guan Y, Lin W, Gu X. Enhanced mechanical properties and biocompatibility of Mg-Gd-Ca alloy by laser surface processing. Surface & Coatings Technology. 2019, 362, 176–84.

[67] Qin H, Zhao Y, An Z, Cheng M, Yuan G. Enhanced antibacterial properties, biocompatibility, and corrosion resistance of degradable Mg-Nd-Zn-Zr alloy. Biomaterials. 2015, 53, 211–20.

[68] Mao L, Zhou H, Chen L, Niu J, Song C, Li Q, Huang GJ, Huang XD, Pan SW, Liu Q. Enhanced biocompatibility and long-term durability in vivo of Mg-Nd-Zn-Zr alloy for vascular stent application. Journal of Alloys and Compounds. 2017, 720, 245–53.

[69] Niu J, Yuan G, Liao Y, Mao L, Ding W. Enhanced biocorrosion resistance and biocompatibility of degradable Mg–Nd–Zn–Zr alloy by brushite coating. Materials Science and Engineering: C. 2013, 33, 4833–41.

[70] Peng F, Li H, Wang D, Tan P, Tian Y, Yuan G, Xu D, Liu X. Enhanced corrosion resistance and biocompatibility of magnesium alloy by Mg–Al-layered double hydroxide. ACS Applied Materials & Interfaces. 2016, 8, 51, 35033–44.

[71] Bornapour M, Muja N, Shum-Tim D, Cerruti M, Pekguleryuz M. Biocompatibility and biodegradability of Mg–Sr alloys: The formation of Sr-substituted hydroxyapatite. Acta Biomaterialia. 2013, 9, 5319–30.

[72] Bornapour M, Mahjoubi H, Vali H, Shum-Tim D, Pekguleryuz M. Surface characterization, in vitro and in vivo biocompatibility of Mg-0.3Sr-0.3Ca for temporary cardiovascular implant. Materials Science and Engineering: C. 2016, 67, 72–84.

[73] Yang Q, Yuan W, Lium X, Zheng Y, Wu S. Atomic layer deposited ZrO2 nanofilm on Mg-Sr alloy for enhanced corrosion resistance and biocompatibility. Acta Biomaterialia. 2017, 58, 515–26.

[74] Gu XN, Zhou WR, Zheng YF, Liu Y, Li YX. Degradation and cytotoxicity of lotus-type porous pure magnesium as potential tissue engineering scaffold material. Materials Letters. 2010, 64, 1871–4.

[75] Liu H. The effects of surface and biomolecules on magnesium degradation and mesenchymal stem cell adhesion. Journal of Biomedical Materials Research. Part A. 2011, 99, 249–60.

[76] Geng F, Tan LL, Jin XX, Yang JY, Yang K. The preparation, cytocompatibility, and in vitro biodegradation study of pure β-TCP on magnesium. Journal of Materials Science. Materials in Medicine. 2009, 20, 1149–57.
[77] Xu L, Yamamoto A. Characteristics and cytocompatibility of biodegradable polymer film on magnesium by spin coating. Colloids and Surfaces. B, Biointerfaces. 2012, 93, 67–74.
[78] Wang Q, Jin S, Lin X, Zhang Y, Yang K. Cytotoxic effects of biodegradation of pure Mg and MAO-Mg on tumor cells of MG63 and KB. Journal of Materials Science & Technology. 2014, 30, 487–92.
[79] Wagener V, Schilling A, Mainka A, Hennig D, Gerum R, Kelch ML, Keim S, Fabry B, Virtanen S. Cell Adhesion on Surface-Functionalized Magnesium. ACS Applied Materials & Interfaces. 2016, 8, 11998–2006.
[80] Li L, Gao J, Wang Y. Evaluation of cytotoxicity and corrosion behavior of alkali-heat-treated magnesium in simulated body fluid. Surface & Coatings Technology. 2004, 185, 92–8.
[81] Tavares DS, Castro LO, Soares GDA, Alves GG, Granjeiro JM. Synthesis and cytotoxicity evaluation of granular magnesium substituted β-tricalcium phosphate. Journal of Applied Oral Science. 2013, 21, 37–42.
[82] Wang Q, Tan L, Yang K. Cytocompatibility and Hemolysis of AZ31B Magnesium Alloy with Si-containing Coating. Journal of Materials Science & Technology. 2015, 31, 845–51.
[83] Wang C, Shen J, Zhang X, Duan B, Sang J. In vitro degradation and cytocompatibility of a silane/Mg(OH)2 composite coating on AZ31 alloy by spin coating. Journal of Alloys and Compounds. 2017, 714, 186–93.
[84] Mochizuki A, Yahata C, Takai H. Cytocompatibility of magnesium and AZ31 alloy with three types of cell lines using a direct in vitro method. Journal of Materials Science. Materials in Medicine. 2016, 27; https://doi.org/10.1007/s10856-016-5762-x.
[85] Zhu B, Wang S, Wang L, Yang Y, Liang J, Cao B. Preparation of hydroxyapatite/tannic acid coating to enhance the corrosion resistance and cytocompatibility of AZ31 magnesium alloys. Coatings. 2017, 7; https://doi.org/10.3390/coatings7070105.
[86] Lopes DR, Silva CLP, Soares RB, Pereira PHR, Oliveira AC, Figueiredo RB, Langdon TG, Lins VFC. Cytotoxicity and corrosion behavior of magnesium and magnesium alloys in Hank's solution after processing by high-pressure torsion. Advanced Materials Engineering. 2019, 21; https://doi.org/10.1002/adem.201900391.
[87] Niederlaender J, Rudi P, Schweizer E. Cytocompatibility of magnesium alloys with adult human endothelial cells. Emerging Materials Research. 2013, 2, 274–82.
[88] Xin Y, Jiang J, Huo K, Tang G, Tian X, Chu PK. Corrosion resistance and cytocompatibility of biodegradable surgical magnesium alloy coated with hydrogenated amorphous silicon. Journal of Biomedical Materials Research. Part A. 2009, 89A, 717–26.
[89] Shi W, Zhao D, Shang P, Nie H, Tang J. Strontium-doped Hydroxyapatite Coatings Deposited on Mg-4Zn Alloy: Physical-chemical Properties and in vitro Cell Response. Rare Metal Materials and Engineering. 2018, 47, 2371–80.
[90] Zhang S, Zheng Y, Zhang L, Bi Y, Li Y. In vitro and in vivo corrosion and histocompatibility of pure Mg and a Mg-6Zn alloy as urinary implants in rat model. Materials Science and Engineering: C. 2016, 68, 414–22.
[91] Ye X, Chen M, Yang M, Wei J, Liu D. In vitro corrosion resistance and cytocompatibility of nano-hydroxyapatite reinforced Mg–Zn–Zr composites. Journal of Materials Science. Materials in Medicine. 2010, 21, 1321–8.
[92] Huan ZG, Leeflang MA, Zhou J. Fratila-APachitei LE, Duszczyk J. In vitro degradation behavior and cytocompatibility of Mg–Zn–Zr alloys. Journal of Materials Science. Materials in Medicine. 2010, 21, 2623–35.

[93] Jin W, Wang G, Kin Z, Feng H, Li W, Peng X, Qasim AM, Chu PK. Corrosion resistance and cytocompatibility of tantalum-surface-functionalized biomedical ZK60 Mg alloy. Corrosion Science. 2017, 114, 45–56.

[94] Hong D, Saha P, Chou D-T, Lee B, Collins BE, Tan Z, Dong Z, Kumta PN. In vitro degradation and cytotoxicity response of Mg–4% Zn–0.5% Zr (ZK40) alloy as a potential biodegradable material. Acta Biomaterialia. 2013, 9, 8534–47.

[95] Yang H, Xia K, Wang T, Niu J, Song Y, Xiong Z, Zheng K, Wei S, Lu W. Growth, in vitro biodegradation and cytocompatibility properties of nano-hydroxyapatite coatings on biodegradable magnesium alloys. Journal of Alloys and Compounds. 2016, 672, 366–73.

[96] Wang B, Huang P, Ou C, Li K, Yan B, Lu W. In vitro corrosion and cytocompatibility of ZK60 magnesium alloy coated with hydroxyapatite by a simple chemical conversion process for orthopedic applications. International Journal of Molecular Science 2013, 14, 23614–28.

[97] Witecka A, Yamamoto A, Idaszek J, Chlanda A, Święszkowski W. Influence of biodegradable polymer coatings on corrosion, cytocompatibility and cell functionality of Mg-2.0Zn-0.98Mn magnesium alloy. Colloids and Surfaces. B, Biointerfaces. 2016, 144, 284–92.

[98] He R, Liu R, Chen Q, Zhang H, Wang J, Guo S. In vitro degradation behavior and cytocompatibility of Mg-6Zn-Mn alloy. Materials Letters. 2018, 228, 77–80.

[99] Li D, Yuan Q, Yu K, Xiao T, Li A. Mg–Zn–Mn alloy extract induces the angiogenesis of human umbilical vein endothelial cells via FGF/FGFR signaling pathway. Biochemical and Biophysical Research Communications. 2019, 514, 618–24.

[100] Du H, Wei Z, Wang H, Zhang E, Du L. Surface microstructure and cell compatibility of calcium silicate and calcium phosphate composite coatings on Mg–Zn–Mn–Ca alloys for biomedical application. Colloids and Surfaces. B, Biointerfaces. 2011, 83, 96–102.

[101] Li H, Peng Q, Li X, Li K, Fang D. Microstructures, mechanical and cytocompatibility of degradable Mg–Zn based orthopedic biomaterials. Materials & Design. 2014, 58, 43–51.

[102] Cipriano AF, Zhao T, Johnson I, Guan R-G, Garcia S, Liu H. In vitro degradation of four magnesium–zinc–strontium alloys and their cytocompatibility with human embryonic stem cells. Journal of Materials Science. Materials in Medicine. 2013, 24, 989–1003.

[103] Cipriano AF, Sallee A, Tayoba M, Cortez Alcaraz MC, Lin A, Guan RG, Zhao ZY, Liu H. Cytocompatibility and early inflammatory response of human endothelial cells in direct culture with Mg-Zn-Sr alloys. Acta Biomaterialia. 2017, 48, 499–520.

[104] Cipriano AF, Sallee A, Guan RG, Lin A, Liu H. A Comparison Study on the Degradation and Cytocompatibility of Mg-4Zn-xSr Alloys in Direct Culture. ACS Biomaterial Science and Engineering 2017, 3, 540–50.

[105] Tian Q, Zhang C, Deo M, Rivera-Castaneda L, Liu H. Responses of human urothelial cells to magnesium-zinc-strontium alloys and associated insoluble degradation products for urological stent applications. Materials Science and Engineering: C. 2019, 96, 248–62.

[106] Anvari-Yazdi AF, Tahermanesh K, Mehdi Hadavi SM, Talaei-Khozani T, Razmkhah M, Abed SM, Mohtasebi MS. Cytotoxicity assessment of adipose-derived mesenchymal stem cells on synthesized biodegradable Mg-Zn-Ca alloys. Materials Science & Engineering. C, Materials for Biological Applications. 2016. 69, 584–97.

[107] Sun Y, Zhang B, Wang Y, Geng L, Jiao X. Preparation and characterization of a new biomedical Mg–Zn–Ca alloy. Materials & Design. 2012, 34, 58–64.

[108] Homayun B, Afshar A. Microstructure, mechanical properties, corrosion behavior and cytotoxicity of Mg–Zn–Al–Ca alloys as biodegradable materials. Journal of Alloys and Compounds. 2014, 607, 1–10.

[109] Xia Y, Zhang B, Wang Y, Qian M, Geng L. In-vitro cytotoxicity and in-vivo biocompatibility of as-extruded Mg–4.0Zn–0.2Ca alloy. Materials Science and Engineering: C. 2012, 32, 665–9.

[110] Pellicer E, González S, Blanquer A, Baró MD, Barrios L, Ibáñez E, Nogués C, Sort J. On the biodegradability, mechanical behavior, and cytocompatibility of amorphous $Mg_{72}Zn_{23}Ca_5$ and crystalline $Mg_{70}Zn_{23}Ca_5Pd_2$ alloys as temporary implant materials. Journal of Biomedicine MaterialvResearch Part A. 2013, 101A, 502–17.

[111] Kang Y, Du B, Li Y, Wang B, Xi T. Optimizing mechanical property and cytocompatibility of the biodegradable Mg-Zn-Y-Nd alloy by hot extrusion and heat treatment. Journal of Materials Science & Technology. 2019, 35, 6–18.

[112] Song X, Chang L, Wang J, Zhu S, Wang L, Feng K, Luo Y, Guan S. Investigation on the *in vitro* cytocompatibility of Mg-Zn-Y-Nd-Zr alloys as degradable orthopaedic implant materials. Journal of Material Science: Material of Medicine. 2018, 29; https://doi.org/10.1007/s10856-018-6050-8

[113] Jiang W, Wang J, Zhao W, Liu Q, Guo S. Effect of Sn addition on the mechanical properties and bio-corrosion behavior of cytocompatible Mg–4Zn based alloys. Journal of Magnesium and Alloys. 2019, 7, 15–26.

[114] Jia ZJ, Li M, Liu Q, Xu XC, Wei SC. Micro-arc oxidization of a novel Mg–1Ca alloy in three alkaline KF electrolytes: Corrosion resistance and cytotoxicity. Applied Surface Science. 2014, 292, 1030–9.

[115] Zhao Y, Jamesh MI, Li WK, Wu G, Wang C, Zheng Y, Yeung KWK, Chu PK. Enhanced antimicrobial properties, cytocompatibility, and corrosion resistance of plasma-modified biodegradable magnesium alloys. Acta Biomaterialia. 2014, 10, 544–56.

[116] Liu Y, Bian D, Wu Y, Li N, Qiu K, Zheng Y, Han Y.Influence of biocompatible metal ions (Ag, Fe, Y) on the surface chemistry, corrosion behavior and cytocompatibility of Mg–1Ca alloy treated with MEVVA. Colloids and Surfaces. B, Biointerfaces. 2015, 133, 99–107

[117] Liu J, Zheng Y, Bi Y, Li Y, Zheng Y. Improved cytocompatibility of Mg-1Ca alloy modified by Zn ion implantation and deposition. Materials Letters. 2017, 205, 87–9.

[118] Neacsu P, Staras AI, Voicu SI, Inoascu I, Soare T, Uzun S, Cojocaru VD, Pandele AM, Croitoru SM, Miculescu F, Cotrut CM, Dan I, Cimpean A. Characterization and In Vitro and In Vivo Assessment of a Novel Cellulose Acetate-Coated Mg-Based Alloy for Orthopedic Applications. Materials (Basel). 2017, 10; doi: 10.3390/ma10070686.

[119] Bakhsheshi-Rad HR, Hamzah E, Jabbarzare KSS, Najafinezhad A. Fabrication, degradation behavior and cytotoxicity of nanostructured hardystonite and titania/hardystonite coatings on Mg alloys. Vacuum. 2016, 129, 9–12.

[120] Bakhsheshi-Rad HR, Hadisi Z, Hamzah E, Ismail AF, Kashefian M. Drug delivery and cytocompatibility of ciprofloxacin loaded gelatin nanofibers-coated Mg alloy. Materials Letters. 2017, 207, 179–82.

[121] Bakhsheshi-Rad HR, Hamzah E, Staiger MP, Dias GJ. Drug release, cytocompatibility, bioactivity, and antibacterial activity of doxycycline loaded Mg-Ca-TiO2 composite scaffold. Materials & Design. 2018, 139, 212–21.

[122] Zeng RC, Cui L, Jiang K, Liu R, Zhao BD, Zheng Y-F. In Vitro Corrosion and Cytocompatibility of a Microarc Oxidation Coating and Poly(L-lactic acid) Composite Coating on Mg–1Li–1Ca Alloy for Orthopedic Implants. ACS Applied Materials & Interfaces. 2016, 8, 10014–28.

[123] Liu Y, Wu Y, Bian D, Gao S, Zhou J. Study on the Mg-Li-Zn ternary alloy system with improved mechanical properties, good degradation performance and different responses to cells. Acta Biomaterialia. 2017, 62, 418–33.

[124] Tie D, Feyerabend F, Müller WD, Schade R, Liefeith K, Kainer KU, Willumeit R. Antibacterial biodegradable Mg-Ag alloys. European Cells & Materials. 2013, 25, 284–98.

[125] Mostofi S, Bonyadi Rad E, Wiltsche H, Fasching U, Szakacs G, Ramskogler C, Srinivasaiah S, Ueçal M, Willumeit R, Weinberg AM, Schaefer U. Effects of Corroded and Non-Corroded Biodegradable Mg and Mg Alloys on Viability, Morphology and Differentiation of MC3T3-E1

Cells Elicited by Direct Cell/Material Interaction. PLoS One. 2016, 11; doi: 10.1371/journal.pone.0159879.

[126] Liu Z, Schade R, Luthringer B, Hort N, Rothe H, Müller S, Liefeith K, Willumeit-Römer R, Feyerabend F. Influence of the microstructure and silver content on degradation, cytocompatibility, and antibacterial properties of magnesium-silver alloys in vitro. Oxidative Medicine and Cellular Longevity. 2017; https://doi.org/10.1155/2017/8091265.

[127] Chou D-T, Hong D, Saha P, Ferrero J, Kumta PN. In vitro and in vivo corrosion, cytocompatibility and mechanical properties of biodegradable Mg–Y–Ca–Zr alloys as implant materials. Acta Biomaterialia. 2013, 9, 8518–33.

[128] Li F, Guo P, Han S, Xu C, Kuan J. A novel magnesium alloy with enhanced mechanical property, degradation behavior and cytocompatibility. Materials Letters. 2019, 244, 70–73.

[129] Guo M, Cao L, Lu P, Liu Y, Xu X, Anticorrosion and cytocompatibility behavior of MAO/PLLA modified magnesium alloy WE42. Journal of Materials Science. Materials in Medicine. 2011, 22, 1735–40.

[130] Smola B, Joska L, Březina V, Stulíková I, Hnilica F. Microstructure, corrosion resistance and cytocompatibility of Mg–5Y–4Rare Earth–0.5 Zr (WE54) alloy. Materials Science and Engineering: C. 2012, 32, 659–64.

[131] Ercetin A, Özgün Ö, Aslantas K, Aykutoğlu G. The microstructure, degradation behavior and cytotoxicity effect of Mg–Sn–Zn alloys in vitro tests. SN Applied Sciences. 2020, 2; https://doi.org/10.1007/s42452-020-1988-9.

[132] Zhou Y-Z, Wu P, Yang Y, Gao D, Feng P, Gao C, Wu H, Liu Y, Bian H, Shuai C. The microstructure, mechanical properties and degradation behavior of laser-melted MgSn alloys. Journal of Alloys and Compounds. 2016, 687, 109–14.

[133] Shuai C, Zhou Y, Lin X, Yang Y, Gao C, Shuai X, Wu H, Liu X, Wu P, Feng P. Preparation and characterization of laser-melted Mg–Sn–Zn alloys for biomedical application. Journal of Materials Science. Materials in Medicine. 2017, 28, 1–8.

[134] Zhao C, Pan F, Zhao S, Pan H, Song K, Tang A. Microstructure, corrosion behavior and cytotoxicity of biodegradable Mg–Sn implant alloys prepared by sub-rapid solidification. Materials Science and Engineering: C. 2015, 54, 245–51.

[135] Levy GK, Ventura Y, Goldman J, Vago R, Aghion E. Cytotoxic characteristics of biodegradable EW10X04 Mg alloy after Nd coating and subsequent heat treatment. Materials Science and Engineering: C. 2016, 62, 752–61.

[136] Grillo CA, Alvarez F, de Mele MAFL. Cellular response to rare earth mixtures (La and Gd) as components of degradable Mg alloys for medical applications. Colloids and Surfaces. B, Biointerfaces. 2014, 117, 312–21.

[137] Weizbauer A, Seitz J-M, Werle P, Hegermann J, Waizy H. Novel magnesium alloy Mg–2La caused no cytotoxic effects on cells in physiological conditions. Materials Science and Engineering: C. 2014, 41, 267–73.

[138] Yang L, Hort N, Laipple D, Höche D, Huang Y, Kainer KU, Willumeit R, Feyerabend F. Element distribution in the corrosion layer and cytotoxicity of alloy Mg–10Dy during in vitro biodegradation. Acta Biomaterialia. 2013, 9, 8475–87.

[139] Niederlaender J, Walter M, Krajewski S, Schweizer E, Post M, Schille C, Geis-Gerstorfer J. Wendel HP. Cytocompatibility evaluation of different biodegradable magnesium alloys with human mesenchymal stem cells. Journal of Materials Science. Materials in Medicine. 2014, 25, 835–43.

[140] Zhang J, Kong N, Niu J, Shi Y, Li H, Zhou Y, Yuan G. Influence of fluoride treatment on surface properties, biodegradation and cytocompatibility of Mg–Nd–Zn–Zr alloy. Journal of Materials Science. Materials in Medicine. 2014, 25, 791–9.

[141] Jin L, Wu J, Yuan G, Chen T. In vitro study of the inflammatory cells response to biodegradable Mg-based alloy extract. PLoS One. 2018, 13: doi: 10.1371/journal.pone.0193276.
[142] Shangguan Y, Sun L, Wan P, Tan L, Yang K. Comparison study of different coatings on degradation performance and cell response of Mg-Sr alloy. Materials Science and Engineering: C. 2016, 69, 95–107.
[143] Zhao C, Pan F, Zhang L, Pan H, Tang A. Microstructure, mechanical properties, bio-corrosion properties and cytotoxicity of as-extruded Mg-Sr alloys. Materials Science and Engineering: C. 2017, 70, 1081–8.
[144] Zhang X, Wu Y, Xue Y, Wang Z, Yang L. Biocorrosion behavior and cytotoxicity of a Mg–Gd–Zn–Zr alloy with long period stacking ordered structure. Materials Letters. 2012, 86, 42–5.
[145] Sanchez AM, Feyerabend F, Laipple D, Willumeit-Römer R, Luthringer BJC. Chondrogenic differentiation of ATDC5-cells under the influence of Mg and Mg alloy degradation. Materials Science and Engineering: C. 2017, 72, 378–88.
[146] Kumar R, Kalmodia S, Nath S, Singh D, Basu B. Phase assemblage study and cytocompatibility property of heat treated potassium magnesium phosphate–silicate ceramics. Journal of Materials Science. Materials in Medicine. 2009, 20. 1689–95.
[147] Ong THD, Yu N, Meenashisundaram GK, Schaller B, Gupta M. Insight into cytotoxicity of Mg nanocomposites using MTT assay technique. Materials Science and Engineering: C. 2017, 78, 647–52.
[148] Del Campo R, Savoini B, Jordao L, Muñoz A, Monge MA. Cytocompatibility, biofilm assembly and corrosion behavior of Mg-HAP composites processed by extrusion. Materials Science and Engineering: C. 2017, 78, 667–73.
[149] Bakhsheshi-Rad HR, Hamzah E, Ismail AF, Aziz M, Chami A. In vitro degradation behavior, antibacterial activity and cytotoxicity of TiO2-MAO/ZnHA composite coating on Mg alloy for orthopedic implants. Surface & Coatings Technology. 2018, 334, 450–60.
[150] Weber M, Steinle H, Golombek S, Hann L, Schlensak C, Wendel HP, Avci-Adali M. Blood-contacting biomaterials: *in vitro* evaluation of the hemocompatibility. Frontiers in Bioengineering and Biotechnology. 2018, 6: https://doi.org/10.3389/fbioe.2018.00099
[151] Liu X, Yuan L, Li D, Tang Z, Wang Y, Chen G, Chen H, Brash JL. Blood compatible materials: state of the art. Journal of Materials Chemistry B. 2014, 2, 5718–38.
[152] https://medical-dictionary.thefreedictionary.com/erythrocyte.
[153] Lu P, Cao L. Liu Y, Xu X, Wu X. Evaluation of magnesium ions release, biocorrosion, and hemocompatibility of MAO/PLLA-modified magnesium alloy WE42. Journal of Biomedical Materials Research. Part B, Applied Biomaterials. 2011, 96, 101–9.
[154] Ma J, Zhao N, Betts L, Zhu D. Bio-adaption between magnesium alloy stent and the blood vessel: a review. Journal of Materials Science & Technology. 2016, 32, 815–26.
[155] Chen Y, Qian H, Wang X, Liu P, Yan G, Huang L, Yi J. To improve corrosion resistance and hemocompatibility of magnesium alloy via cathodic plasma electrolytic deposition combined with surface thiol-ene photopolymerization. Materials Letters. 2015, 158, 178–81.
[156] Kröger N, Kopp A, Staudt M, Rusu M, Schuh A, Liehn EA. Hemocompatibility of plaa electrolytic oxidation (PEO) coated Mg-RE and Mg-Zn-Ca alloys for vascular scaffold applications. Materials Science & Engineering. C, Materials for Biological Applications. 2018, 92, 819–26.
[157] Rezaei, M., Tamjid, E. & Dinari, A. Enhanced cell attachment and hemocompatibility of titanium by nanoscale surface modification through severe plastic integration of magnesium-rich islands and porosification. Scientific Reports. 2017, 7; doi: 10.1038/s41598-017-13169-7.

[158] Wang P, Xion P, Liu J, Gao S, Xi T, Cheng Y. A silk-based coating containing GREDVY peptide and heparin on Mg–Zn–Y–Nd alloy: improved corrosion resistance, hemocompatibility and endothelialization. Journal of Material Chemistry B. 2018, 6, 966–78.
[159] Albrektsson T. Direct bone anchorage of dental implants. Journal Prosthetic Dentistry. 1983, 50, 255–261.
[160] Merritt K, Edwards CR, Brown SA. Use of an enzyme linked immunosorbent assay (ELISA) for quantification of proteins on the surface of materials. Journal of Biomedical Materials Research. 1988, 22, 99–109.
[161] Bothe RT, Beaton LE, Davenport HA. Reaction of bone to multiple metallic implants. Surgery, Gynecology & Obstetrics. 1940, 71, 598–602.
[162] Brånemark P-I, Hansson BO, Adell R, Briene U, Lindstrom J, Hallen O, Ohman A. Osseointegrated implants in the treatment of the edentulous jaw. Experience from a 10-year period. Scandinavian Journal of Plastic and Reconstructive Surgery and Hand Surgery. Supplementum. 1977, 16, 1–132.
[163] Misch CE, Misch CM. Generic root form component terminology. In: Implant Dentistry. Misch CE, editor. Mosby: An Affiliate of Elsevier. 1999. pp.13–15.
[164] Brånemark R, Brånemark P-I, Rydevik B, Myers RR. Osseointegration in skeletal reconstruction and rehabilitation. Journal of Rehabilitation Research and Development. 2001, 38, 175–82.
[165] Zhang X, Zu H, Zhao D, Yang K, Zhang Z. Ion channel functional protein kinase TRPM7 regulates Mg ions to promote the osteoinduction of human osteoblast via PI3K pathway: In vitrosimulation of the bone-repairing effect of Mg-based alloy implant. Acta Biomaterialia. 2017, 63, 369–82.
[166] Castellani C, Lindtner RA, Hausbrandt P, Tschegg E, Stanzl-Tschegg SE, Zanoni G, Beck S, Weinberg AM. Bone-implant interface strength and osseointegration: Biodegradable magnesium alloy versus standard titanium control. Acta Biomaterialia. 2011, 7, 432–40.
[167] Trincă LC, Fântânariu M, Solcan C, Trofin AE, Munteanu C. In vivo degradation behavior and biological activity of some new Mg–Ca alloys with concentration's gradient of Si for bone grafts. Applied Surface Science. 2015, 352, 140–50.
[168] Mushahary D, Wen C, Kumar JM, Lin J, Harishankar N, Hodgson P, Pande G, Li Y. Collagen type-I leads to *in vivo* matrix mineralization and secondary stabilization of Mg–Zr–Ca alloy implants. Colloids Surfaces B: Biointerfaces. 2014, 122, 719–28.
[169] Li H, He W, Pang S, Liaw PK, Zhang T. In vitro responses of bone-forming MC3T3-E1 pre-osteoblasts to biodegradable Mg-based bulk metallic glasses. Materials Science & Engineering. C, Materials for Biological Applications. 2016, 68, 632–41.
[170] Torroni A, Xiang C, Witek L, Rodriguez ED, Coelho PG. Histo-morphologic characteristics of intra-osseous implants of WE43 Mg alloys with and without heat treatment in an in vivo cranial bone sheep model. Journal of Cranio-Maxillofacial Surgery. 2018, 46, 473–8.
[171] Lauterbur PC. Image formation by induced local interactions: Example employing nuclear magnetic resonance. Nature. 1973, 242, 190–1.
[172] Shellock FG, Crues JV. High field strength MR imaging and metallic biomedical implants: an ex vivo evaluation of deflection forces. American Journal of Roentgenology. 1988, 151, 389–92.
[173] Shellock FG, Morisoli S, Kanal E. MR procedures and biomedical implants, materials, and devices, update. Radiology. 1993, 189, 587–99.
[174] Shellock FG, Mink JH, Curtin S, Friesman MJ. MR imaging and metallic implants for anterior cruciate ligament reconstruction: Assessment of ferromagnetism and artifact. Journal of Magnetic Reason Imaging. 1992, 2, 225–8.

[175] Shellock FG. Biomedical implants and devices: Assessment of magenta field interactions with a 3.0 tesla MR system. Journal of Magnetic Reason Imaging. 2002, 16, 721–32.
[176] Shellock FG, Fieno DS, Thompson LJ, Talavage TM, Merman DS. Cardiac pacemaker: In vitro assessment at 1.5 T. American Heart Journal. 2006, 151, 436–43.
[177] Oshida Y, Tuna EB, Aktören O, Gençay K. Dental Implant Systems. International Journal of Molecular Sciences. 2010, 11, 1580–678.
[178] Abbaszadeh K, Heffez LB, Mafee MF. Effect of interference of metallic objects on interpretation of T1-weighted magnetic resonance images in the maxillofacial region. Oral Surgery, Oral Medicine, Oral Pathology, Oral Radiology, and Endodontics. 2000, 89, 759–65.
[179] Hopper TAJ, Vasilić B, Pope JM, Jones CE, Epstein C, Song HK, Wehrli FW. Experimental and computational analyses of the effects of slice distortion from a metallic sphere in an MRI phantom. Magnetic Resonance Imaging. 2006, 24, 1077–85.
[180] Elison JM, Leggitt VL, Thomson M, Oyoyo U, Wycliffe ND. Influence of common orthodontic appliances on the diagnostic quality of cranial magnetic resonance images. American Journal of Orthodontics and Dentofacial Orthopedics : Official Publication of the American Association of Orthodontists, Its Constituent Societies, and the American Board of Orthodontics. 2008, 134, 563–72.
[181] Costa ALF, Appenzeller S, Yasuda CL, Pereira FR, Zanardi VA, Cendes F. Artifacts in brain magnetic resonance imaging due to metallic dental objects. Medicina Oral, Patologia Oral Y Cirugia Bucal. 2009, 14, E278–82.
[182] Blankenstein F, Truong BT, Thomas A, Thieme N, Zachriat C. Predictability of magnetic susceptibility artifacts from metallic orthodontic appliances in magnetic resonance imaging. Journal of Orofacial Orthopedics. 2015, 76, 14–29.
[183] Sonnow L, Könneker S, Vogt PM, Wacker F, von Falck C. Biodegradable magnesium Herbert screw – image quality and artifacts with radiography, CT and MRI. BMC Medical Imaging. 2017, 17; doi:10.1186/s12880-017-0187-7
[184] Ernstberger T, Buchhorn G, Heidrich G. Artifacts in spine magnetic resonance imaging due to different intervertebral test spacers: an in vitro evaluation of magnesium versus titanium and carbon-fiber-reinforced polymers as biomaterials. Neuroradiology. 2009, 51, 525–9.
[185] www.stmri.com/ht_docs/safety-2.html; www.mri.tju.edu/Policies-contraindications.html.

Chapter 18
Biocorrosion and biodegradation

In Section 14.4, we have discussed the corrosion behavior of Mg materials in various environments, excluding biological environments. In this chapter, we discuss the corrosion behavior in biological environments (biocorrosion) and biocorrosion-assisted metal degradation (in short, biodegradation).

18.1 Biocorrosion

In microbiology, it is stated that microorganisms are responsible for decomposition of organic materials accumulated in the environment, which are the recyclers of nutrients in the soil. Biodegradation is the process in which organic compounds are degraded or broken down by the microorganisms. Microorganisms degrade the organic material for their growth and metabolism. As a result, complex organic substances are converted into carbon dioxide and water. There are two modes of biodegradation: aerobic biodegradation and anaerobic biodegradation. Aerobic biodegradation is done by aerobic microorganisms when the adequate supply of oxygen is available for their activity. Aerobic biodegradation is a rapid method that degrades the contaminants completely when compared to anaerobic biodegradation. Anaerobic biodegradation takes place in the absence of oxygen [1]. There is another term called MIC (microbiology-induced corrosion or microbially induced corrosion) [[2-4]]. Therefore, the here-defined biodegradation in microbiology does not refer to any activity related to degradation (or deterioration) of metallic materials, which are exposed to biological corrosive environment. Meanwhile, biocorrosion refers to the corrosion phenomenon under influences of bacteria adhering to surfaces in biofilms. Biocorrosion is a major problem in areas such as cooling systems and marine structures where biofilms can develop. Microorganisms growing on surfaces perform a variety of metabolic reactions, and the products of which may promote the deterioration of the underlying substratum. These reactions refer to biocorrosion when the substratum consists of a metal or metal alloy. The biofilm contains exopolymers that impede the diffusion of solutes and gases between the surface and the bulk aqueous phase. The biofilm also permits the development of highly structured microbial communities on the surface. The various species are able to collectively carry out metabolic activities that are potentially more corrosive to the underlying surface than could be achieved by a single species acting alone [5]. At the same time, as shown in several articles cited in this chapter, the term biocorrosion is used instead of in vivo corrosion, since the corrosion reaction takes place in the biological environment. Therefore, based on aforementioned confusion in terminologies (although each of which is clearly defined for its own), in this chapter we redefine them as follows: biocorrosion include corrosion

https://doi.org/10.1515/9783110676945-018

phenomenon in biological environment (in both in vitro and in vivo manners) but not refer to any deterioration or degradation of metallic substrate or component (which are mainly implants or medical devices), while biodegradation refers to biocorrosion with degradation of substrate metallic materials to some extent.

18.1.1 Mg–Al alloy systems

AE21 (Mg–2Al–1RE) alloy was prepared as a candidate alloy for a coronary stent. Eleven domestic pigs underwent coronary implantation of 20 stents (through overstretch injury) [6]. It was found that (i) no stent caused major problems during implantation or showed signs of initial breakage in the histological evaluation; (ii) there were no thromboembolic events; (iii) quantitative angiography at follow-up showed a significant 40% loss of perfused lumen diameter between days 10 and 35, corresponding to neointima formation seen on histological analysis, and a 25% re-enlargement between days 35 and 56 caused by vascular remodeling (based on intravascular ultrasound) resulting from the loss of mechanical integrity of the stent; and (iv) inflammation and neointimal plaque area depended significantly on injury score. Based on these findings, it was concluded that vascular implants consisting of Mg–Al alloy degradable by biocorrosion seem to be a realistic alternative to permanent implants [6]. Hong et al. [7] investigated the morphology, microstructure, compressive behavior, biocorrosion properties and cytocompatibility of AE42 scaffolds for their potential use in biodegradable biomedical applications, which was synthesized via a camphene-based freeze-casting process with precisely controlled heat treatment. It was reported that (i) the corrosion potential of the Mg alloy scaffold (−1.44 V) was slightly higher than that of bulk AE42 (−1.60 V), but the corrosion rate of the Mg alloy scaffold was faster than that of bulk AE42 due to the enhanced surface area of the Mg alloy scaffold and as a result of cytocompatibility evaluation following ISO10993-5, the concentration of the Mg alloy scaffold extract reducing cell growth rate to 50% (IC_{50}) was 10.7%, which is higher (less toxic) than 5%, suggesting no severe inflammation by implantation into muscle.

18.1.2 Mg–Zn alloy systems

The biocorrosion performance of Mg–3Zn alloy (which was solution-treated and aged at 160 °C) was studied at 37 °C in simulated body fluid (SBF) [8]. It was found that (i) in the solution-treated sample, the dissolution of (α-Mg + MgZn) eutectic phases led to a low corrosion rate (3.05 ± 0.20 mL/cm^2/day) and (ii) the volume fraction of precipitates increases with aging time and causes the corrosion performance to deteriorate because of microcathodic effects, suggesting that the aged sample with the largest volume fraction of precipitates exhibits the worst corrosion resistance (4.65 ±

0.01 mL/cm^2/day). Zhou et al. [9] treated Mg–4Zn alloy by high strain rate rolling and artificial aging to improve mechanical properties and biocorrosion resistance. It was mentioned that (i) the under-aged state is the most corrosion resistant and (ii) biocorrosion resistance of the as-rolled alloy can be improved by double aging of 70 °C × 10 h + 160 °C × 2 h, resulting from stress relief and uniformly distributed nano-scale Guinier-Preston (G.P.) zones and β_1' precipitates. Cheng et al. [10] investigated the effects of minor Sr addition (0, 0.2, 0.6 and 1.0 mass%) on microstructure, mechanical and biocorrosion properties of the as-cast Mg–5Zn-based alloy system. The Sr-free alloy is composed of three phases, that is α-Mg, Mg_7Zn_3 and MgZn, while the alloys with the Sr addition of 0.6% or higher consist of α-Mg, Mg_7Zn_3, MgZn and $Mg_{11}Zn_4Sr_3$. It was mentioned that (i) minor Sr addition can effectively refine grains of the as-cast Mg–5Zn alloy and bring about more grain boundary compounds, (ii) corrosion tests in 0.9% NaCl solution and Hank's solution show that the degradation rate decreases significantly in the following order of Mg–5Zn, Mg–5Zn–0.6Sr, Mg–5Zn–1Sr and Mg–5Zn–0.2Sr and (iii) the as-cast Mg–5Zn–0.2Sr alloy also shows the optimal corrosion resistance both in 0.9%NaCl solution and in Hank's solution. Zhang et al. [11] studied pure Mg and an Mg–6Zn alloy as potential candidates for biodegradable implants for the urinary system in terms of biocorrosion resistance in SBF at 37 °C. The in vivo degradation and histocompatibility were examined through implantation into the bladders of Wistar rats. It was reported that (i) the alloying element Zn elevated the passivation potential and increased the cathodic current density, (ii) both in vitro and in vivo degradation tests showed a faster corrosion rate for the Mg–6Zn alloy and (iii) tissues stained with hematoxylin and eosin suggested that both pure Mg and Mg–6Zn alloy exhibited good histocompatibility in the bladder indwelling implantation and no differences between pure Mg and Mg–6Zn groups were found in the bladder, liver and kidney tissues during the 2 weeks implantation. Zhang et al. [12] investigated effects of pulsed magnetic field treatment on microstructure, mechanical properties and biocorrosion behavior of Mg–7Zn alloy. It was indicated that (i) the solidification microstructure of Mg–7Zn alloy was further refined with increasing discharging voltage, (ii) the second phase was changed from discontinuous reticular to island-like and particle-like morphology, (iii) the pulsed magnetic field treatment was beneficial to the biocorrosion resistance improvement of Mg–7Zn alloy and (iv) the corrosion rate of Mg–7Zn alloy was gradually decreased with increasing discharging voltage.

Mg–1Zn–0.5Ca alloys were prepared by traditional steel mold casting and water-cooled copper mold injection casting at higher cooling rate and were subjected to studies on microstructure, mechanical properties and biocorrosion resistance [13]. The biocorrosion behavior was conducted in 3.5% NaCl and Hank's solution at 37 °C. It was mentioned that (i) the alloy prepared at higher cooling rates has better corrosion resistance in both types of solution, (ii) further mass loss immersion test in Hank's solution reveals the same result and (iii) improved corrosion resistance is attributed to that raising cooling rate brings about homogeneous microstructure, which leads to microgalvanic corrosion alleviation. Kaviani et al.

[14] investigated effect of hot deformation parameters such as temperature and strain rate on mechanical behavior and corrosion properties of Mg-4Zn-0.5Ca-0.75Mn alloy was investigated in SBF solution at room temperature. It was found that (i) the microstructural results and flow curves showed the fine grain microstructure and twinning-free grains as well as fully recrystallized grains achieved at 350 °C and 400 °C at lower strain rates, (ii) polarization curves indicated that the corrosion potential shifts toward more noble potential by increasing the temperature parameter, (iii) the corrosion rate decreased from 0.31 to 0.12 mm/year at 400 °C and 0.001/s due to the fine grain microstructure. Indeed, the protective passive film covered the grain boundaries surface which decreases the corrosion rate and retards the breakdown of passive film and pitting corrosion and (iv) the lowest corrosion rate of the Mg-Zn-Ca-Mn alloy was obtained at 400 °C, which is nearly similar with the coated samples and Mg alloys reinforced with hydroxyapatite. Wang et al. [15] studied the effects of Mn substitution for Mg on the microstructure, mechanical properties and corrosion behavior of $Mg_{69-x}Zn_{27}Ca_4Mn_x$ (x = 0, 0.5 and 1 at%) alloys. It was reported that (i) polarization and immersion tests in the at 37 °C revealed that the Mn-doped Mg–Zn–Ca alloys have significantly higher corrosion resistance than traditional ZK60 and pure Mg alloys, (ii) cytotoxicity test showed that cell viabilities of osteoblasts cultured with Mn-doped Mg–Zn–Ca alloys extracts were higher than that of pure Mg. $Mg_{68.5}Zn_{27}Ca_4Mn_{0.5}$ exhibits the highest biocorrosion resistance, biocompatibility and has desirable mechanical properties, which could suggest to be used as biomedical materials in the future. Wang et al. [16]. investigated the microalloying effects of Y on the microstructure, mechanical properties and biocorrosion behavior of $Mg_{69-x}Zn_{27}Ca_4Y_x$ ($x = 0$, 1, 2 at%) alloys. It was mentioned that (i) electrochemical and immersion tests revealed that these Y-doped Mg–Zn–Ca alloys had good biocorrosion resistance in SBF at 37 °C and (ii) the results of the cytotoxicity test showed high cell viabilities for these alloys, which means good biocompatibility.

Two kinds of Mg-Zn-Mn-Ca alloys with and without Ce addition were prepared to evaluate biocorrosion behavior in Hank's solution at 37 °C [17]. It was mentioned that (i) after Ce adding, the continuous network-distributed $Ca_2Mg_6Zn_3$ phases in Mg-2Zn-0.5Mn-1Ca alloy (alloy I) were separated due to the emerging noncontinuously distributed Mg_2Ca phase and $Mg_{12}CeZn$ phase, leading to corrosion acceleration of Mg matrix at the initial stage but also speed up the formation of compact corrosion products for Mg-2Zn-0.5Mn-1Ca-1.5Ce alloy (alloy II), and therefore enhanced its biocorrosion resistance and (ii) Ce-containing Alloy II has the potential to be used as future biomaterials. Wang et al. [18] added 0.4%Nd (wt%) to into Mg-6Zn-1Mn-0.5Ca alloy to investigate the effect of Nd on the microstructure and corrosion resistance in SBF. It was shown that (i) the grain size decreases with the addition of Nd, (ii) a mixture of secondary phases $Ca_2Mg_6Zn_3 + Mg_{41}Nd_5$ is found in Mg-6Zn-1Mn-0.5Ca-0.4Nd alloy and (iii) after immersion in SBF for 7 d, more such mixture still remains on the Nd-containing alloy surface, whereas few $Ca_2Mg_6Zn_3$ particles remain on the alloy without Nd. Hu et al. [19] coated the extruded Mg-2Zn-1Mn-0.5Ca alloy with a silver and hydroxyapatite (Ag/HA) composite through a chemical conversion process. It was reported that (i) the conversion coating was mainly composed of $Ca_{10}(PO_4)_6(OH)_2$ with limited quantities of Ag/Ag_2CO_3, $CaHPO_4 \cdot 2H_2O$ and $CaSiO_3$, (ii) the electrochemical polarization and EIS tests showed that the conversion coating markedly improved the biocorrosion resistance of the Mg-2Zn-1Mn-0.5Ca alloy in Hank's solution and (ii) the bactericidal activity was assessed with the zone of inhibition method, and the composite coating on the Mg alloy substrates exhibits good antibacterial performance.

The microstructure, mechanical property and in vitro biocorrosion behavior of as-cast single-phase biodegradable Mg–1.5Zn–0.6Zr alloy were studied to compare with a commercial as-cast AZ91D alloy [20]. It was obtained that (i) immersion tests and electrochemical measurements reveal that the alloy displayed lower biocorrosion rate and more uniform corrosion mode than AZ91D in Hank's solution and (ii) the elimination of intensive galvanic corrosion reactions and the formation of a much more compact and uniform corrosion film mainly account for the better biocorrosion properties of the Mg–1.5Zn–0.6Zr alloy than AZ91D.

18.1.3 Mg–Ca alloy system

Mg–1.4Ca (wt%) alloy was treated by soaking in three alkaline solutions (Na_2HPO_4, Na_2CO_3 and $NaHCO_3$) for 24 h, followed by heat treatment at 500 °C for 12 h in order to reduce the biocorrosion rate [21]. It was mentioned that (i) the in vitro corrosion tests in SBF indicated that the corrosion rates of Mg–Ca alloy were effectively decreased after alkaline heat treatments, with the following sequence: $NaHCO_3 < Na_2HPO_4 < Na_2CO_3$ and (ii) the cytotoxicity evaluation revealed that none of the alkaline heat treated Mg–Ca alloy samples induced toxicity to L-929 cells during 7 days culture. Du et al. [22] investigated the effects of the addition of Zn element on the microstructures, mechanical properties and biocorrosion properties of Mg–3Ca alloys. It was reported that (i) as-cast Mg–3Ca alloys are composed of primary Mg and eutectic (α-Mg + Mg_2Ca) phases, while Mg–3Ca–2Zn alloys are constituted of primary Mg and eutectic (α-Mg + Mg_2Ca + $Ca_2Mg_6Zn_3$) phases, (ii) the corrosion resistance is increased by the addition of Zn element and (iii) the presence of $Ca_2Mg_6Zn_3$ phase mainly contributes to these improvements. Binary Mg–*x*Ca alloys and the quaternary Mg-Ca-Mn-*x*Zn were investigated for their biocorrosion in the SBF [23]. It was reported that electrochemical tests show that the corrosion potential of binary Mg–2Ca significantly shifted toward more noble direction from –1,996.8 to –1,616.6 mV (vs SCE) with the addition of 0.5 wt% Mn and 2 wt% Zn content; however, further addition of Zn to 7 wt% into quaternary alloy has the reverse effect. Immersion tests show that the quaternary alloy accompanied by two secondary phases presented higher corrosion resistance compared to binary alloys with single secondary phase. The degradation behavior demonstrates that Mg-2Ca-0.5Mn-2Zn alloy had the lowest degradation rate among quaternary alloys and (iii) in contrast, the binary Mg–2Ca alloy demonstrated higher corrosion rates, with Mg–4Ca alloy having the highest rating.

18.1.4 Mg–Sn alloy system

The as-extruded Mg–Sn–Ca alloys were prepared and investigated for orthopedic applications [24]. It was mentioned that (i) with the addition of 1% Sn and the Ca content of 0.2–0.5%, the microstructure of the as-extruded Mg–Sn–Ca alloys became homogeneous, leading to increased mechanical properties and improved corrosion resistance, (ii) for alloy containing 0.5% Ca, when the Sn content increased from 1% to 3%, the ultimate tensile strength increased with a decreased corrosion resistance, and the lowest yield strength and ductility appeared with the Sn content of 2%, depending on the Sn/Ca mass ratio and (iii) all data indicated that as-extruded Mg–1Sn–0.5Ca alloy was evaluated as a promising biodegradable material for orthopedic implant application.

18.1.5 Mg–Bi alloy system

The corrosion behaviors of as-cast and as-rolled Mg–6Bi–2Sn alloys were investigated in the SBF solution [25]. It was reported that (i) the as-cast alloy mainly consists of α-Mg and Mg_3Bi_2 phases, while a new Mg_2Sn phase can be observed in as-rolledone, (ii) the electrochemical and immersion tests in SBF results indicated that the as-rolled alloy have a lower corrosion rate than the as-cast one, due to refined grain size, finely dispersed secondary phase particles, favorable crystal orientation and the formation of passivity film.

18.1.6 Mg-Nd alloy system

Mg-Nd-Zn-Zr as a potential biodegradable stent material was prepared and subjected to biocorrosion tests in artificial plasma in comparison with the clinical trial Mg alloy WE43 [26]. It was mentioned that (i) the corrosion rate of Mg-Nd-ZN-Zr alloy was much lower than that of WE43 alloy and (ii) this alloy showed a uniform corrosion behavior in artificial plasma, which could avoid stress concentration as well as a rapid reduction in the mechanical integrity, indicating that the as-extruded Mg-Nd-Zn-Zr alloy may be a promising implant material suitable for stent applications. Niu et al. [27] coated Mg-Nd-Zn-Zr alloy with brushite (biodegradable calcium phosphate: $CaHPO_4 \cdot 2H_2O$) for further improvement of biocorrosion resistance and biocompatibility. It was reported that (i) the in vitro corrosion tests indicated that the Ca–P treatment improved the corrosion resistance of the alloy in Hank's solution, (ii) Ca–P treatment significantly reduced the hemolysis rate from 48% to 0.68%, and induced no toxicity to MC3T3-E1 cells, (iii) the in vivo implantation experiment in New Zealand's rabbit tibia showed that the degradation rate was reduced obviously by the Ca–P treatment and less gas was produced from Ca–P-treated Mg-Nd-Zn-Zr bone plates and screws in early stage of the implantation, and at least 10 weeks degradation time can be prolonged by the present coating techniques and (iv) both Ca–P-treated and untreated Mg alloy induced bone growth, indicating that the Ca–P treatment is a promising technique for the degradable Mg-based biomaterials for orthopedic applications. Zhang et al. [28] prepared Mg-2.2Nd-xSr-0.3Zr alloys (x = 0, 0.4 and 0.7 mass%) by gravity casting, followed by the solution treatment to homogenize microstructure and hot extrusion. It was mentioned that (i) the amount of residual eutectic phase of the solution-treated alloys increases with increasing Sr addition, and the grains are significantly refined after hot extrusion and (ii) the biocorrosion resistance in SBF with solution treated alloys deteriorates apparently with increasing Sr addition, while the corrosion resistance of the as-extruded alloys is improved with Sr addition.

18.1.7 Mg–Y alloy system

The biocorrosion behavior of as-extruded Mg-8Y-1Er-2Zn (wt%) alloy containing strip-like 18R long-period stacking ordered (LPSO) phase was studied in a SBF at 37 °C [29]. It was reported that (i) the hydrogen evolution volume per day fluctuates between 0.21 and 0.32 mL/cm^2 in the immersion test for 240 h, and the corresponding corrosion rate is calculated as 0.568 mm/y, (ii) the corrosion product is determined as $Mg(OH)_2$, while a $Ca(H_2PO_4)_2$ compound is also observed on the surface of the samples and (iii) the corrosion site preferentially occurs at the interface between LPSO phase and Mg matrix. Chou et al. [30] evaluated biodegradable Mg-Y-Ca-Zr alloys as orthopedic and craniofacial implant applications. The effects of increasing Y content from 1 to 4 wt% as well as the effects of T4 solution treatment were studied. It was shown that (i) increasing the Y content (from 1 to 4 wt%) contributed to improved corrosion resistance, (ii) the Mg-Y-Ca-Zr alloys demonstrated excellent in vitro cytocompatibility and normal in vivo host response and (iii) the mechanical, corrosion and biological evaluations performed in this study demonstrated that Mg-Y-Ca-Zr alloys, especially with the 4 wt% Y content, would perform well as orthopedic and craniofacial implant biomaterials.

18.1.8 Mg–Li alloy system

Mg–Li alloys were alloyed with Al and RE (rare earth) elements to improve mechanical strength and ductility to form Mg–Li–Al ternary and Mg-Li-Al-RE quaternary alloys [30]. It was mentioned that (i) electrochemical and immersion tests in SBF showed reduced corrosion resistance caused by intermetallic compounds distributed throughout the magnesium matrix in the rare-earth containing Mg–Li alloys, (ii) cytotoxicity assays, hemolysis tests as well as platelet adhesion tests were performed to evaluate in vitro biocompatibilities of the Mg–Li-based alloys and the results of cytotoxicity assays clearly showed that the Mg-3.5Li-2Al-2RE, Mg-3.5Li-4Al-2RE and Mg-8.5Li-2Al-2RE alloys suppressed vascular smooth muscle cell proliferation after 5 days of incubation, while the Mg–3.5Li, Mg–8.5Li and Mg–8.5Li–1Al alloys were proven to be tolerated and (iii) in the case of human umbilical vein endothelial cells, the Mg–Li-based alloys showed no significantly reduced cell viabilities except for the Mg-8.5Li-2Al-2RE alloy, with no obvious differences in cell viability between different culture periods. Based on these finding, it was indicated that (iv) the potential of Mg-Li-(Al)-(RE) alloys as biomaterials for future cardiovascular stent application.

18.1.9 Mg–Dy alloy system

Three Mg–*x*Dy ($x = 10$, 15, 20 wt%) alloys were prepared to investigate the influence of aging treatment on their mechanical and corrosion properties [31]. It was obtained that (i) aging at 250 °C has little influence on the mechanical and corrosion properties, (ii) however, aging at 200 °C significantly increases the yield strength and reduces the ductility and (iii) after aging at 200 °C, the corrosion rate of Mg–20Dy alloy increases largely in 0.9 wt% NaCl solution, but remains unchanged in cell culture medium.

18.1.10 Mg–Gd alloy system

Microstructure, biocorrosion behavior and cytotoxicity of an as-extruded Mg-11.3Gd-2.5Zn-0.7Zr (wt%) alloy were studied to develop new biodegradable magnesium alloy [32]. It was mentioned that the microstructure of the as-extruded alloy mainly consists of the refinement grains, a lamellar X phase with the 14H-type LPSO structure in grain boundaries and the 14H-type LPSO structure within initial grains and refinement grains, and a small amount of β-phase. The corrosion rate in Hanks' solution is only 0.17 mm/year and the corrosion mode of the alloy is uniform corrosion, which is much better than that of as-extruded Mg-10.2Gd-3.3Y-0.6Zr alloy. The cell toxicity grade of the Mg-11.3Gd-2.5Zn-0.7Zr alloy is grade 1, indicating only slightly having cytotoxicity.

18.1.11 Mg–Si alloy system

Biocorrosion behavior of as-cast Mg–Si–(Ca, Zn) alloys were investigated in SBF [33]. It was found that (i) the biocorrosion resistance of Mg–Si alloys was improved by the addition of Ca due to the reduction and refinement of Mg_2Si phase; however, no improvement was observed in the strength and elongation, (ii) the addition of 1.6% Zn to Mg–0.6Si can modify obviously the morphology of Mg_2Si phase from course eutectic structure to a small dot or short bar shape, resulting in significant improvements in tensile strength, elongation and biocorrosion resistance, concluding that (iii) Zn element was one of the best alloying elements of Mg–Si alloy for biomedical application.

18.1.12 Mg–Sr alloy system

Biocorrosion property and cytotoxicity of the as-extruded Mg–Sr alloys were studied for orthopedic application [34]. It was reported that (i) as-extruded Mg–Sr alloys were composed of α-Mg and $Mg_{17}Sr_2$ phases, and the content of $Mg_{17}Sr_2$ phases increased with increasing Sr content, (ii) immersion and electrochemical tests showed that as-extruded Mg–0.5Sr alloy exhibited the best biocorrosion resistance, and the biocorrosion resistance of as-extruded Mg–Sr alloys deteriorated with increasing Sr content, which was greatly associated with galvanic couple effect and (iii) the cytotoxicity test revealed that as-extruded Mg–0.5Sr alloy did not induce toxicity to cells, indicating that (iv) as-extruded Mg–0.5Sr alloy with suitable mechanical properties, biocorrosion resistance and good cytocompatibility was potential as a biodegradable implant for orthopedic application.

18.1.13 Mg composite system

The effect of addition of TiO_2 nanopowders on the corrosion behavior and mechanical properties of Mg/HA-based nanocomposites was investigated [35]. It was found that (i) the corrosion resistance of Mg/HA-based nanocomposites was significantly improved by adding 15 wt% of TiO_2 and decrease HA amount to 5 wt%; this was inferred from the lower corrosion current; 4.8 $\mu A/cm^2$ versus 285.3 $\mu A/cm^2$ for the Mg/27.5 wt%HA, the higher corrosion potential; −1,255.7 versus −1,487.3 mV (vs SCE), the larger polarization resistance; 11.86 versus 0.25 kΩ cm^2 and the significantly lower corrosion rate; 0.1 versus 4.28 mm/year, (ii) the Mg/5HA/15TiO_2 (wt%) nanocomposite possessed high corrosion resistance, cytocompatibility and mechanical properties and can be considered as a promising material for implant applications.

18.2 Biodegradation

Uncontrolled degradation of biomaterials could result in loss of their mechanical integrity, metal contamination in the body and intolerable hydrogen evolution by tissue. As promising applicability of biodegradable Mg materials, it is crucial to understand degradation mechanism in biological environment and to manage its rate when Mg materials are chosen for orthopedic stent or implants, or scaffold frameworks for tissue engineering.

18.2.1 Degradation

A majority of orthopedic implants for repairing fractured bone or joint is normally made of metallic materials including austenitic stainless steels, Co–Cr–Mo alloy, commercially pure Ti and Ti–6Al–4 V or Ti–6Al–7Nb alloys, due to their biocompatibility and adequate mechanical behavior. These are called (semi)permanent implants. Usually, once the patient recovered from a traumatic injury was completely healed, a revision surgery is necessary to remove the implant from the body with careful operation not to cause unwanted problems associated with osteopenia, inflammation of adjacent tissues or sarcoma. Alternatively, to avoid such post-extraction of the implant, intensive efforts are being made in recent years to develop new classes of so-called the biodegradable implants, which are composed of nontoxic materials that become reabsorbed by the human body after a reasonable period of time. Conventionally these implants are polymeric materials. However, there are drawbacks associated with polymeric implants: (i) they are often rather costly, (ii) exhibit relatively low mechanical strength, so biomechanical compatibility will not be able to establish and (iii) polymers can also react with human tissues, leading to osteolysis, particularly unpolymerized monomer would be toxic to surrounding tissues [36, 37]. For these reasons, it is highly desirable to develop cost-effective biodegradable metallic alloys, with better mechanical performance than polymers. Although Fe-based and Mg-based alloys are materials' choice since they exhibit relatively fast biodegradation and strong enough of mechanical performance, Mg alloys are preferred because their stiffness (i.e., Young´s modulus) is closer to that of human bone, leading to established biomechanical compatibility [38].

While semi-permanent metallic implants (such as Ti-based alloys, CoCr alloys and stainless steel) are removed after the completion of the healing process to avoid diverse side effects, long-term disadvantages of this practice include the failure to adapt to rapid growth in young children, bone degradation by stress shielding, microbial implant infections, excessive fibrosis or persistent inflammation [39]. Novel bioresorbable metal implants (such as iron, Zn-based alloys and Mg-based alloys) could provide support during the healing process and then disappear to avoid long-term side effects without requiring surgical removal [40, 41]. Degradation of Mg materials in in vivo environment is compared with other biodegradable materials as follows: it is 0.16 mm/year for pure annealed Fe, 0.2 mm/year for as cast pure Zn and 407 mm/year for pure as cast pure Mg [42]. As Sanchez et al. [43] pointed out, there are several factors influencing degradation rate, including alloy factors (type of material, grain size, alloying element and purity, other metallurgical parameters), in vivo factors (tissue pH value, vascularization of peri-implant zone, chlorine ion concentration and others), and in vitro factors (solution pH and temperature, test methods and others). Since iron and zinc material exhibit slow degradation rate, it would result in (i) complete degradation may require several years or (ii) lifetime by far exceeds expected healing periods [44–46]. On the other hand, due to very rapid degradation rate (in other words, very high corrosion rate) of Mg-based alloys, there is a risk of mechanical failure before the healing process is completed [47–49]. Being metallic materials, Mg and Mg alloys made for scaffolds provide the necessary mechanical support for tissue healing and cell growth in the early stage, while natural degradation and reabsorption by surrounding tissues in the later stage make an unnecessarily follow-up removal surgery. However, uncontrolled degradation may collapse the scaffolds resulting in premature implant failure, and there has been much research in controlling the degradation rates of Mg alloys [50]. To this end, there are mainly two ways: (i) alloying and (ii) surface modification.

18.2.2 Degradation rate, controlled by alloying effect

Degradation behavior of Mg-based alloys are affected by various factors including aqueous corrosive environment and temperature, composition, micro- and macrostructure, surface structure, alloying elements, impurities, heat treatment and secondary phase evolution and manufacturing method and its resultant altered microstructures [51, 52]. Since biodegradable implants become reabsorbed by the human body after a certain period of time, they should be composed of biocompatible alloying elements, so that some alloying element (if alloyed in Mg-based alloys) could exhibit a potential cytotoxicity. For example, elements such as Ni, Cr and V are not suitable to be in contact with human tissues, since these three are well known as heavy toxic metallic elements. As shown in the following table, their substitution by nontoxic elements such as Zn and Ca has permitted the fabrication of biocompatible Mg-based alloys with potential use as biomaterials. Alloying element concentrations: the corrosion behavior of Mg phase can be tuned as a function of the concentration of elements in solid solution. Depending on the nature and distribution of these elements within the matrix phase, the occurrence of microgalvanic cells can be either mitigated or favored. For example, an Al-containing Mg matrix phase becomes more passive as the Al content increases and consequently the corrosion rate decreases. On the contrary, in Zr-containing Al-free Mg alloys, the central areas of the grains (which are enriched in Zr) do not corrode while the grain boundaries severely corrode [36, 37]. Agarwal et al. [53] found that inclusion of alloying elements such as Al, Mn, Ca, Zn and RE elements provides improved corrosion resistance (in other words slowing the degradation rate) of Mg-based alloys. As we have been discussed the corrosion behavior of Mg materials previously (see Chapter 14), various alloying element(s) exhibit controlling influences on chemical and/or electrochemical behavior.

In summarizing all elements affecting corrosion behavior, Table 18.1 lists up the affecting alloying elements.

Table 18.1: Effects of alloying elements for controlling the degradation rate of Mg-based alloys.

First element	Second element	Third element	Others	References
Al	Zn			[54–56]
Al	RE			[57]
Bi	Ca			[58]
Bi	Si			[58]
Ca				[59–64]
Ca	Sr			[65]
Ca	Zn			[66–68]
Cu				[69–71]
Gd	Zn	Zr		[72]
Gd	Y	Sc		[73]
Li	Al			[57, 74]
Li	Al	RE		[57]
Li	Zn			[75]
Mn	Ce			[76]
Si	Sr			[77]
Sn	Mn			[78]
Sr				[79–81]
Si	Ca			[82, 83]
Zn				[84–88]
Zn	Al	Ca		[89]
Zn	Ca			[89–95]

Table 18.1 (continued)

First element	Second element	Third element	Others	References
Zn	Ca	HA		[96]
Zn	Ca	Mg		[97]
Zn	Ca	Mn		[98, 99]
Zn	Ca	Mn	Sr	[99]
Zn	Ca	Pd		[100]
Zn	Ca	Sr		[101]
Zn	Gd			[102]
Zn	Gd	Zr		[103]
Zn	Mn			[104]
Zn	RE	Zr		[105]
Zn	Sr			[106]
Zn	Zr			[107-111]
Zn	Zr	Sc		[112-115]
Zn	Zr	Sr		[116]
Zr	Sr			[117]
Rare earth element group				
Sc	Y			[118]
Y	Er	Zn		[119]
Y	Zn	Zr		[120]
La + Gd				[121]
Gd	Zn	Zr	Mn	[122]
Nd	Zn	Zr		[123-133]
Nd	Y	Zr	Ca	[134]
Dy				[135]
Er	Zn			[136]

RE, rare earth elements; HA, hydroxyapatite.

Figure 18.1 illustrates various alloying effects of metallic elements in terms of decreasing (beneficial) corrosion current density or increasing (adverse) corrosion current density, and increasing (more noble) corrosion potential or decreasing (more less noble) corrosion potential, proving a guideline for appropriate selection of alloying element(s) for Mg-based material [50].

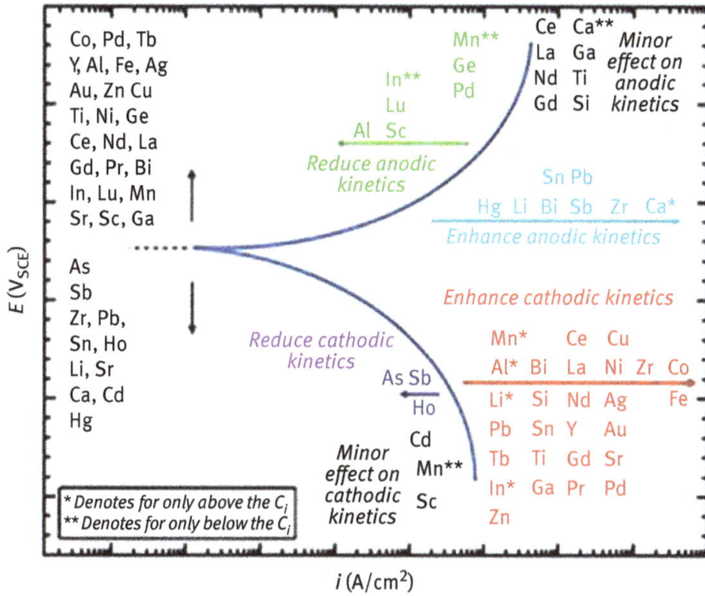

Figure 18.1: Effects of alloying elements for corrosion behaviors [50].

18.2.3 Degradation rate, controlled by surface modification

The crucial problem associated with Mg-based alloys is high corrosion (or degradation) rates in physiological conditions, which makes their biodegradability to be faster than the time required to heal the bone. Hence, it is important to control the degradation rate and to keep their mechanical integrity until the bone heals. Another drawback of magnesium and its alloys is that corrosion is accompanied by intense hydrogen evolution. This gas can be accumulated in pockets next to the implants or can form subcutaneous gas bubbles [51]. Accordingly, a well-balanced property between controlled rate of biodegradation and maintained mechanical integrity during biodegradation becomes extremely important for biodegradable-graded Mg-based alloys. There are two methods principally employed for controlling surface degradation rate, apatite coating and/or surface oxidation treatment. It is believed that preparing stabilized apatite on biodegradable Mg alloy may improve biocompatibility and promote osteointegration and such apatite includes Ca–

P coatings, brushite ($CaHPO_4 \cdot 2H_2O$), hydroxyapatite ($Ca_{10}(PO_4)_6(OH)_2$) and fluoridated hydroxyapatite ($Ca_5(PO_4)_3(OH)_{1-x}F_x$) [137]. If surface layer is subjected to oxidation to form dense and protective oxide film, the degradation rate (in other words, corrosion rate) can be suppressed and such treatment can include PEO (plasma electrolytic oxidation) [138] and MAO (microarc oxidation) [139]. Table 18.2 summarizes these surface coating methods to control the degradation rate.

Table 18.2: Surface modification for controlling the degradation rate of Mg-based alloys.

Alloying system	Surface modification	References
Mg–Al–Zn	CP/chitosan composite coating	[140]
Mg–Al–Zn	Sol–gel-derived HA coating	[141]
Mg–Al–Zn	Phytic acid chemical conversion layer coating	[142]
Mg–Ca–Zn	Composite coating of OCP and HA, overlayer of PCL	[143]
Mg–Mn–Ce	Composite coating of HA and MgO	[144]
Mg-Nd-Zn-Zr	Brushite-derived CP	[145]
Mg-Nd-Zn-Zr	CHP coating	[146]
Mg-Nd-Y-Zr-Ca	Diffusion coating of Nd	[147]
Mg–Sr	MAO treatment and Sr-P coating	[148]
Mg–Zn–Ca	MAO treatment	[149]
Mg–Zn–Ca	β-TCP particle-reinforced Mg matrix composite coating	[150]
Mg–Zn–Gd	CP coating	[151]
Mg-Zn-Gd-Zr	MAO treatment and Sr-P coating, CP coating	[152]
Mg–Zn–Zr	Sr-doped HA coating	[153]
Mg–Zr	MAO treatment and acetic acid containing EPD treatment	[154]
Mg–Y–RE	Al_2O_3-containing oxide layer coating	[155]

CP, calcium phosphate, Ca–P; HA, hydroxyapatite, $Ca_{10}(PO_4)_6(OH)_2$; OCP, octa-calcium phosphate; PCL, polycaprolactone; Brushite, $CaHPO_4 \cdot 2H_2O$; CHP, calcium hydrogen phosphate, $CaHPO_4$; MAO, microarc oxidation; β-TCP, beta-tricalcium phosphate; EPD, electrophoresis deposition.

18.2.4 Biodegradation cases in medicine

18.2.4.1 Orthopedic implants

Fan et al. [156] studied microstructure and degradation and evaluated cytotoxicity of Mg-1.5Y-1.2Zn-0.44Zr alloys for biodegradable metallic implants. The alloys were as-cast state, as-heat treated state and as-extruded state alloys. It was found that (i) the Mg-1.5Y-1.2Zn-0.44Zr alloys are mainly composed of the matrix α-Mg phases and the Mg12ZnY secondary phases; (ii) immersion tests and electrochemical measurements in the SBF indicate that a protective film precipitated on the alloy's surface with the extension of degradation; (iii) the protective film contains $Mg(OH)_2$ and hydroxyapatite which can strengthen the osteoblast activity and promote excellent biocompatibility; and (iv) no significant cytotoxicity toward L-929 cells was detected and the immersion extracts of alloy samples could enhance the cell proliferation with time in the cytotoxicity evaluations, indicating that the Mg-1.5Y-1.2Zn-0.44Zr alloys have the potential to be used for biomedical applications. Mohamed et al. [157] studied degradation assessment of Mg-0.8Ca (wt%) alloy in Hank's balanced salt solution (HBSS). It was reported that (i) degradation in HBSS resulted in the formation of the needle-shaped carbonated hydroxyapatite which was similar to the biological apatite in the human bone, (ii) degradation kinetics showed that Mg–0.8Ca alloy had approximately threefold faster degradation rate than the pure Mg (1.08 ± 0.38 mm/year for Mg–0.8Ca and 0.35 ± 0.17 mm/year for pure Mg), as observed in two independent experiments and (iii) both pure Mg and Mg–0.8Ca alloy were biocompatible, generating no cytotoxic degradation products against human-derived HEK 293 cells. Based on these results, it was concluded that the Mg–0.8Ca alloy was found to be a promising biodegradable implant in terms of bioactivity and compatibility with human cell lines and depending on the application of the implant and the estimated healing time of the bone, the desired degradation rate of an implant can be controlled by the Mg–Ca composition of such alloys. Magnesium-based metals are considered as promising biodegradable orthopedic implant materials due to their potentials of enhancing bone healing and reconstruction, and in vivo absorbable characteristic without second operation for removal. However, the rapid corrosion has limited their clinical applications. Ca–P coating by electrodeposition has been supposed to be effective to control the degradation rate and enhance the bioactivity. Based on this background, Shangguan et al. [158] coated a brushite on the Mg–Sr alloy by pulse electrodeposition (PED) to evaluate its efficacy for orthopedic application. It was mentioned that (i) an inner corrosion layer was observed between the PED coating and the alloy substrate, (ii) the results of in vitro immersion and electrochemical tests showed that the corrosion resistance of the coated alloy was undermined in comparison with the uncoated alloy and (iii) the existence of this corrosion layer was attributed to the worse corrosion performance of the alloy, indicating that the electrodeposition coating should be not suitable for those magnesium alloys with poor corrosion resistance such as the Mg–Sr alloy.

18.2.4.2 Bone repair implants

It was stated that crevice-induced corrosion is not desirable to occur in metallic Mg during many industrial applications; however, orthopedic implants made of Mg alloys have been demonstrated to degrade faster between the joining surface of bone plates and screws after implantation, suggesting the crevice corrosion may occur in the physiological environment [159]. A resin device is designed to parallel high purity Mg plates with closely spaced slits. After a standard corrosion test in the phosphate-buffered saline solution, the paralleled pure Mg samples embedded in the custom-made resin device corrode faster than those without the resin device and it was reported that (i) the corrosion morphology of Mg with the resin device exhibits features of crevice corrosion with many deep holes and river-like texture and (ii) implantation of the bone plate and screws in vivo demonstrates similar corrosion morphology as that of the in vitro test, suggesting the occurrence of crevice-enhanced corrosion in the bone–bone plate interface, as well as the contact area between the bone plate and the screws. Liu et al. [160] investigated the biocorrosion degradation behavior of a Mg–Ca alloy with high Ca content aiming for a potential bone repair material in the SBF. It was mentioned that (i) Mg–30%Ca alloy was composed of α-Mg and Mg_2Ca phases, (ii) during the corrosion process in the SBF, the Mg_2Ca phase acts as an anode and the α-Mg phase acts as a cathode. The final corrosion product of the Mg–30%Ca alloy in SBF includes a small amount of black precipitates and white suspended particles, (iii) the white suspended particles are $Mg(OH)_2$ and the black particles are believed to have a core–shell structure and (iv) the cytotoxicity experiments indicate that these black precipitates do not induce toxicity to cells. Cipriano et al. [161] studied the degradation and biological properties of as-drawn Mg–4Zn–1Sr (ZSr41) and pure Mg wires as bioresorbable intramedullary pins for bone repair. Their cytocompatibility with bone marrow derived mesenchymal stem cells (BMSCs) and degradation in vitro, and their biological effects on peri-implant tissues and in vivo degradation in rat tibiae were also examined. It was reported that (i) the as-drawn ZSr41 pins showed a significantly faster degradation than pure Mg in vitro and in vivo, (ii) the in vivo average daily degradation rates of both ZSr41 and pure Mg intramedullary pins were significantly greater than their respective in vitro degradation rates, likely because the intramedullary site of implantation is highly vascularized for removal of degradation products, (iii) the concentrations of Mg^{2+}, Zn^{2+} and Sr^{2+}ions in the BMSC culture in vitro and their concentrations in rat blood in vivo were all lower than their respective therapeutic dosages, that is, in a safe range and (iv) despite of rapid degradation with a complete resorption time of 8 weeks in vivo, the ZSr41 intramedullary pins showed a significant net bone growth because of stimulatory effects of the metallic ions released; however, proportionally released OH^- ions and hydrogen gas caused adverse effects on bone marrow cells and resulted in cavities in surrounding bone. Zhang et al. [162] fabricated a new hot extruded Mg-3Zn-1Y-4Cu alloy with excellent mechanical properties and rapid degradation behavior by appropriate addition Cu to high-strength Mg–3Zn–1Y alloys, which could be a good candidate materials for degradable fracturing ball. It was mentioned that (i) Mg-3Zn-1Y-4Cu alloy shows a high degradation rate as demonstrated by immersion tests and polarization curves, which is 38 times higher corrosion rates than Mg–3Zn–1Y alloy and (ii) the Mg-3Zn-1Y-4Cu alloy can thus be used as degradable fracturing ball. Niu et al. [163] studied the long-term degradation of Mg-Nd-Zn-Zr screws in the rabbit mandible. It was reported that (i) at 18 months, the screw volume has been reduced by ~90% according to the microcomputed tomography (micro-CT) analysis, and the averaged corrosion rate is 0.122 ± 0.042 mm/year, (ii) the bone–implant interface analysis reveals good osteointegration and (iii) the corrosion products show two-layer structure with Ca and P elements concentrated in the out layer, and the $Mg_{12}Nd$ particles has degraded by Mg element dissolution.

18.2.4.3 Vascular stents

The long-term degradation behavior, hydrogen evolution rates and mechanical properties of three Mg–Li alloys (LA92, LAE912 and LAE922) were investigated in comparison with those of a WE-type alloy [164]. It was shown that (i) immersion tests in Hank's balanced salt solution for 600 days showed that the LA92 alloy degraded much less than the LAE912 and the LAE922 alloys, (ii) it even outperformed the WE-type alloy after immersion for 94 days, (iii) unlike the other three alloys investigated, the LA92 alloy displayed a steady hydrogen evolution rate over the whole period of immersion tests and (iv) it possessed an elongation value of 33%, being much higher than the WE-type alloy, indicating that this alloy has a greater potential of meeting the requirements of radially expandable stents in mechanical properties and degradation performance. Liu et al. [165] evaluated pure Mg and WE43 alloy in human bile to see the corrosion performance as potential biliary stent materials. It was indicated that (i) the weight loss of WE43 after 60 days immersion was only 1.87%, (ii) WE43 performed a superior corrosion resistance to pure Mg, owing to more formation of the secondary reaction product $Mg(H_2PO_4)_2$, (iii) the formation of $H_2PO_4^-$ instead of PO_4^{3-} may be due to the fact that the compositions in the bile can prevent the formation of PO_4^{3-} as it is the main composition of gallstone and (iv) the much slower corrosion rate of the WE43 alloy in human bile indicated that it may be good candidates as biliary stent materials. Peng et al. [166] prepared Mg–Y-based microwire which offers high strength in combination of low degradation rate by a modified melt extraction technique. It was found that (i) a low degradation rate of 0.366 mm/year is attained in a SBF, which is less than 1/10 of that of as-cast sample and (ii) the excellent mechanical properties and low degradation rate provide some prerequisites to develop bio-Mg implants, suggesting that the modified extraction technique is one of effective approaches to prepare microwire, which can be directly used for Mg-based stent self-assembly.

18.2.4.4 Scaffolds

Medical polyporous Mg-Nd-Zn-Zr, $CaHPO_4$-coated Mg-Nd-Zn-Zr and WE43 were manufactured through a mechanical perforation technique, with the porosity of polyporous scaffold of 61.1 ± 2.81% (noncoating) and 49.74 ± 2.11% (coating) [167]. It was reported that (i) SEM examination after 8 weeks of immersion in cells culture environments revealed finer surface topography for Mg-Nd-Zn-Zr than WE43, whereas $CaHPO_4$-coated

Mg-Nd-Zn-Zr presented more uniform, fine-point corrosion pits, (ii) the pH value of the immersion solution with Mg-Nd-Zn-Zr scaffolds was lower than that of WE43, while that of $CaHPO_4$-coated Mg-Nd-Zn-Zr scaffold was the lowest, (iii) the weight of $CaHPO_4$-coated Mg-Nd-Zn-Zr scaffolds decreased 10.13% and 12.76% after 4 weeks and 8 weeks of immersion, respectively, and (iv) the poly-porous scaffold possessed similar elastic modulus and compressive strength to those of human cancellous bone, and $CaHPO_4$-coated Mg-Nd-Zn-Zr foam maintained mechanical integrity while noncoated scaffolds disaggregated over 8 weeks. Based on these results, it was concluded that $CaHPO_4$-coated Mg-Nd-Zn-Zr scaffold possesses great potential in vivo applications compared with Mg-Nd-Zn-Zr and WE43 scaffolds. Zhang et al. [168] developed a new type of scaffold made of a Mg–Zn–Ca alloy with a shape that mimics cortical bone and can be filled with morselized bone to evaluate its durability and efficacy in a rabbit ulna-defect model. Three types of scaffold-surface coating were evaluated: group A, no coating; group B, a 10-µm MAO coating; group C, a hydrothermal duplex composite coating; and group D, an empty-defect control. It was reported that (i) a mechanical stress test indicated that bone repair within each group improved significantly over time, (ii) the degradation behavior of the different scaffolds was assessed by micro-CT and quantified according to the amount of hydrogen gas generated; these measurements indicated that the group C scaffold better resisted corrosion than did the other scaffold types and (iii) calcein fluorescence and histology revealed that greater mineral densities and better bone responses were achieved for groups B and C than for group A, with group C providing the best response, concluding that (iv) Mg–Zn–Ca alloy scaffold effectively aided bone repair and (vi) the group C scaffold exhibited the best corrosion resistance and osteogenesis properties, making it a candidate scaffold for repair of bone defects.

References

[1] https://www.differencebetween.com/difference-between-biodegradation-and-vs-bioremediation/.

[2] Schwermer CU, Lavik G, Abed RMM, Dunsmore B, Ferdelman TG, Stoodley P, Gieseke A, de Beer D. Impact of nitrate on the structure and function of bacterial biofilm communities in pipelines used for injection of seawater into oil fields. Applied and Environmental Microbiology. 2008, 74, 2841–51.

[3] Witecka A, Yamamoto A, Święszkowski W. Influence of SaOS-2 cells on corrosion behavior of cast Mg-2.0Zn0.98Mn magnesium alloy. Colloids and Surfaces. B, Biointerfaces. 2017, 150, 288–96.

[4] Chang J-C, Oshida Y, Gregory RL, Andres CJ, Barco TM, Brown DT. Electrochemical study on microbiology-related corrosion of metallic dental materials. Bio-medical Materials and Engineering. 2003, 13, 281–95.

[5] Geesey G. What is Biocorrosion? In: Flemming HC. et al. ed., Biofouling and Biocorrosion in Industrial Water Systems. Springer, Berlin, Heidelberg, 1991, pp.155–164.

[6] Heublein B, Rohde R, Kaese V, Niemeyer M, Hartung W, Haverich A. Biocorrosion of magnesium alloys: a new principle in cardiovascular implant technology? Heart. 2003, 89, 651–6.
[7] Hong K, Park H, Kim Y, Knapek M, Choe H. Mechanical and biocorrosive properties of magnesium-aluminum alloy scaffold for biomedical applications. Journal of the Mechanical Behavior of Biomedical Materials. 2019, 98, 213–24.
[8] Lu Y, Bradshaw AR, Chiu YL, Jones IP. The role of β′1 precipitates in the bio-corrosion performance of Mg–3Zn in simulated body fluid. Journal of Alloys and Compounds. 2014, 614, 345–52.
[9] Zhou B, Chen J, Yan H, Xia W, Zhu W. To improve strength and bio-corrosion resistance of Mg-4Zn alloy via high strain rate rolling combined with double aging. Materials Letters. 2018, 227, 301–4.
[10] Cheng M, Chen J, Yan H, Su B, Gong X. Effects of minor Sr addition on microstructure, mechanical and bio-corrosion properties of the Mg-5Zn based alloy system. Journal of Alloys and Compounds. 2017, 691, 95–102.
[11] Zhang S, Zheng Y, Zhang L, Bi Y, Li Y. In vitro and in vivo corrosion and histocompatibility of pure Mg and a Mg-6Zn alloy as urinary implants in rat model. Materials Science and Engineering: C. 2016, 68, 414–22.
[12] Zhang L, Hu PH, Zhou Q, Zhan W, Jin F. Effects of pulsed magnetic field on microstructure, mechanical properties and bio-corrosion behavior of Mg-7Zn alloy. Materials Letters. 2017, 193, 224–7.
[13] Wang L-D, Li X-S, Wang C, Wang L-M, Cao Z-Y. Effects of cooling rate on bio-corrosion resistance and mechanical properties of Mg–1Zn–0.5Ca Casting Alloy. Transactions of Nonferrous Metals Society of China. 2016, 26, 704–11.
[14] Kaviani M, Ebrahimi GR, Ezatpour HR. Improving the mechanical properties and biocorrosion resistance of extruded Mg-Zn-Ca-Mn alloy through hot deformation. Materials Chemistry and Physics. 2019, 234, 245–58.
[15] Wang J, Huang S, Li Y, We Y, Xi X, Cai K. Microstructure, mechanical and bio-corrosion properties of Mn-doped Mg-Zn-Ca bulk metallic glass composites. Materials Science and Engineering: C. 2013, 33, 3832–8.
[16] Wang J, Li Y, Huang S, Wei Y, Pan F. Effects of Y on the microstructure, mechanical and bio-corrosion properties of Mg–Zn–Ca bulk metallic glass. Journal of Materials Science & Technology. 2014, 30, 1255–61.
[17] Zhang F, Ma A, Song D, Jiang J, Cen J. Improving in-vitro biocorrosion resistance of Mg-Zn-Mn-Ca alloy in Hank's solution through addition of cerium. Journal of Rare Earths. 2015, 33, 93–101.
[18] Wang Y, Liao Z, Song C, Zhang H. Influence of Nd on microstructure and Bio-corrosion resistance of Mg-Zn-Mn-Ca alloy. Rare Metal Materials and Engineering. 2013, 42, 661–6.
[19] Hu G, Zeng L, Du H, Fu X, Liu X. The formation mechanism and bio-corrosion properties of Ag/HA composite conversion coating on the extruded Mg-2Zn-1Mn-0.5Ca alloy for bone implant application. Surface & Coatings Technology. 2017, 325, 127–35.
[20] Li T, He Y, Zhang H, Wang X. Microstructure, mechanical property and in vitro biocorrosion behavior of single-phase biodegradable Mg–1.5Zn–0.6Zr alloy. Journal of Magnesium and Alloy. 2014, 2, 181–9.
[21] Gun XN, Zheng W, Cheng Y, Zheng YF. A study on alkaline heat treated Mg–Ca alloy for the control of the biocorrosion rate. Acta Biomaterialia. 2009, 5, 2790–99.
[22] Du H, Wei Z, Liu X, Zhang E. Effects of Zn on the microstructure, mechanical property and bio-corrosion property of Mg–3Ca alloys for biomedical application. Materials Chemistry and Physics. 2011, 125, 568–75.

[23] Bakhsheshi HR, Idros MH, Abdul-Kadir MR, Ourdjini A, Hamzah E. Mechanical and bio-corrosion properties of quaternary Mg–Ca–Mn–Zn alloys compared with binary Mg–Ca alloys. Materials & Design. 2014, 53, 283–92.

[24] Zhao C-Y, Pan F-S, Pan H-C. Microstructure, mechanical and bio-corrosion properties of as-extruded Mg–Sn–Ca alloys. Transactions of Nonferrous Metals Society of China. 2016, 26, 1574–82.

[25] Cheng W-L. Ma S-C, Bai Y, Cui Z-Q, Wang H-X. Corrosion behavior of Mg-6Bi-2Sn alloy in the simulated body fluid solution: The influence of microstructural characteristics. Journal of Alloys and Compounds. 2018, 731, 945–54.

[26] Mao L, Yuan G, Wang S, Niu J, Ding W. A novel biodegradable Mg–Nd–Zn–Zr alloy with uniform corrosion behavior in artificial plasma. Materials Letters. 2012, 88, 1–4.

[27] Niu J, Yuan G, Liao Y, Mao L, Ding W. Enhanced biocorrosion resistance and biocompatibility of degradable Mg–Nd–Zn–Zr alloy by brushite coating. Materials Science and Engineering: C. 2013, 33, 4833–41.

[28] Zhang X-B, Ba Z-X, Wang Z-Z, Xue Y-J, Wang Q. Microstructure and biocorrosion behaviors of solution treated and as-extruded Mg–2.2Nd–xSr–0.3Zr alloys. Transactions of Nonferrous Metals Society of China. 2014, 24, 3797–803.

[29] Leng Z, Zhang J, Yin T, Zhang L, Wu R. Influence of biocorrosion on microstructure and mechanical properties of deformed Mg–Y–Er–Zn biomaterial containing 18R-LPSO phase. Journal of the Mechanical Behavior of Biomedical Materials. 2013, 28, 332–9.

[30] Chou D-T, Hong D, Saha P, Ferrero J, Kumta PN. In vitro and in vivo corrosion, cytocompatibility and mechanical properties of biodegradable Mg–Y–Ca–Zr alloys as implant materials. Acta Biomaterialia. 2013, 9, 8518–33.

[30] Zhou WR. Zheng YF, Leeflang MA, Zhou J. Mechanical property, biocorrosion and in vitro biocompatibility evaluations of Mg–Li–(Al)–(RE) alloys for future cardiovascular stent application. Acta Biomaterialia. 2013, 9, 8488–98.

[31] Huang Y, Feyerabend F, Willumeit R, Hort N. Influence of ageing treatment on microstructure, mechanical and bio-corrosion properties of Mg–Dy alloys. Journal of the Mechanical Behavior of Biomedical Materials. 2012, 13, 36–44.

[32] Zhang X, Wu Y, Xue Y, Wang Z. Biocorrosion behavior and cytotoxicity of a Mg–Gd–Zn–Zr alloy with long period stacking ordered structure. Materials Letters. 2012, 86, 42–5.

[33] Zhang E, Yang L, Xu J, Chen H. Microstructure, mechanical properties and bio-corrosion properties of Mg–Si(–Ca, Zn) alloy for biomedical application. Acta Biomaterialia. 2010, 6, 1756–62.

[34] Zhao C, Pan F, Zhang L, Pan H, Tang A. Microstructure, mechanical properties, bio-corrosion properties and cytotoxicity of as-extruded Mg-Sr alloys. Materials Science and Engineering: C. 2017, 70, 1081–8.

[35] Khalajabadi SZ, Ahmad N, Yahya A, Yajid MAM, Abdul Kadir MR. The role of titania on the microstructure, biocorrosion and mechanical properties of Mg/HA-based nanocomposites for potential application in bone repair. Ceramics International. 2016, 42, 18223–37.

[36] González S, Pellicer E, Suriñach, Baró MD, Sort J. Biodegradation and mechanical integrity of magnesium alloys suitable for implants, Biodegradation – Engineering and Technology. 2013; https://www.intechopen.com/books/biodegradation-engineering-and-technology/biodegradation-and-mechanical-integrity-of-magnesium-and-magnesium-alloys-suitable-for-implants.

[37] Sezer N, Evis Z, Kayhan SM, Tahmasebifar A, Koç M. Review of magnesium-based biomaterials and their applications. Journal of Magnesium and Alloys. 2018, 6, 23–43.

[38] Oshida Y, Tuna EB, Aktören O, Gençay K. Dental Implant Systems. International Journal of Molecular Sciences. 2010, 11, 1580–678.

[39] Rahim MI, Ullah S, Mueller PP. Advances and challenges of biodegradable implant materials with a focus on magnesium-alloys and bacterial infections. Metals. 2018, 8, 532; doi:10.3390/met8070532.
[40] Sheikh Z, Najeeb S, Khurshid Z, Verma V, Rashid H, Glogauer M. Biodegradable materials for bone repair and tissue engineering applications. Materials (Basel). 2015, 8, 5744–94.
[41] Middleton JC, Tipton AJ. Synthetic biodegradable polymers as orthopedic devices. Biomaterials. 2000, 21, 2335–46.
[42] Pogorielov M, Husak E, Solodivnik A, Zhdanov S. Magnesium-based biodegradable alloys: Degradation, application, and alloying elements. Interv Medicine Applied Sciemce. 2017, 9, 27–38.
[43] Sanchez AH, Luthringer BJ, Feyerabend F, Willumeit R: Mg and Mg alloys: How comparable are in vitro and in vivo corrosion rates? A review. Acta Biomaterialia. 2015, 13, 16–31.
[44] Pierson D, Edick J, Tauscher A, Pokorney E, Bowen P, Gelbaugh J, Stinson J, Getty H, Lee CH, Drelich J, Goldman J. A simplified in vivo approach for evaluating the bioabsorbable behavior of candidate stent materials. Journal of Biomedical Materials Research. Part B, Applied Biomaterials 2012, 100, 58–67.
[45] Hermawan H, Purnama A, Dube D, Couet J, Mantovani D. Fe-Mn alloys for metallic biodegradable stents: Degradation and cell viability studies. Acta Biomaterialia. 2010, 6, 1852–60.
[46] Yang H, Wang C, Liu C, Chen H, Wu Y, Han J, Jia Z, Lin W, Zhang D, Li W, Yuan W, Guo H, Li H, Yang G, Kong D, Zhu D, Takashima K, Ruan L, Nie J, Li X, Zheng Y. Evolution of the degradation mechanism of pure zinc stent in the one-year study of rabbit abdominal aorta model. Biomaterials. 2017, 145, 92–105.
[47] Zhao D, Wang T, Nahan K, Guo X, Zhang Z, Dong Z, Chen S, Chou DT, Hong D, Kumta PN, Heineman WR. In vivo characterization of magnesium alloy biodegradation using electrochemical H2 monitoring, ICP-MS, and XPS. Acta Biomaterialia. 2017, 50, 556–65.
[48] Zhao D, Witte F, Lu F, Wang J, Li J, Qin L. Current status on clinical applications of magnesium-based orthopaedic implants: A review from clinical translational perspective. Biomaterials. 2017, 112, 287–302.
[49] Staiger MP, Pietak AM, Huadmai J, Dias G. Magnesium and its alloys as orthopedic biomaterials: A review. Biomaterials. 2006, 27, 1728–34.
[50] Li X, Liu X, Wu S, Yeung KWK, Zheng Y, Chu PK. Design of magnesium alloys with controllable degradation for biomedical implants: From bulk to surface. Acta Biomaterialia. 2016, 45, 2–30.
[51] Evis Z, Kayhan SM, Tahmasebifar A, Koç M. Review of magnesium-based biomaterials and their applications. Journal of Magnesium and Alloys. 2018, 6, 23–43.
[52] Hu H, Nie X, Ma Y. Corrosion and Surface Treatment of Magnesium Alloys, Magnesium Alloys – Properties in Solid and Liquid States. 2014; https://www.intechopen.com/books/magnesium-alloys-properties-in-solid-and-liquid-states/corrosion-and-surface-treatment-of-magnesium-alloys.
[53] Agarwal S, Curtin J, Duffy B, Jaiswal S. Biodegradable magnesium alloys for orthopaedic applications: A review on corrosion, biocompatibility and surface modifications. Materials Science and Engineering: C. 2016, 68, 948–63.
[54] Ye SH, et al., Biodegradable zwitterionic polymer coatings for magnesium alloy stents. Langmuir. 2019, 35, 1421–9.
[55] Hernández-Alvarado LA, et al., Phytic acid coating on Mg-based materials for biodegradable temporary endoprosthetic applications. Journal of Alloys and Compounds. 2016, 664, 609–18.

[56] Liu C, et al., Study on biodegradation of the second phase Mg17Al12 in Mg-Al-Zn Alloys: In vitro experiment and thermodynamic calculation. Materials Science and Engineering: C. 2014, 35, 1–7.

[57] Leeflang MA, et al., Long-term biodegradation and associated hydrogen evolution of duplex-structured Mg-Li-Al-(RE) alloys and their mechanical properties Materials Science and Engineering: B. 2011, 176, 1741–5.

[58] Remennik S, et al., New, fast corroding high ductility Mg–Bi–Ca and Mg–Bi–Si alloys, with no clinically observable gas formation in bone implants. Materials Science and Engineering: B. 2011, 176, 1653–9.

[59] Li Z, et al., The development of binary Mg-Ca alloys for use as biodegradable materials within bone. Biomaterials. 2008, 29, 1329–44.

[60] Trincă LC, et al., In vivo degradation behavior and biological activity of some new Mg–Ca alloys with concentration's gradient of Si for bone grafts. Applied Surface Science. 2015, 352, 140–50.

[61] Seong JW, et al., Development of biodegradable Mg-Ca alloy sheets with enhanced strength and corrosion properties through the refinement and uniform dispersion of the Mg2Ca phase by high-ratio differential speed rolling. Acta Biomaterialia. 2015, 11, 531–42.

[62] Desai S, et al., Effect of High Speed Dry Machining on Surface integrity and Biodegradability of Mg-Ca1.0 Biodegradable Alloy. Materials Today: Proceedings. 2017, 4, 6718–27.

[63] Rad HRB, et al., Microstructure analysis and corrosion behavior of biodegradable Mg–Ca implant alloys. Materials & Design. 2012, 33, 88–97.

[64] Fischerauer SF, et al., In vivo degradation performance of micro-arc-oxidized magnesium implants: a micro-CT study in rats. Acta Biomaterialia. 2013, 9, 5411–20.

[65] Berglund IS, et al., Peri-implant tissue response and biodegradation performance of a Mg–1.0Ca–0.5Sr alloy in rat tibia. Materials Science and Engineering: C. 2016, 62, 79–85.

[66] Lee J-H et al., Stability of biodegradable metal (Mg-Ca-Zn alloy) screws compared with absorbable polymer and titanium screws for sagittal split ramus osteotomy of the mandible using the finite element analysis model. Journal of Cranio-Maxillofacial Surgery. 2017, 45, 1639–46.

[67] Bakhsheshi-Rad HR, et al., Synthesis and corrosion behavior of a hybrid bioceramic-biopolymer coating on biodegradable Mg alloy for orthopaedic implants. Journal of Alloys and Compounds. 2015, 648, 1067–71.

[68] Cha PR, et al., Biodegradability engineering of biodegradable Mg alloys: tailoring the electrochemical properties and microstructure of constituent phases. Science Reports 2013, 3: doi: 10.1038/srep02367.

[69] Li Y, et al., Biodegradable Mg–Cu alloy implants with antibacterial activity for the treatment of osteomyelitis: *in vitro* and *in vivo* evaluations. Biomaterials. 2016, 106, 250–63.

[70] Yan X, et al., Improvement of biodegradable and antibacterial properties by solution treatment and micro-arc oxidation (MAO) of a magnesium alloy with a trace of copper. Corrosion Science. 2019, 156, 125–38.

[71] Yan X, et al., Corrosion and biological performance of biodegradable magnesium alloys mediated by low copper addition and processing. Materials Science and Engineering: C. 2018, 93, 565–81.

[72] Zhang X, et al., Microstructures and corrosion behavior of biodegradable Mg–6Gd–xZn–0.4Zr alloys with and without long period stacking ordered structure. Corrosion Science. 2016, 105, 68–77.

[73] Brar HS, et al., The role of surface oxidation on the degradation behavior of biodegradable Mg–RE (Gd, Y, Sc) alloys for resorbable implants. Materials Science and Engineering: C. 2014, 40, 407–17.

[74] Chen X-B et al., Biodegradation of Mg-14Li alloy in simulated body fluid: A proof-of-concept study. Bioactive Materials. 2018, 3, 110–7.
[75] Liu Y, et al., Study on the Mg-Li-Zn ternary alloy system with improved mechanical properties, good degradation performance and different responses to cells. Acta Biomaterialia. 2017, 62, 418–33.
[76] Gnedenkov SV, et al., Composite hydroxyapatite–PTFE coatings on Mg–Mn–Ce alloy for resorbable implant applications via a plasma electrolytic oxidation-based route. Journal of the Taiwan Institute of Chemical Engineers. 2014, 45, 3104–9.
[77] Gil-Santos A, et al., Microstructure and degradation performance of biodegradable Mg-Si-Sr implant alloys. Materials Science and Engineering: C. 2017, 71, 25–34.
[78] Zhen Z, et al., In Vitro Study on Mg–Sn–Mn Alloy as Biodegradable Metals. Journal of Materials Science & Technology. 2014, 30, 675–85.
[79] Wang Y, et al., Microstructures, mechanical properties, and degradation behaviors of heat-treated Mg-Sr alloys as potential biodegradable implant materials. Journal of the Mechanical Behavior of Biomedical Materials. 2018, 77, 47–57.
[80] Shangguan Y, et al., Comparison study of different coatings on degradation performance and cell response of Mg-Sr alloy. Materials Science and Engineering: C. 2016, 69, 95–107.
[81] Bornapour M, et al., Biocompatibility and biodegradability of Mg-Sr alloys: The formation of Sr-substituted hydroxyapatite. Acta Biomaterialia 2013, 9, 5319–30.
[82] Yazici M, et al., Biodegradability and antibacterial properties of MAO coatings formed on Mg-Sr-Ca alloys in an electrolyte containing Ag doped hydroxyapatite. Thin Solid Films. 2017, 644, 92–8.
[83] Bornapour M, et al., Thermal exposure effects on the in vitro degradation and mechanical properties of Mg-Sr and Mg–Ca–Sr biodegradable implant alloys and the role of the microstructure. Materials Science and Engineering: C. 2015, 46, 16–24.
[84] Zhao X, et al., Biodegradable Mg-Zn-Y alloys with long-period stacking ordered structure: Optimization for mechanical properties. Journal of the Mechanical Behavior of Biomedical Materials. 2013, 18, 181–90.
[85] Zhang S, et al., Research on an Mg-Zn alloy as a degradable biomaterial. Acta Biomaterialia. 2010, 6, 626–40.
[86] Song Y, et al., A novel biodegradable nicotinic acid/calcium phosphate composite coating on Mg–3Zn alloy. Materials Science and Engineering: C. 2013, 33, 78–84.
[87] Zhao X, et al., Mg-Zn-Y alloys with long-period stacking ordered structure: In vitro assessments of biodegradation behavior. Materials Science and Engineering: C. 2013, 33, 3627–37.
[88] Manne B, et al., Surface design of Mg-Zn alloy temporary orthopaedic implants: Tailoring wettability and biodegradability using laser surface melting. Surface & Coatings Technology. 2018, 347, 337–49.
[89] Homayun B, et al., Microstructure, mechanical properties, corrosion behavior and cytotoxicity of Mg-Zn-Al-Ca alloys as biodegradable materials. Journal of Alloys and Compounds. 2014, 607, 1–10.
[90] Li W, et al., Preparation and in vitro degradation of the composite coating with high adhesion strength on biodegradable Mg-Zn-Ca alloy. Materials Characterization. 2011, 62, 1158–65.
[91] Lu Y, et al., Tomographic investigation of the effects of second phases on the biodegradation and nano-mechanical performance of a Mg–Zn–Ca alloy. Materialia. 2018, 4, 1–9.
[92] Anvari-Yazdi AF, et al., Cytotoxicity assessment of adipose-derived mesenchymal stem cells on synthesized biodegradable Mg-Zn-Ca alloys. Materials Science and Engineering: C. 2016, 69, 584–597.

[93] Roche V, et al., Degradation of biodegradable implants: The influence of microstructure and composition of Mg-Zn-Ca alloys. Journal of Alloys and Compounds. 2019, 774, 168–81.
[94] Datta MK, et al., Structure and thermal stability of biodegradable Mg-Zn-Ca based amorphous alloys synthesized by mechanical alloying. Materials Science and Engineering: B. 2011, 176, 1637–43.
[95] Amerinatanzi A, et al., Predicting the Biodegradation of Magnesium Alloy Implants: Modeling, Parameter Identification, and Validation. Bioengineering (Basel). 2018, 5; doi: 10.3390/bioengineering5040105.
[96] Liu D, et al., Fabrication of biodegradable HA/Mg-Zn-Ca composites and the impact of heterogeneous microstructure on mechanical properties, in vitro degradation and cytocompatibility. Bioelectrochemistry. 2019, 129, 106–15.
[97] Zhang B, et al., Mechanical properties, degradation performance and cytotoxicity of Mg-Zn-Ca biomedical alloys with different compositions. Materials Science and Engineering: C. 2011, 31, 1667–73.
[98] Cho DH, et al., Effect of Mn addition on grain refinement of biodegradable Mg4Zn0.5Ca alloy. Journal of Alloys and Compounds. 2016, 676, 461–8.
[99] Wang J, et al., Effect of Sr on the microstructure and biodegradable behavior of Mg-Zn-Ca-Mn alloys for implant application. Materials & Design. 2018, 153, 308–16.
[100] González S, et al., Improved mechanical performance and delayed corrosion phenomena in biodegradable Mg-Zn-Ca alloys through Pd-alloying. Journal of the Mechanical Behavior of Biomedical Materials. 2012, 6, 53–62.
[101] Li H, et al., In vitro responses of bone-forming MC3T3-E1 pre-osteoblasts to biodegradable Mg-based bulk metallic glasses. Materials Science and Engineering: C. 2016, 68, 632–41.
[102] Trivedi P, et al., Grain structure dependent self-assembled bioactive coating on Mg-2Zn-2Gd alloy: Mechanism of degradation at biointerfaces. Surface & Coatings Technology. 2017, 315, 250–7.
[103] Chen J, et al. Comparative study on effects of different coatings on biodegradable and wear properties of Mg-2Zn-1Gd-0.5Zr alloy. Surface & Coatings Technology. 2018, 352, 273–84.
[104] He R, et al., In vitro degradation behavior and cytocompatibility of Mg-6Zn-Mn alloy. Materials Letters 2018, 228, 77–80.
[105] Grillo CA, et al., Degradation of bioabsorbable Mg-based alloys: Assessment of the effects of insoluble corrosion products and joint effects of alloying components on mammalian cells. Material Sciemce and Engineering C Materials Biology Applied 2016, 58, 372–80.
[106] Li H, et al., Microstructures, mechanical and cytocompatibility of degradable Mg–Zn based orthopedic biomaterials. Materials & Design. 2014, 58, 43–51.
[107] Gu XN, et al., In vitro degradation performance and biological response of a Mg-Zn-Zr alloy. Materials Science and Engineering: B. 2011, 176, 1778–84.
[108] Hong D, et al., In vitro degradation and cytotoxicity response of Mg-4% Zn-0.5% Zr (ZK40) alloy as a potential biodegradable material. Acta Biomaterialia. 2013, 9, 8534–47.
[109] Wang T, et al., One-pot hydrothermal synthesis, in vitro biodegradation and biocompatibility of Sr-doped nanorod/nanowire hydroxyapatite coatings on ZK60 magnesium alloy. Journal of Alloys and Compounds. 2019, 799, 71–82.
[110] Li T, et al., Microstructure, mechanical property and in vitro biocorrosion behavior of single-phase biodegradable Mg-1.5Zn-0.6Zr alloy. Journal of Magnesium and Alloys. 2014, 2, 181–9.
[111] Wang J, et al., Effects of gas produced by degradation of Mg-Zn-Zr Alloy on cancellous bone tissue. Materials Science and Engineering: C. 2015, 55, 556–61.
[112] Li T, et al., Microstructure, Mechanical Properties and In Vitro Degradation Behavior of a Novel Biodegradable Mg-1.5Zn-0.6Zr-0.2Sc Alloy. Journal of Materials Science & Technology. 2015, 31, 744–50.

[113] Li T, et al., Effects of scandium addition on biocompatibility of biodegradable Mg-1.5Zn-0.6Zr alloy. Materials Letters. 2018, 215, 200–2.
[114] Li T, et al., Microstructure and mechanical property of biodegradable Mg-1.5Zn-0.6Zr alloy with varying contents of scandium. Materials Letters. 2018, 229, 60–3.
[115] Li T, et al., Influence of albumin on in vitro degradation behavior of biodegradable Mg-1.5Zn-0.6Zr-0.2Sc alloy. Materials Letters. 2018, 217, 227–30.
[116] Li Z, et al., The synergistic effect of trace Sr and Zr on the microstructure and properties of a biodegradable Mg-Zn-Zr-Sr alloy. Journal of Alloys and Compounds. 2017, 702, 290–302.
[117] Li Y, et al., Mg-Zr-Sr alloys as biodegradable implant materials. Acta Biomaterialia. 2012, 8, 3177–88.
[118] Brar HS, et al., A study of a biodegradable Mg-3Sc-3Y alloy and the effect of self-passivation on the in vitro degradation. Acta Biomaterialia 2013, 9, 5331–40.
[119] Leng Z, et al., Influence of biocorrosion on microstructure and mechanical properties of deformed Mg-Y-Er-Zn biomaterial containing 18R-LPSO phase. Journal of the Mechanical Behavior of Biomedical Materials. 2013, 28, 332–9.
[120] Fan J, et al., Microstructure, mechanical properties, in vitro degradation and cytotoxicity evaluations of Mg-1.5Y-1.2Zn-0.44Zr alloys for biodegradable metallic implants. Materials Science and Engineering: C. 2013, 33, 2345–52.
[121] Grillo CA, et al., Cellular response to rare earth mixtures (La and Gd) as components of degradable Mg alloys for medical applications. Colloids and Surfaces. B, Biointerfaces. 2014, 117, 312–21.
[122] Gui Z, et al., Mechanical and corrosion properties of Mg-Gd-Zn-Zr-Mn biodegradable alloy by hot extrusion. Journal of Alloys and Compounds. 2016, 685, 222–30.
[123] Liao Y, et al., In vitro degradation and mechanical properties of polyporous CaHPO4-coated Mg-Nd-Zn-Zr alloy as potential tissue engineering scaffold. Materials Letters 2013, 100, 306–8.
[124] Niu J, et al., Enhanced biocorrosion resistance and biocompatibility of degradable Mg-Nd-Zn-Zr alloy by brushite coating. Materials Science and Engineering: C. 2013, 33, 4833–41.
[125] Zhang J, et al., The degradation and transport mechanism of a Mg-Nd-Zn-Zr stent in rabbit common carotid artery: A 20-month study. Acta Biomaterialia. 2018, 69, 372–84.
[126] Zhang J, et al., The degradation and transport mechanism of a Mg-Nd-Zn-Zr stent in rabbit common carotid artery: A 20-month study. Acta Biomaterialia. 2018; doi: 10.1016/j.actbio.2018.01.018.
[127] Li G, et al., Dual modulation of bone formation and resorption with zoledronic acid-loaded biodegradable magnesium alloy implants improves osteoporotic fracture healing: An in vitro and in vivo study. Acta Biomaterialia 2018, 65, 486–500.
[128] Zhang W, et al., Effect of grain refinement and crystallographic texture produced by friction stir processing on the biodegradation behavior of a Mg-Nd-Zn alloy. Journal of Materials Science & Technology. 2019, 35, 777–83.
[129] Niu J, et al., The in vivo degradation and bone-implant interface of Mg-Nd-Zn-Zr alloy screws: 18 months post-operation results. Corrosion Science. 2016, 113, 183–7.
[130] Zhang X, et al., Improvement of mechanical properties and corrosion resistance of biodegradable Mg-Nd-Zn-Zr alloys by double extrusion. Materials Science and Engineering: B. 2012, 177, 1113–19.
[131] Mao L, et al., A novel biodegradable Mg-Nd-Zn-Zr alloy with uniform corrosion behavior in artificial plasma. Materials Letters. 2012, 88, 1–4.
[132] Shi Y, et al., In vitro and in vivo degradation of rapamycin-eluting Mg-Nd-Zn-Zr alloy stents in porcine coronary arteries. Materials Science and Engineering: C. 2017, 80, 1–6.

[133] Liao Y, et al., In vitro response of chondrocytes to a biodegradable Mg-Nd-Zn-Zr alloy. Materials Letters. 2012, 83, 206–8.
[134] Levy GK, et al., Cytotoxic characteristics of biodegradable EW10X04 Mg alloy after Nd coating and subsequent heat treatment. Materials Science and Engineering: C. 2016, 62, 752–61.
[135] Yang L, et al., Influence of Dy in solid solution on the degradation behavior of binary Mg-Dy alloys in cell culture medium. Materials Science and Engineering: C. 2017, 75, 1351–8.
[136] Zhang J, et al., New horizon for high performance Mg-based biomaterial with uniform degradation behavior: Formation of stacking faults. Science Reports 2015, 5: doi: 10.1038/srep13933.
[137] Song Y, Zhang S, Li J, Zhao C, Zhang X. Electrodeposition of Ca-P coatings on biodegradable Mg alloy: In vitro biomineralization behavior. Acta Biomaterialia. 2010, 6, 1736–42.
[138] Matykina E, Garcia I, Arrabal R, Mohedano M, Pardo A. Role of PEO coatings in long-term biodegradation of a Mg alloy. Applied Surface Science. 2016, 389, 810–23.
[139] Cui X-J, Lin X-Z, Liu C-H, Yang R-S, Zheng X-W, Gong M. Fabrication and corrosion resistance of a hydrophobic micro-arc oxidation coating on AZ31 Mg alloy. Corrosion Science. 2015, 90, 402–12.
[140] Zhang J, et al., Degradable behavior and bioactivity of micro-arc oxidized AZ91D Mg alloy with calcium phosphate/chitosan composite coating in m-SBF. Colloids and Surfaces. B, Biointerfaces. 2013, 111, 179–87.
[141] Rojaee R, et al., Controlling the degradation rate of AZ91 magnesium alloy via sol-gel derived nanostructured hydroxyapatite coating. Material Sciemce and Engineering C Materials Biology Applied 2013, 33, 3817–25.
[142] Hernández-Alvarado LA, et al., Phytic acid coating on Mg-based materials for biodegradable temporary endoprosthetic applications. Journal of Alloys and Compounds. 2016, 664, 609–18.
[143] Bakhsheshi-Rad HR, et al., Synthesis and corrosion behavior of a hybrid bioceramic-biopolymer coating on biodegradable Mg alloy for orthopaedic implants. Journal of Alloys and Compounds. 2015, 648, 1067–71.
[144] Gnedenkov SV, et al., Composite hydroxyapatite–PTFE coatings on Mg-Mn-Ce alloy for resorbable implant applications via a plasma electrolytic oxidation-based route. Journal of the Taiwan Institute of Chemical Engineers. 2014, 45, 3104–9.
[145] Niu J, et al., Enhanced biocorrosion resistance and biocompatibility of degradable Mg-Nd-Zn-Zr alloy by brushite coating. Materials Science and Engineering: C. 2013, 33, 4833–41.
[146] Liao Y, et al., In vitro degradation and mechanical properties of polyporous CaHPO4-coated Mg-Nd-Zn-Zr alloy as potential tissue engineering scaffold. Materials Letters. 2013, 100, 306–8.
[147] Levy GK, et al., Cytotoxic characteristics of biodegradable EW10X04 Mg alloy after Nd coating and subsequent heat treatment. Materials Science and Engineering: C. 2016, 62, 752–61.
[148] Shangguan Y, et al., Comparison study of different coatings on degradation performance and cell response of Mg-Sr alloy. Materials Science and Engineering: C. 2016, 69, 95–107.
[149] Fischerauer SF, et al., In vivo degradation performance of micro-arc-oxidized magnesium implants: a micro-CT study in rats. Acta Biomaterialia. 2013, 9, 5411–20.
[150] Yuan Q, et al., Effects of solidification cooling rate on the corrosion resistance of a biodegradable β-TCP/Mg-Zn-Ca composite. Bioelectrochemistry. 2018, 124, 93–104.
[151] Trivedi P, et al., Grain structure dependent self-assembled bioactive coating on Mg-2Zn-2Gd alloy: Mechanism of degradation at biointerfaces. Surface & Coatings Technology. 2017, 315, 250–7.
[152] Chen J, et al., Comparative study on effects of different coatings on biodegradable and wear properties of Mg-2Zn-1Gd-0.5Zr alloy. Surface & Coatings Technology. 2018, 352, 273–84.

[153] Wang T, et al. One-pot hydrothermal synthesis, in vitro biodegradation and biocompatibility of Sr-doped nanorod/nanowire hydroxyapatite coatings on ZK60 magnesium alloy. Journal of Alloys and Compounds. 2019, 799, 71–82.
[154] Tang J, et al., Surface coating reduces degradation rate of magnesium alloy developed for orthopaedic applications. Journal of Orthopaedic Translation. 2013, 1, 41–8.
[155] Uddin MS et al. Surface treatments for controlling corrosion rate of biodegradable Mg and Mg-based alloy implants. Sci and Tech of Advanced Materials. 2015, 16, doi.org/10.1088/1468-6996/16/5/0535021.
[156] Fan J, Qiu X, Niu X, Tuan Z, Meng J. Microstructure, mechanical properties, in vitro degradation and cytotoxicity evaluations of Mg–1.5Y–1.2Zn–0.44Zr alloys for biodegradable metallic implants. Materials Science and Engineering: C. 2013, 33, 2345–52.
[157] Mohamed A, El-Aziz AM, Breitinger H-G. Study of the degradation behavior and the biocompatibility of Mg–0.8Ca alloy for orthopedic implant applications. Journal of Magnesium and Alloys. 2019, 7, 249–57.
[158] Shangguan Y, Wan P, Tan L, Fan X, Qin L, Yang K. Investigation of the inner corrosion layer formed in pulse electrodeposition coating on Mg-Sr alloy and corresponding degradation behavior. Journal of Colloid and Interface Science. 2016, 481, 1–12.
[159] Wu H, Zhang C, Lou T, Chen B, Yi R, Wang W, Zhang R, Zuo M, Zu H, Han P, Zhang S, Ni J, Zhang X. Crevice corrosion – A newly observed mechanism of degradation in biomedical magnesium. Acta Biomaterialia. 2019, 98, 152–9.
[160] Liu Y-C, Liu D-B, Zhao Y, Chen M-F. Corrosion degradation behavior of Mg–Ca alloy with high Ca content in SBF. Transactions of Nonferrous Metals Society of China. 2015, 25, 3339–47.
[161] Cipriano AF, Lin J, Lin A, Sallee A, Le B. Cortez Alcaraz MC, Guan R-G, Botimer G, Inceodlu S, Liu H. Degradation of Bioresorbable Mg-4Zn-1Sr Intramedullary Pins and Associated Biological Responses in Vitro and in Vivo. ACS Appl Mater Interfaces. 2017, 9, 44332–55.
[162] Zhang Y, Wang X, Kuang Y, Liu B, Fang D. Enhanced mechanical properties and degradation rate of Mg-3Zn-1Y based alloy by Cu addition for degradable fracturing ball applications. Materials Letters. 2017, 195, 194–7.
[163] Niu J, Xiong M, Guan X, Zhang J, Yuan G. The in vivo degradation and bone-implant interface of Mg-Nd-Zn-Zr alloy screws: 18 months post-operation results. Corrosion Science. 2016, 113, 183–7.
[164] Leeflang MA, Dzwonczyk JS, Zhou J, Duszczyk J. Long-term biodegradation and associated hydrogen evolution of duplex-structured Mg–Li–Al–(RE) alloys and their mechanical properties. Materials Science and Engineering: B. 2011, 176, 1741–5.
[165] Liu Y, Zheng S, Li N, Guo H, Peng J. Study on the in vitro degradation behavior of pure Mg and WE43 in human bile for 60 days for future usage in biliary. Materials Letters. 2016, 179, 100–3.
[166] Peng Q, Fu H, Pang J, Zhang J, Xiao W. Preparation, mechanical and degradation properties of Mg–Y-based microwire. Journal of the Mechanical Behavior of Biomedical Materials. 2014, 29, 375–84.
[167] Liao Y, Chen D, Niu J, Zhang J, Jiang Y. In vitro degradation and mechanical properties of polyporous CaHPO4-coated Mg–Nd–Zn–Zr alloy as potential tissue engineering scaffold. Materials Letters. 2013, 100, 306–8.
[168] Zhang N, Zhao D, Liu N, Wu Y, Yang J, Wang Y, Xie H, Ji Y, Zhou C, Zhuang J, Wang Y, Yan J. Assessment of the degradation rates and effectiveness of different coated Mg-Zn-Ca alloy scaffolds for in vivo repair of critical-size bone defects. Journal of Materials Science. Materials in Medicine. 2018, 29; 138; https://doi.org/10.1007/s10856-018-6145-2.

Chapter 19 Biomedical applications

19.1 In general

In biomedical applications, the conventionally used metallic materials such as stainless steel (Fe–Ni–Cr), Co-based alloys (Co–Cr) and Ti alloys (Ti–Al–V) exhibit unsatisfactory results such as stress shielding due to mismatching of values of modulus of elasticity and metal ion releases of potential toxic elements including Ni, Cr and V elements. As a result, secondary surgical operation usually becomes inevitable to prevent long-term exposure of body with the toxic implant contents [1, 2]. From the biomedical point of view, magnesium alloys possess appropriate levels of mechanical properties, controllable (to some extent) biodegradation, acceptable biofunctionality as well as biosafety. Magnesium alloys are used for tissue engineering, orthopedic and cardiovascular applications in medicine [3–5] and bone plate and screw or temporary implants in dentistry [6, 7]. Each alloying element exhibits its characteristic influence(s) on specifically aimed properties including mechanical, chemical, physical or combined properties. Although alloying with effective elements improves particularly mechanical properties and corrosion behaviors, there are some limitations due to various factors, for example, thermodynamic limitation such as equilibrium solid solubility, evolution of intermetallics or potential toxicities, including Al for neurotoxicity due to accumulated amount [8, 9] or rare earth (RE) elements such as La and Nd for potential hepatotoxicity [10]. Therefore, the advantage of increasing mechanical properties of some Mg-based alloys cannot be used for biomedical applications, although such modified Mg-based alloys have been successfully employed in nonmedical applications. We have been discussing biological reactions (biocompatibility, cytocompatibility, hemocompatibility) as well as biodegradation of Mg materials. At the same time, there has been extensive research efforts to develop new Mg materials (alloy and composites) with nontoxicity or low toxicity and ideally controllable biodegradation. Various biomedical Mg-based alloy systems such as Mg–Zn series, Mg–Ca series, Mg–Si series and Mg–Sr series have been researched and developed. Magnesium can dissolve in body fluids, which means the implanted Mg can degrade during healing process, and if the degradation is controlled it would leave no debris after the completion of healing. Hence, the need for secondary surgical operation(s) for the implant removal could be eliminated [1]. An additional uniqueness associated with Mg-based biomaterials is its capability of degrading in biological environment (or, in short, biodegradation) [11, 12]. Here the most important issue is how to control the biodegradation rate when administered into the body, since uncontrolled biodegradation could result in loss of mechanical integrity of placed implants, metal contamination in the body and intolerable hydrogen evolution by tissue. Although

https://doi.org/10.1515/9783110676945-019

most of the patients experienced subcutaneous gas cavities caused by hydrogen generated during rapid corrosion of magnesium, they had no pain and almost no infections were observed during the postoperative follow-up [13]. Besides its required biocompatibility, the inherent mechanical properties of Mg are very similar to those of human bone, establishing satisfied biomechanical compatibility [14]. Similar to Figure 2.6, Figure 19.1 illustrates the relationship between strength and rigidity of various Mg biomaterials in comparison with that of cortical bone [14, 15]. In the figure, the predicted zone (with red dotted circle) of hydroxyapatite (HA)-coated Mg (99.9% pure Mg) rod is inserted [16]. The immediate finding from this figure is the fact that strength and rigidity of several types of coated and uncoated Mg materials are close to those values of the receiving hard tissue (cortical bone structure) if such Mg material is implanted. This issue is directly related to the stress shielding effect for bone remodeling process.

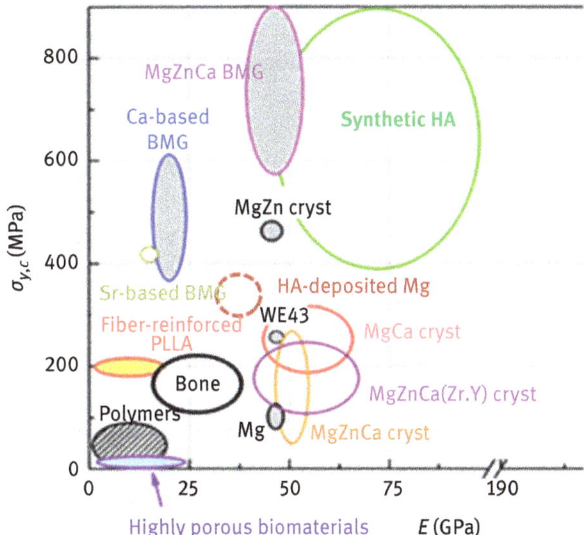

Figure 19.1: Strength versus rigidity of various Mg-based biomaterials, compared with that of cortical bone [14, 15].

Stress shielding (or stress protection) takes place when metal implants are used to repair fractures or in joint replacement surgery and this phenomenon refers to the reduction in bone density (osteopenia) as a result of removal of stress (or load) from the bone implant. According to Wolff's law, bone in a healthy person or animal will remodel in response to the loads it is placed under. Therefore, if the loading on a bone decreases, the bone will become less dense and weaker because there is no stimulus for continued remodeling that is required to maintain bone mass. Such bone remodeling is very sensitive to small changes in cyclic bone stresses. Changes in cyclic bone stresses of less than 1% of the ultimate strength can cause measurable differences in bone remodeling after a period of a few months [17]. Referring to Figure 19.2, the stresses from the body weight on the lower limb skeleton as a steady flow of impulses start at the lower back. In the normal healthy skeleton, the stresses flow symmetrically from there downward through both hip joints, thighbones, knee joints, lower leg bones, and feet into the floor (a). But, as shown in (b), when there is a total hip joint device, the much stiffer shaft component of the total hip takes over the majority of the load stresses. Hence, the stresses of the body weight flow through the total joint center and then through the shaft component of the device. The flow of stresses then enters the thighbone at the tip of the femoral component. The consequences of the changed flow of stresses are as follows: (1) the upper part of the thighbone is unloaded; it contains less bone tissue and it is weaker and more susceptible to fracture. (2) The skeleton around the tip of the femoral component is overloaded; it becomes more thick and stronger. The patients with cementless shafts of total hip devices often claim about the pain in the thigh, especially during the first years after the surgery [18]. Even, macroscopically, the entire implant body of the total hip replacement acts as a stress shielding entity, there should be some differences in the design as seen in (c), where shoulder portions of the implant body seems to be prone to experience the stress shielding [19]. The adverse effect of noticeable differences in rigidity is affecting not only the stress shielding effects but also the interfacial stress development problem. It is obvious that if differences (ΔE) in moduli of elasticity of metallic implant (E_M) and that of bone (E_B) are large, there should be an interfacial stress field developed (σ_{INT}). And if the interfacial stress is larger than the bonding strength of osseointegrated couple of implant and bone, the placed implant could be loose [14].

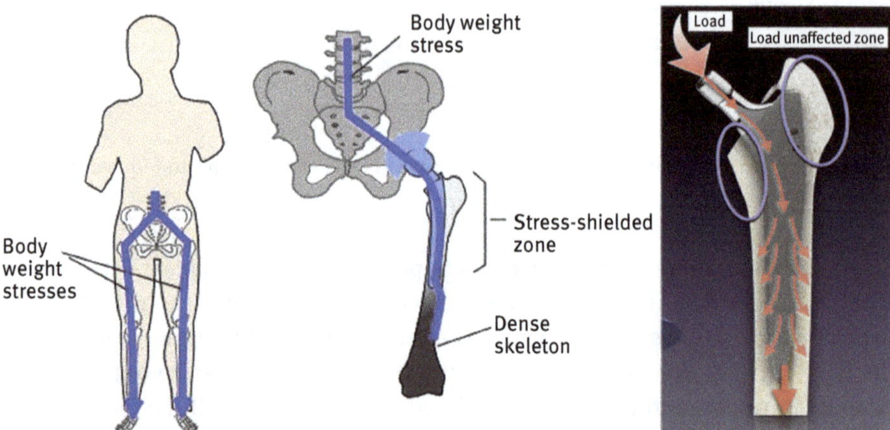

Figure 19.2: Schematic illustration of stress shielding [18, 19]. a: lower limbs bearing body weight b: enlarged view of left side of limb showing the transition body weight through femur c: stress flow line, illustrating load unaffected zone.

In this chapter, we will review medical applications of Mg-based biomaterials in both medicine and dental fields, including already well-established implants and its related devices and those under R&D progress with promised applicability.

19.2 Characterization of Mg biomaterials

As accepted implantable Mg-based biomaterials, Mg bone implants can be characterized as the ones illustrated in Figure 19.3 [20], indicating that after a best combination of fabrication route, material's modification and properties, the acceptable Mg bone material can be selected.

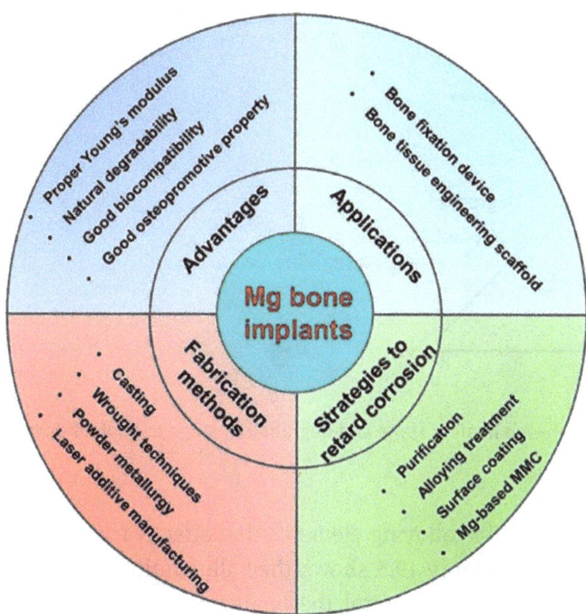

Figure 19.3: Characterization of acceptable Mg bone implant system [20].

There are basically two types of medical implants: permanent implants and temporary implants. Although in medicine, particularly in orthopedics, the temporary implants are dominant, in dentistry both types are frequently employed. For example, dental implants in prosthodontics that serve as an artificial tooth root should remain at the placed position for recovery of normal masticatory function and sometimes additional esthetics, while temporary-type mini-implants are used for an anchorage functioning for orthodontic mechanotherapy and a bone plate and screw-type implant for aggressive corticotomy orthodontic treatment. The low degradation rate of traditional implants has made them unsuitable for temporary implant applications, which has led to the rapid development of biodegradable implants. Polymers and metals are two material classes that have been widely considered for biodegradable temporary applications due to their inherent ability to dissolve away harmlessly within the human body, which eliminates the necessity of the removal of the implant after it has served its purpose [21, 22]. Mg-based biodegradable alloys are expected to degrade with the metabolism at an appropriate degradation rate inside the human body [23–26]. In fact, during the healing process, the mechanical stiffness/strength of the temporary implants slowly decreases, while the surrounding tissue regains stiffness/strength [27], as demonstrated in Figure 19.4 [28]. Harmless dissolution of the implant material eliminates the need for a second surgery that is commonly employed for removal of the implant once the tissue has completely healed [27].

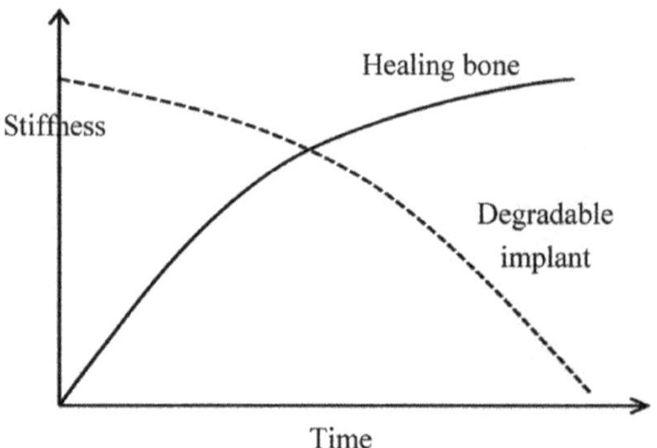

Figure 19.4: Completing processes between healing stage and degradation stage of implant using biodegradable materials [28].

Radha et al. [29] summarized all possible alloying elements that affect various major properties of Mg-based biomaterials. Figure 19.5 shows their illustration [29] along with alloying elements that are effective to control the biodegradation [4, 20, 30]. Development of the biomaterial requires a comprehensive understanding of the biological interaction between the implant and the host tissue, as well as of the behavior in the physiological environment in vivo [31]. In particular, development of innovative Mg biomaterials for implantology requires interdisciplinary approaches covering materials science and engineering, bioscience and biofunction. In addition, due to propensity of corrosion behavior of magnesium, rapid degradation of these materials in physiological environments may lead to gas cavities, hemolysis and osteolysis, thereby hindering their clinical orthopedic applications [32].

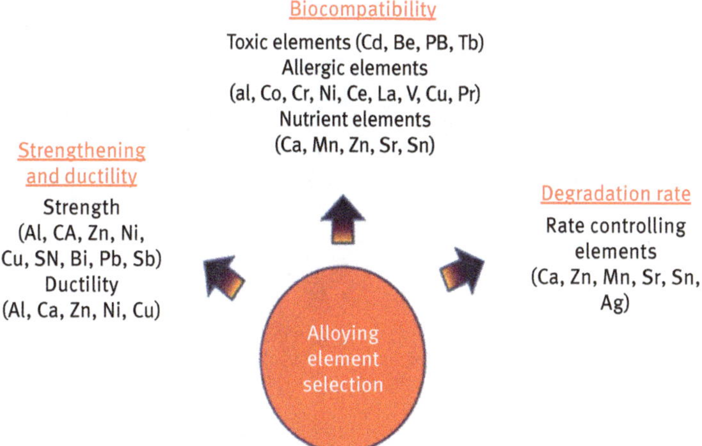

Figure 19.5: Various alloying elements affecting major properties of Mg biomaterials [29].

19.3 Orthopedic bone implants

Orthopedic bone implants represent medical devices that are used to. replace a missing joint or any damaged bone. On the other hand, bone fixation device should include bone screw with self-tapping threads used as fastening elements in prosthetics, bone pin, bone plate, and others which plays a role of consolidation during bone repair.

Marukawa et al. [33] evaluated in vivo the biological responses to implants composed of biodegradable anodized WE43 (Mg-4Y-3-RE-0.4Zr) alloy, untreated WE43 alloy and poly-L-lactic acid (PLLA), which are commonly used materials in clinical settings, and to evaluate the effectiveness of the materials as bone screws. The effectiveness of the magnesium alloy implants in osteosynthesis was evaluated using a bone fracture model involving the tibia of beagle dogs. Referring to Figure 19.6, it was reported that for the untreated WE43 implants, radiological and histological evaluation revealed that bone trabeculae around the implanted monolithic WE43 decreased because of an inflammatory response; however, there was no damage due to hydrogen gas or inflammatory response in the bone tissue around the anodized WE43 implants. After 4 weeks, all the PLLA implants ($n = 3$) had broken but the WE43 implants had not ($n = 6$), which suggests that the WE43 implants had sufficient strength to fix bone fractures at load-bearing sites in orthopedic and oral maxillofacial surgery.

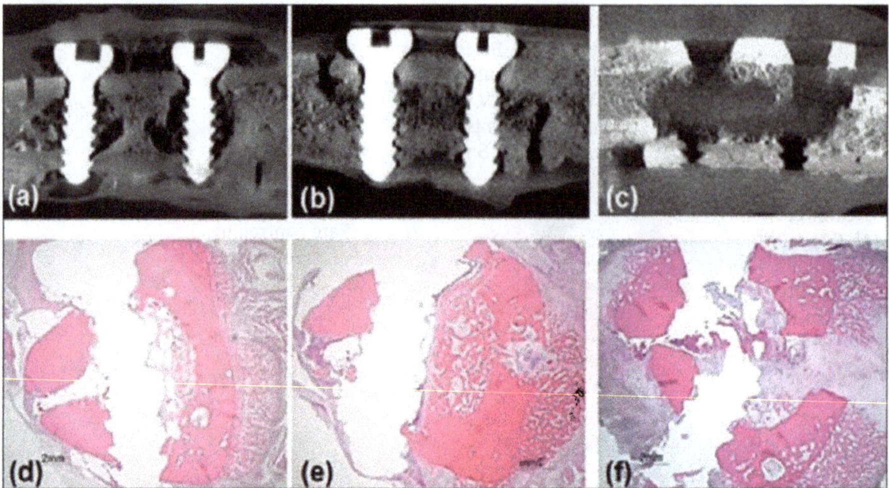

Figure 19.6: X-ray images and stained tissue images of (a, d) anodized WE43, (b, e) untreated WE43 and (c, f) PLLA implants, at 4 weeks after implantation [33].

Using Mg–Y alloy (Mg–3Nd–0.3Zn–0.4Zr) [34], Nie et al. [35] conducted an 18-month implantation. It was observed that, as shown in Figure 19.7, (i) after 4 months, the screw maintained good integrity, with only 16% volume loss, but (ii) a volume reduction of nearly 90% at 18 months.

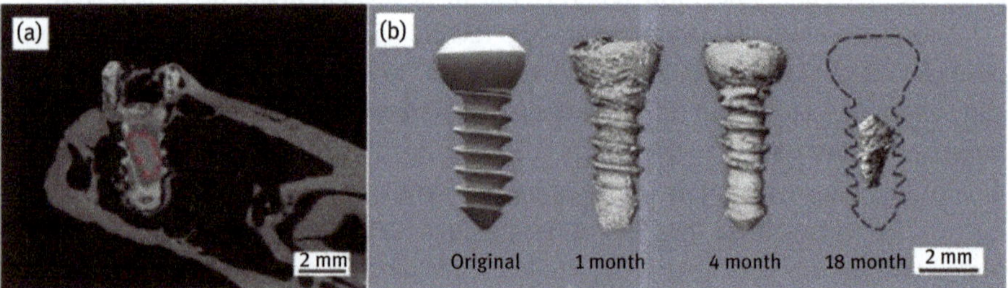

Figure 19.7: Original screw and segmented residual screw at 1, 4 and 18 months postoperation.

Zhang et al. [36] investigated pure Mg and Mg–6Zn alloy as potential candidates for biodegradable implants for the urinary system by conducting the in vitro corrosion behavior by potentiodynamic polarization and immersion tests in simulated body fluid at 37 °C. The in vivo degradation and histocompatibility were examined through implantation into the bladders of Wistar rats. It was reported that (i) Zn elevated the passivation potential and increased the cathodic current density, (ii) both in vitro and in vivo degradation tests showed a faster corrosion rate for the

Mg–6Zn alloy and (iii) tissues stained with hematoxylin and eosin suggested that both pure Mg and Mg–6Zn alloy exhibited good histocompatibility in the bladder indwelling implantation and no differences between pure Mg and Mg–6Zn groups were found in bladder, liver and kidney tissues during the 2 weeks' implantation. Wang et al. [37] investigated the effect of Sr on the microstructure and biocorrosion behavior of $Mg_{65.2-x}Zn_{30}Ca_4Mn_{0.8}Sr_x$ (x = 0, 0.3, 0.5 and 0.8) amorphous matrix composite by electrochemical measurements, immersion test and in vitro cytotoxicity test. It was mentioned that (i) compared with the Mg–Zn–Ca–Mn alloy, the Sr-bearing alloys with minor Sr incorporation improved the glass formation ability and biocorrosion resistance significantly and (ii) the major corrosion products were $Zn(OH)_2$, HA and phosphate after 124 h static immersion test, which were beneficial to the bone growth. This suggests that the Mg–Zn–Ca-based alloy possessed a good corrosion resistance and biocompatibility, showing a promising candidate for the biodegradable implants. Li et al. [38] prepared the Mg–1Zn–xSr (x = 0.2, 0.5, 0.8 and 1 wt%) alloys by zone-purifying solidification followed by backward extrusion. It was found that (i) the grain size was reduced and the hardness was improved with the increased concentration of Sr after backward extrusion, (ii) the extruded Mg–1Zn–0.8Sr alloy was mostly composed of fine precipitates (MgZn and $Mg_{17}Sr_2$) and Mg matrix, (iii) the degradation rate is significantly increased when Sr content is over 0.8 wt%, (iv) the homogeneous degradation rate is achieved and (v) the degradation products show good biocompatibility evaluated by 3-(4,5-dimethylthiazol-2-yl)-2,5-diphenyltetrazolium bromide (MTT) method using L929 cell line, indicating that the microalloying element of Sr is a potential approach to develop novel Mg–Zn-based biomaterials.

Makkar et al. [39] determined the in vitro degradation and in vivo performance of binary Mg–xCa alloy (x = 0.5 or 5.0 wt%) to assess its usability for degradable implant applications. The in vitro degradation tests were conducted via immersion test in phosphate buffer saline solution, and the in vivo performance in terms of interface, biocompatibility and biodegradability of Mg–xCa alloys was examined by implanting samples into the femoral condyle of rabbit for 2 and 4 weeks. It was obtained that (i) the immersion tests revealed that the dissolution rate varies linearly with Ca content exhibiting more hydrogen gas evolution, increased pH and higher degradation for Mg–5.0Ca alloy; (ii) the in vivo studies showed good biocompatibility with enhanced bone formation for Mg–0.5Ca after 4 weeks of implantation compared with Mg–5.0Ca alloy; and (iii) higher initial corrosion rate with prolonged inflammation and rapid degradation was noticed in Mg–5.0Ca compared with Mg–0.5Ca alloy. Based on these findings, it was concluded that Mg–0.5Ca alloy could be used as a temporary biodegradable implant material for clinical applications owing to its controlled in vivo degradation, reduced inflammation and high bone formation capability. Mohamed et al. [40] examined the Mg–0.8Ca alloy as a potential orthopedic biodegradable implant material. The in vitro degradation assessment in Hank's balanced salt solution, hydrogen evolution and electrochemical behavior as well as the cytotoxicity of the degradation products were investigated.

It was reported that (i) degradation in Hank's solution resulted in the formation of the needle-shaped carbonated HA which was similar to the biological apatite in the human bone; (ii) degradation kinetics showed that Mg–0.8Ca alloy had approximately threefold faster degradation rate than the pure Mg (1.08 ± 0.38 mm/year for Mg–0.8Ca and 0.35 ± 0.17 mm/year for pure Mg); and (iii) both pure Mg and Mg–0.8Ca alloy were biocompatible, generating no cytotoxic degradation products against human-derived HEK 293 cells. This indicates that the Mg–0.8Ca alloy was found to be a promising biodegradable implant in terms of bioactivity and compatibility with human cell lines and depending on the application of the implant and the estimated healing time of the bone, the desired degradation rate of an implant can be controlled by the Mg–Ca composition of such alloys. A composite coating composed of octacalcium phosphate (OCP) and HA as an underlayer and polycaprolactone (PCL) as an overlayer was fabricated on an Mg–1.2Ca–2Zn alloy via combination of chemical solution deposition and dip coating methods [41]. It was mentioned that (i) the corrosion current densities of Mg alloy significantly decreased after composite coating from 211.6 to 0.059 $\mu A/cm^2$, indicating that the PCL/OCP/HA composite coating can effectively protect the Mg–1.2Ca–2Zn alloy when used as degradable orthopedic implants.

The Mg–Zr–Sr alloys were prepared by diluting Mg–Zr and Mg–Sr master alloys with pure Mg [42]. The impact of Zr and Sr on the mechanical and biological properties has been thoroughly examined. The in vitro biocompatibility was assessed using osteoblast-like SaOS-2 (sarcoma osteogenic) cells and MTS and hemolysis tests and the in vivo bone formation and biodegradability were studied in a rabbit model. It was mentioned that (i) both Zr and Sr are excellent candidates for Mg alloying elements in manufacturing biodegradable Mg alloy implants; (ii) Zr addition refined the grain size, improved the ductility, smoothed the grain boundaries and enhanced the corrosion resistance of Mg alloys; (iii) Sr addition led to an increase in compressive strength, better in vitro biocompatibility and significantly higher bone formation in vivo; and (iv) Mg–xZr–ySr alloys with x and $y \leqslant 5$ wt% would make excellent biodegradable implant materials for load-bearing applications.

As-extruded Mg–1Sn and Mg–3Sn alloys were prepared and characterized for orthopedic applications [43]. It was reported that (i) the immersion and electrochemical tests indicated that the microstructure of as-extruded Mg–Sn alloys affected their corrosion properties, and the increase of Mg_2Sn phase resulting from the increase of the Sn content led to a higher corrosion rate and (ii) the cytotoxicity test showed that as-extruded Mg–1Sn and Mg–3Sn alloys met the requirement of cell toxicity for orthopedic applications, which indicates that these alloys were promising to be used as biodegradable orthopedic implants.

Proper alloying magnesium with element scandium (Sc) could transform its microstructure from α-phase with hexagonal closed-packed structure into β-phase with body-centered cubic (bcc) structure. Liu et al. [44] developed the Mg–30Sc alloy with single α-phase, dual phases (α + β) or β-phase microstructure by altering the heat-treatment routines and investigated their suitability for usage within the bone. It was reported that (i) the β-phased Mg–30Sc alloy showed the best mechanical performance with ultimate compressive strength of 603 ± 39 MPa and compressive strain of 31 ± 3%; (ii) the in vitro degradation test showed that the element scandium could effectively incorporate into the surface corrosion product layer, form a double-layered structure and further protect the alloy matrix; (iii) no cytotoxic effect was observed for both single α-phased and β-phased Mg–30 wt% Sc alloys on MC3T3 cell line; (iv) the β-phased Mg–30Sc alloy displayed acceptable corrosion resistance in vivo (0.06 mm/year) and maintained mechanical integrity up to 24 weeks; (v) the degradation process did not significantly influence the hematology indexes of inflammation, hepatic or renal functions; and (vi) the bone–implant contact (BIC) ratio of 75 ± 10% after 24 weeks implied satisfactory integration between β-phased Mg–30Sc alloy and the surrounding bone, indicating a potential usage of the bcc-structured Mg–Sc alloy within the bone.

In order to reduce the degradation rate, TiO_2-incorporated microarc oxidation (TO-MAO) coatings were prepared on Mg–Ca alloy using MAO [45]. Subsequently, zinc-doped HA (Zn-HA) coating was deposited by electrophoretic deposition on the MAO coating. The antibacterial activity of the coating against *Escherichia coli* (*E. coli*) tests indicated that the inhibition zone amplified after deposition of TO-MAO and Zn-HA coatings on Mg alloy, whereas more inhibition zone was found around Zn-HA coating. It was further mentioned that (i) the number of *E. coli* colonies reduces to 92% after Zn-HA coating, implying its good antibacterial properties and (ii) the cytotoxicity test indicated that the cell viability of MG63 osteoblast cells cultured with Zn-HA extracts was higher compared with the TO-MOA coating and bare Mg alloy, which suggests that Mg alloy coated with TO-MOA/Zn-HA exhibits high corrosion resistance, antibacterial activity and favorable bioactivity and cytocompatibility, indicating their substantial potentials for biomedical applications. The medical applications of porous Mg scaffolds are limited owing to its rapid corrosion, which dramatically decreases the mechanical strength of the scaffold. Mimicking the bone structure and composition can improve the mechanical and biological properties of porous Mg scaffolds. The Mg structure can also be coated with HA by an aqueous precipitation coating method to enhance both the corrosion resistance and the biocompatibility. However, due to the brittleness of HA coating layer, cracks tend to form in the HA coating layer, which may influence the corrosion and biological functionality of the scaffold. Based on this background, Kang et al. [46] applied hybrid poly(ether imide) (PEI)–SiO_2 layers to the HA-coated biomimetic porous Mg to impart the structure with the high corrosion resistance associated with PEI and excellent bioactivity with SiO_2. The porosity of Mg was controlled by adjusting the concentration of the sodium chloride (NaCl) particles used in the fabrication via the space-holder method. It was found that (i) the mechanical measurements showed that the compressive strength and stiffness of the biomimetic porous Mg increased as the portion of the dense region increased, (ii) HA/(PEI–SiO_2) hybrid-coated biomimetic Mg is a promising biodegradable scaffold for orthopedic applications, (iii) the in vitro testing revealed that the proposed hybrid coating reduced the degradation rate and facilitated osteoblast spreading compared with HA- and HA/PEI-coating scaffolds and (iv) the in vivo testing with a rabbit femoropatellar groove model showed improved tissue formation, reduced corrosion and degradation and improved bone formation on the scaffold.

19.4 Fixation device

The application of implants varies depending on aimed recovery of biofunctionality, including (1) the healing, stabilization and/or consolidation of the fractured bones by using screws with self-tapping threads used as fastening elements in prostheses, bone rods, bone pins and plates; (2) the rectification of deformities such as an abnormal spinal curvature; (3) an improvement in the function of an organ and/or other parts of human body; and (4) the replacement of a damaged and/or diseased part of the anatomy, such as damaged arthritic joints and malfunctioning heart valves [27, 47]. For Mg bone fixation device, its favorable mechanical strength ensures a proper mechanical support at the early stage, and then it undergoes a dynamic degradation with its load-bearing support gradually decreasing, as shown in Figure 19.4. The load bearing of bone tissue at the fracture site gradually increases instead of jumping directly to the stress stimulation at the physiological level, which is conducive to promoting the healing and shaping of new bone tissue [48].

19.4.1 Screws

Yu et al. [49] implanted as-rolled high-purity magnesium (99.99 wt%) screws in tibiae of rabbit for up to 52 weeks in order to investigate their long-term in vivo degradation and the local and systemic effects of their degradation products. A series of long-term monitoring were performed at various time points (4, 12, 26 and 52 weeks) after implantation using numerous investigations such as micro-CT (microcomputed tomography) assay, histomorphometric analysis, local microenvironment testing and biochemical analysis of serum and urine. It was reported that (i) pure Mg screws had a uniform degradation morphology and a slow degradation rate in vivo during the period of 52 weeks, (ii) their degradation products not only increased the local pH values but also changed the local Mg^{2+} ions concentration and gas cavity area in the peri-implant tissues in a dynamic manner, (iii) both the new bone formation and BIC rate were increased at bone–implant interfaces at 26 weeks and 52 weeks postimplantation and (iv) neither abnormal elevation of serum magnesium and urine magnesium level, nor liver and kidney dysfunction were detected during the monitoring period of 26 weeks. This suggests that pure Mg screws possess a slow degradation rate, desirable bone repair capacity and long-term local/systemic biosafety, and consequently may have good potential for application as bone fixation devices. Cha et al. [50] implanted the Mg–5Ca–1Zn alloy bone screw in the femoral condyle of New Zealand white rabbit. Histology using toluidine blue staining at 24 weeks is presented, as shown in Figure 19.8. As mentioned previously, Marukawa et al. [33] evaluated WE32 alloy screws using bone fracture model involving the tibia beagle dogs and Nie et al. [35] examined Mg-Nd-Zn-Zr alloy screws in the mandible of rabbit.

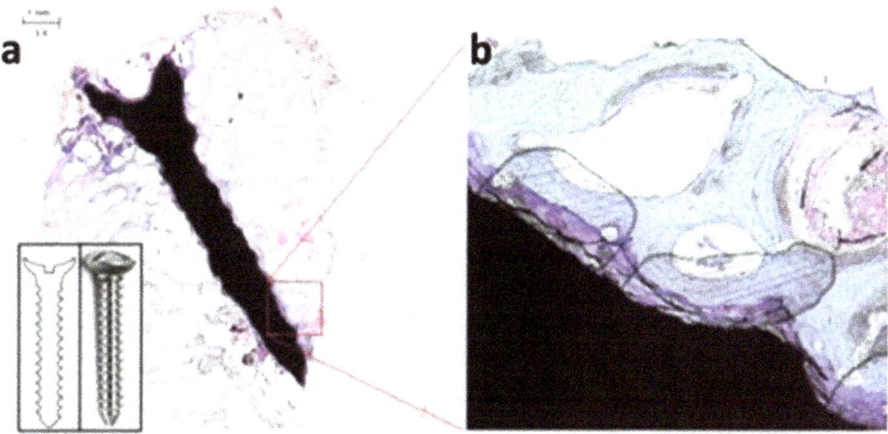

Figure 19.8: Histology of extruded Mg–5Ca–1Zn alloy bone screw in femoral condyle observed at ×33 (a) and ×103 (b) [50].

Waizy et al. [51] investigated the acute, subacute and chronic local effects on bone tissue as well as the systemic reactions to Mg-Y-RE-Zr alloy containing screw. The upper part of the screw was implanted into the marrow cavity of the left femora of 15 adult rabbits (New Zealand white), and animals were euthanized 1 week, 12 weeks and 52 weeks postoperatively. Blood samples were analyzed at set times, and radiographic examinations were performed to evaluate gas formation. It was mentioned that (i) there were no significant increased changes in blood values compared with normal levels; (ii) histological examination revealed moderate bone formation with direct implant contact without a fibrous capsule; and (iii) histopathological evaluation of the lung, liver, intestine, kidneys, pancreas, and spleen tissue samples showed no abnormalities. These indicate that these Mg-based alloy screws containing RE elements have good biocompatibility and osteoconductivity without acute, subacute or chronic toxicity. Windhagen et al. [52] evaluated Mg-Y-RE-Zr alloy screws for fixation during chevron osteotomy in patients with a mild hallux valgus. Patients ($n = 26$) were randomly assigned to undergo osteosynthesis using either titanium or degradable magnesium-based implants of the same design. The

6-month follow-up period included clinical, laboratory and radiographic assessments. It was obtained that (i) no significant differences were found in terms of the American Orthopaedic Foot and Ankle Society score for hallux, visual analog scale for pain assessment or range of motion of the first metatarsophalangeal joint; (ii) no foreign body reactions, osteolysis or systemic inflammatory reactions were detected; and (iii) the groups were not significantly different in terms of radiographic or laboratory results. Based on these results, it was concluded that the radiographic and clinical results demonstrate that degradable magnesium-based screws are equivalent to titanium screws for the treatment of mild hallux valgus deformities.

19.4.2 Staples

Although the application is not for bone fixation, Wu et al. [53] developed biodegradable high-purity magnesium staples for gastric anastomosis. U-shaped staples with two different interior angles, namely original 90° and modified 100°, were designed. It was mentioned that (i) the in vitro tests indicated that the arc part of the original staple ruptured first after 7 days immersion, whereas the modified one was kept intact, demonstrating residual stress greatly affected the corrosion behavior of the pure Mg staples and (ii) the in vivo implantation showed good biocompatibility of the modified Mg staples, without inflammatory reaction 9 weeks postoperation. This indicates that the pure Mg staples kept good closure to the anastomosis, no leaking and bleeding were found and the staples exhibited no fracture or severe corrosion cracks during the degradation, as shown in Figure 19.9.

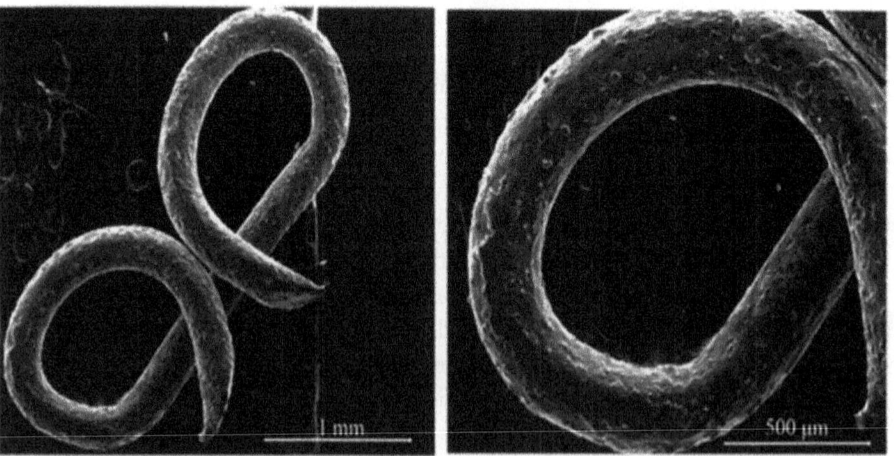

Figure 19.9: Surface morphologies by SEM observation of modified biodegradable surgical staples [53].

Ileocolic anastomoses are commonly performed for right-sided colon cancer and Crohn's disease. The anastomosis may be constructed using a linear cutter stapler or by suturing. Individual trials comparing stapled versus handsewn ileocolic anastomoses have found little difference in the complication rate but they have lacked adequate power to detect potential small difference. Based on this background, Choy et al. [1–54] compared outcomes of ileocolic anastomoses performed using stapling and handsewn techniques to test the hypothesis that stapling technique is associated with fewer complications. After the review, it was found that (i) after obtaining individual data from authors for studies that include other anastomoses, six trials (including one unpublished) with 955 ileocolic participants (357 stapled, 598 handsewn) were included; (ii) the three largest trials had adequate allocation concealment; (iii) stapled anastomosis was associated with significantly fewer anastomotic leaks compared with handsewn ($S = 5/357$, HS = 36/598, OR 0.34 [0.14, 0.82] $p = 0.02$); (iv) one study performed routine radiology to detect asymptomatic leaks; (v) for the subgroup of 825 cancer patients in four studies, stapled anastomosis led to significant fewer anastomotic leaks ($S = 4/300$, HS = 35/525, OR 0.28 [0.10, 0.75] $p = 0.01$); and (v) there were too few Crohn's disease patients to perform subgroup analysis. These indicate that all other outcomes such as stricture, anastomotic hemorrhage, anastomotic time, re-operation, mortality, intra-abdominal abscess, wound infection, length of stay show no significant difference, and stapled functional end-to-end ileocolic anastomosis is associated with fewer leaks than handsewn anastomosis. Qu et al. [55] investigated the biocompatibility and degradation behavior of high-purity magnesium staples with the small intestine. It was reported that (i) pure Mg staples did not affect the relative growth rate, cell cycle and apoptosis of primary rectal mucosal epithelial cells (intestinal epithelial cells, IEC-6) in vitro; (ii) at 1, 2 and 3 days after immersion in intestinal juice, the weight of the 30 rinsed pure Mg staples reduced by 7.5 ± 1.6, 10.6 ± 2.2 and 13.5 ± 2.1 mg, respectively, and those in the Hanks' solution reduced by 3.9 ± 0.8, 6.1 ± 1.2 and 7.1 ± 2.4 mg; and (iii) extracts of pure Mg staples were biosafe for IEC-6, and the corrosion rate of HP staples was faster in the small intestinal juice than in the Hanks' solution. In the in vivo experiments, the small intestine of the minipigs was anastomosed by pure Mg and Ti staples and it was obtained that pure Mg staples neither affected important biochemical parameters nor induced serious inflammation or necrosis in the anastomosis tissues. The residual weight of Mg staples (0.81 ± 0.13 mg) was 89.7% of the original weight (9 ± 0.09 mg) 1 month after surgery. It was further mentioned that the in vivo corrosion rate for one pure Mg staple was determined to be ~0.007 ± 0.001 mm/month, indicating that results of the biocompatibility and degradation of high-purity Mg anastomotic staples are promising. Amano et al. [56] developed a new biodegradable Mg–2.5Nd–1Y alloy staple (whose mechanical properties and biodegradability are similar to those of Mg-Y-RE-Zr and WE43 alloys) and evaluated the safety and feasibility. For the in vitro immersion test, the artificial intestinal juice was used at a ratio of 0.006 g weight of the staple per 1 mL in a humidified atmosphere with 5% CO_2 at 37 °C. It was reported that (i) the immersion test showed satisfactory biodegradable behavior, mechanical durability and biocompatibility in vitro; (ii) hydrogen resulting from rapid corrosion of Mg was observed in small quantities only in the first week of immersion, and most staples maintained their shapes until at least the fourth week, as shown in Figure 19.10; (iii) the tensile force was maintained for more than a week and was reduced to approximately one-half by the fourth week; (iv) the Mg concentration of the intestinal artificial juice was at a low cytotoxic level; (v) in porcine intestinal anastomoses, the Mg alloy staples caused neither technical failure nor such complications as anastomotic leakage, hematoma or adhesion; and (vi) no necrosis or serious inflammation reaction was histopathologically recognized, indicating that the new Mg alloy staple offers a promising alternative to Ti alloy staples.

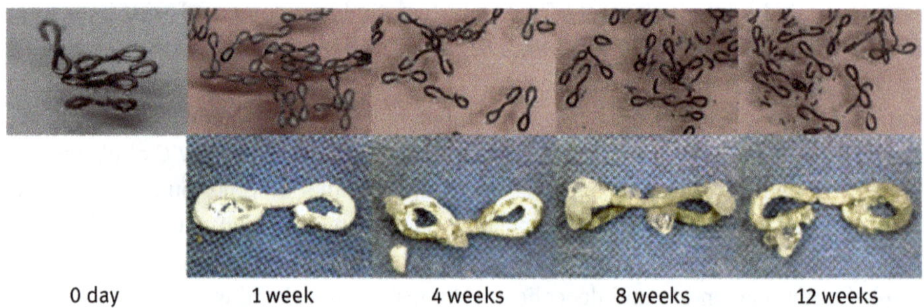

Figure 19.10: Changes in macroscopic views of immersed Mg alloy staples in an artificial intestinal juice for 1, 4, 8 and 12 weeks; (upper) general view kept inside the immersion juice; (lower) typical staple sample removed from the immersion fluid [56].

19.4.3 Clips

Operative clips used to ligate vessels in abdominal operation are usually made of titanium. They remain in the body permanently and form metallic artifacts in CT images, which impair accurate diagnosis. Besides, an allergic reaction case was reported on a breast cancer patient, who received three titanium clips placed at the margin of the excision cavity at the time of surgery [57]. Ikeo et al. [58] developed a biodegradable clip that was equivalent to plastic strain distribution during occlusion. During the development, since the finite element analysis using the material data of pure Mg indicated that a maximum plastic strain of 0.40 is required to allow the Mg clips, the alloying of magnesium with essential elements and the control of microstructure by hot extrusion and annealing were conducted. Hence, this results in developing Mg–Zn–Ca alloy, obtained by double extrusion followed by annealing at 400 °C for 2 h possessing a fracture strain of over 0.40. It was reported that (i) the biocompatibility of the alloy was confirmed here by investigating its degradation behavior and the response of extraperitoneal tissue around the alloy; (ii) small gas cavity due to degradation was observed following implantation of the developed Mg–Zn–Ca clip by in vivo micro-CT; (iii) histological analysis, minimal observed inflammation and an only small decrease in the volume of the implanted Mg–Zn–Ca clip confirmed its excellent biocompatibility and being suitable for biodegradable clips. Bai et al. [59] fabricated a Mg–Zn–Ca alloy biodegradable clip by combining hot extrusion and blanking processing. It was mentioned that the as-extruded Mg–Zn–Ca alloy exhibited a typical fiber microstructure. After blanking, the basal texture intensity increased because of the work-hardening effect and subsequent annealing treatment of the blanking clip can significantly weaken the texture while improving the ductility of the Mg–Zn–Ca alloy. Mg–Zn–Ca clips can maintain closure performance for 2 weeks in in vitro immersion tests while in vivo tests indicated that the Mg–3Zn–0.2Ca alloy clips fabricated by this preparation processing successfully occluded the blood vessels, suggesting that the developed Mg–3Zn–0.2Ca alloy clip is a suitable candidate for biodegradable soft tissue fixation devices such as surgical clips. Yoshida et al. [60] developed a biodegradable Mg–Zn–Ca alloy clip (see Figure 19.11) with good biologic compatibility and enough clamping capability as an operative clip. Nine female beagles were used. Cholecystectomy and ligated the cystic duct by Mg alloy or Ti clips were performed. The chronologic change of clips and artifact formation were compared at 1, 4, 12, 18 and 24 weeks postoperatively by CT. It was reported that the Mg alloy clip formed much fewer artifacts than the titanium clip, and it was almost absorbed at 6 months postoperation. There were no postoperative complications and no elevation of constituent elements such as magnesium, calcium and zinc during the observation period in both groups, concluding that the Mg–Zn–Ca alloy clip demonstrated sufficient sealing capability for the cystic duct and proper biodegradability in canine models and the clip revealed much fewer metallic artifacts in CT than the conventional titanium clip.

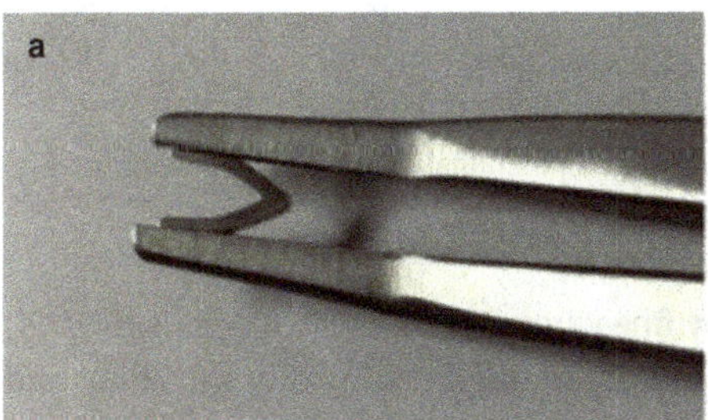

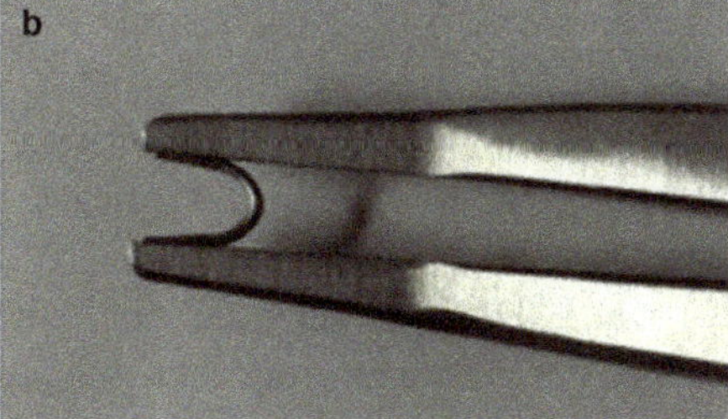

Figure 19.11: Typical Mg alloy clip of V-type (a) and U-type (b) [60].

19.4.4 Wires

Strength and ductility are two essential mechanical properties for successful wires from the standpoint of mechanical requirements. Bian et al. [61] summarized and compared strength and elongation (or ductility) of various biodegradable Mg-based alloys manufactured in different processes, as shown in Figure 19.12.

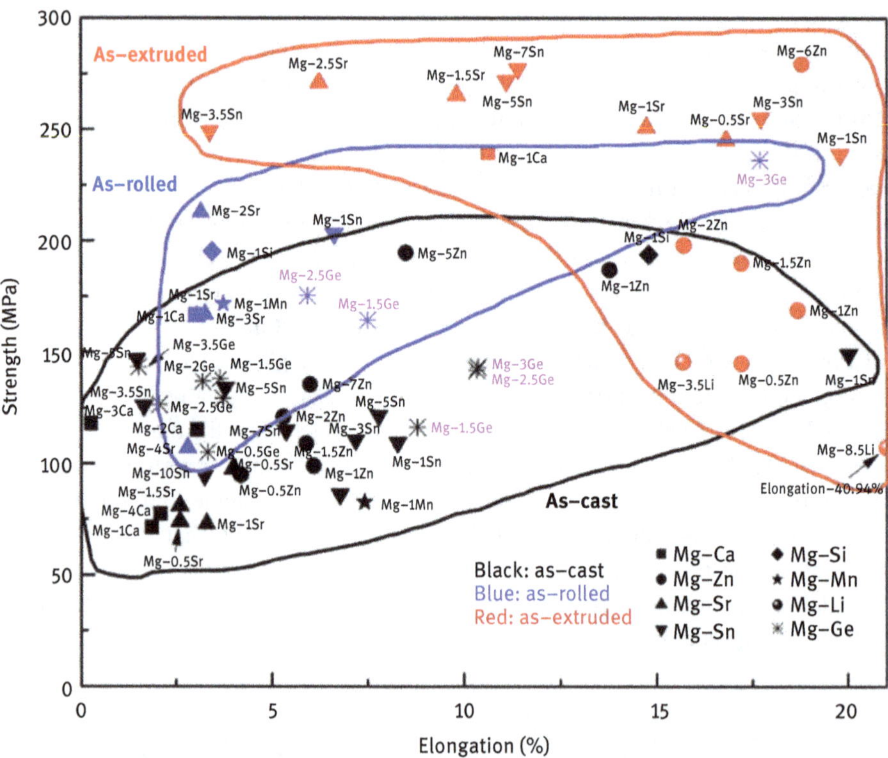

Figure 19.12: Comparative diagram to assess the strength and elongation of various biodegradable Mg-based alloys manufactured in different processes [61].

Bai et al. [62] prepared three kinds of Mg alloy fine wires containing 4 wt% RE(Gd/Y/Nd) and 0.4 wt% Zn with the diameter less than 0.4 μm through casting, hot extruding and multipass cold drawing combined with intermediated annealing process. The degradation test results and surface morphology observations indicate that Mg–4Gd–0.4Zn and Mg–4Nd–0.4Zn fine wires have similar good corrosion resistance and the uniform corrosion behavior in SBF solution. By contrast, Mg–4Y–0.4Zn fine wire shows a poor corrosion resistance and the pitting corrosion behavior. The implantation of intramedullary nails was made of Mg–2Ag alloy into intact and fractured femora of mice [63].

It was reported that prior in vitro analyses revealed an inhibitory effect of Mg–2Ag degradation products on osteoclast differentiation and function with no impair of osteoblast function. In the in vivo tests, Mg–2Ag implants degraded under nonfracture and fracture conditions within 210 and 133 days, respectively (see Figure 19.13). During fracture repair, osteoblast function and subsequent bone formation were enhanced, while osteoclast activity and bone resorption were decreased, leading to an augmented callus formation. A widening of the femoral shaft was observed under steady-state and regenerating conditions, which was at least in part due to an uncoupled bone remodeling; however, Mg–2Ag implants did not cause any systemic adverse effects, suggesting that Mg–2Ag alloy implants might be promising for intramedullary fixation of long bone fractures.

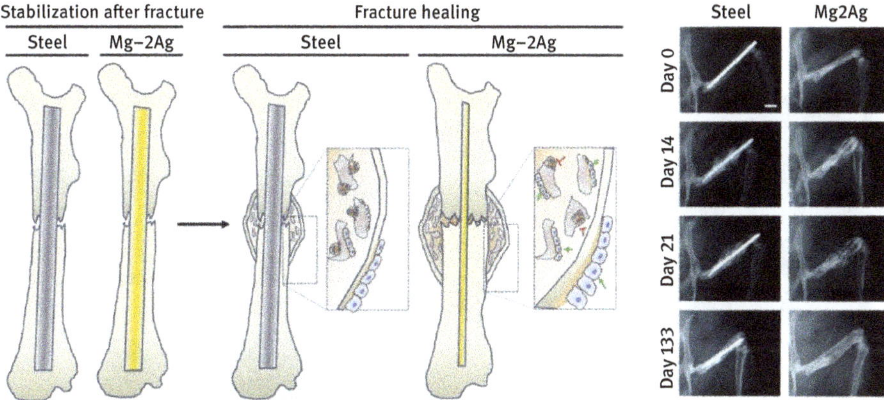

Figure 19.13: X-ray images to determine intramedullary Mg–2Ag alloy wires, with the steel wire, for 133 days in mice when compared with a steel pin (scale bar = 5 mm) [63].

19.4.5 Bone plates

Witte et al. [64] investigated whether the implantation of an open-porous degradable scaffold made of a magnesium alloy (AZ91) could serve as a sufficient temporary replacement of the subchondral bone plate. It was shown that the alloy degrades too rapid in vivo to allow sufficient cartilage repair above the scaffold; however, the surrounding cartilage tissue was not negatively affected by the rapid degradation process and new bone formation was observed at the rim of the degrading implant, indicating that Mg-based alloy scaffolds degrade in vivo but the initial high corrosion rate must be reduced to allow the formation of an appropriate cartilage tissue. To control the early stage of rapid degradation rate of Mg biomaterials in biological environment, there are various methods available including appropriate alloying or heat treatment or surface oxidation (via MAO or PEO), as discussed previously. Based on their previous work observing Mg device degradation, with uninhibited healing and bone formation around degrading Mg, but not titanium, devices, Chaya et al. [65] conducted a more thorough study assessing 99.9% Mg devices in a similar rabbit ulna fracture model to further assess Mg materials' efficacy. Device degradation, fracture healing and bone formation were evaluated using micro-CT, histology and biomechanical tests. It was reported that (i) device degradation was observed throughout, and the calculated corrosion rate was 0.40 ± 0.04 mm/year after 8 weeks; (ii) fracture healing by 8 weeks and maturation after 16 weeks. In accordance with our pilot study, we observed bone formation surrounding Mg devices, with complete overgrowth by 16 weeks, as shown in Figure 19.14 and bend tests revealed no difference in flexural load of healed ulnae with Mg devices compared with intact ulnae, suggesting that Mg devices provide stabilization to facilitate healing, while degrading and stimulating new bone formation.

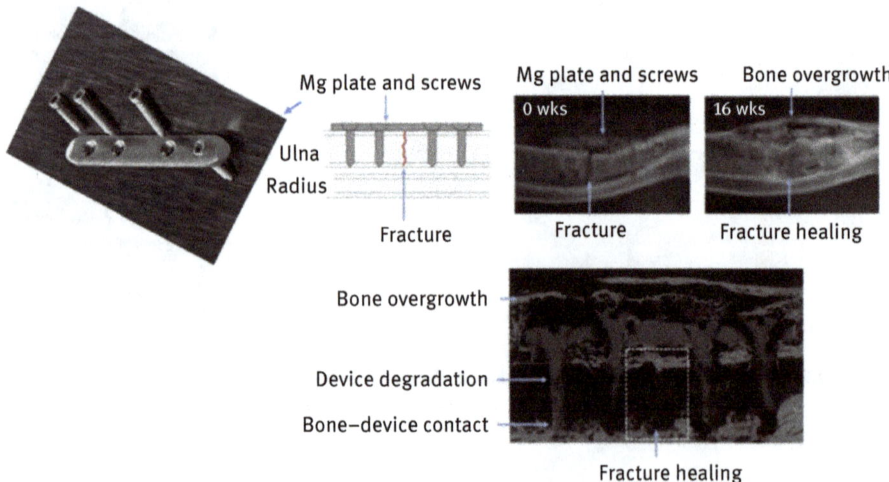

Figure 19.14: Bone healing and overgrowth via Mg bone plates and screws [65].

19.5 Bone grafting and materials

Bone grafting (or transplanting of bone tissue) is a surgical procedure aiming to replace diseased or injured bones with grafting materials. The three common types of bone grafts are (1) autograft which is taken from a bone structure inside the patient such as ribs, hips, pelvis or wrist; (2) allograft (or donors) which uses bone from a deceased donor or a cadaver that has been cleaned and stored in a tissue bank or (3) synthetic materials [66]. Among these bone graft materials, there is an interesting comparison in terms of various parameters concerned. As shown in Figure 19.15 [67], various factors influencing sustainability and long-term graft performance in cardiovascular applications. The treatment of cardiovascular disease often requires the implantation of prosthetic material or insertion of stents. The ideal cardiovascular prosthesis has good functional properties and the ability to regenerate, without activating the immune system of the host organism [67]. In some cases, the implant should only remain in place for a limited period of time in the patient, followed by controlled degradation. Up to date, as shown in Figure 19.15, only biological grafts meet most of the spectrum of these relevant requirements; however, biological prostheses have specific disadvantages, such as insufficient mechanical stability or limited availability [67]. Zhang et al. [68] pointed out that although autograft and allograft possess some advantages, there are some clinical problems such as the necessity of performing additional surgery on the donor site as well as size and geometry limitations of autograft and inconsistency with host tissue, and the possibility of disease transmission from donated allograft and accordingly, a clinical demand for synthetic materials as bone substitutes is ever growing.

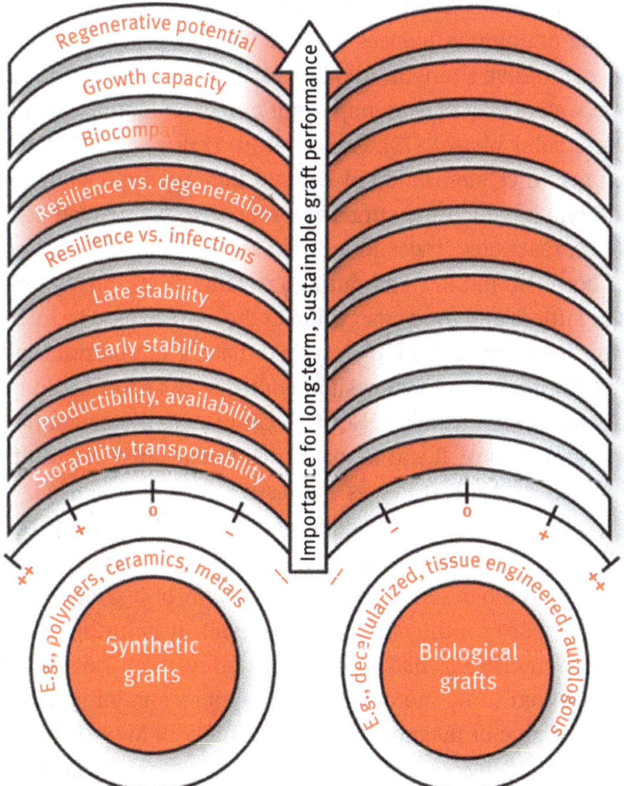

Figure 19.15: Comparison of characterization of synthetic grafts and biological materials in terms of sustainability and long-term performance in cardiovascular applications [67].

Based on the mode of biological actions, bone-grafting materials can also be classified into three classes [69]: (1) autogenous bone is an organic material and forms bone by osteogenesis, osteoinduction and osteoconduction; (2) allografts such as demineralized freeze-dried bone are osteoinductive and osteoconductive and may be cortical and/or trabecular in nature; and (3) alloplasts such as HA and tricalcium phosphate (TCP) may be synthetic or natural, vary in size and are only osteoconductive, and alloplast grafting materials can be further divided into three types based on the porosity of the product, including dense, macroporous and microporous materials. It is also mentioned that alloplastic materials may be crystalline or amorphous and these materials have different properties and therefore indications [69]. Among the wide range of alloplast (synthetic) grafting materials, calcium phosphate cement (CPC) is known to resemble as a good synthetic material to natural bone and is thus clinically suitable to repair bone defects in a variety of orthopedic and dental applications [70, 71]. HA and TCP) are two major materials in the material class of CPC group.

Oshida et al. [72] investigated the alloying effects of various elements and oxides substituted with the HA crystalline structure, and these are summarized in Table 19.1 [72]. As the table indicates, Mg addition influences to promote bone growth, control transform to HA and enhance adhesive strength. Alkaline earth cations present in biological fluids and in natural waters may play an important role in regulating the formation of calcium phosphate solid phases [73]. Amjad et al. [73] investigated the effects of magnesium (Mg) ions on crystallization of HA and fluorapatite (FA) under constant composition conditions in which the supersaturation was maintained constant during the crystallization reactions. It was found that Mg ions markedly retard the rates of precipitation of both HA and FA, and during crystallization, the Mg ions are excluded from the crystal lattices and their adsorption at the surface may be interpreted in terms of a Langmuir isotherm. Li et al. [74] studied that the equilibrium solubility of Mg-containing β-TCP with various magnesium contents was determined by immersing Mg-β-TCP powder for 27 months in a $CH_3COOH–CH_3COONa$ buffer solution at 25 °C under a nitrogen gas atmosphere. It was reported that the negative logarithm of the solubility product (pK_{sp}) of Mg-β-TCP was expressed as $pK_{sp} \sim 28.87432 + 1.40348CMg$, where CMg represents the magnesium concentration in Mg-β-TCP (mol%). The solubility of Mg-β-TCP decreased with increasing magnesium content, owing to the increased structural stability and possible formation of a whitlockite-type [$Ca_9(Mg,Fe)(PO_4)6PO_3OH$] phase on the surface. As a result, it is further mentioned that Mg-β-TCP with 10.1 mol% Mg had a lower solubility than that of HA below pH 6.0. Mg-β-TCP was found to be more soluble than zinc-containing β-TCP given the same molar content of zinc or magnesium. The solubility of Mg-β-TCP and release rate of magnesium from Mg-β-TCP can be controlled by adjusting the Mg content by selecting the appropriate pK_{sp}. Kannan et al. [75] prepared Mg-stabilized TCP by an aqueous precipitation method. The transformation of CDHA into β-TCP has occurred in the range of 700–800 °C. The calculated values for lattice parameters

Table 19.1: Elemental substitutions and their primary influences on HA [72].

	Ag	Zn	Cu	Fe	Sr	Mg	La	Ti	Y	W	Pb	Ba	Na	K	SiC	TiO_2	SiO_2	ZrO_2	Al_2O_3	C	Si	F
Antimicrobial activity	●	●	●		●																	●
Bioactivity		●								●			●					●	●	●		●
Promoting bone growth		●		●	●	●							●				●				●	●
Improve biocompatibility																				●		
Anticancer therapy				●																		
Assisting drug delivery system							●															
Improve radiopacity					●							●										
Control transform to HA						●	●							●								
Improve mechanical strengths							●	●	●						●				●			
Surface energy control																				●		
Enhance adhesive strength						●	●									●						●
Improve corrosion resistance					●											●						●
Control environment											●											

confirm the stabilization role played by Mg, and the thermal stability of the Mg-stabilized β-TCP powders was evident until 1,400 °C, thus broadening the sintering temperature range without transformation into the undesirable α-TCP, concluding that the mechanical properties of the Mg-stabilized β-TCP were improved in comparison with those of pure β-TCP. Mg-HAs were fabricated [76–78]. Ren et al. [76] substituted Mg in HA by the wet chemical precipitation method at 90 °C. It was found that (i) a limited amount of Mg (Mg/(Mg + Ca)) between 5 and 7 mol% could successfully substitute for Ca in HA; (ii) HA crystallites became smaller and more irregular, and they formed greater agglomerates with Mg substitution; and (iii) Mg substitution resulted in decreases in the crystallinity and thermal stability of HA. The incorporation of Mg in HA was investigated using multinuclear solid-state nuclear magnetic resonance and X-ray absorption spectroscopy. It was mentioned that extensive interatomic potential calculations also suggest that a local clustering of Mg within the HA lattice is likely to occur, and such structural characterizations of Mg environments in apatites will favor a better understanding of the biological role of this reaction [77]. Canullo et al. [78] enriched HA with Mg to conduct histological evaluation on postextraction sites that underwent postextraction ridge preservation procedure. It was reported that Mg-enriched HA is a suitable material for socket preservation and ensures early angiogenesis and early osteogenesis.

Mg-HA composite [79] and (Mg,F)-HA composite [80] were fabricated as coating materials. Li et al. [79] compared the effect of Mg-incorporated HA (Mg-HA) (10 mol% Ca^{2+} replaced by Mg^{2+}) coating with that of HA coating on implant fixation in ovariectomized (OVX) rats. Twelve weeks after bilateral ovariectomy, 18 OVX rats received implants in the distal femora; half of the implants were HA coated and the other half were Mg-HA coated. After 12 weeks of healing, rats were selected randomly for histomorphometry, micro-CT evaluation and biomechanical testing. It was reported that (i) surface characterization analysis demonstrated that the addition of Mg did not dramatically change the surface topography or apatite patterns of the coating; (ii) histomorphometry revealed higher BIC and bone area ratio for Mg-HA-coated implants than for HA-coated implants; and (iii) Mg incorporated into an HA coating on titanium implants could improve the biologic fixation of implants in osteoporotic bone. In order to improve the biological properties, Mg and fluorine (F) are simultaneously incorporated in HA to form (Mg,F)-HA coating on titanium alloy via sol–gel process [80]. It was found that (i) after soaking in the SBF solutions for 7 to 28 days, both Mg and F ions are incorporated into the HA crystal structure; (ii) the presence of F promotes Mg incorporation into the HA crystal structure; and (iii) the presence of Mg makes the coatings more bioactive in promoting bone formation; however, at high Mg concentration, formation of Mg-β-TCP takes place. Crespi et al. [81] evaluated the healing of an injectable mixture of nanoparticles of Mg-enriched HA (Mg-HA) in peri-implant defects. Thirty-two dental implants were placed in 16 tibiae of eight female large white pigs. It was reported that (i) the test group exhibited statistically significant higher values for BIC and lower amounts of connective tissue over time, and (ii) the injectable Mg-HA putty could be a useful and suitable bone-grafting material in peri-implant defects. Zhao et al. [82] compared Mg-HA and s-HA coatings on the promotion of osteogenesis in vitro and on the osseointegration in vivo. Electrochemically deposited pure HA or electrochemically deposited magnesium-substituted HA (Mg-HA) coatings were formed on the surface of pure titanium disks or implants. After MC3T3-E1 preosteoblasts culture studies, it was concluded that Mg-HA-coated surfaces promote osteogenic differentiation of preosteoblasts in vitro and may improve implant osseointegration during the early stages of bone healing compared with pure HA-coated surfaces. Caneva et al. [83] evaluated the influence of Mg-HA on bone contour preservation and osseointegration at implants placed immediately into extraction sockets and indicated that the use of Mg-HA to fill the defect around implants placed into the alveolus immediately after tooth extraction did not contribute significantly to the maintenance of the contours of the buccal alveolar bone crest. Dasgupta et al. [84] investigated a dual-doped (Zn,Mg)-HA to control release of protein. Bovine serum albumin (BSA) protein incorporated with HA nanoparticles were synthesized by an in situ precipitation process. Amounts of 2 mol% Zn^{2+} and Mg^{2+} were used as dopants to synthesize Zn^{2+}/Mg^{2+}-doped HA-BSAs. It was shown that the protein release rate from HA nanoparticles can be controlled by the addition of suitable dopants, and doped HA-based nanoparticle systems can be used in bone growth factor and drug release study. Kheradmandfard et al. [85] prepared Mg-doped FA (Mg-FA) nanopowders by the sol–gel method. The designated degree of substitution of Ca^{2+} by Mg^{2+} in the mixture was determined by the x value in the general formula of $[Ca_{10-x}Mg_x(PO_4)_6F_2]$, where $x = 0$, 0.25, 0.5, 0.75 and 1. It was shown that (i) Mg ions entered into the FA lattice and occupied Ca^{2+} sites, and (ii) the incorporation of Mg ions into the FA resulted in the decrease of the lattice parameters. Similarly, Cai et al. [86] prepared Mg-FA and coated on Ti–6Al–4 V via a sol–gel process. It was obtained that (i) the interdiffusion of elements takes place at the coating/substrate interface, and (ii) the incorporation of Mg ions into FA coatings enhances the pull-off adhesion strength between the coating and the substrate, but no significant difference is observed with different Mg concentrations. Gopi et al. [87] prepared (Sr,Mg)-HA/poly(3,4-ethylenedioxythiophene) (PEDOT) and coated on surgical-grade stainless steel (316 L SS). It was reported that (i) the PEDOT/Sr, Mg-HA bilayer exhibited greater adhesion strength than the (Sr,Mg)-HA-coated 316 L SS; (ii) in vitro cell adhesion test of the (Sr, Mg)-HA coating on PEDOT-coated specimen is found to be more bioactive compared with that of the single substituted HA (Sr or Mg-HA) on the PEDOT-coated 316 L SS, concluding that the PEDOT/ (Sr,Mg)-HA bilayer-coated 316 L SS can serve as a prospective implant material for biomedical applications. Similarly, Roy et al. [88] dual-doped HA with Sr and Mg elements and coated on CpTi, using inductively coupled radio frequency (RF) plasma spray. HA powder was doped with 1 wt% Sr (Sr-HA) and 1 wt% Mg (Mg-HA), and heat treated at 800 °C for 6 h. It was reported that (i) in vitro cell material interactions using human fetal osteoblasts (hFOB) showed better cell attachment and proliferation on Sr-HA coatings compared with HA or Mg-HA coatings; (ii) presence of Sr in the coating also stimulated hFOB cell differentiation and alkaline phosphatase (ALP) expression; and (iii) improvement in bioactivity of Sr-doped HA coatings on Ti without compromising its mechanical properties makes it an excellent material of choice for coated implant.

HA and TCP are two major members in Ca–P family and each of these possesses different characters in its composition (Ca/P ratio), solubility behavior, crystallinity, preparation method, bioactivity and so on. Highly dense sintered HA is hard to be dissolved by osteoclast. At the same time, it is stable inside the body which is saturated by HA. Therefore, due to the bone formation by bone modeling (which occurred on the basis of HA resorption by the osteoclast), the major role of HA inside the body is just as a space-making material. On the other hand, TCP is not a rapid self-hardening material, and very slowly resorbed into a body which is already saturated by HA, so that bone reformation is very difficult. TCP has a stoichiometry similar to amorphous bone precursors, whereas HA has a stoichiometry similar to bone mineral [89]. Liu et al. [90] investigated the influences of Ca/P stoichiometry of calcium phosphates on biological performances including osteoblast (bone-forming cell) viability, collagen production, ALP activity and nitric oxide production. A group of calcium phosphates with Ca/P ratios between 0.5 and 2.5 were obtained by intentionally adjusting the Ca/P stoichiometry of the initial reactants necessary for calcium phosphate precipitation. For samples with 0.5 and 0.75 Ca/P ratios, TCP and $Ca_2P_2O_7$ phases were observed. In contrast, for samples with 1.0 and 1.33 Ca/P ratios, the only stable phase was TCP. For samples with a 1.5 Ca/P ratio, the TCP phase was dominant; however, small amounts of the HA phase started to appear. For samples with a 1.6 Ca/P ratio, the HA phase was dominant. Lastly, for samples with 2.0 and 2.5 Ca/P ratios, the CaO phase started to appear in the HA phase which was the dominant phase. It was furthermore reported that (i) the average grain size and the average pore size decreased with increasing Ca/P ratios, (ii) the porosity of calcium phosphate substrates also decreased with increasing Ca/P ratios, (iii) the collagen production by osteoblasts was similar between all the calcium phosphates but slightly lower with a 1.6 Ca/P ratio and (iv) greater ALP activity by osteoblasts was observed in all the cultures with various calcium phosphates (0.5–2.5 Ca/P ratios) than in the control (only cells in culture), suggesting that the Ca/P ratio of calcium phosphate is a very important factor that should be considered when selecting nano-to-micron particulate calcium phosphates for various orthopedic applications [90].

There are several researches to compare osteoblast cell attachment and growth behaviors between HA and TCP. An essential property of bone substitute materials is that they are integrated into the natural bone remodeling process, which involves the resorption by osteoclast cells and the formation by osteoblast cells. When the monocyte cells adhere to a calcium phosphate surface (bone or bone substitute material), they can bind together and form multinucleated osteoclast cells. Detsch et al. [91] showed that osteoclast-like cells derived from a human leukemia monocytic lineage responded in a different way to TCP than to HA ceramics. It was reported that both bioceramics were degraded by resorbing cells; however, HA enhanced the formation of giant cells. The osteoclast-like cells on HA formed a more pronounced actin ring, and larger lacunas could be observed. TCP ceramics are medically used as bone substitute materials because of their high dissolution rate; on the other hand, highly soluble calcium phosphate ceramics like TCP seem to be inappropriate for osteoclast resorption because they produce a high calcium concentration in the osteoclast interface and in the environment. Kasten et al. [92] compared three resorbable biomaterials (CDHA, TCP and demineralized bone matrix (DBM)) in terms of seeding efficacy with human bone marrow stromal cells (BMSCs), cell penetration into the matrix, cell proliferation and osteogenic differentiation. Three biomaterials were seeded with human BMSCs and kept in human serum and osteogenic supplements for 3 weeks. Morphologic and biochemical evaluations were performed on days 1, 7, 14 and 21. It was reported that (i) the allograft DBM and CDHA exhibited both an excellent seeding efficacy while the performance of β-TCP was lower when compared; (ii) the total protein content and the values for specific ALP increased on all matrices and no significant difference was found for these two markers; (iii) BMSCs in monolayer had a significant increase of protein, but not of ALP; (iv) osteocalcin (OC) values increased significantly higher for BMSC in cultures on DBM when compared with CDHA and β-TCP; (v) all three matrices promoted BMSC proliferation and differentiation to osteogenic cells; and (vi) DBM allografts seem to be more favorable with respect to cell ingrowth tested by histology, and osteogenic differentiation ascertained by an increase of OC. Based on the aforementioned findings, it was concluded that CDHA with its high specific surface area showed more favorable properties than β-TCP regarding reproducibility of the seeding efficacy [92].

HA and TCP are also compared in terms of bone formation in sinus augmentations. Hadi et al. [93] compared two different graft materials (bovine HA and β-TCP) associated with platelet-rich plasma in one patient referred for bilateral sinus augmentations. It was reported that (i) the bovine HA and TCP have resulted in bone formation after the sinus lift procedures, and (ii) histomorphometric analysis showed some differences but both biomaterials allowed for stable clinical results. Similarly, Kurkcu et al. [94] compared the biological performance of the bovine HA graft material and the synthetic β-TCP material in sinus augmentation procedure. The study consisted of 23 patients (12 male and 11 female) who were either edentulous or partially edentulous in the posterior maxilla and required implant placement. After average of 6.5 months of healing, bone biopsies were taken from the grafted areas. It was found that (i) the mean new bone formation was 30.13% in bovine HA group and 21.09% in β-TCP group; (ii) the mean percentage of residual graft particle area was 31.88% for bovine HA group and 34.05% for β-TCP group; and (iii) the mean percentage of soft tissue area was 37.99% in bovine HA group and 44.86% in β-TCP group. Based on these clinical data, it was concluded that both graft materials demonstrated successful biocompatibility and osteoconductivity in sinus augmentation procedure, although the bovine HA appears to be more efficient in osteoconduction when compared with β-TCP. Yang et al. [95] compared the bone formation on titanium implant surfaces coated with biomimetically deposited calcium phosphate or electrochemically deposited HA and found that the electrochemically deposited HA coating has good bone formation properties, while the biomimetically deposited Ca–P coating has weaker bone formation properties.

There is development of materials utilizing aforementioned differences between HA and TCP to fabricate biphasic bioceramics. Solubility and degradation profile of HA and TCP varies between very stable, almost insoluble appearance (100% HA) to fast degradation and loss of structure (100% α-TCP). For optimization of the properties of the composite materials for cell seeding and tissue engineering applications, several studies of different ratios of HA/TCP biphase biocomposites have been conducted and reported. Arinzeh et al. [96] prepared 100% HA, 76% HA/24% TCP, 63/37, 56/44, 20/80 and 100% β-TCP (by weight) and seeded human mesenchymal stem cells (hMSCs). The hMSC-loaded implants and cell-free implants were implanted subcutaneously at the backs of 24 severe combined immunodeficient mice. Total porosity of the scaffolds was 60–70%, the pore size ranged between 300 and 600 μm and the grain size ranged between 0.5 and 1.5 mm. Implants were harvested at 6 and 12 weeks and processed for routine decalcified histology. The hMSC-loaded ceramics demonstrated osteogenesis at 6 weeks. It was reported that the composition influenced significantly on bone growth, and 100% HA and 100% TCP promoted the least bone growth. In the compositions of 100% HA, 76/34HA/TCP, 62/37HA/TCP, 56/44HA/TCP and 100% TCP, bone was only present at the peripheral pores of the implant. For hMSC-loaded 20/80HA/TCP implants, bone was detected to be lining all of the pores throughout the ceramic structure, but the phenomenon was similar. The culture media and the donor of cells affected on the amount of bone growth, but it was also shown that the different compositions of HA and TCP were working better than pure 100% HA and 100% TCP alone [96]. Similarly, Jensen et al. [97] prepared three biphasic calcium phosphate bone substitute materials with HA/TCP ratios of 20/80, 60/40 and 80/20 and compared them in terms of reaction to coagulum, particulated autogenous bone and deproteinized bovine bone mineral (DBBM) in membrane-protected bone defects. It was found that (i) 20/80 biphase biocomposite showed bone formation and degradation of the filler material similar to autografts, whereas 60/40 and 80/20 biocomposites rather equaled DBBM; (ii) among the three biphase biocomposites, the amount of bone formation and degradation of filler material seemed to be inversely proportional to the HA/TCP ratio; and (iii) the fraction of filler surface covered with bone was highest for autografts at all time points and was higher for DBBM than 80/20 and 60/40 biocomposites at the early healing phase.

Suzuki et al. [98] prepared 100HA, 80/20, 60/40, 30/70 and 100 β-TCP, and seeded osteoblast-like cells of calvarial cells from neonatal rats and the well-characterized mouse-fibroblast cell line, L-929 (NCTC Clone 929), onto ZrO_2 and LUX plates and the ceramic disk plates (30 mm OD × 2 mm thick) consisting of aforementioned biphase biocomposites of HA and β-TCP with five different ratios. It was reported that (i) the total number of cells on LUX plates at 2 days of culture was higher than that on any TCP-HA plates; (ii) the total number of cells on ZrO_2 plates at 2 days of culture was higher than that on TCP-HA plates, except on the 100% HA plate; (iii) the initial number of cells adhering on the TCP-HA plates after seeding was lower than that found on LUX and ZrO_2 plates, but thereafter, the total number of cells increased rapidly on the TCP-HA plates during the rapid growth phase between 4 and 9 days of culture; and (iv) at 9 days of culture, the numbers of cells on 100% β-TCP/100% HA and composition containing 30/70 (HA/TCP) were higher than those on the reference LUX and ZrO_2 plates. Based on these results, it was suggested that the HA/TCP biphase biocomposites are able to stimulate differentiation of osteoblasts and promote osteogenesis in vivo. Alam et al. [99] prepared five biphasic calcium phosphate ceramics (100HA, 75/25, 50/50, 25/75, 100 β-TCP) and evaluated these ceramics as carriers for recombinant human bone morphogenetic protein 2 (rhBMP-2). These bioceramics impregnated with the different doses of rhBMP-2) (1, 5 and 10 μg) were used for the experimental purpose and the ceramics without rhBMP-2 were used as control. The pellets were placed into subcutaneous pockets on the dorsum of 4-week-old male Wistar rats. The animals were killed at 2 and 4 weeks after implantation. It was found that (i) all experimental pellets exhibited new bone formation, whereas the control pellets produced only fibrous connective tissue; and (ii) 100% HAP ceramic produced more amount of bone, whereas 25HA/75TCP ceramic produced the least amount of bone among different biphasic ceramics at the end of 4 weeks, indicating that the formation of new bone depends on the ceramic content with high HA/TCP ratio and high dose of rhBMP-2. The effects of HA coating and biphasic HA/TCP (50/50) coating on the osseointegration of grit-blasted Ti–6Al–4V implants were compared [100]. Each coated implant was compared with uncoated grit-blasted implants as well. The implants were press fit into the medullary canal of rabbit femora, and their osseointegration was evaluated 3 to 24 weeks after surgery. It was reported that (i) the coated implants had significantly greater new bone ongrowth than the uncoated implants; (ii) unmineralized tissue (cartilage and osteoid) was seen on the uncoated implants but never on the coated implants; (iii) the coated implants had significantly greater interfacial shear strength than the uncoated implants; and (iv) there was no difference between HA and HA/TCP coating in regard to new bone growth or interfacial shear strength [100]. De Kok et al. [101] studied MSC-based alveolar bone regeneration in a canine alveolar saddle defect model, using biphasic HA/TCP (60/40) material with a mean pore size of 300–500 μm. It was reported that (i) histomorphometry analysis showed that equivalent amounts of new bone were formed within the pores of the matrices loaded with autologous MSCs and MSCs from an unrelated donor; and (ii) bone formation in the cell-free HA/TCP matrices was less extensive. Miao et al. [102] investigated the penetration and the attachment of bone marrow stromal stem cells into HA/TCP scaffolds (average pore size: 500 μm; porosity: 87%). The scaffold contained biphasic HA/TCP (80%/20%) and some of them were further processed and coated with polylactide–glycolide copolymer (PLGA) for improvement of the mechanical properties. It was found that (i) the BMSCs were observed to attach well onto the surfaces of the PLGA-coated HA/TCP scaffolds, and (ii) the cells attached well to the exposed ceramic HA/TCP surface and the PLGA coating surface, indicating the biocompatibility of both the ceramic phases and the PLGA phase. Yuan et al. [103] conducted a 2.5-year study in dorsal muscles of dog with porous HA, porous biphasic calcium phosphate ceramic (HA/TCP), porous α-TCP and porous β-TCP. It was reported that (i) normal compact bone with bone marrow was found in HA implants and in HA/TCP implants, 48% pore area was filled with bone in HA implants and 41% in HA/TCP implants; (ii) bone-like tissue, which was a mineralized bone matrix with osteocytes but lacked osteoblasts and bone marrow, was found in β-TCP implants and in one of the four α-TCP implants; and (iii) both normal bone and bone-like tissues were confined inside the pores of the implants, suggesting that calcium phosphate biphasic HA/TCP ceramics are osteoinductive in muscles of dogs.

The skeleton of sea urchin spines is composed of large single crystals of Mg-rich calcite, which have smooth, continuously curved surfaces and form a three-dimensional (3D) fenestrated mineral network. Vecchio et al. [104] converted spines of the echinoids *Heterocentrotus trigonarius* and *Heterocentrotus mamillatus* by the hydrothermal reaction at 180 °C to bioresorbable Mg-substituted TCP (M-TCP). Due to the presence of Mg in the calcite lattice, conversion to M-TCP occurs preferentially to HA formation. The converted M-TCP still maintains the 3D interconnected porous structures of the original spine. The main conversion mechanism is the ion-exchange reaction, although there is also a dissolution–reprecipitation process that forms some calcium phosphate precipitates on the surfaces of the spine network. It was further reported that (i) the average fracture strength of urchin spines and converted spines (M-TCP) in the compression tests are 42 and 23 MPa, respectively, and (ii) the in vivo studies using a rat model demonstrated new bone growth up to and around the M-TCP implants after implantation in rat femoral defects for 6 weeks and some new bone was found to migrate through the spine structural pores, starting from the outside of the implant through the pores at the edge of the implants, indicating good bioactivity and osteoconductivity of the porous M-TCP implants. Similarly, Zhang et al. [105] prepared M-TCP samples either by the solid-state reaction of $CaHPO_4$ (DCPA), $CaCO_3$ and MgO powder at 1,000 °C, or by a two-step process: wet precipitation of a precursor and further calcination of the precursor. It was mentioned that (i) the transition temperature from β-TCP to α-TCP increases with the increase of Mg^{2+} content in M-TCP samples; (ii) an M-TCP sample with 3 mol% Mg^{2+} has β-TCP to α-TCP transition temperature above 1,300 °C, which was then used to fabricate various M-TCP scaffolds; (iii) interconnected porous M-TCP ceramics, with pore size >100 μm and relative density ranging from 81% to 84%, were developed by a replication method using polyurethane foam as a template; micropores were also found in the scaffold struts; (iv) M-TCP ceramics with a porous structure in the center and a dense shell-like structure outside, mimicking the human bone, were fabricated by a molding method; and (v) dense M-TCP ceramic rings were also produced with an average compressive strength of 129 MPa.

19.6 Tissue engineering scaffolds

19.6.1 In general

Tissue engineering and regenerative medicine have arisen as new biomedical fields that bring advanced approaches for restoration, improvement and maintenance of damaged tissue caused by factors such as disease, injury or congenital disabilities [106, 107]. Bone tissue engineering refers to the transplantation of autologous osteoblasts, BMSCs or chondrocytes into an artificial scaffold, which should exhibit good biocompatibility and gradual biodegradation to be absorbed by the human body [20, 108, 109]. Hence, there are several requirements for successful scaffolds, including they should (1) allow cell attachment and migration, (2) deliver and retain cells and biochemical factors, (3) enable diffusion of vital cell nutrients and expressed products and (4) exert certain mechanical and biological influences to modify the behavior of the cell phase. Accordingly, scaffolds provide 3D space to accommodate cell adhesion and in-growth. The scaffold/cell hybrid is then implanted into the defect site. The scaffold gradually degrades in vivo, while the new tissue grows directionally into the scaffolds with cells proliferating, so as to achieve the purpose of reconstruction of the defect bone tissue. In general, an ideal bone tissue engineering scaffold is designed and fabricated to possess similar topological features such as pore size and distribution to those of natural bone [109–111].

19.6.2 Scaffold fabrication and materials

Over time scaffolds should degrade under controlled rate in the human body. They must remain in the organ until all the cells that are delivered become fully integrated. However, they should not linger long enough so that they hinder organ function. A simple solution to this is biodegradability. If the biomaterial used can degrade, then it satisfies all the above necessities a biomaterial should fulfil [112–117]. As a result, effective existing technologies and developed novel methods have been utilized to optimize the scaffold's performance in terms of surface morphology and internal configuration and to produce scaffold's entire structure possessing appropriate porosity (with size and distribution) [112, 118]. The most promising technologies include nanofiber self-assembly [119], solvent casting and particulate leaching [120], gas foaming

[121], emulsification/freeze-drying [122], thermally induced phase separation [123], electrospinning [118], advanced powder metallurgy technique with controlled porosity [124, 125] and CAD/CAM and 3D printing technologies [126–128].

As to scaffold materials, a wide variety of materials has been employed, including natural and synthetic polymers (e.g., proteins, polysaccharides, glycosaminoglycans, poly-lactic acid (PLA), PCL (poly-ε-caprolactone), polypropylene fumarate, polyanhydride, polyphosphazene or polyether ether ketone and poly-glycolic acid (PGA)), inorganic biomaterials, which include metals (e.g., titanium and its alloys and magnesium alloys), bioceramics (e.g., alumina, zirconia, Ca–Ps, CPCs and silicates) and their hybrid combinations [112, 118, 129, 130]. Inorganic biomaterials are recognized for their biocompatibility, osteoconductivity and bioresorbability. To enhance osteoconductivity and mechanical properties of scaffolds, a various combinations of polymers and inorganic materials have been proposed, including polymers of natural origins (collagen, gelatin, silk, chitosan, alginate, hyaluronic acid and gellan gum), synthetic polymers (e.g., PEG, PLA, PGA, PLGA and PCL) and bioceramics, silicates, bioactive glasses and carbon nanotubes [131–133]. All of them exhibit a great impact on mimicking human tissues for regeneration when combating chronic and degenerative diseases [134].

19.6.3 Mg scaffolds

Apart from bone fixation devices, Mg and its alloys are also considered as a kind of promising scaffold materials applied in bone tissue engineering. Among the common metallic biomaterials, pure Mg and a number of its alloys are effective because of their mechanical properties close to those of the human bone, their natural ionic content that may have important functional roles in physiological systems and the in vivo biodegradation characteristics in body fluids. Due to such collective properties, Mg-based alloys can be employed as biocompatible, bioactive and biodegradable scaffolds for load-bearing applications. Recently, porous Mg and Mg alloys have been specially suggested as metallic scaffolds for bone tissue engineering. With further optimization of the fabrication techniques, porous Mg is expected to make a promising hard substitute scaffold [135, 136].

Mg-Ca-Zn-Co alloy scaffolds with high porosity for tissue engineering applications were produced by powder metallurgy with carbamide as a space holder [137]. Fluoride conversion coating was synthesized on the alloy by immersion treatment in hydrofluoric acid. It was reported that (i) increasing Zn content of the alloy increased the elastic modulus, (ii) Ca addition prevented the oxidation of the specimens during sintering, (iii) electrochemical corrosion behavior of the specimens was examined in simulated body fluid and corrosion rate decreased with Zn addition from 1.0% up to 3.0% (mass fraction) and then increased and (iv) mass loss of the specimens initially decreased with Zn addition up to about 3% and then increased. Witte et al. [138] investigated whether the implantation of an open-porous degradable scaffold made of a magnesium alloy (AZ91) could serve as a sufficient temporary replacement of the subchondral bone plate. It was found that (i) AZ91 alloy degrades too rapid in vivo to allow sufficient cartilage repair above the scaffold; however, the surrounding cartilage tissue was not negatively affected by the rapid degradation process and new bone formation was observed at the rim of the degrading implant, concluding that (ii) magnesium scaffolds degrade in vivo but the initial high corrosion rate must be reduced to allow the formation of an appropriate cartilage tissue. Hong et al. [139] studied the morphology, microstructure, compressive behavior, biocorrosion properties and cytocompatibility of Mg–4Al–2.5RE (AE42) alloy scaffolds for their potential use in biodegradable biomedical applications. Mg alloy scaffolds were successfully synthesized via a camphene-based freeze-casting process with precisely controlled heat treatment. It was mentioned that (i) the average porosity was approximately 52% and the median pore diameter was ~13 μm; (ii) the corrosion potential of the Mg alloy scaffold (–1.44 V) was slightly higher than that of bulk AE42 (–1.60 V), but the corrosion rate of the Mg alloy scaffold was faster than that of bulk AE42 due to the enhanced surface area of the Mg alloy scaffold; and (iii) as a result of cytocompatibility evaluation following ISO10993-5, the concentration of the Mg alloy scaffold extract reducing cell growth rate to 50% (IC_{50}) was 10.7%, which is higher (less toxic) than 5%, suggesting no severe inflammation by implantation into the muscle. A product of this program is the SynerMag 410 alloy (equivalent to Mg–4Y–1RE-based) scaffold, which was the first clinically proven magnesium-based bioresorbable scaffold [140].

Figure 19.16 shows a typical example of Mg-based alloy scaffold [141].

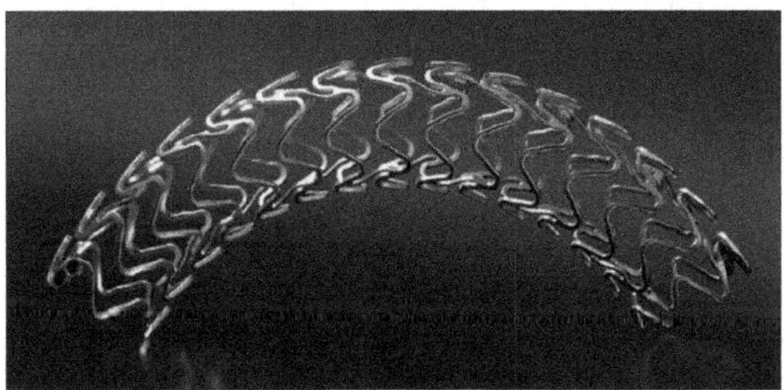

Figure 19.16: The Mg-based alloy scaffold as a key structural backbone of the scaffold [141].

Although Mg based scaffolds are gaining importance in the field of tissue engineering owing to its potential application as a biomaterial, fabrication of porous Mg is still challenging because of its highly reactive nature. Singh et al. [142] fabricated a novel Mg-based open-cell porous structure with pore interconnectivity, and significant strength was successfully fabricated by powder metallurgy approach and Ti-woven wire mesh as a space-holding material. Pore morphology and percentage porosity can be easily altered by adjusting the Ti wire diameter and shape of construct.

It was found that (i) a uniform distribution of pores was obtained with porosity varying in the range of 50–60%; (ii) the measured values of ultimate compressive strength and elastic modulus using quasistatic compression test were found to be 101 MPa and 2 GPa, respectively; and (iii) degradation study as well as cytocompatibility studies using L929 cells was carried out to validate the potential of fabricated scaffold for bone healing/repair applications and it was obtained that fabricated porous structures showed improved corrosion resistance as well as cell viability of more than 90%, suggesting it as a promising development for bone scaffolding applications in future. Wen et al. [143] fabricated porous Mg scaffolds by the foam-forming method and reported that (i) the mechanical strength could reach the range of human cancellous bone by changing the porosity and (ii) when the porosity was 35% with an average pore diameter of 250 μm, the Young's modulus and mechanical strength was 1.8 GPa and 18 MPa, respectively. Yazdimamaghani et al. [135] synthesized porous Mg scaffolds (with a porosity of 35% and a pore size of 150–300 μm) coated by PCL and examined material properties and in vitro biodegradation. It was reported that PCL coating can significantly enhance the compressive strength and degradation resistance of Mg scaffolds. While the uncoated Mg scaffold degrades completely (100% weight loss) after 72 h, the degradation (weight loss) of the Mg scaffolds coated by 3% and 6% PCL is only 36% and 23%, respectively, indicating that PCL-coated Mg scaffolds, as a biodegradable metal scaffold, can potentially have a promising application in bone tissue engineering. Čapek et al. [144] prepared Mg scaffolds using powder metallurgy method with the pore-forming agent and bicarbonate as spacer particles. It was reported that (i) bending strength of these scaffolds with porosity of 12–38% was close to that of human bone and (ii) the porosity of the materials depended on the amount of ammonium bicarbonate and was found to have strong negative effects on flexural strength and corrosion behavior; however, the flexural strength of materials with porosities of up to 28 vol% was higher than the flexural strength of nonmetallic biomaterials and comparable with that of natural bone. Cheng et al. [145] prepared two open-porous magnesium scaffolds with different pore size but in the nearly same porosity with Ti wire as a space holder. Subsequently, the open-porous Mg scaffold was obtained when Ti wires were removed by HF solution. The porosity and pore size can be easily, precisely and individually controlled, as well as the mechanical properties can also be regulated within the range of human cancellous bone by changing the orientation of pores without giving the requisite porous structures. It was reported that (i) the in vitro cell tests indicate that the scaffolds have good cytocompatibility and osteoblastic differentiation properties; (ii) the in vivo findings demonstrate that both scaffolds exhibit acceptable inflammatory responses and can be almost fully degraded and replaced by newly formed bone; and (iii) under the same porosity, the scaffolds with larger pore size can promote early vascularization and upregulate collagen type 1 and osteopontin expression, leading to higher bone mass and more mature bone formation, indicating that open-porous magnesium scaffold with controllable microstructures and mechanical properties was developed, which has great potential clinical application for bone reconstruction in the future.

Jia et al. [146] evaluated the degradation behavior in consideration of the pore strut and the interconnectivity of two Mg scaffolds with different 3D interconnected porous structures. It was mentioned that (i) the interconnectivity of the two scaffolds gradually decreased along with the clogged interconnected pores due to the deposition formation on the pore wall; (ii) Mg scaffold with spherical pores and cambered pore strut degraded faster but exhibited better resistance to the deterioration of the interconnectivity compared with Mg scaffold with irregular pores and polygonal pore struts; and (iii) direct cell culture of MC3T3-E1 osteoblasts on the two scaffolds indicated a promising potential for bone tissue engineering. Mg-based scaffolds have great potential of application for bone defect repair due to their biodegradability and the excellent osteoinductivity, yet currently the fabrication of Mg-based porous materials is still a challenge. Accordingly, Jia et al. [147] produced porous Mg scaffolds by three steps: (1) defectless NaCl open-porous template with enhanced relative density was prepared with NaCl particles by hot press sintering process, (2) green compact of Mg and the NaCl template was produced by infiltration casting and (3) open-porous Mg scaffold was achieved after leaching out the template. By using spherical NaCl particles and irregular polyhedral NaCl particles, respectively, two different types of templates were prepared, and correspondingly Mg scaffolds with spherical and irregular pores were, respectively, fabricated. It was shown that the irregular pore scaffold (I-scaffold) exhibited higher yield strength, while the spherical pore scaffold (S-scaffold) showed superior interconnectivity and more stable compressive deformability due to the uniform spatial structure, as shown in Figure 19.17.

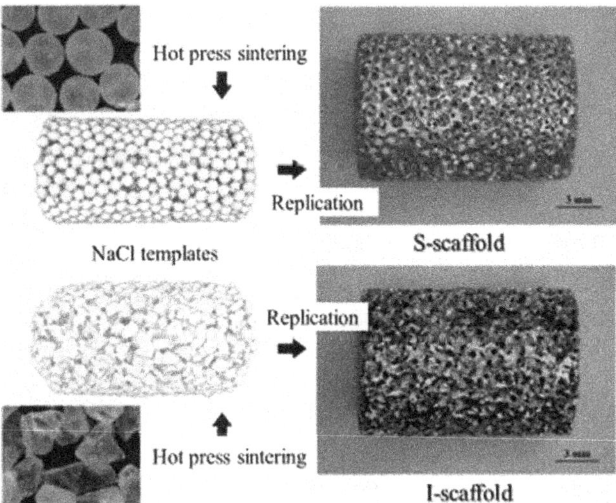

Figure 19.17: Pore-morphology-controlled scaffolds [147].

It should be stated that the aforementioned methods exhibit poor ability to control the pore structure, such as the pore size, shape, spatial orientation or pore connectivity [20]. The capability to fabricate multiple material parts can improve AM (additive manufacturing) technologies by either optimizing the mechanical properties of the parts or providing additional functions to the final parts [148]. Li et al. [149] fabricated topologically ordered porous magnesium (WE43) scaffolds based on the diamond unit cell by selective laser melting and investigated the in vitro biodegradation behavior (up to 4 weeks), mechanical properties and biocompatibility of the developed scaffolds. It was mentioned that the mechanical properties of the additive-manufactured porous WE43 (E = 700–800 MPa) scaffolds were found to fall into the range of the values reported for trabecular bone even after 4 weeks of biodegradation. Electrochemical tests and micro-CT revealed a unique biodegradation mechanism that started with uniform corrosion, followed by localized corrosion, particularly in the center of the scaffolds. Biocompatibility tests performed up to 72 h showed level 0 cytotoxicity (according to ISO 10993-5 and -12), except for one time point (i.e., 24 h). An intimate contact between cells (MG-63) and the scaffolds was also observed in scanning electron microscopic (SEM) images, indicating that (AM of porous Mg may provide distinct possibilities to adjust biodegradation profile through topological design and open up unprecedented opportunities to develop multifunctional bone-substituting materials that mimic bone properties and enable full regeneration of critical-size load-bearing bony defects. For further development of higher functionalized implants (e.g., plate systems or scaffold grafts for bone replacement therapy), Kopp et al. [150] developed the process of laser powder bed fusion (LPBF) for magnesium alloys enabling the production of lattice structures, therefore, allowing for reduction of implant material volume. Magnesium scaffold structures with different pore sizes were therefore manufactured by LPBF and consequently further modified either by thermal heat treatment or plasma electrolytic oxidation (PEO). It was mentioned that the implant performance was assessed by conducting degradation studies and mechanical testing, and PEO-modified scaffolds with small pore sizes exhibited improved long-term stability, while heat-treated specimens showed impaired performance regarding degradation and mechanical stability. Figure 19.18 shows a typical example of Mg-based alloy scaffold [151].

It was mentioned that (i) the combination of biodegradable metals and AM leads to a revolutionary change of metal implants in many aspects including materials, design, manufacturing and clinical applications; (ii) element loss and porosity are common processing problems for AM of biodegradable metals like Zn and Mg, which are mainly caused by evaporation during melting under a high-energy beam; and (iii) the resulting formation quality and properties are closely related to material, design and processing, making AM of biodegradable metals a typical interdisciplinary subject involving biomaterials, mechanical engineering and medicine [152]. Qi et al. [152] introduced an integrated conceptual scaffold design from extensive viewpoints such as material, processing, formation quality, design, microstructure and properties by

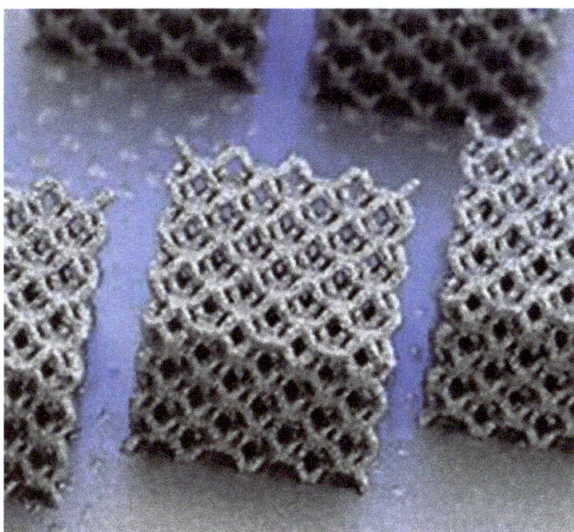

Figure 19.18: Typical scaffold using WE43 Mg alloy [151].

employing beneficial effects of powder properties and processing parameters on formation quality. As a result, Figure 19.19 illustrates an ideal process to fabricate an orthopedic implant scaffold through appropriate processes having hybrid and gradient biofunctionality.

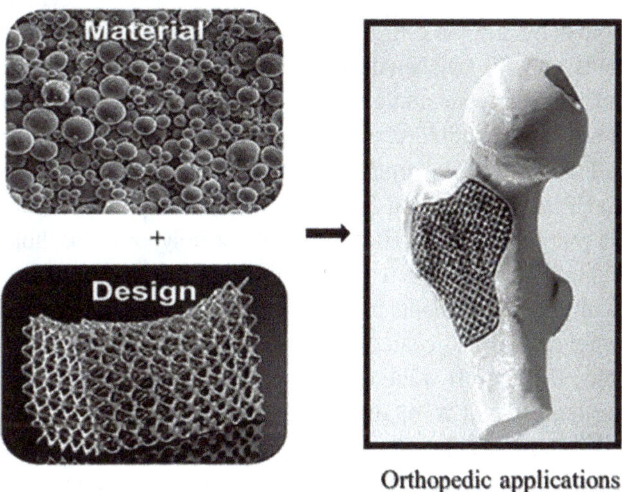

Figure 19.19: Hybrid-type orthopedic implant scaffold [152].

Mg-based composites or hybrids have been fabricated medical-applicable scaffolds. Wong et al. [153] developed a new biodegradable porous scaffold composed of PCL and magnesium (Mg) microparticles. It was found that (i) the compressive modulus of PCL porous scaffold was increased to at least 150% by incorporating 29% Mg particles with the porosity of 74%; (ii) the compressive modulus of this scaffold was further increased to at least 236% when the silane-coupled Mg particles were added; (iii) in terms of cell viability, the scaffold modified with Mg particles significantly convinced the attachment and growth of osteoblasts as compared with the pure PCL scaffold; (iv) the hybrid scaffold was able to attract the formation of apatite layer over its surface after 7 days of immersion in normal culture medium, whereas it was not observed on the pure PCL scaffold, indicating the enhanced bioactivity of the modified scaffold; (v) enhanced bone-forming ability was also observed in the rat model after 3 months of implantation; (vi) high volume of new bone formation could be found in the Mg/PCL hybrid scaffolds when compared with the pure PCL scaffold and both pure PCL and Mg/PCL hybrid scaffolds were degraded after 3 months; however, no tissue inflammation was observed. Based on these findings, it was concluded that the incorporation of Mg microparticles into PCL porous scaffold could significantly enhance its mechanical and biological properties and the modified porous bioscaffold may potentially apply in the surgical management of large bone defect fixation. Cao et al. [154] fabricated magnesium phosphate (MgP)-containing compounds such as newberyite, struvite and brushite 3D porous structures by 3D plotting combining with a two-step cementation process, using magnesium oxide (MgO) as a starting material. It was mentioned that (i) extracts obtained from immersing scaffolds in alpha-modified essential media-induced minimal cytotoxicity and the cells could be attached merely onto newberyite and brushite scaffolds and (ii) newberyite and brushite scaffolds produced through the 3D-plotting and two-step cementation process showed the sustained in vitro degradation and excellent biocompatibility, which could be used as scaffolds for the bone tissue engineering. Liao et al. [155] manufactured medical polyporous magnesium alloys, Mg-Nd-Zn-Zr, $CaHPO_4$-coated Mg-Nd-Zn-Zr and WE43 through a mechanical perforation technique. It was reported that (i) the porosity of polyporous scaffold was 61.1 ± 2.81% (noncoating) and 49.74 ± 2.11% (coating); (ii) SEM examination after 8 weeks of immersion in cell culture environments revealed finer surface topography for Mg-Nd-Zn-Zr than WE43, whereas $CaHPO_4$-coated Mg-Nd-Zn-Zr presented more uniform, fine-point corrosion pits; (iii) the pH value of the immersion solution with Mg-Nd-Zn-Zr scaffolds was lower than that of WE43, while that of $CaHPO_4$-coated Mg-Nd-Zn-Zr scaffold was the lowest (i.e., more acidity); (iv) the weight of $CaHPO_4$-coated Mg-Nd-Zn-Zr scaffolds decreased to 10.13% and 12.76% after 4 and 8 weeks of immersion, respectively; and (v) the polyporous scaffold possessed similar elastic modulus and compressive strength to those of human cancellous bone, and $CaHPO_4$-coated Mg-Nd-Zn-Zr foam maintained mechanical integrity while noncoated scaffolds disaggregated over 8 weeks, concluding that $CaHPO_4$-coated Mg-Nd-Zn-Zr scaffold possesses great potential in in vivo applications when compared with Mg-Nd-Zn-Zr and WE43 scaffolds.

Wilton et al. [156] developed a porous HA structure from waste Kina shell for bone tissue engineering using a hydrothermal process. Kina shells' skeletal plates are composites of organic and inorganic materials with regular pores, and tailored structure, which offers unique characteristics for bone grafting. Cleaned and dried shells were cut to pieces of about 2 × 2 cm and then heated in a furnace at 700 °C to remove organic matter. It was found that the obtained HA had a porous structure with large pores of 300–400 µm and small pores of 10–20 µm, which is an important characteristic for blood and nutrient circulation and bone regeneration. The crystallization of HA was based on reaction time, and 75% conversion was achieved after 8 days. The HA samples had 4.5 ± 0.04 wt% of magnesium (as shown in Figure 19.20), and the nontoxicity and biocompatibility nature of the samples was confirmed using SaOS-2 cell lines through cell cytotoxicity test, indicating that Kina shells were partially converted to Mg-HA with Mg concentration of 4.5 ± 0.04 wt% through a hydrothermal process at 100 °C and at atmospheric pressure.

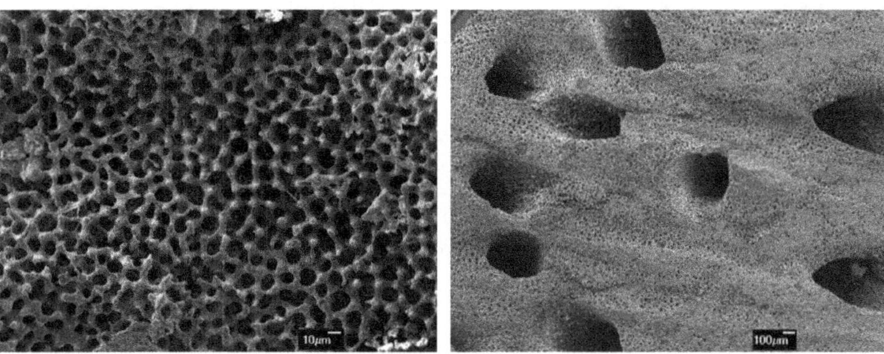

Figure 19.20: SEM images of Kina shell-originated HA incorporated with Mg [156].

19.7 Other medical applications

19.7.1 Stents

A stent is a medical device made of metal or plastic tube or mesh inserted into the lumen of an anatomic vessel or duct to keep the passageway open. There is a wide variety of stents used for different purposes, from expandable coronary, vascular, prostatic and biliary stents to simple plastic stents used to allow the flow of urine between the kidney and the bladder. Coronary stents are placed during a coronary angioplasty. The most common use of coronary stents is in the coronary arteries, into which a bare-metal stent (BMS), a drug-eluting stent, a bioabsorbable stent, a dual-therapy stent (combination of both drug and bioengineered stent) or occasionally a covered stent is inserted. Vascular stents are a common treatment for advanced peripheral and cerebrovascular diseases. Common sites treated with vascular stents include the carotid, iliac and femoral arteries. Ureteral stents are used to ensure the patency of a ureter, which may be compromised, for example, by a kidney stone. This method is sometimes used as a temporary measure to prevent damage to a blocked kidney until a procedure to remove the stone can be performed. Prostatic stents are placed from the bladder through the prostatic and penile urethra to allow drainage of the bladder through the penis. This is sometimes required in benign prostatic hypertrophy. Colon and esophageal stents are a palliative treatment for advanced colon and esophageal cancer. Pancreatic and biliary stents provide pancreatic and bile drainage from the gallbladder, pancreas, and bile ducts to the duodenum in conditions such as ascending cholangitis due to obstructing gallstones. The material for biodegradable stents is requested to have at least the following characteristics: (1) it must be biocompatible, (2) degradation rate must be controlled, (3) degradation products of the material must also be biocompatible, (4) the material must stay in the place for several months before its complete bioabsorption and (5) the radial force of the resultant stent must be enough for the scaffolding effect during the requested period [157, 158]. Based on these requirements, two metallic elements including iron and magnesium have been utilized along with plastics.

Figure 19.4 [28] provides a conceptual idea on two competing processes between healing stage and degradation stage. Among the three stent materials (Mg, Fe and plastics), there are further studies on these two competing processes during the clinical serving as a biostent device [159–161]. Figure 19.21 illustrates an ideal compromise

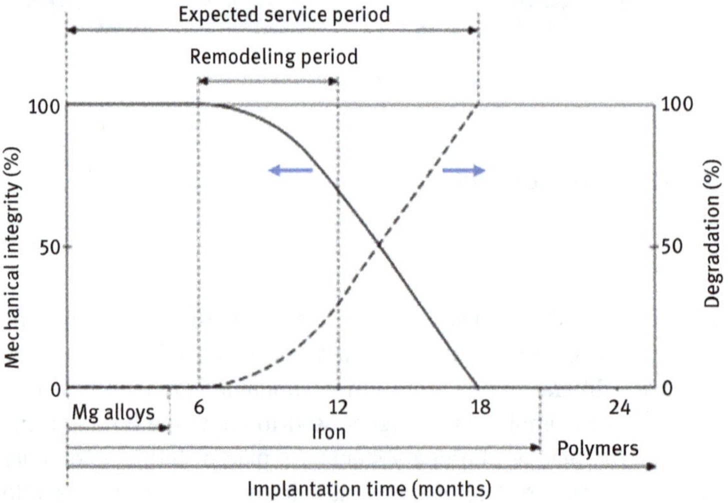

Figure 19.21: The ideal compromise between degradation and mechanical integrity during in vivo implantation of a biodegradable stent [161].

between degradation and mechanical integrity of a biodegradable stent [161]. Times for complete in vivo degradation of current biodegradable stents are mapped at the bottom. Consider a case when the stent is used for arterial vessel, it begins with a very slow degradation rate to keep the optimal mechanical integrity during arterial vessel remodeling. This can be achieved, for example, by coating the stent with a degradable polymer. Thereafter, the degradation progresses while the mechanical integrity decreases. The degradation ideally occurs at a sufficient rate that will not cause an intolerable accumulation of degradation product around the implantation site. Mg alloy stent degrades completely before the remodeling period; conversely, polymeric stents continue their presence thereafter. The degradation of Fe stents, which completes after the remodeling period but is not as long as that of polymeric stents, could be considered as approaching the ideal degradation time [161]. Hence, depending on the anticipated healing period, the stent material type should be accordingly selected.

A variety of biodegradable-grade Mg-based alloys have been developed and clinically used. Coronary stents improve immediate and late results of balloon angioplasty by tacking up dissections and preventing wall recoil. These goals were achieved within weeks after angioplasty but using current technology, stents permanently remain in the artery with many limitations, including the need for long-term antiplatelet treatment to avoid thrombosis. Based on this background, Erbel et al. [162] reported a prospective multicenter clinical trial of coronary implantations of absorbable magnesium stents. A total of 63 patients (44 men; mean age 61.3) in eight centers with single de novo lesions in a native coronary artery in a multicenter nonrandomized prospective were subjected to the study. Follow-up included coronary angiography and intravascular ultrasound at 4 months and clinical assessment at 6 and 12 months. The primary endpoint was cardiac death, nonfatal myocardial infarction or clinically driven target lesion revascularization at 4 months. It was found that (i) 71 stents, 10–15 mm in length and 3.0–3.5 mm in diameter, were successfully implanted after predilatation in 63 patients; (ii) the overall target lesion revascularization rate was 45% after 1 year; (iii) after serial intravascular ultrasound examinations, only small remnants of the original struts were visible, well embedded into the intima; and (iv) neointimal growth and negative remodeling were the main operating mechanisms of restenosis, indicating that biodegradable magnesium stents can achieve an immediate angiographic result similar to the result of other metal stents and can be safely degraded after 4 months [162].

WE 43 (Mg–4Y–3RE) alloy has been developed and manufactured for cardiac stents [163, 164]. Typical stents are shown in Figure 19.22 [165, 166]. Maeng et al. [163] assessed vascular remodeling and neointima formation after implantation of bioabsorbable WE43 Mg alloy stents (AMS) by conducting randomized experimental study. AMS ($n = 11$), sirolimus-eluting stents (Cypher; $n = 11$) and BMS ($n = 9$) were randomly implanted into 31 porcine coronary arteries ($n = 11$ pigs) and it was concluded that coronary implantation of absorbable magnesium stents, when compared with two nonabsorbable stents, was associated with the smallest lumen area at 3-month follow-up because of negative vascular remodeling.

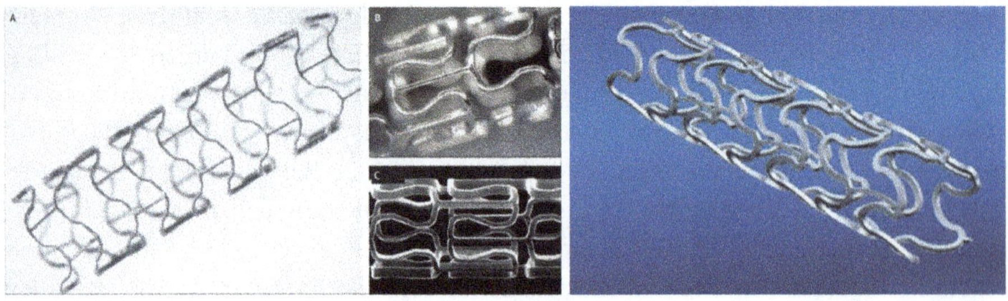

Figure 19.22: Typical intracoronary cardiac WE43 stent for cardiology [165, 166].

Mg–Zn alloy systems are also extensively selected as biodegradable stent materials. Tian et al. [167] investigated a series of four promising Mg alloys that contain zinc (Zn) and strontium (Sr), that is, Mg–4Zn–*x*Sr (ZSr41) alloys for potential ureteral stent application. Specifically, these four alloys have 4 wt% Zn in all and 0.15 wt% Sr in ZSr41 (A), 0.5 wt% Sr in ZSr41 (B), 1.0 wt% Sr in ZSr41 (C) and 1.5 wt% Sr in ZSr41 (D). The cytocompatibility and degradation behaviors of Mg–4Zn–*x*Sr alloys were studied by culturing with human urothelial cells (HUCs) for 24 and 48 h using exposure culture method. It was reported that (i) ZSr41 (B) showed a better cytocompatibility with HUCs among all the Mg–4Zn–*x*Sr alloys in both 24 and 48-h cultures; (ii) the cytocompatibility of insoluble degradation products of Mg (namely, MgO and $Mg(OH)_2$) was also investigated by culturing different concentrations of MgO and $Mg(OH)_2$ nanoparticles with HUCs for 24 and 48 h, and the concentration of MgO and $Mg(OH)_2$ particles at 0.5 mg/mL and above showed a significant decrease of cell density and cell size after 24 and 48-h cultures; and (iii) the concentration of MgO and $Mg(OH)_2$ at 1.0 mg/mL and above showed no viable cells after 24-h culture, recommending to further reduce the degradation rates of Mg alloys in order to control possible side effects of the soluble and insoluble degradation products and to take the benefits of Mg-based biodegradable ureteral stents toward the future clinical translation. Monfared et al. [168] prepared Mg–26Zn–4Ca (in at%) metallic glass ribbon by melt spinning, and structural characteristics were investigated by differential scanning calorimetry and X-ray diffraction. For biocorrosion evaluations, two relaxed and crystallized ribbons were prepared from heat treatment of as-quenched ribbon. MTT assay was used for investigating cytotoxicity of ribbons with Schwann cells for their potential application in nerve regeneration. It was mentioned that (i) relaxed ribbon showed better biocorrosion resistance and biocompatibility than that of crystallized ribbon and (ii) Mg-based metallic glass can be potentially promising candidates for application in nerve tissue regeneration. Ge et al. [169] studied ZM21 (Mg–2Zn–1Mn) by equal-channel angular pressing (ECAP) and extrusion processing to examine its applicability as a candidate material for the manufacturing of biodegradable Mg stents. It was mentioned that (i) ultrafine-grain-sized billets of the ZM21 alloy were obtained by two-stage ECAP, which aimed at achieving an initial refining of the structure at 200 °C and then reaching the submicron grain size range by lowering the processing temperature down to 150 °C; and (ii) a significant improvement in the properties of the ECAP-treated samples was noticed when compared with the starting coarse-grained ZM21 alloy, indicating that processing of biodegradable Mg stent having an ultra-fine-grained microstructure by ECAP and low-temperature extrusion is feasible and that the obtained products feature promising properties. Wang et al. [170] studied the microstructures' mechanical and corrosion properties of three extruded Mg-2Zn-0.46Y-*x*Nd alloys ($x = 0.0$, 0.5, 1.0 wt%) for potential stent applications. It was found that (i) microstructural observations indicated that Nd led to uniformity and variation of morphology of major second phase; (ii) tensile tests showed that Nd can improve the ductility at moderate amount (0.5 wt%) and will be detrimental up to 1.0%; Mg-2Zn-0.46Y-0.5Nd alloy exhibited excellent mechanical properties (σ_B, 269.0 MPa, $\sigma_{0.2}$, 165.6 MPa and elongation, 24%); and (iii) electrochemical tests revealed that Nd can enhance the corrosion resistance and Mg-2Zn-0.46Y-1.0Nd alloy had lowest corrosion current density, hence concluded that the lineshape and rod-like $NdZn_2$ phase might serve as corrosion barriers and the dissolved Nd can raise the electrode potential of the matrix, indicating that Mg-Zn-Y-Nd alloy can be applicable as a stent material. Liu et al. [171] used arginine–leucine-based poly(ester urea urethane)s (Arg–Leu–PEUUs) as protective and biofunctional coatings for bioabsorbable magnesium alloy (Mg-Zn-Y-Nd) in cardiovascular stent applications. It was mentioned that (i) comparing with poly(glycolide-co-lactide) (PLGA) coating, the Arg–Leu–PEUU coating had stronger bonding strength with the substrate; in vitro electrochemical and long-term immersion results verified a significantly better corrosion resistance; (ii) acute blood contact tests proved a better hemocompatibility of Arg–Leu–PEUU coating; (iii) the immunofluorescent staining and cell proliferation test indicated that Arg–Leu–PEUU coating had a far better cytocompatibility; (iv) the Arg–Leu–PEUU coating stimulated human umbilical vein endothelial cells (HUVEC) to release reasonably increased amount of nitric oxide, suggesting its potential in retarding thrombosis and restenosis; and (v) the superior corrosion resistance and biocompatibility as well as the indigenous nitric oxide production biofunctionality of the Arg–Leu–PEUU copolymer family indicate their capability to offer a far better protection of the magnesium-based implantable cardiovascular stent and bring their application closer to clinical reality.

There are still other types of Mg-based alloys used as stents, including Mg–Nd–Zn alloy systems. Nerve injury, especially the large size nerve damage, is a serious problem affecting millions of people. Entubulation of two ends of the injured nerve by using an implantable device, for example, nerve guidance conduit (NGC), to guide the regeneration of nerve tissue is a promising approach for treating the large-size nerve defect. Fei et al. [172] selected NZ20 (Mg–2Nd–Zn), ZN20 (Mg–2Zn–Nd) and Mg–10Li magnesium alloys fabricating the nerve repair implants such as NGC or scaffold. The degradation behavior and biocompatibility were studied by in vitro degradation test and cell adhesion assay, respectively. Specifically, the cytocompatibility to dorsal root ganglion (DRG) neurons, RF/6A choroid–retina endothelial cells and osteoblasts in the cell culture media containing Mg alloy extracts were investigated. It was reported that (i) Mg alloys degraded at different rates in cell culture media and artificial cerebrospinal fluid; (ii) the three alloy extracts showed negligible toxic effects on the endothelial cells and osteoblasts at short term (1 day), while NZ20 extract inhibited the proliferation of these two types of cells; (iii) the effect of Mg alloy extracts on cell proliferation was also concentration dependent; and (iv) for DRG neurons, ZN20 and Mg–10Li alloy extracts showed no neural toxicity compared with control group, indicating a potential and feasibility of Mg–10Li and ZN20 for nerve repair applications. Zhang et al. [173] carried out a 20-month observation after the bare Mg-2.5Nd-0.21Zn-0.44Zr (MgNdZnZr) alloy stent prototype was implanted into the common carotid artery of New Zealand white rabbit in order to evaluate its safety, efficacy and especially degradation behavior. It was shown that the bare Mg-Nd-Zn-Zr stent had good safety and efficacy with a complete re-endothelialization within 28 days. The volume and Ca concentration of the degradation products decreased in the long term, eliminating the clinicians' concern of possible vessel calcification. The alloying elements Mg and Zn in the stent could be safely metabolized as continuous enrichment in any of the main organs were not detected although Nd and Zr showed an abrupt increase in spleen and liver after 1 month implantation. This concludes that the long-term in vivo results showed the rapid re-endothelialization of Mg-Nd-Zn-Zr alloy stent and the long-term safety of the degradation products, indicating its great potential as the backbone of the fully degradable vascular stent. Using the same Mg-Nd-Zn-Zr alloy, Shi et al. [174] prepared rapamycin (RAPA)-eluting poly-(D, L-lactic acid) coating on biodegradable Mg-Nd-Zn-Zr alloy for both in vitro and in vivo investigation of the degradation behaviors of the magnesium alloy stent platform. It was reported that electrochemical tests and hydrogen evolution test demonstrated significant in vitro protection of the polymeric coating against magnesium degradation in both short term and long term. The 3-month in vivo study on the RAPA-eluting Mg alloy stent implanted into porcine coronary arteries confirmed its favorable safety, and in the meanwhile revealed similar neointima proliferation compared with the second-generation DES Firebird 2 with no occurrence of adverse complications. Micro-CT examination indicated a remarkably lower degradation rate and prolonged radial supporting duration of the drug-eluting Mg-Nd-Zn-Zr alloy stent as compared with the bare, which was attributable to the protection of the coating in vivo. This suggests that RAPA-eluting Mg-Nd-Zn-Zr alloy stents exhibit a great potential for clinical application. Mao et al. [175] reported applicability of Mg alloy Mg-2.5Nd-0.21Zn-0.44Zr (wt%) for vascular stent application compared with AZ31 alloy. It was found that the investigation of corrosion properties evaluated by immersion test and electrochemical measurement shows less susceptibility to pitting corrosion and lower corrosion rate of Mg alloy. Its corrosion products do not cause significant adverse effect on the cell viability and growth during in vitro cytotoxicity test of the Mg extract via human vascular endothelial cells (HUVECs). Macrophage response to the Mg extract compromised foreign body reaction determined by human peripheral blood-derived macrophage fusion and inflammatory cytokine and chemokine secretion. The in vivo degradation assessment via implantation of Mg-Nd-Zn-Zr alloy stent in an animal model confirmed a long-term stability and structural integrity of the stent in blood vessel. This suggests that the Mg-Nd-Zn-Zr alloy with excellent biocompatibility and long-term stability and durability in vivo represents a significant advance in the development of biodegradable implants.

Santos-Coquillat et al. [176] coated four bioactive PEO coatings on Mg–0.8Ca alloy using a Ca/P-based electrolyte and adding Si or F as necessary. Direct biocompatibility studies were performed by seeding premyoblastic, endothelial and preosteoblastic cell lines over the coatings. Biocompatibility of the coatings was also evaluated with respect to murine endothelial, preosteoblastic, preosteoclastic and premyoblastic cell cultures using extracts obtained by the immersion degradation of the PEO-coated specimens. It was found that (i) the coatings reduced the degradation of magnesium alloy and released Mg, Ca, P, Si and F; (ii) of all the studied compositions, the Si-containing PEO coating exhibited the optimal characteristics for use in all potential applications, including bone regeneration and cardiovascular applications; (iii) coatings with high F content negatively influenced the endothelial cells; and (iv) RAW 264.7 cell line, MC3T3 cell line and coculture differentiation studies using extracts of PEO-coated Mg–0.8Ca alloy demonstrated improved osteoclastogenesis and osteoblastogenesis processes when compared with the bare alloy.

Bornapour et al. [177] studied the biodegradation mechanism of Mg–0.3Sr–0.3Ca to identify the exact nature of its protective layer and to evaluate the in vitro and in vivo biocompatibility of the alloy for cardiovascular applications. The in vitro biocompatibility evaluated via indirect cytotoxicity assays using HUVECs showed no toxicity effect, and ions extracted from Mg–0.3Sr–0.3Ca in fact increased the viability of HUVECs after 1 week. The in vivo tests were performed by implanting a tubular Mg–0.3Sr–0.3Ca stent along with a WE43 control stent into the right and left femoral arteries of a dog. It was mentioned that (i) postimplantation and histological analyses showed no thrombosis in the artery with Mg 0.3Sr 0.3Ca stent after 5 weeks of implantation while the artery implanted with WE43 stent was extensively occluded and thrombosed and (ii) microscopic observation of the Mg–0.3Sr–0.3Ca implant–tissue interface confirmed the in situ formation of Sr-substituted HA on the surface during in vivo test, indicating that the interfacial layer protects the surface of the Mg–0.3Sr–0.3Ca alloy both in vitro and in vivo, and is the key factor in the biocorrosion resistance of the alloy.

Zhou et al. [178] investigated Mg–Li-based alloy systems for future cardiovascular stent application as they possess excellent ductility. It is known that Mg–Li binary alloys exhibited reduced mechanical strengths due to the presence of lithium, so that it is required to improve the mechanical strengths of Mg–Li binary alloys by adding Al and RE elements to form Mg–Li–Al ternary and Mg-Li-Al-RE quarternary alloys. Six

Mg-Li-Al-RE alloys were fabricated. It was reported that (i) microstructure characterization indicated that grain sizes were moderately refined by the addition of RE elements; (ii) tensile testing showed that enhanced mechanical strengths were obtained, while electrochemical and immersion tests showed reduced corrosion resistance caused by intermetallic compounds distributed throughout the magnesium matrix in the RE-containing Mg–Li alloys; (iii) cytotoxicity assays, hemolysis tests as well as platelet adhesion tests were performed to evaluate in vitro biocompatibilities of the Mg–Li-based alloys and showed that the Mg-3.5Li-2Al-2RE, Mg-3.5Li-4Al-2RE and Mg-8.5Li-2Al-2RE alloys suppressed vascular smooth muscle cell proliferation after 5-day incubation, while the Mg–3.5Li, Mg–8.5Li and Mg–8.5Li–1Al alloys were proven to be tolerated; (iv) in the case of HUVEC , the Mg–Li-based alloys showed no significantly reduced cell viabilities except for the Mg-8.5Li-2Al-2RE alloy, with no obvious differences in cell viability between different culture periods; and (v) with the exception of Mg-8.5Li-2Al-2RE, all of the other Mg-Li-Al-RE alloys exhibited acceptable hemolysis ratios, and no sign of thrombogenicity was found. This indicates the potential of Mg-Li-Al-RE alloys as biomaterials for future cardiovascular stent application.

19.7.2 Suture

For surgical procedures to treat injuries to soft connective tissues, interference screws or suture anchors are needed. A majority of materials used for the devices are nondegradable metals or bioresorbable polymers, potentially leading to complications. Metallic materials suffer from difficulties encountered during revision surgery and interference with MRI, whereas polymeric materials lead to device fracture during implantation, inconsistent degradation rates and poor osteointegration [179]. Sutures that biodegrade and dissolve over a period of several weeks are in great demand to stitch wounds and surgical incisions. These new materials are receiving increased acceptance across surgical procedures whenever permanent sutures and long-term care are not needed. Unfortunately, both inflammatory responses and adverse local tissue reactions in the close-to-stitching environment are often reported for biodegradable polymeric sutures currently used by the medical community [180]. Seitz et al. [180] evaluated biodegradable alloys made of iron, magnesium and zinc as potential materials for the manufacturing of soft and hard tissue sutures and mentioned that (i) in the case of soft tissue closing and stitching, these metals have to compete against currently available degradable polymers and (ii) in the case of hard tissue closing and stitching, biodegradable sternal wires could replace the permanent sutures made of stainless steel or titanium alloys. To search for alternative Mg-based alloy for suture materials with more efficient and low-cost manufacturing process for the fabrication, four existing Mg-based alloys including ZEK100 (Mg-1Zn-0.5RE-0.5Zr), AX30 (Mg–3Al–0.8Ca), AL36 (Mg–3Al–6Li) and Mg–0.8Ca (99.2% Mg) were cast, extruded into 30 mm diameter bars and extruded into 0.5 mm diameter wires [181]. To determine the mechanical properties of the wires, grain size measurements, tensile tests as well as qualitative bending tests were carried out. It was reported that the ZEK100 alloy wires showed the finest microstructure having grains of 1.2 µm in diameter. Coarser microstructures were observed for Mg–0.8Ca, AX30 and AL36. The alloy ZEK100 had the highest tensile stress (367 MPa) also revealing a brittle behavior due to its fine microstructure. The tensile test on AX30 as well as AL36 resulted in comparable high fracture strains (10.6%) and tensile stresses (300 MPa); however, Mg–0.8Ca showed a tensile strength of 315 MPa and a low strain of 1.6%. Within the qualitative bending test, wires made of the alloy AL36 were able to form tight knots, which is a key feature for suture applications, indicating that the comparison of magnesium sutures with commercially available polymeric sutures revealed lower strength and elongation for the magnesium alloys and yet, the wires exhibited mechanical properties that can meet the requirements of a suture material.

19.7.3 Miscellaneous

Magnesium and its alloys were widely investigated in many body fluid microenvironments, including bone, blood, bile, saliva and urine; however, no study has been conducted in the intrauterine microenvironment. Bao et al. [182] investigated the degradation behaviors of pure Mg, Mg–1Ca, and Mg–2Zn alloys in simulated uterine fluid and then the biological response of four kinds of uterine cells to these materials. The gluteal muscle of rat was used as the implantation position to study the in vivo biocompatibility as a mimic of the intrauterine device fixation part. It was found that (i) the 120-day immersion test indicated that the Mg–1Ca alloy had a faster degradation rate than the Mg–2Zn alloy and pure Mg and dissolved entirely in the simulated uterine fluid, (ii) indirect cytotoxicity assay showed that the extracts of pure Mg, Mg–1Ca and Mg–2Zn alloys have positive effects on human uterine smooth muscle cells, human endometrial epithelial cells and human endometrial stromal cells, especially for the Mg–1Ca alloy group and (iii) the in vivo experiment showed that pure Mg, Mg–1Ca and Mg–2Zn alloy implants cause a light inflammatory response in the initial 3 days, but they were surrounded mainly by connective tissue, and lymphocytes were rarely observed at 4 weeks. Based on these findings, it was indicated that it is feasible for using biomedical Mg alloys in obstetrics and gynecology. The long-term biodegradation kinetics of powder metallurgy Mg and AZ31 alloy coated with a phytic acid chemical conversion layer was studied [183]. It was mentioned that (i) the inherent heterogeneity and porosity of the powder metallurgy magnesium specimens, both as-received and coated with phytic acid, promoted rapid hydrogen release and led to their premature fragmentation and complete dissolution before 250 h of immersion tested in a saline phosphate buffer solution at 37 °C and (ii) the phytic acid coating on AZ31 improves corrosion resistance in long-term tests up to 336 h (2 weeks) without affecting biocompatibility, biodegradability and resorbability for use as a temporary endoprosthetic implant.

19.8 Dental applications

19.8.1 Dental implants

The American Dental Association outlines some acceptance guidelines for dental implants: (1) evaluation of physical properties that ensure sufficient strength; (2) demonstration of ease of fabrication and sterilization potential without material degradation; (3) safety and biocompatibility evaluation, including cytotoxicity testing and tissue interference characteristics; (4) freedom from defects; and (5) at least two independent longitudinal prospective clinical studies demonstrating efficacy [184]. Almost all dental implants are made of titanium – a trusted solution, given titanium's ability to integrate with the healthy bone tissue. But because this material may not be a viable option for everyone (people having metal sensitivities), new research showing that magnesium can be a suitable alternative to titanium is encouraging for the implant world [185]. As we have been discussing, magnesium is a material that degrades over time and this behavior does not make the most appealing option for dental implants in its original state. Recently, it was reported that, when WE (Mg–Y–RE) alloy is subjected to T-5 tempering heat treatment (210 °C × 48 h), (i) mechanical properties exhibit similar to those of Ti biomaterials; (ii) its resorbable properties promote bone formation and healing with limited risk of infection; and (iii) retarded degradation rate would prevent damaging bubbles from forming on its surface, so that early deterioration of mechanical integrity can be avoided [186]. Balog et al. [187] studied the titanium–magnesium (Ti–Mg) bioactive metal–metal composite to fabricate dental implants. The biomedical Ti–12 Mg (by vol%) composite was fabricated by extruding a mixture of elemental Ti and Mg powders at low temperature to sound profiles. It was mentioned that the microstructure of composite comprises filaments of biodegradable Mg component, which are arrayed along extrusion direction and are homogeneously distributed within the permanent, bioinert Ti matrix. When compared with Ti grade 4, the reference material used for dental implants, the properties of as-extruded composite include significantly reduced modulus of elasticity (92.1 GPa) and low density (4.12 g/cm^3), while the mechanical strength of Ti grade 4 is maintained. Dynamic testing (following the ISO 14801 standard for endosseous dental implants) confirms fatigue performance of this Ti–Mg composite implants equal to one of the reference materials. Exposure of as-extruded composite samples to Hank's solution yields gradual dilution of Mg from composite surface and volume. Corroded Mg leaves at prior Mg filament site pores within the Ti matrix, which remains intact, resulting in further decrease of modulus of elasticity and enhances macro- and microroughness at implant surface. This indicates that the Ti–Mg composite shows improved mechanical compatibility (namely, reduction of stress shielding) and better osseointegration potential. Figure 19.23 shows a sintered mixture of Ti and Mg powders and a prototype of dental implant using sintered and extruded Ti–12 Mg (by vol%) alloy composite [187].

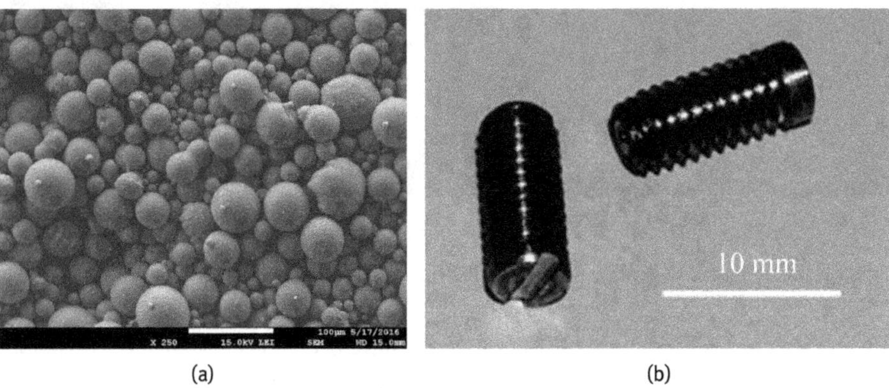

(a) (b)

Figure 19.23: SEM image of sintered mixture of Ti and Mg powders (a) and a prototype of Ti–Mg composite dental implant (b) [187].

19.8.2 Membrane

Treatment of large bone defects represents a great challenge in orthopedic and cranio-maxillofacial surgery. Although there are several methods for bone reconstruction, they all have specific indications and limitations. The concept of using barrier membranes for restoration of bone defects has been developed in an effort to simplify their treatment by offering a single-staged procedure [188]. The application of dental membranes, used in bone reproduction processes, is a standard procedure in the area of dental implant and periodontal surgery. Those membranes are introduced as a barrier to separate cell types like osteoblasts, which have slow proliferation, from epithelial layer and connective tissue, which show rapid proliferation [189]. Bioresorbable polylactide membranes, when applied to bone defects, enhance bone healing by direct osteoconduction, exclusion of nonosseous tissues and enhancing the osteogenic environment for autologous grafts. When combined with appropriate internal fixation and autologous bone graft, bioresorbable polylactide membranes allow for single-step reconstruction of large bone defects [190]. The degradation (including pitting corrosion during immersion tests) and bioactivity behavior (through the Kokubo method [191]) of magnesium foils, as new devices applicable in oral and facial surgery due to their high mechanical stability compared with collagen, were investigated [189]. Mg foils (99.9%; 8 mm ∅ and 0.1 mm thick) were used to allegorize dental membranes. Corrosion tests were carried out in 0.9% NaCl solution for 28, 52 and 72 h. It was found that (i) the progressive degradation in corrosive environment was found, as shown in Figure 19.24 and (ii) the corrosion products are likely magnesium oxide and hydroxide. The bioactivity test shows that magnesium has strong Ca-phosphate layer formation which correlated with high degradation, indicating that magnesium foils appear to hold a great potential for bone implant application.

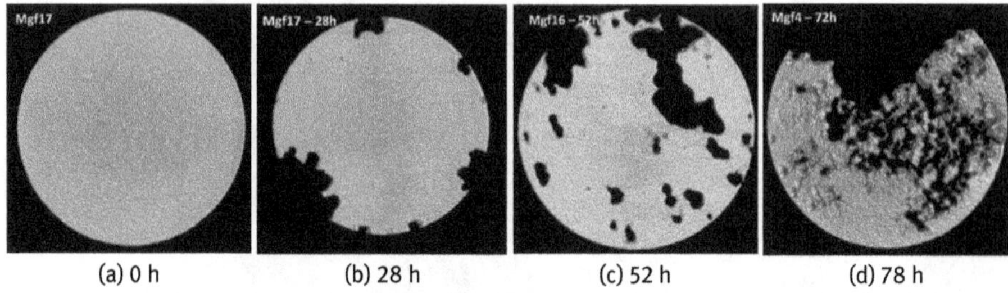

(a) 0 h (b) 28 h (c) 52 h (d) 78 h

Figure 19.24: Progressive degradation of pure Mg foil in NaCl solution [189].

The guided bone regeneration (GBR) procedures have been noted as a reliable periodontal regeneration and alveolar augmentation therapy and have registered high success rates in recent years [192]. Currently, there are two material systems for GBR procedures, namely degradable and nondegradable membrane materials [193]. With degradable regeneration membranes (usually made of PLA or collagen sheets), secondary surgery for implant removal is not required; however, the low mechanical strength and stiffness do not offer sufficient structural strength. In contrast, nondegradable regeneration membranes (e.g., Ti mesh or Teflon mesh) are the most commonly used materials; however, their use requires secondary surgery for membrane removal, which increases the risk of bacterial infection. Based on this background, Lin et al. [194] developed and evaluated Mg–5Zn–0.4Zr alloy for application in dental GBR. Since the microstructure and surface properties of biomedical Mg materials greatly influence anticorrosion performance and biocompatibility, heat treatments and surface coatings were performed to provide varied functional characteristics. The heat-treated Mg regeneration membrane (ARRm-H380) and duplex-treated regeneration membrane group (ARRm-H380-F24 h) were thoroughly investigated to characterize the mechanical properties, as well as the in vitro corrosion and in vivo degradation behaviors. It was reported that significant enhancement in ductility and corrosion resistance for the ARRm-H380 was obtained through the optimized solid solution heat treatment; meanwhile, the corrosion resistance of ARRm-H380-F24 h showed further improvement, resulting in superior substrate integrity. The ARRm-H380 provided the proper amount of Mg ion concentration to accelerate bone growth in the early stage (more than 80% new bone formation), indicating that the heat treatment and duplex treatment could be employed to offer custom functional regeneration membranes for different clinical patients.

19.8.3 Screw and plate

Metal screws and plates that fix the bone and then dissolve upon healing is a new concept in dentistry. Until now, titanium has been the metal of choice for fixing augmented bone. Although titanium plates, screws and nets provide good stability for tissues during the healing phase, these materials have to be removed before further treatment with dental implants [195, 196]. The second operation on screw and plate removal leads to new tissue damage, increased infection risks and high patient costs and suffering [197]. The idea behind magnesium screws is to combine the degradability similar to polymers with good mechanical properties similar to or better than titanium. A review of magnesium as a potential material for temporary metal screws and plates for maxillofacial applications was conducted [197]. It was reported that (i) magnesium alloys (such as Mg–Y–RE and Mg-Y-RE-Zr alloys) have better properties than titanium and are beneficial in fixing bone grafts and (ii) further development and implication of magnesium in the maxillofacial field would be beneficial for patients undergoing dental surgery. Orthodontic mechanotherapy is not limited to adolescents, but an increasing number of adult patients are seeking orthodontic treatment. There are several psychological, biological and clinical differences between the orthodontic treatment of adults and adolescents. Adults have more specific objectives and concerns related to facial and dental aesthetics, the type of orthodontic appliance and the duration of treatment. The development of corticotomy-assisted orthodontic treatment opened doors and offered solutions to many limitations in the orthodontic treatment of adults. This method claims to have several advantages such as a reduced treatment time, enhanced expansion, differential tooth movement, increased traction of impacted teeth and, finally, more postorthodontic stability [198, 199]. These biodegradable magnesium screws and plates can be applied to heal the alveolar bone during the corticotomy-assisted orthodontic treatment.

References

[1] Sezer N, Evis Z, Kayhan SM, Tahmasebifar A, Koç M. Review of magnesium-based biomaterials and their applications. Journal of Magnesium and Alloys. 2018, 6, 23–43.

[2] Persaud-Sharma D, McGoron A. Biodegradable magnesium alloys: a review of material development and applications. Journal of Biomimetics, Biomaterials, and Tissue Engineering. 2012, 12, 25–39.

[3] Prakasam M, Locs J, Salma-Ancane K, Loca D, Largeteau A, Berzina-Cimdina L. Biodegradable materials and metallic implants – a review. Journal of Functional Biomaterials. 2017, 44; DOI: 10.3390/jfb8040044.

[4] Li N, Zheng Y. Novel Magnesium alloys developed for biomedical application: A review. Journal of Materials Science and Technology. 2013, 29, 489–502.

[5] Witte F, Fischer J, Nellesen J, Crostack HA, Kaese V, Pisch A, Beckmann F, Windhagen H. In vitro and in vivo corrosion measurements of magnesium alloys. Biomaterials. 2006, 27, 1013–8.

[6] Ananth H, Kundapur V, Mohammed HS, Anand M, Amarnath GS, Mankar S. A review on biomaterials in dental implantology. International Journal of Biomedical Science. 2015, 11, 113–20.

[7] Wetterlöv Charyeva O. Magnesium screws and plates for bone augmentation: a new concept in dental surgery. JSciMed Dental Surgery. 2017, 2, 1011; https://pdfs.semanticscholar.org/6ed5/9a66297c721d56992c6205cfca35ab840a71.pdf.

[8] Bondy SC. The neurotoxicity of environmental aluminum is still an issue. Neurotoxicology. 2010, 31, 575–81.

[9] Taïr K, Kharoubi O, Taïr OA, Hellal N, Benyettou I, Aoues A. Aluminium-induced acute neurotoxicity in rats: Treatment with aqueous extract of Arthrophytum (Hammada scoparia). Journal of Acute Disease. 2016, 5. 470–82.

[10] Meshram NP, Janbandhu KS. Evaluation of hepatotoxicity of lanthanide complexes of fish Catla catla. International Research Journal of Science & Engineering. 2014, 2, 219–25.

[11] Riaz U, Shabib I, Haider W. The current trends of Mg alloys in biomedical applications – a review. Journal of Biomedical Materials Research. 2018, 107, 1970–96.

[12] Jafari S, Raman RKS, Davies CHJ. Corrosion fatigue of a magnesium alloy in modified simulated body fluid. Engineering Fracture Mechanics. 2015, 137, 2–11.

[13] Witte F. The history of biodegradable magnesium implants – a review. Acta Biomaterialia. 2010, 6, 1680–92.

[14] Oshida Y. Bioscience and Bioengineering of Titanium Materials. Elsevier, London UK, 2007.

[15] Biodegradation Properties of Magnesium Alloys. Total Materia. https://www.totalmateria.com/page.aspx?ID=CheckArticle&site=ktn&NM=370.

[16] Tian Q, Lin J, Rivera-Sastaneda L, Tsanhani A, Dunn ZS, Rodriguez A, Aslani A, Liu H. Nano-to-Submicron Hydroxyapatite Coatings for Magnesium-based Bioresorbable Implants – Deposition, Characterization, Degradation, Mechanical Properties, and Cytocompatibility. Scientific Reports. 2019, 9; https://doi.org/10.1038/s41598-018-37123-3.

[17] Millis DL. 7 – Responses of Musculoskeletal Tissues to Disuse and Remobilization. Canine Rehabilitation and Physical Therapy (Second Edition). 2014, 92–153; https://www.sciencedirect.com/science/article/pii/B9781437703092000077.

[18] http://www.bananarepublican.info/Stress_shielding.htm.

[19] https://seikeigekagaku.info/stress-shielding/.

[20] Yang Y, He C, E D, Yang W, Qi F, Xie D, Shen L, Peng S, Shuai C. Mg bone implant: features, developments and perspectives. Materials & Design. 2020, 185; https://www.sciencedirect.com/science/article/pii/S0264127519306975.

[21] Staiger MP, Pietak AM, Huadmai J, Dias G. Magnesium and its alloys as orthopedic biomaterials: A review. Biomaterials. 2006, 27, 1728–34.

[22] Walker J, Shadanbaz S, Woodfield TBF, Staiger MP, Dias GJ. Magnesium biomaterials for orthopedic application: A review from a biological perspective. Journal of Biomedical Materials Research. Part B, Applied Biomaterials. 2014, 102, 1316–31.

[23] Chen Y, Xu Z, Smith C, Sankar J. Recent advances on the development of magnesium alloys for biodegradable implants. Acta Biomaterialia. 2014, 10, 4561–73.

[24] Schinhammer M, Hänzi AC, Löffler JF, Uggowitzer PJ. Design strategy for biodegradable Fe-based alloys for medical applications. Acta Biomaterialia. 2010, 6, 1705–13.

[25] Witte F, Kaese V, Haferkamp H, Switzer E, Meyer-Lindenberg A, Wirth CJ, Windhagen H. In vivo corrosion of four magnesium alloys and the associated bone response. Biomaterials. 2005, 26, 3557–63.

[26] Zartner P, Cesnjevar R, Singer H, Weyand M. First successful implantation of a biodegradable metal stent into the left pulmonary artery of a preterm baby. Catheterization and Cardiovascular Interventions. 2005, 66, 590–4.

[27] Banerjee PC, Al-Saadi S, Choudhary L, Harandi SE, Singh R. Magnesium implants: prospects and challenges. Materials (Basel) 2019, 12, 136; DOI: 10.3390/ma12010136.
[28] Song G-L. Corrosion of Magnesium Alloys. Woodhead Publishing; Cambridge, UK: 2011.
[29] Radha R, Sreekanth D. Insight of magnesium alloys and composites for orthopedic implant applications – a review. Journal of Magnesium and Alloys. 2017, 5, 286–312.
[30] Witte F, Hort N, Vogt C, Cohen S, Kainer KU, Willumeit R, Feyerabend F. Degradable biomaterials based on magnesium corrosion. Current Opinion in Solid State & Materials Science. 2008, 12, 63–72.
[31] Siefen S, Höck M. Development of magnesium implants by application of conjoint-based quality function deployment. Journal of Biomedical Materials Research. 2019, 107, 2814–34.
[32] Liu C, Ren Z, Xu Y, Pang S, Zhao X, Zhao Y. Biodegradable Magnesium Alloys Developed as Bone Repair Materials: A Review. Scanning. 2018; DOI: 10.1155/2018/9216314.
[33] Marukawa E, Tamai M, Takahashi Y, Hatakeyama I, Sato M, Higuchi Y, Kakidachi H, Taniguchi H, Honda J, Omura K, Harada H. Comparison of magnesium alloys and poly-l-lactide screws as degradable implants in a canine fracture model. Journal of Biomedical Materials Research B. 2016, 104, 1282–9.
[34] Zhang X, Yuan G, Mao L, Niu J, Ding W. Biocorrosion properties of as-extruded Mg-Nd-Zn-Zr alloy compared with commercial AZ31 and WE43 alloys. Materials Letters. 2012, 66, 209–11.
[35] Niu J, Xiong M, Guan X, Zhang J, Huang H, Pei J, Yuan G. The in vivo degradation and bone-implant interface of Mg-Nd-Zn-Zr alloy screws: 18 months post-operation results. Corrosion Science. 2016, 113, 183–7.
[36] Zhang S, Zheng Y, Zhang L, Bi Y, Li Y. In vitro and in vivo corrosion and histocompatibility of pure Mg and a Mg-6Zn alloy as urinary implants in rat model. Materials Science and Engineering: C. 2016, 68, 414–22.
[37] Wang J, Ma Y, Guo S, Jiang W, Liu Q. Effect of Sr on the microstructure and biodegradable behavior of Mg-Zn-Ca-Mn alloys for implant application. Materials & Design. 2018, 153, 308–16.
[38] Li H, Peng Q, Li X, Li K, Fang D. Microstructures, mechanical and cytocompatibility of degradable Mg–Zn based orthopedic biomaterials. Materials & Design. 2014, 58, 43–51.
[39] Makkar P, Sarkar SK, Padalhin AR, Moon BG, Lee YS, Lee BT. In vitro and in vivo assessment of biomedical Mg-Ca alloys for bone implant applications. Journal of Applied Biomaterials & Functional Materials. 2018, 16, 126–36.
[40] Mohamed A, El-Aziz AM, Breitinger H-G. Study of the degradation behavior and the biocompatibility of Mg–0.8Ca alloy for orthopedic implant applications. Journal of Magnesium and Alloys. 2019, 7, 249–57.
[41] Bakhsheshi-Rad HR, Hamzah E, Ismail AF, Sharer Z, Medraj M. Synthesis and corrosion behavior of a hybrid bioceramic-biopolymer coating on biodegradable Mg alloy for orthopaedic implants. Journal of Alloys and Compounds. 2015, 648, 1067–71.
[42] Li Y, Wen C, Mushahary D, Sravanthi R, Hodgson P. Mg–Zr–Sr alloys as biodegradable implant materials. Acta Biomaterialia. 2012, 8, 3177–88.
[43] Zhao C, Pan F, Zhao S, Pan H, Tang A. Preparation and characterization of as-extruded Mg–Sn alloys for orthopedic applications. Materials & Design. 2015, 70, 60–7.
[44] Liu J, Lin Y, Bian D, Wang M, Zheng Y. In vitro and in vivo studies of Mg-30Sc alloys with different phase structure for potential usage within bone. Acta Biomaterialia. 2019, 98, 50–66.
[45] Bakhsheshi-Rad HR, Hamzah E, Ismail AF, Aziz M, Chami A. In vitro degradation behavior, antibacterial activity and cytotoxicity of TiO2-MAO/ZnHA composite coating on Mg alloy for orthopedic implants. Surface & Coatings Technology. 2018, 334, 450–60.

[46] Kang M-H, Lee H, Jang T-S, Seong Y-J, Jung H-D. Mg with tunable mechanical properties and biodegradation rates for bone regeneration. Acta Biomaterialia. 2019, 84, 453–67.
[47] Williams DF. Corrosion of Implant Materials. Annual Reviews of Materials Science. 1976, 6, 237–66.
[48] Romanos GE, Delgado-Ruiz RA, Gómez-Moreno G, López-López PJ, Mate Sanchez de Val JE, Calvo-Guirado JL. Role of mechanical compression on bone regeneration around a particulate bone graft material: an experimental study in rabbit calvaria. Clinical Oral Implants Research. 2018, 29, 612–9.
[49] Yu Y, Lu H, Sun J. Long-term in vivo evolution of high-purity Mg screw degradation – Local and systemic effects of Mg degradation products. Acta Biomaterialia. 2018, 71, 215–24.
[50] Cha P-R, Han H-S, Yang G-F, Kim Y-C, Hong K-H, Lee S-C, Jung J-Y, Ahn J-P, Kim YY, Cho S-Y, Byun JY, Lee -K-S, Yang S-J, Seok H-K. Biodegradability engineering of biodegradable Mg alloys: Tailoring the electrochemical properties and microstructure of constituent phases. Scientific Reports. 2013, 3; DOI: 10.1038/srep02367.
[51] Waizy H, Diekmann J, Weizbauer A, Reifenrath J, Bartsch I, Neubert V, Schavan R, Windhagen H. In vivo study of a biodegradable orthopedic screw (MgYREZr–alloy) in a rabbit model for up to 12 months. Journal of Biomaterials Applications. 2014, 28, 667–75.
[52] Windhagen H, Radtke K, Weizbauer A, Diekmann J, Noll Y, Kreimeyer U, Schavan R, Stukenborg-Colsman C, Waizy H. Biodegradable magnesium–based screw clinically equivalent to titanium screw in hallux valgus surgery: short–term results of the first prospective, randomized, controlled clinical pilot study. Biomedical Engineering. 2013,12; https://doi.org/10.1186/1475-925X-12-62.
[53] Wu H, Zhao C, Ni J, Zhang S, Liu J, Yan J, Chen Y, Zhang X. Research of a novel biodegradable surgical staple made of high purity magnesium. Bioactive Materials. 2016, 1, 122–6.
[54] Choy PYG, Bissett IP, Docherty JG, Parry BR, Merrie AEH.Stapled versus handsewn methods for ileocolic anastomoses. Cochrane Database System Review. 2011, 9; DOI: 10.1002/ 14651858.CD004320.pub2.
[55] Qu S, Xia J, Yan J, Wu H, Wang H, Yi Y, Zhang X, Zhnag S, Zhao C, Chen Y. In vivo and in vitro assessment of the biocompatibility and degradation of high–purity Mg anastomotic staples. Journal of Biomaterials Applications. 2017, 31, 1203–14.
[56] Amano H, Hanada K, Hinoki A, Tainaka T, Shirota C, Sumida W, Yokota K, Murase N, Oshima K, Chiba K, Tanaka Y, Uchida H. Biodegradable surgical staple composed of magnesium alloy. Scientific Reports. 2019, 9; https://www.nature.com/articles/s41598-019-51123-x.
[57] Tamai K, Mitsumori M, Fujishiro S, Kokubo M, Ooya N, Nagata Y, Sasai K, Hiraoka M, Inamoto T. A case of allergic reaction to surgical metal clips inserted for postoperative boost irradiation in a patient undergoing breast-conserving therapy. Breast Cancer. 2001, 8, 90–2.
[58] Ikeo N, Nakamura R, Naka K, Hashimoto T, Yoshida T, Urade T, Fukushima K, Yabuuchi H, Fukumoto T, Ku Y, Mukai T. Fabrication of a magnesium alloy with excellent ductility for biodegradable clips. Acta Biomaterialia. 2016, 29, 468–76.
[59] Bai H, He X, Ding P, Liu D, Chen M. Fabrication, microstructure, and properties of a biodegradable Mg-Zn-Ca clip. Journal of Biomedical Materials Research B: Applied Biomaterials. 2019, 107, 1741–9.
[60] Yoshida T, Fukumoto T, Urade T, Kido M, Toyama H, Asari S, Ajuki T, Ikeo N, Mukai T, Ku Y. Development of a new biodegradable operative clip made of a magnesium alloy: Evaluation of its safety and tolerability for canine cholecystectomy. Surgery. 2017, 161, 1553–60.
[61] Bian D, Zhou W, Deng J, Liu Y, Li W, Chu X, Xiu P, Cai H, Kou Y, Jiang B, Zheng Y. Development of magnesium-based biodegradable metals with dietary trace element germanium as orthopaedic implant applications. Acta Biomaterialia. 2017, 64, 421–36.

[62] Bai J, Yin L, Lu Y, Gan Y, Xue F, Chu C, Yan J, Yan K, Wan X, Tang Z. Preparation, microstructure and degradation performance of biomedical magnesium alloy fine wires. Progress in Natural Science: Materials International. 2014, 24, 523–30.
[63] Jähn K, Saito H, Taipaleenmäki H, Gasser A, Hort N, Feyerabend F, Schlüter H, Rueger JM, Lehmann W, Willumeit-Römer R, Hesse E. Intramedullary Mg2Ag nails augment callus formation during fracture healing in mice. Acta Biomaterialia. 2016, 36, 350–60.
[64] Witte F, Reifenrath J, Müller PP, Crostack H-A, Nellesen J, Bach FW, Bormann D, Rudert M. Cartilage repair on magnesium scaffolds used as a subchondral bone replacement. Materials Science and Engineering Technology. 2006, 37, 504–8.
[65] Chaya A, Yoshizawa S, Verdelis K, Myers N, Costello BJ, Chou D-T, Pal S, Maiti S, Kumta PN, Sfeir C. In vivo study of magnesium plate and screw degradation and bone fracture healing. Acta Biomaterialia. 2015, 18, 262–9.
[66] Moore WR, Graves SE, Bain GI. Synthetic bone graft substitutes. ANZ Journal of Surgery. 2001, 71, 354–61.
[67] Schilling T, Bauer M, LaLonde L, Maier HJ, Haverich A, Hassel T. Cardiovascular applications of magnesium alloys, magnesium alloys. ItechOpen. 2017; https://www.intechopen.com/books/magnesium-alloys/cardiovascular-applications-of-magnesium-alloys.
[68] Zhang J, Liu W, Schnitzler V, Tancret F, Bouler J-M. Calcium phosphate cements for bone substitution: Chemistry, handling and mechanical properties. Acta Biomaterialia. 2014, 10, 1035–49.
[69] Misch CE, Dietsh F. Bone-grafting materials in implant dentistry. Implant Dentistry. 1993, 2, 158–67.
[70] Claes L, Hoellen I, Ignatius A. Biodegradable bone cements. Der Orthopäde. 1997, 26, 459–62.
[71] Geffers M, Groll J, Gbureck U. Reinforcement strategies for load-bearing calcium phosphate biocements. Materials. 2015, 8, 2700–17.
[72] Oshida Y. Hydroxyapatite – Synthesis and Applications. Momentum Press, New York NY, 2015. p/85.
[73] Amjad Z, Koutsoukos PG, Nancollas GH. The crystallization of hydroxyapatite and fluorapatite in the presence of magnesium ions. Journal of Colloid and Interface Science. 1984, 101, 250–6.
[74] Li X, Ito A, Sogo Y, Wang X, LeGeros RZ. Solubility of Mg-containing β-tricalcium phosphate at 25°C. Acta Biomaterialia. 2009, 5. 508–17.
[75] Kannan S, Lemos AF, Rocha JHG, Ferreira JMF. Characterization and mechanical performance of the Mg-stabilized β-$Ca_3(PO_4)_2$ Prepared from Mg-substituted Ca-deficient apatite. Journal of the American Ceramic Society. 2006, 89. 2727–61.
[76] Ren F, Leng Y, Xin R, Ge X. Synthesis, characterization and ab initio simulation of magnesium-substituted hydroxyapatite. Acta Biomaterialia. 2010, 6, 2787–96.
[77] Laurencin D, Almora-Barrios N, de Leeuw NH, Gervais C, Bonhomme C, Mauri F, Chrzanowski W, Knowles JC, Newport RJ, Wong A, Gan Z, Smith ME. Magnesium incorporation into hydroxyapatite. Biomaterials. 2011, 32, 1826–37.
[78] Canullo L, Heinemann F, Gedrange T, Biffar R, Kunert-Keil C. Histological evaluation at different times after augmentation of extraction sites grafted with a magnesium-enriched hydroxyapatite: double-blinded randomized controlled trial. Clinical Oral Implants Research. 2013, 24, 398–406.
[79] Li X. Li Y, Liao Y, Li J, Zhang L, Hu J. The effect of magnesium-incorporated hydroxyapatite coating on titanium implant fixation in ovariectomized rats. International Journal of Oral & Maxillofacial Implants. 2014, 29, 196–202.

[80] Cai Y, Zhang S, Zeng X, Wang Y, Qian M, Weng W. Improvement of bioactivity with magnesium and fluorine ions incorporated hydroxyapatite coatings via sol–gel deposition on Ti6Al4V alloys. Thin Solid Films. 2009, 517, 5347–51.
[81] Crespi R, Capparè P, Addis A, Gherlone E. Injectable magnesium- enriched hydroxyapatite putty in peri-implant defects: a histomorphometric analysis in pigs. International Journal of Oral & Maxillofacial Implants. 2012, 27, 95–101.
[82] Zhao S-F, Jiang Q-H, Peel S, Wang X-X, He F-M. Effects of magnesium-substituted nanohydroxyapatite coating on implant osseointegration. Clinical Oral Implants Research. 2013, 24, 34–41.
[83] Caneva M, Botticelli D, Stellini E, Souza SLS, Salata LA, Niklaus P, Lang NP. Magnesium-enriched hydroxyapatite at immediate implants: a histomorphometric study in dogs. Clinical Oral Implants Research. 2011, 22, 512–7.
[84] Dasgupta S, Banerjee SS, Bandyopadhyay A, Bose S. Zn- and Mg-doped hydroxyapatite nanoparticles for controlled Release of Protein. Langmuir. 2010, 26, 4958–64.
[85] Kheradmandfard M, Fathi MH. Preparation and characterization of Mg-doped fluorapatite nanopowders by sol–gel method. Journal of Alloys and Compounds. 2010, 504, 141–5.
[86] Cai Y, Zhang S, Zeng X, Qian M, Sun D, Weng W. Interfacial study of magnesium-containing fluoridated hydroxyapatite coatings. Thin Solid Films. 2011, 519, 4629–33.
[87] Gopi D, Ramya S, Rajeswari D, Surendiran M, Kavitha L. Development of strontium and magnesium substituted porous hydroxyapatite/poly(3,4-ethylenedioxythiophene) coating on surgical grade stainless steel and its bioactivity on osteoblast cells. Colloids and Surfaces. B, Biointerfaces. 2014, 114, 234–40.
[88] Roy M, Bandyopadhyay A, Bose S. Induction plasma sprayed Sr and Mg doped nano hydroxyapatite coatings on Ti for bone implant. Journal of Biomedical Materials Research B. 2011, 99, 258–65.
[89] Hollinger JO, Brekke J. Role of bone substitutes. Clinical Orthopaedics and Related Research. 1996, 324, 55–65.
[90] Liu H, Yazici H, Ergun C, Webster TJ, Bermek H. An in vitro evaluation of the Ca/P ratio for the cytocompatibility of nano-to-micron particulate calcium phosphates for bone regeneration. Acta Biomaterialia. 2008, 4, 1472–9.
[91] Detsch R, Mayr H, Ziegler G. Formation of osteoclast-like cells on HA and TCP ceramics. Acta Biomaterialia. 2008, 4, 139–48.
[92] Kasten P, Luginbühl R, van Griensven M, Barkhausen T, Krettek C, Bohner M, Bosch U. Comparison of human bone marrow stromal cells seeded on calcium-deficient hydroxyapatite, β-tricalcium phosphate and demineralized bone matrix. Biomaterials. 2003, 24, 2593–603.
[93] Hadi A, Hassan B, Ghizlane A. Bilateral sinus graft with either bovine hydroxyapatite or β tricalcium phosphate, in combination with platelet-rich plasma: a case report. Implant Dentistry. 2008, 17. 350–9.
[94] Kurkcu M, Mehmet Benlidayi E, Cam B, Sertdemir Y. Anorganic bovine-derived hydroxyapatite versus β-tricalcium phosphate in sinus augmentation. A comparative histomorphometric study. Journal of Oral Implants. 2012; DOI: http://dx.doi.org/10.1563/AAID-JOI-D-11-00061.1.
[95] Yang G-L, He F-M, En Song E, Hu J-A, Wang X-X, Zhao S-F. In vivo comparison of bone formation on titanium implant surfaces coated with biomimetically deposited calcium phosphate or electrochemically deposited hydroxyapatite. International Journal of Oral & Maxillofacial Implants. 2010, 25, 669–80.

[96] Arinzeh TL, Tran T, McAlary J, Daculsi G. A comparative study of biphasic calcium phosphate ceramics for human mesenchymal stem-cell-induced bone formation. Biomaterials. 2005, 26, 3631–8.
[97] Jensen SS, Bornstein MM, Dard M, Bosshardt DD, Buser D. Comparative study of biphasic calcium phosphates with different HA/TCP ratios in mandibular bone defects. A Long-term Histomorphometric Study in Minipigs. Journal of Biomedical Materials Research B. 2009, 90, 171–81.
[98] Suzuki T, Hukkanen M, Ohashi R, Yokogawa Y, Nishizawa K, Nagata F, Buttery L, Polak J. Growth and adhesion of osteoblast-like cells derived from neonatal rat calvaria on calcium phosphate ceramics. Journal of Bioscience and Bioengineering. 2000, 89, 18–26.
[99] Alam MI, Asahina I, Ohmamiuda K, Takahashi K, Yokota S, Enomoto S. Evaluation of ceramics composed of different hydroxyapatite to tricalcium phosphate ratios as carriers for rhBMP-2. Biomaterials. 2001, 22, 1643–51.
[100] Jinno T, Davy DT, Goldberg VM. Comparison of hydroxyapatite and hydroxyapatite tricalcium-phosphate coatings. Journal of Arthroplasty. 2002, 17. 902–9.
[101] De Kok IJ, Peter SJ, Archambault M, van den Bos C, Kadiyala S, Aukhil I, Cooper LF. Hydroxyapatite/tricalcium phosphate composites; tissue engineering applications. Clinical Oral Implant Research. 2003, 14, 481–9.
[102] Miao X, Tan DM, Li J, Xiao Y, Crawford R. Mechanical and biological properties of hydroxyapatite/tricalcium phosphate scaffolds coated with poly(lactic-co-glycolic acid). Acta Biomaterialia. 2008, 4. 638–45.
[103] Yuan H, Yang Z, de Bruijn JD, de Groot K, Zhang X. Material-dependent bone induction by calcium phosphate ceramics: a 2.5-year study in dog. Biomaterials. 2001, 22, 2617–23.
[104] Vecchio KS, Massie JB, Wang M, Kim CW. Conversion of sea urchin spines to Mg-substituted tricalcium phosphate for bone implants. Acta Biomaterialia. 2007, 3, 785–93.
[105] Zhang X, Takahashi T, Vecchio KS. Development of bioresorbable Mg-substituted tricalcium phosphate scaffolds for bone tissue engineering. Materials Science and Engineering C. 2009, 6, 2003–10.
[106] Berthiaume F, Maguire TJ, Yarmush ML. Tissue engineering and regenerative medicine: History, progress, and challenges. Annual Review of Chemical and Biomolecular Engineering. 2011, 2, 403–30.
[107] Gregor A, Filová E, Novák M, Kronek J, Chlup H, Buzgo M, Blahnová V, Lukášová V, Bartoš M, Nečas A, Hošek J. Designing of PLA scaffolds for bone tissue replacement fabricated by ordinary commercial 3D printer. Journal of Biological Engineering. 2017, 11; https://doi.org/10.1186/s13036-017-0074-3.
[108] Stevens MM. Biomaterials for bone tissue engineering. Materials Today. 2008, 11, 18–25.
[109] Gupta P, Adhikary M, Kumar M, Bhardwaj N, Mandal BB. Biomimetic, osteoconductive non-mulberry silk fiber reinforced tricomposite scaffolds for bone tissue engineering. ACS Applied Materials & Interfaces. 2016, 8, 30797–810.
[110] Hao Z, Song Z, Huang J, Huang K, Panetta A, Gu Z, Wu J. The scaffold microenvironment for stem cell based bone tissue engineering. Biomaterials Science. 2017, 5, 1382–92.
[111] Yang Y, Wang G, Liang H, Gao C, Peng S, Shen L, Shuai C. Additive manufacturing of bone scaffolds. International Journal of Bioprinting. 2019, 5; http://ijb.whioce.com/index.php/int-j-bioprinting/article/view/148.
[112] Pina S, Ribeiro VP, Marques CF, Maia FR, Silva TH, Reis RL, Oliveira JM. Scaffolding strategies for tissue engineering and regenerative medicine applications. Materials (Basel). 2019, 12, 1824; DOI: 10.3390/ma12111824.
[113] Hubbell JA. Biomaterials in tissue engineering. Biotechnology. 1995, 13, 565–76.
[114] O'brien FJ. Biomaterials & scaffolds for tissue engineering. Materials Today. 2011, 14, 88–95.

[115] Place ES, Evans ND, Stevens MM. Complexity in biomaterials for tissue engineering. Nature Materials. 2009, 8, 457–70.
[116] Ma PX. Biomimetic materials for tissue engineering. Advanced Drug Delivery Reviews. 2008, 60, 184–198.
[117] Furth ME, Atala A, Van Dyke ME. Smart biomaterials design for tissue engineering and regenerative medicine. Biomaterials. 2007, 28, 5068–73.
[118] Eltom A, Zhong G, Muhammad A. Scaffold techniques and designs in tissue engineering functions and purposes: a review. Advances in Science and Materials Engineering. 2019; https://doi.org/10.1155/2019/3429527.
[119] Kumar TS, Chakrapani VY. Electrospun 3D Scaffolds for Tissue Regeneration. In: Chun HJ et. al. ed., Cutting-Edge Enabling Technologies for Regenerative Medicine. Springer; Berlin, Germany: 2018, pp 29–47.
[120] Sola A, Bertacchini J, D'Avella D, Anselmi L, Maraldi T, Marmiroli S, Messori M. Development of solvent-casting particulate leaching (SCPL) polymer scaffolds as improved three-dimensional supports to mimic the bone marrow niche. Materials Science and Engineering C. 2019, 96, 153–65.
[121] Song P, Zhou C, Fan H, Zhang B, Pei X, Fan Y, Jiang Q, Bao R, Yang Q, Dong Z. Novel 3D porous biocomposite scaffolds fabricated by fused deposition modeling and gas foaming combined technology. Composites Part B: Engineering. 2018, 152, 151–9.
[122] Brougham CM, Levingstone TJ, Shen N, Cooney GM, Jockenhoevel S, Flanagan TC, O'brien FJ. Freeze-drying as a novel biofabrication method for achieving a controlled microarchitecture within large, complex natural biomaterial scaffolds. Advanced Healthcare Materials. 2017, 6; DOI: 10.1002/adhm.201700598.
[123] Gay S, Lefebvre G, Bonnin M, Nottelet B, Boury F, Gibaud A, Calvignac B. PLA scaffolds production from thermally induced phase separation: effect of process parameters and development of an environmentally improved route assisted by supercritical carbon dioxide. Journal of Supercritical Fluids. 2018, 136, 123–35.
[124] Xu W, Tian J, Liu Z, Lu X, Hayat MD, Yan Y, Li Z, Qu X, Wen C. Novel porous Ti35Zr28Nb scaffolds fabricated by powder metallurgy with excellent osteointegration ability for bone-tissue engineering applications. Materials Science and Engineering: C. 2019, 105; https://doi.org/10.1016/j.msec.2019.110015.
[125] Sharma P, Pandey PM. A novel manufacturing route for the fabrication of topologically-ordered open-cell porous iron scaffold. Materials Letters. 2018, 222, 160–3.
[126] Lee JM, Yeong WY. Design and printing strategies in 3D bioprinting of cell-hydrogels: A review. Advanced Healthcare Materials. 2016, 5, 2856–65.
[127] Xu Y, Wang X. Application of 3D biomimetic models in drug delivery and regenerative medicine. Current Pharmaceutical Design. 2015, 21, 1618–26.
[128] Ozbolat IT, Moncal KK, Gudapati H. Evaluation of bioprinter technologies. Additive Manufacturing. 2017, 13, 179–200.
[129] Yang Y, Ritchie AC, Everitt NM. Comparison of glutaraldehyde and procyanidin cross-linked scaffolds for soft tissue engineering. Materials Science and Engineering: C. 2017, 80, 263–73.
[130] Roseti L, Parisi V, Petretta M, Cavallo C, Desando G, Bartolotti I, Grigolo B. Scaffolds for bone tissue engineering: state of the art and new perspectives. Materials Science and Engineering: C. 2017, 78, 1246–62.
[131] Azami M, Samadikuchaksaraei A, Poursamar S. Synthesis and characterization of a laminated hydroxyapatite/gelatin nanocomposite scaffold with controlled pore structure for bone tissue engineering. International Journal of Artificial Organs. 2010, 33, 86–95.

[132] Yan L, Salgado A, Oliveira J, Oliveira A, Reis R. De novo bone formation on macro/microporous silk and silk/nano-sized calcium phosphate scaffolds. Journal of Bioactive and Compatible Polymers. 2013, 28, 439–52.
[133] Wang Y, Cui W, Chou J, Wen S, Sun Y, Zhang H. Electrospun nanosilicates-based organic/inorganic nanofibers for potential bone tissue engineering. Colloids and Surfaces. B, Biointerfaces. 2018, 172, 90–7.
[134] Neves LS, Rodrigues MT, Reis RL, Gomes ME. Current approaches and future perspectives on strategies for the development of personalized tissue engineering therapies. Expert Review of Precision Medicine and Drug Development. 2016, 1, 9–108.
[135] Yazdimamaghani M, Razavi M, Vashaee D, Tayebi L. Development and degradation behavior of magnesium scaffolds coated with polycaprolactone for bone tissue engineering. Materials Letters. 2014, 132, 106–10.
[136] Yazdimamaghani M, Razavi M, Vashaee D, Moharamzadeh K, Boccaccini AR, Tayebi L. Porous magnesium-based scaffolds for tissue engineering. Materials Science and Engineering C. 2017, 71, 1253–66.
[137] Mutlu I. Production and fluoride treatment of Mg-Ca-Zn-Co alloy foam for tissue engineering applications. Transactions of Nonferrous Metals Society of China. 2018, 28, 114–24.
[138] Hong K, Park H, Kim Y, Knapek M, Minárik P, Máthis K, Yamamoto A, Choe H. Mechanical and biocorrosive properties of magnesium-aluminum alloy scaffold for biomedical applications. Journal of the Mechanical Behavior of Biomedical Materials. 2019, 98, 213–24.
[139] Polmear I, StJohn D, Niw J-F, Qian M. Magnesium Alloys. Metallurgy of the Light Metals. 2017, 287–367; https://doi.org/10.1016/B978-0-08-099431-4.00006-3.
[140] https://www.medicaldesignbriefs.com/component/content/article/mdb/features/articles/27329.
[141] Singh S, Vashisth P, Shrivastav A, Bhatnagar N. Synthesis and characterization of a novel open cellular Mg-based scaffold for tissue engineering application. Journal of Mechanical Behavior of Biomedical Materials. 2019, 94, 54–62.
[142] Wen C, Yamada Y, Shimojima K, Chino Y, Hosokawa H, Mabuchi M. Compressibility of porous magnesium foam: dependency on porosity and pore size. Materials Letters. 2004, 58, 357–60.
[143] Čapek J, Vojtěch D. Properties of porous magnesium prepared by powder metallurgy. Materials Science and Engineering C. 2013, 33, 564–69.
[144] Cheng M-Q, Wahafu T, Jiang G-F, Liu W, Qiao Y-Q, Peng X-C, Cheng T, Zhang X-L, He G, Liu X-Y. A novel open-porous magnesium scaffold with controllable microstructures and properties for bone regeneration. Scientific Reports. 2016, 6; DOI: 10.1038/srep24134.
[145] Jia G, Chen C, Zhang J, Wang Y, Yue R, Luthringer-Feyerabend BJ, Willumeit-Roemer R, Zhang H, Xiong M, Huang H. In vitro degradation behavior of Mg scaffolds with three-dimensional interconnected porous structures for bone tissue engineering. Corrosion Science. 2018, 144, 301–12.
[146] Jia G, Hou Y, Chen C, Niu J, Zhang H, Huang H, Xiong M, Yuan G. Precise fabrication of open porous Mg scaffolds using NaCl templates: relationship between space holder particles, pore characteristics and mechanical behavior. Materials & Design. 2018, 140–106-13.
[147] Vaezi M, Chianrabutra S, Mellor B, Yang S. Multiple material additive manufacturing–Part 1: a review: this review paper covers a decade of research on multiple material additive manufacturing technologies which can produce complex geometry parts with different materials. Virtual and Physical Prototyping. 2013, 8, 19–50.
[148] Li Y, Zhou J, Pavanram P, Leeflang M, Fockaert L, Pouran B, Tümer K-U, Schröder N, Mol J, Weinans H. Additively manufactured biodegradable porous magnesium. Acta Biomaterila. 2018, 67, 378–92.

[149] Kopp A, Derra T, Müther M, Jauer L, Schleifenbaum JH, Voshage M, Jung O, Smeets R, Kröger N. Influence of design and postprocessing parameters on the degradation behavior and mechanical properties of additively manufactured magnesium scaffolds. Acta Biomaterila. 2019, 98, 23–35.
[150] https://www.ilt.fraunhofer.de/en/media-center/brochures/b-slm-for-medical-implants.html.
[151] Qin Y, Wen P, Guo H, Xia D, Zheng Y, Jauer L, Poprawe R, Voshage M, Schleifenbaum JH. Additive manufacturing of biodegradable metals: current research status and future perspectives. Acta Biomaterialia. 2019, 98, 3–22.
[152] Wong HM, Chu PK, Leung FKL, Cheung KMC, Luk KDK, Yeung KWK. Engineered polycaprolactone–magnesium hybrid biodegradable porous scaffold for bone tissue engineering. Progress in Natural Science: Materials International. 2014, 24, 561–7.
[153] Cao X, Lu H, Liu J, Lu W, Guo L, Ma M, Zhang B, Guo Y. 3D plotting in the preparation of newberyite, struvite, and brushite porous scaffolds: using magnesium oxide as a starting material. Journal of Material Science: Material of Medicine. 2019, 30; https://doi.org/10.1007/s10856-019-6290-2.
[154] Liao Y, Chen D, Niu J, Zhang J, Jiang Y. In vitro degradation and mechanical properties of polyporous $CaHPO_4$-coated Mg–Nd–Zn–Zr alloy as potential tissue engineering scaffold. Materials Letters. 2013, 100, 306–8.
[155] Wilton V, Shavandi A, El-Din A Bekhit A. Synthesis of three dimensional Mg-HA scaffolds from New Zealand sea urchin (Evechinus chloroticus) waste shells. Front. Bioeng. Biotechnol. Conference Abstract: 10th World Biomaterials Congress. 2016. DOI: 10.3389/conf.FBIOE.2016.01.01347.
[156] Saito S. New horizon of bioabsorbable stent. Catheterization and Cardiovascular Interventions. 2005, 66, 595–6.
[157] Moravej M, Mantovani D. Biodegradable metals for cardiovascular stent application: interests and new opportunities. International Journal of Molecular Sciences. 2011, 12, 4250–70.
[158] Bartosch M, Schubert S, Berger F. Magnesium stents – fundamentals, biological implications and applications beyond coronary arteries. BioNanoMaterials. 2015, 16; https://doi.org/10.1515/bnm-2015-0004.
[159] Sankar M, Vishnu J, Gupta M, Manivasagam G. Magnesium-based alloys and nanocomposites for biomedical application. In: Inamuddin et al. ed., Applications of Nanocomposite Materials in Orthopedics. Woodhead Pub. 2019, pp 83–109.
[160] Hernawan H, Dubé D, Mantovani D. Degradable metallic biomaterials for cardiovascular applications. In: Niinomi M. ed., Metals for Biomedical Devices. Woodhead Pub. 2010, pp 379–404.
[161] Erbel R, Di Mario C, Bartunek J, Bonnier J, de Bruyne B, Eberli FR, Erne P, Haude M, Heublein B, Horrigan M, Ilsley C, Böse D, Koolen J, Lüscher TF, Weissman N, Waksman R. Lancet. 2007, 369, 1869–75.
[162] Maeng M, Jensen LO, Falk E, Andersen HR, Thuesen L. Negative vascular remodeling after implantation of bioabsorbable magnesium alloy stents in porcine coronary arteries: a randomized comparison with bare-metal and sirolimus-eluting stents. Heart. 2009, 95, 241–6.
[163] Chen J, Tan L, Yu X, Etim I, Ibrahim M, Yang K. Mechanical properties of magnesium alloys for medical application: A review. Journal of the Mechanical Behavior of Biomedical Materials. 2018, 87, 68–79.
[164] https://kossel-medtech.en.made-in-china.com/product/QvtmUyDEqiYj/China-Manufacturer-of-Mg-Alloy-Intracoronary-Cardiac-Stent-for-Cardiology.html.
[165] Peuster M, Beerbaum P, Bach FW, Hauser H. Are resorbable implants about to become a reality? Cardiology in the Young. 2006, 16, 107–16.

[166] Tian Q, Zhang C, Deo M, Rivera-Castaneda L, Liu H. Responses of human urothelial cells to magnesium-zinc-strontium alloys and associated insoluble degradation products for urological stent applications. Materials Science and Engineering: C. 2019, 96, 248–62.
[167] Monfared A, Ghaee A, Ebrahimi-Barough S. Preparation and characterization of crystallized and relaxed amorphous Mg-Zn-Ca alloy ribbons for nerve regeneration application. Journal of Non-crystalline Solids. 2018, 489, 71–6.
[168] Ge Q, Dellasega D, Demir AG, Vedani M. The processing of ultrafine-grained Mg tubes for biodegradable stents. Acta Biomaterialia. 2013, 9, 8604–10.
[169] Wang B, Guan S, Wang J, Wang L, Zhu S. Effects of Nd on microstructures and properties of extruded Mg–2Zn–0.46Y–xNd alloys for stent application. Materials Science and Engineering: B. 2011, 176, 1673–8.
[170] Liu J, Wang P, Chu C-C, Xi T. Arginine-leucine based poly (ester urea urethane) coating for Mg-Zn-Y-Nd alloy in cardiovascular stent applications. Colloids and Surfaces. B, Biointerfaces. 2017, 159, 78–88.
[171] Fei J, Wen X, Lin X, Saijilafu, Wang W, Ren O, Chen X, Tan L, Yang K, Yamg H, Yang L. Biocompatibility and neurotoxicity of magnesium alloys potentially used for neural repairs. Materials Science and Engineering: C. 2017, 78, 1155–63.
[172] Zhang J, Li H, Wang W, Huang H, Li Y. The degradation and transport mechanism of a Mg-Nd-Zn-Zr stent in rabbit common carotid artery: A 20-month study. Acta Biomaterialia. 2018, 69, 372–84.
[173] Shi Y, Zhang L, Chen J, Zhang J, Yuan G. In vitro and in vivo degradation of rapamycin-eluting Mg-Nd-Zn-Zr alloy stents in porcine coronary arteries. Materials Science and Engineering: C. 2017, 80, 1–6.
[174] Mao L, Zhou H, Chen L, Niu J, Song C. Enhanced biocompatibility and long-term durability in vivo of Mg-Nd-Zn-Zr alloy for vascular stent application. Journal of Alloys and Compounds. 2017, 720, 245–53.
[175] Santos-Coquillat A, Esteban-Lucia M, Martinez-Campos E, Mohedano M, Matykina E. PEO coatings design for Mg-Ca alloy for cardiovascular stent and bone regeneration applications. Materials Science and Engineering: C. 2019, 105; https://doi.org/10.1016/j.msec.2019.110026.
[176] Bornapour M, Mahjoubi H, Vali H, Shum-Tim D, Pekguleryuz M. Surface characterization, in vitro and in vivo biocompatibility of Mg-0.3Sr-0.3Ca for temporary cardiovascular implant. Materials Science and Engineering: C. 2016, 67, 72–84.
[177] Zhou WR, Zheng YF, Leeflang MA, Zhou J. Mechanical property, biocorrosion and in vitro biocompatibility evaluations of Mg–Li–(Al)–(RE) alloys for future cardiovascular stent application. Acta Biomaterialia. 2013, 9, 8488–98.
[178] Kim K. The Development of Biodegradable Metallic Screws and Suture Anchors for Soft Tissue Fixation in Orthopaedic Surgery. 2014, PhD Thesis, University of Pittsburgh.
[179] Seitz JM, Durisin M, Goldman J, Drelich JW. Recent advances in biodegradable metals for medical sutures: a critical review. Advanced Healthcare Materials. 2015, 4, 1915–36.
[180] Seitz J-M, Wulf E, Freytag P, Bormann D, Bach F-M. The Manufacture of Resorbable Suture Material from Magnesium. Advanced Engineering Materials. 2010, 12, 1099–105.
[181] Bao G, Fan Q, Ge D, Sun M, Zheng Y. In vitro and in vivo studies on magnesium alloys to evaluate the feasibility of their use in obstetrics and gynecology. Acta Biomaterialia. 2019, 97, 623–36.
[182] Hernández-Alvarado LA, Hernández LS, Lomelí MA, Miranda JM, Escudero ML. Phytic acid coating on Mg-based materials for biodegradable temporary endoprosthetic applications. Journal of Alloys and Compounds. 2016, 664, 609–18.
[183] Ananth H, Kundapur V, Mohammed HS, Anand M, Amarnath GS, Mankar S. A review on biomaterials in dental implantology. International Journal of Biomedical Sciences. 2015, 11, 113–20.

[184] Koo S, Weil T. Can Magnesium Replace Titanium in Dental Implants? 2017; https://www.pineypointdentalimplants.com/blog/dental-implants-4/.
[185] https://www.perioimplantadvisory.com/dental-implants/lab-consideration/article/16412234/researchers-find-strong-candidate-for-bonefriendly-dental-implants-in-heattempered-magnesium-alloy.
[186] Balog M, Snajdar M, Krizik P, Schauperl Z, Stanec Z, Catic A. Titanium-Magnesium Composite for Dental Implants (BIACOM). TMS 2017 146th Annual Meeting & Exhibition Supplemental Proceedings. 2017; DOI:10.1007/978-3-319-51493-2_26.
[187] Dimitriou R, Mataliotakis GI, Calori GM, Giannoudis PV. The role of barrier membranes for guided bone regeneration and restoration of large bone defects: current experimental and clinical evidence. BMC Medicine. 2012, 10; DOI: 10.1186/1741-7015-10-81.
[188] Hornberger H, Striegl B, Trahanofsky M, Kneissl F, Kronseder M. Degradation and bioactivity studies of Mg membranes for dental surgery. Materials Letters: X. 2019, 2; https://doi.org/10.1016/j.mlblux.2019.100007.
[189] Meinig RP. Clinical use of resorbable polymeric membranes in the treatment of bone defects. Orthopedic Clinics of North America. 2010, 41, 39–47.
[190] Kokubo T, Takadama H. How useful is SBF in predicting in vivo bone bioactivity. Biomaterials. 2006, 27, 2907–15.
[191] Yoshikawa G, Murashima Y, Wadachi R, Sawada N, Suda H. Guided bone regeneration (GBR) using membranes and calcium sulphate after apicectomy: A comparative histomorphometrical study. International Endodontic Journal. 2002, 35, 255–63.
[192] Rakhmatia YD, Ayukawa Y, Furuhashi A, Koyano K. Current barrier membranes: Titanium mesh and other membranes for guided bone regeneration in dental applications. Journal of Prosthodontic Research. 2013, 57, 3–14.
[193] Lin D-J, Hung F-Y, Lee H-P, Yeh M-L. Development of a novel degradation-controlled magnesium-based regeneration membrane for future Guided Bone Regeneration (GBR) therapy. Metals. 2017, 7;https://doi.org/10.3390/met7110481.
[194] Sumitomo N, Noritake K, Hattori T, Morikawa K, Niwa S, Sato K, Niinomi M. Experiment study on fracture fixation with low rigidity titanium alloy: plate fixation of tibia fracture model in rabbit. Journal of Materials Science. Materials in Medicine. 2008, 19, 1581–6.
[195] Waizy H, Seitz J-M, Reifenrath J, Weizbauer A, Bach F-W, Meyer-Lindenberg A, Denkena B, Windhagen H. Biodegradable magnesium implants for orthopedic applications. Journal of Materials Science. 2013, 48, 39–50.
[196] Hassan AH, Al-Fraidi AA, Al-Saeed SH. Corticotomy-assisted orthodontic treatment: review. Open Dentistry Journal. 2010, 4, 159–64.
[197] Farid KA, Mostafa YA, Kaddah MA, El-Sharaby FA. Corticotomy-facilitated Orthodontics Using Piezosurgery Versus Rotary Instruments: An Experimental Study. Journal of International Academy of Periodontology. 2014, 16, 103–8.
[198] Amresh T. et al., Corticotomy Assisted Orthodontic Treatment. J Universal Coll of Med Sci. 2013, 1, 1–6.
[199] Hassan AH. et al., Bone inductive proteins to enhance postorthodontic stability. Angle Orthod. 2010,80, 1051–60.

Chapter 20
Future perspectives

Research and development (R&D) in areas of material design and new manufacturing for magnesium materials possesses twofold natures: seeds oriented and needs oriented. These two R&D activities are progressing concurrently in various engineering and medical sectors. Such R&D activities are aiming at reinforcing and emphasizing advantages of Mg materials and, at the same time, overcoming and improving some disadvantages associated with Mg materials. Well-recognized advantages associated with Mg materials include a lightweight, high specific strength, excellent heat conductivity and dissipation, high damping capacity, high electromagnetic shielding property, recyclability and an abundance of natural resources [1]. In particular, taking advantage of its high electromagnetic shielding property, other than the application for ECU (electronic control unit) housings equipped with automotive, the developments of application have been advancing for several purposes such as surgical instruments, aircrafts and robot structures. Especially for the ECU housings, the adoption of magnesium alloy is expected to increase since high performance in electromagnetic shielding property is required for automotive applications where the number of installed electronics is ever increasing, and more countermeasures for noise will be required in the future [2]. On the other hand, the followings are known as disadvantages with Mg materials: high forming cost, poor formability, poor heat resistance, poor corrosion resistance and bad nonflammability. Mg exhibits crystal anisotropy and can slide only along (0001) and (0012) planes at room temperature, so that it is almost impossible to perform a cold working below the recrystallization temperature of Mg materials. Hence, the high-pressure die casting (HPDC), extrusion with semimelting state (thixomolding) or press forming (combined technique of forging and pressing) have been developed and utilized [3]. Since cold forming is limited, warm or hot forming is normally operated, resulting in high cost forming. Although application of Mg alloys is expected to increase in automobiles, aircrafts or robotics restrained due to poor resistances against heat and corrosion, developments for new Mg alloys are under progress for these measures [4, 5]. For reducing forming cost, developments on sheet can be cold deformed [3] or grain refining by alloying [6] or through the upset forging [7], enabling low-temperature forging. If chips created during lathe machining Mg materials catch fire, it will burn at high temperature and will be exploded under applying water. Hence, nonflammable or flame-retardant Mg-based alloys (basically AM series alloy plus Ca addition) have been developed [8, 9].

The poor corrosion resistance (or with more scientific term, less-noble electromotive force) property should not be considered as unwanted character always. Along with Zn element, Mg is favorably selected and widely employed as a sacrificial anode cathodic protection material and an electrode for Mg–air battery. In addition, excellent biodegradability of Mg biomaterials (which is carefully defined and used; since

https://doi.org/10.1515/9783110676945-020

among various practical Mg alloys, only Mg-based alloys contain any nontoxic or nonharmful elements such as Ca, Zn, Mn, Zr, Sn or Ag can be categorized as Mg biomaterials) can be used to manufacture temporary (bone) implants, tissue engineering scaffolds or drug delivery system material. During the degradation, the control of hydrogen gas evolution and degradation rate should be controlled so that there would not be any risk for inflammation surrounding vital tissues.

It is very important to manage the degradation rate for aforementioned medical applications. It can become more critical for the application of fine biodegradable metallic wires in stress-bearing areas, because the mechanical properties of such wires should be maintained during the expected biofunctioning. For achieving this target, methods such as selection of alloying elements, microstructure adjustments and surface modification will be effective and developments for these controlling techniques are advancing [10–15]. Selecting proper alloying elements in combination with the base metal could adjust the volume degradation rate of the material and concurrently could enhance mechanical properties of an alloy. By employing a proper fabrication process creates a fine and uniform microstructure, which in turn influences the mechanical properties of the material. Various surface modification techniques create a protective layer on the material which resist against corrosion and such layer also increases the osteoinductivity and osteoconductivity of the material. Yang et al. [12] pointed out that (i) the performance of Mg metal might be improved by alloying and further treatment so that the Mg-based metallic materials could be used to design fixation implants for clinical applications; (ii) through affecting the solid/liquid interface instability, alloying and further treatment could affect the morphology and distribution of the primary or secondary phase, and then improve the yield strength, ultimate tensile strength, elongation and corrosion properties of materials; (iii) most of the coatings disappear along with implantation over time, though they can delay the onset of corrosion; (iv) numerous factors should be considered, for example, coating morphology, surface chemistry and adhesion, on their use as biomedical implants in future research; and (v) most of the Mg alloys do not have superior corrosion resistance in vivo that match the physiological environment, indicating that further development in material alloying design is needed. It should also include the design and development of a new paradigm of coatings, mechanical processing techniques, and complete characterization of critical factors including corrosion rate, surface chemistry, near surface residual stress, and coating topography [15]. A hybrid technique combining mechanical processing and coating, along with drug-eluting polymeric layers [16], would be a promising means to control the corrosion rate, hence maintaining the desired mechanical integrity of the implants as they heal and remodel adequately. All of these are expected to potentially widen the applications of Mg-based alloys in revolutionizing the successful development of biomedical devices such as bone fixations and stents [15].

Tissue engineering is an interdisciplinary field constructed on a broad range of areas, so the development of this field has been obtained by numerous biomedical 3D scaffold fabrication techniques comprising conventional and current scaffold manufacturing technologies. The conventional methods are solvent casting and particle leaching, freeze-drying, the thermal-induced phase separation method (to force phase separation via the temperature alternate related to setting the homogeneous polymer solution with a high temperature in a decrease temperature environment to induce phase separation so that a polymer-rich phase, as well as a poor polymer phase) [17], gas foaming and electrospinning [18]. The modern methods (rapid prototyping) have included stereolithography, fused deposition modeling, selective laser sintering and three-dimensional printing [18]. The tissue engineering (TE) technique is a modern technique in the construction of scaffolds to be used in tissue and organ structure. Among prototyping techniques, 3D printing will play an important role in large applications that concern the scaffold-based field. Pore morphology controlling technique has opened an endless possibility of porous Mg scaffolds [19–21].

It is also shown that Mg biomaterials possess a great promise for use in the pharmaceutical sector as a drug-delivery device. Biodegradable polymer coatings on magnesium alloys are attractive, as they can provide corrosion resistance as well as additional functions for biomedical applications, for example, drug delivery. Qi et al. [22] fabricated gelatin nanospheres/chitosan (GNs/CTS) composite coating on WE43 (Mg-4Y-3RE) substrate by electrophoretic deposition with simvastatin (SIM) loaded into the GNs. It was mentioned that (i) apart from a sustained drug release over 28 days, an anticorrosion behavior of the coated WE43 substrates was confirmed by electrochemical tests. Both the degradation and corrosion rates of the coated substrate were significantly minimized in contrast to bare WE43 and (ii) the osteogenic differentiation of MC3T3-E1 cells on SIM-containing coatings was assessed and it was shown that the SIM-loaded composite coating could upregulate the expression of osteogenic genes and related proteins, promote ALP activity and enhance extracellular matrix mineralization, concluding that the SIM-loaded GNs/CTS composite coatings were able to enhance the corrosion resistance of the WE43 substrate and promote osteogenic activity, thus demonstrating a promising coating system for modifying the surface of magnesium alloys targeted for orthopedic applications. Chat et al. [23] electropolymerized a poly(3,4-ethylenedioxythiophene) (PEDOT) and graphene oxide (GO) film directly on Mg surface. GO acted as nano-drug carrier to carry anti-inflammatory drug dexamethasone (Dex). It was reported that (i) PEDOT/GO/Dex coatings improved Mg corrosion resistance and decreased the rate of hydrogen production, (ii) Dex could be released driven by the electrical current generated from Mg corrosion, (iii) the anti-inflammatory activity of the released Dex was confirmed in microglia cultures and (iv) the PEDOT/GO/Dex film displayed the ability to both control Mg corrosion and act as an on-demand release coating that delivers Dex at the corrosion site to minimize detrimental effects of corrosion byproducts, suggesting that the multifunctional smart coating will improve the clinical use of Mg implants and the PEDOT/GO/drug/Mg system may be developed into self-powered implantable drug delivery devices.

Shape-memory alloys (SMAs), which display shape recovery upon heating, as well as superelasticity, offer many technological advantages in various applications. Those distinctive behaviors have been observed in many polycrystalline alloy systems such as NiTi, Cu-, Fe-, Ni-, Co- and Ti-based alloys but not in lightweight alloys such as Mg and Al alloys. Ogawa et al. [24] developed a Mg–20Sc (at%) SMA with superelastic strain of 4.4% at −150 °C and shape recovery upon heating, which is attributed to the reversible martensitic transformation. It was reported that (i) the Mg–Sc has a density of 2 g/cm^3 which is one-third less than that of practical TiNi SMAs, (ii) Mg–20Sc alloy was confirmed to show 6% recoverable strain (including both ordinary elastic and superelastic strain) and (iii) the operation temperature of Mg–Sc SMA can be varied by controlling Sc content, and confirmed that a Mg–Sc alloy with 18.3 at% Sc showed shape recovery upon heating from −30 °C to room temperature. Although this magnesium-scandium alloy is limited to low-temperature applications, development of a new lightweight class of SMAs could be on the horizon. It was also mentioned that this alloy could have significant impact on the aerospace industry such as self-deployable space habitat frames and damping devises on spacecraft systems. Moreover, Mg–Sc SMAs can also be applied in the medical field. Currently, TiNi superelastic alloys are being used as self-expandable stents with great success. However, there is a problem of in-stent restenosis. To overcome the restenosis, biodegradable magnesium alloy stents have recently been proposed. This means that the Mg–Sc superelastic alloy could potentially be applied in biodegradable self-expanding stents [24].

Lastly, it is the first time in this book to mention the AI (artificial intelligence). Design and development of new alloys becoming more complicated and overwhelming tasks if the alloy system is getting higher order (i.e., from binary, ternary, to quaternary or even more multielement alloy systems) and if these new designed alloys were investigated through ordinary laboratory works, it appears to be impossible. Hence, like medicine development conducted at the pharmaceutical companies, new designed alloys should be primarily checked by AI-assisted screening. The AI-assisted screening for new alloy development should be reflected to various factors including limitations from thermodynamics, equilibrium phase diagram, castability and other additional primary properties. As this book proves, amount of information is huge and informatics will be getting more important under the current 5G era. In future, materials science/engineering and applications should be supported by integrated AI-assisted informatics.

References

[1] Monteiro WA, Buso SJ, da Silva LV. Application of Magnesium Alloys in Transport, New Features on Magnesium Alloys. IntechOpen. 2012; https://www.intechopen.com/books/new-features-on-magnesium-alloys/application-of-magnesium-alloys-in-transport.

[2] Friedrich H, Schumann S. Research for a "new age of magnesium" in the automotive industry. Journal of Materials Processing Technology. 2001, 117, 276–81.

[3] Dieringa H, Hort N, Letzig D, Bohlen J, Höche D, Blawert C, Zheludkevich M. Mg Alloys: Challenges and Achievements in Controlling Performance, and Future Application Perspectives. In: Orlov D. et al., ed., Magnesium Technology 2018. TMS 2018. The Minerals, Metals & Materials Series. Springer, 2018, 3–14.

[4] Bettles CJ, Gibson MA, Zhu SM. Microstructure and mechanical behaviour of an elevated temperature Mg-rare earth based alloy. Materials Science and Engineering A. 2009, 505, 6–12.

[5] Zhu S, Easton MA, Abbott TB, Nie J-F, Dargusch MS, Hort N, Gibson MA. Evaluation of magnesium die-casting alloys for elevated temperature applications: microstructure, tensile properties, and creep resistance. Metallurgical and Materials Transactions A. 2015, 46, 3543–54.

[6] Mishra R. Hierarchically Structured Untrafine Grained Magnesium Alloys. Magnesium Technology. In: Jordon J et al., ed., Magnesium Technology 2020. The Minerals, Metals & Materials Series. Springer, Cham, 2020, pp.7–11.

[7] Papenberg NP, Gneiger S, Weißensteiner I, Uggowitzer PJ, Pogatscher S. Mg-Alloys for Forging Applications – A Review. Materials (Basel). 2020, 13; DOI: 10.3390/ma13040985.

[8] Ohara H. Development and application of flame-retardant and heat-resistant magnesium alloys. Journal of the Japan Institute of Light Metals. 2016, 66, 233–9.

[9] Masaki K, Ochi Y, Kakiuchi T, Kurata K, Hirawawa T, Matsumura T, Takigawa Y, Higashi K. High cycle fatigue property of extruded non-combustible Mg alloy AMCa602. Materials Transactions. 2008, 49, 1148–56.

[10] Asgari M, Hang R, Wang C, Yu Z, Li Z, Xiao Y. Biodegradable Metallic Wires in Dental and Orthopedic Applications: A Review. Metals. 2018, 8; https://doi.org/10.3390/met8040212.

[11] Radha R, Sreekanth D. Insight of magnesium alloys and composites for orthopedic implant applications – a review. Journal of Magnesium and Alloys. 2017, 5, 286–312.

[12] Yang Y, He C, E D, Yang W, Qi F, Xie D, Shen L, Peng S, Shuai C. Mg bone implant: Features, developments and perspectives. Materials & Design. 2020, 185; https://www.sciencedirect.com/science/article/pii/S0264127519306975.

[13] Yang Y, He C, E D, Yang W, Qi F, Xie D, Shen L, Peng S, Shuai C. Mg bone Implant: Features, developments and perspectives. Materials & Design. 2020, 185; https://doi.org/10.1016/j.matdes.2019.108259.

[14] Prasadh S, Ratheesh V, Manakari V, Parande G, Gupta M, Wong R. Potential of magnesium based materials in mandibular reconstruction. Metals. 2019, 9; DOI:10.3390/met9030302.

[15] Uddin MS, Hall C, Murphy P. Surface treatments for controlling corrosion rate of biodegradable Mg and Mg-based alloy implants. Science Technology Advanced Materials. 2015, 16: DOI: 10.1088/1468-6996/16/5/053501.

[16] Stefanini GG, Byrne RA, Serruys PW, de Waha A, Meier B, Massberg S, Jüni P, Schömig A, Windecker S, Kastrati A. Biodegradable polymer drug-eluting stents reduce the risk of stent thrombosis at 4 years in patients undergoing percutaneous coronary intervention: a pooled analysis of individual patient data from the ISAR-TEST 3, ISAR-TEST 4, and LEADERS randomized trials. European Heart Journal. 2012, 33, 1214–22.

[17] Li Z, Xie M-B, Li Y, Ma Y, Li J-S, Dai F-Y. Recent progress in tissue engineering and regenerative medicine. Journal of Biomaterials and Tissue Engineering. 2016, 6, 755–66.
[18] Eltom A, Zhong G, Muhammad A. Scaffold techniques and designs in tissue engineering functions and purposes: a review. Advances in Materials Science and Engineering. 2019; https://doi.org/10.1155/2019/3429527.
[19] Jia G, Chen C, Zhang J, Wang Y, Yue R, Luthringer B, Willumeit R, Zhang H, Xiong M, Huang H, Yuan G. Feyerabend F. In vitro degradation behavior of Mg scaffolds with three-dimensional interconnected porous structures for bone tissue engineering. Corrosion Science. 2018, 144, 301–12.
[20] Cerrato E, Barbero U, Gil Romero JA, Quadri G, Mejia-Renteria H, Tomassini F, Ferrari F, Varbella F, Gonzalo N, Escaned J. Magmaris™ resorbable magnesium scaffold: state-of-art review. Future Cardiology. 2019, 15; https://doi.org/10.2217/fca-2018-0081.
[21] EuroPCR 2019: New data confirms future of resorbable magnesium scaffolds. Journal of Invasive Cardiology. 2019; https://www.invasivecardiology.com/news/europcr-2019-new-data-confirms-future-resorbable-magnesium-scaffolds.
[22] Qi H, Heise S, Zhou J, Schuhladen K, Yang Y, Cui N, Dong R, Virtanen S, Chen Q, Boccaccini AR, Lu T. Electrophoretic deposition of bioadaptive drug delivery coatings on magnesium alloy for bone repair. ACS Applied Materials & Interfaces. 2019, 11, 8, 8625–34.
[23] Chat K, Li H, Hoang V, Beard R, Cui T. Self-powered therapeutic release from conducting polymer/graphene oxide films on magnesium. Nanomedicine. 2018, 14, 2495–503.
[24] Ogawa Y, Ando D, Sutou Y, Koike J. A lightweight shape-memory magnesium alloy. Science. 2016, 353, 368–70.

Epilogue

In engineering areas where relatively heavyweight materials such as steels have been used, components or parts have been replaced by Mg materials to reduce total weight, resulting in energy-saving performance and enhancing reliability and safety as well. Mg materials possess easier accessibility for material recycling than plastics. These remarkable advantages are shared with Al materials; hence, in many areas these two light materials are competing. Mg materials have been applied in a wide range of areas due to their unique characteristics as follows: because of their lightweight (2/3 of Al or 1/4 of Fe), they are used for automobile parts and portable machineries; because of their high specific strength and rigidity (compared to plastics), they are used as housing of cellular phone and note-type personal computer and so on; because of their excellent heat conductivity and dissipation, they are used for various types of housing of electric devices; because of their good electromagnetic interference shielding, they are also used for housing of delicate electronics; because of their high damping capacity, they are used as steering core and others; because of their good recyclability, they are used as automobile parts, audiovisual devices and office automation equipment; because of their poor corrosion resistance, they are employed as a sacrificial anode cathodic protection material, an anode electrode for Mg–air battery and various types of biodegradable medical devices. All these applications can be realized by effective and efficient utilizing characteristics and supporting technologies and engineering. The following Mg map, as a product of transdisciplinary study, indicates interrelationships among these characteristics and supporting technologies and almost all of these keywords have been discussed in this book. For those who are conducting research on Mg materials, this Mg map would be useful to find their positioning in entire Mg world. For those who are searching for research topics, this Mg map would be helpful to find it depending on their expertise and research interest(s).

In closing, I admit having a long list of individual names to be mentioned with my memories and appreciation – my mentors who inspired me, friends and colleagues who challenged me, and most importantly, students (some of them are now my colleagues) who continue to both inspire and challenge me. To all of them, I owe my knowledge and capacity to comprehend the cited articles presented in this book. Those who were and are valuable to me and to this book include the late T. Nakayama, the late S. Iguchi, V. Weiss, H.W. Liu, the late J.A. Schwartz, T. Koizumi, A. Kamio, N. Saotome, Y. Miwa, T. Nishihara, F. Farzin-Nia. G.K. Stookey, the late C.J. Andres, the late T.M. Barco. M.J. Kowolik, V. John, D. Brown, D. Burr, D. Morton, A. Zuccari, A. Hashem, A. Wu, M. Yapchulay, S. Isikbay, C. Kuphasuk, C-M. Lin,

https://doi.org/10.1515/9783110676945-021

Y-J. Lim, Z.H. Khabbaz, J. Almeida, I. Katsilieri, E.B. Tuna, O. Aktören, K. Gençay, Y. Güven, T. Miyazaki, Y. Ono and T. Tominaga. Special thanks to H. Yasukawa for comments and editing, and the Japan Magnesium Association (H. Ohara) for providing valuable updated information. Last but not least important, my sincere gratitude goes to excellent editorial team of the De Gruyter Publishing. Thank you all.

Index

https://doi.org/10.1515/9783110676945-022

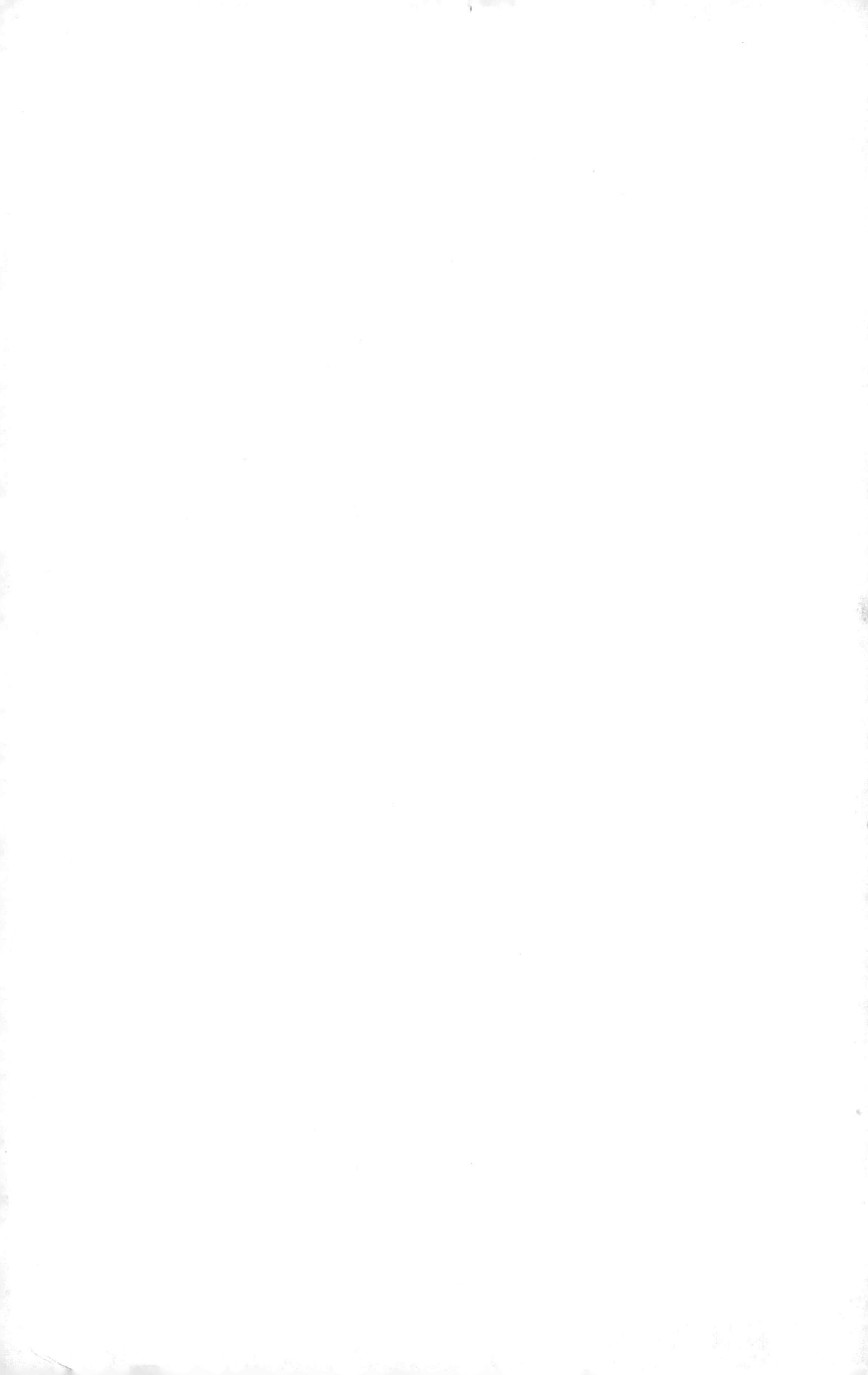

www.ingramcontent.com/pod-product-compliance
Lightning Source LLC
Chambersburg PA
CBHW080334220326
41598CB00030B/4505

* 9 7 8 3 1 1 0 6 7 6 9 2 1 *